T0290511

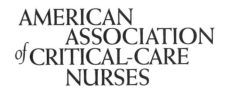

AMERICAN
ASSOCIATION
of CRITICAL-CARE
NURSES

AACN
Procedure Manual *for*
Progressive *and* Critical Care

Edited by

Karen L. Johnson, PhD, RN, FAAN

Director, Nursing Research
Banner Health
Phoenix, Arizona

8th
Edition

ELSEVIER

Elsevier
3251 Riverport Lane
St. Louis, Missouri 63043

AACN PROCEDURE MANUAL FOR PROGRESSIVE AND CRITICAL CARE,   ISBN: 978-0-323-79381-0
EIGHTH EDITION

Notice

Practitioners and researchers must always rely on their own experience and knowledge in evaluating and using any information, methods, compounds or experiments described herein. Because of rapid advances in the medical sciences, in particular, independent verification of diagnoses and drug dosages should be made. To the fullest extent of the law, no responsibility is assumed by Elsevier, authors, editors or contributors for any injury and/or damage to persons or property as a matter of products liability, negligence or otherwise, or from any use or operation of any methods, products, instructions, or ideas contained in the material herein.

Previous editions copyrighted 2017, 2011, 2005, 2001, 1994, 1985.

Executive Content Strategist: Lee Henderson
Content Development Director: Laurie Gower
Content Development Specialist: Casey Potter
Publishing Services Manager: Deepthi Unni
Project Manager: Nayagi Anandan
Designer: Ryan Cook

Printed in India

Last digit is the print number: 9   8   7   6   5   4   3   2   1

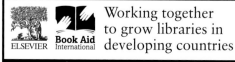

Section Editors

Sonia Astle, MS, RN, CCNS, CCRN, CNRN
Clinical Nurse Specialist
Critical Care
Inova Fairfax Medical Campus
Falls Church, Virginia

Joni L. Dirks, MSN, RN, NPD-BC, CCRN-K
Director
Clinical Education and Professional Development
Providence Inland Northwest Washington
Spokane, Washington

Eleanor Fitzpatrick, DNP, RN, AGCNS-BC, ACNP-BC, CCRN
Clinical Nurse Specialist
Surgical Critical Care
Thomas Jefferson University Hospital
Philadelphia, Pennsylvania

Karen L. Johnson, PhD, RN, FAAN
Director, Nursing Research
Banner Health
Phoenix, Arizona

Marion E. McRae, PhD, RN, ACNP-BC, CCRN-CMC
Nurse Practitioner
Cardiac Surgery
Cedars-Sinai Medical Center
Los Angeles, California

DaiWai M. Olson, PhD, RN, CCRN, FNCS
Professor
Neurology and Neurotherapeutics
University of Texas Southwestern Medical Center
Dallas, Texas

Maureen A. Seckel, MSN, APRN, ACNS-BC, CCNS, CCRN-K, FCCM, FCNS, FAAN
Clinical Nurse Specialist, Medical Critical Care and Sepsis Coordinator
Medical ICU and Department of Medicine
ChristianaCare
Newark, Delaware

Contributors

Anna Alder, DNP, RN, NPD-BC
Clinical Instructor
University of Utah
Salt Lake City, Utah
United States
Procedure 101: *Fecal Microbiota Transplant (Perform)*

Sonia Astle, MS, RN, CCNS, CCRN, CNRN
Clinical Nurse Specialist
Critical Care
Inova Fairfax Medical Campus
Falls Church, Virginia
United States
Procedure 118: *Negative Pressure Wound Therapy*
Procedure 119: *Wound Management With Excessive Drainage*

Andrea Barron, BSN, RN, CNOR
Charge Nurse
University of Texas Southwestern
Dallas, Texas
United States
Procedure 93: *Epidural Catheters: Insertion (Assist) and Pain Management*

Bonjo Batoon, MS, CRNA
Certified Registered Nurse Anesthetist
R Adams Cowley Shock Trauma Center
University of Maryland Medical Systems
Baltimore, Maryland
United States
Procedure 7: *Nasopharyngeal and Oral Airway Insertion*

John Bazil, BSN, RN, BSEE
Staff Nurse
University of Texas Southwestern
Dallas, Texas
United States
Procedure 90: *Pupillometer*

Tracey M. Berlin, MSN, RN, CNRN, CCRN-K
Senior Clinical Specialist and Clinical Research Coordinator
NeurOptics, Inc.
Irvine, California
United States
Procedure 85: *Cerebral Blood Flow Monitoring*

Cynthia Anne Blank-Reid, MSN, RN, CEN, TCRN
Trauma Clinical Nurse Specialist
Department of Trauma and Surgical Critical Care
Temple University Hospital – Main Campus
Philadelphia, Pennsylvania
United States
Procedure 96: *Focused Abdominal Assessment With Sonography*

Heidi Boddeker, BSN, RN, MSN-Ed, CCRN-K
Clinical Education Specialist
Clinical Education–Critical Care
Banner Health
Phoenix, Arizona
United States
Procedure 21: *Closed Chest Drainage System*

Donna C. Bond, DNP, RN, CCNS, AE-C, CTTS, FCNS
Pulmonary Clinical Nurse Specialist
Trauma
Carilion Clinic
Roanoke, Virginia
United States
Procedure 14: *Oxygen Saturation Monitoring With Pulse Oximetry*

Carrie Boom, MSN, ANP-BC, ACNP-BC
Co-Lead Advanced Practice Provider
Senior Lead Advanced Practice Provider
Division of Cardiology
University of Washington Medical Center
Seattle, Washington
United States
Procedure 56: *Central Venous/Right Atrial Pressure Monitoring*
Procedure 61: *Pulmonary Artery Catheter and Pressure Lines, Troubleshooting*

Kim Bowers, MSN, ACNP-BC
Clinical Program Manager, Medical Intensive Care Unit
Clinical Program Manager, Tele Medicine
Lead Nurse Practitioner, APP Float Pool
University of Maryland Medical Center
Baltimore, Maryland
United States
Procedure 23: *Thoracentesis (Perform)*
Procedure 24: *Thoracentesis (Assist)*

Carly D. Byrne, DNP, APRN, PCNS-BC, CCNS, CPN, CCRN-K
Clinical Nurse Specialist
Legacy Health
Portland, Oregon
United States
Procedure 121: *Percutaneous Endoscopic Gastrostomy, Gastrostomy, and Jejunostomy Tube Care*
Procedure 122: *Small-Bore Feeding Tube Insertion and Nursing Care*

Roger M. Casey, MSN, CEN, TCRN, FAEN
Charge RN
Free Standing Emergency Department
Kadlec Regional Medical Center
Richland, Washington
United States
Procedure 9: *Surgical Cricothyrotomy (Perform)*
Procedure 10: *Surgical Cricothyrotomy (Assist)*

Marie Cassalia, MSN, APRN, ACCNS-AG, CCRN-CSC, WTA
Clinical Nurse Specialist CVCCC
ChristianaCare
Newark, Delaware
United States
Procedure 70: *Radial Arterial Sheath Removal*

Alice Chan, MS, RN, CNS, CCRN, NE-BC
Associate Director
Critical Care
Cedars-Sinai Medical Center
Los Angeles, California
United States
Procedure 34: *Emergent Open Sternotomy (Perform) and Defibrillation (Internal) (Perform)*
Procedure 35: *Emergent Open Sternotomy and Internal Defibrillation (Assist)*

Chong Sherry Cheever, MSN, ANP-BC, PhD
Nurse Practitioner, Intensive Care Unit
Pulmonary Medicine
Sacred Heart Medical Center
Spokane, Washington
United States
Procedure 25: *Bronchoscopy (Perform)*
Procedure 26: *Bronchoscopy (Assist)*

Kathleen M. Cox, PhD, DNP, APRN, ACNP-BC, CNE, FAANP
Acute Care Nurse Practitioner
San Antonio, Texas
United States
Procedure 62: *Blood Sampling From a Pulmonary Artery Catheter*
Procedure 77: *Peripherally Inserted Central Catheter and Midline Catheters*

Jacqueline Crawford, MS, CRNP, CNS, ACCNS-P, PCPNP-BC
Magnet Program Specialist
Department of Nursing
Thomas Jefferson University Hospital
Philadelphia, Pennsylvania
United States
Procedure 123: *Small-Bore Feeding Tube Insertion Using Guidance Systems*

Hillary Crumlett, DNP, RN, NEA-BC
Director of Nursing Operations
Northwestern Medicine, Huntley Hospital
Huntley, Illinois
United States
Procedure 52: *Arterial Catheter Insertion (Perform)*
Procedure 53: *Arterial Catheter Insertion (Assist), Care, and Removal*
Procedure 54: *Blood Sampling From an Arterial Catheter*

Katherine Dickerman, MSN, ANP-BC
Instructor
Gastroenterology
University of Colorado
Aurora, Colorado
United States
Procedure 101: *Fecal Microbiota Transplant (Perform)*

Joni L. Dirks, MSN, RN, NPD-BC, CCRN-K
Director
Clinical Education & Professional Development
Providence Inland Northwest Washington
Spokane, Washington
United States
Procedure 63: *Continuous Venous Oxygen Saturation Monitoring*

Marci Ebberts, MSN, APRN, FNP-C, CCRN-K
Clinical Education Specialist
Saint Luke's Hospital
Saint Luke's Health System
Kansas City, Missouri
United States
Procedure 13: *Extracorporeal Membrane Oxygenation*
Procedure 79: *Intraosseous Access*

Heather M. Etzl, MSN, RN, CBC
Clinical Practice Leader
Intensive Care Nursery
Thomas Jefferson University Hospital
Philadelphia, Pennsylvania
United States
Procedure 123: *Small-Bore Feeding Tube Insertion Using Guidance Systems*

Eleanor Fitzpatrick, DNP, RN, AGCNS-BC, ACNP-BC, CCRN
Clinical Nurse Specialist
Surgical Critical Care
Thomas Jefferson University Hospital
Philadelphia, Pennsylvania
United States
Procedure 98: *Endoscopic Therapy*
Procedure 103: *Paracentesis (Perform)*
Procedure 104: *Paracentesis (Assist)*

Nancy Freeland, MS, RN, NPD-BC, CCRN-K
Senior Nurse Educator
Adult Critical Care
University of Rochester Medical Center
Rochester, New York
United States
Procedure 124: *Thermoregulation: Heating, Cooling, and Targeted Temperature Management*

John J. Gallagher, DNP, RN, CCNS, CCRN-K, TCRN, CHSE, RRT, FCCM
Professor / Clinical Nurse Specialist
Director of Simulation Education
University of Pittsburgh School of Nursing
Pittsburgh, Pennsylvania
United States
Procedure 27: *Invasive Mechanical Ventilation (Through an Artificial Airway): Volume and Pressure Modes*

Kellie Girardot, MSN, RN, AGCNS-BC
Trauma & Emergency Department Clinical Nurse Specialist
Parkview Health
Fort Wayne, Indiana
United States
Procedure 125: *Prevention of Immobility-Related Complications: Kinetic Therapy (Continuous Lateral Rotation Therapy and Lateral Rotation Therapy) and Ambulation of Acute and Critically Ill Patients*

Matthew Golbitz, BSN, RN, CCRN
Clinical Nurse
Rapid Response Team
Inova Fairfax Medical Campus
Falls Church, Virginia
United States
Procedure 120: *Fecal Containment Devices and Bowel Management Systems*

Amanda J. Golino, MSN, RN, CCRN, CCNS, RN-BC, TCRN
Clinical Nurse Specialist
Research/Magnet
Inova Loudoun Hospital
Leesburg, Virginia
United States
Procedure 105: *Continuous Renal Replacement Therapies*
Procedure 106: *Hemodialysis*
Procedure 107: *Peritoneal Dialysis*

Faith Newton Good, APRN, AGACNP-BC
Nurse Practitioner
University of Texas Southwestern
Dallas, Texas
United States
Procedure 88: *Lumbar Puncture (Perform)*

Cynthia A. Goodrich, MS, RN, CFRN, CCRN
Adult Clinical Educator and Flight Nurse
Airlift Northwest
University of Washington
Seattle, Washington
United States
Procedure 1: *Endotracheal Intubation (Perform)*
Procedure 2: *Endotracheal Intubation (Assist)*
Procedure 22: *Needle Thoracostomy (Perform)*

Eliza Ajero Granflor, MN, RN, CSN, ACNP-BC, CCRN, CSC
Lead Nurse Practitioner
Critical Care Services
Cedars Sinai Medical Center
Los Angeles, California
United States
Procedure 40: *Atrial Overdrive Pacing (Perform)*

Steven Gudowski, BS, RRT, ASQ, CSSGB
Director of Patient Safety
Hospital of the University of Pennsylvania
Philadelphia, Pennsylvania
United States
Procedure 12: *Continuous End-Tidal Carbon Dioxide Monitoring*

Elizabeth P. Gunter, MSN, RN, CCRN, SCRN
Clinical Educator
University of Texas Southwestern
Dallas, Texas
United States
Procedure 80: *Peripheral Nerve Stimulation: Train-of-Four Monitoring*

Thomas Hagerty, PhD, RN, MSEd, CCRN
Staff Nurse and Adjunct Professor
New York Presbyterian Hospital
New York, New York
United States
Procedure 86: *Cerebral Microdialysis*

Paula Halcomb, DNP, APRN, ACNS-BC, TCRN, FCNS
Clinical Nurse Specialist
Trauma Surgical Services
UK HealthCare;
Adjunct Faculty
University of Kentucky College of Nursing
Lexington, Kentucky
United States
Procedure 126: *Intrahospital Transport of Critically Ill Patients*

Cynthia Hambach, PhD, RN, CCRN-K
Assistant Clinical Professor
College of Nursing and Health Professions
Drexel University
Philadelphia, Pennsylvania
United States
Procedure 32: *Cardioversion*
Procedure 33: *Defibrillation (External)*

Erin Hare, MSN, RN, CCRN
Nursing Professional Development Specialist
Medical ICU and ICU Float Pool
ChristianaCare
Newark, Delaware
United States
Procedure 8: *Suctioning: Endotracheal or Tracheostomy Tube*

Jenna Heaney, DNP, APRN, ACNP-BC, CCRN
Critical Care Advanced Practice Clinician, Fellowship Coordinator
Institute for Learning, Leadership & Development
ChristianaCare
Newark, Delaware
United States
Procedure 6: *Laryngeal Mask Airway*

Kiersten Henry, DNP, ACNP-BC, CCNS, CCRN-CMC
Chief Advanced Practice Clinician
Critical Care
MedStar Montgomery Medical Center
Olney, Maryland
United States
Procedure 31: *Automated External Defibrillation*
Procedure 36: *External Wearable Cardioverter-Defibrillator*
Procedure 42: *Implantable Cardioverter-Defibrillator: Post-insertion Care*

Brandi L. Holcomb, MSN, APRN, AGACNP-BC, CCRN
Advanced Practice Clinician – Lead
Cardiothoracic Surgery
CHRISTUS® Trinity Mother Frances Health System
Tyler, Texas
United States
Procedure 37: *Pericardiocentesis (Perform)*
Procedure 38: *Pericardiocentesis (Assist)*
Procedure 47: *Intraaortic Balloon Pump Management*
Procedure 71: *Pericardial Catheter Management*
Procedure 74: *Central Venous Catheter Insertion (Perform)*

Stephen Hopkins, MSN, RN, CCRN-K
Nursing Faculty
School of Nursing
Spokane Community College
Spokane, Washington
United States
Procedure 30: *Weaning Mechanical Ventilation*

Alexander P. Johnson, MSN, RN, ACNP-BC, CCNS, CCRN
Critical Care Clinical Nurse Specialist
Northwestern Medicine, Huntley Hospital
Huntley, Illinois
United States
Procedure 67: *Esophageal Cardiac Output Monitoring: Perform*
Procedure 68: *Esophageal Cardiac Output Monitoring: Assist, Care, and Removal*

Karen L. Johnson, PhD, RN, FAAN
Director, Nursing Research
Banner Health
Phoenix, Arizona
United States
Procedure 75: *Central Venous Catheter Insertion (Assist), Nursing Care and Removal*

Lisa Koser, DNP, MSN, MS, ACNP-BC, CPNP-AC
Lead Advanced Practice Provider, Trauma, Acute Care Surgery & Burn
Department of Surgery, Division of Trauma, Critical Care & Burn
The Ohio State University Wexner Medical Center
Columbus, Ohio
United States
Procedure 4: *Extubation/Decannulation (Perform)*
Procedure 5: *Extubation/Decannulation (Assist)*

Sandra Kurtin, PhD, ANP-C, AOCN
Director, Advanced Practice
Hematology/Oncology
The University of Arizona Cancer Center;
Assistant Professor of Clinical Medicine
Hematology/Oncology
The University of Arizona;
Adjunct Clinical Assistant Professor of Nursing
The University of Arizona
Tucson, Arizona
United States
Procedure 109: *Bone Marrow Biopsy and Aspiration*
Procedure 110: *Bone Marrow Biopsy and Aspiration (Assist)*

Loudena Lavender, MS, CRNA, APRN
Chief Certified Registered Nurse Anesthetist
Anesthesia Services, PA
New Castle, Delaware
United States
Procedure 6: *Laryngeal Mask Airway*

Rosemary Lee, DNP, APRN, ACNP-BC, CCNS, CCRN
Acute Care Nurse Practitioner
Telehealth Center
Baptist Health South Florida
Coral Gables, Florida
United States
Procedure 95: *Esophagogastric Tamponade Tube*
Procedure 99: *Intraabdominal Pressure Monitoring*

Barbara "Bobbi" Leeper, MN, APRN, CNS M-S, CCRN-K, CV-BC, FAHA
Clinical Nurse Specialist
Cardiovascular & Critical Care Consultant
Dallas, Texas
United States
Procedure 49: *Electrocardiographic Leads and Cardiac Monitoring*

Mary Leier, MSN, NP
Nurse Practitioner
Electrophysiology
Cedars Sinai Smidt Heart Institute
Los Angeles, California
United States
Procedure 43: *Permanent Pacemaker (Assessing Function)*

Emily R. Leiter, DNAP, CRNA, LTC, AN
Chief, Department of Anesthesia
Specialty Deputy Consultant to the Surgeon General
William Beaumont Army Medical Center
Fort Bliss, Texas
United States
Procedure 75: *Central Venous Catheter Insertion (Assist), Nursing Care and Removal*

Kayla Little, MSN, APRN, AGCNS-BC, PCCN
Clinical Nurse Specialist
Cardiovascular Stepdown, Heart & Lung Transplant
Cleveland Clinic
Cleveland, Ohio
United States
Procedure 57: *Blood Sampling From an Arterial Catheter*

Veronica Ann Lock, BSN, RN, CCRN
Clinical Practice Specialist
Intensive Care Unit
Northwestern Huntley Hospital
Huntley, Illinois
United States
Procedure 52: *Arterial Catheter Insertion (Perform)*
Procedure 54: *Blood Sampling From an Arterial Catheter*

Cara Diaz Lomangino, MSN, RN, CRNP
Senior Nurse Practitioner
Trauma Neurosurgery
University of Maryland Medical Center
Baltimore, Maryland
United States
Procedure 91: *Cervical Traction and Stabilization: Assist and Nursing Care*
Procedure 92: *Pin Site and Vest Care*

Amy I. Lucas, MSN, RN, CCRN-K, CCNS
Clinical Nurse Specialist
Nursing Practice
Carilion Roanoke Memorial Hospital
Roanoke, Virginia
United States
Procedure 14: *Oxygen Saturation Monitoring With Pulse Oximetry*

Zoë Maher, MD
Trauma/Surgical Critical Care Attending
Associate Trauma Medical Director
Temple University Hospital – Main Campus;
Associate Professor, Surgery Director, Global Surgery Temple Emergency Action Corps
Temple University;
Faculty Advisor
Lewis Katz School of Medicine at Temple University
Philadelphia, Pennsylvania
United States
Procedure 96: *Focused Abdominal Assessment With Sonography*

Stephanie Maillie, MSN, RN, CCRN, CCNS, WCC
Critical Clinical Nurse Specialist
Medical Intensive Care Unit
Hospital of the University of Pennsylvania
Penn Medicine
Philadelphia, Pennsylvania
United States
Procedure 12: *Continuous End-Tidal Carbon Dioxide Monitoring*

Marc Manley, MSN, RN, NE-BC
Executive Director
Cardiovascular Services
Baptist Health Lexington
Lexington, Kentucky
United States
Procedure 17: *Chest Tube Placement (Perform)*

Gregory Simpson Marler, DNP, APRN, ACNP-BC, FCCP
Assistant Professor, Nursing
Beaver College of Health Sciences
Appalachian State University
Boone, North Carolina
United States;
Critical Care Nurse Practitioner
Wake Forest Baptist Health
Winston-Salem, North Carolina
United States
Procedure: 115 *Wound Closure (Perform)*
Procedure: 117 *Débridement: Pressure Ulcers, Burns, and Wounds*

Sarah R. Martha, PhD, RN
Assistant Professor
College of Nursing
University of Illinois at Chicago
Chicago, Illinois
United States
Procedure 89: *Lumbar Puncture (Assist) and Nursing Care*

Carol Marie McGinnis, DNP, APRN-CNS, CNSC
Clinical Nurse Specialist
Center for Care Management
Sanford USD Medical Center
Sioux Falls, South Dakota
United States
Procedure 100: *Nasogastric and Orogastric Tube Insertion, Nursing Care, and Removal*

Marion E. McRae, PhD, RN, ACNP-BC, CCRN-CMC
Nurse Practitioner
Cardiac Surgery
Cedars-Sinai Medical Center
Los Angeles, California
United States
Procedure 34: *Emergent Open Sternotomy (Perform) and Defibrillation (Internal) (Perform)*
Procedure 35: *Emergent Open Sternotomy and Internal Defibrillation (Assist)*
Procedure 39: *Atrial Electrogram*
Procedure 41: *Temporary Epicardial Pacing Wire Removal*

Dannette A. Mitchell, MSN, ARPN, ACNS-BC, CCRN, FCNS
Clinical Nurse Specialist
Medical Critical Care
ChristianaCare
Wilmington, Delaware
United States
Procedure 15: *Prone Positioning for Acute Respiratory Distress Syndrome Patients*

Kelly Moutray, BSN, MEd, RN, CCRN
Registered Nurse
Cardiovascular Intensive Care Unit
Saint Luke's Hospital
Kansas City, Missouri
United States
Procedure 13: *Extracorporeal Membrane Oxygenation*

Megan T. Moyer, MSN, ACNP-BC, CNRN
Nurse Practitioner
University of Pennsylvania
Philadelphia, Pennsylvania
United States
Procedure 84: *Brain Tissue Oxygen Monitoring: Insertion (Assist), Nursing Care, and Troubleshooting*

Malissa Mulkey, PhD, RN, APN, ACCNS, CCRN, SCRN
Assistant Professor
University of South Carolina College of Nursing
Columbia, South Carolina
United States
Procedure 83: *Signal Processed Electroencephalography*

Angela Muzzy, MSN, RN, CCRN, CNS-BC
Clinical Nurse Specialist
Adult Critical Care
Tucson Medical Center
Tucson, Arizona
United States
Procedure 51: *Twelve-Lead Electrocardiogram With Right and Left Posterior Leads*

Katie Neil, MSN, RN, CCRN-K, NPD-BC
Manager, Office of Professional Practice & Development
Northwestern Medicine, Huntley Hospital
Huntley, Illinois
United States
Procedure 52: *Arterial Catheter Insertion (Perform)*
Procedure 54: *Blood Sampling From an Arterial Catheter*

Jennifer Pesenecker, BSN, RN, PCCN-K
Educational Nurse Coordinator
Cardiothoracic Surgery Step-Down
University of Michigan
Ann Arbor, Michigan
United States
Procedure 44: *Temporary Transcutaneous (External) Pacing*
Procedure 46: *Temporary Transvenous and Epicardial Pacing*

Lynelle N.B. Pierce, MS, RN, CCRN, CCNS, FAAN
Clinical Specialist
Critical Care Nursing
The University of Kansas Health System
Kansas City, Kansas
United States
Procedure 102: *Molecular Adsorbent Recirculating System (MARS)*

Jan Powers, PhD, RN, CCNS, CCRN, NE-BC, FCCM, FAAN
Director, Nursing Research and Professional Practice
Parkview Health
Fort Wayne, Indiana
United States
Procedure 125: *Prevention of Immobility-Related Complications: Kinetic Therapy (Continuous Lateral Rotation Therapy and Lateral Rotation Therapy) and Ambulation of Acute and Critically Ill Patients*

Heather L. Przybyl, DNP, RN, CCRN
RN Certified Specialist
Critical Care
Banner University Medical Center Phoenix
Phoenix, Arizona
United States
Procedure 11: *Tracheostomy Cuff and Tube Care*
Procedure 105: *Continuous Renal Replacement Therapies*
Procedure 106: *Hemodialysis*
Procedure 107: *Peritoneal Dialysis*

Barbara Quinn, DNP, MSN, ACNS-BC, FCNS
Director, Professional Practice & Nursing Excellence
Sutter Health System Office
Sutter Health
Sacramento, California
United States
Procedure 3: *Endotracheal Tube Care and Oral Care Practices for Ventilated and Nonventilated Patients*

Jessica Raymond, MSN, MBA, RN
Nursing Manager, Stroke
Northwestern Medicine Marianjoy Rehabilitation Hospital
Wheaton, Illinois
United States
Procedure 67: *Esophageal Cardiac Output Monitoring: Perform*
Procedure 68: *Esophageal Cardiac Output Monitoring: Assist, Care, and Removal*

Janet Regan-Baggs, DNP, RN, ACNS-BC, CCNS, CCRN-K
Critical Care and Mechanical Circulatory Support Clinical Nurse Specialist
Patient Care Services
University of Washington Medical Center
Seattle, Washington
United States
Procedure 60: *Single-Pressure and Multiple-Pressure Transducer Systems*

Erin Reynolds, BSN, RN, CCRN, CNML
Clinical Director
Medical Surgical Intensive Care Unit
Inova Health System
Falls Church, Virginia
United States
Procedure: 108 *Apheresis and Therapeutic Plasma Exchange (Assist)*
Procedure: 114 *Intracompartmental Pressure Monitoring (Perform)*
Procedure 116: *Cleansing, Irrigating, Culturing, and Dressing an Open Wound*

Melanie Roberts, DNP, RN-BC, CCNS, CCRN-K
Critical Care Clinical Nurse Specialist
Critical Care
UCHealth Medical Center of the Rockies and Poudre Valley Hospital
Loveland, Colorado
United States
Procedure 97: *Gastric Lavage in Hemorrhage and Overdose*

Michael S. Rogers, BSN, RN, CCRN, CNRN, SCRN
Nursing Professional Development Practitioner
Adult Critical Care
University of California at San Francisco
San Francisco, California
United States
Procedure 87: *Intracranial Pressure Monitoring, Nursing Care, Troubleshooting, and Removal*

Cheryl Ruble, MS, RN, CNS
Quality Nurse Consultant
Regional Clinical Quality Programs and Data Analytics
Kaiser Foundation Hospital and Health Plan
Northern California, California
United States
Procedure 3: *Endotracheal Tube Care and Oral Care Practices for Ventilated and Nonventilated Patients*

Thomas A. Santora, MD, MBA
Professor & Vice-Chair
Department of Surgery
Lewis Katz School of Medicine at Temple University
Philadelphia, Pennsylvania
United States
Procedure 96: *Focused Abdominal Assessment With Sonography*

Michael Schnake, MBA, BSN, RN, CFER
Associate Nurse Manager
UCHealth University of Colorado Hospital
Aurora, Colorado
United States
Procedure 101: *Fecal Microbiota Transplant (Perform)*

Susan Scott, PhD, RN, CCRN
Associate Professor
Nursing
Westfield State University
Westfield, Massachusetts
United States
Procedure 55: *Arterial Pressure-Based Cardiac Output Monitoring*
Procedure 65: *Cardiac Output Measurement Techniques (Invasive)*
Procedure 66: *Noninvasive Cardiac Output Monitoring*

Maureen A. Seckel, MSN, APRN, ACNS-BC, CCNS, CCRN-K, FCCM, FCNS, FAAN
Clinical Nurse Specialist, Medical Critical Care and Sepsis
  Coordinator
Medical ICU and Department of Medicine
ChristianaCare
Newark, Delaware
United States
Procedure 8: *Suctioning: Endotracheal or Tracheostomy Tube*

Christine Slaughter, MSN, RN, CCRN-K, CCNS, CV-BC
Clinical Nurse Specialist
Cardiovascular Acute/Progressive and Central Monitoring
  Station
University of Kentucky
Lexington, Kentucky
United States
Procedure 18: *Chest Tube Placement (Assist)*
Procedure 28: *Noninvasive Ventilation*

Valerie Spotts, BSN, RN
Educational Nurse Coordinator
Nursing–Inpatient Cardiology
University of Michigan
Ann Arbor, Michigan
United States
Procedure 44: *Temporary Transcutaneous (External) Pacing*
Procedure 46: *Temporary Transvenous and Epicardial Pacing*

Cynthia Sprinkle, MSN-Ed, RN, CEN, TCRN
Director, Clinical Education
Critical Care
Banner Health
Phoenix, Arizona
United States
Procedure 16: *Autotransfusion*

Mindy Stites, MSN, APRN, ACNS-BC, CCNS, CCNS-AG, CCRN
Clinical Nurse Specialist, Critical Care
The University of Kansas Health System
Kansas City, Kansas
United States
Procedure 73: *Arterial Puncture*

Claire Sutherlin, BSN, RN, CCRN
Clinical Nurse Specialist
Surgical Intensive Care Unit
Thomas Jefferson University Hospital,
Philadelphia, Pennsylvania
United States
Procedure 102: *Molecular Adsorbent Recirculating System (MARS)*

Nikki J. Taylor, BSN, MS, RN, AGCNS-BC
Clinical Nurse Specialist
Cardiothoracic and Vascular Surgery
University of Michigan Health System;
Adjunct Clinical Instructor
School of Nursing
University of Michigan
Ann Arbor, Michigan
United States
Procedure 44: *Temporary Transcutaneous (External) Pacing*
Procedure 45: *Temporary Transvenous Pacemaker Insertion
  (Perform)*
Procedure 46: *Temporary Transvenous and Epicardial Pacing*
Procedure 58: *Pulmonary Artery Catheter Insertion (Perform)*
Procedure 59: *Pulmonary Artery Catheter Insertion (Assist) and
  Pressure Monitoring*
Procedure 64: *Pulmonary Artery Catheter Removal*

Deborah Thorgesen, MSN, RN
Clinical Nurse Manager
Northwestern Medicine, Huntley Hospital
Huntley, Illinois
United States
Procedure 53: *Arterial Catheter Insertion (Assist), Care, and
  Removal*

Misti Tuppeny, MSN, APRN-CNS, CCRN, CNRN, CCNA
Clinical Nurse Specialist
AdventHealth
Orlando, Florida
United States
Procedure 94: *Patient-Controlled Analgesia*

Debra Valdivieso, DNP, CRNA
Nurse Anesthesist
Anesthesia Department
Ascension Health System
Milwaukee, Wisconsin
United States
Procedure 78: *Use of a Massive Infusion Device and a Pressure
  Infuser Bag*

Amanda Virginia, DNP, CRNA
Clinical Education Coordinator
University of Texas Southwestern
Dallas, Texas
United States;
Adjunct Clinical Instructor
School of Nurse Anesthesia
Texas Christian University
Fort Worth, Texas
United States
Procedure 81: *Noninvasive Brain Tissue Monitoring: Near-Infrared
  Cerebral Spectroscopy*

Kathleen M. Vollman, MSN, RN, CCNS, FCCM, FCNS, FAAN
Clinical Nurse Specialist/Consultant
ADVANCING NURSING LLC
Northville, Michigan
United States
Procedure 15: *Prone Positioning for Acute Respiratory Distress Syndrome Patients*

Brooke Wagner, MSN, APN, AGCNS-BC, CNRN, SCRN
Clinical Nurse Specialist
Banner University Medical Center – Phoenix
Phoenix, Arizona
United States
Procedure 82: *EEG Monitoring Assist and Nursing Care*

Shu Wang, MSN, AGACNP
Advanced Practice Nurse
Lymphoma/Myeloma
MD Anderson Cancer Center
Houston, Texas
United States
Procedure 76: *Implantable Venous Access Device: Access, Deaccess, and Care*

Julie M. Waters, MSN, RN, CCRN
Clinical Educator
Cardiac Intensive Care Unit
Providence Sacred Heart Medical Center
Spokane, Washington
United States
Procedure 19: *Chest Tube Removal (Perform)*
Procedure 20: *Chest Tube Removal (Assist)*

Shelley K. Welch, MSN, RN, CCRN-CSC
Professor
Tyler Junior College
Tyler, Texas
United States
Procedure 50: *ST-Segment Monitoring (Continuous)*

Kim Wigen-Dewey, MSN, NPD-BC, CCRN-K, CHSE
Professional Development Specialist
Professional Development Department
Providence Inland Northwest Washington
Spokane, Washington
United States
Procedure 29: *Manual Self-Inflating Resuscitation Bag-Valve-Mask Device*

Laura A. Wilson, MSN, RN, APRN, AACC, CHFN
Faculty
School of Nursing, Graduate Education
The University of Texas at El Paso
El Paso, Texas
United States
Procedure 48: *Ventricular Assist Devices*
Procedure 69: *Femoral Arterial and Venous Sheath Removal*

Marie Woznicki, MSN, APRN, AGACNP-BC
Nurse Practitioner
Cardiology
El Paso Cardiology Associates
El Paso, Texas
United States
Procedure 72: *Transesophageal Echocardiography (Assist)*

Valeda L. Yong, MD
Resident Physician
Department of Surgery
Temple University Hospital
Philadelphia, Pennsylvania
United States
Procedure 96: *Focused Abdominal Assessment With Sonography*

Susan Ziegfeld, MSN, RN, PNP-BC
Manager, Pediatric Trauma and Burn Program, Lead Nurse Practitioner
Johns Hopkins Childrens Center
Baltimore, Maryland
United States
Procedure 111: *Burn Wound Care*
Procedure 112: *Donor-Site Care*
Procedure 113: *Skin-Graft Care*

Reviewers

Lillian Aguirre, DNP, APRN-CNS, CCRN, CCNS
Clinical Nurse Specialist
Orlando Regional Medical Center, Orlando Health
Orlando, Florida
United States

Christine Aiello, MSN, RN, ACCNS-AG, CCRN
Trauma Performance Improvement Coordinator
Penn Presbyterian Medical Center
Philadelphia, Pennsylvania
United States

Kwame Asante Akuamoah-Boateng, DNP, ACNP-BC, RN, FCCM
Assistant Professor
AG-ACNP Nurse Practitioner Program
Murphy Deming College of Health Sciences - Mary Baldwin University
Fishersville, Virginia
United States

Blake Albretsen, BSN, CCRN, RN
Providence Sacred Heart Medical Center
CICU Staff Nurse
Spokane, Washington
United States

Diana Alexander, MSN, RN, CCRN
Manager, Surgical ICU/ICU Float Pool/ECMO Program
Lakeland Regional Health
Lakeland, Florida
United States

Ann Allison, MSN, RN, ACNS-BC
Clinical Nurse Specialist
Intensive Care Unit/Progressive Care Unit
Indiana University Health West
Avon, Indiana
United States

Maighdlin Anderson, DNP, ACNP-BC, FCCM
Assistant Professor and Adult Gerontology Acute Care Nurse Practitioner Program Director
University of Pittsburgh
Pittsburgh, Pennsylvania
United States

Mary Pat Aust, MS, RN, CDE
Equity, Diversity & Inclusion Lead
American Association of Critical-Care Nurses
Aliso Viejo, California
United States

Barbara Bailey, NP, MN, CCN(C)
Nurse Practitioner – Adult Congenital Heart Disease
Toronto Congenital Cardiac Centre for Adults
Peter Munk Cardiac Center
University Health Network
Toronto, Ontario
Canada

Arianna Barnes, DNP, RN, CCRN, PHN
Clinical Nurse Specialist
Barnes Jewish Hospital
St. Louis, Missouri
United States

Gisele Bazan, MSN, RN, CCRN-K
Nursing Professional Development Generalist/Nurse Educator, Cardiac ICU and Nephrology
Covenant Health
Lubbock, Texas
United States

Linda Bell, MSN, RN
Clinical Practice Specialist (retired)
American Association of Critical-Care Nurses
Aliso Viejo, California
United States

Lolita M. Bennett, MSN, RN
Nurse Manager, Medical Intensive Care Unit
Corporal Michael J. Crescenz Veterans Affairs Medical Center
Philadelphia, Pennsylvania
United States

Tracey M. Berlin, MSN, RN, CNRN, CCRN-K
Senior Clinical Specialist & Clinical Research Coordinator
NeurOptics, Inc.
Irvine, California
United States

Bridget Bieber, MSN, RN, CCRN, BC-NPD
Nursing Professional Development Specialist II
Surgical Critical Care
Institute for Learning, Leadership & Development (iLEAD)
ChristianaCare
Newark, Delaware
United States

Debbie Brinker, MSN, RN, CNS
Clinical Practice Specialist
American Association of Critical-Care Nurses
Aliso Viejo, California
United States

Megan E. Brunson, MSN, RN, CCRN-CSC, CNL, FCCM
Rapid Response Nurse/House Supervisor
Medical City Heart Hospital
Dallas, Texas
United States

Kristen Burton-Williams, MSN, APRN, ACCNS-AG, CCRN-K, TCRN, FCNS
Advanced Practice Manager
The Center for Professional Practice and Innovation
Rhode Island Hospital
Providence, Rhode Island
United States

Kimberly R. Bush, MSN, RN, PCCN, CCCTM
Clinical Practice Leader
Intermediate Surgical ICU
Thomas Jefferson University Hospital
Philadelphia, Pennsylvania
United States

Jaime Byrne, MSN, RN, CCRN-CSC, CCCTM
Clinical Practice Leader, CVICU
Thomas Jefferson University Hospital
Philadelphia, Pennsylvania
United States

Cindy Cain, DNP, RN, CNS, CCRN-K
Clinical Practice Specialist
American Association of Critical-Care Nurses
Aliso Viejo, California
United States

Leah Riggs Capra, MSN, AGACNP-BC
Nurse Practitioner – Cardiac Catheterization
  Lab
Mount Sinai Morningside
New York, New York
United States

**Marie L. Cassalia, MSN, APRN,
  ACCNS-AG, CCRN-CSC, WTA**
Clinical Nurse Specialist
Nursing
ChristianaCare
Newark, Delaware
United States

**Jose Chavez, MSN, RN, ACCNS-AG,
  CCRN, AACC**
Clinical Nurse Specialist
Critical Care Services
  (Coronary ICU)
Cedars-Sinai Medical Center
Los Angeles, California
United States

**Mary Ann "Cammy" Christie, APRN,
  MSN, CCRN, PCCN, CSC**
APRN, Division of Critical Care Medicine,
  CVICU
University of Florida
Gainesville, Florida
United States

Lawrence Chyall, CNS, RN
Neuroscience Nurse Manager
San Francisco General Hospital
San Francisco, California
United States

Alexa Collins, BSN, RN, SCRN
Nurse Manager
UT Southwestern Medical Center
Dallas, Texas
United States

Chris Robert Cornachione, CRNP
Surgical Critical Care
University of Maryland Medical System
Baltimore, Maryland
United States

**Ginnie Covey, BSN, RN, CV-BC,
  CHFN**
Magnet Program Director
CHRISTUS® Trinity Mother Frances
  Hospital – Tyler
Tyler, Texas
United States

Haley Culbertson, BSN, RN, CCRN, CSC
RN V, Cardiovascular Intensive Care Unit
Banner University Medical Center
Tucson, Arizona
United States

Monica Cummins, MSN, RN, PCCN
Clinical Nurse Specialist Intern
Cardiovascular Surgery Stepdown
Thoracic Surgery Stepdown
Cleveland Clinic
Cleveland, Ohio
United States

Hina N. Dave, MD
Associate Professor, Neurology
McGovern Medical School
University of Texas Health Sciences
Houston, Texas
United States

**Michelle Ann Dedeo, DNP,
  ARNP-CNS, ACCNS-AG, CCRN,
  CNRN, SCRN**
Neuroscience Clinical Nurse Specialist
Swedish Health Services
Everett, Washington
United States

Francine Dehaan, MSN, RN
Clinical Educator
Inova Fairfax Medical Campus
Falls Church, Virginia
United States

**Kate Deis, MSN, RN CEN ACNS-BC,
  TCRN, NE-BC**
Nurse Manager, Emergency Department
Thomas Jefferson University
  Hospital
Philadelphia, Pennsylvania
United States

**Sonia B. Depina, MSN, RN, PCCN-K,
  BPD, BC**
Advanced Practice Manager (MICU, RICU,
  ICCU)
Lifespan Healthcare System
Rhode Island Hospital
Providence, Rhode Island
United States

**Marcia Depolo, DNP, CCRN, CNRN,
  TCRN, NPD-BC**
Clinical Instructor
Academic Nursing Program
Ballad Health
Johnson City, Tennessee
United States

**Justin DiLibero, DNP, APRN,
  CCRN-K, CCNS, ACCNS-AG,
  FCNS**
Interim Dean
Zvart Onanian School of Nursing
Rhode Island College
RI Nursing Education Center
Providence, Rhode Island
United States

**Marci Ebberts, MSN, APRN, FNP-C,
  CCRN-K**
Clinical Education Specialist
Saint Luke's Hospital
Saint Luke's Health System
Kansas City, Missouri
United States

**Margaret M. Ecklund, MS, RN,
  CCRN-K, ACNP-BC, WTA-C**
Clinical Nurse Specialist
Clinical Practice Support
Wound & Ostomy & Skin Care
Legacy Health
Portland, Oregon
United States

**John Emberger, RRT-ACCS, FAARC,
  CPHQ, LSSBB**
Director, Respiratory Care
ChristianaCare
Newark, Delaware
United States

Stephen Figueroa, MD
Associate Professor of Neurology
University of Texas Southwestern
Dallas, Texas
United States

**R. Denise Filiatrault, DNP, MN, RN,
  NPD-BC**
Sr. Director
Clinical Education & Practice
Swedish Hospital System
Seattle, Washington
United States

**Kathleen Flarity, DNP, PhD, CEN,
  CFRN, FAEN, FAAN, Brigadier
  General (ret) USAF**
Deputy Director
Colorado University Anschutz Center for
  COMBAT Research & Associate Professor
Department of Emergency Medicine
University of Colorado School of Medicine
Research Nurse Scientist
UCHealth
Aurora, Colorado
United States

**Mary Beth Flynn Makic, PhD, RN,
  CCNS, CCRN-K, FAAN, FNAP, FCNS**
Professor
Research Scientist
Specialty Director, Adult-Gerontology
  Clinical Nurse Specialist Program
University of Colorado Anschutz Campus
College of Nursing
Denver Health
Aurora, Colorado
United States

Nikki Galaviz, MSN, RN, CCRN-K, NPD-BC
Nursing Professional Development Specialist
Surgical Intensive Care Unit
Covenant Health
Lubbock, Texas
United States

John J. Gallagher, DNP, RN, CCNS, CCRN-K, TCRN, CHSE, RRT, FCCM
Professor/Clinical Nurse Specialist
Director of Simulation Education
University of Pittsburgh School of Nursing
Pittsburgh, Pennsylvania
United States

Rebecca Garber, MSN, RN
Nurse Practitioner
Greely Burn Clinic
Greely, Colorado
United States

James A. Gerding, PA-C
R Adams Cowley Shock Trauma Center
Baltimore, Maryland
United States

Jean Gima, MN, NP
Nurse Practitioner-Electrophysiology
Ronald Reagan UCLA Medical Center
Los Angeles, California
United States

Robynn Goldstein, MSN, RN, ACNP-C, CNS
Congenital Electrophysiology NP
Ronald Reagan UCLA Medical Center
Los Angeles, California
United States

Jennifer Gosztyla-Borzoni, MSN, RN, NPD-BC
Manager, Nursing Center of Excellence
Queen of the Valley Medical Center
Napa, California
United States

Joel M. Green, MSN, RN, CCRN-CSC-CMC
Interim Nurse Manager, CT-ICU
University of Washington MCMontlake;
Harborview Medical Center
Seattle, Washington
United States

Ami Grek, DNP, APRN
Lead APP, Critical Care
Mayo Clinic Florida
Jacksonville, Florida
United States

Sara Grieshop, MHI, BSN, RN
Practice Excellence Supervisor
American Association of Critical-Care Nurses
Aliso Viejo, California
United States

Ryan Gunn, MSN, APRN, ACNP-BC
Nurse Practitioner – Cardiothoracic Surgery
CHRISTUS® Mother Frances Hospital
Tyler, Texas
United States

Christian Guzman, MS, ACNP-AG, APRN, CCRN
Advanced Practice Provider, Critical Care Medicine
University of Florida Health
Gainesville, Florida
United States

Heather Hall, BSN, DVM, CCRN-K
Clinical Educator
Inova Health System
Falls Church, Virginia
United States

Erin Hare, MSN, RN, CCRN
Nursing Professional Development Team Leader
Medical Intensive Care
ChristianaCare
Newark, Delaware
United States

Emily Hart, MSN, ACNP-BC
Senior Nurse Practitioner
Critical Care Resuscitation Unit
R Adams Cowley Shock Trauma Center
Baltimore, Maryland
United States

Tonja Hartjes-Cubbellotti, DNP, CNS, APRN, CCRN, CNEcl, FAANP
CEO
Coastal Consultants and Education LLC
Keystone Heights, Florida
United States

Jan Healey, BS, RN
Principal
Consultants in Acute & Critical Care
Miami, Florida
United States

P. Christine High, MSN, RN, CCRN-K
Clinical Nurse Educator
Baptist Health South Florida
Miami, Florida
United States

Angela Hinman, MSN, RN, CCRN
Critical Care RN
Providence St. Patrick Hospital
Missoula, Montana
United States

Mary Eng Huntsinger, MSN, ACNP-BC, CNS
Electrophysiology Nurse Practitioner, Cardiovascular Medicine
Keck Hospital of USC
University of Southern California
Los Angeles, California
United States

Wendy Hansen Ibarra, BSN, RN
RN Education Specialist, Medical Imaging & Cath Lab
Banner Health
Phoenix, Arizona
United States

Flerida Imperial-Perez, PhD, RN, CNS-BC, CCNS-P
Manager and CNS, Cardiothoracic ICU
Children's Hospital Los Angeles
Los Angeles, California
United States

Robin Jackson, MSN, RN
Clinical Nurse Specialist
Inova Alexandria Hospital
Alexandria, Virginia
United States

Katherine Janaszek, MSN, NP-BC
Nurse Practitioner, Cardiovascular Medicine
Health Texas Employee Network, Baylor Scott & White Legacy Heart Center
Plano, Texas
United States

Brian Jefferson, DNP
Hepato-Pancreato-Biliary Surgery
Atrium Health HPB Surgery Cabarrus
Concord, North Carolina
United States

Rachael Alexis Jividen, MSN, APRN, ACCNS-AG, CCRN-CSC
ECLS/ECMO Coordinator
Acute Care Clinical Nurse Specialist
Cardiothoracic ICUs
Cleveland Clinic
Cleveland, Ohio
United States

Steven B. Johnson, MD, FCCM, FACS
Trauma/Critical Care Surgeon
Scottsdale, Arizona
United States

Renee Johnson, MS, APRN, CCRN, CCNS
Cardiovascular Surgery Clinical Nurse Specialist
Northside Hospital
Lawrenceville, Georgia
United States

Dawn Johnston, MSN-Ed, RN
System Clinical Education Specialist
Critical Care Education Team
Banner Health
Phoenix, Arizona
United States

Ashlee Jontz, MS, ACNP-BC, ANP
Surgical Trauma Nurse Practitioner
Lead Nurse Practitioner
Banner University Medical Center – Phoenix
Phoenix Arizona
United States

Abdulkadir Kamal II., BSN, RN
Neurocritical Care Staff Nurse
University of Texas Southwestern
Dallas, Texas
United States

Emily Kelly, PA-C
Critical Care Physician Assistant
Medical University of South Carolina
Charleston, South Carolina
United States

Bridget Kelly, MSN, RN-BC, CCCTM
Clinical Practice Leader
Transplant Unit
Thomas Jefferson University Hospital
Philadelphia, Pennsylvania
United States

Michelle Kidd, DNP, APRN, ACNS-BC, CCRN-K, FCNS
Clinical Nurse Specialist
Indiana University Health Ball Memorial Hospital
Muncie, Indiana
United States

Deborah Klein, MSN, APRN, ACNS-BC, CCRN-K, FAHA, FAAN
Clinical Nurse Specialist (retired), Cardiac Critical Care
Cleveland Clinic
Cleveland, Ohio
United States

Karin Kloppel, BSN, RN, CCRN, CEN
Clinical Educator, ED & ICU
Providence Holy Family Hospital
Spokane, Washington
United States

Sara Knippa, MS, RN, CCRN, ACCNS-AG
Clinical Nurse Specialist/Educator
Cardiac Intensive Care Unit
UC Health
University of Colorado Hospital
Aurora, Colorado
United States

Lisa Koser, DNP, MSN, MS, ACNP-BC, CPNP-AC
Lead Advanced Practice Provider
Trauma, Burn & Acute Care Surgery
Department of Surgery
Division of Trauma, Critical Care & Burn
The Ohio State University Wexner Medical Center
Columbus, Ohio;
Flight Nurse Practitioner
Cleveland Clinic Critical Care Transport
Cleveland, Ohio
United States

Yasmine Lee, DNP, ANP-BC
Nurse Practitioner – Arrhythmia Program
Hoag Memorial Hospital Presbyterian
Newport Beach, California
United States

Louie Lee, MSN, RN, CCRN, CEN, TCRN
Senior Clinical Nurse II
Critical Care Resuscitation Unit & Biocontainment Team
R Adams Cowley Shock Trauma Center
University of Maryland Medical Center
Baltimore, Maryland
United States

Shamma LeGrand, MSN, CCRN
Clinical Risk Manager/Patient Safety Officer
Baptist Health South Florida
Coral Gables, Florida
United States

Emily R. Leiter, DNAP, CRNA, LTC, AN
Chief, Department of Anesthesia
Specialty Deputy Consultant to the Surgeon General
William Beaumont Army Medical Center
Fort Bliss, Texas
United States

Andrea Lever, BSN, RN, CCRN, CPAN
Clinical Nurse III, Cardiac PACU
Cedars-Sinai Medical Center
Los Angeles, California
United States

Cathleen Lindauer, DNP, RN
Nursing Practice & Professional Development Specialist
Centralized Nursing, Johns Hopkins Health Systems
Baltimore, Maryland
United States

Vicki Lindgren, MSN, RN, CCNS
Clinical Nurse Specialist
Inova Fair Oaks Hospital
Fair Oaks, Virginia
United States

Kayla Little, MSN, APRN, AGCNS-BC, PCCN
Clinical Nurse Specialist
Cardiovascular Stepdown
Heart & Lung Transplant
Cleveland Clinic
Cleveland, Ohio
United States

Andrea Ma Lupera, MSN, RN, CCRN
Nursing Professional Development Practitioner
Critical Care Services
Cedars-Sinai Medical Center
Los Angeles, California
United States

Melani Mangum-Williams, MSN, RN, CCRN-K, NPD-BC
Senior Program Manager, Critical Care, Stepdown/Progressive Care, Emergency
Providence Nursing Institute Clinical Academy
Walla Walla, Washington
United States

Stephanie Maniquis, AG-ACNP, CCRN-CSC
Nurse Practitioner II – Cardiothoracic ICU
Ronald Reagan UCLA Medical Center
Los Angeles, California
United States

Lynne Martin, MSN, RN, PHN, PCCN-K
House Support Manager
Loma Linda Medical Center Murrieta
Murrieta, California
United States

Nikki Matos, DNP, APRN
Lead Advanced Practice Provider,
    Cardiovascular Thoracic ICU
Mayo Clinic
Jacksonville, Florida
United States

Ann Matta, MSN, ACNP-BC
Acute Care Nurse Practitioner
University of Maryland Medical Center
Baltimore, Maryland
United States

Eileen C. McDonald-Karcz, MSN, NP
Nurse Practitioner – Cardiology
Halton Heathcare Services – Oakville
    Trafalgar Memorial Hospital
Oakville, Ontario
Canada

Connor McLaughlin, BSN, RN
Artificial Heart & Mechanical Circulatory
    Support Coordinator
Banner University Medical Center – Phoenix
Phoenix, Arizona
United States

Molly M. McNett, PhD, RN, CNRN,
**   FNCS, FAAN**
Professor of Nursing
The Ohio State University
Columbus, Ohio
United States

Teresa Ann Meeks, BSN, RN, CCRN
Clinical Educator II
CHRISTUS® Trinity Mother Frances
    Health System
Louis and Peaches Owen Heart Hospital
Tyler, Texas
United States

Julie Miller, BSN, RN, CCRN-K
Clinical Practice Specialist
American Association of Critical-Care Nurses
Aliso Viejo, California
United States

Ashifa Moledina, DNP, AG-ACNP,
**   ACCNS**
Critical Care Nurse Practitioner
R Adams Cowley Shock Trauma Center
Baltimore, Maryland
United States

Jessica Montanaro, MSN, RN, ANCC
Critical Care Nurse
Mount Sinai Morningside Hospital
New York, New York
United States

Donna Mursch, BSN, RN, CCRN
Nurse Manager
University of Maryland
R Adams Cowley Shock Trauma Center
Baltimore, Maryland
United States

Russell Neptune, BSN, RN
Manager, Kidney Center
Banner University Medical Center
Tucson, Arizona
United States

Christopher Noel, MSN, NP-C, CWS
Nurse Practitioner
Kaiser Permanente
Lafayette, Colorado
United States

Amber O'Conner, BSN, RN, CCRN-K
Learning Consultant
Critical Care Team
Orlando Health
Orlando, Florida
United States

Meredith Padilla, PhD, RN,
**   CCRN-CMC/CSC**
Clinical Practice Specialist
American Association of Critical-Care
    Nurses
Aliso Viejo, California
United States

Angela D. Pal, PhD, APRN, ACNP-BC,
**   CHSE**
Assistant Professor
Specialty Director, Adult Gerontology
    Acute Care NP Program
College of Nursing
University of Colorado Anschutz Medical
    Campus
Aurora, Colorado
United States

Sarah H. Peacock, DNP, APRN,
**   ACNP-BC**
Department of Critical Care Medicine
Mayo Clinic
Jacksonville, Florida
United States

Matthew Piper, BSN, BS, RN, TCRN,
**   PHRN**
Senior Clinical Nurse II
Trauma Resuscitation Unit
R Adams Cowley Shock Trauma Center
University of Maryland Medical Center
Baltimore, Maryland
United States

Patricia Radovich, PhD, CNS, FCCM
Director, Nursing Research
Loma Linda University Health System
Loma Linda, California
United States

Darlene M. Rebeyka, MSN, RN,
**   ACNP, CCN(C)**
Nurse Practitioner, Adult Cardiovascular
    Surgery
Mazankowski Alberta Heart Institute
Edmonton, Alberta
Canada

Tamera Reichert, BSN, RN
Clinical Education Specialist
Critical Care Education Team
Banner Health
Phoenix, Arizona
United States

Holly Rodgers, MSN, CRNP,
**   ACNPC-AG, CCRN**
SICU Nurse Practitioner
Corporal Michael J. Crescenz VA Medical
    Center
Philadelphia, Pennsylvania
United States

Emily Rogers, DNP, AGACNP-BC,
**   APRN**
Advanced Practice Provider
Mayo Clinic Florida, Department of Critical
    Care
Jacksonville, Florida
United States

Alicia Roth, DNP, AG-ACNP, CNRN
Nurse Practitioner
Pulmonary Critical Care
Banner University Medical Center
Phoenix, Arizona
United States

Christan Santos, DNP, APRN
Nurse Practitioner
Department of Critical Care Medicine
Mayo Clinic Florida;
Adjunct Faculty
School of Nursing
University of North Florida
Jacksonville, Florida
United States

Erin Sarsfield, MSN, RN
Clinical Coordinator, Head and Neck
    Surgery
Penn State Hershey Medical Center
Hershey, Pennsylvania
United States

Kelsey Sawyer, MSN, RN, CCRN, NPD-BC
Nursing Professional Development
Specialist, MICU
Covenant Health
Lubbock Texas
United States

Mary Scott-Herring, DNP, MS, CRNA
Assistant Professor
Doctor of Nurse Anesthesia Practice
(DNAP) Program
Georgetown University
Washington, DC
United States

Ashley Seawright, DNP, ACNP-BC
Executive Director of Advanced Practice
Providers
Chief of APPs, Department of Surgery
Clinical Director of Transplant and Surgical
Oncology
University of Mississippi Medical Center
Jackson, Mississippi
United States

Casey Shaouni, MSN, RN, CCRN-K
Learning Consultant
Critical Care Team
Orlando Health
Orlando, Florida
United States

Heizel Aloida Singson, MSN, RN, BSN, Gero-BC, CCRN-K
Nurse Educator
NYC Health & Hospital Woodhull
Bergenfield, New Jersey
United States

Althea Sment, MSN, RN, ACCNS, CCRN-CSC
Nurse Educator
Zablocki VA Medical Center
Mukwonago, Wisconsin
United States

Susan Smith, DNP, RN, CEN, CCRN, CNLCP, COWCN
Faculty
St. Francis University
Warriors Mark, Pennsylvania
United States

Nancy Colobong Smith, MN, ANP-BC, CNN
Renal, Dialysis & Transplant Clinic Nurse
Specialist
University of Washington Medical Center;
Affiliate Instructor
Department of Biobehavioral Nursing &
Health Informatics
University of Washington School of Nursing
Seattle, Washington
United States

Cynthia Sprinkle, MSN-Ed, RN, CEN, TCRN
Director
Clinical Education
Banner University Medical Center
– Phoenix
Phoenix, Arizona
United States

Mary Stahl, MSN, RN, CCNS, CCRN-K
Clinical Practice Specialist
American Association of Critical-Care
Nurses
Aliso Viejo, California
United States

Robyn Strauss, ACNS-BC, RN, MSN, WCC
Lead CNS, CV Service Line
CNS VI H & V ICU
Hospital of the University of Pennsylvania
Philadelphia, Pennsylvania
United States

Megan Swanson, RN
CICU Staff Nurse
Providence Sacred Heart Medical Center
Spokane, Washington
United States

Mihaela D. te Winkel, ACNP-BC, CSC, RNFA
Nurse Practitioner–Cardiology
Raluca B. Arimie Cardiology Private Practice
West Hills, California
United States

Lindsay Thomas, BA, MS, RN, CNS, CCNS
Interventional Cardiology CNS
Stanford Hospital and Clinics
Stanford, California
United States

Sonia Thomas, BSN, RN
Clinical Informatics Nurse Specialist
UT Southwestern Medical Center
Dallas, Texas
United States

Denise Thomas, DNP, APN, ACNS-BC, CCNS, CCRN-CMC, CEN
Clinical Nurse Specialist, Critical Care
Enterprise Clinical Specialist
Critical Care
Centura Health
Lakewood, Colorado
United States

Ashley N. Thompson, DNP, AGACNP-BC
Nurse Practitioner
Acute Care Track Coordinator
Clinical Assistant Professor
UF Health
University of Florida College of
Nursing
Gainesville, Florida
United States

Paul Thurman, PhD, RN, ACNPC, CCNS, CCRN
Nurse Scientist in Trauma and Critical Care
R Adams Cowley Shock Trauma Center
University of Maryland Medical Center;
Assistant Professor
University of Maryland School of
Nursing
Baltimore, Maryland
United States

Judy Tipton, MSN, RN, CNE
Clinical Nurse Educator
Inova Fairfax Medical Campus
Falls Church, Virginia
United States

Sherry VanHoy, MSN, APRN, ACNS-BC, FNP-BCN
Clinical Nurse Specialist
ChristianaCare
Newark, Delaware
United States

Brooke Wagner, MSN, APN, AGCNS-BC, CNRN, SCRN
Clinical Nurse Specialist
Banner University
Medical Center – Phoenix
Phoenix, Arizona
United States

Joan Walsh, DNP, APRN, CNS, CCNS-BC, CNRN, SCRN
Assistant Professor
Rhode Island College;
Nursing Education Partner
Rhode Island Hospital
Providence, Rhode Island
United States

Jacqueline Wavelet, MSN, RN, CNE
Clinical Nurse Educator
Inova Fairfax Medical
Campus
Falls Church, Virginia
United States

Michelle Weaver, DNP, ACNP-BC, CCRN, CHFN
Wexner Medical Center
The Ohio State University
Columbus, Ohio
United States

Mary Jane Willard, PhD, MBA, MA, BSN, RNP, CCRN, CNRN
Nurse Educator
Central Arkansas Veterans Healthcare System
Little Rock, Arkansas
United States

Stephanie Yoakum, MSN, RN, ACNP-BC
Electrophysiology Nurse Practitioner
University of California, San Diego
La Jolla, California
United States

Mary Zellinger, APRN, MN, ANP-BC, CCRN-CSC, CCNS, FCCM, FAAN
Consultant
Cardiovascular Critical Care Nursing
  Education
Emory University Hospital
Atlanta, Georgia
United States

Cindy Zerfoss, DNP, RN, ACNP-BC, FCCM
Adjunct Faculty, RN-BSN Program
Centra College
Centra Medical Group
Acute Care Nurse Practitioner
Psychiatric and Behavioral
  Health
Lynchburg, Virginia
United States

Elizabeth K. Zink, PhD, RN, CCNS, CNRN
Clinical Nurse Specialist
Johns Hopkins Hospital
Baltimore, Maryland
United States

Preface

The eighth edition of the *AACN Procedure Manual* has a new title: the *AACN Procedure Manual for Progressive and Critical Care*. I have worked closely with the section editors, clinical experts, and key AACN and Elsevier staff members to revise and update this edition. We have removed procedures no longer common and added procedures for new technologies, devices, and interventions. Although every attempt was made to capture current clinical practice, we recognize that progressive and critical care clinical practice is dynamic, and therefore that any resource to support that practice must be considered a work in progress. In addition to the updated expert content, I hope you will enjoy the full-color illustrations, boxes, and tables!

AACN's vision is of a healthcare system driven by the needs of patients and families where acute and critical care nurses make their optimal contribution. It is that mission that was the driving force for this edition of the *AACN Procedure Manual for Progressive and Critical Care*.

This edition will be an asset for nurses and other critical care providers across the spectrum of progressive and critical care practice. The manual includes a comprehensive review of state-of-the-art information on procedures needed to provide care to these patients. The following procedures related to new and emerging trends have been added:

- Bronchoscopy (Perform) **AP**
- Bronchoscopy (Assist)
- Noninvasive Brain Tissue Monitoring
- EEG Monitoring Assist and Nursing Care
- Signal Processed EEG
- Fecal Microbiota Transplant
- Thermoregulation: Heating, Cooling, and Targeted Temperature Management
- Prevention of Immobility-Related Complications: Kinetic Therapy and Ambulation of Patients in Acute and Critical Care Settings
- Intrahospital Transport of Critically Ill Patients

All procedures have been revised to reflect changes in practice. This edition contains not only procedures commonly performed by critical care nurses but procedures performed by advanced practice providers as well. Each advanced practice procedure has an **AP** designation in the Table of Contents and a special **AP** icon and explanatory footnote on the first page of the procedure.

Because we recognize that these procedures are only a portion of the repertoire needed by today's acute and critical care practitioners to skillfully care for critically ill patients, we recommend that it be used in conjunction with the *AACN Core Curriculum for Progressive and Critical Care Nursing* and *AACN Advanced Critical Care Nursing*.

The *AACN Procedure Manual for Progressive and Critical Care* is designed so that information within each procedure can be found quickly. To provide high-quality care to patients, we need resources that provide us with readily available, need-to-know information. The book is organized into units, with most including multiple sections. All procedures are designed in the same style and begin with the following:

- Purpose of the Procedure
- Prerequisite Nursing Knowledge, which includes information the nurse needs before performing the procedure
- Equipment List, which includes equipment necessary to perform the procedure (some of the procedures identify additional equipment that may be necessary based on individual situations)
- Patient and Family Education, which identifies essential information that should be taught to patients and their families
- Patient Assessment and Preparation, which includes specific assessment criteria that should be obtained before the procedure and describes how the patient should be prepared for the procedure

Each step-by-step procedure includes the following:

- Steps, Rationales, and, for some steps, Special Considerations
- Associated Research and appropriate figures and tables
- Expected Outcomes, including the anticipated results of the procedure
- Unexpected Outcomes, including potential complications or untoward outcomes of the procedure
- Patient Monitoring, which includes information related to assessments and interventions that should be completed (the rationale for each item is described, and conditions that necessitate notification of an advanced practice nurse, physician, or other health care professional are identified)
- Explanations about what should be documented after the procedure is performed
- References are included, and the majority of procedures also include Additional Readings

This edition of the *AACN Procedure Manual for Progressive and Critical Care* includes several icons that are common to many of the procedures. These icons include the following:

AP This procedure should be performed only by clinicians who have demonstrated competence and are credentialed to perform it. In addition, the procedure must be within the scope of practice defined by their professional licensure, and in accordance with professional practice acts. Physicians, advanced practice nurses, and physician assistants may be credentialed to perform this procedure.

HH A procedure step with the HH icon designates that hand hygiene should be performed. This step is essential to reduce the transmission of microorganisms and is part of Standard Precautions.

PE A procedure step with the PE icon designates that personal protective equipment should be applied. Personal protective equipment may include gloves, protective eyeglasses, masks, gowns, and any additional equipment needed to protect the nurse or provider performing the procedure. The application of personal protective equipment reduces the transmission of microorganisms, minimizes splash, and is part of Standard Precautions.

This edition of the *AACN Procedure Manual for Progressive and Critical Care* uses AACN's current levels of evidence system. Therefore, whenever it is available, this evidence-based information is provided to indicate the strength of recommendation for various interventions. AACN's levels of evidence system is as follows:

Level A: Meta-analysis of quantitative studies or meta-synthesis of qualitative studies with results that consistently support a specific action, intervention, or treatment (including systematic review of randomized controlled trials).

Level B: Well-designed, controlled studies with results that consistently support a specific action, intervention, or treatment.

Level C: Qualitative studies, descriptive or correlational studies, integrative reviews, systematic reviews, or randomized controlled trials with inconsistent results.

Level D: Peer-reviewed professional and organizational standards with the support of clinical study recommendations.

Level E: Multiple case reports, theory-based evidence from expert opinions, or peer-reviewed professional organizational standards without clinical studies to support recommendations.

Level M: Manufacturer's recommendations only.

The references and additional readings for the eighth edition are provided online. To access the references and additional readings for each Procedure, simply scan the QR code found at the end of the procedure using your smartphone.

Finally, many of the included procedures use electrical equipment. This manual makes the assumption that all equipment is maintained by the institution's bioengineering department according to accepted national and state regulations for the individual piece of equipment.

I hope that you find this book an essential resource for clinical practice.

Karen L. Johnson

Acknowledgments

This edition of the *AACN Procedure Manual for Progressive and Critical Care* could not have been developed without the help of numerous dedicated people. I would like to thank AACN for giving me the opportunity to edit this edition. AACN's leadership and staff are totally committed to AACN's mission: "Acute and critical care nurses rely on AACN for expert knowledge and the influence to fulfill their promise to patients and families. AACN drives excellence because nothing less is acceptable." That commitment is reflected in the contributions to this edition. I would like to express my sincere appreciation and gratitude to Michael Muscat, Publishing Manager AACN, for his unwavering support and guidance. I would also like to thank the AACN Clinical Practice Specialists who served as expert clinical content reviewers: Linda Bell, MSN, RN; Meredith Padilla, PhD, RN, CCRN-CMC-CSC; Cindy Cain, DNP, RN, CNS, CCRN-K; Debbie Brinker, MSN, RN, CNS; Mary Stahl, MSN, RN, CCNS, CCRN-K; Julie Miller, BSN, RN, CCRN-K; Sara Grieshop, MHI, BSN, RN; and Mary Pat Aust, MS, RN, CDE.

This edition was largely written by nurses during the COVID-19 pandemic. While working the front lines during extraordinary circumstances, everyone remained dedicated to AACN's mission and to this book. I want to extend a huge thank-you to each of the section editors: Maureen Seckel, MSN, APRN, ACNS-BC, CCNS, CCRN-K, FCCM, FCNS, FAAN; Joni L. Dirks, MSN, RN, NPD-BC, CCRN-K; Marion E. McRae, RN, PhD, ACNP-BC, CCRN-CMC; DaiWai M. Olson, PhD, RN; Eleanor Fitzpatrick, DNP, RN, AG-CNS, ACNP, CCRN, CCCTM; and Sonia Astle, MS, RN, CCNS, CCRN, CNRN. The section editors coordinated the development and revision of each procedure within their sections. They worked with the contributors and reviewers as each procedure was developed, reviewed, revised, and edited. I am truly appreciative of their commitment to a quality product and enjoyed working with such an expert team.

This book would not have been possible without the contributors who shared their knowledge and expertise. The contributors are the staff nurses and advanced practice providers who developed new procedures and revised existing procedures. Each contributor worked diligently to ensure that each procedure included all of the information needed so that acute and critical care nurses would have the most helpful information at their fingertips.

I also want to thank the staff nurses and advanced practice nurses who reviewed each of the procedures. At least two reviewers critiqued each procedure and provided important feedback to the contributors. The reviewers' critiques improved the quality of each procedure.

I am very grateful that I had the opportunity to work with the talented and dedicated editorial staff at Elsevier. I want to extend a special thank-you to Lee Henderson, Executive Content Strategist, Nursing Content. Lee provided essential leadership, guidance, and support throughout the entire publication process. He was so understanding that the nurses who contributed to this book were working in the most stressful times of a pandemic. I also extend my sincere gratitude to Casey Marie Potter, Content Development Specialist, for coordinating the day-to-day progress of the book, despite a pandemic! She provided important behind-the-scenes help as references were double-checked, figures were drawn/redrawn, permissions were obtained, and all of the key aspects of the book were pulled together. She worked closely with Ryan Cook, who designed the updated cover and color sections. Nayagi Anandan, as project manager, orchestrated the final pages of the manual, and Muthukumaran Thangaraj, the senior graphics artist, coordinated the beautiful artwork. This Elsevier team worked very hard to produce this quality textbook.

They say, "it takes a village," and this edition of the *AACN Procedure Manual for Progressive and Critical Care*, surely reflects that. Everyone on this team was committed to AACN's mission to provide acute and critical care nurses with expert knowledge to fulfill their promise to patients and families, because nothing less is acceptable.

Contents

PROCEDURE

1

Endotracheal Intubation [AP] (Perform)

Cynthia A. Goodrich

PURPOSE: Endotracheal intubation is performed to establish and maintain a patent airway, facilitate oxygenation and ventilation, reduce the risk of aspiration, and assist with the clearance of secretions.

PREREQUISITE NURSING KNOWLEDGE

- Anatomy and physiology of the airway and pulmonary system.
- Knowledge of rapid-sequence intubation (RSI).
  - RSI is a common method used to reduce the risk for aspiration in patients with full stomachs when emergent airway control with intubation is indicated.[8]
  - This involves almost simultaneous administration of a rapid-acting induction agent followed by a neuromuscular (paralytic) blocking agent to facilitate optimal conditions for intubation.[3,8]
  - The goal is to induce unconsciousness and paralysis, which will facilitate intubation as well as decrease the risk for gastric regurgitation and aspiration as well as damage to the airway.[3]
  - Medications that are given for RSI should have a rapid onset and short duration. Induction agents induce sedation and unconsciousness. Commonly use drugs include ketamine, etomidate, propofol, and midazolam. Neuromuscular agents cause muscular relaxation and induce paralysis. Commonly used agents includes rocuronium and succinylcholine.[3,9]
  - During RSI, the provider is totally responsible for oxygenation, ventilation, and providing an airway for the patient.[8]
  - RSI is sometimes used in patients with predicted difficult airways as long as there is immediate access to

additional equipment necessary to restore oxygenation and ventilation including bag-valve-mask (BVM) devices, extraglottic airways, and surgical airway tools.[3]
  - The "Seven Ps" mnemonic is a useful tool outlining the key steps for RSI planning and performance. These include preparation, preoxygenation, preintubation optimization, paralysis and induction, positioning, placement proof, and postintubation management.[3]
- Indications for endotracheal intubation include the following[4,16]:
  - Inadequate oxygenation and ventilation
  - Altered mental status (e.g., head injury, drug overdose) who are unable to protect their own airway
  - Anticipated airway obstruction (e.g., facial burns, epiglottitis, major facial or oral trauma)
  - Upper airway obstruction (e.g., from swelling, trauma, tumor, bleeding)
  - Apnea
  - Ineffective clearance of secretions (i.e., inability to maintain or protect airway adequately)
  - High risk of aspiration
  - Respiratory distress, respiratory failure
- Pulse oximetry should be used during intubation so that oxygen desaturation can be quickly detected and treated (see Procedure 14, Oxygen Saturation Monitoring with Pulse Oximetry).[3,4,14,18]
- Two types of laryngoscope blades exist: straight and curved (Fig. 1.1). The straight (Miller) blade is designed so that the tip extends below the epiglottis, to lift and expose the glottic opening. The straight blade is recommended for use in obese patients, pediatric patients, and patients with short necks because the trachea may be located more anteriorly. When a curved (Macintosh) blade is used, the tip is advanced into the vallecula (the space

[AP] This procedure should be performed only by clinicians who have demonstrated competence and are credentialed to perform it. In addition, the procedure must be within the scope of practice defined by their professional licensure, and in accordance with professional practice acts. Physicians, advanced practice nurses, and physician assistants may be credentialed to perform this procedure.

between the epiglottis and the base of the tongue), resulting in indirect elevation of the epiglottis and exposure of the glottic opening. The wide flange of this blade helps retract the tongue from the field of view, increasing the space available to pass the endotracheal tube. This blade is often chosen because it provides a better view for placement and manipulation of the tube.[16]

- There are also two types of laryngoscopes: reusable and disposable. The disposable products have incorporated batteries that cannot be accessed.
- Laryngoscope blades are available with bulbs or with a fiberoptic light delivery system. Fiberoptic light delivery systems provide a brighter light, but the bulbs are prone to becoming scratched or covered with secretions.
- Videolaryngoscopy is gaining increased popularity as a method for oral intubation. This involves the use of fiberoptics or a micro video camera encased in the laryngoscope that provides a wide-angle view of the glottic opening while attempting oral intubation. Emerging literature supports this highly effective tool as a method to increase first-pass success by providing a superior view of the glottis compared with traditional direct laryngoscopy.[5,9,11,12,15,17] This method also requires minimal lifting force, resulting in less movement of the cervical spine during intubation.[11]

- Endotracheal tube size reflects the internal diameter of the tube. Tubes range in size from 2.0 mm for neonates to 9.0 mm for large adults. Endotracheal tubes that range in size from 7.0 to 7.5 mm are used for average-sized adult women, whereas endotracheal tubes that range in size from 7.5 to 8.0 mm are used for average-sized adult men (Fig. 1.2).[1,8,9,16] The tube with the largest clinically acceptable internal diameter should be used to minimize airway resistance and assist in suctioning.
- Endotracheal intubation can be done via oral or nasal routes. Orotracheal intubation is the preferred route, but nasal intubation may be done under certain circumstances in the ICU. The route selected will depend on the skill of the practitioner performing the intubation and the patient's clinical condition.[4]
  - ❖ Nasal intubation is rarely performed and requires a patient who is breathing spontaneously. It is relatively contraindicated in trauma patients with facial fractures or suspected fractures at the base of the skull and after cranial surgeries such as transnasal hypophysectomy.[4] Complications include epistaxis, pressure necrosis, meningitis, and sinusitis.[4,9]
- Improper intubation technique may result in trauma to the teeth, soft tissues of the mouth or nose, vocal cords, trachea, and posterior pharynx.
- The patient's airway should be assessed before intubation. The LEMON mnemonic can be used to determine whether a difficult intubation is anticipated.[3,4]
  - ❖ L = Look Externally: Look for features associated with a difficult intubation such as a short neck, prominent incisors, broken teeth, a large protruding tongue, a narrow or abnormally shaped face, a receding jaw, or a prominent overbite.[4]

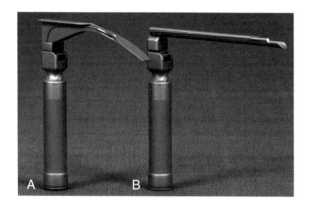

Figure 1.1 Types of blades for direct laryngoscopy. **A,** Macintosh *(curved).* **B,** Miller *(straight). (From Driver BE, Reardon RF: Tracheal intubation. In: Roberts JR, Custalow CB, Thomsen TW, editors. Roberts and Hedges' clinical procedures in emergency medicine and acute care, ed 7, Philadelphia, PA, 2019, Elsevier, p 69.)*

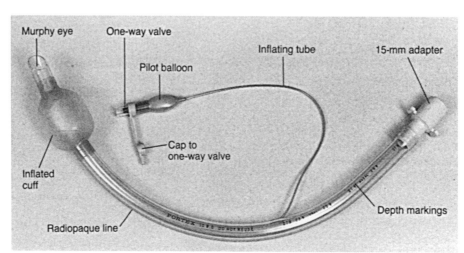

Figure 1.2 Parts of an endotracheal tube (soft-cuffed Tube by Smiths Industries Medical Systems, Valencia, CA). *(From Kersten LD:* Comprehensive respiratory nursing, *Philadelphia, 1989, Saunders, 1989, p 637.)*

❖ E = Evaluate using the 3-3-2 rule: These three rules help determine whether there will be alignment of the pharyngeal, laryngeal, and oral axes.[4]

❖ Three fingers: distance between upper and lower incisors in the mouth opening

❖ Three fingers: distance between tip of chin and chin-neck junction (hyoid bone)

❖ Two fingers: distance between thyroid cartilage and mandible

❖ M = Mallampati Score: This scoring system provides an estimate of the space available for oral intubation using direct laryngoscopy. It relates the amount of mouth opening to the size of the tongue. Classes I and II predict a routine laryngoscopy, class III predicts difficulty, and class IV predicts extreme difficulty. While sitting up, the patient is asked to open the mouth as wide as possible, sticking the tongue out. While looking into the mouth, a light is used to assess the amount of visible hypopharynx (Fig. 1.3).[4] Mallampati scores may not be an option for patients who are unconscious, uncooperative, or unable to sit up.

❖ O = Obstruction: Look for causes that might interfere with intubation, such as tonsillar abscess, epiglottitis, trauma, tumors, swollen tongue, and obesity.[4]

❖ N = Neck Mobility: Look for conditions that might limit neck range of motion, such as a hard cervical collar (trauma), ankylosing spondylitis, previous neck surgery, or rheumatoid arthritis. If trauma is not suspected, ask the patient to touch the chin to the chest and to extend the neck to the ceiling.[4]

• Proper positioning of the patient is critical for successful intubation. Placing the patient supine with the head of the bed at 20 to 25 degrees or alternatively in the reverse Trendelenburg position at 30 degrees for those with suspected or confirmed spinal injuries improves preoxygenation and provides better visualization of airway structures during intubation.[3,8,9,16,23]

• Apneic oxygenation involves passive movement of oxygen from the upper airways into the alveoli without respiratory effort. A commonly used method involves the use of a standard nasal cannula set at 15 L/minute. The nasal cannula is placed during preoxygenation and continued until the patient is intubated. Apneic oxygenation has been shown to prolong the period of safe apnea, thereby reducing the incidence of critical desaturation during a prolonged or difficult intubation.[16,19,20,21,24]

• Visualization of the vocal cords can be aided by using external laryngeal manipulation. This is accomplished by applying backward, upward, and rightward pressure (BURP) on the thyroid cartilage to move the larynx to the right while the tongue is displaced to the left by the laryngoscope blade (Fig. 1.4).[4]

• The routine application of cricoid pressure is controversial, and it is no longer being recommended in many settings.[18,25] This procedure is accomplished by applying firm downward pressure on the cricoid ring, pushing the vocal

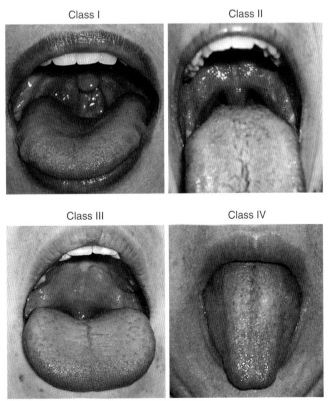

Class I   Class II

Class III   Class IV

Figure 1.3 The Mallampati classification predicts intubation difficulty based on the visibility of intraoral structures. Classes III and IV predict difficult intubation. *(From Kryger MH: Sleep breathing disorders: examination of the patient with suspected sleep apnea. In Kryger MH, editor:* Kryger atlas of clinical sleep medicine. *Philadelphia, 2010, Elsevier, p 66.)*

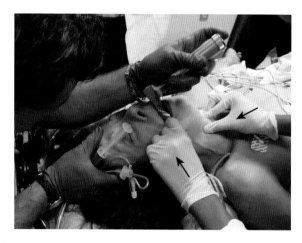

Figure 1.4 Note the assistant manipulating the anterior part of the neck and retracting the cheek *(arrows)* for better visualization. *(From Driver BE, Reardon RF: Tracheal intubation. In: Roberts JR, Custalow CB, Thomsen TW, editors.* Roberts and Hedges' clinical procedures in emergency medicine and acute care, *ed 7, Philadelphia, PA, 2019, Elsevier, p 77.)*

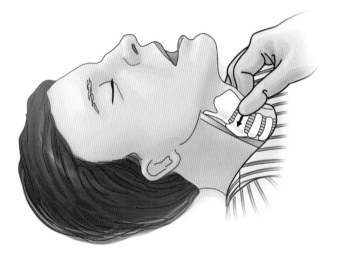

Figure 1.5 Cricoid pressure. Firm downward pressure on the cricoid ring pushes the vocal cords downward toward the field of vision while sealing the esophagus against the vertebral column.

cords downward so they are more easily visualized (Fig. 1.5).[2,14,18] In non–cardiac arrest patients, there is limited evidence that it may help protect against gastric insufflation and aspiration into the lungs during bag-valve-mask ventilation.[8,18] If applied incorrectly, it may interfere with ventilation and make laryngoscopy intubation more difficult. Once begun, cricoid pressure must be maintained until intubation is completed unless there is difficulty intubating or ventilating the patient. In cardiac arrest patients, there is no evidence that it reduces the risk of aspiration, and its use is not recommended.[2,14,18]

• In trauma patients with suspected spinal cord injuries and those who are not completely evaluated, manual in-line cervical immobilization of the head and neck must be maintained during the entire endotracheal intubation procedure to keep the head in a neutral position. An assistant should be directed to manually immobilize the head and neck

by placing his or her hands on either side of the patient's head, with thumbs along the mandible and fingers behind the head on the occipital ridge. Gentle but firm stabilization should be maintained throughout the procedure.[4,9] The front of the cervical collar may be opened or removed to allow for increased mandibular displacement as long as spinal precautions are maintained during the procedure.[4,9,16]

• The Cormack-Lehane grading system of laryngeal views (Fig. 1.6) can be used to score the view of the glottic opening during laryngoscopy. Patients with grades I and II are usually easy to intubate, whereas those with grades III and IV are more difficult to intubate.[8]

• Confirmation of endotracheal tube placement should be done immediately after intubation to protect against unrecognized esophageal intubation. This includes using both clinical findings and end-tidal carbon dioxide ($ETco_2$).[4,8,14,18]

❖ Clinical findings consistent with tracheal placement include visualization of the tube passing through the vocal cords, absence of gurgling over the epigastric area, auscultation of bilateral breath sounds, symmetrical chest rise and fall during ventilation, and mist in the tube.[8,14,16,18]

❖ The most accurate method for confirmation of endotracheal tube placement into the trachea is $ETco_2$ determination using colorimetric or quantitative capnography (see Procedure 12, Continuous End-Tidal Carbon Dioxide Monitoring) in the non–cardiac arrest patient. The presence of CO_2 in the expired air indicates that the airway has been successfully intubated but does not ensure the correct position of the endotracheal tube.[2,14,16,18]

❖ Disposable $ETco_2$ detectors are chemically treated with a nontoxic indicator that changes color in the presence of CO_2. In general, color changes from purple (no CO_2) to yellow (positive CO_2).

❖ Continuous $ETco_2$ (capnography) assists in confirming proper placement of the endotracheal tube into the trachea as well as allowing for detection of future tube dislodgment.

❖ During cardiac arrest (nonperfusing rhythms), low pulmonary blood flow may cause insufficient expired CO_2.[14,18] If CO_2 is not detected using $ETco_2$, an esophageal detector device may be used for confirmation of proper placement into the trachea.[2,14,16,18]

❖ At least five to six exhalations with a consistent CO_2 level must be assessed to confirm endotracheal tube placement in the trachea, because the esophagus may yield a small but detectable amount of CO_2 during the first few breaths.[16]

❖ Esophageal detector devices work by creating suction at the end of the endotracheal tube by compressing a flexible blub or pulling back on a syringe plunger. When the tube is placed correctly in the trachea, air allows for reexpansion of the bulb or movement of the syringe plunger. If the tube is in the esophagus, no movement of the syringe plunger or reexpansion of the bulb is seen. These devices may be misleading in patients who are morbidly obese, in status asthmaticus, late in pregnancy, or in patients with large amounts of tracheal secretions.[1,14,16,18]

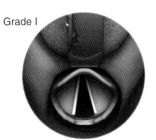 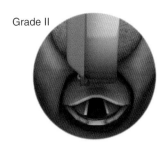 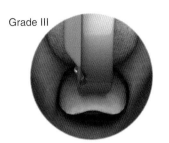 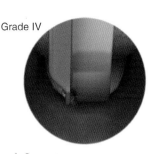

Grade I Grade II Grade III Grade IV

Figure 1.6 Cormack-Lehane grading of laryngeal views during laryngoscopy. **A,** In grade I, most of the glottis is visible. **B,** In grade II, the posterior aspect of the glottis is visible. **C,** In grade III, only the epiglottis is seen; no part of the laryngeal inlet is visible. **D,** In grade IV, the epiglottis is not vis Patients with grades I and II are usually easy to intubate with direct laryngoscopy, whereas those with grades III and IV are often difficult; the ability to see the arytenoid cartilage is the important difference. *(From Driver BE, Reardon RF: Tracheal intubation. In: Roberts JR, Custalow CB, Thomsen TW, editors.* Roberts and Hedges' clinical procedures in emergency medicine and acute care, *ed 7, Philadelphia, PA, 2019, Elsevier, p 67.)*

- Endotracheal tube cuff pressure should be checked after verifying correct endotracheal tube position. The cuff pressure recommended for assistance in preventing both microaspiration and tracheal damage is 20 to 30 cm H_2O (see Procedure 3, Endotracheal Tube Care and Oral Care Practices for Ventilated and Nonventilated Patients).[6,9,10,13,22]
- Intubation attempts should take no longer than 15 to 20 seconds. If more than one intubation attempt is necessary, ventilation with 100% oxygen using a self-inflating manual resuscitation bag device with a tight-fitting face mask for 3 to 5 minutes before each attempt. If intubation is not successful after three attempts, consider using another airway adjunct, such as a laryngeal mask airway (LMA) (see Procedure 6, Laryngeal Mask Airway) or other supraglottic devices.
- It is important to have a clearly defined institutional difficult/failed airway plan. This should include a process to obtain alternative airway equipment in case of unsuccessful intubation. This may consist of a gum elastic bougie, supraglottic device, and videolaryngoscope. Surgical airway equipment such as that needed for a cricothyroidotomy should also be readily available along with trained providers in case of a failed airway.[16]

EQUIPMENT

- Personal protective equipment (PPE): Intubation is considered an aerosol-generating procedure, and appropriate respiratory PPE should be used based on patient presentation and past medical history.
- Appropriately sized endotracheal tube with intact cuff and 15 mm connector (women, 7.0-mm to 7.5-mm tube; men, 7.5-mm to 8.0-mm tube).
- Laryngoscope handle with fresh batteries if nondisposable
- Laryngoscope blades (straight and curved)
- Spare bulb for nondisposable laryngoscope blades
- Flexible stylet
- Magill forceps (to remove foreign bodies obstructing the airway if present)
- Self-inflating manual resuscitation bag-valve-mask device with tight-fitting face mask connected to supplemental oxygen (15 L/min)

- Assortment of oropharyngeal airways and nasopharyngeal airways
- Oxygen source (will need two oxygen sources if doing apneic oxygenation)
- Luer-tip 10-mL syringe for cuff inflation or commercially available cuff inflation device
- Water-soluble lubricant
- Rigid pharyngeal suction-tip (Yankauer) catheter
- Suction apparatus (portable or wall) and second suction source if using ETT with continuous subglottic suctioning
- Suction catheters
- Bite-block
- Endotracheal tube–securing apparatus or appropriate tape
  ❖ Commercially available endotracheal tube holder
  ❖ Adhesive tape (6 to 8 inches long)
  ❖ Hydrocolloid dressing if indicated
- Stethoscope
- Monitoring equipment: cardiac monitor, pulse oximetry, and sphygmomanometer or noninvasive blood pressure (NIBP)
- Disposable $ETco_2$ detector, continuous $ETco_2$ monitoring device, or esophageal detection device
- Rescue airway including supraglottic device such as LMA (see Procedure 6, Laryngeal Mask Airway)
- Emergency airway equipment: gum elastic bougie, videolaryngoscope, optical stylet fiberoptic scope, and cricothyroidotomy kit should be readily available in case of a failed airway
- Drugs for intubation as indicated (induction agent, sedation, paralyzing agents, lidocaine, atropine)
- Ventilator

Additional equipment, to have available as needed, includes the following:
- Anesthetic spray (nasal approach)
- Local anesthetic jelly (nasal approach)

PATIENT AND FAMILY EDUCATION

- If time permits, assess the patient's and family's level of understanding about the condition and rationale for endotracheal intubation. *Rationale:* This assessment identifies the patient's and the family's knowledge deficits concerning the patient's condition, the procedure, the expected benefits, and the potential risks. It also allows time for questions to clarify information and voice concerns. Explanations decrease patient anxiety and enhance cooperation.

- Explain the procedure and the reason for intubation if the clinical situation permits. If not, explain the procedure and reason for the intubation after it is completed. *Rationale:* This explanation enhances patient and family understanding and decreases anxiety.
- If indicated and the clinical situation permits, explain the patient's role in assisting with insertion of the endotracheal tube. *Rationale:* This explanation elicits the patient's cooperation, which assists with insertion.
- Explain that the patient will be unable to speak while the endotracheal tube is in place, but that other means of communication will be provided. *Rationale:* This information enhances patient and family understanding and decreases anxiety.
- Explain that the patient will be unable to eat or drink while the endotracheal tube is in place, but that other nutrition and fluids will be provided. *Rationale:* This information enhances patient and family understanding and decreases anxiety.
- Explain the importance of not pulling at or touching the endotracheal tube and risk of inadvertent removal. The patient will be assessed and treated as needed for pain, anxiety, and delirium during the stages of intubation, postintubation, and readiness for extubation. *Rationale:* This information enhances patient and family understanding and decreases anxiety.

PATIENT ASSESSMENT AND PREPARATION

Patient Assessment

- Verify the correct patient with two identifiers. *Rationale:* Before performing a procedure, the nurse should ensure the correct identification of the patient for the intended intervention.
- Assess for recent history of trauma with suspected spinal cord injury or cranial surgery. *Rationale*: Knowledge of pertinent patient history allows for selection of the most appropriate method for intubation, which helps reduce the risk of secondary injury.
- Assess nothing-by-mouth status when expected use of a self-inflating manual resuscitation bag-valve-mask device before intubation, and for signs of gastric distention. *Rationale:* Increased risk of aspiration and vomiting occurs with accumulation of air (from the use of a self-inflating manual resuscitation bag-valve-mask device), food, or secretions.
- Assess level of consciousness, level of anxiety, and respiratory difficulty. *Rationale:* This assessment assists in determining the most appropriate medications to be used for intubation.
- Assess the oral cavity for presence of dentures, loose teeth, or other possible obstructions, and remove if appropriate. *Rationale:* Ensures that the airway is free from any obstructions.

- Perform an airway assessment before intubation using a tool such as the LEMON. *Rationale:* Assist in identifying if a difficult intubation should be anticipated.[3,4,8]
- Assess vital signs, and assess for the following: tachypnea, dyspnea, shallow respirations, hypoxia, apnea, altered level of consciousness, tachycardia, cardiac dysrhythmias, hypertension, and headache. *Rationale:* Any of these conditions may indicate a problem with oxygenation, ventilation, or both.
- Assess patency of nares (for nasal intubation) and presence of septal deviation. *Rationale:* Selection of the most appropriate naris facilitates insertion and may improve patient tolerance of the tube.
- Assess need for premedication. *Rationale:* Various medications provide sedation or paralysis as needed.

Patient Preparation

- Perform a preprocedural verification and time out. *Rationale:* Ensures patient safety and improves communication.
- Ensure that the patient understands preprocedural teaching, if appropriate. Answer questions as they arise, and reinforce information as needed. *Rationale:* Understanding of previously taught information is evaluated and reinforced.
- Before intubation, initiate intravenous or intraosseous access or verify patency of existing access. *Rationale:* Readily available intravenous or intraosseous access is required to administer medications for intubation.
- Position the patient appropriately.
  - Positioning of the nontrauma patient is as follows: place the patient supine with the head in the sniffing position, in which the head is extended and the neck is flexed. Placement of a small towel or pillow under the occiput elevates it several inches, allowing for proper flexion of the neck (Fig. 1.7). *Rationale:* Placement of the head in the sniffing position allows for better visualization of the larynx and vocal cords by aligning the axes of the mouth, pharynx, and trachea.
  - In nontrauma patients, consider placing the patient supine with the head of the bed at 20 to 25 degrees or alternatively in the reverse Trendelenburg position at 30 degrees. *Rationale*: Elevating the head of the bed helps improve preoxygenation and improves visualization of the glottis.[3,4,8,9,16,23]
  - Trauma patients can be placed in the reverse Trendelenburg position at 30 degrees, with manual in-line cervical spinal immobilization maintained during the entire process of intubation to minimize cervical spine motion.[3,4,8,9,16,23] *Rationale:* Because cervical spinal cord injury must be suspected in all trauma patients until proven otherwise, this position helps prevent secondary injury should a cervical spine injury be present.
- Prepare and administer medications necessary for intubation including induction and paralytic agents as indicated. *Rationale:* Appropriate intubation medications allow for a more controlled intubation, reducing the incidence of insertion trauma, aspiration, laryngospasm, and improper tube placement.
- Notify the respiratory therapy department of impending intubation so a ventilator can be set up. *Rationale:* The ventilator is set up before intubation.

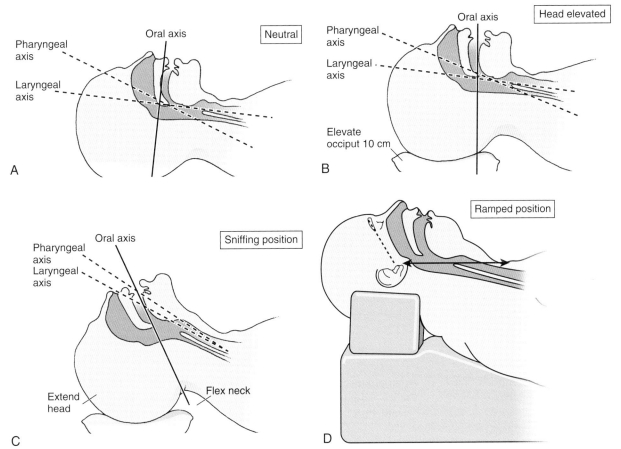

Figure 1.7 Head positioning for tracheal intubation. **A,** Neutral position. **B,** Head elevated. **C,** "Sniffing" position with a flexed neck and extended head. Note that flexing the neck while extending the head lines up the various axes and allows direct laryngoscopy. **D,** Morbidly obese patients are best intubated in a ramped position with elevation of the upper part of the back, neck, and head; the ideal position aligns the external auditory canal and the sternum. *(From Driver BE, Reardon RF: Tracheal intubation. In: Roberts JR, Custalow CB, Thomsen TW, editors.* Roberts and Hedges' clinical procedures in emergency medicine and acute care, *ed 7, Philadelphia, PA, 2019, Elsevier, p 71.)*

Procedure	for Performing Endotracheal Intubation		
Steps	Rationale		Special Considerations
General Setup			
1. **HH**			
2. **PE**			Intubation is considered an aerosol-generating procedure, and additional respiratory PPE based on the patient's presentation and past medical history may be required for all providers involved in the intubation procedure.
3. Establish intravenous or intraosseous access if not present.	Provides access to deliver indicated medications.		Consider placing a second line that can be dedicated for administration of drugs during intubation and as a backup line in case of catheter dislodgement of the primary line.

Procedure continues on following page

Procedure for Performing Endotracheal Intubation—*Continued*

Steps	Rationale	Special Considerations
4. Attach the patient to monitoring equipment including cardiac and blood pressure monitors and a pulse oximeter. Consider continuous $ETco_2$ monitoring (capnography) if available.	Provides continuous patient monitoring during intubation.	
5. Set up suction apparatus, and connect rigid suction-tip catheter to tubing.	Prepares for oropharyngeal suctioning as needed.	
6. Have a self-inflating manual resuscitation bag-valve-mask device connected to a 100% oxygen source and face mask ready for hyperoxygenation and manual ventilation.	Intubation attempts should not take longer than 30 seconds. Patients must be hyperoxygenated and ventilated between intubation attempts.[1,4,8]	If intubation is unsuccessful within 30 seconds or the patient's oxygen saturation falls below 90% during the attempt, remove the tube.[16] Ventilate with 100% oxygen with a bag-valve-mask device before another intubation attempt is made. Before reattempting intubation, correct problems related to positioning, procedure, or equipment.
7. Check equipment.		
A. Choose an appropriate-sized endotracheal tube.	Appropriate-sized endotracheal tubes facilitate both intubation and ventilation.	Generally, a 7.0- to 7.5-mm internal diameter tube is used for adult females, and a 7.5- to 8.0-mm internal diameter tube is used for adult males.[1,8,9,16]
B. Use a 10-mL syringe to inflate the cuff on the tube, assessing for leaks. Completely deflate the cuff once its integrity has been checked.	Verifies that equipment is functional and that the tube cuff is patent without leaks; prepares the tube for insertion.	Once the endotracheal tube cuff has been checked for leaks and it is completely deflated, place it back into its packaging to avoid contamination.
C. Insert the stylet into the endotracheal tube, ensuring that the tip of the stylet does not extend past the end of the endotracheal tube.	Provides structural support for the flexible endotracheal tube during insertion. Maintaining the tip of the stylet within the lumen of the endotracheal tube prevents damage to the vocal cords and trachea.	The stylet must be recessed by at least 0.5 inch from the distal end of the tube so it does not protrude beyond the end of the tube.
D. Connect the laryngoscope blade to the handle, and ensure that the blade's bulb is securely seated.	Verifies that the equipment is functional.	Check the bulb for brightness. Replace the bulb if it is dull or burnt out for nondisposable products.
8. Assess the patient's airway to determine whether a difficult intubation is anticipated. (**Level E***)	The LEMON assessment tool can be used to identify potentially difficult airways.[3,4,]	

Procedure for Performing Endotracheal Intubation—*Continued*

Steps	Rationale	Special Considerations
9. Position the patient's head by flexing the neck forward and extending the head into the sniffing position (only if neck trauma is not suspected (see Fig. 1.7). If spinal trauma is suspected, request that an assistant maintain the head in a neutral position with in-line spinal immobilization. *This is performed by manually immobilizing the head and neck by placing your hands on either side of the patient's head, with thumbs along the mandible and fingers behind the head on the occipital ridge. Use gentle but firm stabilization throughout the procedure.*[4,9] The front of the cervical collar may be opened or removed, allowing for increased mandibular displacement as long as spinal precautions are maintained during the procedure.[4,9,16]	Allows for visualization of the vocal cords with alignment of the mouth, pharynx, and trachea.[4,8,9,16]	The ear (external auditory meatus) and sternal notch should be aligned when the patient is examined from the side. This allows for flexion of the cervical spine.[8,16,18] Placement of a small towel under the occiput elevates it, allowing for proper neck flexion. *Do not flex or extend the neck of a patient with suspected spinal cord injury; the head must be maintained in a neutral position with manual in-line cervical spine immobilization.*[4,6]
10. Check the mouth for dentures, and remove if present.	Dentures should be removed before oral intubation is attempted but may remain in place for nasal intubation or bag-valve-mask ventilation before oral intubation.	
11. Suction the mouth and pharynx as needed if secretions are visualized.	Provides a clear view of the posterior pharynx and larynx.	
12. Insert an oropharyngeal or nasopharyngeal airway if indicated (see Procedure 7, Nasopharyngeal and Oral Airway Insertion).	Assists in maintenance of upper airway patency. Helps improve ability to ventilate during bag-valve-mask ventilation.	Only use oral airways in unconscious patients with an absent gag reflex.
13. Preoxygenate for 3–5 minutes, with 100% oxygen via a nonrebreather mask if ventilations are adequate or via a self-inflating manual resuscitation bag-valve-mask device (see Procedure 29, Manual Self-inflating Resuscitation Bag-Valve Device) if ventilations are inadequate.	Helps prevent hypoxemia. Gentle breaths reduce the incidence of air entering the stomach (leading to gastric distention, aspiration), decrease airway turbulence, and distribute ventilation more evenly within the lungs. Preoxygenation ensures that nitrogen is washed out of the lungs and will extend the allowable apneic time until the oxygen in the lungs is used up.[4,8,16]	Bag-valve-mask ventilation may not be needed in a spontaneously breathing patient. Avoid aggressive positive-pressure ventilation with a self-inflating manual resuscitation bag because this may increase the risk for gastric distension and vomiting.[3,8,9,16]

Procedure continues on following page

Procedure	for Performing Endotracheal Intubation—*Continued*	
Steps	**Rationale**	**Special Considerations**
14. Administer intubation medications including induction and paralytic agents as indicated. After medication administration, assess the patient for jaw relaxation, apnea, and lack of movement.	Sedates and relaxes the patient, allowing for easier intubation. Jaw relaxation and apnea indicate that the patient is adequately medicated.	This may require a second assistant to administer and document medications given before, during, and after intubation.
15. Remove the oropharyngeal airway if present. For nasotracheal intubation, proceed to Step 36.	Clears the airway for advancement of the laryngoscope blade and endotracheal tube.	
Orotracheal Intubation		
16. Grasp the laryngoscope (with the blade in place and illuminated light on) in the left hand.	Prepares for efficient blade placement.	Grasp the handle as low as possible, and keep the wrist rigid to prevent using the upper teeth as a fulcrum.
17. Use fingers of the right hand to open the mouth. Having an assistant pull the lip/right cheek laterally will increase the space in the mouth to insert the laryngoscope blade (see Fig. 1.4).[8]	Provides access to the oral cavity.	A scissor-like motion with the thumb and second finger of the right hand can be used to gently open the mouth in paralyzed patients. Hold the tips of the thumb and middle finger of the right hand together. Insert them between the upper and lower incisors. Using a scissor-like motion, move the fingers past one another by flexing each finger.[16]
18. Using a controlled motion, slowly insert the blade into the right side of the patient's mouth, using it to push the tongue to the left (Fig. 1.8). Advance the blade inward and toward midline past the base of the tongue.	Displaces the tongue to the left, increasing visualization of the glottic opening.	Avoid pressure on the teeth and lips. Inserting the blade smoothly and quickly obtaining an optimal view of the glottic opening will help increase first-pass success.[16] If the patient's chest is obstructing placement of the laryngoscope handle, consider placing blankets or towels under the head and upper back to elevate the head relative to the chest. Do not do this if cervical spine injury is suspected.[4,16] In trauma victims, consider turning the handle 90 degrees to insert the blade into the mouth and rotate to midline as the blade is advanced.

Procedure	**for Performing Endotracheal Intubation—*Continued***	
Steps	**Rationale**	**Special Considerations**
19. Visually identify the base of the tongue and the epiglottis.	Identification of anatomical landmarks facilitates successful intubation.	External laryngeal manipulation with the BURP (backward, upward, rightward pressure) technique may assist with visualization of the vocal cords (see Fig. 1.4).[4] Apply BURP on the thyroid cartilage to move the larynx to the patient's right while the tongue is displaced to the left by the laryngoscope blade and bring the cords into the intubator's view.[4] This may be done by the intubator or by an assistant. Cricoid pressure (Sellick maneuver) may provide increased visualization of the vocal cords by moving the trachea posteriorly. This is accomplished by applying firm downward pressure on the cricoid ring, pushing the vocal cords downward so they are visualized more easily (see Fig. 1.5). *Once cricoid pressure is applied, it must be maintained until the intubation is completed.* The routine use of cricoid pressure is not recommended during cardiac arrest.[2,14,18]
20. Carefully advance the blade toward the epiglottis in a well-controlled manner (Fig. 1.9).	Identification of the epiglottis is key for successful direct laryngoscopy intubation.	The Cormack-Lehane grading system of laryngeal views may assist in identifying if a difficult intubation is anticipated[8] (see Fig 1.6).
A. With a curved blade, advance the tip into the vallecula (space between the base of the tongue and the epiglottis), and exert outward and upward gentle traction at a 45-degree angle (decreases the risk of dental injury from using the teeth as a fulcrum). Lift the laryngoscope in the direction of the handle to lift the tongue and posterior pharyngeal structures out of the way, allowing for exposure of the glottic opening. Do not allow the handle to lever back, causing the blade to hit the teeth.	Exposes the glottic opening. This lifting motion elevates the epiglottis, keeping the tongue out of the way, allowing for maximal exposure of the glottis.	Levering back on the laryngoscope handle will impair the view and may cause dental trauma. Touching the teeth indicates excessive levering or ineffective lift.[16]

Procedure continues on following page

Procedure for Performing Endotracheal Intubation—*Continued*

Steps	Rationale	Special Considerations
B. With a straight blade, advance the tip just beneath the epiglottis, and exert an outward and upward motion at a 45-degree angle to the bed. The blade may be inserted to the right of the tongue into the natural gutter between the lower molars (paraglossal technique) or midline.[16] Do not allow the handle to lever backward, causing the blade to cause dental injury.	Exposes the glottic opening. Using the paraglossal technique allows for a better view by displacing the tongue with minimal effort.[16]	Levering back on the laryngoscope handle will impair the view and may damage the teeth. Touching the teeth indicates excessive levering or ineffective lift.[16] Using a straight blade may provide a better view when the larynx is more anterior or in patients with a receding chin.[16] Midline insertion of the blade often results in difficulty in controlling the tongue, which may obscure the view, particularly in unconscious adults.
21. Lift the laryngoscope handle up and away from the operator (at a 45- to 55-degree angle from the trachea) until the vocal cords are visualized (Fig. 1.10).	Allows for correct placement of the tube into the trachea.	Do not use the blade as a fulcrum; this may result in oral and/or dental injury.[15] The BURP technique may assist with visualization of the vocal cords.[4]
22. Hold the top end of the tube in the right hand with the curved portion downward.	The tube is placed with the right hand.	
23. Under direct visualization, gently insert the tube from the right corner of the mouth (Fig. 1.11) through the vocal cords (Fig. 1.12) until the cuff is no longer visible and has passed through the vocal cords (Fig. 1.13). Do not apply pressure on the teeth or oral tissues.	The tube must be seen passing through the vocal cords to ensure proper placement. Advance the tube 1.25–2.5 cm farther into the trachea. When correctly positioned, the tip of the tube should be halfway between the vocal cords and the carina.[16]	Having an assistant pull the lip/right cheek laterally will increase the space in the mouth to place the endotracheal tube (see Fig. 1.4). The front teeth or gums should be aligned between the 19-cm and 23-cm depth markings on the tube to ensure that the tip of the tube is above the carina.[9,16] Common tube placement at the teeth or gums is 20–21 cm for women and 22–23 cm for men.[9,16] If intubation is unsuccessful within 30 seconds, or the patient's oxygen saturations falls below 90% during the attempt, remove the tube.[16] Ventilate with 100% oxygen with a bag-valve-mask device before another intubation attempt is made (repeat steps 13–20). Before reattempting intubation, correct any identified problems related to positioning, procedure, or equipment. This may include placement of an oropharyngeal airway to facilitate optimal bag-valve-mask ventilation (see Procedure 7, Nasopharyngeal and Oral Airway Insertion).

Procedure	for Performing Endotracheal Intubation—*Continued*	
Steps	**Rationale**	**Special Considerations**
24. When the tube is correctly placed, continue to hold it securely in place at the lips with the right hand. Withdraw the laryngoscope blade and then the stylet with the left hand.	Firmly holding the tube at the lips provides stabilization and prevents inadvertent extubation.	An assistant may remove the stylet while the intubator firmly holds the endotracheal tube in place, preventing dislodgement of the tube.
25. Inflate the cuff with 5–10 mL of air depending on the manufacturer's recommendations. Do not overinflate the cuff. **(Level M*)**	Inflation volumes vary depending on the manufacturer and size of the tube. If a manometer is available, keep cuff pressure between 20 and 30 mm Hg to decrease the risk of aspiration and prevent ischemia and decreased blood flow.[8,9,14]	In adults, decreased mucosal capillary blood flow (ischemia) results when pressure is greater than 30 mm Hg.[8,14,22] Consider using a manometer to measure cuff pressure and increase or decrease pressure as indicated to achieve cuff pressure of 20–30 mm Hg.[6,8,9,13,14,22]
26. Confirm endotracheal tube placement while manually bagging with 100% oxygen.	Ensures correct placement of the endotracheal tube.	
A. Auscultate over the epigastrium. **(Level D*)**	Allows for identification of esophageal intubation.[2,4,9,14]	If air movement or gurgling is heard, esophageal intubation has most likely occurred. The tube must be immediately removed with suction readily available, and intubation reattempted after oxygenating the patient with 100% FiO_2 via bag-valve-mask ventilation. Improper insertion may result in hypoxemia, gastric distention, vomiting, and aspiration.
B. Auscultate lung bases and apices for bilateral breath sounds. **(Level D*)**	Assists in verification of correct tube placement into the trachea. A right mainstem bronchus intubation results in diminished left-sided breath sounds.[1,4,8,16]	
C. Observe for symmetrical chest wall movement. **(Level D*)**	Assists in verification of correct tube placement.[1,4,8,16]	Asymmetrical or absent breath sounds may indicate right main stem or esophageal intubation.
D. Attach disposable $ETco_2$ detector. Watch for color change, which indicates the presence of CO_2. **(Level D*)**	A disposable CO_2 detector may be used to assist with identification of proper tube placement.[1,8,16] Detection of CO_2 confirms proper endotracheal tube placement into the trachea.[1,4,8,16]	CO_2 detectors are placed between the self-inflating manual resuscitation bag-valve-mask device and the endotracheal tube. It should be used in conjunction with physical assessment findings. At least five to six exhalations with a consistent color change must be assessed to confirm endotracheal tube placement in the trachea because the esophagus may yield a small but detectable amount of CO_2 during the first few breaths.[16]

Procedure continues on following page

Procedure for Performing Endotracheal Intubation—*Continued*		
Steps	**Rationale**	**Special Considerations**
and/or Attach a continuous $ETCO_2$ monitor, and observe for detection of CO_2 (see Procedure 12, Continuous End-tidal Carbon Dioxide Monitoring). **(Level D*)**	Continuous $ETCO_2$ monitoring is a reliable indicator of proper tube placement and allows for detection of future tube dislodgment.[1,4,8,16]	At least five to six exhalations with a consistent CO_2 level must be assessed to confirm endotracheal tube placement in the trachea because the esophagus may yield small but detectable amounts of CO_2 during the first few breaths.[16]
Or Consider use of an esophageal detection device in cardiac arrest. **(Level D*)**	During cardiac arrest (nonperfusing rhythms), low pulmonary blood flow may cause insufficient expired CO_2.[1,14,16] If CO_2 is not detected, use of an esophageal detector device is recommended.[1,14,16]	

*Level D: Peer-reviewed professional and organizational standards with the support of clinical study recommendations.
*Level M: Manufacturer's recommendations only.

E. Evaluate oxygen saturation (SpO_2) with noninvasive pulse oximetry (see Procedure 14, Oxygen Saturation Monitoring with Pulse Oximetry). **(Level D*)**	SpO_2 decreases if the esophagus has been inadvertently intubated. The value may or may not change in a right mainstem bronchus intubation.[1,16]	SpO_2 findings should be used in conjunction with physical assessment findings.
27. If CO_2 detection, assessment findings, or SpO_2 reveals that the tube is not correctly placed into the trachea, deflate the cuff, and remove the tube immediately. Ventilate and hyperoxygenate with 100% oxygen for 3–5 minutes, and then reattempt intubation, beginning with Step 13. Consider placing an oropharyngeal airway to facilitate optimal bag-valve-mask ventilation (see Procedure 7, Nasopharyngeal and Oral Airway Insertion). **(Level D*)**	Esophageal intubation results in gas flow diversion and hypoxemia.[1,2,16]	
28. If breath sounds are absent on the left, deflate the cuff and withdraw tube 1.2 cm. Reevaluate for correct tube placement (Step 26) after tube manipulation.	Absence of breath sounds on the left may indicate right mainstem intubation, which is common because of the anatomical position of the right mainstem bronchi.[1,4,8,16]	When correctly positioned, the tube tip should be halfway between the vocal cords and the carina.[2]
29. Connect the endotracheal tube to the oxygen source via a self-inflating manual resuscitation bag-valve-mask device, or mechanical ventilator, using a swivel adapter.	Use of a swivel adapter reduces motion on the tube and the mouth or nares.	
30. If indicated, insert a bite-block or oropharyngeal airway (to act as a bite-block) along the endotracheal tube.	Prevents the patient from biting down on the endotracheal tube.	If used, the bite-block should be secured separately from the tube to prevent dislodgment of the tube.

Procedure for Performing Endotracheal Intubation—*Continued*

Steps	Rationale	Special Considerations
31. Secure the endotracheal tube in place (according to institutional standards). Note the position of the tube at the teeth or gums (use centimeter markings on the tube). **(Level D*)**	Prevents inadvertent dislodgment of the tube.[1,4,8,16] Establishes a baseline for future assessment of possible endotracheal tube migration, in or out.	The commercial tube holder or tape should not cause compression on the sides or front of the neck, which may result in impaired cerebral venous return.[1,16] Consider manually holding the endotracheal tube when moving the patient to prevent inadvertent dislodgement of the tube. Common tube placement at the teeth or gums is 20–21 cm for women and 22–23 cm for men.[9,16]

Use of Commercially Available Endotracheal Tube Holder

A. Apply according to manufacturer's recommendations. **(Level M*)**	Allows for secure stabilization of the tube, decreasing the likelihood of inadvertent extubation.[1,14]	Commercially available tube holders (Fig. 1.14) are often more comfortable for patients and easier to manage if the endotracheal tube is manipulated.[16]

Use of Adhesive Tape

A. Prepare tape as shown in Fig. 1.15.		
B. Secure the tube by wrapping double-sided tape around the patient's head and torn tape edges around the endotracheal tube.	Secures the endotracheal tube in place.	Tape should not cause compression on the sides or front of the neck, which may impair venous return from the brain.[1,16]
32. Reevaluate for correct tube placement (Step 26).	Verifies that the tube was not inadvertently displaced during securing of the tube.	
33. Reconfirm the position of the tube at the teeth or gums (use centimeter markings on the tube).	Establishes a baseline for future assessment of possible endotracheal tube migration, in or out.	Common tube placement at the teeth or gums is 20–21 cm for women and 22–23 cm for men.[9,16]
34. Hyperoxygenate, and suction the endotracheal tube and pharynx as indicated (see Procedure 8, Suctioning: Endotracheal or Tracheostomy) as needed.	Removes secretions that may obstruct the tube or accumulate on top of the cuff.	
35. Confirmation of correct tube position should be verified with a chest radiograph.	Chest radiograph documents actual tube location (distance from the carina). The endotracheal tube should be noted approximately 2 cm above the carina.[16]	Because a chest radiograph is not immediately available, it should not be used as the primary method of tube assessment.[4,9,16]

Nasotracheal Intubation

36. Follow steps 1–15.	Steps necessary to initiate nasal intubation.	Dentures may be left in place for nasotracheal intubation. A stylet is not used for nasal intubation.
37. Spray the nasal passage with anesthetic and vasoconstrictor, as indicated or ordered.	Anesthetizes and vasoconstricts nasal mucosa to decrease the incidence of trauma and bleeding.[8]	
38. Lubricate the tube with local anesthetic jelly. Water soluble is an alternative if an anesthetic jelly is not available.	Allows for smooth passage of the tube.	Endotracheal tubes that range in size from 7.0–7.5 mm are commonly used for adults.[8]

Procedure continues on following page

Procedure for Performing Endotracheal Intubation—*Continued*

39. Slowly insert the tube into the selected naris, and guide the tube through the naris, then backward and down into the nasopharynx.	The tube is introduced into the airway channel.	

*Level D: Peer-reviewed professional and organizational standards with the support of clinical study recommendations.

40. Gently advance the tube into the posterior pharynx until maximal sound of moving air is heard through the tube.	The tube is located at the opening of the trachea.	Breath sounds become maximal just before entering the glottis.
41. While listening, continue to advance the tube during inspiration.	Facilitates movement of the tube through the glottic opening.	
42. When the endotracheal tube is placed, inflate the cuff (Step 25).	A properly inflated cuff will minimize secretion aspiration and facilitate stabilization in the trachea.	
43. Follow Steps 26–29 and 31–35 to evaluate tube placement and secure the tube in place.	For nasotracheal intubation, note the position of the tube at the nares.	The usual distance from the external nares to the tip of the tube is 26 cm in females and 28 cm in males.[8]
44. Remove **PE**.	Reduces transmission of microorganisms and body secretions.	
45. **HH**		

Expected Outcomes

- Placement of patent artificial airway
- Properly positioned and secured airway
- Improved oxygenation and ventilation
- Facilitation of secretion clearance

Unexpected Outcomes

- Intubation of esophagus or right mainstem bronchus (improper tube placement)
- Accidental extubation
- Cardiac dysrhythmias because of hypoxemia and vagal stimulation
- Cardiac arrest
- Broken or dislodged teeth
- Leaking of air from the endotracheal tube cuff
- Oral or nasal trauma with bleeding
- Tracheal injury at the tip of the tube or at the cuff site
- Laryngeal edema
- Vocal cord trauma
- Suctioning of gastric contents or food from endotracheal tube (aspiration)
- Obstruction of endotracheal tube
- Device related pressure injury

Patient Monitoring and Care

Steps	Rationale	Reportable Conditions
		These conditions should be reported to the provider if they persist despite nursing interventions.
1. Auscultate breath sounds on insertion, with every manipulation of the endotracheal tube and every 2–4 hours and as needed.	Allows for detection of tube movement or dislodgment.	- Absent, decreased, or unequal breath sounds

Patient Monitoring and Care —*Continued*

Steps	Rationale	Reportable Conditions
2. Maintain tube stability, with use of specially manufactured holder, twill tape, or adhesive tape.	Reduces the risk of movement and dislodgment of the tube. See manufacturer's recommendations for repositioning the tube.	• Unplanned extubation
3. Monitor and record the position of the tube at the teeth, gums, or nares (in reference to centimeter markings on tube) per institutional policy.	Provides for identification of tube migration.	• Tube movement from original position • This is often a shared responsibility between nursing and respiratory therapy.
4. Maintain an endotracheal tube cuff pressure of 20–30 mm Hg (see Procedure 3, Endotracheal Tube Care and Oral Care Practices for Ventilated and Nonventilated Patients).[8,9,14,22]	Provides adequate inflation to decrease aspiration risk and prevents overinflation of the cuff to avoid tracheal injury.[8,9,14,22]	• Cuff pressure less than 20 mm Hg or higher than 30 mm Hg that persists despite nursing interventions. • This is often a shared responsibility between nursing and respiratory therapy.
5. Hyperoxygenate and suction the endotracheal tube, as indicated (see Procedure 8, Suctioning: Endotracheal or Tracheostomy).	Prevents obstruction of the tube and subsequent hypoxemia.	• Inability to pass a suction catheter • Copious, frothy, or bloody secretions • Significant change in amount or character of secretions
6. Assess for pain, agitation/sedation, delirium, immobility, and sleep disruption (PADIS).[7]	Allows for early identification of PADIS related to intubation and mechanical ventilation.	• Pain, agitation, or delirium not controlled by medications or nursing interventions • Observed ventilator dyssynchrony
7. Inspect oral cavity, face, securement devices, and nares (if nasally intubated) once per shift or per institutional guidelines while the patient is intubated. Consider hydrocolloid dressings as needed or other prevention dressings (see Procedure 3, Endotracheal Tube Care and Oral Care Practices for Ventilated and Nonventilated Patients).	Allows for detection of potential skin breakdown and incorporation of preventive measures.	• Redness, drainage, and skin breakdown

Documentation

Documentation should include the following:
- Patient and family education
- Indication for intubation
- Time out performed per institutional standards
- Vital signs before, during, and after intubation, including oxygen saturation and $ETco_2$.
- Size of endotracheal tube
- Type of intubation: oral or nasal (include location)
- Type and size of blade used
- Number of intubation attempts
- Depth of endotracheal tube insertion in centimeters at teeth, gums, or nares
- Confirmation of tube placement, including chest radiograph, $ETco_2$ detector, and capnography (method of placement confirmation)
- Clinical confirmation of tube placement including assessment of breath sounds
- Measurement of cuff pressure
- Use of any medications including RSI (sedation and neuromuscular blockade agents)
- Patient response to procedure
- Occurrence of unexpected outcomes
- Pain assessment, interventions, and effectiveness

References and Additional Readings

For a complete list of references and additional readings for this procedure, scan this QR code with your smartphone, or visit https://www.elsevier.com/__data/assets/pdf_file/0010/1319779/Chapter0004.pdf

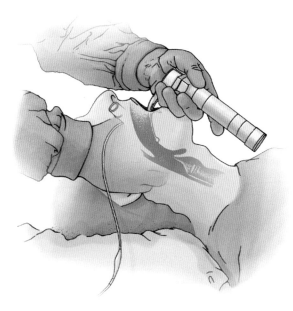

Figure 1.8 Technique of orotracheal intubation. The laryngoscope blade is inserted into the oral cavity from the right, pushing the tongue to the left as it is introduced.

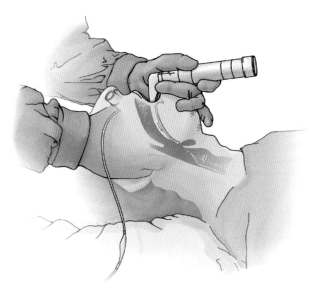

Figure 1.9 The blade is advanced into the oropharynx, and the laryngoscope is lifted to expose the epiglottis.

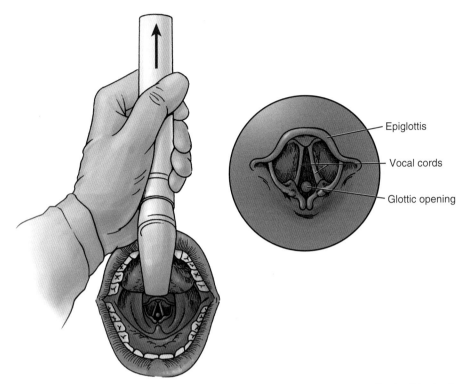

Epiglottis

Vocal cords

Glottic opening

Figure 1.10 The vocal cords are visualized. (*From Driver BE, Reardon RF.* Tracheal intubation. In: Roberts JR, Custalow CB, Thomsen TW, eds. *Roberts and Hedges' clinical procedures in emergency medicine and acute care.* 7th ed. Philadelphia, PA: Elsevier. 2019, 67)

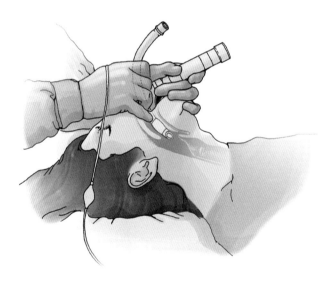

Figure 1.11 The tip of the blade is placed in the vallecula, and the laryngoscope is lifted further to expose the glottis. The tube is inserted through the right side of the mouth.

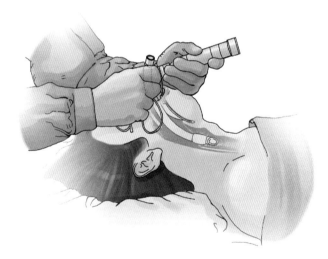

Figure 1.12 The tube is advanced through the vocal cords into the trachea.

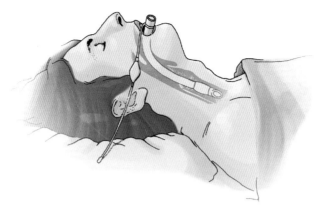

Figure 1.13   The tube is positioned so the cuff is below the vocal cords, and the laryngoscope is removed.

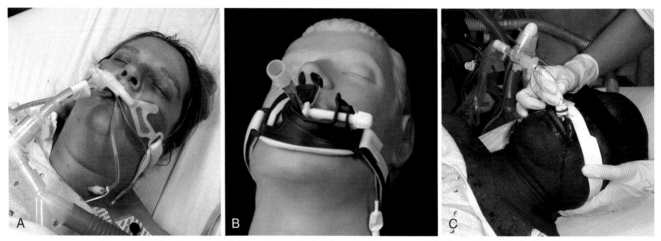

Figure 1.14   Commercial disposable tube holders. **A,** A commercial disposable tube holder is ideal and preferred to secure an endotracheal (ET) tube without the use of messy tape. **B,** A plastic disposable ET holder firmly secures the ET tube with a small clamp. **C,** When positioning a patient for transfer to another bed or for a chest radiograph, ensure the integrity of the ET tube by placing the right hand firmly against the right side of the face while holding the tube securely with the same hand. The other hand immobilizes the neck. (**B,** *Image used courtesy of Laerdal Medical.*) (*From Driver BE, Reardon RF: Tracheal intubation. In Roberts JR, Custalow CB, Thomsen TW, editors. Roberts and Hedges' clinical procedures in emergency medicine and acute care, ed 7, Philadelphia, PA, 2019, Elsevier, p 82.*)

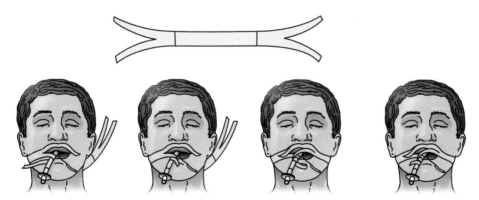

Figure 1.15   Methods of securing adhesive tape. Example protocol for securing the endotracheal tube with adhesive tape. 1. Clean the patient's skin with mild soap and water. 2. Remove oil from the skin with alcohol and allow to dry. 3. Apply a skin adhesive product to enhance tape adherence. (When the tape is removed, an adhesive remover is necessary.) 4. Place a hydrocolloid membrane over the cheeks to protect friable skin. 5. Secure with adhesive tape as shown. (*From Henneman E, Ellstrom K, St John RE: AACN protocols for practice: care of the mechanically ventilated patient series, Aliso Viejo, CA, 1999, American Association of Critical-Care Nurses, p 56.*)

2

Endotracheal Intubation (Assist)

Cynthia A. Goodrich

PURPOSE: Endotracheal intubation is performed to establish and maintain a patent airway, facilitate oxygenation and ventilation, reduce the risk of aspiration, and assist with the clearance of secretions.

PREREQUISITE NURSING KNOWLEDGE

- Anatomy and physiology of the airway and pulmonary system.
- Knowledge of rapid-sequence intubation (RSI)
  - RSI is a common method used to reduce the risk for aspiration in patients with full stomachs when emergent airway control with intubation is indicated.[8]
  - This involves almost simultaneous administration of a rapid-acting induction agent followed by a neuromuscular (paralytic) blocking agent to facilitate optimal conditions for intubation.[3,8]
  - The goal is to induce unconsciousness and paralysis, which will facilitate intubation as well as decrease the risk for gastric regurgitation and aspiration as well as damage to the airway.[3]
  - Medications that are given for RSI should have a rapid onset and short duration. Induction agents induce sedation and unconsciousness. Commonly used drugs include ketamine, etomidate, propofol, and midazolam. Neuromuscular agents cause muscular relaxation and induce paralysis. Commonly used agents include rocuronium and succinylcholine.[3,9]
  - During RSI, the provider is totally responsible for oxygenation, ventilation, and providing an airway for the patient.[8]
  - RSI is sometimes used in patients with predicted difficult airways as long as there is immediate access to additional equipment necessary to restore oxygenation and ventilation including bag-valve-mask (BVM) devices, extraglottic airways, and surgical airway tools.[3]
  - The "Seven Ps" mnemonic is a useful tool outlining the key steps for RSI planning and performance. These include preparation, preoxygenation, preintubation optimization, paralysis and induction, positioning, placement proof, and postintubation management.[3]
- Indications for endotracheal intubation include the following[4,16]:
  - Inadequate oxygenation and ventilation
  - Altered mental status (e.g., head injury, drug overdose) who are unable to protect their own airway
  - Anticipated airway obstruction (e.g., facial burns, epiglottitis, major facial or oral trauma)
  - Upper airway obstruction (e.g., from swelling, trauma, tumor, bleeding)
  - Apnea
  - Ineffective clearance of secretions (i.e., inability to maintain or protect airway adequately)
  - High risk of aspiration
  - Respiratory distress, respiratory failure
- Pulse oximetry should be used during intubation so oxygen desaturation can be quickly detected and treated (see Procedure 14, Oxygen Saturation Monitoring with Pulse Oximetry).[3,4,14,18]
- Two types of laryngoscope blades exist: straight and curved (Fig. 2.1). The straight (Miller) blade is designed so the tip extends below the epiglottis to lift and expose the glottic opening. The straight blade is recommended for use in obese patients, pediatric patients, and patients with short necks because the tracheas may be located more anteriorly. When a curved (Macintosh) blade is used, the tip is advanced into the vallecula (the space between the epiglottis and the base of the tongue), resulting in indirect elevation of the epiglottis and exposure of the glottic opening. The wide flange of this blade helps retract the tongue from the field of view, increasing the space available to pass the endotracheal tube. This blade is often chosen because it provides a better view for placement and manipulation of the tube.[16]
- There are also two types of laryngoscopes: reusable and disposable. The disposable products have incorporated batteries that cannot be accessed.
- Laryngoscope blades are available with bulbs or with a fiberoptic light delivery system. Fiberoptic light delivery systems provide a brighter light, but the bulbs are prone to becoming scratched or covered with secretions.
- Videolaryngoscopy is gaining increased popularity as a method for oral intubation. This involves the use of fiber-optics or a micro video camera encased in the

laryngoscope that provides a wide-angle view of the glottic opening while attempting oral intubation. Emerging literature supports this highly effective tool as a method to increase first-pass success by providing a superior view of the glottis, compared with traditional direct laryngoscopy.[5,9,11,12,15,17] This method also requires minimal lifting force, resulting in less movement of the cervical spine during intubation.[11]

- Endotracheal tube size reflects the size of the internal diameter of the tube. Tubes range in size from 2.0 mm for neonates to 9.0 mm for large adults. Endotracheal tubes that range in size from 7.0 to 7.5 mm are used for average-sized adult women, whereas endotracheal tubes that range in size from 7.5 to 8.0 mm are used for average-sized adult men (Fig. 2.2).[1,8,9,16] The tube with the largest clinically acceptable internal diameter should be used to minimize airway resistance and assist in suctioning.
- Endotracheal intubation can be done via oral or nasal routes. Orotracheal intubation is the preferred route, but nasal intubation may be done under certain circumstances in the ICU. The route selected will depend on the skill of the practitioner performing the intubation and the patient's clinical condition.[4]
    - ❖ Nasal intubation is rarely performed and requires a patient who is breathing spontaneously. It is relatively contraindicated in trauma patients with facial fractures or suspected fractures at the base of the skull and after cranial surgeries such as transnasal hypophysectomy.[4] Complications include epistaxis, pressure necrosis, meningitis, and sinusitis.[4,9]
- Improper intubation technique may result in trauma to the teeth, soft tissues of the mouth or nose, vocal cords, trachea, and posterior pharynx.
- Proper positioning of the patient is critical for successful intubation. Placing the patient supine with the head of the bed at 20 to 25 degrees or alternatively in the reverse Trendelenburg position at 30 degrees for those with suspected or confirmed spinal injuries improves preoxygenation and provides better visualization of airway structures during intubation.[3,8,9,16,23]
- Apneic oxygenation involves passive movement of oxygen from the upper airways into the alveoli without respiratory effort. A commonly used method involves the use of a standard nasal cannula set at 15 L/min. The nasal cannula is placed during preoxygenation and continued until the patient is intubated. Apneic oxygenation has been shown to prolong the period of safe apnea, thereby reducing the incidence of critical desaturation during a prolonged or difficult intubation.[16,19,20,21,24]
- Visualization of the vocal cords can be aided by using external laryngeal manipulation. This is accomplished by applying backward, upward, and rightward pressure (BURP) on the thyroid cartilage to move the larynx to the right while the tongue is displaced to the left by the laryngoscope blade (Fig. 2.3).[4]
- The routine application of cricoid pressure is controversial, and it is no longer being recommended in many settings.[18,25] This procedure is accomplished by applying firm downward pressure on the cricoid ring,

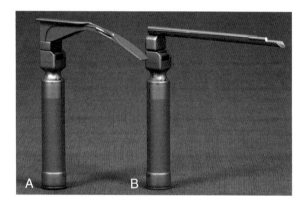

Figure 2.1 Types of blades for direct laryngoscopy. **A,** Macintosh *(curved)* and **B,** Miller *(straight). (From Driver BE, Reardon RF: Tracheal intubation. In Roberts JR, Custalow CB, Thomsen TW, editors.* Roberts and Hedges' clinical procedures in emergency medicine and acute care, *ed 7, Philadelphia, PA, 2019, Elsevier, p 69.)*

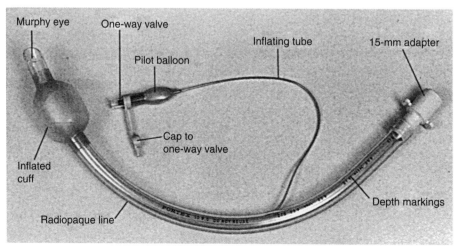

Figure 2.2 Parts of an endotracheal tube (soft-cuffed tube by Smiths Industries Medical Systems, Valencia, CA). *(From Kersten LD:* Comprehensive respiratory nursing, *Philadelphia, 1989, Saunders, p 637.)*

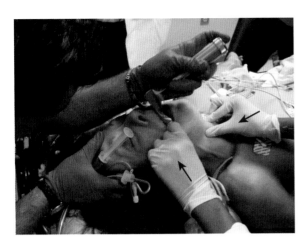

Figure 2.3 Note the assistant manipulating the anterior part of the neck and retracting the cheek *(arrows)* for better visualization. *(From Driver BE, Reardon RF: Tracheal intubation. In Roberts JR, Custalow CB, Thomsen TW, editors.* Roberts and Hedges' clinical procedures in emergency medicine and acute care, *ed 7, Philadelphia, PA, 2019, Elsevier, p 77.)*

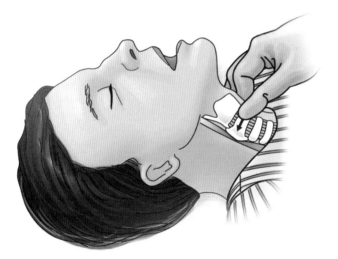

Figure 2.4 Cricoid pressure. Firm downward pressure on the cricoid ring pushes the vocal cords downward toward the field of vision while sealing the esophagus against the vertebral column.

pushing the vocal cords downward so they are more easily visualized (Fig. 2.4).[2,14,18] In non–cardiac arrest patients, there is limited evidence that it may help protect against gastric insufflation and aspiration into the lungs during bag-valve-mask ventilation.[8,18] If applied incorrectly, it may interfere with ventilation and make laryngoscopy intubation more difficult. *Once begun, cricoid pressure must be maintained until intubation is completed* unless there is difficulty intubating or ventilating the patient. In cardiac arrest patients, there is no evidence that it reduces the risk of aspiration, and its use is not recommended.[2,14,18]

- In trauma patients with suspected spinal cord injuries and those who are not completely evaluated, manual in-line cervical immobilization of the head and neck must be maintained during the entire endotracheal

intubation procedure to keep the head in a neutral position. An assistant should be directed to manually immobilize the head and neck by placing his or her hands on either side of the patient's head, with thumbs along the mandible and fingers behind the head on the occipital ridge. Gentle but firm stabilization should be maintained throughout the procedure.[4,9] The front of the cervical collar may be opened or removed to allow for increased mandibular displacement as long as spinal precautions are maintained during the procedure.[4,9,16]

- Confirmation of endotracheal tube placement should be done immediately after intubation to protect against unrecognized esophageal intubation. This includes using both clinical findings and end-tidal carbon dioxide ($ETco_2$).[4,8,14,18]
  - Clinical findings consistent with tracheal placement include visualization of the tube passing through the vocal cords, absence of gurgling over the epigastric area, auscultation of bilateral breath sounds, symmetrical chest rise and fall during ventilation, and mist in the tube.[8,14,16,18]
  - The most accurate method for confirmation of endotracheal tube placement into the trachea is $ETco_2$ determination using colorimetric or quantitative capnography (see Procedure 12, Continuous End-Tidal Carbon Dioxide Monitoring) in the non–cardiac arrest patient. The presence of CO_2 in the expired air indicates that the airway has been successfully intubated but does not ensure the correct position of the endotracheal tube.[2,14,16,18]
  - Disposable $ETco_2$ detectors are chemically treated with a nontoxic indicator that changes color in the presence of CO_2. In general, color changes from purple (no CO_2) to yellow (positive CO_2).
  - Continuous $ETco_2$ (capnography) assists in confirming proper placement of the endotracheal tube into the trachea as well as allowing for detection of future tube dislodgment.
  - During cardiac arrest (nonperfusing rhythms), low pulmonary blood flow may cause insufficient expired CO_2.[14,18] If CO_2 is not detected using $ETco_2$, an esophageal detector device may be used for confirmation of proper placement into the trachea.[2,14,16,18]
  - At least five to six exhalations with a consistent CO_2 level must be assessed to confirm endotracheal tube placement in the trachea, because the esophagus may yield a small but detectable amount of CO_2 during the first few breaths.[16]
  - Esophageal detector devices work by creating suction at the end of the endotracheal tube by compressing a flexible bulb or pulling back on a syringe plunger. When the tube is placed correctly in the trachea, air allows for reexpansion of the bulb or movement of the syringe plunger. If the tube is in the esophagus, no movement of the syringe plunger or reexpansion of the bulb is seen. These devices may be misleading in patients who are morbidly obese, in status asthmaticus, late in pregnancy, or in patients with large amounts of tracheal secretions.[1,14,16,18]

- Endotracheal tube cuff pressure should be checked after verifying correct endotracheal tube position. The cuff pressure recommended for assistance in preventing both microaspiration and tracheal damage is 20 to 30 cm H_2O (see Procedure 3, Endotracheal Tube Care and Oral Care Practices for Ventilated and Nonventilated Patients).[6,9,10,13,22]
- Intubation attempts should take no longer than 15 to 20 seconds. If more than one intubation attempt is necessary, ventilate with 100% oxygen using a self-inflating manual resuscitation bag device with a tight-fitting face mask for 3 to 5 minutes before each attempt. If intubation is not successful after three attempts, consider using another airway adjunct, such as a laryngeal mask airway (LMA) (see Procedure 6, Laryngeal Mask Airway) or other supraglottic devices.
- It is important to have a clearly defined institutional difficult/failed airway plan. This should include a process to obtain alternative airway equipment in case of unsuccessful intubation. This may consist of a gum elastic bougie, supraglottic device, and videolaryngoscope. Surgical airway equipment such as that needed for a cricothyroidotomy should also be readily available along with trained providers in case of a failed airway.[16]
- Those assisting with intubation should have additional knowledge, skills, and demonstrated competence per professional licensure and institutional standards.

EQUIPMENT

- Personal protective equipment (PPE): Intubation is considered an aerosol-generating procedure, and appropriate respiratory PPE should be used based on patient presentation and past medical history.
- Appropriately sized endotracheal tube with intact cuff and 15-mm connector (women, 7.0-mm to 7.5-mm tube; men, 7.5-mm to 8.0-mm tube)
- Laryngoscope handle with fresh batteries if nondisposable
- Laryngoscope blades (straight and curved)
- Spare bulb for nondisposable laryngoscope blades
- Flexible stylet
- Magill forceps (to remove foreign bodies obstructing the airway if present)
- Self-inflating manual resuscitation bag-valve-mask device with tight-fitting face mask connected to supplemental oxygen (15 L/min)
- Assortment of oropharyngeal airways and nasopharyngeal airways
- Oxygen source (will need two oxygen sources if doing apneic oxygenation)
- Luer-tip 10-mL syringe for cuff inflation or commercially available cuff inflation device
- Water-soluble lubricant
- Rigid pharyngeal suction-tip (Yankauer) catheter
- Suction apparatus (portable or wall) and second suction source if using ETT with continuous subglottic suctioning

- Suction catheters
- Bite-block
- Endotracheal tube–securing apparatus or appropriate tape
  - ❖ Commercially available endotracheal tube holder
  - ❖ Adhesive tape (6 to 8 inches long)
  - ❖ Hydrocolloid dressing if indicated
- Stethoscope
- Monitoring equipment: cardiac monitor, pulse oximetry, and sphygmomanometer or noninvasive blood pressure (NIBP)
- Disposable $ETco_2$ detector, continuous $ETco_2$ monitoring device, or esophageal detection device
- Rescue airway including supraglottic device such as LMA (see Procedure 6, Laryngeal Mask Airway)
- Emergency airway equipment: gum elastic bougie, videolaryngoscope, optical stylet fiberoptic scope, and cricothyroidotomy kit should be readily available in case of failed airway
- Drugs for intubation as indicated (induction agent, sedation, paralyzing agents, lidocaine, atropine) as ordered per provider
- Ventilator

Additional equipment, to have available as needed, includes the following:
- Anesthetic spray (nasal approach)
- Local anesthetic jelly (nasal approach)

PATIENT AND FAMILY EDUCATION

- If time permits, assess the patient's and family's levels of understanding about the condition and rationale for endotracheal intubation. ***Rationale:*** This assessment identifies the patient's and family's knowledge deficits concerning the patient's condition, the procedure, the expected benefits, and the potential risks. It also allows time for questions to clarify information and voice concerns. Explanations decrease patient anxiety and enhance cooperation.
- Explain the procedure and the reason for intubation if the clinical situation permits. If not, explain the procedure and reason for the intubation after it is completed. ***Rationale:*** This explanation enhances patient and family understanding and decreases anxiety.
- If indicated and the clinical situation permits, explain the patient's role in assisting with insertion of the endotracheal tube. ***Rationale:*** This explanation elicits the patient's cooperation, which assists with insertion.
- Explain that the patient will be unable to speak while the endotracheal tube is in place, but that other means of communication will be provided. ***Rationale:*** This information enhances patient and family understanding and decreases anxiety.
- Explain that the patient will be unable to eat or drink while the endotracheal tube is in place but that other nutrition and fluids will be provided. ***Rationale:*** This information enhances patient and family understanding and decreases anxiety.
- Explain the importance of not pulling at or touching the endotracheal tube and risk of inadvertent removal. The

patient will be assessed and treated as needed for pain, anxiety, and delirium during the stages of intubation, post-intubation, and readiness for extubation. ***Rationale:*** This information enhances patient and family understanding and decreases anxiety.

PATIENT ASSESSMENT AND PREPARATION

Patient Assessment

- Verify the correct patient with two identifiers. ***Rationale:*** Before performing a procedure, the nurse should ensure the correct identification of the patient for the intended intervention.
- Assess for recent history of trauma with suspected spinal cord injury or cranial surgery. ***Rationale:*** Knowledge of pertinent patient history allows for selection of the most appropriate method for intubation, which helps reduce the risk of secondary injury.
- Assess nothing-by-mouth status when expected use of a self-inflating manual resuscitation bag-valve-mask device before intubation, and for signs of gastric distention. ***Rationale:*** Increased risk of aspiration and vomiting occurs with accumulation of air (from the use of a self-inflating manual resuscitation bag-valve-mask device), food, or secretions.
- Assess level of consciousness, level of anxiety, and respiratory difficulty. ***Rationale:*** This assessment assists in determining the most appropriate medications to be used for intubation.
- Assess the oral cavity for presence of dentures, loose teeth, or other possible obstructions, and remove if appropriate. ***Rationale:*** Ensures that the airway is free from any obstructions.
- Assess vital signs, and assess for the following: tachypnea, dyspnea, shallow respirations, hypoxia, apnea, altered level of consciousness, tachycardia, cardiac dysrhythmias, hypertension, and headache. ***Rationale:*** Any of these conditions may indicate a problem with oxygenation, ventilation, or both.
- Assess need for premedication. ***Rationale:*** Various medications provide sedation or paralysis as needed.

Patient Preparation

- Perform a preprocedural verification and time out. ***Rationale:*** Ensures patient safety and improves communication.

- Ensure that the patient understands preprocedural teaching, if appropriate. Answer questions as they arise, and reinforce information as needed. ***Rationale:*** Understanding of previously taught information is evaluated and reinforced.
- Before intubation, initiate intravenous or intraosseous access, or verify patency of existing access. ***Rationale:*** Readily available intravenous or intraosseous access is required to administer medications for intubation.
- Position the patient appropriately.
  - ❖ Positioning of the nontrauma patient is as follows: place the patient supine with the head in the sniffing position, in which the head is extended and the neck is flexed. Placement of a small towel or pillow under the occiput elevates it several inches, allowing for proper flexion of the neck (Fig. 2.5). ***Rationale:*** Placement of the head in the sniffing position allows for better visualization of the larynx and vocal cords by aligning the axes of the mouth, pharynx, and trachea.
  - ❖ In nontrauma patients, consider placing the patient supine with the head of the bed at 20 to 25 degrees or alternatively in the reverse Trendelenburg position at 30 degrees. ***Rationale:*** Elevating the head of the bed helps improve preoxygenation and improves visualization of the glottis.[3,4,8,9,16,23]
  - ❖ Trauma patients can be placed in the reverse Trendelenburg position at 30 degrees, with manual in-line cervical spinal immobilization maintained during the entire process of intubation to minimize cervical spine motion.[3,4,8,9,16,23] ***Rationale:*** Because cervical spinal cord injury must be suspected in all trauma patients until proven otherwise, this position helps prevent secondary injury should a cervical spine injury be present.
- Prepare and administer medications necessary for intubation including induction and paralytic agents as ordered. ***Rationale:*** Appropriate intubation medications allow for a more controlled intubation, reducing the incidence of insertion trauma, aspiration, laryngospasm, and improper tube placement.
- Notify the respiratory therapy department of impending intubation so a ventilator can be set up. ***Rationale:*** The ventilator is set up before intubation.

Procedure for Performing Endotracheal Intubation

Steps	Rationale	Special Considerations
General Setup		
1. HH		
2. PE		Intubation is considered an aerosol-generating procedure, and additional respiratory personal protective equipment based on the patient's presentation and past medical history may be required for all providers involved in the intubation procedure.
3. Establish intravenous or intraosseous access if not present.	Provides access to deliver indicated medications.	Consider placing a second line that can be dedicated for administration of drugs during intubation and as a backup line in case of catheter dislodgement of the primary line.
4. Attach the patient to monitoring equipment, including cardiac and blood pressure monitor and pulse oximeter. Consider continuous $ETco_2$ monitoring if available.	Provides continuous patient monitoring during intubation.	
5. Set up suction apparatus, and connect rigid suction-tip catheter to tubing.	Prepares for oropharyngeal suctioning as needed.	
6. Have a self-inflating manual resuscitation bag-valve-mask device connected to a 100% oxygen source and face mask ready for hyperoxygenation and manual ventilation.	Intubation attempts should not take longer than 30 seconds. Patients must be hyperoxygenated and ventilated between intubation attempts.[1,4,8]	If intubation is unsuccessful within 30 seconds or the patient's oxygen saturation falls below 90% during the attempt, remove the tube.[16] Ventilate with 100% oxygen with a bag-valve-mask device before another intubation attempt is made. Before reattempting intubation, correct problems related to positioning, procedure, or equipment.
7. Check equipment as directed by individual performing the intubation.		
A. Choose an appropriate-sized endotracheal tube.	Appropriate-sized endotracheal tubes facilitate both intubation and ventilation.	Generally, a 7.0- to 7.5-mm internal diameter tube is used for adult females and a 7.5- to 8.0-mm internal diameter tube is used for adult males.[1,8,9.16]
B. Use a 10-mL syringe to inflate the cuff on the tube, assessing for leaks. Completely deflate the cuff once its integrity has been checked.	Verifies that equipment is functional and that the tube cuff is patent without leaks; prepares the tube for insertion.	Once the endotracheal tube cuff has been checked for leak and it is completely deflated, place it back into its packaging to avoid contamination.
C. Insert the stylet into the endotracheal tube, ensuring that the tip of the stylet does not extend past the end of the endotracheal tube.	Provides structural support for the flexible endotracheal tube during insertion. Maintaining the tip of the stylet within the lumen of the endotracheal tube prevents damage to the vocal cords and trachea.	The stylet must be recessed by at least 0.5 inch from the distal end of the tube so it does not protrude beyond the end of the tube.

Procedure | for Performing Endotracheal Intubation—*Continued*

Steps	Rationale	Special Considerations
D. Connect the laryngoscope blade to the handle, and ensure that the blade's bulb is securely seated.	Verifies that the equipment is functional.	Check the bulb for brightness. Replace the bulb if it is dull or burned out for nondisposable products.
8. Assist in positioning the patient's head by flexing the neck forward and extending the head into the sniffing position (only if neck trauma is not suspected (see Fig. 2.5). If spinal trauma is suspected, assist in maintaining the head in a neutral position with in-line spinal immobilization. *This is performed by manually immobilizing the head and neck by placing your hands on either side of the patient's head, with thumbs along the mandible and fingers behind the head on the occipital ridge. Use gentle but firm stabilization throughout the procedure.*[4,9,] The front of the cervical collar may be opened or removed, allowing for increased mandibular displacement as long as spinal precautions are maintained during the procedure.[4,9,16] **(Level D*)**	Allows for visualization of the vocal cords with alignment of the mouth, pharynx, and trachea.[4,8,9,16]	The ear (external auditory meatus) and sternal notch should be aligned when the patient is examined from the side. This allows for flexion of the cervical spine.[8,16,18] Placement of a small towel or pillow under the occiput elevates it, allowing for proper neck flexion. *Do not flex or extend the neck of a patient with suspected spinal cord injury; the head must be maintained in a neutral position with manual in-line cervical spine immobilization.*[4,6]
9. Check the mouth for dentures, and remove if present.	Dentures should be removed before oral intubation is attempted but may remain in place for nasal intubation or bag-valve-mask ventilation before oral intubation.	
10. Suction the mouth and pharynx as needed if secretions are visualized.	Provides a clear view of the posterior pharynx and larynx.	
11. Insert an oropharyngeal or nasopharyngeal airway if indicated (see Procedure 7, Nasopharyngeal and Oral Airway Insertion).	Assists in maintenance of upper airway patency. Helps improve ability to ventilate during bag-valve-mask ventilation.	Only use oral airways in unconscious patients with an absent gag reflex.
12. Preoxygenate for 3–5 minutes, with 100% oxygen via a nonrebreather mask if ventilations are adequate or via a self-inflating manual resuscitation bag-valve-mask device (see Procedure 29, Manual Self-inflating Resuscitation Bag-Valve Device) if ventilations are inadequate.	Helps prevent hypoxemia. Gentle breaths reduce the incidence of air entering the stomach (leading to gastric distention, aspiration), decrease airway turbulence, and distribute ventilation more evenly within the lungs. Preoxygenation ensures that nitrogen is washed out of the lungs and will extend the allowable apneic time until the oxygen in the lungs is used up.[4,8,16]	Bag-valve-mask ventilation may not be needed in a spontaneously breathing patient. Avoid aggressive positive-pressure ventilation with a self-inflating manual resuscitation bag because this may increase the risk for gastric distension and vomiting.[3,8,9,16]

Procedure continues on following page

Procedure for Performing Endotracheal Intubation—*Continued*

Steps	Rationale	Special Considerations
13. Administer intubation medications including induction and paralytic agents as directed by the practitioner intubating the patient.	Sedates and relaxes the patient, allowing for easier intubation. Jaw relaxation and apnea indicate that the patient is adequately medicated.	This may require a second assistant to administer and document medications given before, during, and after intubation.
14. Remove the oropharyngeal airway if present.	Clears the airway for advancement of the laryngoscope blade and endotracheal tube.	
15. Apply external laryngeal manipulation (BURP) and/or cricoid pressure **ONLY** as directed by the practitioner performing the intubation.	External laryngeal manipulation (BURP) may assist with visualization of the vocal cords.[4] Apply BURP on the thyroid cartilage to move the larynx to the right while the tongue is displaced to the left by the laryngoscope blade.[4] Cricoid pressure moves the trachea toward the posterior, which may provide better visualization of the vocal cords by the practitioner.	In some cases, the intubator may perform the BURP manipulation by themselves to initially visualize the vocal cords. The assistant should be prepared to take over for the intubator once the cords are visualized. Once cricoid pressure (Sellick maneuver) is applied, it must be maintained until the intubation is completed. The intubator may request the assistant to retract the corner of the patient's right lip/cheek to increase the field of view (see Fig. 2.3).
16. Once the tube has been correctly placed, assist with cuff inflation as directed. Inflate cuff with 5–10 mL of air depending on the manufacturer's recommendations. Do not overinflate the cuff. **(Level M*)**	Inflation volumes vary depending on manufacturer and size of tube. If a manometer is available, keep cuff pressure between 20 and 30 mm Hg to decrease risk of aspiration and prevent ischemia and decreased blood flow.[8,9,14]	In adults, decreased mucosal capillary blood flow (ischemia) results when pressure is greater than 30 mm Hg.[8,14,22] Consider using a manometer to measure cuff pressure and increase or decrease pressure as indicated to achieve cuff pressure of 20–30 mm Hg.[6,8,9,13,14,22]
17. Once the endotracheal tube has been placed, assist with confirmation of tube placement as directed by the intubator. Continue ventilating with 100% oxygen self-inflating manual resuscitation bag.	Ensures correct placement of endotracheal tube into the trachea.	If requested, hold the endotracheal tube securely at the lip, making note of how far the tube has been placed into the trachea by noting the markings on the endotracheal tube. Avoid hyperventilation; gently ventilate with 10–12 breaths per minute watching for visible chest rise.[1]
Auscultate over epigastrium. **(Level D*)**	Allows for identification of esophageal intubation.[2,4,9,14]	If air movement or gurgling is heard, esophageal intubation has most likely occurred. The tube must be immediately removed with suction readily available, and intubation reattempted after oxygenating the patient with 100% Fio_2 via bag-valve-mask ventilation. Improper insertion may result in hypoxemia, gastric distention, vomiting, and aspiration.
B. Auscultate lung bases and apices for bilateral breath sounds. **(Level D*)**	Assists in verification of correct tube placement into the trachea. A right mainstem bronchus intubation results in diminished left-sided breath sounds.[1,4,8,16]	

Procedure for Performing Endotracheal Intubation—*Continued*		
Steps	Rationale	Special Considerations
C. Observe for symmetrical chest wall movement. (**Level D***)	Assists in verification of correct tube placement.[1,4,8,16]	Asymmetrical or absent breath sounds may indicate right mainstem or esophageal intubation.
D. Attach disposable $ETCO_2$ detector. Watch for color change, which indicates the presence of CO_2. (**Level D***)	Disposable CO_2 detectors may be used to assist with identification of proper tube placement.[1,8,16] Detection of CO_2 confirms proper endotracheal tube placement into the trachea.[1,4,8,16]	CO_2 detectors are placed between the self-inflating manual resuscitation bag-valve-mask device and the endotracheal tube. CO_2 detectors should be used in conjunction with physical assessment findings. At least five to six exhalations with a consistent color change must be assessed to confirm endotracheal tube placement in the trachea because the esophagus may yield small but detectable amounts of CO_2 during the first few breaths.[16]
and/or Attach continuous $ETCO_2$ monitor, and observe for detection of CO_2 (see Procedure 12, Continuous End-tidal Carbon Dioxide Monitoring). (**Level D***)	Continuous $ETCO_2$ monitoring is a reliable indicator of proper tube placement and allows for detection of future tube dislodgment.[1,4,8,16]	At least five to six exhalations with a consistent CO_2 level must be assessed to confirm endotracheal tube placement in the trachea because the esophagus may yield small but detectable amounts of CO_2 during the first few breaths.[16]
Or Consider use of esophageal detection device in cardiac arrest. (**Level D***)	During cardiac arrest (nonperfusing rhythms), low pulmonary blood flow may cause insufficient expired CO_2.[1,14,16] If CO_2 is not detected, use of an esophageal detector device is recommended.[1,14,16]	

*Level D: Peer-reviewed professional and organizational standards with the support of clinical study recommendations.
*Level M. Manufacturer's recommendations only.

E. Evaluate oxygen saturation (Spo_2) with noninvasive pulse oximetry (see Procedure 14, Oxygen Saturation Monitoring with Pulse Oximetry). (**Level D***)	Spo_2 decreases if the esophagus has been inadvertently intubated. The value may or may not change in a right mainstem bronchus intubation.[1,16]	Spo_2 findings should be used in conjunction with physical assessment findings.

Procedure continues on following page

Procedure for Performing Endotracheal Intubation—*Continued*

18. If CO_2 detection, assessment findings, or SpO_2 reveals that the tube is not correctly placed into the trachea, deflate the cuff and assist with tube removal as directed by the intubator. Ventilate and hyperoxygenate with 100% oxygen for 3–5 minutes, then assist with reattempt at intubation, beginning with Step 11. Consider placing an oropharyngeal airway to facilitate optimal bag-valve-mask ventilation (see Procedure 7, Nasopharyngeal and Oral Airway Insertion). (**Level D***)

    Esophageal intubation results in gas flow diversion and hypoxemia.[1,2,16]

19. If breath sounds are absent on the left, cuff should be deflated and withdrawn by 1–2 cm. Reevaluate for correct tube placement (Step 17) as directed by the intubator.

    Absence of breath sounds on the left may indicate right mainstem intubation, which is common because of the anatomical position of the right mainstem bronchi.[1,4,8,16]

    When correctly positioned, the tube tip should be halfway between the vocal cords and the carina.[2]

20. Connect the endotracheal tube to the oxygen source via a self-inflating manual resuscitation bag-valve-mask device or a mechanical ventilator, using a swivel adapter.

    Use of a swivel adapter reduces motion on the tube and mouth or nares.

21. If indicated, insert a bite-block or oropharyngeal airway (to act as a bite-block) along the endotracheal tube.

    Prevents the patient from biting down on the endotracheal tube.

    If used, the bite-block should be secured separately from the tube to prevent dislodgment of the tube.

22. Secure the endotracheal tube in place as directed (according to institutional standards). Note the position of the tube at the teeth, gums, or nares (use centimeter markings on the tube). (**Level D***)

    Prevents inadvertent dislodgment of the tube.[1,4,8,16]

    The commercial tube holder or tape should not cause compression on the sides or front of the neck, which may result in impaired cerebral blood flow.[1,16] Consider manually holding the endotracheal tube when moving the patient to prevent inadvertent dislodgement of the tube.

Use of Commercially Available Endotracheal Tube Holder

A. Apply according to manufacturer's directions. (**Level M***)

   Allows for secure stabilization of the tube, decreasing the likelihood of inadvertent extubation.[1,14]

   Commercially available tube holders (Fig. 2.6) are often more comfortable for patients and easier to manage if the endotracheal tube is manipulated.[16]

---

*Level D: Peer-reviewed professional and organizational standards with the support of clinical study recommendations.
*Level M: Manufacturer's recommendations only.

Use of Adhesive Tape

A. Prepare tape as shown in Fig. 2.7.

Procedure for Performing Endotracheal Intubation—*Continued*

B. Secure the tube by wrapping double-sided tape around the patient's head and torn tape edges around endotracheal tube.

Secures the endotracheal tube in place.

Tape should not cause compression on sides or front of the neck, which may impair venous return to the brain.[1,16]

23. Reevaluate for correct tube placement (Step 17).

Verifies that the tube was not inadvertently displaced during the securing of the tube.

24. Reconfirm the position of the tube at the teeth or gums (use centimeter markings on the tube).

Establishes a baseline for future assessment of possible endotracheal tube migration, in or out.

Common tube placement at the teeth or gums is 20–21 cm for women and 22–23 cm for men.[9,16] If nasal intubation, the usual distance from the external nares to the tip of the tube is 26 cm in females and 28 cm in males.[8]

25. Hyperoxygenate and suction the endotracheal tube and the pharynx (see Procedure 8, Suctioning: Endotracheal or Tracheostomy) as needed.

Removes secretions that may obstruct the tube or accumulate on top of the cuff.

26. Confirmation of correct tube position should be verified with a chest radiograph.

Chest radiograph documents actual tube location (distance from the carina). The endotracheal tube tip should be noted approximately 2 cm above the carina.[16]

Because a chest radiograph is not immediately available, it should not be used as the primary method of tube assessment.[4,9,16]

27. Remove **PE**

Reduces transmission of microorganisms and body secretions.

28. **HH**

Expected Outcomes
- Placement of patent artificial airway
- Properly positioned and secured airway
- Improved oxygenation and ventilation
- Facilitation of secretion clearance

Unexpected Outcomes
- Intubation of esophagus or right mainstem bronchus (improper tube placement)
- Accidental extubation
- Cardiac dysrhythmias because of hypoxemia and vagal stimulation
- Cardiac arrest
- Broken or dislodged teeth
- Leaking of air from the endotracheal tube cuff
- Oral or nasal trauma with bleeding
- Tracheal injury at the tip of the tube or at the cuff site
- Laryngeal edema
- Vocal cord trauma
- Suctioning of gastric contents or food from endotracheal tube (aspiration)
- Obstruction of endotracheal tube
- Device-related pressure injury

Procedure continues on following page

Patient Monitoring and Care

Steps	Rationale	Reportable Conditions
		These conditions should be reported to the provider if they persist despite nursing interventions.
1. Auscultate breath sounds on insertion, with every manipulation of the endotracheal tube and every 2–4 hours and as needed.	Allows for detection of tube movement or dislodgment.	• Absent, decreased, or unequal breath sounds
2. Maintain tube stability, with use of a specially manufactured holder, twill tape, or adhesive tape.	Reduces the risk of movement and dislodgment of the tube. See manufacturer's recommendations for repositioning the tube.	• Unplanned extubation
3. Monitor and record the position of the tube at the teeth, gums, or nares (in reference to centimeter markings on the tube) per institutional standards.	Provides identification of tube migration.	• Tube movement from the original position • This is often a shared responsibility between nursing and respiratory therapy.
4. Maintain an endotracheal tube cuff pressure of 20–30 mm Hg (see Procedure 3, Endotracheal Tube Care and Oral Care Practices for Ventilated and Nonventilated Patients).[8,9,14,22]	Provides adequate inflation to decrease aspiration risk and prevents overinflation of the cuff to avoid tracheal injury.[8,9,14,22]	• Cuff pressure less than 20 mm Hg or higher than 30 mm Hg that persists despite nursing interventions. • This is often a shared responsibility between nursing and respiratory therapy.
5. Hyperoxygenate and suction the endotracheal tube, as indicated (see Procedure 8, Suctioning: Endotracheal or Tracheostomy).	Prevents obstruction of the tube and subsequent hypoxemia.	• Inability to pass a suction catheter • Copious, frothy, or bloody secretions • Significant change in amount or character of secretions
6. Assess for pain, agitation/sedation, delirium, immobility, and sleep disruption (PADIS).[7]	Allows early identification of PADIS related to the intubation and mechanical ventilation.	• Pain, agitation, or delirium not controlled by medications or nursing interventions • Observed ventilator dyssynchrony
7. Inspect the oral cavity, face, securement devices, and nares (if nasally intubated) once per shift or per institutional standards while the patient is intubated. Consider hydrocolloid dressings as needed or other prevention dressings (see Procedure 3, Endotracheal Tube Care and Oral Care Practices for Ventilated and Nonventilated Patients).	Allows for detection of potential skin breakdown and incorporation of preventive measures.	• Redness, drainage, and skin breakdown.

Documentation

Documentation should include the following:

- Patient and family education
- Time-out performed per institutional standards
- Vital signs before, during, and after intubation, including oxygen saturation and $ETCO_2$
- Size of endotracheal tube
- Type of intubation: oral or nasal (include location)
- Depth of endotracheal tube insertion centimeters at teeth, gums, or nares
- Confirmation of tube placement, including chest radiograph, $ETCO_2$ detector, capnography (method of placement confirmation)
- Clinical confirmation of tube placement including assessment of breath sounds
- Measurement of cuff pressure
- Number of intubation attempts
- Use of any medications including RSI (sedation and neuromuscular blockade agents)
- Patient response to procedure
- Occurrence of unexpected outcomes
- Pain assessment, interventions, and effectiveness

References and Additional Readings

For a complete list of references and additional readings for this procedure, scan this QR code with your smartphone, or visit https://www.elsevier.com/__data/assets/pdf_file/0010/1319779/Chapter0002.pdf

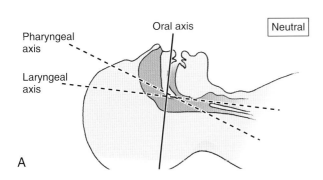

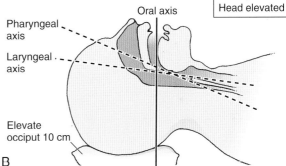

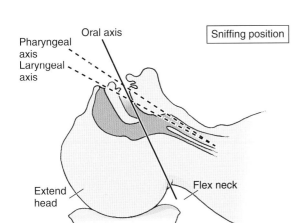

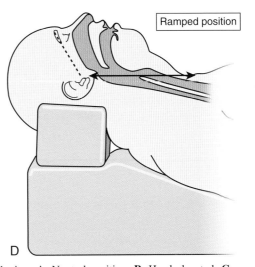

Figure 2.5   Head positioning for tracheal intubation. **A,** Neutral position. **B,** Head elevated. **C,** "Sniffing" position with a flexed neck and extended head. Note that flexing the neck while extending the head lines up the various axes and allows direct laryngoscopy. **D,** Morbidly obese patients are best intubated in a ramped position with elevation of the upper part of the back, neck, and head; the ideal position aligns the external auditory canal and the sternum. *(From Driver BE, Reardon RF: Tracheal intubation. In Roberts JR, Custalow CB, Thomsen TW, editors.* Roberts and Hedges' clinical procedures in emergency medicine and acute care, *ed 7, Philadelphia, PA, 2019, Elsevier, p 71.)*

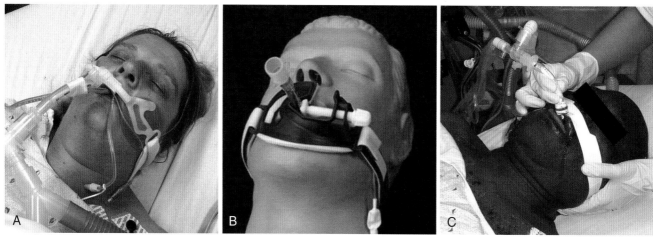

Figure 2.6 Commercial disposable tube holders. **A,** A commercial disposable tube holder is ideal and preferred to secure an endotracheal (ET) tube without the use of messy tape. **B,** A plastic disposable ET holder firmly secures the ET tube with a small clamp. **C,** When positioning a patient for transfer to another bed or for a chest radiograph, ensure the integrity of the ET tube by placing the right hand firmly against the right side of the face while holding the tube securely with the same hand. The other hand immobilizes the neck. (**B,** Image used courtesy of Laerdal Medical.) *(From Driver BE, Reardon RF: Tracheal intubation. In Roberts JR, Custalow CB, Thomsen TW, editors.* Roberts and Hedges' clinical procedures in emergency medicine and acute care, *ed 7, Philadelphia, PA, 2019, Elsevier, p 82.)*

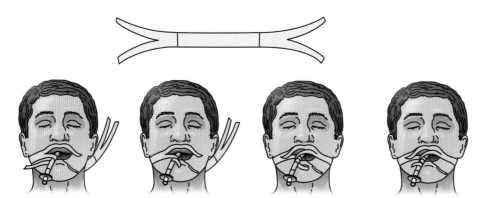

Figure 2.7 Methods of securing adhesive tape. Example protocol for securing the endotracheal tube with adhesive tape. 1. Cleanse the patient's skin with mild soap and water. 2. Remove oil from the skin with alcohol, and allow to dry. 3. Apply a skin adhesive product to enhance tape adherence. (When the tape is removed, an adhesive remover is necessary.) 4. Place a hydrocolloid membrane over the cheeks to protect friable skin. 5. Secure with adhesive tape as shown. *(From Henneman E, Ellstrom K, St John RE:* AACN protocols for practice: Care of the mechanically ventilated patient series, *Aliso Viejo, CA, 1999, American Association of Critical-Care Nurses, p 56.)*

PROCEDURE

3

Endotracheal Tube Care and Oral Care Practices for Ventilated and Nonventilated Patients

Barbara Quinn and Cheryl Ruble

PURPOSE: Endotracheal tube (ETT) management and oral care are performed to prevent buccal, oropharyngeal, and tracheal trauma from the tube and cuff; to provide oral hygiene; to promote ventilation; and to decrease the risk of healthcare-acquired pneumonia (HAP), which includes ventilator-associated pneumonia (VAP) and nonventilator healthcare-acquired pneumonia (NV-HAP).

PREREQUISITE NURSING KNOWLEDGE

- Anatomy and physiology of the pulmonary system.
- ETTs are used to maintain a patent airway or to facilitate mechanical ventilation. The presence of artificial airways, especially ETTs, prevents effective coughing and secretion removal, necessitating periodic removal of secretions (see Procedure 8, Suctioning: Endotracheal and Tracheostomy).
- The oropharynx and the upper gastrointestinal tract are the main reservoirs for pathogens associated with VAP and NV-HAP, and aspiration can result in pneumonia.[16,31,64,67]
- Appropriate cuff management (see Procedure 11, Tracheostomy Cuff and Tube Care) helps prevent major aspirations of pulmonary secretions, prepares for tracheal extubation, and decreases the risk of iatrogenic infection.[21,34,36]
- Constant pressure from the ETT securement device or tape and ETT on the mouth or nose can cause skin breakdown. Assessment and device-related pressure injury prevention strategies should be used.[22,23,48]
- If the patient is anxious or uncooperative, use of two caregivers for retaping and/or repositioning the ETTs may help prevent accidental dislodgment of the tube. Management of the patient's pain and delirium will decrease patient anxiety, decrease agitation, facilitate rest, and reduce intragenic risk.[15]
- VAP and NV-HAP increase the risk of ventilator and intensive care unit (ICU) days and hospital length of stay, overall morbidity, and mortality.[6,12,18,27,45]
- Oral hygiene

AP This procedure should be performed only by clinicians who have demonstrated competence and are credentialed to perform it. In addition, the procedure must be within the scope of practice defined by their professional licensure, and in accordance with professional practice acts. Physicians, advanced practice nurses, and physician assistants may be credentialed to perform this procedure.

- ❖ The importance of evidence-based oral hygiene procedures as the standard of care should be understood.[26,30,50]
- ❖ The oral cavity is a significant source of bacterial colonization. Even short-term hospitalization and illness contribute to dysbiosis and a microbial shift of the oral microbiome with an increase in respiratory pathogens not normally found in healthy individuals, resulting in adverse clinical outcomes.[32,63,69] There is a documented association between pathogens in oral biofilm and trach secretions in patients who develop VAP, including *Staphylococcus aureus*, *Klebsiella pneumoniae*, *Candida albicans*, *Pseudomonas aeruginosa*, *Enterobacter gergoviae*, *Streptococcus* spp., and *Serratia marcescens*.[59,66]
- ❖ Salivary flow is a natural host defense in facilitating the removal of plaque and microorganisms and acts as a protective barrier to pathogenic bacteria, fungi, and viruses. Immunoglobulin A (IgA) in saliva can inhibit absorption and adhesion of bacteria to the upper airways.[40]
- ❖ The equipment used to remove oral secretions as well as suctioning of the ETT may contribute to colonization of the oral cavity.[62]
- ❖ Many medications and withholding food and oral fluids may contribute to dry mouth in hospitalized patients, including those not on a ventilator. Reduced salivary flow with the subjective feeling of thirst is one of the ten most distressful patient experiences in the ICU.[8,33,68]
- ❖ Comprehensive oral hygiene for ventilated and nonventilated patients is associated with reduced risk for VAP and NV-HAP.[17,20,26,30,47,56]
- Oral care practices for ventilator patients
  - ❖ The purpose of comprehensive oral care for ventilated patients is to decrease bacterial colonization in the oropharyngeal cavity. Mechanical toothbrushing is recommended as part of an effective oral care program and an essential element of a VAP prevention bundle.[9,17]
  - ❖ Toothbrushing and swabbing have been found to be effective to remove plaque, and toothbrushing combined with use of an antiseptic oral rinse may be

35

more effective than using an oral rinse alone to reduce VAP.[43,46,75]

❖ Many types of oral rinses have been tested, including but not limited to povidone-iodine, sodium bicarbonate, hydrogen peroxide (H_2O_2), cetylpyridinium chloride (CPC), and variable concentrations of chlorhexidine gluconate (CHG).

❖ Research has shown that oral care with CHG rinses have not shown impact on ICU length of stay or mortality.[26,37] Additionally, there has been an association noted between CHG oral use and higher mortality rates.[14,35,37,54] Recent VAP guidelines have recommended the use of oral care including toothbrushing without CHG.[34] Oral CHG use as a VAP prevention strategy is no longer recommended.

❖ Optimal frequency of oral care in the ventilated patient is every 2 to 4 hours, which appears to provide a greater improvement in oral health.[1,19]

❖ Routine oral care with alcohol-free, antiseptic mouthwash and application of oral mucosa and lip moisturizer increases patient comfort and decreases perceived patient thirst.[55,60,72]

• Oral care practices for nonventilated patients

❖ Patients not on a ventilator are still at risk for pneumonia, and studies indicate that oral care can reduce this risk. Currently, NV-HAP occurs more often than VAP, with high mortality rates, costing more lives and dollars than VAP.[12,18]

❖ Oral care two to three times a day for nonventilated adult hospitalized patients can reduce NV-HAP by 37% to 92%.[47,56]

❖ Perioperative oral care can prevent postoperative pneumonia, and lack of oral care before surgery may lead to increased risk.[29,44,51,65]

❖ There are no documented studies that show the optimal frequency of oral care for nonventilated patients in the hospital. For the general public, the American Dental Association (ADA) recommends brushing for 2 minutes twice daily with a soft-bristled toothbrush using toothpaste with fluoride, rinsing with an antiseptic mouthwash, and moisturizing the lips and mouth, as needed.[5] An ADA-approved oral care protocol for hospitalized adult patients recommends oral care four times a day.[12] Successful NV-HAP prevention studies have documented oral hygiene two to three times a day.[47,56]

❖ If a nonventilated patient cannot manage oral secretions and is at high risk for aspiration, the caregiver may consider using a suction toothbrush, like those used in the ventilated-patient setting.[67]

❖ Dentures are also a reservoir for pathogens and require routine cleaning to reduce the risk of translocation and lung infection.[49]

EQUIPMENT

• Nonsterile gloves
• A combination of goggles or glasses, mask, and/or face shield to protect mucous membranes.
• Soft pediatric/adult toothbrush or suction toothbrush
• Foam oral swab or oral suction swab
• Oral cleansing solution

• Oral moisturizer for lips and mouth

Additional equipment, to have available as needed, includes the following:

❖ Bite-block or oral airway
❖ Adhesive or twill tape; commercial ETT holder (design must ensure ability to provide oral care and suctioning)
❖ 2 × 2 gauze or cotton swab for cleansing around the nares
❖ Suction catheters for oral and subglottal secretion suctioning
❖ Two sources of suction or a bifurcated connection device attached to a single suction source
❖ Connecting tube(s) (4 to 6 feet)
❖ Sterile 0.9% normal saline, sterile or distilled water (for rinsing the reusable suction catheter)

PATIENT AND FAMILY EDUCATION

• Explain to the patient and family the procedure, the purpose of ETT care, and the importance of comprehensive oral care in prevention of infection in both intubated and nonintubated patients. **Rationale:** This step identifies patient and family knowledge deficits concerning patient condition, procedure, expected benefits, and potential risks and allows time for questions to clarify information and voice concerns. Explanations decrease patient and family anxiety and enhance cooperation.[11,24]

• If indicated, explain the patient's role in assisting with ETT care. **Rationale:** Eliciting the patient's cooperation assists with care.

• Explain how the patient's family may participate in care, with nurse instruction and according to their comfort level. **Rationale:** Family participation in care has been shown to improve patient outcomes and increase patient and family satisfaction.[7,11,24]

• Explain that the patient will be unable to speak while the ETT is in place but that other means of communication will be provided. **Rationale:** This information enhances patient and family understanding and decreases anxiety.[11,74]

• Remind the patient and family to refrain from touching or pulling on the tube to prevent accidental dislodgment of the ETT. **Rationale:** This information enhances patient and family understanding and decreases anxiety.[11,24,74]

PATIENT ASSESSMENT AND PREPARATION

Patient Assessment

• Verify the correct patient with two identifiers. **Rationale**: Before performing a procedure, the nurse should ensure the correct identification of the patient for the intended intervention.

• Assess for signs and symptoms that indicate oral cavity and ETT care is necessary in between routine care.[61] **Rationale**: Assessment provides for early recognition that oral or ETT care is needed.

❖ Excessive secretions (oral or tracheal)
❖ Dry oral mucosa
❖ Debris in the oral cavity
❖ Plaque buildup on teeth
❖ Soiled tape or ties or commercial device

❖ Patient biting or kinking ETT
❖ Pressure areas on the nares, corner of mouth, or tongue
❖ ETT moving in and out of the mouth
❖ Patient able to verbalize or audible air leak around ETT
❖ Presence of course crackles on tracheal auscultation
❖ Decline in oxygen saturation
❖ Changes in ventilator assessment such as presence of a sawtooth pattern on the ventilator monitor, increase in pressure mode ventilation peak inspiratory pressure, or decrease in pressure-controlled tidal volume.

• Assess level of pain, consciousness and level of anxiety using a validated tool such as the Richmond Agitation-Sedation Scale (RASS) or Sedation Agitation Scale (SAS). *Rationale:* This assessment determines the need for pain medication or sedation during ETT care and the number of care providers needed to perform the activities safely.[15]

Patient Preparation

• Ensure that the patient understands the preprocedural teaching. Answer questions as they arise, and reinforce information as needed. *Rationale*: This process evaluates and reinforces understanding of previously taught information.[11]
• Increase the head of the bed to a 30- to 45-degree position before performing care if not contraindicated or the head of the bed is not already in position. *Rationale:* This position promotes comfort, reduces physical strain, and maintains head of bed elevation to reduce the risk of aspiration.[1,34,73]

Procedure   for Endotracheal Tube and Oral Care for Ventilated Patients

Steps	Rationale	Special Considerations
1. **HH**		
2. **PE**		
3. Ensure that the ETT is connected to the ventilator with a swivel adapter.	Decreases pressure exerted by ventilator tubing on the ETT, thereby minimizing the risk of pressure injury.	
4. Support the ETT and tubing as needed.	Prevents inadvertent displacement or dislodgement of the tube.	If the patient is at risk for inadvertent or sudden movements, obtain an assistant to manually support the ETT and tubing.
5. If ETT suctioning is clinically indicated, hyperoxygenate via the ventilator before ETT suction and between attempts[61] (see Procedure 8, Suctioning: Endotracheal and Tracheostomy).	Removes secretions that may obstruct the tube.	Suctioning of airways should be performed only for a clinical indication and not as a routine fixed-schedule treatment.[61]
6. If the patient is nasally intubated, cleanse around the ETT with saline solution–soaked gauze or cotton swabs.	Removes secretions that could cause pressure and subsequent skin breakdown.	Assess nasal skin and folds for skin breakdown from ETT, tape, and securement device.[22,23,48]
7. If the patient is intubated orally, remove the bite-block or oropharyngeal airway (acting as a bite-block) before proceeding with oral hygiene, if feasible.	The bite-block or oropharyngeal airway prevents the patient from biting down on the ETT and occluding airflow. It also allows access to the oral cavity by preventing the patient from biting on suction and oral care equipment.	The bite-block should be secured separately from the tube to prevent dislodgment of the ETT. The bite-block or ETT securing mechanism may be a barrier to providing good oral care. Removal of the ETT securing mechanism may result in dislodgement of the ETT. Removal of a bite block should be performed with caution because of the danger of the patient obstructing the ETT, snapping oral swabs in half, and impediment of cleansing item use due to patient biting. Staff should not insert fingers into patient's oral cavity because of the risk of staff injury from bite.

Procedure continues on following page

Procedure **for Endotracheal Tube and Oral Care for Ventilated Patients—*Continued***

Steps	Rationale	Special Considerations
8. Raise the head of the bed to 30 to 45 degrees unless contraindicated and if not already in position.	Reduces the risk of aspiration.	Ensure that the ETT and other equipment is secure when positioning the patient to prevent dislodgement.
9. Initiate oral hygiene with a pediatric or adult (soft) toothbrush for 2 minutes, at least twice a day.[5] Gently brush the patient's teeth, gums, tongue, and outer surface of the ETT.[25] **(Level D*).**	Mechanical cleansing and oral hygiene reduce oropharyngeal colonization and dental plaque, which is associated with VAP.[13,42]	Toothbrushing is superior to no toothbrushing to prevent VAP.[13,43,46,60] When brushing with good technique, a dentifrice such as toothpaste may not be necessary.[71]
10. In addition to brushing twice daily, use oral swabs with a therapeutic oral cleansing solution such as hydrogen peroxide or cetylpyridinium chloride for 30 seconds to cleanse the mouth every 2–4 hours.[75]	Oral cleansing, suctioning, and moisturizing every 2–4 hours is a part of comprehensive oral care that has shown to improve oral health and reduce the risk of HAP.[55] Studies support the safety and efficacy of hydrogen peroxide (>1%– <3%) and cetylpyridinium chloride (0.07%–1%) as mouthwashes for effective plaque removal and maintaining overall gingival health.[58,75] Povidone-iodine may reduce VAP, but its effectiveness remains unclear.[70]	Foam swabs are effective in stimulating mucosal tissue and removing plaque.[13,43,46]
11. Suction oropharyngeal secretions after each cleansing, and apply a mouth moisturizer to the oral mucosa and lips to keep the tissue moist. **(Level C*)**	Saliva serves a protective function. Mechanical ventilation causes drying of the oral mucosa, affecting salivary flow, and contributing to mucositis, bacterial deposits, and growth.[8,33,68]	Implementation of a comprehensive oral care program is recommended by the U.S. Centers for Disease Control and Prevention (CDC) and the Society for Healthcare Epidemiology of America (SHEA) to reduce VAP.[34]
12. Suction the oral cavity and pharynx (subglottic) at a minimum frequency of every 4 hours.[61] **(Level C*)** *Or* Perform continuous subglottic suctioning[41,53] **(Level A*)**	Removes secretions that may accumulate on top of the cuff and cause microaspiration.[41,53] Continuous subglottic suctioning with a specially designed ETT has been shown to reduce VAP.[10]	Continuous subglottic suctioning is recommended by CDC and SHEA guidelines.[34] Oral suction equipment and suction tubing should be changed every 24 hours. Nondisposable, noncovered oral suction apparatus has been shown to be colonized with microorganisms present in the oral cavity.[62] Covered oral suction apparatus should be rinsed with a sterile solution and the cover put back in place.[62] Placement of nonrinsed oral suction back into the package is associated with greater colonization.[62] Disconnection of a closed suction system to provide oral suctioning may contribute to increased bacterial colonization at the point of the disconnection.[62]

*Level A: Meta-analysis of quantitative studies or meta-synthesis of qualitative studies with results that consistently support a specific action, intervention, or treatment (including systematic review of randomized controlled trials).
*Level C: Qualitative studies, descriptive or correlational studies, integrative reviews, systematic reviews, or randomized controlled trials with inconsistent results.
*Level D: Peer-reviewed professional and organizational standards with the support of clinical study recommendations.

Procedure	for Endotracheal Tube and Oral Care for Ventilated Patients—*Continued*	
Steps	**Rationale**	**Special Considerations**
13. Move the oral tube to the other side of the mouth, per organization policy. Replace the bite-block along the ETT if necessary, to prevent biting. If deflation of the cuff is necessary to move from one side of the mouth to the other, perform deep oral suctioning before deflation.[23] **(Level C*)**	Redistribution of pressure prevents or minimizes the mechanical load on the lips, tongue, and oral cavity.[52] Deep oral suctioning above the cuff before deflation or position change can reduce the risk of colonized oral secretions being aspirated.[61]	Care is needed when removing ETT tapes or adjusting the ETT securement device to prevent ETT dislodgement.
14. After oral hygiene is completed, change the ETT securing mechanism with new tape, ties, or a commercial device, as needed, according to institutional standards (see Procedure 2, Endotracheal Intubation [Assist]). **(Level C*)**	The securing mechanism should be changed if using tape and/or moved at least once daily to provide an opportunity for assessment and repositioning of the ETT to reduce the risk of a pressure skin injury. If the securing mechanism loosens, more frequent change may be necessary.[23] Commercial ETT securement devices may have a lower risk of lip ulcers, facial skin tears, and ETT dislodgement compared with adhesive and cloth tape.[38,39]	If the method to secure the ETT obstructs the ability to provide effective oral care, consider changing the securement method. Prone positioning may require additional intervention to prevent ETT dislodgement and skin and tissue injury (see Procedure 15, Pronation Therapy).
15. Ensure proper cuff inflation to maintain 20–30 cm H_2O (see Procedure 2, Endotracheal Intubation [Assist]).	Helps prevent air leaks during ventilation and avoid microaspiration of oral secretions.[36]	
16. Reconfirm tube placement (see Procedure 1), and note the position of the tube at the teeth, gumline, or nares.	Common tube placement at the teeth is 20 to 21 cm for women and 22 to 23 cm for men.	
17. Remove **PE**, and discard supplies.		
18. **HH**		

*Level C: Qualitative studies, descriptive or correlational studies, integrative reviews, systematic reviews, or randomized controlled trials with inconsistent results.

Procedure	for Oral Care: Nonventilated Patients	
Steps	**Rationale**	**Special Considerations**
Independent Self-Care		
1. Instruct the patient to brush gently for 1 to 2 minutes and swish with alcohol-free, therapeutic oral rinse with antimicrobial ingredients for 30 seconds. Moisturize lips and mouth as needed for dryness.	Removes buildup of plaque and bacteria that coat the teeth and mouth, while therapeutic oral rinse achieves areas toothbrushing cannot reach, further reducing oral pathogens and bad breath.[4]	Consider using the following tools: soft-bristled toothbrush, toothpaste with fluoride, alcohol-free antiseptic oral rinse such as 1% hydrogen peroxide (H_2O_2) or 0.075%–1% cetylpyridinium (CPC), and non–petroleum-based moisturizer.[4,5,57] Lemon glycerin swabs are contraindicated due to irritation and drying of the mucosa and serve to worsen xerostomia.[55]

Procedure continues on following page

Procedure	for Oral Care: Nonventilated Patients—*Continued*	
Steps	**Rationale**	**Special Considerations**
2. Encourage toothbrushing at least two times a day, to include the gums and tongue.[5,57] **(Level C*)**	Toothbrushing removes plaque, which provides a microbiome for bacteria, including those that cause lung infection.[1]	Consider performing oral care more frequently for patients at highest risk for aspiration.

Dependent, Unable to Manage Own Oral Care or Secretions Safely

1. 🅷🅷		
2. 🅿🅴		
3. Brush with a suction toothbrush and toothpaste or gel for 2 minutes, suctioning frequently. Brush or swab the teeth and mouth with therapeutic alcohol-free oral rinse containing antimicrobial ingredients for 30 seconds, and moisturize as needed.[57]	Removes buildup of plaque and bacteria that coat the teeth and mouth, and therapeutic oral rinse achieves areas toothbrushing cannot reach, further reducing oral pathogens and bad breath.[4] Suctioning during and after toothbrushing may reduce the risk of aspiration and prevent pneumonia.[67]	Consider using the following tools: suction toothbrush, toothpaste or gel, alcohol-free therapeutic oral rinse preparations such as 1%–1.5% hydrogen peroxide (H_2O_2) or 0.075%–1% cetylpyridinium chloride (CPC), and non–petroleum-based moisturizer.[4,5]
4. Remove 🅿🅴, and discard supplies.		
5. 🅷🅷		

Edentulate Patients, Dentures

1. 🅷🅷		
2. 🅿🅴		
3. If the patient has no teeth or dentures, gently brush the gums and tongue for 1–2 minutes at least two times a day. If the patient is allowed nothing by mouth or is on tube feedings, oral care can be performed every 6–8 hours. Apply a therapeutic alcohol-free oral rinse containing antimicrobial ingredients for 30 seconds with a moistened swab, and suction. Apply moisturizer with a swab as needed.[4,5,57] **(Level C*)**	Cleansing the gums, tongue, and roof of the mouth removes plaque and stimulates circulation.[5]	Consider using the following tools: soft-bristled toothbrush and swab, toothpaste/gel, alcohol-free antimicrobial oral rinse preparations such as 1%–1.5% hydrogen peroxide (H_2O_2) or 0.075%–1% cetylpyridinium chloride (CPC), and non–petroleum-based moisturizer.[4,5,57]
4. If the patient is wearing dentures, care of the appliance includes rinsing and brushing with a soft bristle or denture brush and a nonabrasive cleanser. Remove and store dentures, covered with water at night and when not wearing to prevent misshaping.[5,57] **(Level C*)**	Removes plaque and bacteria from the surface of the dentures.	Dentures can be a reservoir for pathogens, and wearing dentures during sleep is a significant risk factor for pneumonia.[28,49]
5. Remove 🅿🅴, and discard supplies.		
6. 🅷🅷		

*Level C: Qualitative studies, descriptive or correlational studies, integrative reviews, systematic reviews, or randomized controlled trials with inconsistent results.

Expected Outcomes

- Patent airway
- Secured ETT
- Removal of oral secretions
- Intact oral and nasal mucous membranes
- Reduced oral colonization
- Moist pink oral cavity

Unexpected Outcomes

- Dislodged ETT
- Occluded ETT
- ETT cuff leak
- Pressure ulcers in the mouth or on the lips or nares
- Aspiration
- HAP

Patient Monitoring and Care

Steps	Rationale	Reportable Conditions
		These conditions should be reported to the provider if they persist despite nursing interventions.
1. Keep the head of the bed elevated at least 30 degrees, unless contraindicated.[1,2,34,36] (**Level C***)	Maintaining the head of the bed in an elevated position decreases the risk of aspiration. Contraindications include hemodynamic instability, decreased cerebral perfusion pressure, and patient in the prone position.	
2. Suction ETT if clinically indicated.[61]	Maintains a patent airway.	• Inability to pass the suction catheter
3. Monitor the amount, type, and color of secretions.	Monitors for signs of infection.	• Change in quantity or characteristics of secretions
4. If the patient is nasally intubated, recommend reintubation in the oral cavity. (**Level C***)	Nasal intubation is associated with an increased risk for sinusitis and the potential development of VAP.[3,34]	• Purulent drainage from the nares or present in the back of the throat
5. Assess the oral cavity and lips every 2 hours, and perform oral care based on patient type: independent, dependent, edentulate, or ventilated. (**Level C***)	Early recognition of pressure injury or drainage allows for prompt intervention.[41,53] Promotes good oral hygiene.[5]	• Breakdown of lips, tongue, or oral cavity • Presence of mouth sores • Bleeding of the gums during brushing
6. With oral care, assess the oral cavity for buildup of plaque on the teeth or potential infection related to oral abscess.	Oral assessment can identify abnormalities.	• Continued plaque buildup on teeth; presence of an abscess or sore
7. Avoid reusing devices unless covered or protected (e.g., in-line suction or covered Yankauer).	Apparatuses exposed to the oral cavity or secretions in the lungs when left unprotected within the environment have been shown to be colonized with bacteria in the oral cavity.[62]	
8. Assess tube placement and securement devices once per shift or per institutional guidelines while the patient is intubated (see Procedure 2, Endotracheal Intubation [Assist]).	Ensures a secured tube and allows for detection of mucosal and skin breakdown and incorporation of preventive measures.	• Tube migration from previous placement position
9. For ETT with subglottic suctioning, assess the patency of the irrigation port with oral care every 2–4 hours. Irrigate with air per the manufacturer's recommendations if the tube becomes clogged. Do not increase suction pressure beyond what is recommended by the manufacturer. (**Level M***)	Consider routine irrigation with air to prevent clogging.	• Clogged subglottic suction port

*Level C: Qualitative studies, descriptive or correlational studies, integrative reviews, systematic reviews, or randomized controlled trials with inconsistent results.
*Level M: Manufacturer's recommendations only.

Procedure continues on following page

Documentation

Documentation should include the following:
- Patient and family education
- Patient tolerance to suctioning
- Aspirate amount, type, and color
- Presence of nasal drainage
- Repositioning of ETT and new position
- Retaping of ETT
- Oral care, moisturizing, and oral suctioning
- Condition of the lips, mouth, and tongue
- Absence of a cuff leak
- Pressure in the cuff (20–30 mm Hg)
- Depth of endotracheal tube insertion centimeters at the teeth, gums, or nares

References and Additional Readings

For a complete list of references and additional readings for this procedure, scan this QR code with your smartphone, or visit https://www.elsevier.com/__data/assets/pdf_file/0009/1319778/Chapter0003.pdf

4

Extubation/Decannulation (Perform)

Lisa Koser

PURPOSE: The purpose of extubation or decannulation is to remove the artificial airway, allowing the patient to breathe through the upper airway.

PREREQUISITE NURSING KNOWLEDGE

- *Extubation* refers to removal of a translaryngeal endotracheal tube, whereas *decannulation* refers to removal of a tracheostomy tube.
- Indications for extubation and decannulation include the following[1,7,8]:
  - ❖ The underlying condition that led to the need for an artificial airway is reversed or improved.
  - ❖ Hemodynamic stability is achieved, with no new reasons for continued artificial airway support.
  - ❖ The patient is able to effectively clear pulmonary secretions.
  - ❖ Adequate muscle strength is achieved.
  - ❖ The ability to protect airway and minimal risk for aspiration exists.
  - ❖ Mechanical ventilatory support is no longer needed (i.e., adequate spontaneous ventilation and oxygenation is achieved, or palliative extubation is planned) (see Procedure 30, Weaning Mechanical Ventilation).
- Most extubations and decannulations are planned. Planning allows for preparation of the patient physically and emotionally, decreasing the likelihood of reintubation and hypoxic sequelae. Unintentional or unplanned extubation complicates a patient's overall recovery and increases the risk of inpatient death.[2,5,7]
- Extubation may occur in a rapid fashion when the previous indications are met, whereas decannulation generally occurs in a stepwise fashion.[10] The patient with a tracheostomy tube may be weaned gradually from the tracheostomy tube, including downsizing the tube diameter, using fenestrated tubes and inner cannulas, changing to cuffless tubes, using speaking valves, and capping the tracheostomy tube.[9,11,12] The tracheostomy tube is removed when the patient[9,11,12] is able to breathe comfortably, maintain adequate ventilation and oxygenation,

and manage secretions through the normal anatomical airway.

EQUIPMENT

- Cardiopulmonary monitoring (preprocedure, during procedure, and postprocedure)
- Personal protective equipment (including eye protection)
- Self-inflating manual resuscitation bag-valve-mask device connected to a 100% oxygen source
- Oxygen delivery device (i.e., nasal cannula, face mask, high flow nasal cannula, or non-invasive ventilator) connected to humidified oxygen
- Established intravenous site
- Suctioning equipment with sterile suction catheter or kit
- Rigid pharyngeal suction-tip (Yankauer) catheter
- Scissors (for tape or ties)
- 10-mL syringe (if cuff present)
- Stethoscope
- Endotracheal intubation supplies and access to emergency cart
- Decannulation only:
  - ❖ Sterile dressing for tracheal stoma
  - ❖ Spare tracheostomy tube at bedside

PATIENT AND FAMILY EDUCATION

- Explain the purpose of and procedure for removing the endotracheal or tracheostomy tube. ***Rationale:*** Identifies knowledge deficits of the patient and family concerning the patient's condition, the procedure, and the expected benefits. This step also allows time for questions to clarify information and voice concerns. Explanations decrease patient anxiety and enhance cooperation.
- Explain the suctioning process and the importance of coughing and deep breathing after the tube is removed. ***Rationale:*** Understanding therapy encourages cooperation with the follow-up procedures necessary to maintain a patent airway.
- Explain that the patient's voice may be hoarse after extubation or decannulation. Following the removal of the tracheostomy tube, occlusion of the stoma may be necessary to facilitate normal speech and coughing. ***Rationale:*** Knowledge minimizes the patient's and family's fear and anxiety.

- Explain that the patient may need continued oxygen or humidification support. ***Rationale:*** Many patients continue to need supplemental oxygen after extubation. Continued humidification often helps decrease hoarseness and liquefies secretions.
- Explain that reinsertion of the endotracheal tube or cannula may be necessary if the patient develops respiratory failure. ***Rationale:*** Patients may require mechanical ventilation if respiratory failure develops after extubation or decannulation.
- After extubation, a swallow screening or evaluation is often necessary. ***Rationale:*** Patients who are intubated for 48 hours or more are at risk for postextubation dysphagia and aspiration with oral intake.

PATIENT ASSESSMENT AND PREPARATION

Patient Assessment

- Assessment for the patient's readiness for extubation[2,6,7] (see Procedure 30, Weaning Mechanical Ventilation).
  - ❖ Desired level of consciousness (most patients are awake and able to follow commands)
  - ❖ Absence of respiratory distress and other indications for intubation
  - ❖ Consider a cuff leak test in patients at high risk for airway edema and postextubation stridor (listen over the trachea for presence of airflow around the ETT after cuff deflation)
  - ❖ Negative inspiratory force (NIF) pressure less than or equal to −20 to −30 cm H_2O

- ❖ Spontaneous tidal volume between 4 and 6 mL/kg ideal body weight
- ❖ Fraction of inspired oxygen (Fio_2) less than or equal to 50%
- ❖ Normal or baseline pH and partial pressure of carbon dioxide ($Paco_2$)
- ❖ Positive end-expiratory pressure <8 cm H_2O
- ❖ Hemodynamic stability and absence of serious cardiac dysrhythmias

Rationale: Patients who are not ready for extubation are at high risk for the need for reintubation and complications.
- Assess the patient's ability to cough. ***Rationale:*** The ability to cough and clear secretions is important for successful airway management after extubation.

Patient Preparation

- Verify the correct patient with two identifiers. ***Rationale:*** Before performing a procedure, the nurse should ensure the correct identification of the patient for the intended intervention.
- Ensure that the patient and family understand preprocedural teachings. Answer questions as they arise, and reinforce information as needed. ***Rationale:*** This process evaluates and reinforces understanding of previously taught information.
- Place the patient in the high Fowler's (>60 degrees) or semi-Fowler's (>30 degrees) position if not contraindicated and does not contribute to restriction of breathing (i.e., obesity). ***Rationale:*** Respiratory muscles are more effective in an upright position versus a supine or prone position. This position facilitates coughing and minimizes the risk of vomiting and consequent aspiration.

Procedure	for Performing Extubation and Decannulation		
Steps	**Rationale**		**Special Considerations**
1. **HH**			
2. **PE**			• Extubation is considered an aerosol-generating procedure. Additional personal protective equipment based on the patient's symptoms and past medical history may be required for all providers present in the room.
3. Hyperoxygenate and suction the endotracheal tube or tracheostomy[1] (see Procedure 8, Suctioning: Endotracheal or Tracheostomy).	Removes secretions in the artificial airway and oral cavity.[1]		
4. Remove tape or securement device.	Frees the tube for removal.		
5. Insert syringe into the one-way valve of the pilot balloon.	Prepares for cuff deflation.		Some tracheostomy tubes may not be cuffed.

Procedure for Performing Extubation and Decannulation—*Continued*		
Steps	Rationale	Special Considerations
6. Suction the oral cavity, hypopharynx, and, supraglottic secretions[1] (see Procedure 3, Endotracheal Tube Care and Oral Care Practices for Ventilated and Nonventilated Patients).	Removes secretions above the cuff and reduces the risk of aspiration of secretions.[1]	Alternative methods to facilitate removal of supraglottic secretions while an endotracheal tube is removed include application of positive pressure while the cuff is deflated, insertion of a suction catheter 1–2 inches (5 cm) below the distal end of the tube, and application of suction while the cuff is deflated and the tube is removed.[2]
7. Deflate the tube cuff (if it is inflated) over 2–3 seconds.	Readies the tube for removal.	
8. Ask the patient to take a deep breath and remove the tube on inspiration, while monitoring and supporting the patient.[1]	Promotes hyperinflation. Vocal cords are maximally abducted at peak inspiration. Assists in a smooth, quick, less traumatic removal. In addition, the initial cough response expected after extubation should be more forceful if started from maximal inspiration versus expiration.[1]	A self-inflating manual resuscitation bag-valve-mask device can assist in hyperinflation.
9. Encourage the patient to cough and breathe deeply.	Initial cough response expected after extubation should be more forceful if started from maximal inspiration versus expiration.[1]	
10. Suction the oropharynx.[1]	Removes secretions.[1]	
11. Apply supplemental oxygen and aerosol, as appropriate.[1]	Promotes moisture and prevents oxygen desaturation.[1]	Cool humidification is usually preferred after extubation to help minimize upper airway swelling.[8]
12. Decannulation ONLY: place a dry, sterile, 4 × 4 dressing over the stoma when the tracheostomy tube is removed.	Contains secretions that may leak out of the stoma.	Tracheostomy stoma closure usually occurs within a few days but may take longer with a long-term tracheostomy.
13. Discard used supplies and remove PE.		

Expected Outcomes

- Smooth atraumatic extubation or decannulation
- Stable respiratory status
- Stable hemodynamics
- Stable neurological status

Unexpected Outcomes

- Need for reintubation or recannulation
- Fatigue and respiratory failure
- Postextubation stridor
- Persistent hoarseness
- Vocal cord dysfunction
- Tracheal stoma narrowing
- Aspiration
- Laryngospasm
- Trauma to soft tissue
- Upper airway obstruction
- Cardiopulmonary or neurological decline

Procedure continues on following page

UNIT I

Patient Monitoring and Care

Steps	Rationale	Reportable Conditions
		These conditions should be reported if they persist despite nursing interventions.
1. Monitor vital signs, respiratory status, oxygenation, neurological status, and phonation immediately after extubation, within 1 hour, and per institutional standards.	Change in vital signs and oxygenation after extubation or decannulation may indicate respiratory compromise, which necessitates reintubation.	• Tachycardia • Tachypnea • Blood pressure significantly greater than baseline • Oxygen saturation (SpO_2) less than or equal to 90% (unless otherwise ordered) • Stridor • Breathing difficulty • Respiratory dyssynchrony • Increased agitation (may indicate early signs of hypoxemia)
2. Provide supplemental oxygen as needed.	Decreases incidence of oxygen desaturation immediately after extubation.	• SpO_2 less than or equal to 90% (unless otherwise ordered) • Increasing oxygen requirement • Decreased level of consciousness (may indicate elevated $PaCO_2$) • Inability to auscultate adequate air exchange • Increased agitation (could indicate early sign of hypoxemia)
3. Monitor for aspiration related to pooled secretions.	Failure to suction or ineffective suctioning of the pharynx allows accumulated secretions to advance farther into the trachea on cuff deflation.	• Inability to handle secretions
4. Encourage frequent coughing and deep breathing and use of other respiratory devices as indicated.[3]	Prevents atelectasis and secretion accumulation.	• Ineffective cough
5. Frequent oral care (see Procedure 3, Endotracheal Tube Care and Oral Care Practices for Ventilated and Nonventilated Patients).	Maintains oral mucosa and keeps oral cavity clear of dried secretions.	
6. Assess swallowing ability. Consider use of a postextubation dysphagia screening tool for patients who are alert and able to follow commands.[4]	Presence of tube over extended periods may result in impaired swallowing ability.	• Inability to handle secretions • Inability to swallow without coughing • Failure of postextubation dysphagia (PED) screening tool
7. Follow institutional standards for assessing pain. Administer analgesia as indicated.	• Identifies need for pain interventions.	• Continued pain despite pain interventions

Documentation

Documentation should include the following:
- Patient and family education
- Respiratory and vital signs assessment before and after procedure
- Date and time when procedure is performed
- Breath sounds and upper airway sounds, ability to cough
- Neurological status
- Patient response to procedure
- Unexpected outcomes and complications
- Other interventions taken
- Pain assessment, interventions, and effectiveness
- Ability to phonate, presence of wet, gurgling, or poor voice quality

References and Additional Readings

For a complete list of references and additional readings for this procedure, scan this QR code with your smartphone, or visit https://www.elsevier.com/__data/assets/pdf_file/0010/1319779/Chapter0004.pdf

5 Extubation/Decannulation (Assist)

Lisa Koser

PURPOSE: The purpose of extubation or decannulation is to remove the artificial airway, allowing the patient to breathe through the upper airway.

PREREQUISITE NURSING KNOWLEDGE

- *Extubation* refers to removal of a translaryngeal endotracheal tube, whereas *decannulation* refers to removal of a tracheostomy tube.
- Indications for extubation and decannulation include the following[1,7,8]:
  - ❖ The underlying condition that led to the need for an artificial airway is reversed or improved.
  - ❖ Hemodynamic stability is achieved, with no new reasons for continued artificial airway support.
  - ❖ The patient is able to effectively clear pulmonary secretions.
  - ❖ Adequate muscle strength is achieved.
  - ❖ The ability to protect the airway and minimal risk for aspiration exists.
  - ❖ Mechanical ventilatory support is no longer needed (i.e., adequate spontaneous ventilation and oxygenation are achieved or palliative extubation is planned) (see Procedure 30, Weaning Mechanical Ventilation).
- Most extubations and decannulations are planned. Planning allows for preparation of the patient physically and emotionally, decreasing the likelihood of reintubation and hypoxic sequelae. Unintentional or unplanned extubation complicates a patient's overall recovery and increases the risk of inpatient death.[2,5,7]
- Extubation may occur in a rapid fashion when the previous indications are met, whereas decannulation generally occurs in a stepwise fashion.[10] The patient with a tracheostomy tube may be weaned gradually from the tracheostomy tube, including downsizing the tube diameter, using fenestrated tubes and inner cannulas, changing to cuffless tubes, using speaking valves, and capping the tracheostomy tube.[9,11,12] The tracheostomy tube is removed when the patient is able to breathe comfortably, maintain adequate ventilation and oxygenation, and manage secretions through the normal anatomical airway.

EQUIPMENT

- Cardiopulmonary monitoring (preprocedure, during the procedure, and postprocedure)
- Personal protective equipment (including eye protection)
- Self-inflating manual resuscitation bag-valve-mask device connected to a 100% oxygen source
- Oxygen delivery device (i.e., nasal cannula, face mask, high-flow nasal cannula, or noninvasive ventilator) connected to humidified oxygen
- Established intravenous site
- Suctioning equipment with sterile suction catheter or kit
- Rigid pharyngeal suction-tip (Yankauer) catheter
- Scissors (for tape or ties)
- 10-mL syringe (if cuff present)
- Stethoscope
- Endotracheal intubation supplies and access to emergency cart
- Decannulation only:
  - ❖ Sterile dressing for tracheal stoma
  - ❖ Spare tracheostomy tube at bedside

PATIENT AND FAMILY EDUCATION

- Explain the purpose of and procedure for removing the endotracheal tube or tracheostomy. ***Rationale:*** This step identifies knowledge deficits of the patient and family concerning the patient's condition, the procedure, and the expected benefits. This step also allows time for questions to clarify information and voice concerns. Explanations decrease patient anxiety and enhance cooperation.
- Explain the suctioning process and the importance of coughing and deep breathing after the tube is removed. ***Rationale:*** Understanding therapy encourages cooperation with the follow-up procedures necessary to maintain a patent airway.
- Explain that the patient's voice may be hoarse after extubation or decannulation. After the removal of the tracheostomy tube, occlusion of the stoma may be necessary to facilitate normal speech and coughing. ***Rationale:*** Knowledge minimizes the patient's and family's fear and anxiety.

- Explain that the patient may need continued oxygen or humidification support. ***Rationale:*** Many patients continue to need supplemental oxygen after extubation or decannulation. Continued humidification often helps decrease hoarseness and liquefies secretions.
- Explain that reinsertion of the endotracheal tube or cannula may be necessary if the patient develops respiratory failure. ***Rationale:*** Patients may require mechanical ventilation if respiratory failure develops after extubation or decannulation.
- After extubation, a swallow evaluation is often necessary. ***Rationale:*** Patients who are intubated for 48 hours or more are at risk for postextubation swallowing dysfunction and aspiration with oral intake.

PATIENT ASSESSMENT AND PREPARATION

Patient Assessment

- Assessment for the patient's readiness for extubation[2,6,7] (see Procedure 30, Weaning Mechanical Ventilation).
  - ❖ Desired level of consciousness (most patients are awake and able to follow commands)
  - ❖ Absence of respiratory distress and other indications for intubation
  - ❖ Consider a cuff leak test in patients at high risk for airway edema and postextubation stridor (listen over the trachea for presence of airflow around the ETT after cuff deflation)
  - ❖ Negative inspiratory force (NIF) less than or equal to −20 to −30 cm H_2O

- ❖ Spontaneous tidal volume between 4 and 6 mL/kg ideal body weight
- ❖ Fraction of inspired oxygen (Fio_2) less than or equal to 50%
- ❖ Normal or baseline pH and partial pressure of carbon dioxide ($Paco_2$)
- ❖ Positive end-expiratory pressure <8 cm H_2O
- ❖ Hemodynamic stability and absence of serious cardiac dysrhythmias

  Rationale: Patients who are not ready for extubation are at high risk for the need for reintubation and complications.
- Assess the patient's ability to cough. ***Rationale:*** The ability to cough and clear secretions is important for successful airway management after extubation.

Patient Preparation

- Verify the correct patient with two identifiers. ***Rationale:*** Before performing a procedure, the nurse should ensure the correct identification of the patient for the intended intervention.
- Ensure that the patient and family understand preprocedural teachings. Answer questions as they arise, and reinforce information as needed. ***Rationale:*** This process evaluates and reinforces understanding of previously taught information.
- Place the patient in the high Fowler's (>60 degrees) or semi-Fowler's (>30 degrees) position if not contraindicated and does not contribute to restriction of breathing (i.e., obesity). ***Rationale:*** Respiratory muscles are more effective in an upright position versus a supine or prone position. This position facilitates coughing and minimizes the risk of vomiting and aspiration.

Procedure	**for Assisting With Extubation and Decannulation**	
Steps	**Rationale**	**Special Considerations**
1. 🅗🅗		
2. 🅟🅔		• Extubation is considered an aerosol-generating procedure. Additional respiratory personal protective equipment based on the patient's symptoms and past medical history may be required for all providers present in the room.
3. Hyperoxygenate and suction the endotracheal tube or tracheostomy[1] (see Procedure 8, Suctioning: Endotracheal or Tracheostomy).	Removes secretions in the artificial airway and oral cavity.[1]	
4. Remove tape or securement device.	Frees the tube for removal.	
5. Insert syringe into the one-way valve of the pilot balloon.	Prepares for cuff deflation.	Some tracheostomy tubes may not be cuffed.

Procedure for Assisting With Extubation and Decannulation—*Continued*

Steps	Rationale	Special Considerations
6. Assist with suctioning of the oral cavity, hypopharynx, and supraglottic secretions[1] (see Procedure 3, Endotracheal Tube Care and Oral Care Practices for Ventilated and Nonventilated Patients).	Removes secretions above the cuff and reduces the risk of aspiration of secretions.[1]	Alternative methods to facilitate removal of supraglottic secretions while an endotracheal tube is removed include application of positive pressure while the cuff is deflated, insertion of a suction catheter 1–2 inches (5 cm) below the distal end of the tube, and application of suction while the cuff is deflated and the tube is removed.[2]
7. Deflate the tube cuff (if it is inflated) as directed over 2–3 seconds.	Readies the tube for removal.	
8. Ask the patient to take a deep breath while the provider removes the tube on inspiration. Monitor and support the patient.[1]	Promotes hyperinflation. Vocal cords are maximally abducted at peak inspiration. Assists in a smooth, quick, less traumatic removal. In addition, the initial cough response expected after extubation should be more forceful if started from maximal inspiration versus expiration.[1]	A self-inflating manual resuscitation bag-valve-mask device can assist in hyperinflation.
9. Encourage the patient to cough and breathe deeply.	Initial cough response expected after extubation should be more forceful if started from maximal inspiration versus expiration.[1]	
10. Suction the oropharynx.[1]	Removes secretions.[1]	
11. Apply supplemental oxygen and aerosol, as ordered.	Promotes moisture and prevents oxygen desaturation.	Cool humidification is usually preferred after extubation to help minimize upper airway swelling.[8]
12. Decannulation ONLY: place a dry, sterile, 4 × 4 dressing over the stoma when the tracheostomy tube is removed.	Contains secretions that may leak out of the stoma.	Tracheostomy stoma closure usually occurs within a few days but may take longer with a long-term tracheostomy.
13. Discard used supplies and remove **PE**.		

Expected Outcomes

- Smooth atraumatic extubation or decannulation
- Stable respiratory status
- Stable hemodynamics
- Stable neurological status

Unexpected Outcomes

- Need for reintubation or recannulation
- Fatigue and respiratory failure
- Postextubation stridor
- Persistent hoarseness
- Vocal cord dysfunction
- Tracheal stoma narrowing
- Aspiration
- Laryngospasm
- Trauma to soft tissue
- Upper airway obstruction
- Cardiopulmonary or neurological decline

Procedure continues on following page

Patient Monitoring and Care

Steps	Rationale	Reportable Conditions
		These conditions should be reported to the provider if they persist despite nursing interventions.
1. Monitor vital signs, respiratory status, oxygenation, neurological status, and phonation immediately after extubation, within 1 hour, and per institutional standards.	Change in vital signs and oxygenation after extubation or decannulation may indicate respiratory compromise, which necessitates reintubation.	• Tachycardia • Tachypnea • Blood pressure significantly greater than baseline • Oxygen saturation (SpO_2) less than or equal to 90% (unless otherwise ordered) • Stridor • Breathing difficulty • Respiratory dyssynchrony • Increased agitation (may indicate early signs of hypoxemia)
2. Provide supplemental oxygen as needed.	Decreases incidence of oxygen desaturation immediately after extubation.	• SpO_2 less than or equal to 90% (unless otherwise ordered) • Increasing oxygen requirement • Decreased level of consciousness (may indicate elevated $PaCO_2$) • Inability to auscultate adequate air exchange • Increased agitation (may indicate early sign of hypoxemia)
3. Monitor for aspiration related to pooled secretions.	Failure to suction or ineffective suctioning of the pharynx allows accumulated secretions to advance farther into the trachea on cuff deflation.	• Inability to handle secretions
4. Encourage frequent coughing and deep breathing and other respiratory devices as indicated.[3]	Prevents atelectasis and secretion accumulation.	• Ineffective cough
5. Frequent oral care (see Procedure 3, Endotracheal Tube Care and Oral Care Practices for Ventilated and Nonventilated Patients)	Maintains oral mucosa and keeps oral cavity clear of dried secretions.	
6. Assess swallowing ability. Consider use of a postextubation dysphagia screening tool for patients who are alert and able to follow commands.[4]	Presence of tube over extended periods may result in impaired swallowing ability.	• Inability to handle secretions • Inability to swallow without coughing • Failure of postextubation dysphagia (PED) screening tool
7. Follow institutional standards for assessing pain. Administer analgesia as indicated.	Identifies need for pain interventions.	• Continued pain despite pain interventions

Documentation

Documentation should include the following:
• Patient and family education
• Respiratory and vital signs assessment before and after procedure
• Date and time when procedure is performed
• Breath sounds and upper airway sounds, ability to cough
• Neurological status
• Patient response to procedure
• Unexpected outcomes and complications
• Other interventions taken
• Pain assessment, interventions, and effectiveness
• Ability to phonate, presence of wet, gurgling, or poor voice quality

References and Additional Readings

For a complete list of references and additional readings for this procedure, scan this QR code with your smartphone, or visit https://www.elsevier.com/__data/assets/pdf_file/0003/1319781/Chapter0005.pdf

PROCEDURE

6

Laryngeal Mask Airway AP

Loudena Lavender and Jenna Heaney

PURPOSE: This procedure focuses on the use of the laryngeal mask airway (LMA) as an emergency airway device when an airway is compromised in the unconscious patient or when endotracheal intubation is not readily available or has failed. LMAs have less risk of gastric insufflation and are easier to use than a bag-valve-mask device in emergency situations (e.g., cardiac arrest, failed intubation, difficult airway, prehospital airway management) and have become more widely used in the intensive care unit, emergency department, and in prehospital field settings. They can be used as an alternative to endotracheal intubation in advanced cardiac life support, are better able to assist basic life support providers in establishing an airway, and can also assist in being a conduit for facilitating elective endotracheal intubation outside of the operating room. LMAs have been indicated for use in patients with severe facial deformity or in patients with excessive facial hair or in any other situation in which bag-valve-mask ventilation would be challenging. LMAs are a type of supraglottic airway device and come in a variety of models including early first-generation devices. Although second-generation LMAs offer better protection against aspiration, it should be understood that the LMA is not a definitive airway.[1,4,6,8,9,11]

PREREQUISITE NURSING KNOWLEDGE

- The requirements for rapid airway management in an unconscious patient.
- The anatomy and physiology of the upper airway.
- The design available should be understood (Figs. 6.1 to 6.3):
  - ❖ An airway tube connects the mask and the 15-mm male adapter.
  - ❖ The mask's cuff, when inflated, conforms to the contours of the hypopharynx, with the opening of the air tube positioned directly over the laryngeal opening (Fig. 6.4).
  - ❖ A cuff inflation line with a valve and a pilot balloon leads to the mask's cuff.
- As there are many versions of the LMA, it is critical to develop a working knowledge of your institution's version of the LMA that is readily available in an emergency situation (Tables 6.1 to 6.3).
- The ability to ventilate an unconscious patient adequately with a mouth-to-mask or bag-valve-mask device.
- The underlying risks associated with use of the LMA.

- ❖ Because of the potential risk of regurgitation and aspiration, do not use the LMA as a "first-choice airway" in the following elective or difficult airway patients on a nonemergency pathway[12]
  - ○ Patients who have not fasted, including patients whose fasting cannot be confirmed.[12]
  - ○ Patients who are morbidly obese, are more than 14 weeks pregnant, have multiple or massive injury or acute abdominal or thoracic injury, have any condition associated with delayed gastric emptying, or have used opiate medication before fasting. However, in all of these clinical scenarios, the LMA

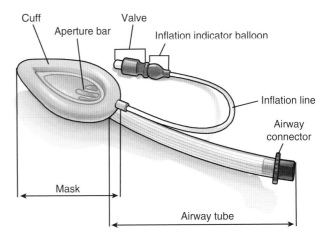

Figure 6.1 Components of a first-generation laryngeal mask airway (LMA; *LMA Classic shown*). *(Image courtesy of Teleflex Incorporated. © 2022 Teleflex Incorporated. All rights reserved.)*

Supreme (second-generation supraglottic device) is ideally suited to serve as an "airway rescue device" in preference to the LMA Classic or the LMA Unique (first-generation supraglottic device) (Table 6.1).[5,12]

❖ The LMA Supreme is contraindicated in the following patients:

○ Patients with fixed decreased pulmonary compliance, such as in pulmonary fibrosis caused by an inadequate seal around the larynx[12]

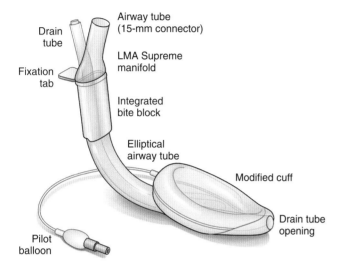

Figure 6.2 Components of a second-generation laryngeal mask airway *(LMA Supreme shown)*. Manifold with an integral bite block, an anatomically shaped airway tube enclosing a drain tube, a modified cuff that is inflated via the pilot cuff. *(From Hagberg C. Benumof and Hagberg's Airway Management. 3rd ed. Philadelphia: 2013. Elsevier.)*

○ Adult patients who have had radiotherapy to the neck involving the hypopharynx (risk of trauma, failure to seal effectively)[12]

○ Patients with a mouth opening that is not adequate to permit insertion[12]

○ Patients with suspected acute intestinal obstruction or ileus or patients who were injured shortly after ingesting a substantial meal[12]

○ Patients who have ingested caustic substances[12]

❖ LMA Supreme usage precautions include the following:

○ The LMA Supreme is a single use–only device.[12]

○ Oropharyngeal tissue is vulnerable to swelling and bleeding with mild to moderate traumatic forces (potentially resulting in dire consequences). Excessive force should not be used at any time during insertion of the LMA Supreme or insertion of a gastric tube through the drain tube of the LMA Supreme.[2,12]

○ Never overinflate the cuff after insertion. An appropriate intracuff pressure is 60 cm H_2O. Excessive intracuff pressure can result in malposition and sore throat, dysphagia, or nerve injury.[3,12]

○ If airway problems persist or ventilation is inadequate, the LMA Supreme should be removed, and an airway should be established by another means.[12]

○ The LMA Supreme is made of medical-grade polyvinyl chloride that can be torn or perforated. Avoid contact with sharp or pointed objects at all times. Do not insert the device unless the cuff is fully deflated, as described in the instructions for insertion.[12]

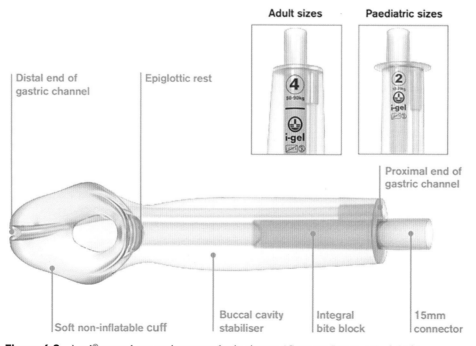

Figure 6.3   i-gel® second-generation supraglottic airway. *(Courtesy Intersurgical, Ltd.)*

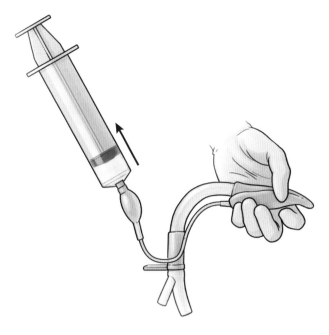

Figure 6.4 Dorsal view of a laryngeal mask airway showing the position in relation to pharyngeal anatomy (LMA Classic shown.) *(From The Laryngeal Mask Company Limited: Instruction manual: LMA-Classic. San Diego: 2005. Laryngeal Mask Company Limited;)*

TABLE 6.1	Improvements to Second-Generation Supraglottic Airway Devices Compared With First-Generation Devices
Design Improvements	**Rationale**
Improved pharyngeal seal	Controlled ventilation at higher airway pressures (and hence in a wider range of patients and clinical situations)
Increased esophageal seal	Lessens the likelihood of regurgitant fluids entering the pharynx and leading to aspiration
Integrated bite block	Impedes the patient's ability to bite and potentially occludes the airway, risking hypoxia and negative pressure pulmonary edema
Gastric port	May be used to confirm correct device positioning, enable access to the stomach, alert the user to the presence of regurgitation, and enable gastric contents to safely bypass the oropharynx and exit the patient (e.g., LMA Supreme and LMA Proseal)

From Cook T, Woodall N, Frerk C. Major complications of airway management in the UK: The Fourth National Audit Project of the Royal College of Anaesthetists; 2011. Available at www.rcoa.ac.uk/nap4.

TABLE 6.2	Types of Laryngeal Mask Airways With Their Corresponding Generation and Features	
Type of Supraglottic Device (LMA)	**Generation LMA**	**Features**
LMA Classic (see Fig. 6.1)	1st	Early prototype nondisposable LMA
LMA Unique	1st	Disposable standard LMA
LMA Proseal	2nd	Inflatable cuff with improved pharyngeal seal = ventilation tolerances, gastric port, and an integrated bite block
LMA Supreme (see Fig. 6.2)	2nd	
Air-Q LMA	2nd	Designed to facilitate endotracheal intubation through the LMA device; no gastric port
AMBU Aura-I LMA	2nd	
LMA Fastrach	2nd	
LMA CTrach	2nd	Incorporates a camera to facilitate passage of an endotracheal tube; no gastric port

Adapted From Hagberg C. *Benumof and Hagberg's Airway Management*. 6th ed. Philadelphia: Elsevier; 2018; Butterworth J, Mackey DC, Wasnick J. *Morgan & Mikhail's Clinical Anesthesiology*. 6th ed. New York: McGraw Hill; 2018; Nagelhout JJ, Elisha S. *Nurse Anesthesia*. 6th ed. St. Louis: Elsevier; 2018.

- ○ Store the device in a dark, cool environment, avoiding direct sunlight or extremes of temperature.[12]
- The LMA may provide a more viable means of ventilation than a bag-valve-mask device in patients with a beard or without teeth.[5]
- Initial and ongoing training is necessary to maximize insertion success and minimize complications.[5,6,9,12]
- This procedure refers specifically to the LMA Supreme, a second-generation LMA. Other types of second-generation LMA devices are available and provide additional features, such as use as a conduit for endotracheal intubation through the LMA (e.g., LMA Fastrach, which is designed to facilitate blind intubation).[11]

- An understanding of the different models now available will aid in LMA selection (Table 6.2).
- Understand the advantages and disadvantages of LMAs compared with face mask ventilation and endotracheal tube intubation (Table 6.3).

EQUIPMENT

- LMA Supreme size selection (Table 6.4)
  - ❖ A #4 LMA is the first choice for adults weighing 50 to 70 kg.[6] A #5 LMA is usually suitable for an adult weighing 70 to 100 kg.[4]
- Water-soluble lubricant

TABLE 6.3   Advantages and Disadvantages of the Laryngeal Mask Airway Compared With Face Mask Ventilation and Tracheal Intubation

	Advantages	Disadvantages
LMA compared with face mask	• Hands-free operation • Better seal in bearded patients • Often easier to maintain airway • Protects against airway secretions • Less facial nerve and eye trauma	• More invasive • More risk of airway trauma • Requires new skill • Multiple contraindications
LMA compared with tracheal intubation	• Less invasive • Very useful in difficult intubations • Less tooth and laryngeal trauma • Less laryngospasm and bronchospasm • Does not require neck mobility • No risk of esophageal or endobronchial intubation	• Increased risk of gastrointestinal aspiration • Limits maximum positive pressure ventilation • Less secure airway • Can cause gastric distention • Not designed for prolonged use; maximum period of 10–24 hours has been studied without adverse effects[4]

From Butterworth J, Mackey DC, Wasnick J. *Morgan & Mikhail's Clinical Anesthesiology*. 6th ed. New York: McGraw-Hill; 2018.

TABLE 6.4   Laryngeal Mask Airway Supreme Selection Guide

Airway Size	Patient Weight	Maximum-Size Nasogastric Tube	Recommended Maximum Inflation Volume	Optimum Intracuff Pressure (Do Not Exceed)
1	<5 kg	6 Fr	5 mL	60 cm H_2O
1.5	5–10 kg	6 Fr	8 mL	
2	10–20 kg	10 Fr	12 mL	
2.5	20–30 kg	10 Fr	20 mL	
3	30–50 kg	14 Fr	30 mL	
4	50–70 kg	14 Fr	45 mL	
5	70–100 kg	14 Fr	45 mL	

From Teleflex Medical Incorporated, Morrisville, NC.

- Gloves, mask, and eye protection
- Suction equipment (suction canister with control head, tracheal suction catheters, Yankauer suction tip)
- Mouth-to-mask or bag-valve-mask device attached to a high-flow oxygen source
- Tape
- 60-mL syringe with Luer-lock connection
- Pulse oximetry
- Capnography
- Additional alternative airway options available should LMA insertion fail. Refer to institutional protocols for emergency airway management.

Additional equipment, to have available as needed, includes the following:
- Nasogastric (NG) tube (for sizing, see Table 6.4). The drain port of the LMA Supreme can facilitate the passage of an appropriate-sized NG tube after correct positioning of an LMA Supreme.
- Medications such as sedatives and paralytics to facilitate intubation if planning for endotracheal tube insertion

PATIENT AND FAMILY EDUCATION

- If time allows, provide the family with information regarding the LMA and the reason for insertion. *Rationale:* This

information assists the family in understanding why the procedure is necessary and decreases family anxiety.

PATIENT ASSESSMENT AND PREPARATION

Patient Assessment

- Assess the level of consciousness and responsiveness. *Rationale:* In an emergency situation, the LMA should be inserted only into a patient who is profoundly unconscious and unresponsive.[12] Laryngospasm and/or vomiting may result, causing the inability to ventilate if an LMA is introduced into a conscious or semiconscious patient. There is a risk of aspiration with the LMA.
- Assess for pregnant patients >14 weeks and patients with obesity; these may be considered relative contraindications as these patients are considered to have a "full" stomach.[11]
- Assess history and patient information for the possibility of delayed gastric emptying (e.g., hiatal hernia, recent food ingestion, poorly controlled diabetes). *Rationale:* In a patient with delayed gastric emptying, the benefits of LMA insertion must be weighed against the possibility of regurgitation.[12]
- Assess history and patient information for possibility of decreased pulmonary compliance (i.e., pulmonary

fibrosis, obesity). ***Rationale:*** The high pressures needed to ventilate a patient with decreased pulmonary compliance may override the occlusive pressure of the LMA.[12]

- Assess predictors of difficult LMA insertion.[8] Consider the mnemonic "RODS":
  - ❖ R = restricted mouth opening
  - ❖ O = obstruction/obesity
  - ❖ D = disrupted or distorted airway
  - ❖ S = stiff, as in asthma, pulmonary fibrosis, or pulmonary edema[8]

Patient Preparation

- Verify the correct patient with two identifiers. ***Rationale:*** Before performing a procedure, the inserter should ensure the correct identification of the patient for the intended intervention.
- If time permits, assess the patient's and family's level of understanding about the condition and rationale for use of the LMA. ***Rationale:*** This assessment identifies the patient's and family's knowledge deficits concerning the patient's condition.
- Ensure adequate ventilation and oxygenation with either a mouth-to-mask or bag-valve-mask device (see

Procedure 29, Manual Self-Inflating Resuscitation Bag-Valve Device). ***Rationale:*** The patient is nonresponsive and apneic without assisted ventilation before the LMA insertion.[12]

- Ensure that the suction equipment is assembled and in working order. ***Rationale:*** The patient may regurgitate during the insertion or while the LMA is in place and may require oropharyngeal or tracheal suctioning.[12]
- Anything that is not permanently affixed in the patient's mouth (e.g., dentures, partials, jewelry) should be removed. ***Rationale:*** Inadvertent dislodgment and aspiration might occur with placement of the LMA.[12] Significant time should not be wasted in removing such oral appliances if significant hypoxia is being experienced.
- Placement is most successful with the patient positioned supine with the head in the neutral or sniffing position.[12] ***Rationale:*** Proper head positioning facilitates successful placement of an LMA.
- May need to consider LMA placement in the lateral decubitus position for patients in certain uncommon clinical situations (e.g., posterior neck or back mass). ***Rationale:*** In patients requiring lateral decubitus positioning, LMA insertion was superior to endotracheal intubation.[7]

Procedure for Laryngeal Mask Airway (LMA Supreme) Blind Insertion		
Steps	Rationale	Special Considerations
1. 🄷🄷		
2. 🄿🄴		Follow institutional standards for potential exposure of aerosolization and secretions, don appropriate personal protective equipment.
3. Ensure that a spare LMA of the same type is immediately available. (**Level M***)	Provides for a "backup" device should the initial device fail.	
4. Remove the LMA from the package, and inspect it. (**Level M***)	Ensures that the device is not defective and will work as indicated.	
A. Inspect the exterior of the mask for any cuts, tears, or scratches.	Ensures that the exterior surface of the device has not been damaged in any way.	
B. Inspect the interior of the airway tube for any particles.	Particles in the airway tube may be inhaled when the device is used.	Discard the device if any evidence of damage is found, and open the backup device.
C. Examine the 15-mm male connector at the end of the airway tube, and ensure that it fits tightly into the tube.	The 15-mm male connector is essential for ventilation with a bag-valve-mask device or ventilator.	Discard the device if any particles cannot be removed from the tube, and open the backup device.
5. Perform the deflation and inflation tests. (**Level M***)		
A. Expel the air from the 60-mL syringe, and connect it to the pilot balloon valve.	Ensures that the device is not defective and will work as indicated.	
B. Pull back the syringe plunger to deflate the cuff fully. Remove the syringe, and expel air.	The appropriate-sized syringe is needed to inflate the cuff to the proper test level.	Discard the device if the connector does not fit tightly into the airway tube, and open the backup device.[12]
C. Examine the cuff to ensure that it remains fully deflated.	Full deflation of the cuff helps ensure its patency.	Discard the device if the cuff does not remain fully deflated, and open the backup device.[12]

Procedure continues on following page

Procedure	for Laryngeal Mask Airway (LMA Supreme) Blind Insertion—*Continued*		
Steps	**Rationale**	**Special Considerations**	
D. Using the 60-mL syringe previously obtained, pull back on the syringe to the volume required for each LMA size, reattach it to the valve, and inflate the cuff with the appropriate volume for the size (see Table 6.4). Remove syringe,	Ensures that the device is not defective and will work as indicated.	Discard the device if the cuff does not remain fully deflated, and open the backup device.[12]	
E. Examine the inflated cuff to ensure that it is symmetrical without bulges.	Ensure that the device is not defective and will work as indicated.	Discard the device if the cuff bulges asymmetrically, and open the backup device.[12]	
F. Examine the pilot balloon to ensure that its inflated shape is elliptical.	Ensures that the device is not defective and will work as indicated.	Discard the device if the pilot balloon is spherical or bulges, and open the backup device.[12]	

Insertion Technique

Preoxygenate patients with 100% oxygen for several minutes before insertion of any advanced airway adjunct intervention.[3,6,8,9] **(Level E*)**	Facilitates replacing nitrogen with oxygen in the lungs. Increases the duration of apnea without desaturation, which facilitates more time to place the airway adjunct and improves patient safety	Conditions that increase oxygen demand (e.g., sepsis, pregnancy) and decrease functional residual capacity (e.g., morbid obesity, pregnancy) reduce the apnea period before desaturation ensues.[3]	
6. Fully deflate the cuff by holding the device so the distal end is curled slightly anteriorly. Attach a syringe. Compress the distal tip of the mask with the thumb and index finger. **(Level M*)**	Facilitates smooth insertion and avoids deflection of the epiglottis.		
7. Lubricate the posterior surface of the cuff and airway tube with a small amount of water-soluble lubricant. **(Level M*)**	Facilitates smooth insertion.	Avoid excessive lubrication on the anterior portion (aperture side) of the cuff because it may be aspirated or occlude the lumen. Do not use lidocaine lubricants because they may delay the return of protective reflexes and may cause an allergic reaction.[10]	
8. Stand behind or beside the patient's head. Place the patient's head in the neutral or sniffing position (see Fig. 6.5, step A).	Facilitates proper body position for the person inserting the device and the patient's head during insertion.	The patient's head may be left in a neutral position if cervical spine injury is possible.[12] If cervical instability is suspected, manual stabilization should be maintained by the assistant during the placement procedure.	
9. Hold the device as shown in Fig. 6.5, steps B and C. Press the distal tip against the inner aspect of the upper teeth or gums (see Fig. 6.5, step B).	Facilitates smooth insertion.		
10. Slide inward using a slightly diagonal approach (direct the tip away from the midline). Continue to slide inward, rotating the hand in a circular motion so the device follows the curvature behind the tongue (see Fig. 6.5, step C).	Assists in maneuvering the LMA into the proper position	Do not use force. If the LMA does not advance, remove, reventilate, and reinsert.[12] The mask must be pressed up against the hard palate to be inserted correctly.[12] If the cuff becomes obstructed by the tonsils, a diagonal maneuver is often successful.[12]	

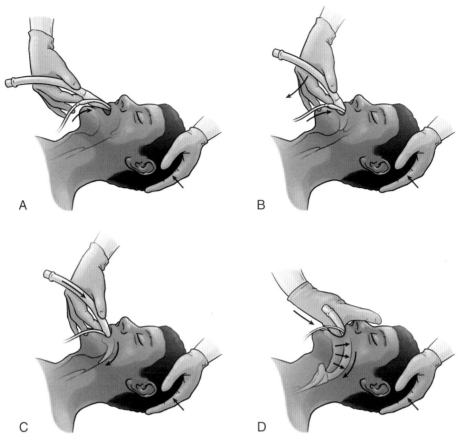

Figure 6.5 Classic technique for insertion of a laryngeal mask airway. *(From Ramachandran SK, Kumar AM. Supraglottic airway devices.* Resp Care. *2014;59[6]:920–932. Image courtesy of Teleflex Incorporated. © 2022 Teleflex Incorporated. All rights reserved.)*

Procedure	for Laryngeal Mask Airway (LMA Supreme) Blind Insertion—*Continued*	
Steps	**Rationale**	**Special Considerations**
11. Resistance should be felt when the distal end of the device meets the upper esophageal sphincter. The device is now fully inserted (see Fig. 6.5, step D).	Continues moving the LMA into the proper final position.	
12. Inflate with the minimal amount of air needed to achieve an effective seal. For further details on successful insertion, see Box 6.1.	The recommended intracuff pressure should not exceed 60 cm H_2O.	

Procedure continues on following page

UNIT I

Procedure	for Laryngeal Mask Airway (LMA Supreme) Blind Insertion—*Continued*	
Steps	Rationale	Special Considerations
13. Check the end-tidal carbon dioxide device to confirm placement.[4,10] **(Level D*)**	Confirms proper placement of LMA	
14. Connect the bag-valve-mask apparatus to the tube, and begin ventilation at 8–10 breaths/minute. Confirm ventilation by lung auscultation and chest rise.[4]	Allows for ventilation with established airway	
Securing the LMA (Fixation)[7]		
15. Use a piece of adhesive tape 30–40 cm long, holding it horizontally by both ends	Facilitates the approximate length necessary to secure the LMA.	
16. Press the adhesive tape transversely across the fixation tab (if present) or an area 2–3 cm above the lips on the LMA airway tube.	The fixation tab is located above the bite block on the LMA Supreme. Other first- and second-generation devices *do not* possess fixation tabs.	The fixation tab should be located 1–2 cm above the lips if placement and sizing is appropriate. The fixation tab should not be applied with downward pressure to the lips/teeth or be located >3 cm above the lips (may indicate improper sizing or improper LMA placement).
17. Continue to press downward so the ends of the tape adhere to each of the patient's cheeks and the device itself is gently pressed inward by the tape.	Secures the LMA with slight inward pressure. This assists in maintaining the LMA seal.	Without securing the LMA in place, displacement or migration of the device from the airway is probable.
18. Bite block may be considered if utilizing a first-generation LMA.	The patient may bite down on a first-generation LMA airway, collapsing the tube and thus compromising the airway.	Second-generation LMAs incorporate bite blocks within the device.
19. Dispose of supplies.		
20. 🅷🅷		

*Level D: Peer-reviewed professional and organizational standards with the support of clinical study recommendations.
*Level E: Multiple case reports, theory-based evidence from expert opinions, or peer-reviewed professional organizational standards without clinical studies to support recommendations.
*Level M: Manufacturer's recommendations only.

BOX 6.1	**Successful Insertion of a Laryngeal Mask Airway Depends on Attention to Several Details**

1. Choose the appropriate size (see Table 6.4), and check for leaks before insertion.
2. The leading edge of the deflated cuff should be wrinkle free and face away from the aperture.
3. Lubricate the back side of the cuff.
4. The patient must be vastly unresponsive and relaxed before attempting insertion.
5. Place the patient's head in sniffing position (see Fig. 6.6).
6. Correct positioning can be aided by using your index finger to guide the cuff along the hard palate and down into the hypopharynx until an

increased resistance is felt. The longitudinal black line should be facing the patient's upper lip.
7. Inflate with the correct amount of air (see Table 6.4).
8. Ensure adequate sedation or anesthesia.
9. Obstruction after insertion is usually caused by a down-folded epiglottis or transient laryngospasm.
10. Avoid pharyngeal suction, cuff deflation, or laryngeal mask removal until the patient is awake (e.g., opening mouth on command) unless removing to facilitate a more secure airway.

From Butterworth J, Mackey DC, Wasnick J. *Morgan & Mikhail's Clinical Anesthesiology.* 6th ed. New York: McGraw-Hill; 2018.

Procedure for Laryngeal Mask Airway (LMA Supreme) Correct Positioning

Steps	Rationale	Special Considerations
1. Correct placement should produce a leak-free seal against the glottis, with the mask tip at the upper esophageal sphincter.	Maintenance of low ventilator pressures prevents overriding the pressure in the cuff, creating a leak, or forcing air into the stomach.	If sounds are heard in the epigastrium on auscultation, remove the device and manually ventilate the patient with a bag-valve-mask device. Limit tidal volumes to <8 mL/kg.
2. The bite-block portion of the LMA Supreme should lie between the teeth.	Helps confirm the correct depth with the primary assessment.	
3. A drop of water-soluble lubricant (1–2 mL) can be placed on the proximal end of the gastric drainage tube port.		
4. Observe a slight up-down meniscus movement of the lubricant after the application and release of gentle pressure on the suprasternal notch.	Confirms proper placement with the tip of the LMA sealed in the esophagus. Indicates that the distal end of the drain tube is correctly placed so it seals around the upper esophageal sphincter.	Observe a slight up-down meniscus movement of the lubricant after the application and release of gentle pressure on the suprasternal notch[12] (also called the *suprasternal notch test*).[12] This is more important if the rescuer plans to pass an NG tube of appropriate size down the LMA for gastric decompression purposes. Increased risk of laryngospasm and airway occlusion can result if the LMA is malpositioned, resulting in NG placement down the bronchi.

Procedure for Laryngeal Mask Airway (LMA Supreme) Removal

Steps	Rationale	Special Considerations
1. **HH**		
2. **PE**		Follow institutional standards for potential exposure of aerosolization and secretions; don appropriate personal protective equipment.

Procedure continues on following page

Procedure	for Laryngeal Mask Airway (LMA Supreme) Removal—*Continued*	
Steps	**Rationale**	**Special Considerations**
3. Remove the LMA as follows: 　A. Gently assist with ventilations when the patient begins spontaneously breathing. 　B. Observe for signs of swallowing. When the patient can open his or her mouth on command, deflate the cuff and remove the LMA.[12] 　C. Continue to assess for airway and breathing effectiveness: 　　i. Establishment of an effective airway in an emergency situation 　　ii. Maintenance of adequate ventilation 　　iii. Recovery of spontaneous ventilation	Removal may prevent agitation, regurgitation, and laryngeal spasm. Prevents excess ventilator pressures. Indicates a return of some protective reflexes. If the LMA is removed before effective swallowing and coughing, secretions may enter the larynx, causing bronchospasm. Maintains monitoring of the airway and the patient's ability to breathe on his or her own.	Removal of the LMA is often to facilitate the placement of a more secure and definitive airway such as an endotracheal tube. This is usually accomplished by personnel specifically trained in airway emergencies (e.g., anesthesiologists and certified registered nurse anesthetists). The tape or tube-securing device may be removed at this time. Unless overt secretions are noted after LMA removal, avoid suctioning because it may cause laryngeal spasm. The cuff should remove excess secretions when removed and prevent aspiration.[12] Potential complications related to LMA use appear to be inversely proportional to the experience and skill level of the operator and to patient-related factors (e.g., placement in a semiconscious individual or a patient with a full stomach).[6,12] • Regurgitation • Aspiration • Laryngospasm • Gagging • Retching • Trauma to tissues • Damage to various nerves • Sore or dry mouth • Hoarseness, stridor
4. Dispose of supplies 5. ▣▣		

Expected Outcome

- Establishment of an emergent artificial airway
- Properly positioned and secured airway
- Adequate oxygenation and ventilation
- Improved or stabilized patient condition

Unexpected Outcomes

- Aspiration of gastric contents
- Trauma to oral and pharyngeal tissue potentially leading to worsening ventilation, nerve damage, and aspiration of blood
- Inability to ventilate lungs effectively secondary to:
1. Improper sizing or position of the LMA
2. High airway and thoracic pressures (e.g., obese and asthmatic patients)
3. Obstruction: secretion or foreign body
4. Semiconscious patient
5. Poor seal of LMA cuff (overinflated or underinflated)
6. Anatomical mismatch of the patient and device (uncommon anatomical airway variants can result in a poor seal and fit of the LMA)[3,6,9]

Patient Monitoring and Care

Steps	Rationale	Reportable Conditions
1. Monitor the patient and LMA during ventilation for potential problems. A. Attach a pulse oximeter, and monitor for trends. B. Watch for air leaks around the cuff that may be caused by malposition. If suspected, assess for normal smooth oval swelling around the cricothyroid membrane. If absent, in conjunction with a prolonged expiratory phase, remove the LMA, reventilate the patient, and reinsert the device.[12] C. If regurgitation occurs, as indicated by fluid in the airway tube, immediately tilt the patient's head down, turn the patient's body to one side, remove the bag-valve-mask device, and suction through the airway tube.	Ensures proper ventilation and airway management. Pressure-controlled and volume-controlled ventilation may be used but should be minimized or avoided because LMAs are not designed for long-term airway management. Pressure-controlled ventilation may require lower peak airway pressures.[6,12] Efforts should be made to secure a definitive airway (endotracheal intubation) as soon as possible. With mechanical ventilation, tidal volume, respiratory rate, and inspiratory-to-expiratory ratios must be adjusted to prevent high peak airway pressures.[4,6,12] Monitors adequate oxygenation. May indicate problems with LMA positioning. Do not add more air to the cuff because it may force the soft cuff off the larynx.[12] Allows drainage and clearance of fluid from the airway tube. If airway problems, difficulty with ventilation, or regurgitation continue, remove the LMA, and establish an airway by other means.[12]	*These conditions should be reported to the provider if they persist despite nursing interventions.* • Inability to ventilate the patient • Decreased oxygen levels despite adequate oxygen delivery • Indications of an air leak, especially with a prolonged expiratory phase or lack of normal smooth oval swelling around the cricothyroid membrane[6,12] • The LMA's cuff pressures may need to be adjusted during the ascent and descent portions of air transport for unpressurized cabins • Monitor for signs of excessive or deficient LMA cuff pressures, namely, ventilation difficulties and excessive air leaks • Airway problems, difficulty with ventilation, or regurgitation

Documentation

Documentation should include the following:
• Initial patient assessment that indicates a need for LMA insertion
• Performance of visual inspection, inflation, and deflation tests
• After insertion, assessment of end-tidal carbon dioxide for placement confirmation, chest rise and fall, and continuous pulse oximetry.
• Before removal, presence of swallowing and ability to open the mouth
• Any complications while the LMA is in place (e.g., regurgitation or air leaks)
• Preoxygenation and ventilation before LMA insertion
• Insertion technique
• Initial cuff inflation pressure
• Signs of correct placement and cuff inflation
• Securing of the LMA
• After removal, patency of airway, effectiveness of breathing, pulse oximetry and vital sign readings, patient symptoms, or signs of complications

References and Additional Readings

For a complete list of references and additional readings for this procedure, scan this QR code with your smartphone, or visit https://www.elsevier.com/__data/assets/pdf_file/0003/1319781/Chapter0006.pdf

7

Nasopharyngeal and Oral Airway Insertion

Bonjo Batoon

PURPOSE: Nasopharyngeal airways (NPAs) and oropharyngeal airways (OPAs) are essential airway management adjuncts used to establish and maintain short-term airway patency in patients with the inability to protect their airway or who are at risk for airway obstruction. Additionally, these airway adjuncts can ease bag-valve-mask ventilation and facilitate oropharyngeal/tracheobronchial suctioning; however, they do not protect against aspiration. Finally, placement of definitive airway via endotracheal intubation should be considered if these devices fail to relieve obstruction or the need for prolonged airway assistance is suspected.

PREREQUISITE NURSING KNOWLEDGE

Nasopharyngeal Airway

- The NPA is designed to facilitate airway patency by creating space between the base of the tongue and the posterior oropharynx.[2]
- Partial or complete airway obstruction can result from alterations in mental status, oversedation, or narcosis.[11,14,33]
- The NPA consists of three parts: flange, body (cannula), and beveled tip (Fig. 7.1). The flange prevents the patient from aspirating the NPA into the airway, and the body is a cuffless tube that allows airflow to pass between the base of the tongue and the posterior oropharynx. Finally, the soft beveled tip allows for ease of insertion from the nasal passage to the posterior oropharynx.
- To determine the proper length, the NPA is measured from the tip of the patient's nose to the patient's earlobe or the tragus of the ear (Fig. 7.2). Select an NPA with an external diameter that is slightly smaller than the patient's external naris to avoid difficulty entering the nasal cavity. NPAs that are too small may result in failure to relieve obstruction, increased airway resistance, and/or reduced airflow, while an NPA that is too large may result in soft tissue damage of the oropharyngeal and nasopharyngeal structures, bleeding, coughing, gagging, vomiting, and aspiration.[2,31]
- Proper placement is confirmed when the flange is resting on the patient's naris (Fig. 7.3) with the tip of the NPA resting in the posterior oropharynx beyond the pharyngeal edge of the soft palate, relief of airway obstruction, and/or improved air exchange has occurred.[11] Optimally, the tip of the NPA should rest just beyond the soft palate between the tongue and the soft palate, but should not overlay the epiglottis (Fig. 7.4).[8,12,35]
- Unlike oropharyngeal airways, NPAs can be easily placed and tolerated in patients who are conscious with intact airway reflexes. Additionally, NPAs can facilitate the removal of oropharyngeal and tracheobronchial secretions

while reducing damage to the soft tissues of the nasopharynx and oropharynx during frequent suctioning. Finally, NPAs can be used to relieve airway obstruction in patients with limited mouth opening or trismus.[7,35]

- Although most NPAs are designed to be inserted into the right naris with the bevel tip facing medially toward the nasal septum (see Fig. 7.3), either naris can be used for NPA placement.[30] Before insertion, the nasal passages should be inspected for deformity, obstruction, bleeding, and patency. The NPA should be placed in the naris with the best airflow with no obvious obstructions. If unable to pass through the originally selected naris, placement should be attempted in the opposite naris. For left naris insertion, the lubricated NPA should be rotated 180 degrees with the bevel facing medially toward the nasal

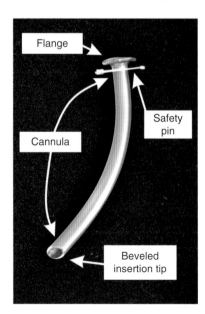

Figure 7.1 Parts of a nasopharyngeal airway (NPA). NPA shown with an optional safety pin inserted perpendicular to the proximal cannula just below the flange,[30] which can be used as a securement device to prevent aspiration of the NPA.

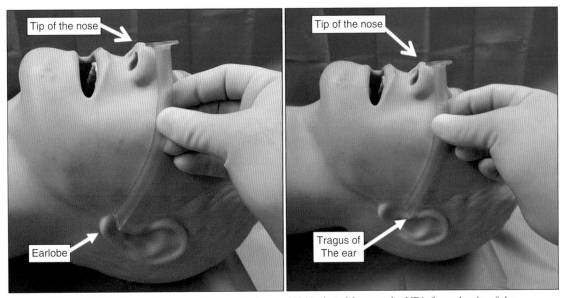

Figure 7.2 Estimating nasopharyngeal airway (NPA) size. Measure the NPA from the tip of the nose to either the earlobe or the tragus of the ear.

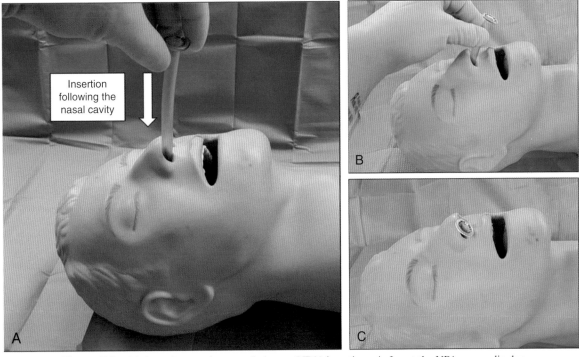

Figure 7.3 Right naris nasopharyngeal airway (NPA) insertion. **A,** Insert the NPA perpendicular to the patient's face with the beveled tip facing the nasal septum. **B,** Advance using gentle forward pressure following the natural curvature of the nasal passage. **C,** Advance until the flange rests on the naris.

septum; advance with gentle forward pressure through the left naris until firmly into the nasal cavity; again, rotate the NPA 180 degrees and gently advance the NPA following the natural curvature of the nasopharynx into the posterior oropharynx until the flange rests on the patient's nostril (Fig. 7.5).

- Contraindications
  - ❖ Facial trauma and midface fracture[2]
  - ❖ Basal skull or cribriform plate fracture[2,23]
  - ❖ Obstructed nasal passages
  - ❖ Patients with coagulation disorders or on anticoagulants (relative contraindication)[2,7]
- Complications
  - ❖ Epistaxis[2,31,34]
  - ❖ Nasopharyngeal soft tissue trauma[26,31]
  - ❖ Failure to relieve airway obstruction
  - ❖ Gagging, which can result in vomiting and aspiration[34]
  - ❖ Migration of unsecured NPA into the upper airway[6,15,31]

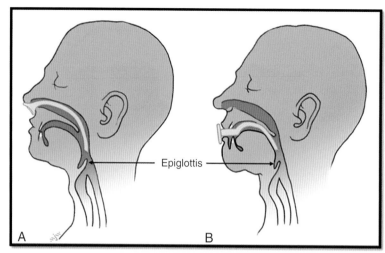

Figure 7.4   Placement of a nasopharyngeal airway (NPA) and oropharyngeal airway (OPA). **A,** The NPA flange rests on the nostril with the tip resting in the posterior oropharynx just above the epiglottis. **B,** The OPA flange rests at the lips with the tip resting in the posterior oropharynx just above the epiglottis.

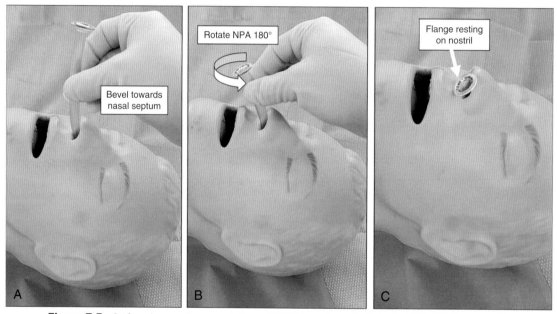

Figure 7.5   Left naris nasopharyngeal airway (NPA) insertion. **A,** Spin the NPA 180 degrees with the bevel facing the nasal septum, and apply gentle forward pressure. **B,** Once firmly in the nasal cavity, rotate the NPA 180 degrees, and advance it following the natural curvature of the nasal passage. **C,** Advance the NPA until the flange rests on the nostril.

Oropharyngeal Airway

- Oropharyngeal airways are curved, rigid, plastic airway adjuncts use to relieve airway obstruction by preventing the tongue from obstructing the airway and/or covering the epiglottis.[9,17]
- The four parts of the OPA include the tip, body, flange, and channel (Fig. 7.6). When fully inserted, the tip of the OPA will face the base of the tongue. The body follows the curvature of the tongue and creates space between the tongue and the oropharynx, and the flange prevents the device from being aspirated by the patient.[9,10,13]
- OPAs come in a variety of sizes for infants, children, and adults. Typically, the size is determined by placing the

OPA on the patient's face with the flange positioned at the corner of the mouth and the tip of the OPA aligned with the angle of the mandible. Measuring from the maxillary incisors to the angle of the mandible is another method for proper sizing of the OPA (Fig. 7.7).[16]
- If the OPA is too small, failure to relieve obstruction may occur, but if the OPA is too large, the patient may gag, cough, vomit, and/or aspirate. For male and female patients of average height, a size 5 (10-cm) oral airway for male patients and a size 4 (9-cm) oral airway for female patients may be appropriate (Table 7.1).[18] A smaller and larger OPA should be immediately available in case the initial OPA fails to relieve airway obstruction.

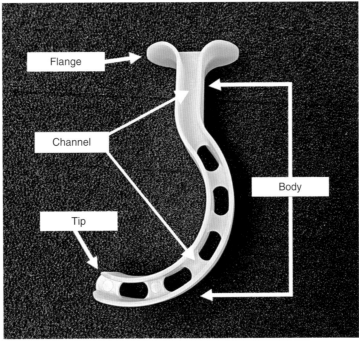

Figure 7.6 Parts of the oropharyngeal airway (OPA).

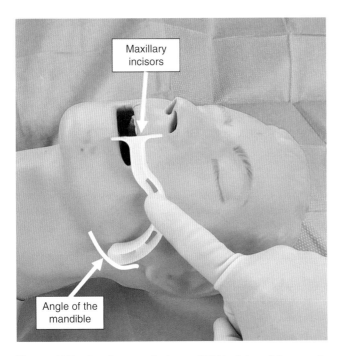

Figure 7.7 Oropharyngeal airway (OPA) sizing. Measure the OPA from the maxillary incisors to the angle of the mandible.

TABLE 7.1	Oral Pharyngeal Airway Size Chart
Size	Length (Flange to Tip)
0	5 cm
1	6 cm
2	7 cm
3	8 cm
4*	9 cm*
5**	10 cm**

*Ideal for average-sized female patients.
**Ideal for average-sized male patients.[12]
Note: An OPA one size above and below should be immediately available if the original OPA fails to relieve airway obstruction.
Modified from: https://www.teleflex.com/usa/en/product-areas/anesthesia/airway-management/oral-and-nasal-airways/oral-airways/index.html#guedel.

- OPAs can be used facilitate bag-valve-mask ventilation in patients with poor or absent respiratory effort, in the absence of a gag reflex. Additionally, the air channel within the OPA facilitates suctioning of the oropharynx and hypopharynx.[10]
- Placement of an OPA is contraindicated in patients who are conscious, actively seizing, and have intact airway or gag reflexes.[9]
- If the patient has trismus or limited mouth opening, an NPA should be considered.
- Complications
  - Failure to relieve airway obstruction[9]
  - Gagging/coughing resulting in possible aspiration[9,18,31]
  - Laryngospasm[18]
  - Oral cavity injury[19,24]
  - Airway trauma and/or bleeding[10,24]
- Contraindications
  - Conscious patients[9]
  - Intact airway reflexes[9,27]
  - Actively seizing patients
  - Use as a bite block[22]
  - Trismus[30,31]

❖ Oral trauma (relative contraindication)[27,30]
❖ Limited mouth opening (relative contraindication)
❖ Airway obstruction caused by a foreign body[9]

EQUIPMENT

• Appropriate personal protective equipment (PPE)
  ❖ Gloves, mask, gown, and eye protection
• Appropriate-sized NPA or OPA
  ❖ Various sizes immediately available
• Water-soluble lubricant or local anesthetic gel (NPA)
• Tongue depressor (OPA)
• Tape, safety pin, and endotracheal tube adaptor (NPA)[22,32]
• Suction equipment
• Oxygen source
• Bag-valve-mask device
• Standard monitoring equipment (if available): pulse oximeter, noninvasive blood pressure cuff, and EKG
• Capnography equipment (if available) to continuously monitor respiratory/ventilatory function, detect early respiratory compromise, and determine adequacy of bag-valve-mask device[2,5,20,25]

PATIENT AND FAMILY EDUCATION

• If the patient's condition allows and/or the family is present, the need for placement of the airway adjunct should be explained. This discussion should include the expected benefits, potential risks associated with the performance of the procedure, and what they should they expect to see. **Rationale:** This addresses the patient's and family's potential knowledge deficit related the patient's current condition and need for an airway adjunct. Additionally, this allows the opportunity for the patient and family to ask questions and voice concerns related to the procedure, which may reduce anxiety and encourage communication among the patient, family, and healthcare team.
• Discuss with the patient, if conscious, the sensory experiences they may experience during and after insertion of the airway adjunct, which may include pain on insertion (NPA), presence of the NPA or OPA, gagging, coughing, epistaxis (NPA), and/or sore throat (OPA). **Rationale:** Information regarding the expected sensory experiences may reduce anxiety and distress related to the insertion and presence of an NPA or OPA.

PATIENT ASSESSMENT AND PREPARATION

• Assess the patient's respiratory status by noting the patient's respiratory rate, effort, quality, oxygen saturation, and oxygen requirements. **Rationale:** This baseline assessment will determine the need and immediacy for the placement of an NPA or OPA.
• If possible, review the patient's medication list, and avoid placing an NPA in coagulopathic patients and patients taking anticoagulant medications (e.g., ASA, warfarin, heparin, and/or direct/indirect thrombin inhibitors) **Rationale:** There is an increased risk for epistaxis (NPA), and it is a relative contraindication.
• Assess the patient's neurological status and ability to protect the airway including the presence or absence of the gag reflex. **Rationale:** Placement of OPA in patients with intact airway reflexes may lead to coughing, gagging, vomiting, and/or pulmonary aspiration. The nurse should consider an NPA in the presence of intact airway reflexes.
• If the patient requires an NPA or OPA, the need for definitive airway placement should be considered and continually reevaluated. **Rationale:** OPAs and NPAs are considered short-term airway adjuncts, and they do not offer protection against pulmonary aspiration.
• Assessment for NPA placement should include inspection of the nasal passages for deformity, obstruction, bleeding, and patency. Visualize the nasal passages using a flashlight, looking for any obstruction that may impede insertion of an NPA. To assess for patency, occlude one nostril at a time, and check for air movement from the contralateral nostril. **Rationale:** Preprocedural nasal passage assessment can reduce the number of attempts needed for passage of the NPA, which may reduce bleeding and trauma to the nasopharyngeal passages.
• To reduce trauma, bleeding, and discomfort associated with the placement and presence of an NPA, contact the provider and obtain an order for a topical anesthetic, with or without a vasoconstrictor, to lubricate the NPA. **Rationale:** The topical anesthetic can reduce pain, while the vasoconstrictor can reduce bleeding within the nasal passages before insertion.[19]
• Before insertion of an OPA, assess the patient's oral airway including the lips, teeth, gums, oral mucosa, presence of dentures, partial plates, or foreign objects (e.g., piercings/jewelry), presence of airway contaminants (secretions, vomitus, and/or blood), and absence of airway reflexes. **Rationale:** Allows the nurse to identify and remove any materials that can be aspirated before OPA insertion, and allows nurses to compare the baseline assessment to their subsequent assessments.

Patient Preparation

• Verify the correct patient with two identifiers. **Rationale:** Preprocedural identification and confirmation ensures that the right procedure is being performed in the right patient.
• Along with appropriate-sized airway adjuncts as described earlier in the "Prerequisite Nursing Knowledge" section, proper patient monitoring should be in place, with suction and emergency equipment immediately available.
• An NPA can be placed with the patient in the supine, semi-Fowler's or high Fowler's position, while the supine position is preferred for OPA placement. **Rationale:** Proper positioning provides optimal conditions for placement of an NPA or OPA while ensuring comfort for the patient and the nurse.

Procedure | **for Nasopharyngeal Airway Insertion**

Steps	Rationale	Special Considerations
1. [HH]		
2. [PE]		Follow institutional guidelines regarding potential for aerosolization of secretions, and don appropriate PPE.
3. Assess need for an NPA.	Proper assessment confirms the need for an invasive airway technique.	Assess the patient's respiratory rate and effort, baseline vital signs including oxygen saturation, and any interventions attempted to improve ventilation (e.g., attempted OPA).
4. Assess need to suction secretions, blood, vomitus, or foreign material. **(Level D*)**	Clears the airway and may reduce risk of aspiration.[8,28,29]	
5. Gather equipment, and select the appropriate-sized NPA using external landmarks (see Fig 7.2).		Have a size larger NPA in case the originally inserted NPA fails to relieve obstruction and a smaller NPA in case the originally placed NPA is too large causing coughing, gagging, vomiting, or aspiration.[11,34,35]
6. Lubricate the outer tip of the NPA with a water-soluble lubricant or topical local anesthetic, if ordered. **(Level D*)**	Facilitates passage and reduces friction damage during insertion of the NPA.[11,31,34]	Avoid lubricating of the inner lumen of the NPA. Consider obtaining an order for a topical vasoconstrictor to reduced bleeding.
7. If no cervical spine injury is suspected, place the patient in the sniffing position (Fig. 7.11), and determine which naris is wider or has better airflow.	The sniffing position can be used to relieve airway obstruction while providing a means to examine the site for insertion.[2]	Choose an NPA slightly smaller than the chosen naris.
8. Insert the NPA perpendicular to the patient's face, along the nasal cavity, using gentle forward pressure until the flange rests on the nostril (see Fig. 7.3).	Reduces trauma and allows the NPA to follow the natural contour of the nasal passage.[6]	Avoid inserting the NPA in a cephalad direction. For right naris insertion, gently advance the NPA with the beveled tip facing the nasal septum, and slightly rotate the NPA side to side if resistance is met during insertion (see Fig. 7.3). If unable to advance the NPA, insertion through the opposite naris should be attempted. For left naris insertion, rotate the NPA 180 degrees with the bevel facing medially toward the nasal septum, apply gentle forward pressure until firmly in the nasal cavity, and rotate the NPA 180 degrees to allow the NPA to follow the natural curvature of the nasal airway until the flange rests on the nostril (see Fig. 7.5).

*Level D: Peer-reviewed professional and organizational standards with the support of clinical study recommendations

Procedure continues on following page

Procedure for Nasopharyngeal Airway Insertion—*Continued*

Steps	Rationale	Special Considerations
9. Refer to your institution's policy for securement of NPAs. **(Levels E*)**	May prevent caudal displacement and/or aspiration of NPA. Although several securement methods are described in the literature, including the use of safety pins (see Fig. 7.1), tape (Fig. 7.12A), and endotracheal tube connectors (see Fig. 7.12B), securement is optional because no standards currently exist.[3,4,32]	Optional securement techniques: 1. Place a safety pin through the cannula of the NPA just below the flange (see Fig. 7.1). 2. Just below the flange of the NPA, wrap a thin piece of tape around the cannula, and secure the NPA to the patient's nose similar to securing a nasogastric tube (see Fig 7.12A). 3. Remove the endotracheal adapter from the endotracheal tube, and insert it into the proximal end of the NPA[4] (see Fig. 7.12B).
10. If possible, visually confirm proper placement by opening the patient's mouth and looking for the NPA resting on the posterior oropharynx beyond the pharyngeal edge of the soft palate.[12]	Visually verifies proper placement of NPA and provides a means to assess the airway for excessive bleeding or damage to oropharyngeal tissues.	
11. Assess airway patency and relief of airway obstruction.	Proper placement relieves airway obstruction, improves air exchange, facilitates oropharyngeal and tracheobronchial suctioning, and can ease bag-valve-mask ventilation.	
12. Suction oropharyngeal secretion as needed.	Maintains airway patency and prevents aspiration (see Procedure 3, Endotracheal Tube Care and Oral Care Practices for Ventilated and Nonventilated Patients)	
13. Assess the need for bag-valve-mask ventilation and/or the need for advanced airway placement.	Failure to improve air exchange and/or ineffective ability to clear secretions may necessitate endotracheal intubation.	NPAs are not intended for long-term use.
14. Assess tolerance of the NPA, including the need for analgesia.	Identifies the need for analgesia.	Consider a local or nonopioid analgesic for patients with tenuous respiratory status.
15. Dispose of used supplies and equipment.	Reduces unnecessary exposure to body fluids.	
16. Discard PPE, and perform hand hygiene.		

*Level E: Multiple case reports, theory-based evidence from expert opinions, or peer-reviewed professional organizational standards without clinical studies to support recommendations.

Procedure	**for Oropharyngeal Airway Insertion**	
Steps	**Rationale**	**Special Considerations**
1. HH		
2. PE		Follow institutional guidelines regarding the potential for aerosolization of secretions, and don appropriate PPE.
3. Assess the need for an OPA.	Avoids unnecessary invasive procedures.	Assess the patient's respiratory rate and effort, baseline vital signs including oxygen saturation, and any interventions attempted to improve ventilation (e.g., chin-lift or jaw-thrust).
4. Gather equipment, and select an appropriate-sized OPA using external landmarks[9,16,18] (Fig. 7.7). **(Level D*)**		Various styles and manufacturers exist. Become familiar with your manufacturer and institutional guidelines. For average-sized male and female patients, consider 9-cm and 10-cm OPAs, respectively.[6]
5. Using the scissor technique, open the patient's mouth, and suction the oropharynx of blood, secretions, or vomitus before insertion.	Clears airway before insertion and reduces risk for pulmonary aspiration.[9]	
6. Assess the airway, noting the condition of teeth and the presence of dentures or other foreign objects before inserting the OPA.	Teeth can be chipped during and after placement of an OPA, while loose teeth can be dislodged and potentially aspirated. Poorly fitting dentures may impede placement of the OPA and worsen airway obstruction.	
7. There are three OPA insertion techniques. A. Insert the OPA with the tip pointed toward the roof of the mouth, and advance until the OPA slides off the hard palate; then spin the OPA 180 degrees so the tip faces the base of the tongue (Fig. 7.8). or B. Use a tongue depressor to displace the tongue caudally, and slide the OPA with the tip facing the tongue along the length of the tongue blade until it curves around the base of the tongue into the posterior oropharynx (Fig. 7.9). or C. Open mouth, insert the OPA sideways toward the corner of the mouth, then rotate 90 degrees and advance toward the posterior oropharynx[9] (Fig. 7.10).	Proper placement of the OPA follows the natural curvature of the tongue and displaces the tongue off the posterior oropharynx.[9]	A tongue depressor can be used to control the tongue during insertion. Intact airway reflexes, including coughing and gagging, should preclude OPA insertion.

Procedure continues on following page

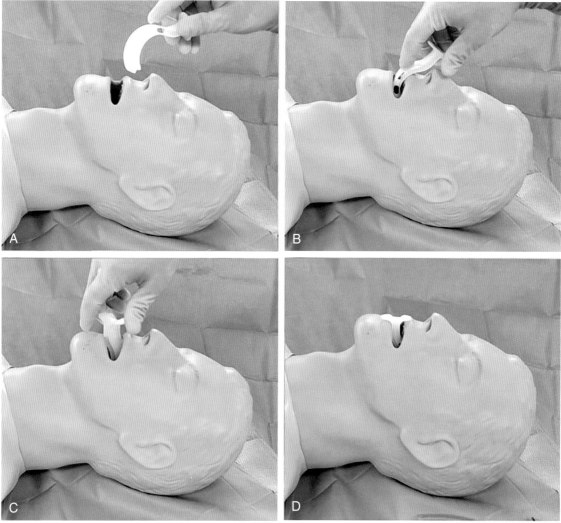

Figure 7.8 Oropharyngeal airway (OPA) insertion. **A,** Insert the OPA with the tip facing the roof of the mouth. **B,** Advance the OPA along the hard palate. **C,** Once off of the hard palate, carefully rotate the OPA 180 degrees, and advance it until it is firmly seated at the base of the tongue. **D,** Final resting position of the OPA.

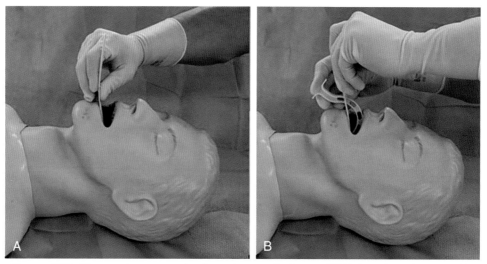

Figure 7.9 Tongue depressor–assisted oropharyngeal airway (OPA) insertion. **A,** Insert the tongue depressor to displace the tongue caudally. **B,** Slide the OPA along the shaft of the tongue depressor.

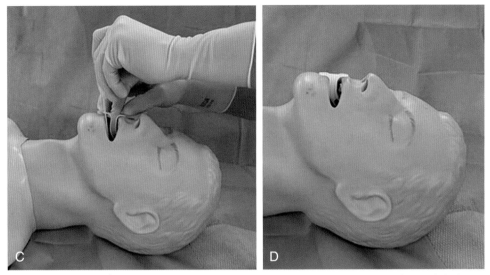

Figure 7.9, cont'd **C,** Slide the OPA until it slides off the tongue depressor and around the base of the tongue. **D,** Final resting position of the OPA.

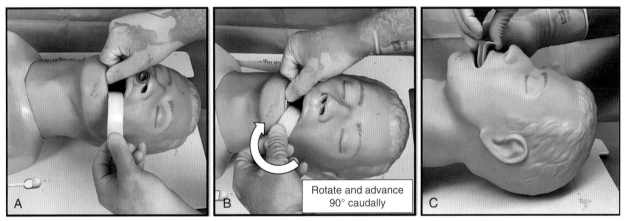

Figure 7.10 Lateral oropharyngeal airway (OPA) insertion. **A,** Open the patient's mouth and insert the OPA into the side of the mouth. **B,** Gently rotate and advance the OPA 90 degrees caudally until the tip of the OPA rests in the posterior oropharynx. **C,** Final resting position of the OPA.

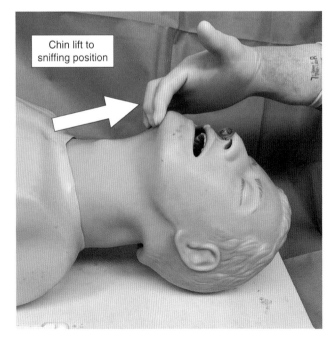

Figure 7.11 Technique for placing the patient in the sniffing position. With the fingers under the mandible, gently tilt the patient's chin and head back.

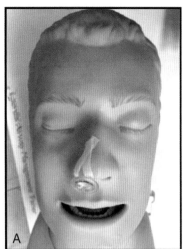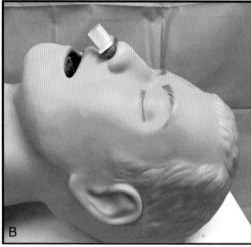

Figure 7.12   Optional nasopharyngeal airway (NPA) securement techniques. **A,** Wrap a thin strip of tape around the cannula of the NPA, and tape it to the patient's nose just below the flange. **B,** Insert an endotracheal tube adaptor into the proximal end of the NPA (known as the *modified nasal trumpet*[3]).

Procedure for Oropharyngeal Airway Insertion—*Continued*

Steps	Rationale	Special Considerations
8. Verify correct placement and airway patency by attempting bag-valve-mask ventilation.	Correct placement should improve airway patency and/or ease bag-valve-mask ventilation.	Securement and taping are not encouraged as they may increase the risk of aspiration when airway reflexes return or the patient regains consciousness.
9. Suction the oropharynx as needed. **(Level D*)**	Maintains airway patency and reduces risk of aspiration.[28,29]	
10. Continuous and ongoing assessment of respiratory status.	Failure to relieve obstruction or effectively ventilate after placement necessitates definitive airway management.	
11. Dispose of used supplies and equipment.	Reduces unnecessary exposure to body fluids.	
12. Discard PPE, and perform hand hygiene.		

*Level D: Peer-reviewed professional and organizational standards with the support of clinical study recommendations

Expected Outcomes

- Relief of airway obstruction and improved air exchange
- Improved oxygenation
- Ability to effectively remove secretions from the oropharynx, hypopharynx, and tracheobronchial tree
- Improved bag-valve-mask ventilation
- Forward displacement of the base of the tongue away from the posterior oropharynx

Unexpected Outcomes

- Failure to relieve or worsening of airway obstruction
- Worsening hypoxia
- Pulmonary aspiration
- Aspiration of NPA
- Damage to teeth and oropharyngeal and/or nasopharyngeal structures
- Laryngospasm
- Epistaxis (NPA)

Patient Monitoring and Care

Steps	Rationale	Reportable Conditions
1. In the case of prolonged use, assessment of the skin and mucosa in contact with the airway adjunct should occur every 8–12 hours or per institutional guidelines. If a securement device is used for an NPA (e.g., safety pin), contact points should be more frequently assessed.	Alterations in tissue integrity including skin, mucosa of the nasopharyngeal and oropharyngeal passages, teeth, and gums can be detected by frequent and thorough inspection.	*These conditions should be reported to the provider if they persist despite nursing interventions.* Redness Swelling Drainage Bleeding Skin or mucosal breakdown Dislodgement of airway adjunct
2. Prolonged use of an OPA in a nonintubated patient requires definitive airway management.	Obtunded patients without airway reflexes are at risk for pulmonary aspiration.	Failure to ventilate Hypoventilation Hypoxia Aspiration
3. Provide thorough oral care every 2–4 hours, as needed.[1]	Assessment of the oral cavity can take place while providing complete oral hygiene.	Redness Swelling Drainage Bleeding Skin or mucosal breakdown
4. Assess the need for suctioning and supplemental oxygen.		Inability to clear secretions Increasing oxygen requirements
5. Evaluate respiratory status every 2–4 hours.	Provides early identification of respiratory failure.	Increased work of breathing Increasing oxygen requirements Stridor Crowing Agonal respirations Continued airway obstruction Mental status changes
6. Assess pain, and provide analgesia as indicated.	Identifies patient discomfort and the need for intervention.	Unrelieved pain despite intervention. Consider local anesthetics and/or nonopioid analgesics to avoid respiratory depressant effects of opioids.

Documentation

- Date and time of insertion
- Description for the need of an OPA or NPA
- Education provided to the patient and/or family
- Location, type, and size of airway inserted (inserter)
- Respiratory assessment before and after airway insertion
- Adjuncts used: lubrication, local anesthetic, and/or tongue depressor (inserter)
- Number of insertion attempts, any difficulties with insertion and how resolved (inserter)
- Complications and/or adverse outcomes (inserter)
- Airway securement type, if used
- Vitals signs and patient's tolerance to the procedure
- Consults with other services such as critical care, anesthesia, and/or surgical team (inserter)
- Date and time of removal

References and Additional Readings

For a complete list of references and additional readings for this procedure, scan this QR code with your smartphone, or visit https://www.elsevier.com/__data/assets/pdf_file/0004/1319782/Chapter0007.pdf

8 Suctioning: Endotracheal or Tracheostomy Tube

Erin Hare and Maureen A. Seckel

PURPOSE: Endotracheal or tracheostomy tube suctioning is performed to maintain patency of an artificial airway and to improve gas exchange, decrease airway resistance, prevent obstruction, and reduce infection risk by removing secretions from the trachea and mainstem bronchi. Suctioning also may be performed to obtain samples of tracheal secretions for laboratory analysis.

PREREQUISITE NURSING KNOWLEDGE

- Endotracheal and tracheostomy tubes are used to maintain a patent airway and to facilitate mechanical ventilation. The presence of an artificial airway may prevent the patient from being able to effectively cough and clear secretions, necessitating periodic removal of pulmonary secretions with suctioning. In acute-care settings, suctioning is always performed as a sterile procedure to prevent hospital-acquired infections.
- There are two methods to perform suctioning: open and closed. The open-suction technique requires disconnecting the patient's airway from the ventilator circuit or oxygen source to insert a single-use suction catheter via the open end of the tube. The closed-suction technique, also referred to as *in-line suctioning,* involves attachment of a sterile, in-line suction catheter inside a sterile plastic sleeve, which is inserted through a special diaphragm continuously attached to the end of the endotracheal or tracheostomy tube (Fig. 8.1). The closed-suction technique facilitates continuous oxygenation and ventilation support during the suctioning procedure. The closed-suction technique decreases the risk for suctioning-induced lung derecruitment, hypoxemia, and aerosolization of tracheal secretions, and it may reduce equipment cross-contamination.[6,10,25] Use of the closed-suction technique is preferred in patients who experience cardiopulmonary instability during suctioning with the open-suction technique, require high levels of positive end-expiratory pressure (PEEP; >10 cm H_2O) or inspired oxygen (>80%), are at risk for derecruitment, or have grossly bloody pulmonary secretions.[6,25] The closed-suction technique minimizes the risk of airborne transmission to the healthcare worker during suctioning.[42]
- Suctioning of artificial airways should only be performed based on clinical indication and not as a routine fixed-schedule treatment.[6,40,41,44]
- Indications for suctioning include the following[6,40]:
  - ❖ Visible or audible secretions in the artificial airway
  - ❖ Suspected aspiration of gastric or upper airway secretions
  - ❖ Auscultation of adventitious lung sounds (rhonchi or crackles) over the trachea and/or mainstem bronchi

- ❖ Increased peak inspiratory pressure during volume-controlled ventilation or decreased tidal volume during pressure-controlled ventilation
  - ❖ Sawtooth pattern on the flow-volume loop on a ventilator monitor (indicator of retained pulmonary secretions)[40] (Fig. 8.2)
  - ❖ Acute respiratory distress, including increased respiratory rate and/or frequent coughing
  - ❖ Deterioration in oxygen saturation and/or arterial blood gas values (Pao_2, Sao_2, Spo_2)
  - ❖ Patient inability to generate effective cough and/or airway patency is questioned
- Suctioning is a necessary procedure for patients with an artificial airway when clinical indicators are present and there is no absolute contraindication to suctioning. In situations in which suctioning would be poorly tolerated by the patient, a specific plan for suctioning that is developed with the healthcare team should be implemented.
- Complications associated with suctioning of artificial airways include the following:
  - ❖ Hypoxemia
  - ❖ Respiratory arrest
  - ❖ Cardiac dysrhythmias (premature contractions, tachycardias, bradycardias, heart blocks)
  - ❖ Cardiac arrest
  - ❖ Hypertension or hypotension
  - ❖ Decreases in mixed venous oxygen saturation (Svo_2)
  - ❖ Increased intracranial pressure
  - ❖ Bronchospasm
  - ❖ Pulmonary hemorrhage or bleeding
  - ❖ Pain and anxiety
- Hyperoxygenation should always be provided before and after each pass of the suction catheter into the artificial airway, whether via open- or closed-suction technique. Use of the ventilator to hyperoxygenate is preferred over manual ventilation to hyperoxygenate, as it is more effective at delivering a fraction of inspired oxygen (Fio_2) of 1.0.[6,43,44] Note that the majority of research regarding suctioning has been performed with patients on mechanical ventilation via endotracheal tube or tracheostomy. For tracheostomy patients who are not on mechanical ventilation, the need to preoxygenate or hyperventilate should be

based on institutional protocol and individualized patient assessment, including level of consciousness, ability to cough and manage secretions, SpO_2, and FiO_2.

- Tracheal mucosal damage (epithelial denudement, hyperemia, loss of cilia, edema) occurs during suctioning when tissue is pulled into the catheter tip holes. These areas of damage increase the risk of infection and bleeding.[19,25] Although special-tipped catheters may cause less injury, all suction catheters have the potential of producing some damage to tracheal mucosa. Repetition of suctioning, vigor and depth of insertion, level of suction applied, and continuous versus intermittent suction all potentially contribute to mucosal damage.

- The correct suction depth has continued to be controversial. There is no conclusive evidence to support the practice of minimally invasive suctioning versus deep suctioning because of inconsistencies in definitions and outcomes. There are multiple definitions of minimally invasive or shallow suctioning in the literature, including the following examples: insertion of the suction catheter without the catheter passing beyond the end of the endotracheal tube,[3,17,18,33,35] insertion of the suction catheter to a predetermined length of the airway and connector,[6] or insertion of the suction catheter 2 cm beyond the endotracheal tube.[5,6,18] *Deep suctioning* has been defined as insertion of the suction catheter beyond the length of the ETT or tracheostomy tube until resistance is met with withdrawal of 1 cm before applying suction.[6,17]

- Postural drainage and percussion may improve secretion mobilization from small to large airways in chronic respiratory diseases with large mucus production (e.g., cystic fibrosis, bronchiectasis) but has not been shown in the literature to be effective for routine use in all patients.[30,38]

- Adequate systemic hydration and supplemental humidification of inspired gases assist in thinning secretions for easier aspiration from airways. Instillation of a bolus of normal saline solution is not effective in thinning or liquifying mucous or secretions and may cause patient harm. Instillation of normal saline may decrease arterial and mixed venous oxygenation and may potentially contribute to lower-airway contamination from the mechanical dislodgment of bacteria within the artificial airway or from contamination of saline solution during instillation.[4,6,17,30] Saline solution should not be instilled into the artificial airway before suctioning.[4,6,8,15,16,34,38,41,44]

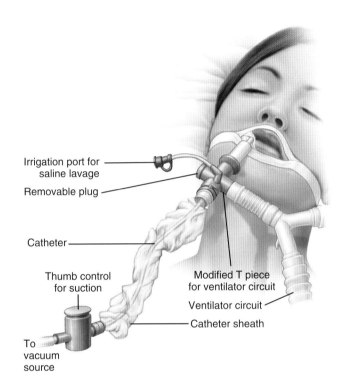

Figure 8.1 Closed-suction technique. *(From Sills JR: Entry-level respiratory therapist exam guide, ed 3, St Louis, 2000, Mosby.)*

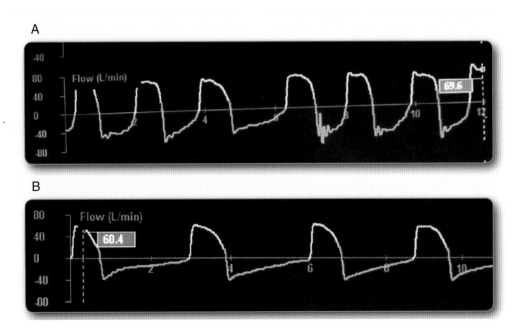

Figure 8.2 Ventilator flow-time waveform. **A,** Sawtooth waveform. **B,** Normal waveform.

- The suction catheter should not be any larger than half of the internal diameter of the endotracheal or inner cannula of the tracheostomy tube (Table 8.1).
- Directional catheters are available for selective right or left mainstem bronchus suctioning. Straight catheters usually enter the right mainstem bronchus.[18,20,22]

EQUIPMENT

- Open technique
  - Suction catheter of appropriate size (see Table 8.1)
  - Sterile saline or sterile water solution
  - Sterile gloves
  - Sterile solution container
  - Source of suction (wall mounted or portable)
  - Suction canister
  - Connection tubing, generally 4 to 6 feet
  - Goggles and mask, or mask with eye shield. Open-suction technique is an aerosolizing procedure. Refer to institutional guidelines for isolation precautions and necessary personal protective equipment (PPE).

Additional equipment to have available as needed includes the following:

  - Self-inflating manual resuscitation bag-valve-mask device connected to an oxygen flow meter, set at 15 L/min (not recommended for patients on mechanical ventilation as a routine method to deliver hyperoxygenation breaths)
  - Positive end-expiratory pressure (PEEP) valve (for patients on >5 cm H_2O PEEP and who must be hyperoxygenated with a self-inflating manual resuscitation bag)
- Closed technique
  - Closed suction setup with a catheter of appropriate size (see Table 8.1)
  - Sterile saline solution (prepackaged bullets or syringes) (5 to 10 mL)
  - Individually packaged suction catheters for oral care
  - Source of suction (wall mounted or portable)
  - Suction canister
  - Connecting tube, generally 4 to 6 feet
  - Nonsterile gloves
  - Goggles and mask, or mask with eye shield. Although suctioning using the closed technique is not directly an aerosolizing procedure, there is potential for ventilator

disconnect. Refer to institutional guidelines for isolation precautions and necessary PPE.

PATIENT AND FAMILY EDUCATION

- Explain the procedure for endotracheal or tracheostomy tube suctioning to the patient and family. ***Rationale:*** The explanation reduces anxiety and allows for family members to step out if uncomfortable with the procedure.
- Explain that suctioning may be uncomfortable and could cause the patient to experience shortness of breath. ***Rationale:*** This information reduces anxiety and elicits patient cooperation.
- Explain the patient's role in assisting with secretion removal by coughing during the procedure. ***Rationale:*** This information encourages cooperation and facilitates removal of secretions. Participation in the procedure provides a sense of control for the patient.

PATIENT ASSESSMENT AND PREPARATION

Patient Assessment

- Assess for signs and symptoms of airway obstruction, including secretions in the airway, inspiratory wheezes, expiratory crackles, restlessness, ineffective coughing, decreased level of consciousness, decreased breath sounds, tachypnea, tachycardia or bradycardia, cyanosis, hypertension or hypotension, and shallow respirations. ***Rationale:*** Physical signs and symptoms result from inadequate gas exchange associated with airway obstruction.
- Note increased peak inspiratory pressures during volume ventilation, decreased tidal volume during pressure ventilation, or sawtooth pattern on the ventilator flow-time waveform. ***Rationale:*** These pressure changes may indicate potential secretions in the airway, increasing resistance to gas flow.
- Evaluate Spo_2 and Sao_2 levels. ***Rationale***: These values indicate potential secretions in the airway and impaired gas exchange.
- Assess signs and symptoms of inadequate breathing patterns, including dyspnea, shallow respirations, nasal flaring, intercostal and suprasternal retractions, frequent triggering of ventilator alarms, and increased respiratory rate. ***Rationale:*** Respiratory distress is a late sign of lower-airway obstruction.

TABLE 8.1	Guideline for Catheter Size for Endotracheal and Tracheostomy Tube Suctioning*			
Patient Age	Endotracheal Tube Size (mm)	Tracheostomy Tube Size (mm, Inner Diameter)	Suction Catheter Size
Small child (2–5 years)	4.0–5.0	3.0–5.5	6F to 8F
School-age child (6–12 years)	5.0–6.0	4.0–6.5	8F to 10F
Adolescent to adult	7.0–9.0	5.0–9.0	10F to 16F

*This guide should be used as an estimate only. Actual sizes depend on the size and individual needs of the patient. Always follow the manufacturer's recommendations.
Modified from St John RE, Seckel M: Airway management. In *AACN Protocols for Practice: Care of the Mechanically Ventilated Patient Series*. Sudbury, MA, 2007, Jones and Bartlett, p 41.

Patient Preparation

- Verify the correct patient with two identifiers. ***Rationale:*** Before performing a procedure, the nurse should ensure the correct identification of the patient for the intended intervention.
- Ensure that the patient understands preprocedural teachings. Answer questions as they arise, and reinforce information as needed. ***Rationale:*** This communication evaluates and reinforces understanding of previously taught information.

- Assist the patient in achieving a position that is comfortable for the patient and nurse, generally 30 degrees or higher, with the head of the bed elevated to the nurse's waist level. ***Rationale:*** This positioning promotes comfort, oxygenation, and ventilation, and it reduces strain.
- Secure additional personnel to assist with the self-inflating manual resuscitation bag-valve-mask device to provide hyperoxygenation (open-suction technique only) if utilized. ***Rationale:*** Two hands are necessary to inflate the self-inflating manual resuscitation bag-valve-mask device for adult tidal volume levels (>600 mL).

Procedure	for Endotracheal or Tracheostomy Tube Suctioning	
Steps	**Rationale**	**Special Considerations**
1. 🔲 HH		
2. 🔲 PE		Follow institutional guidelines regarding potential for aerosolization of secretions, and don appropriate PPE.
3. Turn on the suction apparatus, and set the vacuum regulator to 80–120 mm Hg. **(Level D*)**	The amount of suction applied should be only enough to remove secretions effectively. High negative-pressure settings >150 mm Hg may increase tracheal mucosal damage.[6,7,28,29,40]	Follow manufacturer's recommendations for suction pressure levels with closed-suction catheter systems. **(Level M*)**
4. Secure one end of the connection tubing to the suction source, and place the other end in a convenient location within reach.	Prepares suction apparatus.	
5. Monitor the patient's cardiopulmonary status before, during, and after the suctioning period. **(Level B*)**	Observes for signs and symptoms of complications: decreased arterial and mixed venous oxygen saturation, cardiac dysrhythmias, bronchospasm, respiratory distress, derecruitment, cyanosis, increased blood pressure or intracranial pressure, anxiety, pain, agitation, or changes in mental status.[4,6,11,16,17,21,23-27,29,32,33,36,45]	Development of cardiopulmonary instability, particularly cardiac dysrhythmias, or arterial desaturation, necessitates immediate termination of the suctioning procedure.
6a. Open-suction technique only A. Open the sterile catheter package on a clean surface, with the inside of the wrapping used as a sterile field.	Prepares catheter and prevents transmission of microorganisms.	
B. Depending on manufacturer, set up the sterile solution container on the sterile field. Use a prefilled solution container or an open empty container, taking care not to touch the inside of the container. Fill with approximately 100 mL of sterile normal saline solution or sterile water.	Prepares catheter flush solution.	

*Level D: Peer-reviewed professional and organizational standards with the support of clinical study recommendations.
*Level B: Well-designed, controlled studies with results that consistently support a specific action, intervention, or treatment.
*Level M: Manufacturer's recommendations only.

UNIT I

Procedure for Endotracheal or Tracheostomy Tube Suctioning—*Continued*		
Steps	Rationale	Special Considerations
C. Don sterile gloves.	Prevents contamination of the open sterile suction catheter.	If one sterile glove and one nonsterile glove are used, apply the nonsterile glove to the nondominant hand and the sterile glove to the dominant hand. Handle all nonsterile items with the nondominant (nonsterile) hand.
D. Pick up the suction catheter with care to avoid touching nonsterile surfaces. With the nondominant hand, pick up the connection tubing. Secure the suction catheter to the connection tubing.	Maintains catheter sterility. Connects the suction catheter and connecting tubing.	The dominant (sterile) hand should not come into contact with the nonsterile connecting tubing. Wrapping the suction catheter around the sterile dominant hand helps prevent inadvertent contamination of the catheter.
E. Check equipment for proper functioning by suctioning a small amount of sterile solution from the container. Proceed to **Step 7.**	Ensures that equipment is functioning properly.	
6b. Closed-suction technique only		
A. Connect the suction tubing to the closed-system suction port if not already connected, and unlock the thumb valve according to manufacturer and institutional guidelines. Proceed to **Step 7.**	Readies the suction setup for suctioning.	
7. Hyperoxygenate the patient for at least 30 seconds with one of the following three methods. **(Level B*)**	Hyperoxygenation with 100% oxygen is used to prevent a decrease in arterial oxygen levels during the suctioning procedure.[6,15-17,28,43]	Use of the ventilator to deliver the hyperoxygenation may be more effective in increasing arterial oxygen levels.[6,7,22,31]
A. Press the suction hyperoxygenation button on the ventilator with the nondominant hand. **(Level B)**	Hyperoxygenation with 100% oxygen is used to prevent a decrease in arterial oxygen levels during the suctioning procedure.[6,15-17,43]	
or		
B. Increase the baseline Fio$_2$ level on the mechanical ventilator to 100%. **(Level B)**	Hyperoxygenation with 100% oxygen is used to prevent a decrease in arterial oxygen levels during the suctioning procedure.[6,12,15-17,28,43]	With this method, caution must be used to return the Fio$_2$ to baseline levels after completion of suctioning.

*Level B: Well-designed, controlled studies with results that consistently support a specific action, intervention, or treatment.

Procedure continues on following page

Procedure for Endotracheal or Tracheostomy Tube Suctioning—*Continued*		
Steps	Rationale	Special Considerations

or

C. Disconnect the ventilator or gas-delivery tubing from the end of the endotracheal or tracheostomy tube, attach the self-inflating manual resuscitation bag-valve-mask device to the tube with the nondominant hand, and administer five to six breaths over 30 seconds. **(Level B*)**	Attach a PEEP valve to the self-inflating manual resuscitation bag-valve-mask device for patients on greater than 5 cm H_2O PEEP. Verify 100% oxygen delivery capabilities of manual resuscitation bag-valve-mask device by checking manufacturer's recommendations or with direct measurement with an in-line oxygen analyzer when baseline ventilator oxygen delivery to the patient is greater than 60%. Some self-inflating manual resuscitation bag-valve-mask device models entrain room air and deliver less than 100% oxygen.	Use of a second person to deliver hyperoxygenation breaths with the self-inflating manual resuscitation bag-valve-mask device significantly increases tidal volume delivery.[7,12-14,17,43] One-handed bagging rarely achieves adult tidal volume breaths (>500 mL).[12-14]
8. Open-suction technique and/or hyperoxygenation with self-inflating manual resuscitation bag-valve-mask device: Remove the ventilator circuit or self-inflating manual resuscitation bag-valve-mask device with the nondominant hand. Both open-suction and closed-suction techniques: With the control vent of the suction catheter open to air, gently but quickly insert the catheter with the dominant hand into the artificial airway until resistance is met, then pull back 1 cm before applying suction.[7,17,23,32,37,41] **(Level E*)**	Suction should be applied only as needed to remove secretions and for as short a time as possible to minimize decreases in arterial oxygen levels.	Minimally invasive suctioning has not been determined to be superior to current definitions of deep suctioning.[3,5,17,18,25,33,35] Deep suctioning has been defined as insertion of the suction catheter until resistance is met.[5,6,17]
9. Place the nondominant thumb over the control vent of the suction catheter to apply continuous or intermittent suction. Place and maintain the catheter between the dominant thumb and forefinger as you completely withdraw the catheter for less than or equal to 10 seconds into the sterile catheter sleeve (closed-suction technique) or out of the open airway (open-suction technique). **(Level B)**	Tracheal damage from suctioning is similar with intermittent or continuous suction.[9,17,19,22,24,31,32] **(Level C*)** Decreases in arterial oxygen levels during suctioning can be kept to a minimum with brief suction periods.[6,7,17,24,41] **(Level B)**	
10. Hyperoxygenate for 30 seconds as described in **Step 7. (Level B*)**	Hyperoxygenation with 100% oxygen is used to prevent a decrease in arterial oxygen levels during the suctioning procedure.[6,11,15-17,24,28,43]	

*Level B: Well-designed, controlled studies with results that consistently support a specific action, intervention, or treatment.
*Level C: Qualitative studies, descriptive or correlational studies, integrative reviews, systematic reviews, or randomized controlled trials with inconsistent results.

Procedure for Endotracheal or Tracheostomy Tube Suctioning—*Continued*		
Steps	**Rationale**	**Special Considerations**
11. One or two more passes of the suction catheter, as delineated in **Steps 8 and 9,** may be performed if secretions remain in the airway and the patient is tolerating the procedure. Provide 30 seconds of hyperoxygenation before and after each pass of the suction catheter (see **Step 7**).	The number of suction passes should be based on the amount of secretions and the patient's clinical assessment because of the risk of complications including pain and discomfort.[4,6,7,24,37,40,41] **(Level E*)** Hyperoxygenation with 100% oxygen is used to prevent a decrease in arterial oxygen levels during the suctioning procedure.[6,11,15-17,24,28,43] **(Level B*)**	Consider allowing the patient rest and hemodynamic recovery time after several suction catheter passes. Discuss with the team the treatment plan for excessive secretions.
12. If the patient does not tolerate suctioning despite hyperoxygenation, try the following steps:		
A. Ensure secure and correct connections in equipment and ensure that 100% oxygen is being delivered.	Hyperoxygenation with 100% oxygen is used to prevent a decrease in arterial oxygen levels during the suctioning procedure.[6,11,15-17,28,43] **(Level B*)**	
B. Ensure that the PEEP valve is attached properly to the self-inflating manual resuscitation bag-valve-mask device with use of that method for hyperoxygenation.	Maintenance of PEEP prevents collapse of alveoli during suctioning.	
C. Allow longer recovery intervals between suction passes.	Allows the patient to regain prior oxygenation levels.	
D. Hyperventilation may be used in situations in which the patient does not tolerate suctioning with hyperoxygenation alone, with either the self-inflating manual resuscitation bag-valve-mask device or the ventilator.	Because of the possibility of barotrauma, hyperventilation should be used only if the patient does not tolerate suctioning with hyperoxygenation alone.	Hyperinflation should be delivered by the ventilator to control pressures and avoid disconnection.[6,7] **(Level C*)**
13. When the airway has been cleared adequately of secretions, perform oropharyngeal suctioning as indicated or per institutional protocol. **(Level D*)** A. A separate suction catheter must be opened for this step with the closed-suction technique.	Suctioning of the oropharyngeal area if secretions are present may enhance patient comfort and should be part of an oral hygiene program.[1-3,39] After oropharyngeal suctioning, the suction catheter is contaminated with bacteria present in the oral cavity, potentially gram-negative bacilli, and should not be used for lower-airway suctioning[6,7,15,16,21] (see Procedure 3, Endotracheal Tube Care and Oral Care Practices for Ventilated and Nonventilated Patients)	Care should be taken to avoid oropharyngeal tissue trauma and gagging during suctioning.

*Level B: Well-designed, controlled studies with results that consistently support a specific action, intervention, or treatment.

*Level D: Peer-reviewed professional and organizational standards with the support of clinical study recommendations.

Procedure continues on following page

Procedure for Endotracheal or Tracheostomy Tube Suctioning—*Continued*

Steps	Rationale	Special Considerations
14. Rinse the catheter and connecting tubing with sterile saline or sterile water solution until clear. A. Open-suction technique: suction the unused sterile solution until tubing is clear. B. Closed-suction technique: instill sterile saline or water solution into the side port of the in-line suction catheter, taking care not to lavage down the endotracheal tube, while applying continuous suction until the catheter is clear.	Removes buildup of secretions in the connecting tubing and, with the closed-suction catheter system, in the in-line suction catheter.	
15. Open-suction technique only: on completion of upper-airway suctioning, wrap the catheter around the dominant hand. Pull the glove off inside out. The catheter should remain in the glove. Pull off the other glove in the same fashion, and discard it. Turn off the suction device.	Reduces transmission of microorganisms.	
16. Suction collection tubing and canisters may remain in use for multiple suctioning episodes.	Solutions and catheters that come in direct contact with the lower airways during suctioning must be sterile to decrease the risks for hospital-acquired pneumonia. Devices that are not in direct contact with the lower airways have not been shown to increase infection risk.[17] (**Level D***)	Refer to institutional standards on discarding multiuse sterile solution containers and equipment.
17. Remove PE and discard used supplies.		
18. HH		

*Level D: Peer-reviewed professional and organizational standards with the support of clinical study recommendations.

Expected Outcomes

- Removal of secretions from the large airways
- Improved gas exchange
- Airway patency
- Identification of clinical signs or symptoms of need for suctioning (e.g., adventitious breath sounds, coughing, high airway pressures)
- Sample for laboratory analysis

Unexpected Outcomes

- Cardiac dysrhythmias (premature atrial or ventricular contractions, tachycardias, bradycardias, heart blocks, asystole)
- Hypoxemia
- Bronchospasm
- Excessive increases in arterial blood pressure or intracranial pressure
- Hospital-acquired infections
- Cardiopulmonary distress
- Decreased level of consciousness
- Airway obstruction
- Pain or discomfort

Patient Monitoring and Care

Steps	Rationale	Reportable Conditions
		These conditions should be reported to the provider if they persist despite nursing interventions.
1. Monitor the patient's cardiopulmonary status before, during, and after the suctioning period. **(Level B*)**	Observes for signs and symptoms of complications.[4,6,7,11,16-19,21,23-27,29,32,33,35,38,44]	Decreased arterial or mixed venous oxygen saturation Cardiac dysrhythmias Bronchospasm Respiratory distress Cyanosis Increased blood pressure or intracranial pressure Anxiety, agitation, pain, or changes in mental status Diminished breath sounds Decreased oxygenation Increased peak airway pressures Coughing Increased work of breathing
2. Reassess the patient for signs of suctioning effectiveness.	Assesses effectiveness of intervention and the possible indications for further suctioning.	
3. Follow institutional guidelines for assessing pain. Administer analgesia as indicated.	Identifies the need for pain interventions.	Continued pain despite pain interventions

Documentation

Documentation should include the following:
- Patient and family education
- Presuctioning assessment, including clinical indication for suctioning
- Suctioning of endotracheal or tracheostomy tube
- Size of endotracheal or tracheostomy tube
- If a nonstandard suction catheter is required, it should be documented in the plan of care
- Pain assessment, interventions, and effectiveness
- Volume, color, consistency, and odor of secretions obtained
- Any difficulties during catheter insertion or hyperoxygenation
- Tolerance of suctioning procedure, including development of any unexpected outcomes during or after the procedure
- Nursing interventions
- Postsuctioning assessment

References and Additional Readings

For a complete list of references and additional readings for this procedure, scan this QR code with your smartphone, or visit https://www.elsevier.com/__data/assets/pdf_file/0005/1319783/Chapter0008.pdf

9 Surgical Cricothyrotomy (Perform)

Roger M. Casey

PURPOSE Surgical cricothyrotomy is an emergent procedure that is performed by making a skin incision that extends through the cricothyroid membrane to facilitate placement of an endotracheal or tracheostomy tube to provide effective oxygenation and ventilation.[2,3,5,6,11]

PREREQUISITE NURSING KNOWLEDGE

- Surgical cricothyrotomy is used only when the airway cannot be obtained or maintained by standard means such as bag-valve-mask device ventilation, the use of airway adjuncts (oropharyngeal or nasopharyngeal airway), endotracheal intubation, or rescue airways (supraglottic airway, esophageal-tracheal airway, or laryngeal mask airway [LMA]; Procedures 29, 7, 1, and 6, respectively). This procedure is often the last step of a difficult airway/cannot intubate/cannot ventilate algorithm.[5,6,8]
- A surgical cricothyrotomy may be preferable to an emergency tracheostomy as it is easier to perform, has less bleeding associated with it, and requires less time to perform.[1]
- Surgical cricothyrotomy may be necessary in patients with extensive facial and/or neck trauma. Injury to the facial structure may prevent control of the airway with a bag-valve-mask device as a result of an inadequate seal. Injuries may cause the airway to be obstructed or disrupted, making endotracheal intubation difficult or ineffective.
- An inability to obtain or maintain an airway may result from upper airway obstruction caused by trauma including surgery, allergic reactions with swelling and angioedema, foreign bodies, anatomical variations, tumors, or bleeding.[1]
- The need for emergent surgical cricothyrotomy must be determined quickly. This intervention is potentially life-saving, and implementation cannot be delayed.
- Commercially prepared cricothyrotomy kits are available and often use a specially designed airway and a modified Seldinger or percutaneous technique for insertion.
- This procedure is a low-volume, high-risk skill and requires continual training for successful completion.

 This procedure should be performed only by clinicians who have demonstrated competence and are credentialed to perform it. In addition, the procedure must be within the scope of practice defined by their professional licensure, and in accordance with professional practice acts. Physicians, advanced practice nurses, and physician assistants may be credentialed to perform this procedure.

Contraindications

Absolute
- Airway can be managed effectively with a bag-valve-mask device, intubation, or rescue airway such as a supraglottic airway, esophageal-tracheal airway, or LMA.[6,11]

Relative
- Complete transection of trachea[5,6,11]
- Laryngotracheal disruption with retraction of distal trachea[5,6,11]
- Anterior neck hematoma—preexisting pathology of larynx or trachea including hematoma, infection, tumor, or abscess occurring at or near the incision site[11]
- Coagulopathies[6]
- Fractured larynx with inability to identify anatomical landmarks[6,8,11]
- Lacerations of the structures of the neck[11]
- Massive neck swelling[11]
- Children younger than 12 years of age[2,5,6,11]

EQUIPMENT[3,6,11]

- Personal protective equipment (mask, eye protection, gown)
- Sterile surgical gloves
- Sterile surgical drape/towels
- Topical antiseptic solution (chlorhexidine preferred)[7,9,10,12]
- Topical/injectable anesthetic (e.g., lidocaine)
- Sedation and analgesic medications
- No. 10, 11, 15, or 20 scalpel blades
- 4 × 4 gauze sponges
- Suction and suction catheters (including Yankauer)
- Curved hemostats
- Tracheal hook
- Tracheal (Trousseau) dilator or nasal speculum
- Tracheal tube introducer (e.g., gum elastic bougie or guide wire)
- 5.0-mm to 6.0-mm cuffed endotracheal tube or 4.0-mm to 6.0-mm cuffed tracheostomy tube
- 14-gauge (or larger) over-the-needle intravenous catheter[2,6]

- 10-mL syringe
- Tracheostomy ties, sutures, or other securement devices
- Self-inflating manual resuscitation bag-valve-mask device with oxygen source
- Oxygen source and tubing
- Cardiac and pulse oximeter monitors
- End-tidal carbon dioxide ($ETCO_2$) detector
- Stethoscope

Additional equipment, to have available as needed, includes the following:

- Commercially prepared cricothyrotomy kit
- Ultrasound equipment (for use by experienced providers to identify the cricothyroid membrane)[11]
- Emergency airway cart and equipment determined by institutional procedure

PATIENT AND FAMILY EDUCATION

- As time permits, assess the patient's and family's level of understanding about the condition and rationale for the procedure. Often the emergent conditions in which this procedure is performed will preclude a discussion of the procedure, risks, benefits, and complications. These discussions may be held with the patient and/or family in patients who are predicted to have a difficult airway.[11] *Rationale:* This assessment identifies the patient's and family's knowledge deficits concerning the patient's condition, the procedure, the expected benefits, and the potential risks. It also allows time for questions to clarify information and discuss concerns, with the goal of decreasing patient anxiety and enhancing cooperation.
- Family members should be provided with a quick and concise explanation of the emergent need to obtain an airway. This information may be explained by another member of the healthcare team to prevent delay in establishing the airway. If possible, obtain consent for the procedure from the family member. *Rationale:* This explanation enhances patient and family understanding and decreases anxiety.
- A patient who needs emergency surgical cricothyrotomy is likely unresponsive from the inability to maintain the airway and adequate oxygenation and ventilation; therefore patient education may not be possible. *Rationale:* The emergency nature of the procedure may preclude patient education.

PATIENT ASSESSMENT AND PREPARATION

Patient Assessment

- Assess airway patency.
  - ❖ Open the airway with the jaw-thrust or chin-lift maneuver. If traumatic injury is suspected, maintain cervical stabilization. *Rationale:* Allows for visualization of the airway for foreign bodies, secretions, or other obstructions.
  - ❖ Assess for presence of foreign bodies, secretions, or other obstructions. Use suction, basic life support (BLS) maneuvers, or Magill forceps to clear and maintain the airway. *Rationale:* Often airway patency can be achieved

and maintained with simple maneuvers such as patient positioning, use of an airway maneuver, suction, or insertion of an oral or nasal pharyngeal airway. If the patient has potential for airway compromise (i.e., bleeding, swelling, or traumatic injuries) but is alert and able to maintain the airway, allow the patient to maintain a position of comfort and suction to maintain a patent airway.
  - ❖ If the airway is maintained, do not attempt to place the patient in the supine position, because this may cause significant airway compromise. *Rationale:* If the patient has the ability to maintain an airway, allowing the patient to remain in an upright position, with suction provided, if necessary, assist the patient in maintaining the airway. If the patient is placed in the supine position for packaging or transport, this move may cause significant airway compromise.
- Assess respiratory effort.
  - ❖ Assess rate, depth of respirations, accessory muscle use, chest wall motion, and breath sounds. *Rationale:* This process is to identify inadequate respiratory efforts quickly and determine the optimal method for oxygenation and ventilation.
  - ❖ Monitor oxygen saturation and end-tidal carbon dioxide ($ETCO_2$), if available. If respiratory efforts are inadequate, attempt ventilation with a bag-valve-mask device and supplemental oxygen. If an airway cannot be maintained or oxygenation and ventilation with a bag-valve-mask device are inadequate, prepare for endotracheal intubation. *Rationale:* This process is to identify inadequate respiratory efforts quickly to determine the optimal method for oxygenation and ventilation.
  - ❖ If intubation is not possible and other means to manage an airway are not effective, prepare for emergent surgical cricothyrotomy. *Rationale:* This process is to identify inadequate respiratory efforts quickly and determine the optimal method for oxygenation and ventilation.
  - ❖ Assess the patient's neurological status. *Rationale:* The patient may require sedation or analgesia depending on neurological status and the emergent nature of the procedure.

Patient Preparation

- Verify the correct patient with two identifiers. *Rationale:* Before performing a procedure, the nurse should ensure the correct identification of the patient for the intended intervention.
- Perform a pre-procedure verification and time out, if non-emergent. *Rationale:* Ensures patient safety.
- Position the patient supine, and maintain cervical spine stabilization if indicated. Once manual stabilization is in place, the anterior portion of the collar can be removed for the procedure. *Rationale:* Patients who need emergent surgical cricothyrotomy often have traumatic injuries that necessitate cervical spine stabilization.
- Continue attempts to ventilate and oxygenate the patient with a bag-valve-mask device by any means possible if the patient is apneic or respiratory efforts are inadequate. *Rationale:* This action can mitigate further hypoxia and hypercarbia.

Procedure	for Surgical Cricothyrotomy	
Steps	**Rationale**	**Special Considerations**
1. 🅷🅷		
2. 🅿🅴		In addition to sterile drapes, gowns, and gloves, the use of a face mask and eye protection is recommended because of the increased risk of airborne blood or body fluids during this procedure.
3. Consider local anesthesia, sedation, and/or analgesia		Under emergency situations, there may not be time to administer medications. However, if the patient is agitated or struggling, sedation and/or analgesia may be necessary to secure the airway.
4. Place the patient in the supine position with the head and neck in neutral position.	Positions the patient to expose the neck and larynx.	Maintain manual cervical spine stabilization for patients with suspected cervical spine injury. Once manual stabilization is in place, the anterior portion of the collar can be removed for the procedure.
5. Identify the cricothyroid membrane (Fig. 9.1). First, identify the thyroid prominence, or Adam's apple. The cricothyroid membrane is a depression that is palpated in the midline, approximately one fingerbreadth below the thyroid prominence between the cricoid and thyroid cartilage. **(Level D*)**	Identifies the correct location for incision and endotracheal tube placement. The cricothyroid membrane is preferred over the trachea because it is more anterior than the lower trachea, and less thyroid and soft tissue are found between the membrane and the skin. Additionally, there is less vascularity, leading to less significant chance of bleeding.[1,2,6,11]	The incision is just inferior to the vocal cords and superior to the thyroid gland.[1,2,6,11]

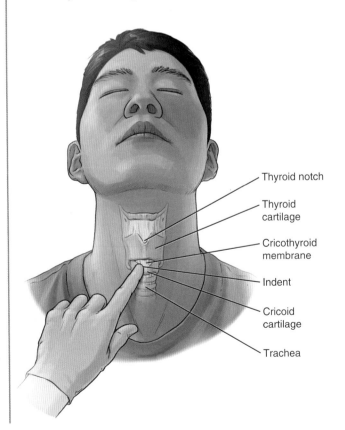

Thyroid notch

Thyroid cartilage

Cricothyroid membrane

Indent

Cricoid cartilage

Trachea

Figure 9.1 Anatomy of the neck and location of the cricothyroid membrane. *(From Committee on Advanced Trauma Life Support: ATLS of the American College of Surgeons [ACS]. ATLS advanced trauma life support: Student course manual, ed 10, 2018. American College of Surgeons.)*

Procedure continues on following page

Procedure for Surgical Cricothyrotomy—*Continued*

Steps	Rationale	Special Considerations
6. Prepare the skin with a topical antiseptic solution. **(Level A*)**	Decreases potential for wound infection.	Evidence suggests that chlorhexidine is a better topical antiseptic than povidone iodine[7,9,10,12]
7. Immobilize the larynx by placing the thumb and middle finger on both sides of the trachea and stretching the skin with the thumb and middle finger to make it taut and stabilize the larynx.	Allows for ease in creating an incision in the skin and keeps the larynx from shifting.	Throughout the procedure, the larynx must be immobilized.
8. Make a 2-cm vertical midline incision through the dermis, over the cricothyroid membrane.	Overly deep or long incisions risk damage to the larynx, cricoid cartilage, and trachea.	Avoid directing the scalpel toward the head, as this may cause laceration of the vocal cords.[6,11] Some references recommend an additional horizontal skin incision[5,6,11]; however, care should be taken as a horizontal incision may cause injury to lateral vascular structures.[3]
9. Dab the wound with sterile gauze to control any bleeding from the incision.	Use a dabbing technique to minimize further tissue trauma and bleeding.	Use an assistant, if available, to control bleeding and minimize interruptions in the procedure.
10. Identify the cricothyroid membrane. Palpate the cricothyroid membrane through the skin incision with the index finger. If necessary, use the curved hemostats to bluntly dissect along the vertical incision and visualize the cricothyroid membrane. **(Level D*)**	Blunt dissection is preferred over sharp dissection to minimize further tissue trauma and bleeding.	The index finger can be placed on the inferior aspect of the thyroid cartilage to identify the superior border of the cricothyroid membrane.[1,2,6,11]
11. Make a horizontal stab incision, palpate the membrane, and then incise horizontally (Fig. 9.2).	Incising the lower half of the membrane is preferred to avoid the superior cricothyroid artery and vein. The opening must be large enough to accommodate a 5- to 6-mm cuffed endotracheal or No. 4 to No. 6 tracheostomy tube. A stablike incision may also puncture the posterior wall of the trachea and lacerate the esophagus and could lacerate or damage the vocal cords.	The incision should be approximately 1–1.5 cm in length. Do not attempt to puncture the cricothyroid membrane. Use the scalpel to gently incise only the membrane.
12. Dab the wound with sterile gauze to control any bleeding from the incision.	Use a dabbing technique to minimize further tissue trauma and bleeding.	Use an assistant, if available, to control bleeding and minimize interruptions in the procedure.
13. Consider utilizing the tracheal hook to maintain the opening and insert the tracheal dilator or nasal speculum into the opening in the cricothyroid membrane. Direct the tip of the speculum toward the patient's feet.	Avoids further trauma to the cricothyroid membrane or vocal cords and guides the tube into the airway.	
14. Carefully spread the dilator or speculum vertically, and advance the tube into the opening. If resistance is met, do not force the tube into the opening.	The dilator or speculum enlarges the opening vertically, but caution should be used to avoid further trauma to the cricothyroid membrane. Care must be taken to ensure that there is an instrument in the airway at all times so as not to allow the cricothyroid incision to close.	The tube should advance easily into the tracheal opening.

Procedure	for Surgical Cricothyrotomy—*Continued*	
Steps	**Rationale**	**Special Considerations**

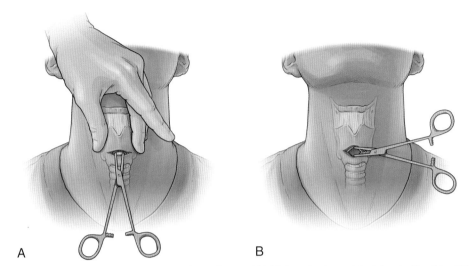

Figure 9.2 Incising the cricothyroid membrane. (A) Make a horizontal incision to the skin. (B) Make a horizontal incision in the cricothyroid membrane. *(From Committee on Advanced Trauma Life Support: ATLS of the American College of Surgeons [ACS]. ATLS advanced trauma life support: Student course manual, ed 10, 2018. American College of Surgeons, p 37.)*

Steps	Rationale	Special Considerations
15. Carefully remove the tracheal hook and tracheal dilator or nasal speculum once the tube has been placed in the trachea, taking care not to break the balloon.	Use caution to avoid inadvertent removal of the tube along with the dilator or speculum.	
16. Inflate the tube cuff with the syringe to a minimal occlusive pressure.	Prevents air leak and optimizes oxygenation and ventilation.	
17. Attach the bag-valve-mask device to the tube, and oxygenate and ventilate the patient.		
18. Auscultate for the presence of equal breath sounds and the absence of epigastric sounds with a stethoscope. Observe chest rise and fall.	The tube position may be confirmed with the same methods as used for oral or nasal endotracheal tube placement (see Procedure 1, Endotracheal Intubation).	Primary confirmation relies on physical examination techniques to confirm correct tube placement.[6,11]
19. Confirm correct placement such as an exhaled CO_2 detector or monitoring device. Obtain chest radiography.	Tube position may be confirmed with the same methods as oral or nasal endotracheal tube placement.	Confirmation verifies correct tube placement.[6,11]
20. Secure the tube with tracheostomy ties or another securement device. Apply dressing with gauze and tape or per institutional guidelines (see Procedure 11, Tracheostomy Cuff and Tube Care).	Prevents dislodgment or movement of tube.	Use a square knot to secure the tracheostomy ties.
21. Dispose of supplies.		
22. **HH**		

*Level A: Meta-analysis of quantitative studies or metasynthesis of qualitative studies with results that consistently support a specific action, intervention, or treatment (including systematic review of randomized controlled trials.)

*Level D: Peer-reviewed professional and organizational standards with the support of clinical study recommendations.

Expected Outcomes

- Establishment of emergent surgical airway access
- Adequate oxygenation and ventilation
- Improved or stabilized patient condition

Unexpected Outcomes[4,6,11]

- Blood loss or hemorrhage
- Aspiration or asphyxia
- False passage of the endotracheal tube into the subcutaneous tissue or esophagus [6,11]
- Tracheal perforation
- Esophageal perforation
- Subcutaneous emphysema
- Mediastinal emphysema
- Vocal cord injury or paralysis
- Tracheal stenosis (delayed)

Patient Monitoring and Care[6,11]

Steps	Rationale	Reportable Conditions
		These conditions should be reported to the provider if they persist despite nursing interventions.
1. Monitor breath sounds, adequacy of oxygenation and ventilation, and oxygen saturation (SpO_2). Consider continuous capnography.	Monitors effectiveness of airway, oxygenation, and ventilation.	Decreased or absent breath sounds Sudden or progressive decrease in SpO_2 Inability to ventilate Decrease or loss of $ETCO_2$
2. Monitor endotracheal or tracheostomy tube position and securement. Note the centimeter (cm) mark on the tube.	Prevents movement or dislodgment of the tube.	Change in position or measurement of the tube Dislodgment or removal of the tube
3. Observe the insertion site for bleeding, swelling, or subcutaneous air.	Identifies injury, malposition, or air leak.	Excessive bleeding from the site Swelling or subcutaneous air at the insertion site
4. Follow institutional standards for assessing pain. Administer analgesia as indicated.	Identifies the need for pain interventions.	Continued pain despite pain interventions

Documentation

Documentation should include the following:
- Assessment findings to support the need for an emergent surgical airway
- Inability to obtain or maintain an airway and provide oxygenation and ventilation by any other means
- Size and type of endotracheal/tracheostomy tube inserted and centimeter mark at skin opening
- Confirmation of proper tube placement with both primary and secondary means
- Pain and sedation assessments, interventions, and effectiveness to include any sedative agents or analgesic agents used
- Documentation of the procedure including obtaining consent, if possible, and confirming patient identification, the procedure being performed, and the procedure date and time[11]
- Vital signs before, during, and after procedure
- Ventilator settings
- Any complications encountered during the procedure

References and Additional Readings

For a complete list of references and additional readings for this procedure, scan this QR code with your smartphone, or visit https://www.elsevier.com/__data/assets/pdf_file/0006/1319784/Chapter0009.pdf

10 Surgical Cricothyrotomy (Assist)

Roger M. Casey

PURPOSE Surgical cricothyrotomy is an emergent procedure that is performed by making a skin incision that extends through the cricothyroid membrane to facilitate placement of an endotracheal or tracheostomy tube to provide effective oxygenation and ventilation.[2,3,5,6,11]

PREREQUISITE NURSING KNOWLEDGE

- Surgical cricothyrotomy is used only when the airway cannot be obtained or maintained by standard means such as bag-valve-mask device ventilation, the use of airway adjuncts (oropharyngeal or nasopharyngeal airway), endotracheal intubation, or rescue airways (supraglottic airway, esophageal-tracheal airway, or laryngeal mask airway [LMA]; Procedures 29, 7, 1, and 6, respectively). This procedure is often the last step of a difficult airway/cannot intubate, cannot ventilate algorithm.[5,6,8]
- A surgical cricothyrotomy may be preferable to an emergency tracheostomy, as it is easier to perform, has less bleeding associated with it, and requires less time to perform.[1]
- Surgical cricothyrotomy may be necessary in patients with extensive facial and/or neck trauma. Injury to the facial structure may prevent control of the airway with a bag-valve-mask device as a result of inadequate seal. Injuries may cause the airway to be obstructed or disrupted, making endotracheal intubation difficult or ineffective.
- An inability to obtain or maintain an airway may result from upper airway obstruction as a result of trauma including surgery, allergic reactions with swelling and angioedema, foreign bodies, anatomical variations, tumors, or bleeding.[1]
- The need for emergent surgical cricothyrotomy must be determined quickly. This intervention is potentially lifesaving, and implementation cannot be delayed.
- Surgical cricothyrotomy requires specialized training and should be performed only by physicians, advanced practice nurses, and other healthcare professionals (including critical care nurses and trained transport personnel) with additional knowledge, skills, and demonstrated competence per professional licensure or institutional/organizational standards.[4,8]
- Commercially prepared cricothyrotomy kits are available and often use a specially designed airway and modified Seldinger or percutaneous technique for insertion.
- This procedure is a low-volume, high-risk skill and requires continual training for successful completion.

Contraindications

Absolute
- Airway can be managed effectively with a bag-valve-mask device, intubation, or rescue airway such as a supraglottic airway, esophageal-tracheal airway, or LMA.[6,11]

Relative
- Complete transection of trachea[5,6,11]
- Laryngotracheal disruption with retraction of distal trachea[5,6,11]
- Anterior neck hematoma—preexisting pathology of larynx or trachea including hematoma, infection, tumor, or abscess occurring at or near the incision site[11]
- Coagulopathies[6]
- Fractured larynx with inability to identify anatomical landmarks[6,8,11]
- Lacerations of the structures of the neck[11]
- Massive neck swelling[11]
- Children younger than 12 years of age[2,5,6,11]

EQUIPMENT[3,6,11]

- Personal protective equipment (mask, eye protection, gown)
- Sterile surgical gloves
- Sterile surgical drape/towels
- Topical antiseptic solution (chlorhexidine preferred)[7,9,10,12]
- Topical/injectable anesthetic (e.g., lidocaine)
- Sedation and analgesic medications
- No. 10, 11, 15, or 20 scalpel blades
- 4 × 4 gauze sponges
- Suction device and suction catheter (including Yankauer)
- Curved hemostats
- Tracheal hook
- Tracheal (Trousseau) dilator or nasal speculum
- Tracheal tube introducer (e.g., gum elastic bougie or guide wire)
- 5.0-mm to 6.0-mm cuffed endotracheal tube or 4.0-mm to 6.0-mm cuffed tracheostomy tube
- 14-gauge or larger over-the-needle intravenous catheter[2,6]
- 10-mL syringe
- Tracheostomy ties, sutures, or other securement devices
- Self-inflating manual resuscitation bag-valve-mask device

- Oxygen source and tubing
- Cardiac and pulse oximeter monitors
- End-tidal carbon dioxide ($ETco_2$) detector
- Stethoscope
Additional equipment, to have available as needed, includes the following:
- Commercially prepared cricothyrotomy kit
- Ultrasound equipment (for use by experienced providers to identify the cricothyroid membrane)[11]
- Emergency airway cart and equipment determined by institutional procedure

PATIENT AND FAMILY EDUCATION

- As time permits, assess the patient's and family's level of understanding about the condition and rationale for the procedure. Often the emergent conditions in which this procedure is performed will preclude a discussion of the procedure, risks, benefits, and complications. These discussions may be held with the patient and/or family in patients who are predicted to have a difficult airway.[11] *Rationale:* This assessment identifies the patient's and family's knowledge deficits concerning the patient's condition, the procedure, the expected benefits, and the potential risks. It also allows time for questions to clarify information and discuss concerns, with the goal of decreasing patient anxiety and enhancing cooperation.
- Family members should be provided with a quick and concise explanation of the emergent need to obtain an airway. This information may be explained by another member of the healthcare team rather than the provider performing the procedure to prevent delay in establishing the airway. If possible, obtain consent for the procedure from the family member. *Rationale:* This explanation enhances patient and family understanding and decreases anxiety.
- A patient who needs emergency surgical cricothyrotomy is likely unresponsive from the inability to maintain the airway and adequate oxygenation and ventilation; therefore patient education may not be possible. *Rationale:* The emergent nature of the procedure may preclude patient education.

PATIENT ASSESSMENT AND PREPARATION

Patient Assessment

- Assess airway patency.
  - Open the airway with the jaw-thrust or chin-lift maneuver. If traumatic injury is suspected, maintain cervical stabilization. *Rationale:* Allows for visualization of the airway for foreign bodies, secretions, or other obstructions.
  - Assess for presence of foreign bodies, secretions, or other obstructions. Use suction, basic life support (BLS) maneuvers, or Magill forceps to clear and maintain the airway. *Rationale:* Often airway patency can be achieved and maintained with simple maneuvers

such as patient positioning, use of an airway maneuver, suction, or insertion of an oral or nasal pharyngeal airway. If the patient has potential for airway compromise (i.e., bleeding, swelling, or traumatic injuries) but is alert and able to maintain the airway, allow the patient to maintain a position of comfort, and suction to maintain a patent airway.
  - If airway is able to be maintained, do not attempt to place the patient in the supine position because this may cause significant airway compromise. *Rationale:* If the patient has the ability to maintain an airway, allowing the patient to remain in an upright position, with suction provided, if necessary, assists the patient in maintaining the airway. If the patient is placed in the supine position for transport, this move may cause significant airway compromise.
- Assess respiratory effort.
  - Assess rate, depth of respirations, accessory muscle use, chest wall motion, and breath sounds. *Rationale:* This process is to identify inadequate respiratory efforts quickly and determine the optimal method for providing oxygenation and ventilation.
  - Monitor oxygen saturation and end-tidal carbon dioxide ($ETco_2$), if available. If respiratory efforts are inadequate, attempt ventilation with a self-inflating manual resuscitation bag-valve-mask device and supplemental oxygen. *Rationale:* This process is to identify inadequate respiratory efforts quickly to determine the optimal method for providing oxygenation and ventilation.
  - If intubation is not possible and other means to manage an airway are not effective, prepare for emergent surgical cricothyrotomy. *Rationale:* This process is to identify inadequate respiratory efforts quickly and determine the optimal method for providing oxygenation and ventilation.
  - Assess the patient's neurological status. *Rationale:* The patient may require sedation or analgesia depending on neurological status and the emergent nature of the procedure.

Patient Preparation

- Verify the correct patient with two identifiers. *Rationale:* Before performing a procedure, the nurse should ensure the correct identification of the patient for the intended intervention.
- Perform a preprocedure verification and time out, if nonemergent. *Rationale:* Ensures patient safety.
- Position the patient supine, and maintain cervical spine stabilization if indicated. Once manual stabilization is in place, the anterior portion of the collar can be removed for the procedure. *Rationale:* Patients who need emergent surgical cricothyrotomy often have traumatic injuries that require cervical spine stabilization.
- Continue attempts to ventilate and oxygenate the patient with a self-inflating manual resuscitation bag-valve-mask device if the patient is apneic or respiratory efforts are inadequate. *Rationale:* This action can prevent further hypoxia and hypercarbia.

Procedure for Assisting With Surgical Cricothyrotomy		
Steps	Rationale	Special Considerations
1. [HH]		
2. [PE]		In addition to sterile drapes, gowns, and gloves, the use of a face mask and eye protection is recommended because of the increased risk of airborne blood or body fluids during this procedure.
3. Consider local anesthesia, sedation, and/or analgesia		Under emergency situations, there may not be time to administer medications. However, if the patient is agitated or struggling, sedation and/or analgesia may be necessary to secure the airway.
4. Place the patient in the supine position, with the head and neck in neutral position.	Position the patient to expose the neck and larynx.	Maintain manual cervical spine stabilization for patients with suspected cervical spine injury. Once manual stabilization is in place, the anterior portion of the collar can be removed for the procedure.
5. If one assistant (assistant A) is available, continue attempts to oxygenate and ventilate the patient with a bag-valve-mask device.	Prevents further hypoxia and hypercarbia. Use of an assistant minimizes interruptions in the procedure.	Maintain a sterile field, and anticipate the needs of the person performing the procedure. Use caution when handling equipment to prevent contamination or inadvertent injury.
6. If a second assistant (assistant B) is available, assist the person performing the procedure.		
7. The person performing the procedure locates the cricothyroid membrane (Fig. 10.1), prepares the skin with a topical antiseptic solution, and makes an incision through the skin. (**Level A***)	Identifies the correct location for incision and tube placement. The cricothyroid membrane is preferred over the trachea because it is more anterior than the lower trachea, and less thyroid and soft tissue are found between the membrane and the skin.[1,2,11,6,11]	The incision is just inferior to the vocal cords and superior to the thyroid gland.[1,2,6,11] Evidence indicates that chlorhexidine is a better topical antiseptic than povidone iodine.[7,9,10,12]
8. Assistant B uses gauze sponges and a dabbing technique to control any bleeding from the incision, when asked by the person performing the procedure.	A dabbing technique minimizes further tissue trauma and bleeding. Only assist with blood loss control when asked to avoid contact with the scalpel.	If a second assistant is not available, the primary assistant should continue to attempt to ventilate the patient.
9. The person performing the procedure makes a stab incision in the cricothyroid membrane with the scalpel. Assistant B prepares the curved hemostats that may be needed to bluntly dissect the skin to locate and visualize the cricothyroid membrane.	Discontinuing ventilations minimizes airborne contamination when the cricothyroid membrane is incised. Blunt dissection is preferred over sharp dissection to minimize further tissue trauma and bleeding.	Assistant A stops ventilations just before the incision is being made.
10. Assistant B prepares the endotracheal or tracheostomy tube and tracheal dilator or nasal speculum for the person performing the procedure.	Enlarging the opening in the cricothyroid membrane allows passage of the tube.	Assistant A continues to hold ventilation attempts until the tube is placed.

Procedure continues on following page

Procedure **for Assisting With Surgical Cricothyrotomy—***Continued*

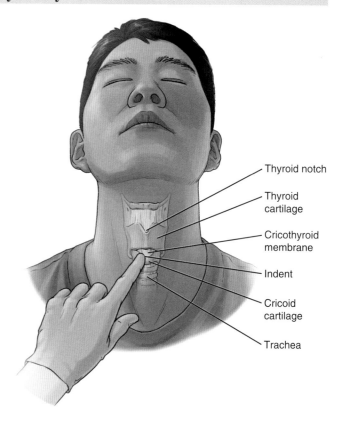

Thyroid notch

Thyroid cartilage

Cricothyroid membrane

Indent

Cricoid cartilage

Trachea

Figure 10.1 Anatomy of the neck and location of the cricothyroid membrane. *(From Committee on Advanced Trauma Life Support. ATLS of the American College of Surgeons [ACS].* ATLS advanced trauma life support: Student course manual, *ed 10, 2018. American College of Surgeons, p 37.)*

Procedure **for Assisting With Surgical Cricothyrotomy—***Continued*

Steps	Rationale	Special Considerations
11. Assistant B uses the syringe to inflate the tube cuff to a minimal occlusive pressure once the tube is placed.	Prevents an air leak and optimizes oxygenation and ventilation.	
12. Assistant A attaches the bag-valve-mask device to the tube and oxygenates and ventilates the patient. Assistant B manually stabilizes the tube.	Prevents inadvertent movement or displacement of the tube.	
13. Auscultate for the presence of equal breath sounds and the absence of epigastric sounds with a stethoscope. Observe chest rise and fall.	The tube position may be confirmed with the same methods as oral or nasal endotracheal tube placement (see Procedure 2, Endotracheal Intubation).	Primary confirmation relies on physical examination techniques to confirm correct tube placement.[6,11]
14. Confirm correct placement such as an exhaled CO_2 detector or monitoring device. Obtain chest radiography.	The tube position may be confirmed with the same methods as used for oral or nasal endotracheal tube placement.	Confirmation verifies correct tube placement.[6,11]
15. Secure the tube with tracheostomy ties or other securement device. Apply dressing with gauze and tape or per institutional guidelines (see Procedure 11, Tracheostomy Cuff and Tube Care).	Prevents dislodgment or movement of tube.	Use a square knot to secure the tracheostomy ties.
16. Dispose of supplies.		
17. 🄷🄷		

*Level A: Meta-analysis of quantitative studies or metasynthesis of qualitative studies with results that consistently support a specific action, intervention, or treatment (including systematic review of randomized controlled trials.

Expected Outcomes

- Establishment of emergent surgical airway access
- Provision of adequate oxygenation and ventilation
- Improved or stabilized patient condition

Unexpected Outcomes[4,6,11]

- Blood loss or hemorrhage
- Aspiration or asphyxia
- False passage of the endotracheal tube into the subcutaneous tissue or esophagus[6,11]
- Tracheal perforation
- Esophageal perforation
- Subcutaneous emphysema
- Mediastinal emphysema
- Vocal cord injury or paralysis
- Tracheal stenosis (delayed)

Patient Monitoring and Care[6,11]

Steps	Rationale	Reportable Conditions
		These conditions should be reported to the provider if they persist despite nursing interventions.
1. Monitor breath sounds, adequacy of oxygenation and ventilation, and oxygen saturation (SpO_2). Consider continuous capnography.	Monitors effectiveness of airway, oxygenation, and ventilation.	Decreased or absent breath sounds Sudden or progressive decrease in SpO_2 Inability to ventilate Decrease or loss of $ETCO_2$
2. Monitor endotracheal or tracheostomy tube position and securement. Note the centimeter (cm) mark on the tube.	Prevents movement or dislodgment of the tube.	Change in position or measurement of the tube Dislodgment or removal of the tube
3. Observe the insertion site for bleeding, swelling, or subcutaneous air.	Identifies injury, malposition, or air leak.	Excessive bleeding from the site Swelling or subcutaneous air at the insertion site
4. Follow institutional standards for assessing pain. Administer analgesia as indicated.	Identifies the need for pain interventions.	Continued pain despite pain interventions

Documentation

Documentation should include the following:

- Assessment findings to support the need for an emergent surgical airway
- Inability to obtain or maintain an airway and provide oxygenation and ventilation by other means
- Size and type of endotracheal/tracheostomy tube inserted and centimeter mark at skin opening
- Confirmation of proper tube placement by both primary and secondary means
- Pain and sedation assessments, interventions, and effectiveness to include and sedative agents or analgesic agents used
- Documentation of the procedure including obtaining consent, if possible, confirming patient identification, the procedure being performed, and the procedure date and time[11]
- Vital signs before, during, and after the procedure
- Ventilator settings
- Any complications encountered during the procedure

References and Additional Readings

For a complete list of references and additional readings for this procedure, scan this QR code with your smartphone, or visit https://www.elsevier.com/__data/assets/pdf_file/0007/1319785/Chapter0010.pdf

11 Tracheostomy Cuff and Tube Care

Heather L. Przybyl

PURPOSE: Tracheostomy tube care including care of the tracheal tube cuff, inner cannula, and outer cannula of the tracheal tube; site care including tracheal dressing and securement; and prevention of complications.

- Care of the tracheostomy tube maintains an adequate airway seal (if a cuffed tube is needed), tracheal tube patency, and patency of the stoma.[5]
- Adequate cuff inflation may decrease the risk of aspiration of some particles.
- Site care includes assessing the tracheal dressing and changing it to maintain skin integrity, prevent device-related pressure injuries, and decrease the risk of infection.
- Securement devices such as sutures, a tracheostomy tube holder, and ties help maintain stability of the tracheal tube and prevent tube dislodgement.

PREREQUISITE NURSING KNOWLEDGE

- *Tracheotomy* refers to a procedure that directly connects the trachea to the exterior neck.[9,30]
- *Tracheostomy* refers to a procedure to create a temporary or permanent opening (stoma) made by the incision. The tracheostomy creates an opening below the cricoid cartilage through the second to fourth tracheal rings (Fig. 11.1), producing a more permanent fistula or opening.[9,21,33,35]
- The terms *tracheotomy* and *tracheostomy* are often used interchangeably.[28]
- Tracheostomies are one of the most commonly performed procedures in critical care.[5,8,28,35,46]
- A *tracheostoma* is a permanent opening in the trachea through the neck. This term usually refers to the permanent opening that is made after a permanent laryngectomy.[9]
- A *tracheostomy tube* is an artificial airway inserted into the tracheotomy (Fig. 11.2).
- Surgical access to the trachea can be accomplished the following ways[30]:
  - Surgical tracheostomy.[15,16,30,37]
    - Elective or emergent tracheotomy may be performed in the operating room or at the bedside
  - Percutaneous tracheostomy (PT) or percutaneous dilational tracheostomy (PDT).[15,16,37]
    - These procedures are commonly performed at the bedside in a nonemergent basis for patients receiving mechanical ventilation.[30]
    - A flexible or rigid video-endoscope is used to visualize the airway and aid in placement of the tracheotomy.[30]

- Tracheostomy: indications, benefits, surgical approaches, and complications
  - Compared with endotracheal tubes, tracheostomy tubes provide added benefits to patients. (Box 11.1).
  - A tracheotomy is performed as either an elective or emergent procedure. Box 11.2 provides indications for tracheotomy. There is no standard time frame when a tracheotomy should be performed. The decision is based on the projected length of time that mechanical ventilation or an artificial airway is required to remain in place.
  - A tracheostomy tube is the preferred method of airway maintenance in patients who may require long-term mechanical ventilation for more than 10 to 21 days.[3,7,9,17,28,33,35,41,51]
  - Studies have been conflicted about whether early tracheostomy improves outcomes such as mortality, ventilator days, and so on, but may decrease the need for sedation.[3,7,9,28,34,41,51]
  - Surgical placement is performed under general anesthesia. Using an open surgical technique, a stoma is created. The trachea is visualized by the surgeon. Landmarks are identified by the surgeon, and an incision is made below the cricoid cartilage. The isthmus of the thyroid gland is exposed, cross-clamped, and ligated.[7,9,16,21,30]
  - A Bjork flap may be created. The flap is created when a small portion of the tracheal cartilage is pulled down and sutured to the skin. The flap helps facilitate reinsertion of the tracheostomy tube if it is dislodged, especially in patients who may be obese or have difficult anatomy.[7,19,21,28,30]
  - Percutaneous tracheotomy has been proven to be a safe alternative to surgical tracheostomy on mechanically ventilated patients.[15,24,37] Unlike surgical tracheotomy, percutaneous tracheotomy can be performed without direct visualization of the trachea.[9,15,30] A bronchoscope may or may not be used to assist with visualization during the procedure. A needle is passed into the trachea. A J-tipped guidewire is placed into the trachea, the incision is then the dilated, and the tracheostomy tube is placed.[9,30]
  - Initial tracheostomy securement can be achieved using commercial securement devices or sutures to secure the

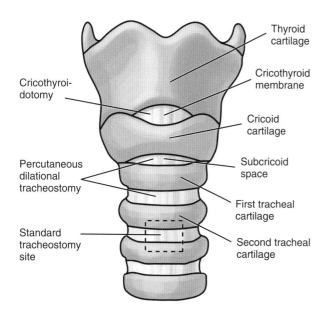

Figure 11.1 Sites for tracheostomy insertion. *(From Serra A: Tracheostomy care. Nurs Stand 14[42]:45–55, 2000.)*

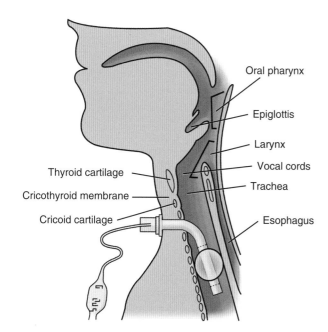

Figure 11.2 A tracheostomy (sometimes called a *tracheotomy*) is created surgically by making an opening through the skin of the neck into the trachea. *(From Serra A: Tracheostomy care. Nurs Stand 14[42]:45–55, 2000.)*

tracheostomy flange to the patient's skin. There are no recommendations related to the type of suture, number of sutures to utilize, or technique, and it is the provider's preference.[14]

- Most commonly the four-quadrant technique is utilized, which essentially is two sutures placed on each side of the flange.[14]
- Sutures should be removed per institutional protocol to minimize pressure injuries once the stoma is healed; this is typically between 7 to 10 days for a percutaneous stoma and 4 days for a surgical stoma.[14,15,28]

Compared With Endotracheal Tubes, Tracheostomy Tubes Provide Added Benefits[22,23,30,31,53]

- Prevention of laryngeal injury from the endotracheal tube
- Improved patient comfort, acceptance, and tolerance
- Ease of oral care
- Decreased work of breathing due to decreased airflow resistance
- Facilitation of weaning from mechanical ventilation
- Decreased requirements for sedation
- Provision of a speech mechanism that enhances communication
- Increased patient mobility
- Facilitation of removal of secretions
- Reduced risk for unintentional airway loss

Indications for Tracheostomy[15,22,23]

- Bypass of acute upper airway obstruction
- Prolonged need for an artificial airway
- Prophylaxis for anticipated airway problems
- Reduction of anatomic dead space
- Prevention of pulmonary aspiration
- Retained tracheobronchial secretions
- Chronic upper airway obstruction

- Tracheostomies are not without complications and include infection, bleeding, tracheomalacia, stenosis, device-related skin breakdown, and transesophageal fistula (TAF; Table 11.1)).[7,8,9,31,35,37,46]
- Postoperative tracheostomy emergencies are tracheostomy decannulation, obstruction, and hemorrhage.[6] Hemorrhage can occur at the stoma site or into the trachea.[6] A small amount of postprocedure bleeding is expected and is limited to a short period. Postoperative bleeding that continues over 48 hours to 3 weeks or is moderate to large in volume could be caused by a bleeding vessel or a tracheoinnominate artery fistula (TIAF). Bleeding vessels may need to be ligated by the provider.[6,30]
- Tube obstruction can occur from secretions or from the tracheostomy tube being displaced into the anterior portion of the trachea within a false passage (Fig. 11.3). If the tube is obstructed from secretions, it should be suctioned. If the tube is felt to be dislodged into a false passage, treatment depends on how mature the stoma is. If the stoma is mature, the tube should be replaced. If the stoma is immature (i.e., the stoma is less than 1 week old), mask ventilation should be employed with the cuff deflated, and an orotracheal tube should be inserted. Once the airway is secure, the tracheostomy can be revised.[24] The provider should be notified if the tube becomes obstructed and aggressive measures other than routine suctioning are needed to clear the cannula or secretions of debris. Airway emergency procedures should be implemented per institutional guidelines.

TABLE 11.1	Complications Related to Tracheostomies[7,8,9,13,35,37,46,49]	
Immediate Postoperative Complications	Early Complications(Less than 48 Hours)	Late Complications (Beyond 48 Hours)
<ul><li>Bleeding<ul><li>Postoperative minor bleeding (controlled by compression) is expected[49]</li><li>Major: >7 gauze sponges or >20 mL</li></ul></li><li>Loss of airway</li><li>Hypoxemia/hypercarbia</li><li>Structural damage to the trachea or surrounding areas</li><li>Pneumothorax</li><li>Death</li></ul>	<ul><li>Bleeding<ul><li>Minor: <20 mL</li><li>Major: >7 gauze sponges or >20 mL</li></ul></li><li>Tube displacement/ decannulation</li><li>Pneumothorax</li><li>Pneumomediastinum</li><li>Subcutaneous emphysema</li><li>Infection</li><li>Ulceration of the stoma</li><li>Pressure injury[14]</li></ul>	<ul><li>Tracheoinnominate artery fistula (TIAF)</li><li>Surgical site infection</li><li>Stenosis</li><li>Tracheomalacia</li><li>Pneumonia</li><li>Aspiration</li><li>Tracheoesophageal fistula (TEF)</li><li>Pressure injury[14]</li></ul>

Modified from Cheung NH, Napolitano LM: Tracheostomy: epidemiology, indications, timing, technique, and outcomes. *Respir Care* 59(6):895–919, 2014.

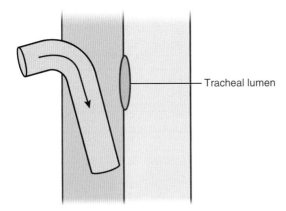

Figure 11.3 Dislodgement of a tracheostomy tube within a false passage anterior to the trachea (airway). *(From Morris LL, Afifi MS, editors:* Tracheostomies: The complete guide, *New York, 2010, Springer.)*

- ❖ TIAF is a rare complication, affecting less than 1% of patients with an estimated mortality rate over 90%.[6] In this complication, the innominate artery has eroded into the trachea, which can result in exsanguination. This is more common when a tracheostomy tube is subject to traction to one side or the other, away from the midline. Any concerns over bleeding should be reported to the provider immediately.
- ❖ Follow facility specific protocols related to tracheostomy emergencies. The National Tracheostomy Safety Project (NTSP) recommends basic and advanced airway supplies needed for emergencies to be placed in every room of patients with a tracheostomy.[5,15]
- Tracheostomy management
  - ❖ An initial tracheotomy tube change varies depending on whether the tracheotomy was placed via standard surgical procedure or via the percutaneous approach; this is referred to as *downsizing* the tracheotomy tube and may assist with the weaning process. Currently there is no evidence to justify when the initial or subsequent tracheotomy tubes should be changed; it typically occurs by provider preference. The first tube change most commonly occurs around 7 to 10 days postoperatively.[15,28,46] Some reports state that for a percutaneous tracheotomy, initial change should not occur until

postoperative day 10 to allow the stoma to mature.[15,46] After the initial change, the tracheotomy should be changed approximately every 14 days thereafter. The first change is performed by the provider.[19,24,28,29,46]

- ❖ Caution should be used to ensure that the tracheostomy tube is not accidently dislodged or decannulated. The stoma takes approximately 1 week to heal posttracheotomy.[14,15] Dislodgment of the tube in the first week is considered an emergency; the tissue may collapse, and it may not be possible to replace the tracheal tube. Predisposing factors to tube dislodgement or decannulation include an underinflated cuff, loose ties, neck or airway edema, excessive coughing, agitation or undersedation, morbid obesity, downward traction caused by the weight of the ventilator circuit, and an improperly sized tracheostomy tube.
- ❖ Tracheostomy tubes should be secured with sutures and/or commercial devices or ties. Weight or traction from the ventilator circuit should be minimized; when transporting or mobilizing the patient, the tube should remain in the neutral midline position. Tube position should be noted before and after the patient is moved to ensure safety. Individual institutions usually have protocols to manage new tracheostomy tubes and accidental dislodgment to ensure patient safety.[5,7,9,19,24,49,51]
- Variations of tracheostomy tubes
  - ❖ A tracheostomy tube is shorter than but similar in diameter to an endotracheal tube. Tracheostomy tubes may have both outer and inner cannulas or a single lumen (no inner cannula). The outer cannula forms the body of the tracheostomy tube with a cuff if present. The neck flange, attached to the outer cannula, assists in stabilizing the tube in the trachea and provides the holes necessary for securing the tube (Fig. 11.4).
  - ❖ Most tracheostomy tubes have both an inner cannula and outer cannula. The inner cannula is inserted into the outer cannula and is removable for cleaning and may be either reusable or disposable. The 15-mm connector that connects the tracheostomy tube to the ventilator is located on the inner cannula for dual-lumen tubes.
  - ❖ Tracheostomy tubes are available in various materials, sizes, and styles from several manufacturers. It is important for the clinician to understand the differences

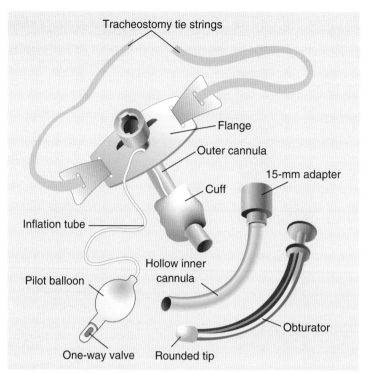

Figure 11.4 Parts of a tracheostomy tube. *(From Eubanks DH, Bone RC: Comprehensive respiratory care, ed 2, St. Louis, 1990, Mosby, 570.)*

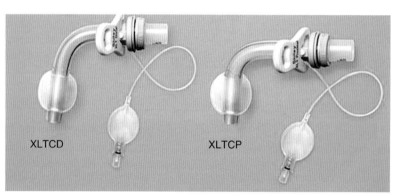

Figure 11.5 (Left) Shiley™ adult extended-length tracheostomy tube with distal extension. (Right) Shiley™ adult extended-length tracheostomy tube with proximal extension. *(© 2023 Medtronic. All rights reserved. Used with the permission of Medtronic.)*

between the various tracheostomy tubes to ensure the appropriate features, fit, and size for the patient. The tube should be selected with the goal of minimizing damage to the tracheal wall, allowing adequate ventilation and, when indicated, promoting translaryngeal airflow for communication to assist with future rehabilitation and therapy. Several associations have published guidelines to guide users in selecting the appropriate tube and size.[28,33,46] Routine patient care and tube maintenance may be affected based on tube size, style, and construction.

❖ Tracheostomy tubes can be constructed of metal (silver or stainless steel) or plastic (polyvinyl chloride or silicone). Metal tubes are rarely used due to cost, rigid construction, lack of cuff, the possibility of damage by cleaning with hydrogen peroxide or enzymatic cleaners, and lack of a 15-mm connector needed to attach the tracheostomy tube to a ventilator or bag-valve-mask device.[9,24] Polyvinyl chloride softens with the patient's body temperature, which helps the tube conform to the patient's anatomy and assists in centering the distal tip in the trachea. Silicone tubes are naturally soft and are not affected by the patient's body temperature.[9]

❖ Tracheostomy tubes may be angled or curved to improve the fit in the trachea, and they come in standard or extra length, fenestrated, and cuffed or uncuffed. A curved tube may be too short for the trachea and cause anterior compression of the trachea. Extra-length tubes increase the length proximally, which facilitates placement in large necks or distally, which may be useful in patients with tracheomalacia[7,24,35,36] (Fig. 11.5).

❖ An extra-long tracheostomy tube (XLT) can be beneficial in patients with large necks (e.g., obese patients), tracheal anomalies, or tracheomalacia. An improper tube size selection can result in an occlusion of the distal end of the tracheostomy tube.[24]

❖ Fenestrated tracheostomy tubes are standard tracheostomy tubes with an added opening(s) located in the posterior portion of the tube above the cuff. Fenestrated tubes come with an inner cannula and a plastic plug. When the inner cannula is removed, the cuff is deflated, and the tracheostomy tube is occluded with the plastic plug, the patient can breathe through the fenestration(s) and around the tube using the normal anatomic airway. When a fenestrated tracheostomy tube is occluded in this manner, the patient can speak, as air can pass over the vocal cords. Additional oxygen can be provided to the patient via nasal cannula if needed.[24]

• Tracheostomy Tube with cuff and cuff pressures[15,24,35,36,40,46,52]

❖ Tracheostomy tubes may be used with or without a cuff. The tracheal tube cuff is an inflatable balloon that surrounds the shaft of the tracheal tube near its distal end. When inflated, the cuff presses against the tracheal wall to prevent air leakage and pressure loss from the lungs during positive pressure ventilation. The tracheal tube cuff is usually inflated by injecting air through a pilot balloon with a one-way inflation valve. The air in the pilot balloon is used to assess of the amount of pressure in the tracheal tube cuff (see Fig. 11.4).[24]

❖ Cuffed tubes are generally used in patients requiring mechanical ventilation. Cuffed tubes allow for airway clearance, and the cuff limits aspiration of oral and gastric secretions in ventilated patients.[25]

❖ The amount of pressure and volume necessary to obtain a seal and prevent mucosal damage depends on tube size and design, cuff configuration, and mode of ventilation.[24]

❖ Cuff pressure for most tracheostomy tubes should be less than 20 to 25 mm Hg (34 cm H_2O) to minimize the risk of tracheal wall injury and decrease the risk of microaspiration.[15,24,34,35,40,46] Maintain the cuff pressure at the minimum pressure necessary to prevent a cuff leak.[40]

❖ Most cuffed tubes have high-volume, low-pressure cuffs (Fig. 11.6). These tubes allow a large surface area to meet the tracheal wall, distributing the pressure over a much greater area.[15,24,35,36,46]

○ A small number of specialty tubes have low-volume, high-pressure cuffs (see Fig.11.6), or tight-to-shaft cuffed tubes that are filled with sterile water. These cuffs should be measured with the minimum occlusive volume (MOV) technique, and the number of milliliters needed to achieve an airtight seal should be

SOFT CUFF
• High volume
• Exerts low and equal lateral tracheal wall pressure (TWP) (arrows)
• Minimizes tracheal inury

HARD CUFF
• Low volume
• Exerts high and unequal lateral TWP (arrows)
• Causes tracheal inury

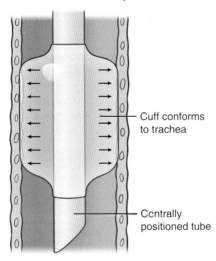
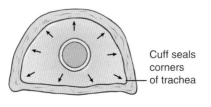
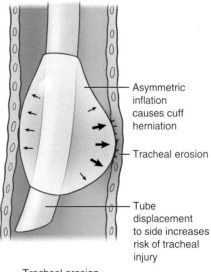
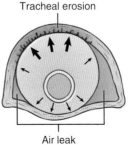

Figure 11.6 Cross-sectional view in a D-shaped trachea. Effects of soft and hard cuff inflation on the tracheal wall. *(From Kersten LD: Comprehensive respiratory nursing. Philadelphia, 1989, Saunders, 648.)*

recorded. An additional specialty tracheostomy tube has a foam cuff that fills passively to atmospheric air.
- Uncuffed tubes are commonly used in children, in non–mechanically ventilated patients with laryngectomies, and during weaning from the tracheostomy. Uncuffed tubes may also be used in selected long-term mechanically ventilated patients who have adequate pulmonary compliance and sufficient oropharyngeal muscle strength for functional swallowing and articulation and laryngeal strength to achieve glottis closure.[7,24,27,35]
- Complications that could occur when cuff pressures are too high include mucosal ischemia, inflammation or necrosis, tracheal stenosis, tracheomalacia, tracheoesophageal fistula, and tracheoinnominate artery fistula.[11,24,25,44]
  - Damage typically occurs when the cuff pressure does not allow for the normal delivery of oxygen to the capillaries. Normal tracheal capillary pressure ranges from 20 to 30 mm Hg. Higher cuff pressure impedes blood flow to those capillaries.[11,24]
  - Common causes of high cuff pressures include a tracheostomy tube that is too small, overfilling of the balloon, a malpositioned tracheostomy tube, and tracheal dilation.
- Complications that can occur when the cuff pressure is too low include silent aspiration or microaspiration, inadvertent decannulation, and difficulty managing adequate ventilation. Aspiration of oral or gastric contents could result in ventilator-acquired complications such as pneumonia.[25]
- Two major mechanisms are mainly responsible for airway damage: tube movement and cuff pressure.
- Cuff pressures should be measured and documented at minimum every 4 to 8 hours following facility-specific guidelines.[11,15,39,40,46]
  - Measurement of tracheal tube cuff pressures can be achieved to assess pressure via a bedside manometer. An advantage to direct cuff pressure monitoring is that there is no need to deflate then reinflate the cuff, thus decreasing the potential risk for aspiration. Disadvantages are that these devices are designed for high-volume, low-pressure cuffs that are air filled.[37]
- Minimizing pressure injuries related to tracheostomy tubes
  - Prolonged exposure to mechanical devices that exert pressure on the patient's skin and tissue can result in pressure injuries. Mechanical devices are usually constructed with stiff polymer materials (secured with tape or strapping) that produce a microclimate where the device meets the skin. Methods should be implemented to reduce skin breakdown at the site of the tracheostomy tube:[14,18]
    - Regularly monitor the tension of the device on the skin and surrounding areas to reduce pressure.[18]
    - Assess skin for pressure injuries surrounding the device with routine assessments.[18]
    - Ensure suture removal per institutional protocol to minimize pressure injuries once the stoma is healed. This is typically between 7 and 10 days for a percutaneous stoma and 4 days for a surgical stoma.[14]
      - Consider the use of prophylactic dressings under medical devices.[12,18]
- Consideration should be given to obtaining assistance with tracheostomy care, especially when tracheal ties are changed or when the patient is agitated. An assistant can minimize risk for accidental dislodgement.

EQUIPMENT

- Personal protective equipment (PPE) including goggles and mask or mask with eye shield.
  - Open-technique suctioning and ventilator disconnect are aerosolizing procedures. Refer to institutional guidelines for isolation precautions and necessary PPE.
- Cuff pressure manometer
- Stethoscope
- Self-inflating manual resuscitation bag-valve-mask device
- Oxygen source and tubing
- Suction supplies (see Procedure 8, Endotracheal or Tracheostomy)
- Sterile normal saline solution
- Two to three sterile containers to place supplies (cotton swabs, sterile saline)
- Sterile cotton-tipped applicators
- Sterile nylon brush (for reusable inner canula only)
- Sterile 4 × 4 gauze
  - Foam dressings may be used as alternative to manage moisture and minimize associated skin damage.[12,18]
- Some institutions have prepackaged tracheostomy cleaning kits to ease the collection of supplies for the procedure.
- Commercial tracheostomy tube holder or tracheostomy ties
- Sterile precut tracheostomy dressing or dressing used by institutional preference
  - Use only precut tracheostomy dressings to minimize the chance of fibers from gauze being introduced in the airway or a potential source of infection.[12]
- If the inner cannula is disposable, a new sterile disposable inner cannula of the same size
- Extra sterile tracheostomy kit at the bedside or obturator per institutional policy

Additional equipment to have available as needed includes the following:
- Scissors
- 10-mL syringe
- Three-way stopcock
- Padded hemostats
- Short 18-gauge or 23-gauge blunt needle
- Tongue depressor
- Tape (1 inch wide)
- Reintubation equipment, in case of accidental extubation

PATIENT AND FAMILY EDUCATION[50]

- Explain the procedure and the reason for tracheal tube cuff care, tracheal tube care, and/or tracheostomy dressing change. ***Rationale:*** This communication identifies patient and family knowledge deficits concerning the patient's condition, procedure, expected benefits, and potential risks, and it allows time for questions to clarify information and voice concerns. Explanations decrease patient anxiety, increase knowledge, and enhance cooperation.

- Explain that the procedure may cause the patient to cough. *Rationale:* This explanation prepares the patient for what to expect.

PATIENT ASSESSMENT AND PREPARATION

Patient Assessment

- Assess the presence of bilateral breath sounds. *Rationale:* This assessment provides baseline data.
- Assess the signs and symptoms of cuff leakage, including an audible or auscultated inspiratory leak over the larynx, audible patient vocalizations, inflation (pilot) valve balloon, and loss of inspiratory and expiratory volume on patients with mechanical ventilation. *Rationale:* An adequate seal of the cuff to the tracheal wall does not permit air to flow past the cuff.
- Assess signs and symptoms of inadequate ventilation, including increasing $Paco_2$ chest-abdominal dyssynchrony, patient-ventilator dyssynchrony, dyspnea, headache, restlessness, confusion, lethargy, increasing (early sign) or decreasing (late sign) arterial blood pressure, and activation of expiratory or inspiratory volume alarms on the mechanical ventilator. *Rationale:* These signs and symptoms guide needed interventions.
- Assess the size of the tracheal tube and the size of the patient. *Rationale:* The volume and pressure of air needed to seal the airway depends on the relationship between the tracheal tube and the diameter of the trachea.
- Assess the amount of air or pressure currently used to inflate the cuff by collaborating with respiratory therapy or reviewing previous documentation. *Rationale:* The amount of air previously used to inflate the cuff can be used as a guideline to determine changes in volume, pressure, or both.
- Assess the amount of secretions. *Rationale:* This may increase the frequency of suctioning and tube care.
- Assess the stoma site for the presence of tracheal sutures. *Rationale:* After 7 days (when the tracheostomy is mature), the sutures may no longer be required. If they remain in place, notify the physician, and query for removal. The sutures increase the risk of decannulation because of difficulty with maneuvering to care for the site and dressing. Prolonged suture retention may also promote skin breakdown.[33] Refer to institutional policy for suture removal.
- Assess the stoma and surrounding skin for signs and symptoms of skin breakdown or infection, and consider preventive dressings. *Rationale:* A device-related pressure injury may occur from prolonged pressure, shearing, or moisture, and the risk is increased with comorbidities. Localized skin infections may also occur because of this breakdown.[14]

Patient Preparation

- Ensure that the patient and family understand preprocedural teachings. Answer questions as they arise, and reinforce information as needed. *Rationale:* This communication evaluates and reinforces understanding of previously taught information.
- Verify the correct patient with two identifiers. *Rationale:* Before performing a procedure, the nurse should ensure the correct identification of the patient for the intended intervention.
- Consider placing the patient in the semi-Fowler's position. *Rationale:* This positioning promotes general relaxation, oxygenation, and ventilation. It also reduces stimulation of the gag reflex and risk of aspiration.

Procedure for Tracheostomy Cuff and Tube Care		
Steps	Rationale	Special Considerations
Measurement of Cuff Pressure		
1. 🅷🅷		
2. 🅿🅴		Includes goggles and mask or mask with eye shield. (Open technique suctioning and ventilator disconnect are aerosolizing procedures. Refer to institutional guidelines for isolation precautions and necessary PPE.)
3. Hyperoxygenate and suction the tracheobronchial tree and pharynx (subglottic) before cuff deflation if there are positive indications of secretions. (More information regarding subglottic suctioning is provided in Procedure 8, Endotracheal or Tracheostomy). **(Level D*)**	Clears secretions above the tracheostomy cuff and in the lower airway and decreases the incidence of aspiration.	If an open suction system is used, a sterile catheter is needed for suctioning the tracheobronchial tree. When suctioning of the tracheobronchial tree is complete, the same catheter may be used to suction the oropharynx. If a closed suction system is used in suctioning the tracheobronchial tree, an additional catheter is needed for suctioning the oropharynx.

*Level D: Peer-reviewed professional and organizational standards with the support of clinical study recommendations.

Procedure continues on following page

Procedure for Tracheostomy Cuff and Tube Care—*Continued*

Steps	Rationale	Special Considerations
4. Attach a commercial pressure gauge to the tracheal cuff.[11]	Allows for measurement of cuff pressure.	Determine via the facility's protocol as to whose responsibility it is to measure tracheal cuff pressures. Often there is close collaboration with respiratory therapy for shared responsibilities.
5. Read the measurement.[11,26]	Intracuff pressure measurement provides an approximation of cuff–to–tracheal wall pressure.[25,26]	
6. If the cuff pressure is >25 cm H$_2$O, press the pressure-release button on the pressure gauge until the pressure reaches 20–25 cm H$_2$O. If the pressure is <20 cm H$_2$O, add air by squeezing the bulb to increase the pressure.[11,26] **(Level D*)**	Provides optimal pressure to seal the cuff without causing excessive tracheal pressure.	Hazards of cuff inflation include cuff overinflation, distention, and rupture. The patient who is alert and cooperative may be asked to speak. If the trachea is sealed, vocalization is not possible.[11]
7. If unable to maintain appropriate pressures, notify the provider.	Elevated cuff pressures have been associated with tracheal stenosis and necrosis. Inadequate cuff pressures may lead to impaired ability to provide ventilation and increase the risk for aspiration.[11]	
8. Dispose of used supplies and equipment, and remove **PE**.		
9. **HH**		
Troubleshooting Tracheal Cuff Problems *Faulty Inflation Valve*		
1. **HH**		
2. **PE**		Includes goggles and mask or mask with eye shield. (Open technique suctioning and ventilator disconnect are aerosolizing procedures. Refer to institutional standards for isolation precautions and necessary PPE.)
3. Identify the faulty inflation valve by determining that the cuff continually deflates, despite the addition of air to the cuff (Fig. 11.7).	Determines the need for repair.	If the inflation valve becomes faulty and reintubation is undesirable, consider instituting an emergency cuff-inflation technique. There are commercial cuff inflation–valve repair kits available. Follow institutional standards regarding who is responsible for repairing a faulty inflation valve.
4. Clamp the inflation tube with the padded hemostat.	Prevents further air loss through the faulty inflation valve.	
5. Insert a three-way stopcock into the inflation valve.	Provides access to the cuff.	

*Level D: Peer-reviewed professional and organizational standards with the support of clinical study recommendations.

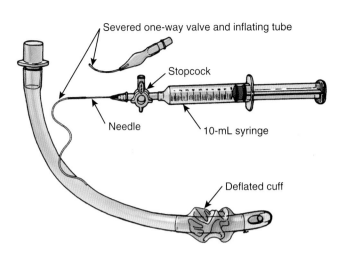

Severed one-way valve and inflating tube

Stopcock

Needle

10-mL syringe

Deflated cuff

Figure 11.7 Attachments for emergency cuff inflation for a faulty inflation line. *(From Sills J: An emergency cuff inflation technique.* Respir Care *31:200, 1986.)*

Procedure for Tracheostomy Cuff and Tube Care—*Continued*

6. Inflate the cuff with the MOV technique.	Allows for cuff inflation; restores the tracheal wall and cuff seal.	
7. Turn the stopcock off to the inflation valve, and leave it in place; remove the hemostat.	Temporarily maintains cuff pressure.	Check the connection between the valve and three-way stopcock frequently as the inflation valve is not a Luer lock and could loosen over time
8. Discard used supplies and remove **PE**.		
9. **HH**		
Faulty Inflation Tube		
1. **HH**		
2. **PE**		Includes goggles and mask or mask with eye shield. (Open technique suctioning and ventilator disconnect are aerosolizing procedures. Refer to institutional standards for isolation precautions and necessary PPE.)
3. Identify malfunctioning of the inflation tube by determining that an air leak is present in the tube (see Fig. 11.7).	Determines the need for and method of repair.	Commercial inflation tube repair kits are available. Follow institutional standards regarding who is responsible for repairing a faulty inflation tube. Collaborate with respiratory therapy and the provider.
4. Clamp the inflation tube below the leak with the padded hemostat.	Prevents further air loss through the faulty inflation line.	Placement of the padded hemostat should allow adequate inflation tube length to accept the blunt needle.
5. Cut the inflation line above the padded hemostat but below the identified leak.	Allows introduction of the blunt needle for repair.	
6. Insert a short 18-gauge to 23-gauge blunt needle into the inflation tube.	Provides inflation access.	Maintain care to avoid puncture or severing of inflation line or clinician's skin.

Procedure continues on following page

UNIT 1

Procedure	for Tracheostomy Cuff and Tube Care—*Continued*

7. Attach a three-way stopcock to a blunt needle with the "OFF" position facing the cuff inflation tube).	Provides control of airflow in and out of the inflation tube.	
8. Attach a 10-mL syringe, turn the stopcock to allow inflation, and inflate the cuff using the MOV technique.	Allows cuff inflation; restores tracheal wall and cuff seal.	
9. Turn the stopcock back to "OFF" position facing the cuff inflation tube.	Provides for temporary use of the tracheal tube while maintaining cuff pressure.	
10. Secure the assembled device with tape to a tongue depressor.	Provides for stabilization and protection.	
11. Assemble equipment for tracheal tube replacement.	Prepares for tracheal tube replacement.	Plan to change the tube as a more permanent solution.
12. Discard used supplies, and remove **PE**.	Reduces transmission of microorganisms and body secretions; standard precautions.	

13. **HH**

Tracheostomy Tube Care

1. **HH**		
2. **PE**		Includes goggles and mask or mask with eye shield. (Open technique suctioning and ventilator disconnect are aerosolizing procedures. Refer to institutional standards for isolation precautions and necessary PPE.)
3. Hyperoxygenate and suction the trachea and oropharynx as needed (see Procedure 8, Suctioning: Endotracheal or Tracheostomy).	Reduces the risk of hypoxemia and arrhythmias; removes secretions and diminishes the patient's need to cough during the procedure.	Sterile saline solution should not be instilled into the artificial airway before suctioning (see Procedure 8, Suctioning: Endotracheal or Tracheostomy). Saline flushes do not loosen secretions but may potentiate infection. **(Level D*)**
4. Remove and discard soiled tracheostomy dressing **PE**.	Provides access and visibility of the tracheostomy site.	
5. With dressings removed and the stoma site visible, assess the skin surrounding the stoma and under the medical device.	Assesses for potential skin-related issues and implements prevention measures as appropriate	Document as appropriate.
6. **PE**		
7. **HH**		Replace soiled PPE
8. For a disposable inner cannula: A. Open the prepackaged inner cannula. B. Apply clean gloves. C. Remove the soiled inner cannula. D. Replace with the prepackaged cannula.	Replaces the inner cannula. Hold the inner cannula (soiled and replacement) by the connector to avoid contamination. Stabilize the neck plate with your free hand during the unlocking and locking procedure to avoid pressure on the patient's neck and stoma.	

*Level D: Peer-reviewed professional and organizational standards with the support of clinical study recommendations.

Procedure for Tracheostomy Cuff and Tube Care—*Continued*

Steps	Rationale	Special Considerations
9. For a nondisposable inner cannula (open prepackaged commercial tracheostomy care kit): A. Prepare sterile saline on a sterile field.[43] B. Apply sterile gloves. C. Remove the oxygen source and then the inner cannula, placing it in sterile saline.	Prepares for cleaning the tracheostomy.	Sterile saline should be used for cleaning tracheostomy tubes. There are conflicting data regarding the use of hydrogen peroxide (H_2O_2); follow manufacturer recommendations or facility-specific guidelines.[10,27,43,47,48] H_2O_2 may cause pitting of metal tracheostomy tubes.[10,27,47,48]
8. Place oxygen over or near the outer cannula.	Maintains oxygen supply.	If the patient cannot tolerate disconnection from a ventilator for the time needed to clean the inner cannula, replace the existing inner cannula with a clean one, and reattach the ventilator. Then, clean the cannula just removed from the patient, and store it in a sterile container for the next inner cannula change.
9. Clean the inner cannula with a small brush.	Assists in removal of debris and thick secretions.	
10. Rinse the inner cannula by pouring sterile saline over the cannula. Remove excess solution by tapping on the inside edge of the sterile container. Do not dry the outside portion of the inner cannula.	Removes any remaining debris from the cannula. Excess solution left on the inside of the inner cannula may lead to aspiration. Solution on the outside portion of the inner cannula may help act as a lubricant for insertion.[10,27,43,47,48]	
11. Remove the oxygen source from over the outer cannula.	Allows access to the opening of the outer cannula.	
12. Insert the inner cannula, and lock it into place.	Secures the inner cannula.	
13. Reapply the oxygen source to the inner cannula hub.	Reestablishes oxygen supply.	
14. Moisten 4 × 4 gauze pads with sterile saline, and clean the stoma site, outer cannula, and neck plate surface by wiping with cotton-tipped swabs and 4 × 4 gauze.	Removes debris and secretions from the stoma area.	There are conflicting data regarding the use of H_2O_2; follow manufacturer recommendations or facility-specific guidelines.[10,27,43,47,48] H_2O_2 could cause irritation to skin or increase the risk of infection.[47]
15. Dry the skin around the stoma by gently patting it dry.	Decreases the likelihood of microorganism growth and skin breakdown.	

Procedure continues on following page

Procedure   **for Tracheostomy Cuff and Tube Care—*Continued***

16. If needed, prepare to attach a new tracheostomy tube holder.	The tracheostomy tube holder may need to be replaced if it is soiled.	Review individual institutional polices regarding the use of twill tape or commercial tracheostomy tie devices. Twill tape is often used during the initial insertion of the tracheostomy tube. Institutions may prohibit tracheostomy tube holders from being changed for up to 72 hours after tracheostomy tube placement because of the risk of dislodgement. Consideration should be given to obtaining assistance with tracheostomy care, especially when tracheal ties are changed or when the patient is agitated. An assistant can minimize risk for accidental dislodgement.[12]
17. Remove the current tracheostomy tube holder or twill tape.	Prepares for replacement.	Ensure that an assistant securely holds the tracheostomy in place.
18. *Tracheostomy tube holder:* Connect one side of the neck plate to the new tracheostomy tube holder, and then connect the other side of the neck plate to secure the tube holder. *Twill tape:* Cut a length long enough to encircle the patient's neck two times. Cut ends diagonally. Insert one end through the faceplate eyelet, and pull the ends even. Pass both ends of the tie around the patient's neck, and insert one end through the faceplate's second eyelet. Pull snugly to allow space between the tie and the patient's neck, and tie the ends securely with a double square knot on the side of the patient's neck (Fig. 11.8).	Removes the soiled holder or tape. Whether using a commercial holder or twill tape, the tracheostomy tube should be positioned midline to minimize movement of the tube while not being too tight and causing pressure on the neck.[15]	A variety of commercial tracheostomy tube holders are available. In some instances, a newly placed tracheostomy tube may be sutured into place, and no holder or ties are used (e.g., for patients with a new laryngectomy and flap). If this occurs, the provider should document in an order if a tracheostomy holder or twill tape should not be used.
19. Apply a clean, precut tracheostomy dressing under the neck plate or other preventive dressing.	Provides a dressing between the tracheostomy and the neck plate.	Apply a dressing according to institution-specified protocol. Any precut surgical gauze is sufficient. Never cut a 4 × 4 gauze pad because cut edges fray and provide a potential source for infection.[10,27,43,47,48] **(Level D*)**
20. Provide oral care (see Procedure 3, Endotracheal Tube Care and Oral Care Practices for Ventilated and Nonventilated Patients).	Increases patient comfort.	
21. Discard used supplies, and remove 🄿🄴.		
22. 🄷🄷		

---

*Level D: Peer-reviewed professional and organizational standards with the support of clinical study recommendations.

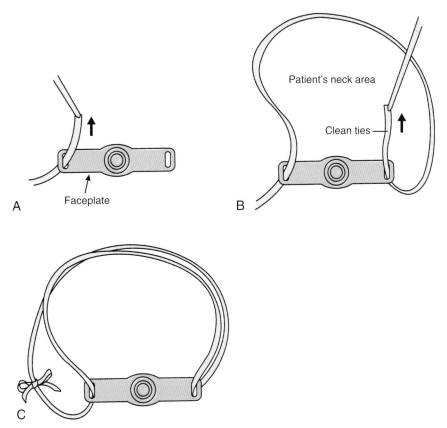

A   Faceplate

B   Patient's neck area

Clean ties

C

Figure 11.8 Placement of tracheostomy twill tape. **A,** Faceplate with threading of twill tape (for prevention of decannulation, an additional person needs to stabilize the faceplate). **B,** Advancing of the twill tape around the back of the neck and looping through the other side of the faceplate. **C,** Doubling the twill tape and securing it in a knot at side of neck.

Expected Outcomes	Unexpected Outcomes
• Tracheal tube remains in correct position • Cuff pressure is kept at a level to maintain a seal between the cuff and the tracheal wall (usually between 20 and 25 mm Hg). • Cuff remains intact • Airway remains patent • Stoma site is free from infection and without device-related pressure injury	• Decannulation or tube dislodgment • Tracheal mucosal ischemia from cuff overinflation • Faulty inflation valve or tube • Cuff overinflation and distention over the end of the tube • Cuff rupture • Prolonger apnea, increasing hypoxemia, or cardiopulmonary arrest • Hemorrhage • Interstitial air: subcutaneous emphysema, pneumothorax, pneumopericardium, pneumomediastinum • Thyroid gland injury • Cardiac dysrhythmias • Tube tip erosion into the innominate artery • Skin breakdown, pressure areas, stomatitis • Signs of stoma infection • Device-related pressure injury • Bronchopulmonary infection • Displacement or dislodgement out of the trachea • Excessive cuff pressure • Leaking airway cuff • Airway obstruction from misalignment, cuff overinflation, or dried or excessive secretion • Tracheal stenosis, tracheomalacia, or tracheoesophageal fistula

Patient Monitoring and Care

Steps	Rationale	Reportable Conditions
		These conditions should be reported if they persist despite nursing interventions.
1. Assess respiratory status for optimal ventilation.[20]	Inadequate interface between the tracheal cuff and tracheobronchial mucosa decreases inspiratory flow.	• Increasing $Paco_2$ • Chest-abdominal dyssynchrony • Patient-ventilator dyssynchrony • Dyspnea • Headache • Restlessness • Confusion • Lethargy • Increasing (early sign) or decreasing (late sign) arterial blood pressure • Activation of expiratory or inspiratory volume alarms on the mechanical ventilator
2. Measure cuff pressure every 4–8 hours per institutional requirements, maintaining cuff pressure between 20 and 25 mm Hg.[11,15,39,40,46] **(Level D*)**	Prevents tracheal injury and aspiration. Excessive cuff pressure is cited as the most frequent problem of tracheal intubation and the best predictor of tracheolaryngeal injury.[11,24] If the volume (milliliters) needed to seal the airway increases, evaluate the patient for tracheal dilation with chest radiography of cuff diameter/tracheal diameter ratio. Increasing volumes also may indicate a leak in the cuff, inflation valve, or tube. Some institutions may use continuous cuff manometry devices.[26]	• Cuff pressure <20 mm Hg or >25 mm Hg • Inability to maintain cuff pressure
3. Maintain tracheal tube cuff integrity.	Manipulation of the tracheal tube increases the likelihood of cuff disruption. Cuff leak or rupture is evident when the pressure on the manometer continues to decrease.	• Inability to maintain cuff inflation • Audible air through the patient's nose or mouth • Low-pressure or low-volume alarm sounds on the mechanical ventilator • Audible or auscultated inspiratory leak over the larynx • Patient able to vocalize audibly • Pilot balloon deflation • Loss of inspiratory and expiratory volume on patients with mechanical ventilation
4. Hyperoxygenate and suction the patient based on assessment (see Procedure 8, Suctioning: Endotracheal or Tracheostomy).	Removal of secretions reduces the chance for partial or complete airway obstruction.	

*Level D: Peer-reviewed professional and organizational standards with the support of clinical study recommendations.

Patient Monitoring and Care *—Continued*		
Steps	**Rationale**	**Reportable Conditions**
5. Compare the patient's cardiopulmonary status before, during, and after tracheal tube cuff care.	Identifies the effects of tracheal tube cuff care on the cardiovascular system.	• Decreased arterial oxygen saturation • Cardiac dysrhythmias • Bronchospasm • Respiratory distress • Cyanosis • Increased blood pressure or intracranial pressure • Anxiety, agitation, or changes in level of consciousness
6. Reassess cuff pressure and volume when transporting the patient from one altitude to another (i.e., air transport) or during hyperbaric therapy without environmental pressurization.	Changes in altitude may change the volume of gas in the cuff; volume and pressure must be reevaluated during and after transport.	
7. Provide continuous humidified air or use a heat moisture exchanger (HME) and/or oxygen with warm or cool air as appropriate.[4,20,38,46] **(Level D*)**	Artificial airways bypass the nose and mouth, preventing normal warming, humidification, and filtering.[4,39]	
8. Maintain the tracheostomy tube in a neutral position, midline with the patient's body.	Traction on the tracheostomy from ventilator circuits, oxygen, or suction tubing may result in decannulation, displacement into a false passage, tracheal fistula, tracheal stenosis, or granuloma from movement of the tube. Traction on sutures if present may also lead to extension of the incision and/or infection.	• Tracheostomy tube that is unable to be maintained midline or has changed position • Sutures that prevent adequate stoma care contributing to pressure injuries or are tight due to edema.
9. Auscultate lung sounds to check proper placement of the tracheostomy tube, and ensure that the tube is securely in place.[20]	Displacement into the subcutaneous tissue or decannulation can occur and lead to inadequate ventilation. Follow facility-specific guidelines for emergency equipment and procedures for an airway emergency.[4,15] A trained inserter should reinsert the tracheostomy tube for mature stomas as per individual facility policy.[30] For stomas that are present for less than 7 days, consider ETT intubation.[24,30]	• Decreased chest wall motion • Unilateral breath sounds • Audible expiratory wheeze • Bilateral decreased breath sounds • Oxygen desaturation • Dyspnea and respiratory distress • Stridor • Ventilator alarms • Inability to insert suction catheter greater than 5–7 cm
10. Inspect and palpate for an increase in subcutaneous air under the skin.	Air may escape into the incision on insertion, causing some initial subcutaneous emphysema. Changes or increase in subcutaneous air (emphysema) may be sign of fistula development or movement of the tracheostomy tube into a false passage.[20]	• Subcutaneous emphysema

*Level D: Peer-reviewed professional and organizational standards with the support of clinical study recommendations.

Procedure continues on following page

Patient Monitoring and Care —*Continued*

Steps	Rationale	Reportable Conditions
11. Assess for bleeding or a constant ooze of blood.	Surgical procedures increase the risk of potential injury to adjacent tissue or structures. Stoma placement below the second and third cartilaginous rings results in an increased incidence of innominate artery erosion.	• Frank bleeding or constant oozing of blood
12. Gently palpate the tube for pulsation.	Pulsation felt on the tracheal tube is suggestive of potential erosion of major blood vessels.	• Pulsation of the tracheal tube
13. Follow institutional standards for assessing pain and administering analgesia as prescribed.	Identifies pain and the need for appropriate interventions.	• Continued pain despite interventions
14. Tracheostomy care should be minimally done twice daily and as needed or per institutional policy depending on the type and volume of secretions produced.[5,12,33,40,42,46] **(Level E*)**	Keeps the tube free from secretions, mucus, and plugs that may impede airway patency. Inner cannula changes should take place twice a day per manufacturer guidelines or institutional standards.	• Frequent plugs • Copious drainage • Change in color, odor, or tenacity of secretions
15. Assess the stoma for signs of infection, inflammation, or pressure from tension by tracheostomy ties or equipment.	Skin irritation or breakdown may occur from the neck plate, tracheostomy tube holder, or sutures, if present.	• Elevated temperature • Swelling • Excoriated or open areas • Redness
16. Monitor secretions for color, consistency, odor, and amount.	Change in secretion characteristic may indicate infection or inadequate hydration.	• Purulent drainage • Excessively thick secretions • Copious or purulent secretions
17. Elevate the head of the bed for patients receiving enteral nutrition or mechanical ventilation unless contraindicated.[2,32,41,45] **(Level D*)**	Promotes oropharyngeal and nasopharyngeal drainage and minimizes the risk of aspiration. Helps prevent ventilator-associated or hospital-acquired pneumonia. Follow institutional guidelines for monitoring gastric residuals and related actions.	• Signs and symptoms of aspirations including nausea and vomiting, increased secretions, and fever
18. Perform oral care every 2–4 hours and as needed[1,20] (see Procedure 3, Endotracheal Tube Care and Oral Care Practices for Ventilated and Nonventilated Patients).	Prevents bacterial overgrowth and promotes patient comfort.	
19. Promote effective patient-provider communication (paper and pencil, letter or word boards, electronic devices such as a tablet, or one-way speaking valves, if appropriate).	The patient cannot talk, which may result in fear and anxiety. Patients need an established communication mechanism. A speaking valve may be used to facilitate speech.	

*Level E: Multiple case reports, theory-based evidence from expert opinions, or peer-reviewed professional organizational standards without clinical studies to support recommendations.

Documentation

Documentation should include the following:

- Patient and family education
- Vital signs
- Date, time, and frequency of tracheostomy care
- Type and size of tracheostomy tube, changing of inner cannula, replacement of tracheostomy tube holder, and general condition of stoma, dressing if present, and skin
- Nursing interventions in response to assessed complications
- Patient and family education
- Method of cuff inflation
- Cuff inflation volume and cuff pressure
- Patient's tolerance of the procedure
- Expected and unexpected outcomes
- Type and amount of secretions; frequency of suctioning
- Oral care
- Pain assessment interventions and effectiveness
- Evidence that the securing device is adequate without being excessively tight

References and Additional Readings

For a complete list of references and additional readings for this procedure, scan this QR code with your smartphone, or visit https://www.elsevier.com/__data/assets/pdf_file/0008/1319786/Chapter0011.pdf.

PROCEDURE

12 Continuous End-Tidal Carbon Dioxide Monitoring

Stephanie Maillie and Steven Gudowski

PURPOSE: End-tidal carbon dioxide monitoring, also referred to as *patient end-tidal carbon dioxide (CO₂)* or *$Petco_2$*, provides a noninvasive continuous measurement of exhaled CO_2 concentration commonly referred to as *capnometry*. A capnograph is a graphic depiction of a waveform tracing of each respiratory cycle. The partial pressure of end-tidal CO_2 is representative of alveolar CO_2 ($Paco_2$), which under normal ventilation/perfusion matching in the lungs closely parallels arterial levels of CO_2 ($Paco_2$).

PREREQUISITE NURSING KNOWLEDGE

- There are three broad categories of indications for capnography/capnometry: verification of artificial airway placement, assessment of circulation and respiratory status, and optimization of mechanical ventilation.[3,11]
- Capnography provides the clinician with a direct measure of airway respiratory rate (RR), and the combination of both $Petco_2$ and RR can provide clinicians with one of the earliest indications that ventilation is compromised.[11] Capnography can detect respiratory depression before changes in pulse oximetry occur. $Petco_2$ monitoring allows clinicians to identify a patient's clinical changes and rapidly correct abnormal ventilatory concerns, such as airway obstruction, over-sedation/analgesia, congestive heart failure, pulmonary embolism, or asthma and chronic obstructive pulmonary disease (COPD) exacerbations.[3,11,13]
- The principles of arterial blood gas sampling (see Procedure 54, Blood Sampling From Arterial Catheter) and comparison between $Paco_2$ with $Petco_2$ should be understood.
- Ventilation is the bulk movement of gases into and out of the lung during the respiratory cycle and is composed of two distinct processes: inspiration and expiration.
  - ❖ During inspiration, gas is drawn into the alveoli, at which time it participates in gas exchange. Oxygenation occurs when the oxygen diffuses across the alveolar membrane into the capillary bed. CO_2 exchange occurs during this time as it diffuses across the alveolar membrane into the alveoli. Oxygenated blood is then distributed to and metabolized by the cells of the body. Oxygen saturation can be evaluated with a blood gas analyzer (oxygen saturation [Sao_2]) or pulse oximetry (Spo_2).
  - ❖ During expiration, alveolar gas is exhaled, which results in elimination of CO_2. Cells produce CO_2 as a byproduct of metabolism; this CO_2 is transported by the vascular system to the lungs, where it is eliminated through exhalation. CO_2 elimination can also be evaluated with a blood gas analyzer or capnometer.

- In intubated patients, $Petco_2$ can be monitored through a sensor that is placed directly into the ventilator circuit.
- In nonintubated patients, capnography can be performed with a specialized nasal cannula that delivers supplemental oxygen while measuring $Petco_2$ and respiratory rate. Breath samples are obtained from both nostrils, and oxygen is delivered through the nasal prongs (design depends on manufacturer). For patients who breathe either partially or fully through their mouths, a specially designed nasal cannula can be used that allows for exhaled gas to be captured for analysis.
- The $Petco_2$ monitor may be a standalone system or a module incorporated into the patient's bedside physiological monitor or the mechanical ventilator. An infrared capnometer passes light through an expiratory gas sample and, with a photodetector, measures light absorption by CO_2 in the exhaled gas. The capnograph determines the amount of CO_2 in the gas sample based on the absorption properties of CO_2. The capnograph provides a display called a capnogram or *$Petco_2$ waveform*.
- The capnograph samples exhaled CO_2 by one of two methods: aspiration (sidestream) or nonaspiration (mainstream) sampling. In the sidestream method, a sample of gas is transported via small-bore tubing to the bedside monitor for analysis. In the mainstream system, analysis occurs directly at the patient-ventilator circuit.
- Normal $Petco_2$ concentration in a patient with healthy lungs and airway conditions is 35 to 45 mm Hg. As the patient breathes, a characteristic waveform is created that can be divided into two segments: inspiration and expiration.[9] The $Paco_2$ (partial pressure of arterial carbon dioxide)-$Petco_2$ gradient is the difference between the $Paco_2$ obtained from an arterial blood gas and the $Petco_2$ measure by the capnometer. A normal gradient is 2 to 5 mm Hg with the $Paco_2$ always higher. A widened gradient can result from increasing dead space ventilation such as is seen in patients with COPD and acute respiratory distress syndrome (ARDS). Additionally, a widened gradient can result from low perfusion disease states and pulmonary embolism.

- The normal capnographic waveform has the following characteristics (Fig. 12.1):
    - The zero baseline (phase I, A to B) is seen during inspiration of fresh gas and the beginning of exhalation as CO_2-free gas from anatomical dead space is expelled. This gas comes from the nonperfused areas of the respiratory circuit, such as the large airways and either the artificial airway (if present) or the oropharynx, and nasopharynx
    - A rapid sharp upstroke (phase II, B to C) occurs as the gas from the intermediate airways, containing a mixture of nonperfused gas and CO_2-rich gas, is expired from the lungs
    - A nearly flat expiratory plateau (phase III, C to D) occurs as exhaled flow velocity slows and mixed gas is displaced by alveolar gas. Alveolar exhalation of CO_2 is nearing completion.
    - A distinct end-tidal point (D) most closely reflects the maximal concentration of exhaled CO_2 and the end of exhalation.
    - A rapid downstroke (phase 0, D to E) occurs as the patient begins inspiration of fresh gas that is relatively devoid of CO_2 and returns to baseline.
    - The orientation of the capnogram is commonly confused because the positive aspect of the waveform occurs with exhalation, whereas the negatively deflected limb occurs with inhalation. This is opposite from other respiratory waveforms, including the respirogram, spirogram, and flow-volume loop. The capnogram deviates from normal whenever physiological or mechanical disruption of the breath occurs.
    - A waveform with a curved upslope with loss of expiratory plateau is an indication of airway obstruction such as is seen in COPD and asthma exacerbations, obstruction in the ventilator circuit, foreign body in upper airway, or kinked or occlude airway (Fig. 12.2).
- Waveform capnography allows the provider to do the following:
    - Monitor CPR quality and optimize chest compressions. High-quality chest compressions are achieved when the $Petco_2$ value is between 10 and 20 mm Hg (Fig. 12.3).[7,8,9,10]
    - Detect return of spontaneous circulation (ROSC) (Fig. 12.4).[7,8,9,10,14]

EQUIPMENT

- Personal protective equipment
- Capnometer
- Airway adapter or $Petco_2$ nasal cannula

PATIENT AND FAMILY EDUCATION

- Discuss with the patient and family the reason for implementation of capnography. ***Rationale:*** Discussing the purpose of monitoring reduces anxiety for the patient and/or family associated with an additional monitor, related interventions, and unfamiliar procedures.
- If the patient is alert, explain the procedure to the patient and family; if the patient is not alert, explain the procedure to the family. ***Rationale:*** Communication informs the patient and/or the family of procedure expectations, reduces anxiety, and improves cooperation with interventions.

PATIENT ASSESSMENT AND PREPARATION

Patient Assessment

- Assess for indications for $Petco_2$ monitoring, including general anesthesia,[1] monitored anesthesia care, procedural sedation and analgesia,[3,4,7,12] confirmation of endotracheal tube placement,[9] adequacy of chest compressions in cardiopulmonary arrest,[9,11,14] detection of ROSC,[9] analysis/

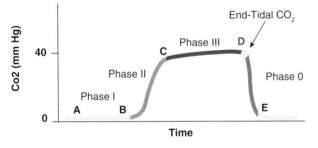

Figure 12.1 Essentials of the normal capnographic waveform. Phase I (A–B): baseline; phase II (B–C): rapid sharp expiratory upstroke; phase III (C–D): expiratory plateau; D: end-tidal concentration; phase 0 (D–E): rapid downstroke, inspiration. *(From Gallagher JJ: Capnography monitoring during procedural sedation and analgesia. AACN Adv Crit Care 26(4):405-414. © 2018 by the American Association of Critical-Care Nurses. All rights reserved. Used with permission.)*

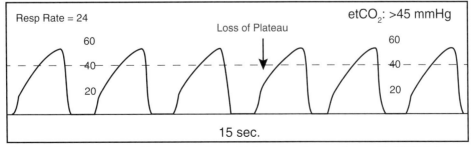

Figure 12.2 Waveform with curved upslope with loss of expiratory plateau. *(© 2023 Medtronic. All rights reserved. Used with the permission of Medtronic.)*

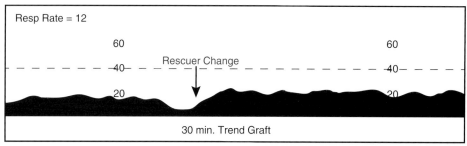

Figure 12.3 Cardiac arrest Petco₂ waveform demonstrating cardiopulmonary resuscitation. *(© 2023 Medtronic. All rights reserved. Used with the permission of Medtronic.)*

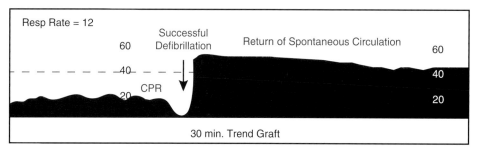

Figure 12.4 Cardiac arrest Petco₂ waveform showing return of spontaneous circulation (ROSC). *(© 2023 Medtronic. All rights reserved. Used with the permission of Medtronic.)*

monitoring of ventilation in mechanical ventilation,[11] obstructive sleep apnea,[1] and neuromuscular disease. Additional indications (actual or potential) include acute airway obstruction or apnea, dead space ventilation, and incomplete alveolar emptying. ***Rationale:*** Assessment for initiation of Petco₂ monitoring ensures that patients at risk for inadequate ventilation and gas exchange receive monitoring for such occurrences, allowing for early implementation of appropriate interventions.

Patient Preparation

- Verify the correct patient with two identifiers. ***Rationale:*** Before performing a procedure, the nurse should ensure the correct identification of the patient for the intended intervention.
- Ensure that the patient understands preprocedural teaching. Answer questions as they arise, and reinforce information as needed. ***Rationale:*** Understanding of previously taught information is evaluated and reinforced.

Procedure for Continuous End-Tidal Carbon Dioxide Monitoring

Steps	Rationale	Special Considerations
1. **HH**		
2. **PE**		
3. Obtain order or follow institutional protocol for continuous Petco₂ monitoring with capnography.	Order provides guideline for duration of monitoring, acceptable parameters for results, and appropriate interventions for abnormal results.	
4. Assess for proper functioning of capnograph, including electronic equipment, self-start, autocalibration, airway adapter, sensor, and display monitor, and secure connections. (**Level M***)	Ensures reliability of Petco₂ values and waveforms obtained.	
5. Connect the capnometer into a grounded wall outlet, connect the appropriate patient cable into the display monitor, and turn on the instrument. (**Level M***)	Decreases the incidence of electrical interference.	Check capnograph's battery capacity and charging time, if applicable.

Procedure for Continuous End-Tidal Carbon Dioxide Monitoring—*Continued*		
Steps	Rationale	Special Considerations
6. Perform the calibration routine as per manufacturer's recommendations for use. The calibration procedure should occur most often when the instrument is in clinical use.[3,9] **(Level M*)**	Accurate measurement for devices depends on proper calibration. Improper calibration may lead to erroneous $Petco_2$ values.	All monitors have some type of calibration procedure; see operator's manual for exact steps.
7. If the patient is not intubated, apply the $Petco_2$ nasal cannula and connect it to the capnograph.		$Petco_2$ nasal cannula does not require supplemental oxygen to measure $Petco_2$.
8. For intubated patients, assemble the airway adapter, sensor, and display monitor; connect to the patient's circuit as close as possible to the patient's ventilation connection.	Decreases the incidence of improper gas sampling.	Sampling errors and gas leaks in the system are major causes of inaccurate readings. Placing the sensor or sampling port as close as possible to the patient's airway decreases response time to detect a change in CO_2.
9. Ensure that the light source is on top of the circuit so condensation and secretions do not pool and obstruct the light transmission in the mainstream sensor. **(Level M*)**	Decreases condensation and secretion accumulation on the CO_2 port, where gas is drawn for sampling.	
10. Set appropriate alarms. Alarm limits should include respiratory rate, apnea default, high and low $Petco_2$, and minimal levels of inspiratory CO_2. The alarm limit should be set according to institutional policy. **(Level M*)**	Alerts the nurse to potentially life-threatening problems.	The $Petco_2$ alarm is set 5% above and below acceptable parameter or per institutional standards. If the monitor is interfaced with other equipment (electrocardiogram monitor, mechanical ventilator, pulse oximeter), ensure that alarms are set consistently among all monitors.
11. Discard **PE** and used supplies in appropriate receptacles.		
12. **HH**		

*Level M: Manufacturer's recommendations only.

Expected Outcomes
- Early significant changes in ventilatory status are detected
- Alterations in the alveolar-arterial carbon dioxide gradient are identified

Unexpected Outcomes
- Inaccurate measurements of $Petco_2$ are displayed
- Inaccurate measurements from calibration drift or contamination of optics with moisture or secretions are displayed
- Equipment malfunction occurs
- Inadvertent extubation from weight of sensor

Procedure continues on following page

UNIT I

Patient Monitoring and Care

Steps	Rationale	Reportable Conditions
		These conditions should be reported if they persist despite nursing interventions.
1. **HH**		
2. **PE**		
3. Observe the artificial airway for patency.[11]	The airway adapter often adds weight to the airway and increases the risk of dislodgment or kinking. If kinking occurs, support the airway with an artificial support or towel.	Endotracheal or tracheal tube dislodgment
4. If the patient is not intubated, check the nasal cannula or mouthpiece for proper placement, and ensure that it is clear of secretions.	Poor placement or occlusion of the nasal cannula or mouthpiece interferes with accurate $Petco_2$ monitoring.	
5. Observe waveform for quality. **(Level M*)**	If the waveform is of poor quality, the numerical $Petco_2$ value should not be accepted. If the $Petco_2$ waveform is acceptable and the $Petco_2$ numerical reading is questionable, obtain arterial blood gas measurement to confirm changes in $Petco_2$.	Poor-quality waveform Questionable $Petco_2$ reading
6. Observe waveform for gradually increasing $Petco_2$ (Fig. 12.5).[14]	Increasing $Petco_2$ occurs from increased CO_2 production, absorption of CO_2 from exogenous sources, increased circulatory delivery of CO_2 to the lungs, and increased elimination of CO_2. Clinical conditions in which increasing $Petco_2$ results from increased metabolism include hyperthermia (usually indicated by a rapid increase in $Petco_2$), pain, shivering, malignant hyperthermia, sepsis, and diabetic ketoacidosis. Clinical conditions that include increased circulator delivery of CO_2 include bradypnea, hypoventilation, sedation, analgesia, ingestion of respiratory depressant drugs, inadequate minute ventilation, neuromuscular blockade, decreased alveolar ventilation, partial airway obstruction, and conditions that cause metabolic alkalosis. Clinical conditions with a sudden increase in cardiac output such as ROSC and passive leg raise also result in increase in CO_2.	$Petco_2$ increase of greater than 10% of baseline

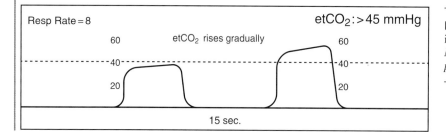

Figure 12.5 Waveform with gradually increasing $Petco_2$ or hypoventilation. *(© 2023 Medtronic. All rights reserved. Used with the permission of Medtronic.)*

Patient Monitoring and Care —*Continued*

Steps	Rationale	Reportable Conditions
7. Observe for an increase in both baseline CO_2 and $Petco_2$ values (Fig. 12.6).[14]	Reflects rebreathing of previously exhaled gas. Clinical conditions in which a gradual increase in both baseline CO_2 and $Petco_2$ levels is found include a defective exhalation valve on the mechanical ventilator, excessive mechanical dead space in the ventilator circuit, insufficient expiratory time, or partial rebreathing.	Malfunction of the ventilator

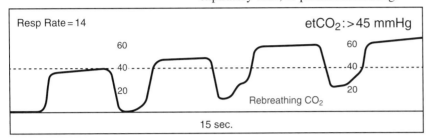

Resp Rate = 14   etCO$_2$:>45 mmHg

Rebreathing CO$_2$

15 sec.

Figure 12.6 Waveform with rebreathing CO_2 without return to baseline. *(© 2023 Medtronic. All rights reserved. Used with the permission of Medtronic.)*

8. Observe for an exponential decrease in $Petco_2$ (Fig. 12.7).[14]	Indicates an increase in dead space ventilation or hyperventilation or seen in clinical conditions with a decrease in pulmonary blood flow such as cardiopulmonary bypass, pulmonary embolism, or severe pulmonary hypoperfusion.[12]	$Petco_2$ decrease by greater than 10% of baseline

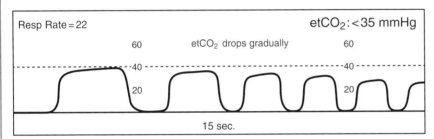

Resp Rate = 22   etCO$_2$:<35 mmHg

etCO$_2$ drops gradually

15 sec.

Figure 12.7 Waveform with gradual decrease in $Petco_2$ or hyperventilation. *(© 2023 Medtronic. All rights reserved. Used with the permission of Medtronic.)*

9. Observe for decreased $Petco_2$ (with a normal waveform) (Fig. 12.8).[14]	Gradual decreases indicate a decrease in perfusion such as patients with high minute volumes, hyperventilation, decreased cardiac output, and hypovolemia or a decrease in CO_2 production such as sedation, hypothermia, sleep, and compensated metabolic acidosis.	$Petco_2$ decreased by greater than 10% of baseline

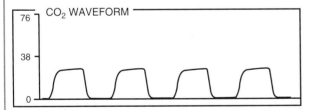

CO$_2$ WAVEFORM

Figure 12.8 Decreased $Petco_2$. *(Reprinted with permission from Nellcor Puritan Bennett LLC, Boulder, CO, part of Covidien.)*

10. Observe for a sudden decrease in $Petco_2$ to low values (Fig. 12.9).[14]	Incomplete sampling or full exhalation is not detected in the system. This may be seen in patients with a leak in the airway system, partial airway obstruction, mechanical ventilator malfunction, malpositioning/dislodgement of the airway, or partial disconnection of a ventilator circuit.	$Petco_2$ decreased by greater than 10% of baseline

Procedure continues on following page

Patient Monitoring and Care —*Continued*

Steps	Rationale	Reportable Conditions

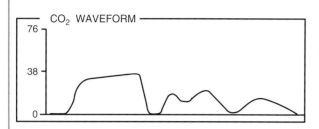

Figure 12.9 Sudden decrease in Petco₂ values. (*Reprinted with permission from Nellcor Puritan Bennett LLC, Boulder, CO, part of Covidien.*)

11. Observe for a sudden decrease in Petco₂ to near zero (Fig. 12.10).[14]

Drop in waveform to baseline or near baseline (baseline equals zero) implies that no respirations are present. A decrease in waveform may also occur within the case of significant ventilation/perfusion changes such as pulmonary emboli, airway disconnect, or an unplanned extubation.

Dislodged endotracheal tube
Complete airway obstruction
Mechanical ventilator malfunction
Airway disconnection
Esophageal intubation
Apnea

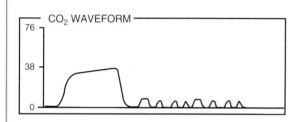

Figure 12.10 Sudden decrease in Petco₂ to near zero. (*Reprinted with permission from Nellcor Puritan Bennett LLC, Boulder, CO, part of Covidien.*)

12. Observe for a sustained low Petco₂ without an alveolar plateau (Fig. 12.11).[14]

Sustained low Petco₂ values are indicative of incomplete alveolar emptying, such as in a partially kinked endotracheal tube, bronchospasm, mucous plugging, improper exhaled gas sampling, or insufficient expiratory time on the ventilator.

Complete airway obstruction that necessitates reintubation
Petco₂ decreased by greater than 10% of baseline

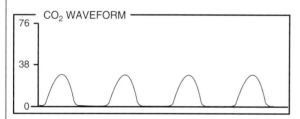

Figure 12.11 Low Petco₂, without an alveolar plateau. (*Reprinted with permission from Nellcor Puritan Bennett LLC, Boulder, CO, part of Covidien.*)

13. Routinely monitor the airway adapter or sampling port for signs of obstruction.[14]

If the adapter or the port becomes obstructed, the quality of the capnographic waveform will be poor, and Petco₂ is not reliable.

Obstruction in the airway adapter or sampling port

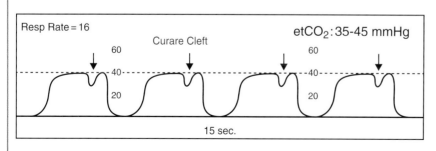

Figure 12.12 Waveform with cleft suggestive of attempts at spontaneous breathing while paralytics are used. (*© 2023 Medtronic. All rights reserved. Used with the permission of Medtronic.*)

Patient Monitoring and Care —*Continued*

Steps	Rationale	Reportable Conditions
14. Evaluate the patient's response to activities that may positively or negatively affect ventilation (e.g., sedation, analgesia, suctioning, repositioning, change in mechanical support, nutritional supplementation, cardiopulmonary resuscitation (CPR), neuromuscular blockade, verification of endotracheal tube placement·).[2,5,6,8,10] **(Level A*)**	The impact of activities (e.g., suctioning, repositioning, change in mechanical support, nutritional supplementation, CPR, neuromuscular blockade, verification of endotracheal tube placement) on ventilation can be evaluated with $Petco_2$ monitoring. Waveform capnography allows the provider to monitor CPR quality, optimize chest compressions, and detect ROSC. High quality chest compressions are achieved when the $Petco_2$ value is between 10 and 20 mm Hg.[7]	$Petco_2$ values increased or decreased by more than 10% of baseline During CPR for an intubated patient, measurement of a $Petco_2$ <10 mm Hg would indicate that the quality of chest compressions need improvement. When ROSC occurs, there will be a significant increase in $Petco_2$ (35–45 mm Hg).[7] Curare cleft is a patient's attempt at a spontaneous breath suggestive of inadequate paralysis or sedation (Fig. 12.12).
15. Discontinue and discard supplies	Once clinical indication for continuous $Petco_2$ is no longer needed, continuous $Petco_2$ can be discontinued.	
16. ㏊		

*Level A: Meta-analysis of quantitative studies or metasynthesis of qualitative studies with results that consistently support a specific action, interventions, or treatment (including systematic review of randomized controlled trials).Well-designed, controlled studies with results that consistently support a specific action, intervention, or treatment.
*Level M: Manufacturer's recommendations only.

Documentation

Documentation should include the following:
- Patient and family education
- Mechanical ventilator settings
- $Petco_2$ value and capnogram
- $Paco_2$-$Petco_2$ gradient (special attention should be given to this gradient as an indication of dead space ventilation)
- Arterial blood gases
- Times of calibration
- Respiratory therapies
- Medications that may affect the respiratory system (e.g., neuromuscular blockers, sedatives, bronchodilators)
- Respiratory assessment (e.g., respiratory rate, breathing patterns, adventitious sounds)
- Unexpected outcomes
- Assessment findings and nursing interventions
- Patient teaching

For a complete list of references and additional readings for this procedure, scan this QR code with any freely available smartphone code reader app, or visit https://www.elsevier.com/__data/assets/pdf_file/0009/1319787/Chapter0012.pdf.

13 Extracorporeal Membrane Oxygenation

Kelly Moutray and Marci Ebberts

PURPOSE: Extracorporeal membrane oxygenation (ECMO) is a mechanical circulatory assist device used to support the heart or the heart and lungs when conventional means prove inadequate or when their delivery proves more damaging (i.e., high-dose vasopressors or high ventilator settings) than therapeutic. When oxygen delivery cannot meet oxygen demand, ECMO is used to pump blood out of the body through an external membrane (oxygenator), where carbon dioxide is removed and replaced with oxygen, then pumped back to the tissues and organs of the body.[6] There are multiple indications for ECMO in adults with acute severe heart and/or lung failure with high mortality risk despite optimal conventional therapy.[4,15]

PREREQUISITE NURSING KNOWLEDGE

- Advanced cardiac life support skills.
- Cardiac anatomy and physiology including central venous and arterial anatomy, arterial and venous blood gas interpretation, cardiac and respiratory failure, and ventilator management.
- Fundamental understanding of ECMO equipment and mechanics.[14]
- Participation in a specialized ECMO curriculum and annual competency.[16]
- An understanding of the possible causes of cardiac and/or respiratory failure.
- Drug properties may influence the degree of bioavailability in the ECMO-supported patient. An understanding of pharmacokinetics is important.
- ECMO physiology differs significantly based on cannula location, even though the circuit configuration that delivers oxygenated blood under pressure remains the same.
  - ❖ Venous-to-venous (VV) cannulation provides gas exchange (oxygenation of blood and removal of carbon dioxide) and is used exclusively for respiratory failure (Fig. 13.1).[20]
  - ❖ Venous to arterial (VA) cannulation also provides mechanical circulatory support by introducing the oxygenated blood under pressure into the arterial system (providing circulatory support as well as gas exchange) (Fig. 13.2).
- There are many possible cannulation sites.[5,26] Deoxygenated blood is mechanically pumped out of the body with a drainage cannula most commonly placed in the femoral or internal jugular vein or sometimes directly from the right atrium (central cannulation) into an exchanger, where blood is oxygenated and carbon dioxide is removed.
- In VV ECMO, the oxygenated blood is then pumped back via the return cannula into the right atrium (VV). A single dual-lumen bicaval cannula for VV cannulation is also available.[4]

- In instances of right ventricular failure, the ECMO cannulation may be configured to return the oxygenated blood to the pulmonary artery, thereby using ECMO as a right ventricular assist device (RVAD).
- In VA ECMO, the oxygenated blood is returned via a cannula placed in the aorta, thereby bypassing the weak left ventricle. Other cannula configurations might be considered, depending on patient need and physician preference.[8] Connection of a plasmapheresis device or renal replacement with the ECMO circuit is possible, but elevated pressures can be problematic.[19]
- Indications:

There are multiple indications for extracorporeal membrane oxygenation (ECMO) in adults with acute severe heart and/or lung failure with high mortality including cardiac arrest.[6,15]
  - ❖ Indications for VV ECMO: Respiratory failure, including acute hypoxic respiratory failure of any etiology[4,18] when the risk of mortality is greater than 50% (Pao_2/Fio_2 <150 on Fio_2 >90%). The Murray lung injury score, which considers consolidation on chest x-ray, Pao_2/Fio_2 ratio, positive end-expiratory pressure (PEEP), and compliance (calculated with tidal volume, peak inspiratory pressure, and PEEP) may also be used to determine when ECMO should be considered.[21] When the risk of mortality is greater than 80% (Pao_2/Fio_2 <100 on Fio_2 >90% and/or a Murray lung injury score of 3 to 4), ECMO is indicated. Other indications for VV ECMO include hypercarbic respiratory failure refractory to traditional mechanical ventilator support, despite plateau pressure (Pplat) >30 cm H_2O, severe air leak syndromes (such as from a bronchopleural fistula after a pulmonary resection), bridge to lung transplantation, or immediate respiratory collapse (pulmonary emboli, blocked airway).[15,18]
  - ❖ Indications for VA ECMO: Cardiogenic shock, as a bridge to a ventricular assist device (VAD), transplant, or recovery caused by inadequate tissue perfusion

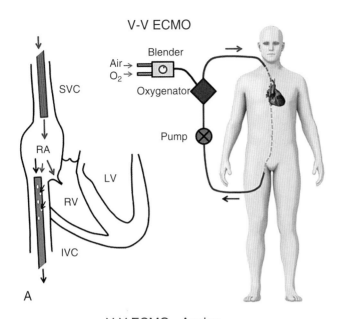

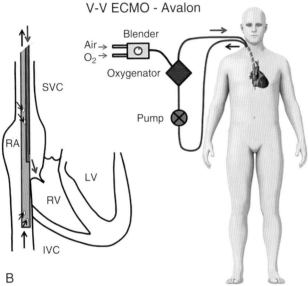

Figure 13.1 **A,** Venous-to-venous (VV) cannulation using two catheters. **B,** VV cannulation using a single-lumen single catheter. *IVC,* inferior vena cava; *LV,* left ventricle; *PA,* pulmonary artery; *RA,* right ventricle; *SVC,* superior vena cava. (*Image reproduced with permission from http://icuecmo.ca.*)

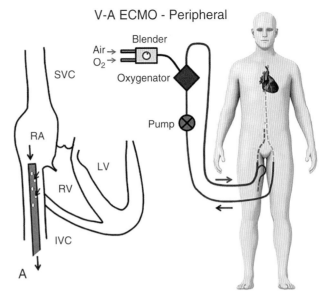

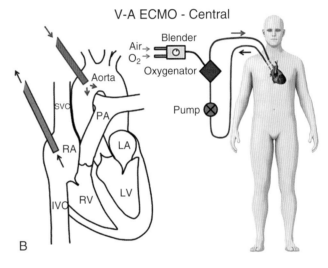

Figure 13.2 **A,** Venous-to-arterial (VA) cannulation —peripheral. **B,** VA cannulation. *IVC,* inferior vena cava; *LV,* left ventricle; *PA,* pulmonary artery; *RA,* right ventricle; *SVC,* superior vena cava. (*Image reproduced with permission from http://icuecmo.ca.*).

from low cardiac output despite adequate volume resuscitation, refractory to inotropes, vasopressors, and intraaortic balloon pump counterpulsation. This typically occurs secondary to acute myocardial infarction, myocarditis, peripartum cardiomyopathy, decompensated chronic heart failure, or postcardiotomy shock.[15]

- Indication for extracorporeal cardiopulmonary resuscitation (ECPR): Witnessed arrest with refractory pulselessness despite advanced cardiac life support and continuous CPR with an easily reversible etiology[15,28]

• Contraindications: Most contraindications are relative, balancing the potential benefits with the risks involved[8,15]:
  - Irreversible central nervous system damage
  - Multiple organ dysfunction syndrome

- Unrecoverable native heart in a patient who is not a candidate for a VAD, total artificial heart, or cardiac transplant
- Chronic organ dysfunction (i.e., liver failure, renal failure requiring dialysis)
- Prolonged CPR with unknown downtime and unknown neurological status[27]
- Preexistent illness affecting overall quality of life, such as terminal malignancy
- Mechanical ventilation with high airway pressures and/ or high levels of FiO_2 greater than 7 days or more.[15] The most favorable outcomes are associated with early ECMO support, within 1 to 2 days.[15]
- Contraindication to anticoagulation
- Advanced age with risk of complications and mortality increasing with age[31]
- Pharmacological immunosuppression (absolute neutrophil count <400/mm³)[15]
- Recent or expanding central nervous system hemorrhage

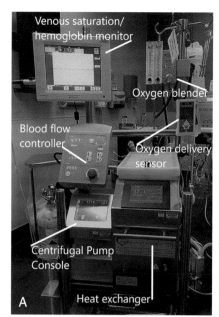
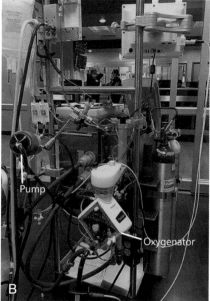

Figure 13.3 **A,** Complete extracorporeal membrane oxygenation (ECMO) circuit *(front).* **B,** Complete extracorporeal membrane oxygenation (ECMO) circuit *(back).*

- Obesity is not a contraindication to ECMO, and there is no specific maximum weight or body mass index.[33]

Considerations:
- VV cannulation reduces the risk of arterial thrombus and limb ischemia, but the patient must have adequate circulatory function (may be supported with vasoactive medications and inotropes).[5,15]
- In a VV configuration, mixed venous oxygenation saturation measurements are elevated, reflecting that the venous return blood is fully saturated from the exterior oxygenator.[8,15]
- Cannula placement should be assessed on initial placement with echocardiography, radiographs, or fluoroscopy, and serially by measuring and documenting the length from the skin puncture to the end of the cannula.

EQUIPMENT

- Nonsterile gloves, masks, and caps
- Sterile gloves, gowns, and drapes
- Central venous catheter insertion supplies (see Procedure 75, Central Venous Catheter Insertion [Assist], Nursing Care and Removal)
- Arterial catheter insertion supplies (see Procedure 53, Arterial Catheter Insertion [Assist], Nursing Care and Removal)
- Normal saline intravenous solutions
- Tape
- Sutures
- Commercial tube securement device
- Cannulas
    - VV: either large dual lumen cannula or two large venous cannulas (see Fig. 13.1)
    - VA: large venous drainage and arterial return cannulas. May need a small catheter for antegrade distal

femoral artery perfusion to prevent lower extremity ischemia.[27] The distal perfusion cannula returns a small portion of the oxygenated arterial return blood to the lower extremity, distal to the large arterial cannula (see Fig. 13.2A).
- Equipment needed (Fig. 13.3):
    - ECMO device, including components:
    - Pump
    - Oxygenator
    - Heat exchanger
    - Oxygen delivery sensor
    - Blood flow controller
    - Centrifugal pump console
    - Venous saturation and hemoglobin monitor if available

Additional equipment to have available as needed includes the following:
- Emergency cart (defibrillator, respiratory equipment, cardiac medications)
- Extra intravenous pumps
- Ultrasound/echocardiography equipment
- Mechanical ventilator

PATIENT AND FAMILY EDUCATION

- Answer questions and address concerns from the family regarding ECMO therapy. *Rationale:* Explanation may decrease patient and family anxiety.
- Explain the environment and plan of care to the patient and family on an ongoing basis, including but not limited to the frequency of assessment; sounds and function of equipment; placement of the cannulas; explanation of alarms, dressings, and additional therapies; diagnosis; and prognosis. *Rationale:* This communication provides information to the patient and family and may alleviate some of the apprehension they experience.[30,32]

PATIENT ASSESSMENT AND PREPARATION

Patient Assessment

- Assess the patient's medical history, including cardiac, pulmonary, renal, and other chronic and acute illnesses. *Rationale:* Provides important baseline data.
- Perform a hemodynamic, cardiovascular, peripheral vascular, pulmonary, and neurological assessment. *Rationale:* Provides baseline data.
- Assess the current laboratory profile specifically including complete blood count (CBC), chemistry panel, partial thromboplastin time (PTT), international normalization ratio (INR), liver function panel, arterial blood gas (ABG), type and crossmatch, and central or mixed venous oxygen saturation if access is available. *Rationale:* Provides baseline data and prepares to anticipate complications, including possible blood transfusion.
- Assess for active bleeding, *Rationale:* The inner surface of the cannulas, the tubing, and the oxygenator are thrombogenic, and the patient will require anticoagulation to prevent thrombus formation. Severe bleeding is a contraindication to anticoagulation and thus is problematic for patients requiring ECMO.

Patient Preparation

- Verify the correct patient with two identifiers. *Rationale:* Before performing a procedure, the physician, advanced practice nurse, or other healthcare professional should ensure the correct identification of the patient for the intended intervention.
- Ensure that the patient and/or family understands the pre-procedural information. Answer questions as they arise, and reinforce information as needed. *Rationale:* Understanding of previously taught information is evaluated and reinforced.
- Perform a pre-procedure verification and time out. *Rationale:* Ensures patient safety.
- Administer prescribed sedation or analgesics as needed. *Rationale:* Sedation and analgesics minimize anxiety and discomfort.
- Ensure that an echocardiogram has been performed as prescribed. *Rationale:* This study documents heart function.

Procedure	for Extracorporeal Membrane Oxygenation	
Steps	Rationale	Special Considerations
Assisting with Initial Cannulation (if not already cannulated)		
1. Gather equipment; type of equipment will depend on the type of cannulas to be placed (**Level M***)	VV vs. VA configurations require different types of cannulas.[5]	Intraoperative or emergent bedside central cannulation by sternotomy approach may be required but is not a first-line approach.
2. Plug the pump controller into an electrical outlet with an emergency power backup	Provides the power supply. Battery life may vary.	Have heparin available to be administered by bolus and continuous infusion at the time of cannulation.[15]
3. Prime the ECMO circuit with sterile saline.	The circuit should be free from air to prevent air embolism.	
1. 🅷🅷		
2. 🅿🅴		ECMO is not considered an aerosol-generating procedure, but patients on a ventilator may require droplet and/or airborne precautions depending on the underlying diagnosis.
4. Assist as needed with clipping hair and preparing the skin with an antiseptic solution (e.g., 2% chlorhexidine-based preparation).	Limits the introduction of potentially infectious skin flora into the vessel during the puncture.	
5. Discard used supplies, perform hand hygiene, and apply sterile gown and gloves if assisting with cannulation.	Reduces the transmission of microorganisms and prepares for the procedure.	Cap and mask are required for everyone in the room. Sterile gown and gloves are required for those performing or directly assisting with cannulation.
6. Assist as needed with placing sterile drapes.	Prepares sterile field.	

*Level M: Manufacturer's recommendations only

UNIT I

Procedure	for Extracorporeal Membrane Oxygenation—*Continued*	
Steps	Rationale	Special Considerations
7. If ultrasound is to be used, assist as needed with equipment, and ensure that the probe is covered with a sterile sheath.	Maintenance of sterile technique is essential to prevent bacteremia and device colonization and reduces contamination risk.[6]	Ultrasound will not provide useable images without adequate conduction gel. Sterile ultrasound gel must be inside and outside the sheath.
8. Assist with cannulation as directed by the provider.	Provides needed assistance.	Ensure that sterility is maintained throughout the procedure.
9. Before initiation of the pump, the cannulas are connected to the ECMO circuit with a wet-to-wet connection to ensure an airless seal. (**Level D***)	A wet-to-wet connection ensures an airless seal, preventing air bubbles from entering the system and preventing air embolism.[15]	
10. Assess for dark venous blood draining from the drainage cannula and return of bright red oxygenated blood to the return cannula. Label the ends of the cannulas as *drainage* and *return*. (**Level D***)	Drainage cannula (deoxygenated blood to the ECMO circuit). Return cannula (oxygenated blood returning to the patient).[15,22]	Poor color change means the cannulas may be positioned too closely and should prompt further investigation for signs of recirculation.
11. Some patients may require placement of an additional distal perfusion catheter (**Level E***)	Some VA configurations may require a second, smaller return line to provide distal antegrade perfusion because the large arterial cannula often blocks flow.[8]	This may be placed during the initial cannulation or at a later date. Assessment of a third cannula will be required.
12. Assist as needed with applying sterile, transparent dressings.	Decreases the risk of infection.	According to institutional protocols.
13. Assist the insertion team as radiographs, fluoroscopy, or bedside echocardiography are obtained.	Aids in determining proper positioning of the cannulas.	
14. Measure the length of exposed cannula, from insertion site to metal end. Mark the skin, secure tightly with both tape and sutures, and document. (**Level E***)	Ensures that the system is secure; maintains safety.[7]	Consider also utilizing a commercial tube attachment device.
15. Imaging postcannulation may include chest and abdominal x-rays and formal echocardiogram.	Ensures proper placement of cannulas and patient response to ECMO.	
16. Reassessment of patient following ECMO initiation may require rapid titration of vasopressors, inotropes, and pulmonary vasodilators as well as changes to ventilator settings.	As patient responds to ECMO, hemodynamic parameters and perfusion may change rapidly.	Clear communication of changing assessment findings with the provider and other team members is critical to meet the needs of the patient.
17. Obtain laboratory samples, including arterial and venous blood gases and response to anticoagulation.	Titrations to ECMO and ventilator settings are determined by blood gases. Anticoagulation is necessary to prevent clotting, but bleeding becomes a greater risk.	Pre- and postoxygenator gases may be obtained to determine functionality of the oxygenator.
18. Remove 🄿🄴 and sterile equipment, and discard used supplies.		
19. 🄷🄷		

*Level E: Multiple case reports, theory-based evidence from expert opinions, or peer-reviewed professional organizational standards without clinical studies to support recommendations

*Level D: Peer-reviewed professional and organizational standards with the support of clinical study recommendations

Procedure continues on following page

Procedure   for Troubleshooting

Steps	Rationale	Special Considerations
1. **HH**		
2. **PE**		
3. High pressure alarms (>300–400 mm Hg) if available on the pump controller. Check the circuit distal to the pump for kinks or occlusions. Check the patient's blood pressure. **(Level D*)**	The high-pressure alarm indicates increased pressures on the (arterial) return side of the oxygenator. Small clots caught in the oxygen exchanger or pump may impede blood flow, resulting in a high-pressure alarm. In a VA configuration, this alarm may result from an elevated blood pressure.[15]	Notify the provider if unable to resolve high pressure alarms.

4. Assess for chatter/chugging of the ECMO circuit tubing, and report to provider immediately
A. Assess the patient's volume status.
    i. Decreasing the flow rate (if hemodynamically appropriate) can temporarily reduce chatter, but the flow setting should be returned to previous settings when possible.
    ii. Flow should be noted before and after decreasing support.
B. Assess cannula position and patient positioning by comparing with the baseline cannula position measurement for evidence of catheter migration. Radiographic confirmation may also be necessary.
	Relative or absolute volume depletion will require administration of fluids or blood. Chatter can lead to hemolysis.[6,15] A malpositioned or kinked cannula may create turbulent staccato flow leading to chatter.	Decreasing the flow rate is a temporary solution; correcting the underlying fluid deficiency must be addressed. When the drainage cannula sucks up against the venous wall, turbulent staccato flow through the circuit may cause the tubes to shake.

5. Assess for clots or fibrin deposits within the circuit tubing and oxygenator (clots typically have a dark maroon appearance, and fibrin deposits are white), and notify the provider if they are found. **(Level D*)**	Deposits on the oxygenator can decrease its efficiency and lead to decreased gas exchange. Deposits distal to the oxygenator (arterial) in the return cannula may embolize, causing pulmonary embolus, stroke, or organ damage from ischemia. Large deposits may cause hemodynamically significant alterations in flow rate, turbulent flow, and hemolysis.	Turbulent swirling of the blood near clots or fibrin deposits may be seen through the tubing. Clots may require exchange of the affected part of the circuit. Notify the perfusionist or ECMO specialist if a clot is noted.[15] Ensure that anticoagulation is therapeutic (patient-specific PTT goal). Therapeutic anticoagulation reduces the risk of developing these deposits. Typically heparin (but alternatively a direct thrombin inhibitor such as argatroban or bivalirudin) may be used if heparin-induced thrombocytopenia is suspected.

*Level D: Peer-reviewed professional and organizational standards with the support of clinical study recommendations

Procedure for Troubleshooting—*Continued*		
Steps	**Rationale**	**Special Considerations**

6. Electrical or mechanical failure
  A. Ensure pump switches to battery power.
  B. Switch off the water bath/heater.
  C. If the battery loses power, hand crank the pump:
    i. Remove the pump from its electronic power source.
    ii. Attach the manufacturer-supplied hand crank, and turn. Notify the physician. **(Level M*)**
	ECMO machines typically have a short battery life.
	Switching off less essential components such as the heater can conserve power (if both the controller and heater are receiving power from the same source). Hand-cranking the pump can prevent low-flow thrombosis and continue to provide some support until power is restored.
		Some pumps may not have a hand-cranking backup feature. Summon assistance as this will be fatiguing if done for an extended period.
		Be aware of the expected battery duration at your institution, and take this into consideration when planning to move the patient (e.g., for CT scanning).

7. Assess for hyperthermia. If the patient's temperature is higher than the target:
  A. Use the ice bath.
  B. Use the heater, and adjust the temperature knob to the desired temperature.
	Fevers can be controlled by utilizing an ice bath within the circuit to cool the blood as it passes through.	If the patient's condition warrants, workup for infection should be completed and empiric antibiotics initiated.

8. Assess for hypothermia.[4]	Due to the large volume of blood circulating outside the body, patients are susceptible to heat loss.[6]	The ECMO circuit will have a temperature exchanger with a heater and ice bath, and the desired temperature may be adjusted with a dial and utilization of an ice bath. The ECMO circuit may be utilized to maintain normothermia in hypothermic patients. The ECMO circuit may be utilized to induce and maintain hypothermia/targeted temperature management (e.g., post–cardiac arrest).

9. Assess for inadequate oxygenation.
  A. If the outlet saturation (determined by drawing a blood gas from the return cannula of the circuit, postoxygenator) is <95%, venous saturation (before the oxygenator) is ≥70–75%, and Hgb is ≥12, the oxygenator may need to be exchanged.
  B. Check for water in the gas phase.
  C. Assess hematocrit. In general, a hematocrit greater than 40% will optimize oxygen delivery. **(Level D*)**
	Because of the altered cardiopulmonary physiology in ECMO patients, oxygenation can provide clues to device malfunction or the need to titrate oxygen delivery. Suggests failure of the oxygenator itself, as opposed to a problem with the patient. Optimizing hematocrit improves the oxygen-carrying capacity of the blood.[15]	Maximizing gas flow through the oxygenator will improve hypoxemia, but further evaluation is typically warranted. Increasing RPMs can cause hemolysis over time. Address patient conditions contributing to increased oxygen consumption. Exchange of components in the ECMO circuit is typically performed by a perfusionist or ECMO specialist. Hematocrit targets may vary by center; follow institutional standards.

*Level M: Manufacturer's recommendations only

*Level D: Peer-reviewed professional and organizational standards with the support of clinical study recommendations

Procedure continues on following page

Procedure **for Troubleshooting—*Continued***

10. Assess for hypercarbia (pH <7.35, pCO_2 >45).	Normalized Pco_2 contributes to acid-base balance and cerebral perfusion. Elevated Pco_2 typically requires adjustment to ECLS settings.	Increasing the sweep gas flow through the oxygenator will remove CO_2 from the blood. If the initial systemic Pco_2 is >70, it may take several hours to normalize. Avoid adjusting too rapidly, and follow arterial blood gas (ABG) trends.[15]
11. Assess for any air bubbles in the circuit. A. If air is found in the circuit, immediately clamp the lines, and notify the provider. B. Support the patient by increasing ventilator support and vasoactive support as prescribed. C. Check the circuit proximal to the pump for an open stopcock, leaky connection, tubing compromise, dislodged cannula, or decannulation. Correct the problem identified, and notify the physician. D. Check the intravenous lines for air in the line, and remove the air if found.	If air is allowed to enter the pulmonary artery or aorta, it may obstruct blood flow, causing organ ischemia.	Exercise caution with all venous lines and catheters and central line sites to avoid accidental entrainment of air into the circuit.
12. Assess extremities for inadequate perfusion including compartment syndrome: A. Diminished pulses, cool, mottled skin, or slow capillary refill. B. Pain, particularly with passive muscle stretch of the affected compartment, tautness of a muscular compartment C. Increasing girth of extremity.	Patients on VA ECMO are at higher risk for cannula-related limb complications. Ischemia from embolus or mechanical occlusion of the artery may cause compartment syndrome of the extremity distal to arterial cannulation.	A technique used to improve perfusion to the distal limb is placement of a distal perfusion cannula. An introducer sheath is inserted into the superficial femoral artery (SFA) just distal to the insertion point of the ECMO cannula and then attached to the side port of the arterial cannula. This provides the leg with retrograde perfusion, reducing risk of limb ischemia.[5] The presence of distal pulses does not rule out compartment syndrome. Consider obtaining an ABG from the right upper extremity and oxygen saturation in either the right upper extremity or the right earlobe, and compare with the left lower extremity or the lower extremities. Regional oxygenation saturation sensors may be helpful in detecting unilateral decreases in oxygenation.

Procedure	for Troubleshooting—*Continued*

13. In VA ECMO patients, evaluate for Harlequin syndrome, also known as *north-south syndrome* (flow competition in the aorta caused by left ventricular recovery with upper body hypoxia). **(Level D*)**	Harlequin syndrome[6,7] can occur as a result of flow competition in the aorta between the native left ventricle output and the ECMO return cannula output, leading to poorly oxygenated blood from the left ventricle entering the brachiocephalic and coronary arteries and well-oxygenated blood from the ECMO circuit only going to the more distal arteries.	Measurement of ABG should be from the right radial artery. Oxygen saturation is best monitored from the forehead, earlobe, or right finger. The presence of Harlequin syndrome can signal circulatory recovery. Consider change to VV if lung failure persists despite cardiac recovery.
14. In VA ECMO, assess for left ventricular (LV) strain. A pulmonary artery diastolic pressure greater than 25 mm Hg and an elevated PCWP suggests the LV is not properly decompressed. (For PA catheter troubleshooting, see Procedure 61, Pulmonary Artery Catheter and Pressure Lines, Troubleshooting)	The return cannula may create a marked increase in afterload that may lead to LV distention.[9]	A strategy to "vent" the left ventricle may need to be used, such as a temporary left ventricular assist device.
15. Assess for hemolysis. A. Check plasma-free hemoglobin and lactate dehydrogenase (LD). B. Assess urine color. C. Check the inlet suction. D. Check for clots in the pump chamber. E. Notify the physician. **(Level D*)** 16. Remove **PE**, and discard used supplies. 17. **HH**	Turbulence from rapid blood flow through a small opening can cause hemolysis.[3,6] Hemolysis may be a sign of device malfunction, turbulent flow, or excessive negative pressures, and it may require flow adjustment or cannula position adjustment.	Plasma-free hemoglobin >10 indicates hemolysis. Pink-tinged urine may be caused by hemolysis. Inlet suction >300 mm Hg can cause hemolysis.

*Level M: Manufacturer's recommendations only
*Level D: Peer-reviewed professional and organizational standards with the support of a clinical study recommendations

Expected Outcomes

- Rapid increase in oxygenation and gas exchange
- Circulatory stabilization
- Signs of adequate tissue perfusion

Unexpected Outcomes

- Related to initial cannulation: Perforation, rupture, tear, or dissection of femoral vein, vena cava, femoral artery, or aorta. Retroperitoneal hemorrhage. Cannula malposition. Inability to cannulate.
- Secondary: Distal limb ischemia, left ventricular distension, thrombosis, maldistribution of oxygenated blood (VA),[7] coagulopathy, hemorrhage (anticoagulation), organ failure, hemorrhagic stroke, hemolysis, bleeding, sepsis, air embolism skin breakdown, renal failure, cannula dislodgement.[23]
- Equipment failure: pump malfunction, oxygenator failure
- Hemolysis (membrane failure, turbulence in cannula or pump from hypovolemia)

Procedure continues on following page

Patient Monitoring and Care

Steps	Rationale	Reportable Conditions
		These conditions should be reported to the provider if they persist despite nursing interventions.
1. Assess vital signs and pulmonary artery pressures (if a PA catheter is present) frequently as the patient's status dictates. Titrate vasopressors and inotropic medications per provider orders. Follow institutional standards.	Demonstrates the effectiveness of ECMO therapy.	Unstable vital signs Abnormal pulmonary artery pressures
2. Assess level of consciousness.	Monitors for cerebral perfusion. Thrombi may develop and dislodge during ECMO therapy. Sudden neurological changes may be an indication of intracerebral hemorrhage.	Change in level of consciousness Changes in pupillary response Increased agitation or confusion Change in saturation levels (per device instructions for use) if utilizing cerebral oxygenation monitors
3. Perform pupil checks every 2–4 hours (more often if administering neuromuscular blockade).	Assess for adequacy of cerebral perfusion.[10,15]	Change in pupil size and reactivity
4. Follow institutional standards for assessing pain. Administer analgesia as needed.	Identifies the need for pain interventions.[1]	Continued pain despite pain interventions
5. Assess agitation and sedation using a validated scale (e.g., RASS), and administer anxiolytics as prescribed.	Identifies the need for medications and support.[11,30]	Continued anxiety despite anxiety interventions
6. If neuromuscular blockade is used, assess muscle relaxation with a peripheral nerve stimulator (e.g., Train of 4) according to institutional policy.[29] If available, may use bispectral index (BIS) monitoring to quantify depth of sedation (see Procedures 80, Peripheral Nerve Stimulation: Train of Four Monitoring and 83, Signal Processed EEG). (**Level D***)	Identifies the percent of nerve receptors blocked. Monitoring the depth of sedation during neuromuscular blockade ensures patient comfort while chemically paralyzed.[7,10,11,29]	Change in assessment findings
7. Assess circulation to the extremities at least every 2 hours.	Demonstrates adequate peripheral perfusion.[15] Changes may indicate thrombotic or embolic obstruction of perfusion to extremity. A rare but serious complication could be compartment syndrome of the extremity.	Capillary refill >3 seconds Diminished or absent pulses (pulses may be absent on VA support at high flow rates) Pale color or color change, mottled or cyanotic Diminished or absent sensation Pain Diminished or absent movement Cold or cool to touch
8. Assess for the presence or increase in edema. Position the patient to promote optimal perfusion of the extremities, and minimize dependent edema. (**Level D***)	Edema of extremities may indicate poor perfusion and concern for compartment syndrome.[15]	Change in skin integrity Increase in edema Signs or symptoms of compartment syndrome
9. Assess cardiac status by auscultating heart tones, evaluating for jugular venous distention, and assessing heart rhythm.	Demonstrates adequate perfusion and cardiac function. Provides baseline for weaning parameters.	Change in heart tones (e.g., new murmur) Change in heart rhythm

Patient Monitoring and Care —*Continued*		
Steps	Rationale	Reportable Conditions
10. Assess respiratory status by auscultating breath sounds and evaluating respiratory rate and effort, ABG, and peak inspiratory pressure if mechanically ventilated.	Demonstrates adequacy of respiratory/ventilator support (gas exchange is controlled primarily by the membrane oxygenator).	Abnormal ABG results Abnormal pulse oximetry values Abnormal breath sounds and pulmonary assessment
11. Assess for hypercarbia (Pco_2 >70). **(Level D*)**	Pco_2 contributes to acid-base balance and cerebral perfusion. Elevated Pco_2 typically requires adjustment to ECLS settings. Increasing the airflow through the "sweep" part of the oxygenator removes more CO_2 from the blood. If the initial systemic Pco_2 is >70, it may take several hours to normalize, so avoid adjusting too rapidly.[15]	Pco_2 >70
12. Perform gastrointestinal assessment (bowel sounds, bowel movements, abdominal assessment). Maintain nasogastric/orogastric tube for feeding and/or decompression as prescribed.	Monitors gastrointestinal status.	Changes in gastric tube drainage Abnormal bowel sounds Abdominal distention and tenderness Changes in bowel activity
13. Measure urine output hourly.	Demonstrates adequate perfusion to the kidneys.	Urine output <0.5 mL/kg/hour
14. Obtain daily weights.	Daily weights assist in assessment of fluid balance.	Change in weight of more than 2 kg/day
15. Maintain normothermia. Temperature is usually maintained close to 37°C. Core temperature should be monitored. If the patient was cannulated during or after a resuscitation event or has other conditions that could lead to hypoxic ischemic brain injury, it is reasonable to maintain mild hypothermia (32–34°C) for the first 24–72 hours to minimize brain injury. **(Level D*)**	Temperature can be regulated by adjusting the temperature of the water bath. Mild hypothermia after an anoxic event may improve the odds of neurological recovery.[13,15]	Difficulty maintaining targeted temperature
16. For patients with femoral cannulation, consider elevating the head of the bed by placing the patient in the reverse Trendelenburg position.	Elevation and maintaining the patient's head in midline position encourage venous return. Placing the patient in the reverse Trendelenburg position elevates the patient's head without compromising femoral lines.	Change in venous return as evidenced by change in flow rates
17. Encourage regular sleep-wake cycles by providing periods of stimulation and quiet time.[15] **(Level D*)**	Clustering of care, intermittent periods of darkness, and promoting prolonged periods of rest can promote neurological recovery.[2]	Lack of response to therapy, disruption of sleep-wake cycle, or increased delirium

Procedure continues on following page

Patient Monitoring and Care —*Continued*

Steps	Rationale	Reportable Conditions
18. Monitor platelet count, hematocrit, activated clotting time (ACT), CBC count, prothrombin time (PT), PTT, and INR as ordered. Consider measurement of thromboelastography (TEG) in the setting of profound coagulopathy.	Anticoagulation increases the risk of intracranial hemorrhage and excessive bleeding.[25] Hematocrit should be >40%.[15]	Abnormal laboratory values; follow institutional standards
19. Monitor daily laboratory values and chest x-rays.	Identify changes to baseline data.	Abnormal laboratory values
20. Monitor for systemic evidence of bleeding or coagulation disorders.	Hematological and coagulation profiles may be altered as a result of blood loss during ECMO insertion, anticoagulation therapy, platelet dysfunction, and hemolysis.[15,20,23]	Bleeding from ECMO insertion site Bleeding from incisions or mucous membranes Petechiae/ecchymosis Guaiac-positive nasogastric aspirate or stool Hematuria Decreased hemoglobin/hematocrit
21. Frequent repositioning with close examination of the back of the head, heels, and sacrum. Consider utilizing a specialty bed with low air loss and continuous lateral rotation; also consider utilizing products to decrease the risk of friction injuries such as a turning and positioning glide sheet.	Promotes comfort and skin integrity as well as enhanced pulmonary perfusion.	Skin breakdown Inability of patient to tolerate movement and repositioning
22. Assess the ECMO circuit at least every hour. Fdo$_2$ (fraction of delivered oxygen) Sweep (L/min) Flow rates (L/min) Motor rate (RPM) Color of blood in lines Observe for clots or fibrin strands on oxygenator Pressures: pre- and postoxygenator, venous drainage line pressure Svo$_2$ and Hgb Follow institutional standards	Demonstrates adequate ECMO therapy.	Abnormal ECMO circuit findings, such as air in the line or clots in the oxygenator
23. Assess insertion sites, and maintain sterile dressings on all invasive lines and cannula sites. Using chlorhexidine gluconate–impregnated dressing reduces the frequency of dressing changes to every 7 days. **(Level D*)**	Decreases the incidence of infection, and allows for site assessment.[22]	Signs and symptoms of infection
24. For internal jugular cannulations, when patient is hemodynamically stable and condition allows, ambulate progressively. Use of a multidisciplinary team is essential. Follow institutional standards.	Prevents hazards of immobility and begins rehabilitation. Ensures that all lines are secure when the patient is ambulating.[17]	Postural hypotension Decrease in flow with position change Unrelieved dizziness Prolonged deconditioning

UNIT I

Patient Monitoring and Care —*Continued*

Steps	Rationale	Reportable Conditions
25. In VV ECMO patients, assess for readiness to wean from mechanical ventilation. VV ECMO is weaned by Fio_2 and sweep, with careful attention to oxygenation. Early tracheostomy may be considered[12] (see Procedure 30, Weaning Mechanical Ventilation).	Prolonged mechanical ventilation may lead to increased morbidity such as pneumonia, barotrauma, respiratory weakness, and musculoskeletal deconditioning.[12,24]	Ventilator settings of Fio_2 40% and PEEP of 5 cm H_2O with Pao_2/Fio_2 ≥200, pH >7.35, minute ventilation <10 L/min while receiving a sweep gas flow of <6 L/min on ECMO would be acceptable to consider extubation.
26. In VA ECMO, sweep and flow are weaned, with careful attention to hemodynamic parameters. Follow institutional parameters.	ECMO support is limited and temporary, and it is used as a bridge to a more permanent solution (i.e., VAD, transplant) or palliation. Collaborative planning for next steps should be considered daily.	Improvement or deterioration Increasing vasopressor requirements may indicate that the patient is not ready to wean
27. Evaluate the family's coping mechanism, strengths, and needs on a continual basis, and provide support. Consult pastoral care, palliative care, and/or bereavement specialists per institutional guidelines.	Promotes family involvement in care and decision making. Team assists with meeting family and patient needs.[30,32]	Family's inability to cope
28. Ensure safe transport of the patient and equipment to tests and procedures.	Ensures entire team, including nurses, providers, respiratory therapists, and perfusionist or ECMO specialist, is prepared for transport.[15]	Patient's inability to be transported, such as unstable vital signs or instability of ECMO circuit

*Level D: Peer-reviewed professional and organizational standards with the support of clinical study recommendations

Documentation

Documentation should include the following:

- Patient and family education
- Plan of care
- Universal protocol requirements, sterile procedure/protocol
- Informed consent
- Patient response to ECMO
- Confirmation of placement
- Hemodynamic status
- Pain assessment, interventions, and effectiveness
- Activity level
- Additional interventions
- ECMO parameters (pump flow, Fio_2, and sweep flow)
- Cannula site and cannula measurements
- Securement of cannulas
- Dressing changes and site assessment
- Skin integrity
- Patient tolerance
- Unexpected outcomes

References and Additional Readings

For a complete list of references and additional readings for this procedure, scan this QR code with your smartphone, or visit https://www.elsevier.com/__data/assets/pdf_file/0010/1319788/Chapter0013.pdf

14 Oxygen Saturation Monitoring With Pulse Oximetry

Amy I. Lucas and Donna C. Bond

PURPOSE: Pulse oximetry is a noninvasive monitoring technique used to estimate arterial oxygen saturation. Pulse oximetry is indicated in patients at risk for hypoxemia, such as during conscious sedation procedures, transport, and adjustment of fraction of inspired oxygen (Fio_2). Continuous monitoring of pulse oximetry provides a more accurate assessment of oxygenation than intermittent spot checks.[15]

PREREQUISITE NURSING KNOWLEDGE

- Oxygen saturation is an indicator of the percentage of hemoglobin saturated with oxygen at the time of the measurement. This procedure will focus on the oxygen saturation of arterial blood. The sensor measures the differences in light absorption between oxygenated and deoxygenated hemoglobin using red and infrared light transmitted through the tissues. The amount and type of light transmitted through the tissue is converted to a digital value that represents the percentage of hemoglobin saturated with oxygen (Fig. 14.1).[8]
- Trending oxygen saturation values obtained with pulse oximetry (Spo_2) represent one part of a complete assessment of a patient's oxygenation status and is not a substitute for measurement of arterial saturation of oxygen (Sao_2). A complete assessment of oxygenation includes evaluation of oxygen content and delivery, which includes the following parameters: arterial partial pressure of oxygen (Pao_2), Sao_2, hemoglobin, cardiac output, and, when available, mixed venous oxygen saturation (Svo_2). Spo_2

trends blood oxygen content and can alert the nurse to changes in oxygenation.
- Tissue oxygenation is not reflected by arterial oxygen saturation obtained with pulse oximetry. Pulse oximetry reflects the adequacy of oxygen delivery, but will not indicate whether the tissues are able to access and use the oxygen. The affinity of hemoglobin with oxygen may impair or enhance oxygen release at the tissue level.
  - ❖ Oxygen is more readily released to the tissues when pH is decreased (acidosis), body temperature is increased, arterial pressure of carbon dioxide ($Paco_2$) is increased, and 2,3-diphosphoglycerate (2,3-DPG) levels are increased (decreased oxygen affinity). 2,3-DPG is a byproduct of glucose metabolism that facilitates the dissociation of oxygen from the hemoglobin molecule to tissue.
  - ❖ When hemoglobin has greater affinity for oxygen, less is released to the tissues (increased oxygen affinity). Conditions such as increased pH (alkalosis), decreased temperature, decreased $Paco_2$, and decreased 2,3-DPG (as found in stored blood products) increase oxygen binding to the hemoglobin and limit its release to the tissue.
- Normal oxygen saturation values are approximately 95% to 100% in a healthy individual breathing room air at sea level. An oxygen saturation value of 95% is clinically accepted in a patient with a normal hemoglobin level. With a normal blood pH and body temperature, an oxygen saturation value of 90% is generally equated with a Pao_2 of 60 mm Hg.[8] Patients living at higher altitudes may have lower oxygen saturation levels at baseline.[21]
  - ❖ Anemic patients will have normal oxygen saturation levels but may be hypoxic because there is less hemoglobin to carry oxygen, even if it is highly saturated.
  - ❖ Oxygen saturation values may vary with the amount of oxygen usage or uptake by the tissues. In some patients, a difference is seen in Spo_2 values at rest compared with values during activity, such as ambulation, motion, or positioning.[12,14,17]
- Oxygen saturation does not directly reflect the patient's ability to ventilate. The true measure of ventilation is determination of the arterial partial pressure of carbon dioxide [$Paco_2$] and can be estimated noninvasively using

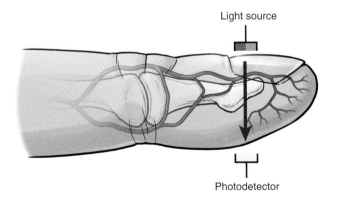

Light source

Photodetector

Figure 14.1 A sensor device that contains a light source and a photodetector is placed around a pulsating arteriolar bed, such as the finger, great toe, nose, or earlobe. Red and infrared wavelengths of light are used to determine arterial saturation. *(© 2022 Medtronic. All rights reserved. Used with the permission of Medtronic.)*

end-tidal CO_2 (Etco$_2$) or by arterial blood gas to measure PaCO$_2$ (see Procedure 12, Continuous End-Tidal Carbon Dioxide Monitoring).

- ❖ Patients at risk of respiratory depression may have a normal Spo$_2$ despite inadequate ventilation, especially if they are receiving supplemental oxygen.[11]
- ❖ The normal baseline Spo$_2$ for a patient with known severe restrictive disease and more definitive methods of determination of the effectiveness of ventilation must be assessed before consideration of interventions that enhance oxygenation. Use of Spo$_2$ in a patient with obstructive pulmonary disease may result in erroneous clinical assessments of a condition. Enhancing the patient's oxygenation and increasing the Spo$_2$ may limit the ability to ventilate (Box 14.1).
- Oxygen saturation is also unable to detect significant hyperoxia unless correlated by an arterial blood gas measurement of Pao$_2$.[15] This is because of relatively small changes that are reflected in Spo$_2$ with large changes in Pao$_2$ at higher values of oxygen saturation. Maintaining high levels of Spo$_2$ (98% to 100%) has the potential to worsen outcomes.[7,10]
- Discoloration of the nail bed or obstruction of the nail bed (i.e., blood under the fingernail or bruising) can potentially affect the transmission of light through the digit and result in an artificially decreased Spo$_2$ value. Pulse oximetry has not been shown to be affected by the presence of an elevated bilirubin.[2]
- Caution should be used when there are nail enhancements. Dark nail polish, such as blue, green, brown, or black, has been previously reported to affect the Spo$_2$, although more recent studies, including a systematic review, showed that nail polish does not cause a clinically significant change in the pulse oximeter readings.[3] The presence of acrylic fingernails may impair the accuracy of the pulse oximetry reading, and removal of the nail covering may be necessary to ensure accurate measurement, although unpolished acrylic nails have been proven not to affect pulse oximetry readings.[22] Gel polish may also affect the accuracy of the pulse oximetry reading. A recent study compared 10 colors and 2 different oximeters and found that there was a trend in overestimating the oxygen saturation that varied by color. These changes were not always clinically significant. Because of the difficulty in removing gel polish, an alternate site was recommended.[24] If the nail polish cannot be removed and is believed to be affecting the accuracy of the reading, the sensor can be placed in the lateral position on the finger to obtain readings so the light shines through the sides of the finger instead of through the nail if no other site such as the earlobe or nose is available.[21]
- Standard pulse oximetry equipment should never be used in suspected cases of carbon monoxide exposure. Standard pulse oximeters are unable to differentiate between oxygen and carbon monoxide bound to hemoglobin. This can lead to the oximeter reporting a normal Spo$_2$ measurement when in reality the patient is hypoxic, with carbon monoxide bound to the hemoglobin instead of oxygen. An arterial blood gas always should be obtained to determine the accurate oxygen saturation, and measurement of carboxyhemoglobin and methemoglobin should also be obtained if a carbon monoxide (CO) oximeter is available.[6,23]

BOX 14.1 Causes of Inaccurate SpO$_2$ Readings

INABILITY TO READ SpO$_2$
- Poor perfusion–examples include:
  - Cold digits
  - Arterial compression due to a pumped-up blood pressure cuff
  - Blockages due to peripheral vascular disease

FALSE ELEVATION OR FALSE NORMAL READING
- Dyshemoglobinemias–examples include:
  - Carboxyhemoglobinemia
  - Methemoglobin
  - Sulfhemoglobin
- Glycohemoglobin A1c (>7%)
- Skin pigmentation

FALSELY LOW READING
- Anemias or abnormal hemoglobin–examples include:
  - Sickle cell anemia
  - Inherited forms of abnormal hemoglobin
  - Hb Lansing
  - Hb Bonn
  - Severe anemia
- Methemoglobinemia
- Excessive movement–examples include:
  - Agitation
  - Shivering
- Intravenous dyes–examples include:
  - Methylene blue
- Fingernail enhancements
  - Polish
  - Acrylics
  - Gels
- Venous pulsations–may be caused by:
  - Venous engorgement
  - Fluid overload
- Discoloration or obstruction of nail bed–examples:
  - Bruising
  - Onychomycosis

MAY CAUSE FALSE HIGH OR LOW READING
- Poor probe positioning–examples:
  - Probe too loose
  - Incorrectly positioned so that light is detected at the photodetector before passing through the tissue
- Sickle cell anemia

From Chan ED, Chan MM, Chan MM: Pulse oximetry: understanding its basic principles facilitates appreciation of its limitations. Respir Med 107(6):789-799, 2013; Jubran A: Pulse oximetry. Crit Care 19(272):1-7, 2015; Nazik H, Nazik S, Gül FC, Demir B, Mülayim MK: Effect of onychomycosis on pulse oximeter. Egypt J Dermatol Venerol 38(2):85-88, 2018.

- Dark skin has been suggested to possibly affect the ability of the pulse oximeter to accurately monitor arterial oxygen saturation by interfering with the transmission of light and thus the accuracy of the readings. In a recent large cohort study, adult black patients had nearly three times the frequency of occult hypoxemia as white patients that was not detected by pulse oximetry.[18] If there are concerns that the pulse oximetry is not accurately reporting the oxygen saturation, a blood gas should be done to verify the accuracy.

- Certain dyes used intravenously may interfere with the accuracy of measurements, although the impact is limited as a result of rapid clearance. Dyes include methylene blue, indigo carmine, indocyanine green, and fluorescein.[4,9]
- A pulse oximeter should not be used as a predictive indicator of the actual arterial blood gas saturation; however, pulse oximetry does provide information about changes in the patient's oxygenation. Continuous pulse oximetry monitoring in critical care settings can allow clinicians to recognize early signs of deterioration and provide early interventions that may prevent rescue events such as cardiac arrest or respiratory arrest.[20]
  - ❖ A pulse oximeter should never be used during a cardiac arrest situation because of the extreme limitations of blood flow during cardiopulmonary resuscitation and the pharmacological action of vasoactive agents administered during the resuscitation effort.[13]
  - ❖ Low-perfusion states such as hypotension, vasoconstriction, hypothermia, or administration of vasoconstrictive agents limit the ability of the oximeter to distinguish arterial pulsation. In monitors that show a waveform, the pulsations in the waveform should match the patient's heart rate. Discrepancies can mean that the device is not providing an accurate reading of either the heart rate or SpO_2.
- The oxygen saturation value from the finger of an arm that has been physically restrained has been shown to be significantly different from the finger of an unrestrained arm. Therefore if physical restraints are being used, it is recommended that the pulse oximetry sensor not be placed on the finger of a restrained arm.[2]
- In vasoconstrictive states, oxygen saturation may be measured with a finger sensor, but in patients with significant shifts in hemodynamic stability, the ear, forehead, or nasal alar has been shown to be reasonably resistant to the vasoconstrictive effects of the sympathetic nervous system.[14,16]
- Forehead sensors use reflectance and are more accurate in low-flow states but may be affected by venous congestion. Forehead sensors used in patients placed in the Trendelenburg position may require up to 20 mm Hg of external pressure to achieve accurate readings, which may be accomplished with the headband supplied by the manufacturer[1] (see Fig. 14.3). Disposable pulse oximeters intended for use on fingers should not be used on the forehead because they are often inaccurate.[19]

EQUIPMENT

- Oxygen saturation monitor
- Oxygen saturation cable and sensor (disposable or nondisposable)
- Manufacturer's recommended germicidal agent for cleaning the nondisposable sensor and cables (used for cleaning between patients)

PATIENT AND FAMILY EDUCATION

- Explain the need for determination of oxygen saturation with a pulse oximeter and that it is part of the overall assessment of respiratory status. *Rationale:* This explanation informs the patient of the purpose of monitoring, enhances patient cooperation, decreases patient anxiety, and prepares the patient and family for other possible diagnostic tests of oxygenation (e.g., arterial blood gas).
- Explain the equipment, including sensor positioning, displayed values, and alarms as well as how patient movement and sensor position can affect the reading. *Rationale:* This information decreases patient and family anxiety and facilitates patient cooperation in maintaining sensor placement.

PATIENT ASSESSMENT AND PREPARATION

Patient Assessment

- Signs and symptoms of decreased oxygenation, including dyspnea, tachypnea, increased work of breathing, agitation, confusion, disorientation, decreased level of consciousness, cyanosis, tachycardia, and bradycardia. Clubbing of the digit tips is a sign of long-term oxygenation issues and may be seen in patients with chronic lung diseases such as chronic obstructive pulmonary disease (COPD). *Rationale:* Patient assessment determines the need for continuous pulse oximetry monitoring. Anticipation of conditions in which hypoxia could be present allows earlier intervention before unfavorable outcomes occur. Changes in mentation, such as confusion or agitation, may be the earliest signs of hypoxia.
- Assess the extremity (digit) or area where the sensor will be placed for decreased peripheral pulses, peripheral cyanosis, decreased body temperature, decreased blood pressure, exposure to excessive environmental light sources (e.g., examination lights), excessive movement or tremor in the digit, presence of dark nail polish or bruising under the nail, presence of artificial nails, and blood under the fingernails. *Rationale:* Assessment of factors that may inhibit accuracy of the measurement of oxygenation before attempting to obtain the SpO_2 reading enhances the validity of the measurement and allows for correction of factors as is possible.

Patient Preparation

- Verify the patient with two identifiers. *Rationale:* Before performing a procedure, the nurse should ensure the correct identification of the patient for the intended intervention.
- Ensure that the patient understands preprocedural teachings. Answer questions as they arise, or use teach-back methods, and reinforce information as needed. *Rationale:* This communication evaluates and reinforces understanding of previously taught information.

UNIT I

Procedure for Oxygen Saturation Monitoring With Pulse Oximetry		
Steps	Rationale	Special Considerations

1. ▣ **HH**
 2. ▣ **PE**
 3. Prepare equipment:
   A. Plug the oximeter power cord into a grounded wall outlet if the unit is not portable. If the unit is portable, ensure sufficient battery charge by turning it on before use.
   B. Plug the patient cable into the monitor and the sensor into the oximeter patient cable (if indicated).
   C. Turn the instrument power switch on.
	A. With use of electrical outlets, grounded outlets decrease the occurrence of electrical interference.
	 B. Connects the sensor to the oximeter, which allows SpO_2 measurement and analysis of waveforms.
	 C. Applies power to the device.
		A. Portable systems have rechargeable batteries and depend on sufficient time plugged into an electrical outlet to maintain the proper level of battery charge. When the system is used in the portable mode, always check battery capacity.
		 B. Allow adequate time for self-testing procedures and for detection and analysis of waveforms before values are displayed. The time required to perform the self-test and adequately warm depends on the specific manufacturer.

4. Select the desired sensor site. If digits are chosen, assess for warmth and capillary refill. Confirm the presence of arterial blood flow to the area monitored.	Adequate arterial pulse strength is necessary for obtaining accurate SpO_2 measurements.	Avoid sites distal to indwelling arterial catheters, blood pressure cuffs, arteriovenous fistulas, or venous engorgement.
5. Select the appropriate pulse oximeter sensor for the area with the best pulsatile vascular bed to be sampled (Figs. 14.2 to 14.4). **(Level C*)**	The correct sensor optimizes signal capture and minimizes artifact-related difficulties. The digits are the most common site because of ease of application of the sensor. Consideration of other sites may produce more accurate results in conditions of extreme peripheral vasoconstriction or decreased perfusion.[1,4,9,16,19]	Several different types of sensors are available, including disposable and nondisposable sensors, which may be applied over a variety of vascular beds, including digits, the earlobe, nasal bridge, septum, nasal alae, or forehead. Follow manufacturer's recommendations for the appropriate site for each type of sensor. Do not use a sensor designed for the finger on the forehead or ear.[19] Do not use one manufacturer's sensor with another manufacturer's pulse oximeter unless compatibility has been verified.

6. Apply the sensor in a manner that allows the light source (LEDs) to be:
   A. Directly opposite the light detector (photodetector). **(Level C*)**
 	
   B. Shielded from excessive environmental light.
	To determine a pulse oximetry value properly, the light sensors must be in opposing positions directly over the area of the sample. The exception is the sensor designed for the forehead.[1,4]
	
	 Light from sources such as examination lights or overhead lights can cause falsely elevated oximetry values.[9]
		
		 If the oximeter sensor fails to detect a pulse when perfusion seems adequate, excessive environmental light (overhead examination lights, phototherapy lights, infrared warmers) may be blinding the light sensor. Troubleshoot by reapplying the sensor, shielding the sensor with a towel or blanket, or moving the sensor to a different monitoring site.

*Level C: Qualitative studies, descriptive or correlational studies, integrative reviews, systematic reviews, or randomized controlled trials with inconsistent results.

Procedure | **for Oxygen Saturation Monitoring With Pulse Oximetry—*Continued***

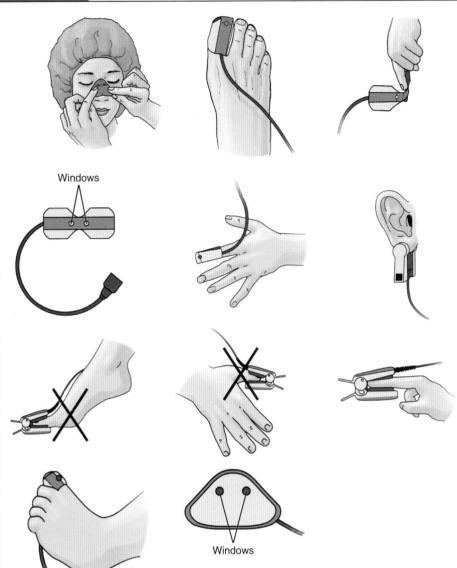

Figure 14.2 Sensor types and sensor sites for pulse oximetry monitoring. Use "wrap" or "clip" style sensors on the fingers (including thumb), great toe, and nose. The windows for the light source and photodetector must be placed directly opposite each other on each side of the arteriolar bed to ensure accuracy of Spo₂ measurements. Choice of the correct size of the sensor helps decrease the incidence of excess ambient light interference and optical shunting. "Clip" style sensors are appropriate for fingers (except the thumb) and the earlobe. Ensuring that the arteriolar bed is well within the clip with the windows directly opposite each other decreases the possibility of excess ambient light interference and optical shunting. *(Reprinted with permission from Nellcor Puritan Bennett LLC, Boulder, CO, part of Covidien.)*

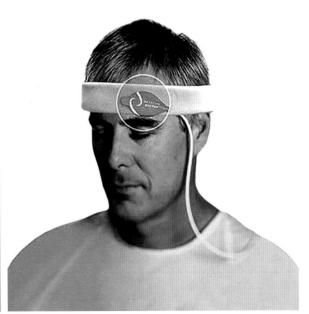

Figure 14.3 Nellcor™ MAXFAST forehead sensor. *(© 2023 Medtronic. All rights reserved. Used with the permission of Medtronic.)*

Procedure continues on following page

Procedure for Oxygen Saturation Monitoring With Pulse Oximetry—*Continued*		
Steps	**Rationale**	**Special Considerations**

Figure 14.4 Nasal alar pulse oximeter sensor. *(Courtesy of Royal Philips.)*

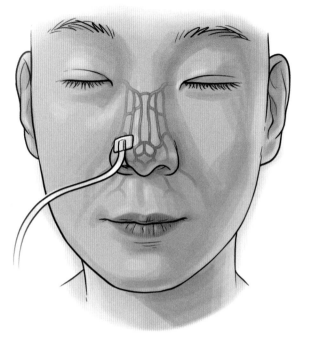

Steps	Rationale	Special Considerations
C. Positioned so all sensor-emitted light comes into contact with perfused tissue beds and is not seen by the other side of the sensor or without coming into contact with the area to be read.	If the light from the sensor's LEDs bypasses the tissue bed and is detected at the photodetector, the result is either a falsely high reading or no reading.	Known as *optical shunting,* the light bypasses the vascular bed; shielding the sensor does not eliminate this if the sensor is too large or not properly positioned.
7. Gently position the sensor so it does not cause restriction to arterial flow or venous return. (Level C*)	The pulse oximeter is unable to distinguish between true arterial pulsations and fluid waves (e.g., venous engorgement or fluid accumulation).[4]	Restriction of arterial blood flow can cause a falsely low value and lead to vascular compromise, causing potential loss of viable tissues. Edema from restriction of venous return can cause venous pulsation. Elevation of the site above the level of the heart reduces the possibility of venous pulsation. Moving the sensor to another site on a routine schedule also reduces tissue compromise. Never place the sensor on an extremity that has decreased or absent sensation because the patient may not be able to identify discomfort or the signs and symptoms of loss of circulation or tissue compromise. Assess for development of medical device–related pressure injury and assess site every 2–4 hours or per facility guidelines or manufacturer recommendations. Rotate the site of a reusable sensor per manufacturer's recommendations.

*Level C: Qualitative studies, descriptive or correlational studies, integrative reviews, systematic reviews, or randomized controlled trials with inconsistent results.

Procedure for Oxygen Saturation Monitoring With Pulse Oximetry—*Continued*

Steps	Rationale	Special Considerations
8. Determine the accuracy of the detected waveform by comparing the numeric heart rate value with that of a monitored heart rate, an apical heart rate, or both. (Level M*)	If arterial blood flow through the sensor is insufficient, the heart rate values may vary significantly. If the pulse rate detected with the oximeter does not correlate with the patient's heart rate, the oximeter is not detecting sufficient arterial blood flow for accurate values.	This problem occurs particularly with the use of the fingers and toes in conditions of low blood flow. Consider moving the sensor to another site, such as the earlobe or forehead (be sure the sensor type is appropriate for the monitoring site).
9. Set appropriate alarm limits.	Alarm limits should be set appropriate to the patient's condition.	Oxygen saturation limits should be 5% less than the patient's acceptable baseline or per facility policy. Heart rate alarms should be consistent with the cardiac monitoring limits (if monitored).
10. Clean the nondisposable sensor, if used, between patients with manufacturer's recommended germicidal agent.	Reduces transmission of microorganisms to other patients.[5]	
11. Discard used supplies and remove **PE**		
12. **HH**		

Expected Outcomes

- Changes in oxygen saturation are detected
- Periods of oxygen desaturation are addressed quickly
- The need for invasive techniques for monitoring oxygenation is reduced
- False-positive pulse oximeter alarms are reduced

Unexpected Outcomes

- Inaccurate or inability to obtain oxygen saturation (see Box 14.1)
- Medical device–related pressure injury

Patient Monitoring and Care

Steps	Rationale	Reportable Conditions
		These conditions should be reported to the provider if they persist despite nursing interventions.
1. Evaluate laboratory data along with the patient for evidence of reduced arterial oxygen saturation or hypoxemia.	Spo_2 values are one segment of a complete evaluation of the patient's oxygenation status and supplemental oxygen therapy. Data should be integrated into a complete assessment to determine the overall status of the patient. If Spo_2 is used as an indicator of Sao_2, an arterial blood gas with CO oximetry should be done to determine whether the values correlate consistently.	Inability to maintain oxygen saturation levels as desired
2. Assess sensor site every 2–4 hours or per facility guidelines or manufacturer's recommendations. Rotate the site of a reusable sensor per manufacturer's recommendations. **(Level M*)**	Assessment of the skin and tissues under the sensor identifies skin breakdown or loss of vascular flow, allowing appropriate interventions to be initiated. Application of additional tape may constrict blood flow at the monitoring site and result in both inaccurate monitor readings and further compromised local skin perfusion.	Change in skin color\nLoss of warmth of tissue unrelated to vasoconstriction\nLoss of blood flow to the digit\nEvidence of skin breakdown from the sensor\nChange in color of the nail bed, which indicates compromised circulation to the nail\nMedical device–related pressure injury

*Level M: Manufacturer's recommendations only.

Procedure continues on following page

Patient Monitoring and Care —*Continued*

Steps	Rationale	Reportable Conditions
3. Monitor the sensor site for excessive movement, which results in motion artifact.	Excessive movement at the monitoring site may result in unreliable saturation values. Moving the sensor to a less physically active site may reduce the risk of motion artifact; use of an adhesive versus reusable sensor may also help as a result of better fit. If the digits are used, ask the patient to rest the hand on a flat or secure surface.	Inability to obtain pulse oxygen saturation levels
4. Compare and monitor the actual heart rate with the pulse rate value from the pulse oximeter to determine accuracy of values.	The two numeric heart rate values should correlate closely. A difference in pulse rate values reported with the pulse oximeter may be from excessive movement, poor peripheral perfusion at the monitoring site, or loss of pulsatile flow detection.	Inability to correlate actual heart rate and pulse rate from the oximeter

Documentation

Documentation should include the following:
- Patient and family education
- Indications for use of pulse oximetry
- Heart rate with SpO_2 measurement
- FiO_2 delivered (if patient is receiving oxygen)
- Arterial blood gases (if available)
- Hemoglobin measurement (if available)
- Skin assessment at sensor site
- Pulse oximeter monitor alarm settings
- Events precipitating acute desaturation
- Unexpected outcomes
- Nursing interventions

References and Additional Readings

For a complete list of references and additional readings for this procedure, scan this QR code with your smartphone, or visit https://www.elsevier.com/__data/assets/pdf_file/0011/1319789/Chapter0014.pdf

15 Prone Positioning for Acute Respiratory Distress Syndrome Patients

Kathleen M. Vollman and Dannette A. Mitchell

PURPOSE: Prone positioning is used as an adjunct short-term supportive therapy to recruit alveoli to improve gas exchange and reduce ventilator injury in critically ill, mechanically ventilated patients diagnosed with acute respiratory distress syndrome (ARDS), including patients with COVID-19 with severe hypoxemia. Severe hypoxemia can be defined as a partial pressure of arterial oxygen (Pao_2)/fraction of inspired oxygen (Fio_2) ratio of <150 mm Hg, Fio_2 of at least 60%, positive end-expiratory pressure (PEEP) of at least 5 cm H_2O, and a tidal volume close to 6 mL/kg of predicted body weight.

PREREQUISITE NURSING KNOWLEDGE

- Knowledge of the physiological effect of prone positioning on gas exchange is critical to understanding the importance of the procedure as an early strategy for managing ARDS patients.[1,6,7,11,23] The improvement in oxygenation is likely the result of three physiological effects: a change in pressure gradient, reduced lung compression, and improved lung perfusion matching[7,11,23] (Fig. 15.1).
    - ❖ The transpulmonary pressure (PTP) gradient is reduced, resulting in a decrease in overinflation of the anterior portions of the lung with less posterior alveolar collapse. This results in less ventilator-induced lung injury from overdistension and the repetitive opening and closing of the alveoli reducing shear stress.[7,10,15,23]
    - ❖ The heart structures are not compressing the lungs and the diagrams is displaced resulting in less compression leading to improved overall ventilation.[7,10,11,23]
    - ❖ Although perfusion is relatively unchanged, an increase in recruited alveoli available to match with perfusion results in improved oxygenation.[11,23]
- Prone positioning in patients with ARDS and severe hypoxemia should be initiated early, and patients must be maintained in the position for at least 16 consecutive hours a day to see the greatest impact on mortality.[4,8,12,19,25,36] The American Thoracic Society, the European Society of Intensive Care Medicine, and the Society of Critical Care Medicine 2017 guidelines for ventilation of the ARDS patients give a strong recommendation for using prone therapy for patients with severe ARDS.[6]
- Prone ventilation may require an increase in pain and sedation medications. The use of neuromuscular blocking agents is warranted if ventilator asynchrony continues after maximum pain and sedative medications are used.[16,23]

- The major complications seen with prone positioning include airway complications and pressure injuries.[19,36] Airway complications were defined as unplanned extubation or endotracheal tube obstruction. The area of greatest risk for pressure injuries in the prone patient is the face including the chin and cheeks.[21] Additional pressure injury risk areas include other part of the face including the lips and forehead, the chest/clavicles, area over the iliac crest, knees, and feet.[26] Other complications noted are peripheral nerve injuries, dislodging of tubes and lines, vomiting, and transient arrythmias.[12,13,23]
- Suggested criteria for use of prone positioning:
    - ❖ After 12 to 24 hours of optimization of mechanical ventilation with lung-protective strategies, consider use of the prone position for patients with ARDS with severe hypoxemia defined as a Pao_2/Fio_2 ratio <150 mm Hg, Fio_2 >60%, PEEP at least 5 cm H_2O, and tidal volume close to 6 mL/kg of predicted body weight.[12]
- Precautions for prone positioning include the following[10,23,24,34,37]:
    - ❖ Absolute contraindications
        - ○ Unstable cervical, thoracic, or lumbar fractures
        - ○ Goal of care: allow for natural death (comfort care)
    - ❖ Relative contraindications
        - ○ Uncontrolled intracranial pressure or poorly controlled seizures
        - ○ Massive bleeding or hemoptysis
        - ○ Venous thrombosis treated <48 hours
        - ○ Increased intracranial pressure
        - ○ Patient with hemodynamically unstable condition (as defined by a systolic blood pressure <90 mm Hg or MAP <60) with fluid and vasoactive support in place
        - ○ Cardiac abnormalities: life-threatening arrhythmias, ventricular-assist devices, intra-aortic balloon pump, ECMO, fresh pacemaker
        - ○ Unstable chest wall, open abdomen
        - ○ Bronchopleural fistula, Unstable airway, tracheal surgery within 2 weeks

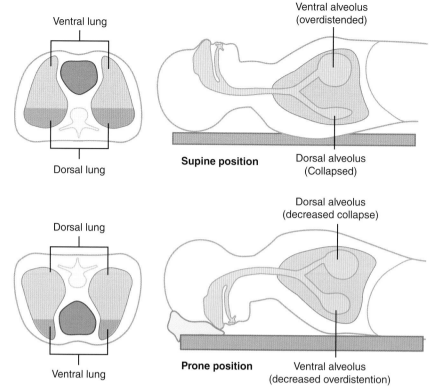

Figure 15.1 Physiology of prone positioning in ARDS. Prone positioning decreases the difference between dorsal and ventral transpulmonary pressure *(PTP).* This leads to a decrease in ventral alveolar overinflation, dorsal alveolar collapse, and recruitment of collapsed alveoli. *(From Harding MM. Lewis's medical-surgical nursing: assessment and management of clinical problems, 12th edition, Philadelphia: Elsevier, 2023.)*

- ○ Second or third trimester pregnancy or extremely distended abdomen (padding above and below the distension may offset unnecessary pressure)
- ○ Weight 160 kg or greater (weigh the risk/benefit ratio for the patient and staff)
- ○ Burns >20% of the ventral body surface
- ○ Advanced arthritis
- Prone positioning should be discontinued when the patient no longer shows a positive response to the position change or when the following criteria were met:[12]
  - ❖ Improvement in oxygenation, defined as Pao_2/Fio_2 ratio >150 mm Hg, with Fio_2 <60% with PEEP ≤10 cm H_2O after a minimum of 4 hours in the supine position.
  - ❖ Complications occurring during a prone session leading to its immediate interruption.
  - ❖ When improvements in oxygenation are no longer occurring or the goals of care have changed to palliative care or end of life.

PERSONNEL AND EQUIPMENT FOR PRONE POSITIONING

Personnel

- Recommend five clinicians: Add additional members in accordance with institutional policy or needs related to patient size. These should include the following:
  - ❖ Four clinicians for the turning process: One should be the primary nurse caring for the patient. The other roles

can be a combination of nurses, respiratory therapists, physical therapists, or other personnel.
  - ❖ One clinician at the head of the bed: If the respiratory therapist or other provider at the head of the bed is not a designated intubator, an additional provider able to intubate should be available in case of accidental extubation.

Equipment

- Patient gown
- Pillows (3 to 6), fluidizers, or foam positioners
- ECG leads and pads
- 2 flat sheets for positioning
- Absorbent pads
- Multilayer soft silicone foam prophylactic dressings
- Resuscitation bag-valve-mask device connected to an oxygen source and additional emergency equipment
- Consider use of lateral rotation therapy feature while supine if available on the bed

Additional equipment to have available as needed includes the following:
- Transfer devices, friction-reducing devices
- Mechanical lift and lift sheet
- Capnography monitor

Special Considerations

- Additional devices and accompanying procedures may be utilized during prone positioning for patient and healthcare worker safety, such as mechanical lift devices, friction-reducing sheets, prone wedges, and positioners[41] (Fig. 15.2). Please follow the manufacturer's recommendations

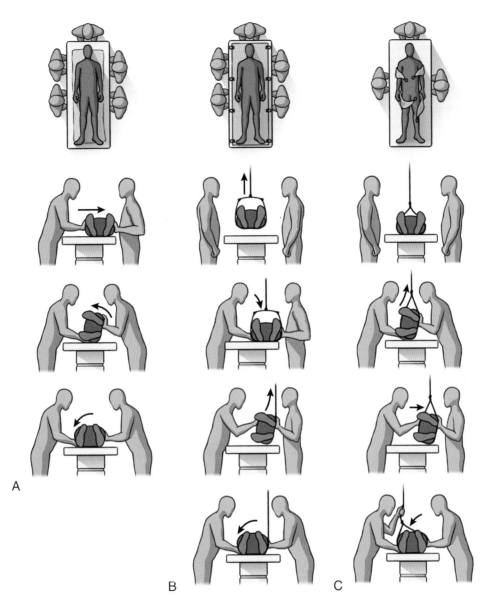

Figure 15.2 Various prone positioning strategies using safe patient-handling techniques. **A,** Manual prone positioning using a positioning sheet. **B,** Prone positioning using a mechanical lift device and a positioning sheet. **C,** Prone positioning using a mechanical lift device with a lift sheet with straps. In all scenarios, the patient is lifted, moved horizontally to the side, carefully lowered to the side-lying position, and then placed in the prone position. Thoughtful consideration must be given to airway, lines, tubes, wounds, and so on. *(From Wiggermann N, Zhou J, Kumpar D: Proning patients with COVID 19: a review of equipment and methods.* Hum Factors *62[7]:1069–1076, 2020.)*

when utilizing devices during the prone positioning procedure. Follow institutional guidelines for safe patient handling. It is recommended to seek consultation of experts in safe patient handling at your facility such as physical therapists to determine best practices for incorporating your institution's devices into the prone positioning process.[41]

PATIENT AND FAMILY EDUCATION

• Explain the procedure for prone positioning to the patient and family (if available), including the positioning procedure, perceived benefit, frequency of assessments, expected response, appearance while in the prone position,

and parameters for discontinuation of the positioning technique and equipment (if a special bed is initiated). Assess understanding of education via use of the teach-back method or another validated tool. ***Rationale:*** Although consent is not required for this procedure, providing full explanation of the problem and the intervention will aid in decreasing patient and family anxiety. This communication provides an opportunity to set expectations and allows the patient and family to verbalize concerns and ask questions about the procedure. The teach-back method is a validated tool used to assess understanding of information provided to learners (in this process, the patient, family, and/or caregivers).[38]

PATIENT ASSESSMENT AND PREPARATION FOR PRONE POSITIONING

Patient Assessment

- Assess the time interval from the initial diagnosis to the first position change. *Rationale:* Prone positioning should be performed within the first 24 hours of the diagnosis of severe ARDS. Prone positioning should occur for at least 16 hours in a 24-hour period.[12,24]
- Assess the patient for any contraindications to prone positioning (see contraindications earlier in this chapter). *Rationale:* Ensure that the patient does not have any contraindications to prevent possible injury. If the patient has a relative contraindication, the interdisciplinary team should conduct a risk-benefit discussion.
- Assess pain, agitation and anxiety, and delirium with validated tools before using the prone position. *Rationale:* Assessing pain, agitation, and delirium using a reliable and valid scale and ensuring appropriate management before, during, and after the turn are key to providing a safe environment for use of the prone position.
- Assess the size and weight load to determine the ability to turn within the critical care bed frame being utilized and to weigh the potential risk of injury to healthcare workers. *Rationale:* For morbidly obese patients, the team must consider the potential for injury to healthcare workers and the patient when making the decision to turn the patient prone and must ensure appropriate equipment before attempting the turn.
- Evaluate the patient for any history of contraindications for arm, neck, and leg positions while in the prone position (e.g., previous injuries, surgeries, or hereditary conditions). *Rationale:* Identifies patients with arm, neck, shoulder, or leg injuries that may require modifications of patient positioning to prevent injury.

Patient Preparation

- Verify the order for prone positioning.
- Verify the patient with two identifiers. *Rationale:* Before performing a procedure, the nurse should ensure the correct identification of the patient for the intended intervention.
- If feeding via the enteral route, consider turning off the tube feeding, and disconnect from the NGT/OGT 1 hour before the prone and supine turns are made.[17] Prone positioning should not be delayed if unable to hold the feeding for gastric emptying. *Rationale:* This action assists with gastric emptying and reduces the risk of aspiration during the turning procedure.[17,24] Enteral feeding should be continued during prone positioning; use of prokinetic agents or transpyloric feedings should be considered to prevent complications associated with vomiting or high gastric residual volumes.[3,33]
- Before placing patient in the prone position, the following care activities should be performed. *Rationale:* These activities help prevent areas of pressure and potential skin breakdown; avoid complications related to pressure injury, accidental extubation, or dislodgement of other lines and

tubes; and promote the delivery of comprehensive care before, during, and after positioning.[5,21,22,24]

- ❖ Perform eye care including lubrication, and consider taping the eyelids closed if possible. Tape the eyes in a horizontal fashion using paper tape (or per institutional guidelines).[14]
- ❖ Ensure that the tongue is inside the patient's mouth. If the tongue is swollen or protruding, consider a dental mouth-prop or device. The dental mouth-prop fits between the teeth (upper and lower) holding the mouth open to prevent the teeth from digging into the tongue. Other bite blocks may be used, but do not use bite blocks that fit over the tongue as this will cause undue pressure and increase the risk of tongue breakdown.
- ❖ If a commercial ETT securement device is in use, consider switching to tape or ties before executing the turn.[9] Commercial ETT securement devices are not recommended for use during prone positioning because of the potential for increased skin breakdown and breakdown of adhesive from increased salivary drainage.[26] If using a commercial ETT securement device, take precautions to protect the skin from pressure injury and to assess the stability of the device with repositioning. When using tape or ties to secure the airway, ensure that the ETT or tracheotomy tube is secure. If adhesive tape is used to secure the ETT, consider double-taping or wrapping completely around the head because increased salivary drainage during prone positioning may loosen the adhesive.[26]
- ❖ Central venous and arterial lines should be sutured or a securement device in place. The securement device should be assessed for potential pressure injury while in the prone position. Dressings should be secured; replace if nonocclusive. Consider not disconnecting intravenous lines because of the potential risk of infection. Follow institutional standards for infection prevention related to central and arterial lines.
- ❖ If a wound dressing on the anterior body is scheduled for change during the prone session, perform the dressing change before the turn. Evaluate all dressings on return to the supine position. The patient may require additional changes beyond what is ordered.
- ❖ If the patient has an open abdomen, discuss the plan for wound dressing with providers. Consider covering the abdomen with a synthetic material, vacuum dressing, or support, such as an abdominal binder, before positioning. Identify a positioning strategy that allows the abdomen to be free from restriction.
- ❖ Apply soft silicone multilayer prophylactic foam dressings to all bony prominences and other areas that may be affected by pressure during prone positioning, such as the face, shoulders, chest, breasts, penis, elbows, pelvic bones, knees, or anterior feet.[5,24,26,27]
- ❖ Consider an indwelling urinary drainage device and fecal containment device for patients with increased stool to minimize moisture-related skin concerns before the position change.[5] Remove the securement devices from anterior placement, and place them laterally once the patient is in the prone position to prevent pressure injury.

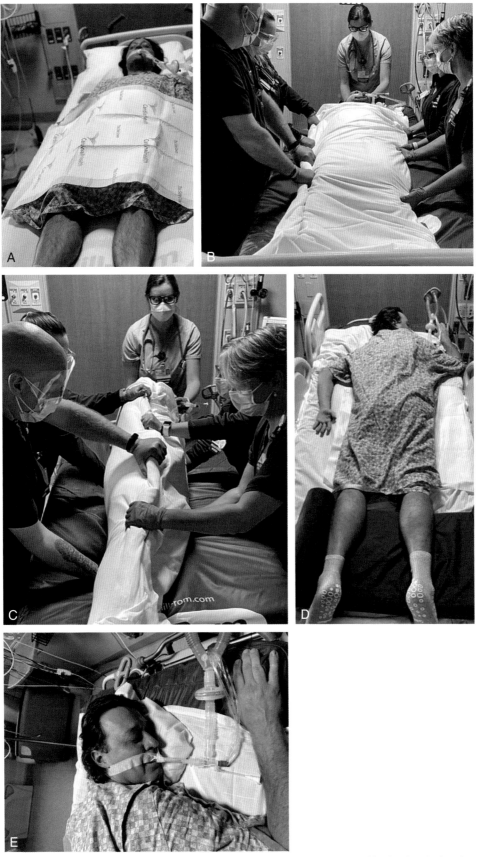

Figure 15.3 The burrito method. **A,** The patient is prepared for prone positioning by placing the positioner or pillows at the chest, pelvis, or legs. *Note:* The patient's gown should be removed before the procedure. **B,** A positioning sheet is placed on top of the patient and rolled tight to sandwich the patient and positioning pillows for security during the turn. **C,** The patient is moved to the side of the bed away from the ventilator and then turned 45 degrees, tubes and lines are assessed, and the patient is moved to the prone position. **D,** Prone position with arms in the swimmer position. **E,** Head position on gel or other cushions. *(Photos courtesy ChristianaCare.)*

❖ Empty ileostomy/colostomy bags before positioning. To prevent direct pressure on the stoma, placing the drainage bag to gravity drainage and padding around the stoma are recommended.

❖ Consider use of capnography monitoring to help ensure proper positioning of the ETT and additional monitoring during the turning procedure and while in the prone position.[18]

Special Patient Populations

Tracheostomies

• Patients with tracheostomies present challenges but are not considered absolute contraindications for prone positioning. Tracheostomies placed less than 24 hours and tracheal surgeries 2 weeks before prone positioning have been listed as relative contraindications and should be evaluated more closely.[23] Special care must be taken to ensure that the tracheostomy tube and ventilator tubing are unencumbered. Additionally, minimizing neck extension and rotation of the neck will be important. Before prone positioning, ensure stability and placement of the tube. Additional chest and head support may be required to keep the tube from touching the bed or other devices utilized. Consultation of providers and those performing the prone procedure should be considered to evaluate the risk versus the benefit.

Pregnancy

• Pregnancy is not an absolute contraindication to prone positioning. Few cases have been reported noting the efficacy of prone positioning in pregnant patients with severe ARDS.[28] Careful consideration must be made when attempting to place a pregnant patient in the prone position. Notably, the abdomen must not be compressed in patients with obese abdomens, abdominal surgeries, or open abdomens. Additional supports to the chest and pelvic area are required to provide ample elevation to minimize abdominal compression. Additionally, continuous fetal monitoring will be necessary during prone positioning.[31] Consultation of all providers and those performing the prone procedure should be considered to evaluate the risk versus the benefit.

Procedure	**Immediately Before Manual Prone Positioning***	
Steps	Rationale	Special Considerations
1. 🄷🄷		
2. 🄿🄴		
3. Pre-prone huddle with team members.[24] Recommend five staff members as minimum and add additional members in accordance with your institutional guidelines for safe patient handling. Two nurses	Team should huddle to plan the procedure and assign roles. An initial huddle pre-prone to determine what must be done to prepare the patient for prone positioning. When ready to physically prone, consider a brief second huddle to verify the roles and plan.	A provider should be available for huddle in person or virtually for guidance and in the event of emergencies.
• One respiratory therapist		
• One provider-physician or APP (if available)		
• Two to three additional staff members (e.g., nurses, nursing technicians, physical therapists, occupational therapists, or wound ostomy continence nurses)		
4. Two staff members are positioned on each side of the bed, with another staff member (preferably, respiratory therapist [RT]) positioned at the head of the bed to manage the airway, manage the ventilator, and turn the patient's head. (**Level D***)	A minimum of five individuals are needed to manually place the patient safely in the prone position. Additional personnel may be necessary, based on the weight and body habitus of the patient.[17,24]	The RT at the head of the bed is responsible for managing the ETT, ventilator, and positioning of the patient's head. For increased airway security, the RT should hold the ETT and patient's head during the turn.[24] If the respiratory therapist or other provider at the head of the bed is not a designated intubator, an additional provider able to intubate should be available in case of accidental extubation.

Procedure	Immediately Before Manual Prone Positioning—*Continued*	
Steps	**Rationale**	**Special Considerations**
5. Position all tubes and invasive lines.	All intravenous tubing and invasive lines are adjusted to prevent kinking, disconnection, and dislodgement during the turning procedure and while the patient remains in the prone position.[17,24,39]	The nurse adjacent to the RT monitors the intravenous lines located near the patient's head. If the patient is in skeletal traction, one individual should apply traction to the leg while the lines and weights are removed for the turn. If a skeletal pin comes into contact with the bed, a pillow should be placed in the correct position to alleviate pressure points.
6. Intravenous lines inserted in the upper torso are aligned with either shoulder, and excess tubing is placed at the head of the bed. *Exception is for chest tubes or other large-bore tubes (e.g., for ECMO).[24,39] **(Level D*)**	Consider not disconnecting intravenous lines, if possible, to reduce infection risk.	Follow institutional standards for infection prevention.
7. Chest tubes and lines or tubes placed in the lower torso are aligned with either leg and extend off the end of the bed.[24,39] **(Level D*)**	Consider addition of an extension tube to lines that are too short to be placed at the head of the bed or the end of the bed.	Consider emptying chest tube drainage or marking the level before turning.
8. If the patient has a large, pregnant, or open abdomen (adequately dressed), identify a positioning strategy that allows the abdomen to be free from restriction.	Large, pregnant, or open abdomens are not a contraindication for use of the prone position.[17,23]	Consult with providers. Utilize pillows/foam or fluidized positioners in the chest area and in the pelvic area to offload the abdomen.
9. If the patient is on a low air-loss surface, maximally inflate the surface before the initial move.[39] **(Level E*)**	Maximally inflating the surface firms up the mattress, making all movements easier to perform.	Consider use of additional devices such as positioning sheets, static overlay mattresses, slings to ease movement and reduce risk to patient and staff, with or without use of maximum inflate function.[41]
10. Preoxygenate the patient with FiO_2 of 100% before prone or supine positioning.[39] **(Level E*)**	Maximize oxygenation before turning.	
11. Remove any nonessential monitoring (e.g., continuous cardiac output) before the position change.		
12. Discard used supplies, and remove **PE**		
13. **HH**		

*Level D: Peer-reviewed professional and organizational standards with the support of clinical study recommendations.

*Level E: Multiple case reports, theory-based evidence from expert opinions, or peer-reviewed professional organizational standards without clinical studies to support recommendations.

*Note that prone positioning may be accomplished by manual turning using several different although similar methodologies. Additionally, positioning may be accomplished with the use of commercial beds. Although this procedure is specific to manual prone positioning using the burrito method, steps may be adapted per your facility's guidelines.

Procedure   for Prone Positioning: Burrito Method (Fig. 15.3)

1. Start with the patient in the supine position on a clean, flat sheet.

   This initial positioning sheet will be used to move the patient and will become the top sheet.

2. Remove the patient's gown, ECG leads, and pads; and replace to the posterior chest with wires toward the head: RA and LA leads to upper posterior shoulders, RL and LL to right and left lower back positions. Place the V1 lead once in position.

   Ensure ECG monitoring throughout the process unless there are other means to evaluate patient response to position changes (e.g., arterial line, end tidal CO_2). To minimize pressure to the posterior chest, move the leads just before the turn.

3. Place absorbent pads over the perineal area. Place pillows positioning foam/fluidizer in the chest area, pelvic area, and shins (see Fig. 15.3A).

   Use pillows/foam/fluidizer to protect pressure points. Use as needed based on the patient's anatomy. May double-stack pillows (consider the same pillowcase) for patients with increased weight and to off-load the abdomen as needed, or use prone design foam or fluidizer to provide better support.

4. Tuck the patient's arms and hands under the buttocks on either side.

   This maneuver protects the arm and allows them to be pulled from under the patient after completing the turn.

5. Cover the patient and all supports fully with a second flat sheet. This will be the bottom sheet once in the prone position.

6. The RT should be positioned at the head of the bed holding the head, ETT, and tubing, with the head turned away from the ventilator.

   The RT should hold the head and ETT for increased airway security.[39]

7. Two persons on both sides will roll the top and bottom sheets together: team members on the side of the ventilator (receiving team) will roll the sheets under (down) and tuck. Team members on the side of the patient away from the ventilator (delivering team) will roll sheets over (up), getting as close to the patient as possible (see Fig. 15.3B).

   Rolling positioning sheets on both sides to ensure a controlled hold of patient, supports dressings, and so on.
   Positioning sheets are rolled under and over for ease of grasping during the turn and settling the patient into position (prone or supine).

8. With the RT holding the patient's head and ETT, on their count, move the patient laterally away from the ventilator.

   The RT should hold the head and ETT for increased airway security.[39] The person managing the airway should initiate the count to ensure readiness and prevent accidental dislodgement of the ETT. If the team leader initiates the count, readiness should be determined by the person managing the airway.

| Procedure | for Prone Positioning: Burrito Method (Fig. 15.3)—*Continued* |

9. Turn the patient onto the full side-lying position facing the ventilator, allowing the receiving team to position hands on the patient and sheets to prepare for prone positioning (see Fig. 15.3C).
10. The team furthest away from the ventilator (delivering team) will pull the positioning sheets under the patient while the receiving team on the other side lowers the patient into the complete prone position.
11. The patient is now prone.Use the sheet to center the patient.
- Straighten all lines and tubes.
- Position the head to prevent pressure areas.
- Gently place extremities in swimmer's position if not contraindicated. Avoid any overextension, overabduction, or overrotation of the neck and arms (see Fig. 15.3D)
- Place the patient in the reverse Trendelenburg position if not contraindicated; consider between 10 and 30 degrees
- Elevate the feet to protect toes from pressure by placing pillows under the shins
- Plan for post-prone ABG after 30 minutes to 1 hour
- Prepare to reposition the patient (rotation of head and arm positions) every 2 hours (or more frequently based on assessments in conjunction with RT*: to manage airway and head while repositioning.[26],[35] (see Fig.15.3D,E) (**Level D***)

Provides team time to reposition the hands on the patient and sheets to lower the patient into position.

Every attempt is made to prevent pressure areas to the face, around lines and tubes, and over bony prominences. The head should be placed in the side-lying position directly on the bed or on foam, fluidizer, or gel pillow of choice with the ETT visible at all times.
Head side-lying and reverse Trendelenburg positioning decreases orbital pressure and minimizes facial edema.
Arms are positioned for comfort by placing them in the swimmer's position: The face should be turned to the raised limb (arm abducted approximately 70 degrees or less, the elbow flexed at about 60 degrees, and the contralateral arm should remain at the side of the body.
Ensure not to overextend the neck, and avoid extensive rotation.
Support the chest with pillows or positioners so the shoulders are forward versus depressed and the abdomen (add pillows in the pelvic region) is offloaded, minimizing compression.[17],[26],[35]

Patients may have limitations in shoulder rotation, increasing the risk for injury.
The patient should be repositioned every 2 hours or more frequently based on assessments with skin inspection to pressure areas, the same as a patient in the supine position. The head and arms should also be rotated from side to side at this time.[22]

*Level D: Peer-reviewed professional and organizational standards with the support of clinical study recommendations.

| Procedure | for the Burrito Method for Return to Supine |

Review rationale and special considerations for process steps
From prone process unless otherwise noted

1. Start with the patient in the prone position on a positioning sheet. Return both arms to the patient's sides. Remove additional bedding and positioning aids around the patient.

Procedure continues on following page

UNIT I

2. Remove the patient's gown. Remove ECG leads and pads, and replace to the anterior chest with wires toward the head: place RA and LA leads to the upper chest and RL and LL to the right and left lower abdomen. Place the V1 lead once in the supine position.

3. Place the absorbent pad over buttocks.

4. Tuck the patient's arms and hands under the anterior thighs on either side.

5. Cover the patient fully with the second sheet. This will be the bottom sheet once in supine position.

6. The RT should be positioned at head of the bed holding the patient's head, ETT, and tubing with the head turned toward the ventilator.

7. Two persons on both sides will roll top and bottom positioning sheets together: team members on the side of the ventilator (delivering team) will roll sheets over (up). Team members on the side of the patient away from the ventilator (receiving team) will roll sheets under (down), getting as close to the patient as possible.

8. With the RT holding the patient's head and ETT, on their count, move the patient horizontally *toward* the ventilator.

9. Turn the patient onto the full side-lying position facing the ventilator, allowing the receiving team to position the hands on the patient and positioning sheets to prepare for supine positioning.

10. The team closest to the vent (delivering team) will pull sheets under the patient, while the receiving team lowers patient into the complete supine position.

11. The patient is now supine. Use the sheet to center the patient.
   - Straighten all lines and tubes.
   - Position the patient's head on the pillow to prevent pressure areas if not contraindicated.
   - Elevate the head of the bed 30 degrees unless contraindicated.
   - Elevate the legs/feet to float the heel using a heel suspension device.
   - Plan for post-supine ABG after 30 minutes to 1 hour.
   - Continue to reposition patient every 2 hours while supine.

12. Complete a full skin assessment.

To minimize pressure to the anterior chest, move the leads just before the turn.

Create a tight cocoon to reduce patient movement and help them feel more secured during the turn.

Place the legs/feet in heal-elevating device/boots to free-float the heels and reduce edema. Place the arms on pillows to reduce edema and prevent pressure. Place the head on a pillow, if not contraindicated. Provide range of motion. The patient should be repositioned every 2 hours or more often as determine by assessment unless contraindicated.

Examine the skin under the dressings as part of your complete skin assessment.

Procedure for Every-2-Hour Repositioning and Head Rotation

1. Upon completion of prone positioning, ensure that the RT and two other members are aware of timing for every-2-hour repositioning of the patient and head rotation.

   Set expectations with clear communication to team. Every-2-hour turns are necessary to protect the patient from pressure areas as well as strain to the neck and shoulders. Frequent repositioning and assessment are necessary to minimize nerve injuries[35] and pressure injuries.[26]

2. Lower the patient's bed to flat if the head of the bed is elevated or in reverse Trendelenburg. Place the patient's arm to the side out of the swimmer's position.

3. The RT should be positioned at the head of the bed holding the patient's head and ETT. On RT count (or team leader count), nurses should lift the patient by the shoulders
   - Gently turn the head to desired side
   - Inspect the ETT, and ensure proper positioning
   - Rest the head onto a bed or pillow on the side
   - Inspect the face on the side the patient was lying

   May consider alternate process for repositioning the head if unable to lift the patient by the shoulders.
   RT at the head of the bed holding the patient's head and ETT. On RT count (or team leader count), team members on either side of the patient move the patient up in bed with a draw sheet to where the head is slightly hanging over the mattress. Gently turn head to desired side. Slide the patient back onto the mattress. Rest the patient's head onto the bed or pillow.

4. Place extremities in the swimmer's position (see Fig. 15.3).

   Arms are positioned for comfort by placing them in the swimmer's position: The face should be turned to the raised limb (arm abducted approximately 70 degrees or less, the elbow flexed at about 60 degrees, and the contralateral arm should remain at the side of the body.[35]
   Ensure not to overextend the neck, and avoid extensive rotation.
   Support the chest with pillows or positioners so shoulders are forward versus depressed and the abdomen (add pillows in pelvic region) is offloaded, minimizing compression.[17,35]

   Consider tilting the patient to side approximately 20 degrees to offload the abdomen or lines, tubes, or drains.

5. Once the position change is complete, return the patient to the reverse Trendelenburg position.

   Head side-lying and reverse Trendelenburg positioning decreases orbital pressure and minimizes facial edema 10 to 30 degrees.

   Ensure that the patient does not slide while in reverse as this may cause overextension of the neck and displacement of lines, tubes, and devices.

Expected Outcomes

- Increased oxygenation
- Improved secretion clearance
- Improved compliance of the lungs and alveolar recruitment
- Improved mortality
- Increased oxygenation

Unexpected Outcomes

- Agitation
- Pressure injuries
- Disconnection or dislodgment of airway, tubes, and lines
- Peripheral arm nerve injury
- Periorbital and conjunctival edema
- Corneal abrasions
- Eye pressure or injury

Patient Monitoring and Care

Steps	Rationale	Reportable Conditions
		These conditions should be reported if they persist despite nursing interventions.
1. Assess the patient's tolerance to the turning procedure: • Respiratory rate and effort • Heart rate and blood pressure	Oxygen saturation is not used as a measure of intolerance to the turning procedure because patients often have desaturation with a deep lateral turn; however, if the patient responds to the prone position, the condition stabilizes quickly when settled into the prone position. If respiratory rate and effort, heart rate, and blood pressure do not return to normal within 10 minutes of the turn, the patient may be displaying initial signs of intolerance.[40.]	Failure of the respiratory rate, respiratory effort, heart rate, and blood pressure to return to normal 5–10 minutes after the turn.[40]
2. Assess the patient's response to the prone position: • Pulse oximetry (SpO_2) • Mixed venous oxygenation saturation if available and hemodynamics • Arterial blood gases 30 minutes after position change • PaO_2/FiO_2 ratio	Of all patients with ARDS turned prone, more than 70% had improvement in oxygenation.[12,19,36] A response is defined by an increase in PaO_2/FiO_2 ratio >20% or a PaO_2 >10 mm Hg of pre-prone position. The time response varies among patients. Some patients immediately respond, whereas others may take a longer time to show maximal response to the position change. Hemodynamic measurements are accurate in the prone position compared with the supine position as long as the zero-reference point is calibrated at the phlebostatic axis.[39]	Decrease from baseline in the SpO_2 or failure of mixed venous oxygenation saturation to return to baseline after 5–10 minutes
3. Assess for pain, agitation, and delirium before repositioning and before/after administering medications as ordered to provide relief. Additionally, continue to assess for pain and agitation every 4 hours, and assess for delirium every 8 hours.	The act of turning to the prone position or back to a supine position can be a frightening and potentially anxiety-provoking experience for the patient.	
4. Refer to prone procedure for every-2-hour limb repositioning and head rotation.	The face, chin, and ears have minimal structural padding to reduce the risk of skin breakdown. Patients with short necks or limited neck range of motion have difficulty assuming a head side-lying position. These patients are more likely to have facial breakdown develop, making micro-turning the patients head more frequently critical to prevent breakdown.[24,26]	Pressure injuries of high-risk areas, including the face, chest, pelvis, patella, and pretibial areas.

Patient Monitoring and Care —*Continued*

Steps	Rationale	Reportable Conditions
5. Assess pressure points before placing the patient in the prone position (anterior surfaces) and before returning the patient to the supine position (posterior surfaces). Assess pressure points when alternating arm and head positions. Apply soft silicone multilayer prophylactic foam dressings to all bony prominences and other areas that may be affected by pressure during prone position (e.g., face, shoulders, chest, breasts, penis, elbows, pelvic bones, knees, anterior feet).[5,24,26] Assess under the dressing on return to the supine position. **(Level D*)**	Greater than 2 hours on a standard surface without changing position increases the patient's risk for breakdown. If the patient is on a pressure-reduction surface, the time remaining in a stationary position can be lengthened.[26] The use of a soft silicone multilayer foam dressing serves as a protective barrier, reducing the risk of pressure, shearing, and friction injuries.[5,24,26]	Nonblanchable redness Pressure, shear, and friction injuries
6. Provide frequent oral care and suctioning of the airway as needed (see Procedure 3, Endotracheal Tube Care and Oral Care Practices for Ventilated and Nonventilated Patients and Procedure 8, Suctioning: Endotracheal or Tracheostomy).	The prone position promotes postural drainage through the natural use of gravity. Drainage from the nares may be a clinical sign of an undetected sinus infection. With excessive oral or nasal secretions, the skin of the face and neck are at risk for moisture injuries.[26]	Drainage from the nares Change in amount or character of secretions
7. Maintain eye care to prevent corneal abrasions.	It is important to maintain lubrication via institutional standards to prevent dryness leading to corneal abrasions.[32] To ensure protection, provide eye lubrication, and consider closed eyes, taping horizontally if applicable.[32]	Changes in the conditions of the eyes
8. Resume tube feeding after positioning the patient prone. Maintain tube feeding as tolerated per institutional standards. In the published studies to date, patients received similar amounts with no differences in complications between the prone and supine positions. In these studies, enteral nutrition was delivered via a nasogastric or orogastric tube.[20,29,30,33] **(Level C*)**	To reduce the risk of aspiration, place the bed in a 10- to 30-degree reverse Trendelenburg position.[3,29,30,33] **(Level C*)** Use of prokinetic agents or transpyloric feedings is suggested to prevent complications associated with vomiting or high gastric residuals.[3]	Evidence of tube feeding material when suctioning
9. Consider fecal containment strategies while prone to reduce incontinence, associated dermatitis, and potential contamination of the urinary catheter.[5]	The prone position creates gravity movement of fecal matter, which may cause areas beneath to be difficult to clean and protect.	Catheter-associated urinary tract infection Incontinence-associated dermatitis

Procedure continues on following page

UNIT I

Patient Monitoring and Care —*Continued*

Steps	Rationale	Reportable Conditions
10. Scheduling frequency: the positioning schedule is based on the largest RCT, which suggests at least 16 hours of prone positioning per day.[12] A. Time spent in the supine position is based on the length of time the patient can sustain or maintain the improvement in gas exchange that occurred while prone.[12,24] **(Level B*)**	The literature demonstrates that longer times in the prone position within a 24-hour period is better, however, it is important that the healthcare team weigh other physiological factors when a patient remains in any stationary position for an extended period.[40]	Clinically significant decreases in oxygenation (>10 mm Hg) or oxygen saturation (<88%)
11. Prone positioning should be discontinued if the following criteria have been met:Improvement in oxygenation defined as Pao_2/Fio_2 ratio >150 mm Hg, Fio_2 <60%, and PEEP ≤10 cm H_2O[12] **(Level B*)**	Consider use of lateral rotation therapy when the patient is in the supine position. The therapy has been associated with a reduction in pulmonary complications.[24]	Complications occurring during a prone session leading to its immediate interruption, including accidental extubation or ETT obstruction, sustained decreases in oxygen saturation, massive hemoptysis, and any other life-threatening reason.[2,12] **(Level B*)**

*Level B: Well-designed, controlled studies with results that consistently support a specific action, intervention, or treatment.

*Level C: Qualitative studies, descriptive or correlational studies, integrative reviews, systematic reviews, or randomized controlled trials with inconsistent results.

*Level D: Peer-reviewed professional and organizational standards with the support of clinical study recommendations.

Documentation

Documentation should include the following:

- Patient and family education
- Ability to tolerate the turning procedure
- Length of time in the prone position: Prone start time, return to supine time
- Maximal oxygenation response in the prone position
- Oxygenation response when returned to the supine position
- Pain, agitation, and delirium assessments
- Full skin assessment
- Positioning schedule used: institutional protocol (prone/supine lengths of time)
- Complications noted during or after the procedure
- Use of continuous lateral rotation therapy or other devices
- Amount and type of secretions
- Unexpected outcomes

References and Additional Readings

For a complete list of references and additional readings for this procedure, scan this QR code with your smartphone, or visit https://www.elsevier.com/__data/assets/pdf_file/0003/1319790/Chapter0015.pdf.

PROCEDURE

16 Autotransfusion

Cynthia Sprinkle

PURPOSE: Autotransfusion is the collection of the patient's own blood from an active bleeding source within the thoracic cavity, caused by trauma or surgery, which is then reinfused to maintain the patient's blood volume.

PREREQUISITE NURSING KNOWLEDGE

- Understanding of infusion therapy and fluid balance is necessary.
- Autotransfusion is commonly used for trauma victims and for patients undergoing cardiothoracic procedures, reducing the need for bank blood transfusions and the associated risks of transfusion reactions and disease transmission.[3,8,9]
- Indications for autotransfusion include patients that are losing blood into a collection system. It must be reinfused within 4 to 6 hours.[2]
- A variety of autotransfusion devices are available. Autotransfusion may be a component of a standard water-seal or dry-chest-drainage system (Fig. 16.1) or a separate system, and it may be continuous or intermittent.
  - ❖ In-line systems utilize an autotransfusion bag that collects the blood from the patient prior to the chest-drainage collection unit.
  - ❖ Self-filling systems utilize a vacuum bag that attaches to the chest-drainage system and pulls blood directly from the chest drainage collection unit. The autotransfusion bag is disconnected from the chest-drainage collection unit connected to a saline-primed blood administration infusion set for delivery to the patient (see Fig. 16.1A).
  - ❖ Continuous systems have an intravenous line connected directly to the patient from the chest-drainage collection unit, via an intravenous pump (see Fig. 16.1B).
- Nurses should be familiar with their institution's autotransfusion system, policies, and procedures.
- Contraindications to autotransfusion include the following:[5]
  - ❖ Contamination of the blood in the thoracic cavity, possibly caused by penetrating trauma with involvement of the gastrointestinal tract, or other possible fluid contamination
  - ❖ Septicemia
  - ❖ Malignant cells in the blood shed
  - ❖ Renal or hepatic insufficiency
  - ❖ Coagulopathies
  - ❖ Blood that has been in the collection system for longer than institutional standards allow
  - ❖ Any of these contraindications may be overruled if the patient is exsanguinating and there is not an adequate supply of banked blood available.[3]

- Patient (or surrogate) consent should always be obtained before any blood infusion in a nonemergent setting. Patients have the right to know the risks and benefits of receiving transfusions of any kind. Emergent transfusions will usually include allogeneic blood transfusions and should be administered per institutional protocol.[8]
- Patients (or their surrogate) may decline autotransfusions because of religious or personal beliefs. Jehovah's Witnesses will not accept a transfusion of whole blood nor the primary components that make up whole blood. Many Jehovah's Witnesses will however accept blood through autotransfusion or cell salvage. They may also agree to products like cryoprecipitate, fibrinogen, and prothrombin complex concentrate. It is ultimately a matter of individual choice.[7]

EQUIPMENT

- Personal protective equipment (i.e., gloves, mask, and eye shield)
- Chest-drainage unit
- Autotransfusion collection system
- Blood administration set
- 40-μm microemboli filter
- Normal saline solution
- Wall suction and regulator
- Anticoagulation as indicated

PATIENT AND FAMILY EDUCATION

- If time permits, assess the patient's and family's level of understanding about the condition and rationale for the procedure. *Rationale:* This assessment identifies the patient's and family's knowledge deficits concerning the patient's condition, the procedure, the expected benefits, and the potential risks. It also allows time for questions to clarify information and voice concerns. Explanations decrease patient anxiety and enhance cooperation.
- Explain the procedure and the reason for the procedure, if the clinical situation permits. If not, explain the procedure and reason for the transfusion after it is completed. *Rationale:* This explanation enhances patient and family understanding and decreases anxiety.

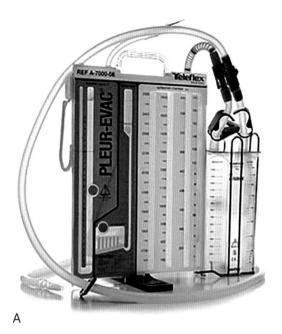

A

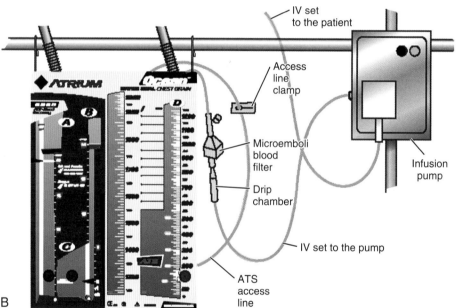

B

Figure 16.1 **A,** Intermittent autotransfusion. Blood is collected in a bag attached to the chest drainage system and then reinfused when enough volume is obtained. **B,** Continuous autotransfusion. Blood is continuously reinfused into the patient as it collects in the chest drainage system. *(A, Image courtesy of Teleflex Incorporated. © 2022 Teleflex Incorporated. All rights reserved. B, Courtesy Atrium Medical Corporation, Hudson, NH.)*

PATIENT ASSESSMENT AND PREPARATION

Patient Assessment

- The patient should be assessed for signs and symptoms of hypovolemia and shock, which include the following[3,4,8]:
  - Pale, cool, clammy skin
  - Dyspnea
  - Tachycardia
  - Hypotension
  - Decreased cardiac output or index
  - Narrowing pulse pressure
  - Oliguria
  - Decreased hemoglobin and/or hematocrit
  - Decreased central venous pressure, pulmonary artery pressure, or pulmonary wedge pressure.

  Rationale: Significant blood loss, related systemic hypoperfusion, and the associated decrease in oxygen-carrying capacity, with its effect on hypoxemia, often require the replacement of blood with whole blood or packed red blood cells. In appropriate patient populations (trauma or cardiovascular), autotransfusion should be considered as the need to replace blood becomes apparent.[3,6,8]

Patient Preparation

- Ensure that the patient (or his or her surrogate) understands the procedural education. Answer questions as they arise, and reinforce information as needed. *Rationale:* This communication evaluates and reinforces understanding of previously provided education.

Procedure for Autotransfusion

Steps	Rationale	Special Considerations
1. 🄷🄷		
2. 🄿🄴		
3. Assemble the collection system.	Prepares the equipment.	Wall suction will be required to facilitate drainage into chest-drainage system.
4. Addition of anticoagulant into the autotransfusion bag before collecting the blood may be considered, depending on institutional protocol or manufacturer's recommendations. **(Level E*)**	There are various anticoagulants that can be used during the transfusion process, including citrate phosphate dextrose, acid citrate dextrose, or heparin, depending on the collection system.	Follow institutional protocol and collection system manufacturer's recommendations for dosing.
5. Connect the patient's drainage system or chest tube to the collection bag directly or via a water-seal system.	Allows for collection of shed blood.	
6. Before disconnecting the filled collection bag for infusion, prepare a new collection bag.	Prevents infection by keeping the transfusion system closed and sterile.	For continuous infusion, follow the manufacturer's guidelines.
7. Close the clamp or clamp tubes on the new collection bag.	Prevents air from entering the system.	
8. Close the clamp on the chest-drainage system.	Stops drainage while changing the tubing and adding a new collection bag, again decreasing the chance for infection and exposure to blood-borne pathogens.	If the collection bag is part of the water-seal system, close the clamps to the water-seal drainage unit. Prepares the system for changing of collection bags and prevents infection or air entering the system.
9. Disconnect the filled bag from the patient system, taking care to always maintain sterility.	Prepares the filled bag for administration of the shed blood to the patient.	
10. Take the previously prepared new collection bag; attach it to the water-seal unit or to the patient's chest tube or drainage tube.	Prepares the chest-drainage system for the collection of further shed blood, if necessary.	
11. Confirm that all connections are secured; open clamps on the autotransfusion bag and patient drainage tubing.	Ensures integrity of the system.	
12. Prime the blood-administration tubing with normal saline.	Prepares the blood-administration set for shed blood infusion.	Do not apply pressure or use with a pressure device during transfusion.
13. Add the microfilter to the blood side of the tubing, and connect the filled collection bag.[1,2,5] **(Level E*)**	Prevents microembolization from the shed blood.	A 40-µm filter is always used when transfusing salvaged blood to prevent microembolization.[5]
14. Initiate infusion of the shed blood. **(Level D*)**	Restores blood volume.	Reinfuse blood within 6 hours of collection, and ensure that it is complete within 4 hours of starting the infusion.[1,2]
15. Repeat this procedure as needed based on reassessment of the patient following the initial transfusion.	Restores blood volume.	
16. Discard supplies and equipment, and remove 🄿🄴		
17. 🄷🄷		

*Level D: Peer-reviewed professional and organizational standards with the support of clinical study recommendations.

*Level E: Multiple case reports, theory-based evidence from expert opinions, or peer-reviewed professional organizational standards without clinical studies to support recommendations.

Expected Outcomes

- Patient infused with own blood in a timely manner
- Improved hemoglobin and hematocrit
- Improved oxygenation
- Hemodynamic stability

Unexpected Outcomes

- Blood transfusion reaction
- Fluid overload
- Infection; septicemia

Patient Monitoring and Care

Steps	Rationale	Reportable Conditions
		These conditions should be reported to the provider if they persist despite nursing interventions.
1. Assess cardiopulmonary status and vital signs every 15 minutes, until 1 hour after transfusion is completed as per institutional protocol.	Provides baseline and ongoing assessment of the patient's condition.	Tachycardia Hypoxia or hypoxemia Jugular vein distention Hypotension Dysrhythmias Fever
2. Evaluate and maintain chest tube patency every 2 hours as per institutional protocol.	Obstruction of the drainage interferes with drainage of blood from the chest.	Inability to establish patency
3. Monitor the amount of blood accumulation in the chest-drainage unit, and mark the drainage on the outside of the unit in hourly or shift increments, as necessary.	Volume loss can cause patients to become hypovolemic.	Blood accumulation of >100 mL/hour New onset of clots Sudden decrease or absence of drainage
4. Monitor for a blood-transfusion reaction.	A patient receiving autotransfusion is unlikely to experience a blood-transfusion reaction.	Fever >101°F (38.5°C) Chills Tachycardia Abdominal or back pain Hypotension Hematuria
5. Monitor patient coagulation laboratory values. Anticipate infusion of fresh-frozen plasma, platelets, and cryoprecipitate as indicated.	Hemothorax blood is not the same as fresh whole blood. It is depleted in coagulation factor V and fibrinogen and has a high concentration of fibrin-degradation products.[10]	Hypotension Tachycardia Obvious signs of bleeding Increased output in chest tube Abnormal laboratory values
6. Monitor ionized calcium levels.	If citrate is utilized, it lowers ionized calcium levels.	Low ionized calcium levels Signs and symptoms of citrate toxicity Hypernatremia Metabolic alkalosis Low magnesium Arrhythmias

Documentation

Documentation should include the following:

- Patient and surrogate education
- Amount of drainage
- Amount of transfusion volume (continuous infusions)
- Date and start time of collection, volume, and when it was infused (intermittent infusions)
- Patient response, including vital signs
- Nursing interventions
- Unexpected outcomes

References and Additional Readings

For a complete list of references and additional readings for this procedure, scan this QR code with your smartphone, or visit https://www.elsevier.com/__data/assets/pdf_file/0004/1319791/Chapter0016.pdf

17 Chest Tube Placement 🅰🅿 (Perform)

Marc Manley

PURPOSE: Chest tube placement, also known as *tube thoracostomy,* is performed for the removal or drainage of air, blood, or fluid from the thorax, whether emergent, elective, life-saving, or palliative.[9] In addition, chest tubes may be used to introduce sclerosing agents into the pleural space for chemical pleurodesis.

PREREQUISITE NURSING KNOWLEDGE

- The thoracic cavity is a closed airspace in normal conditions. Any disruption results in the loss of negative pressure within the intrapleural space. Air or fluid that enters the space competes with the lung, resulting in collapse of the lung. Associated conditions are the result of disease, injury, surgery, or iatrogenic causes.
- Chest tubes are sterile flexible polyvinyl chloride (PVC) or silicone nonthrombogenic catheters approximately 20 inches (51 cm) long, varying in size from 8F to 40F. The size of the tube placed is determined by the indication and viscosity of the drainage.[6] The side of the chest tube usually has a radiopaque strip to assist in visualization on chest radiographs.
- Indications for chest tube placement include but are not limited to the following[11]:
  - Removal of an air collection in the pleural space
    - Pneumothorax
    - Tension pneumothorax
    - Hemopneumothorax
  - Removal of fluid collection or accumulation between visceral and parietal pleura
    - Hemothorax
    - Pleural effusion
    - Chylothorax
    - Empyema
  - Use as a conduit for the delivery of medication or fluid into the pleural space
    - Delivery of warmed fluid into the thoracic space as a method of internal warming of the core and circulating blood volume
    - Delivery of anesthetic solutions, sclerosing agents, or fibrinolytic therapy
    - Delivery of chemotherapeutic agents directly into the thoracic space

🅰🅿 This procedure should be performed only by clinicians who have demonstrated competence and are credentialed to perform it. In addition, the procedure must be within the scope of practice defined by their professional licensure, and in accordance with professional practice acts. Physicians, advanced practice nurses, and physician assistants may be credentialed to perform this procedure.

- Chest tubes inserted for traumatic hemopneumothorax or hemothorax (blood) should be large (36F to 40F). Medium tubes (24F to 36F) should be used for fluid accumulation (pleural effusions). Tubes inserted for pneumothorax (air) should be small (≤24F).[3,10]
- A pneumothorax may be classified as an *open, closed,* or *tension* pneumothorax.
  - *Open pneumothorax:* The chest wall and the pleural space are penetrated, which allows air to enter the pleural space, as in a penetrating injury or trauma; a surgical incision in the thoracic cavity (i.e., thoracotomy); or a complication of surgical treatment (e.g., unintentional puncture during invasive procedures, such as thoracentesis or central venous catheter insertion).
  - *Closed pneumothorax:* The pleural space is penetrated, but the chest wall is intact, which allows air to enter the pleural space from within the lung, as in spontaneous pneumothorax. A closed pneumothorax occurs without apparent injury and often is seen in patients with chronic lung disorders (e.g., emphysema, cystic fibrosis, tuberculosis, necrotizing pneumonia) and in young, tall men who have a greater than normal height-to-width chest ratio; after blunt traumatic injury; or iatrogenically, occurring as a complication of medical treatment (e.g., intermittent positive-pressure breathing, mechanical ventilation with positive end-expiratory pressure, lung biopsy, bronchoscopy, central line insertion, pacemaker placement).
  - *Tension pneumothorax:* Air leaks into the pleural space through a tear in the lung and has no means to escape from the pleural cavity, creating a one-way valve effect. With each breath the patient takes, air accumulates and pressure within the pleural space increases, and the lung collapses. This condition causes the mediastinal structures (i.e., heart, great vessels, and trachea) to be compressed and shift to the opposite or unaffected side of the chest. Venous return and cardiac output are impeded, and collapse of the unaffected lung is possible. This life-threatening emergency requires prompt recognition and intervention.
- *Absolute contraindications:* There is no absolute contraindication in an emergency situation.[2] In a nonemergent situation, a lung that is densely adherent to the chest wall

throughout the hemithorax is considered to be an absolute contraindication to chest tube placement.[12]

- *Relative contraindications:* Use of chest tubes in patients with multiple adhesions, giant blebs, or coagulopathies should be carefully considered. However, these relative contraindications are superseded by the need to reexpand the lung. When possible, any coagulopathy or platelet defect should be corrected before chest tube insertion. The differential diagnosis between a pneumothorax and bullous disease necessitates careful radiological assessment.[12]
- Ultrasound guidance for localizing fluid and/or air during chest tube placement is strongly recommended and may decrease the risk of complications.[4]
- Chest tubes should be inserted into the "triangle of safety." This is an area bordered inferiorly by a horizontal line at the level of the fifth intercostal space, anteriorly by the lateral border of the pectoralis major, and posteriorly by the lateral border of the latissimus dorsi.[4]
- The tube size and insertion site selected for the chest tube are determined by the indication.[8,127] If draining air, the tube is optimally placed near the apex of the lung (second intercostal space); if draining fluid, the tube is optimally placed near the base of the lung (fourth or fifth intercostal space; Fig. 17.1).
  - ❖ Once the tube is in place, it should be sutured to the skin to prevent displacement and a dry occlusive dressing applied (Fig. 17.2). The chest tube should also be connected to a chest drainage system (see Procedure 21, Closed Chest-Drainage System) to remove air and fluid from the pleural space, which facilitates reexpansion of the collapsed lung. Secure all tube connections from the chest tube to the drainage system, using either tape (Fig. 17.3) or zip ties (Parham-Martin bands) (Fig. 17.4).
  - ❖ The water-seal chamber should bubble gently immediately on insertion of the chest tube during expiration and with coughing. Continuous bubbling in this chamber indicates a leak within the patient or in the chest-drainage system. Fluctuations in the water level in the water-seal chamber of 5 to 10 cm, rising during inhalation and falling during expiration (also known as *tidaling*), should be observed with spontaneous respirations. If the patient is on mechanical ventilation, the pattern of fluctuation is just the opposite. Depending on the chest drainage system used, it may be necessary to disconnect suction temporarily to assess correctly for fluctuations in the water-seal chamber.

EQUIPMENT

- Caps, masks, sterile gloves, gowns, drapes
- Protective eyewear (goggles)
- Antiseptic swab and/or solution: 2% chlorhexidine or povidone-iodine
- Local anesthetic: 1% or 2% lidocaine solution (with or without epinephrine)
- 10-mL syringe with 20-gauge 1½-inch needle
- 5-mL syringe with 25-gauge 1-inch needle
- Tube thoracostomy insertion tray
  - ❖ Sterile towels, 4 × 4 sterile gauze
  - ❖ Scalpel with No. 10 or 11 blade
  - ❖ Two Kelly clamps
  - ❖ Needle holder
  - ❖ Monofilament or silk suture material (No. 0 or 1-0)
  - ❖ Sterile basin or medicine cup
  - ❖ Suture scissors
  - ❖ Two hemostats

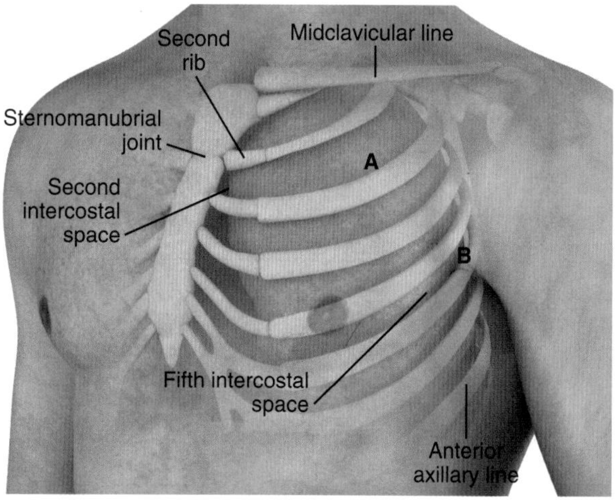

Figure 17.1 Entry sites for tube thoracostomy. The second intercostal space, the midclavicular line, is the preferred site for needle aspiration or catheter insertion (**A**). To find the second intercostal space, first palpate the sternomanubrial joint. The second rib articulates with this structure. The second intercostal space is found below the second rib. The fourth or fifth intercostal space, midaxillary to anterior axillary line (lateral to the pectoralis muscle and breast tissue), is preferred for a chest tube (**B**). The fifth intercostal space is usually at the level of the nipple. In an obese person, an assistant may need to retract the breast upward to identify landmarks and avoid low placement. *(From Margolis AM, Kirsch TD:* Roberts and Hedges' clinical procedures in emergency medicine and acute care, *ed 7, Philadelphia, 2019, Elsevier.)*

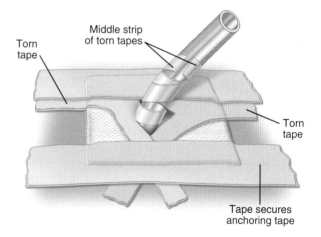

Figure 17.2 Occlusive chest tube dressing. After securing the tube to the skin with sutures, apply an occlusive dressing to cover the defect around the tube. A wide piece of tape is longitudinally split into three pieces; the two outside pieces are placed on the skin on either side of the tube, and the center strip is wrapped around the chest tube. A similar piece of tape can be secured to the tube at a 90-degree angle to the first piece. The tape is secured to the skin with an anchoring piece of tape. *(From Fonseca RJ, Barber HD, Powers MP, et al:* Oral and maxillofacial trauma, *ed 4, St. Louis, 2013, Elsevier.)*

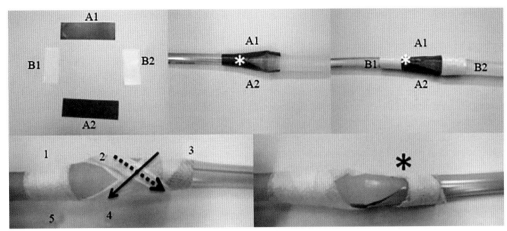

Figure 17.3 The securing of connection points with tape utilizing one of three different methods (straight method and cross method) for junction connection. Straight method: Two longer tapes (A1 and A2, measured 2.5 × 9 cm) are applied longitudinally; another two shorter tapes (B1 and B2, measured 2.5 × 5 cm) are applied making circumferential turns; the connection junction *(*)* is not covered by the tapes. Cross (X) method: One single long tape measured 2.5 × 40 cm is used; one complete circumferential turn is made at one end; a diagonal turn is made; a complete circumferential turn is made at the other end; another diagonal turn is made, making an *X* shape with step 2; completed with a final circumferential turn; a "window" is created so that the connection junction *(*)* is visible to detect any disconnection or subtle loosening. *(From Li KK, Wong KS, Wong YH, et al: How to secure the connection between thoracostomy tube and drainage system?* World J Emerg Med *5[4]:259–263, 2014.)*

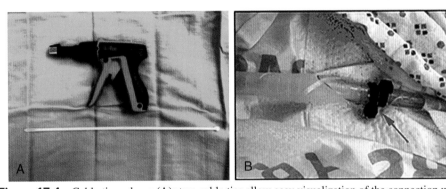

Figure 17.4 Cable tie and gun **(A)**; two cable ties allow easy visualization of the connection with complete assurance that the connection will not be dislodged **(B).** *(From Pieracci FM, Burlew CC, Spain D, et al: Tube thoracostomy during the COVID-19 pandemic: guidance and recommendations from the AAST Acute Care Surgery and Critical Care Committees.* Trauma Surg Acute Care Open *5[1]:e000498, 2020.)*

- Thoracostomy tubes (8F to 40F, as appropriate)
- Closed chest-drainage system
- Suction source
- Suction connector and connecting tubing (usually 6 feet for each tube)
- 1-inch adhesive tape or zip ties
- Occlusive dressing materials:
  ❖ 4 × 4 gauze pads or slit drain sponges
  ❖ Tape or a commercial securing device

Additional equipment to have available as needed includes the following:

- Ultrasound machine, ultrasound gel, and sterile probe cover

PATIENT AND FAMILY EDUCATION

- If time permits, assess the patient's and family's level of understanding about the condition and rationale for the procedure. *Rationale:* This assessment identifies the patient's and family's knowledge deficits concerning the

patient's condition, the procedure, the expected benefits, and the potential risks. It also allows time for the patient and/or family to pose questions to clarify information and voice concerns. Explanations may decrease patient anxiety and enhance cooperation.

- Explain the procedure and the reason for the procedure if the clinical situation permits. If not, explain the procedure and reason for it after it is completed. *Rationale:* This explanation may enhance patient and family understanding and decrease anxiety.
- Explain to the patient that their only participation during the procedure is to remain as immobile as possible and maintain relaxed breathing. *Rationale:* This explanation facilitates insertion of the chest tube and prevents complications during insertion.
- After the procedure, instruct the patient to sit in the semi-Fowler's position (unless contraindicated). *Rationale:* This position facilitates drainage, if present, from the pleural space by allowing air to rise and fluid to settle to be

removed via the chest tube. This position may also make breathing easier.

- Instruct the patient to turn and/or change position every 2 hours. The patient may lie on the side with the chest tube but should keep the tubing free from kinks. ***Rationale:*** Turning and changing position may prevent complications related to immobility and retained pulmonary secretions. Keeping the tube free from kinks maintains patency of the tube, facilitates drainage, and prevents accumulation of pressure within the pleural space that interferes with lung reexpansion.
- Instruct the patient to cough and deep breathe, with splinting of the affected side. ***Rationale:*** Coughing and deep breathing increase pressure within the pleural space, facilitating drainage, promoting lung reexpansion, and preventing respiratory complications associated with retained secretions. The application of firm pressure over the chest tube insertion site (i.e., splinting) may decrease pain and discomfort.
- Encourage active or passive range-of-motion exercises of the arm on the affected side. ***Rationale:*** The patient may limit movement of the arm on the affected side to decrease discomfort at the insertion site, which may result in joint discomfort and potential joint contractures.
- Instruct the patient and family about activity as prescribed while maintaining the drainage system below the level of the chest. ***Rationale:*** This activity facilitates gravity drainage and prevents backflow and potential infectious contamination into the pleural space.
- Instruct the patient about the availability of prescribed analgesic medication and other pain-relief strategies. ***Rationale:*** Pain relief ensures comfort and facilitates coughing, deep breathing, positioning, range of motion, and recuperation.

PATIENT ASSESSMENT AND PREPARATION

Patient Assessment

- Assess for significant medical history or injury, including chronic lung disease, spontaneous pneumothorax, hemothorax, pulmonary disease, therapeutic procedures, lung surgery, and mechanism of injury. ***Rationale:*** Medical history or injury may provide the etiological basis for the occurrence of pneumothorax, empyema, pleural effusion, or chylothorax.
- Evaluate diagnostic test results (if the patient's condition does not necessitate immediate intervention), including chest radiograph, coagulation tests, and arterial blood gases. ***Rationale:*** Diagnostic testing confirms the presence of air or fluid in the pleural space, a collapsed lung, hypoxemia, and respiratory compromise.
- Assess baseline cardiopulmonary status for signs and symptoms that necessitate chest tube insertion.[12] ***Rationale:*** Accurate assessment of signs and symptoms allows for prompt recognition and treatment. Baseline assessment provides comparison data for evaluation of changes and outcomes of treatment.
  - ❖ Tachypnea
  - ❖ Decreased or absent breath sounds on the affected side
  - ❖ Crackles adjacent to the affected area
  - ❖ Shortness of breath, dyspnea

- ❖ Asymmetrical chest excursion with respirations
- ❖ Cyanosis
- ❖ Decreased oxygen saturation
- ❖ Hyperresonance on the affected side (pneumothorax)
- ❖ Subcutaneous emphysema (pneumothorax)
- ❖ Dullness or flatness on the affected side (hemothorax, pleural effusion, empyema, chylothorax)
- ❖ Sudden, sharp chest pain
- ❖ Anxiety, restlessness, apprehension
- ❖ Tachycardia
- ❖ Hypotension
- ❖ Dysrhythmias
- ❖ Tracheal deviation to the unaffected side (tension pneumothorax)
- ❖ Neck vein distention (tension pneumothorax)
- ❖ Muffled heart sounds (tension pneumothorax)

Patient Preparation

- Verify the correct patient with two identifiers. ***Rationale:*** Before performing a procedure, the nurse should ensure the correct identification of the patient for the intended intervention.
- Ensure that the patient understands preprocedural teachings. Answer questions as they arise, and reinforce information as needed. ***Rationale:*** This communication evaluates and reinforces understanding of previously taught information.
- Obtain informed consent if circumstances allow. ***Rationale:*** Invasive procedures, unless performed with implied consent in a life-threatening situation, require written consent of the patient or significant other.
- Ensure that the patient has a patent intravenous access. ***Rationale:*** This access provides a route for procedural analgesic, sedation, and emergency medications.
- Determine the insertion site, and mark the skin with an indelible marker. ***Rationale:*** The insertion site is determined by the indication for the chest tube and diagnostic images. For a pneumothorax, the tube may be directed anterior and apical. For fluid drainage, it may be aimed posterior and basilar.[10]
- Determine the size of chest tube needed. ***Rationale:*** Evacuation of air necessitates a smaller tube; evacuation of fluid necessitates a larger tube.
- Assist the patient to the most appropriate position based on the reason for the chest tube insertion. If the tube placement is for removal of an air collection, place the patient in the lateral supine position with the patient's forearm raised above their head and the hand tucked behind the head. If the tube placement is for removal of a fluid collection, assist the patient to the semi-Fowler's position, or consider having them sit upright, leaning over an overbed table with a pillow under their arms for comfort.[7,13] ***Rationale:*** Appropriate positioning enhances accessibility to the insertion site specifically needed for the chest tube.
- Administer prescribed analgesics or sedatives as needed; follow institutional policy for procedural sedation. ***Rationale:*** Analgesics and sedatives reduce the discomfort and anxiety experienced and facilitate patient cooperation.
- Administer supplemental oxygen, as needed. Monitor the pulse oximeter and/or end-tidal carbon dioxide level. ***Rationale:*** Real-time assessment of patient's respiratory status during the procedure is provided.

Procedure	for Performing Pleural Chest Tube Placement		
Steps	**Rationale**		**Special Considerations**
1. ▉▉			
2. ▉▉			
3. Don sterile gloves, sterile gown, mask, eye protection, and head covering.	Chest tube insertion is a sterile procedure and requires full surgical attire, unless performed in a life-threatening situation.		
4. Have an assistant open the outer wrapper of the tube thoracostomy insertion tray, remove the tray from the wrapper, and open it using sterile technique.	Reduces transmission of microorganisms.		

5. Prepare equipment.
   A. Check that all equipment is present before beginning the procedure.
   B. Have an assistant open antiseptic solution and pour it into a basin or medicine cup using aseptic technique, or open an antiseptic swab packet and stand by.
   C. Have an assistant open the chest tube package and empty it onto the open tray.
   D. Grasp the suture needle with the needle holder.
   E. Remove and discard the trocar from the chest tube, and grasp the proximal end of the chest tube with a large Kelly clamp (Fig. 17.5). Prepare the syringe with lidocaine solution.
	Facilitates insertion of the tube.		Insertion of the chest tube with a trocar is not recommended, since this is associated with a higher incidence of iatrogenic injury.[10]

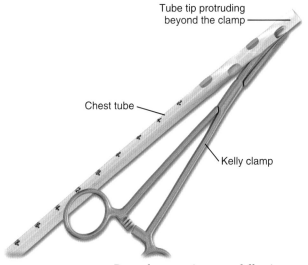

Figure 17.5 Hold the tube with the tip of the tube protruding beyond the tip of the clamp to reduce the risk for pulmonary injury. *(From Margolis AM, Kirsch TD:* Roberts and Hedges' clinical procedures in emergency medicine and acute care, *ed 7, Philadelphia, 2019, Elsevier.)*

Tube tip protruding beyond the clamp

Chest tube

Kelly clamp

Procedure continues on following page

Procedure | for Performing Pleural Chest Tube Placement—*Continued*

Steps	Rationale	Special Considerations
6. Identify the insertion site, and have an assistant position the patient. **(Level E*)**	Assists in preparation of the area for insertion and proper placement of the tube.[12]	The insertion site for air removal is the right or left second intercostal space. The insertion site for fluid removal is the right or left fifth or sixth intercostal space, midaxillary line. The incision site is one rib below the insertion site.
7. Perform a preprocedural verification and time out, if nonemergent.	Ensures patient safety.	
8. Surgically prepare the skin with antiseptic solution, and drape the area surrounding the insertion site. **(Level E*)**	Inhibits growth of bacteria at the insertion site; maintains sterility.[3,124]	Prepare the area from the clavicle to the umbilicus, mid-chest to anterior axillary line.
9. Anesthetize the skin, subcutaneous tissue, muscle, and periosteum one intercostal space below the intercostal space that will be used to place the tube with lidocaine solution. A. With a 5-mL syringe (25-gauge needle), inject a subcutaneous wheal of lidocaine at the insertion site. B. With a 10-mL syringe (20-gauge, 1½-inch needle), advance the needle/syringe, aspirating as you go, until air or pleural fluid is confirmed. C. Inject the lidocaine deeper, and slowly withdraw the syringe, generously anesthetizing the rib periosteum, subcutaneous tissue, and pleura (Fig. 17.6). **(Level E*)**	Results in loss of sensation and decreased pain during insertion.[3,124]	When infiltrating with lidocaine, aspirate repeatedly as the needle is inserted to identify the presence of air or fluid; up to 30–40 mL of lidocaine may be needed for anesthesia.

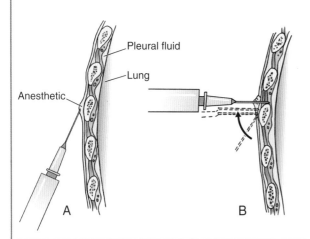

Figure 17.6 Insertion of a chest tube can be relatively painless with proper infiltration of the skin and pleura with local anesthetic. **A,** The anesthetic is first injected subcutaneously over the rib at the insertion site. **B,** The needle is then advanced slowly over the top of the rib while aspirating until air or fluid confirm the pleura is entered. The liberal use of buffered 1% lidocaine without epinephrine (maximal lidocaine dose, 5 mg/kg) is recommended. *(From Margolis AM, Kirsch TD: Roberts and Hedges' clinical procedures in emergency medicine and acute care, ed 7, Philadelphia, 2019, Elsevier.)*

*Level E: Multiple case reports, theory-based evidence from expert opinions, or peer-reviewed professional organizational standards without clinical studies to support recommendations.

Procedure	for Performing Pleural Chest Tube Placement—*Continued*		
Steps	Rationale	Special Considerations
10. An incision should be made, similar to the diameter of the tube being inserted, directly over the inferior aspect of the anesthetized rib below the insertion site (Fig. 17.7). **(Level E*)**	Allows for the diameter of the chest tube.[3,12]	When making the incision, incise down through the subcutaneous tissue; the space should be large enough to admit a finger.

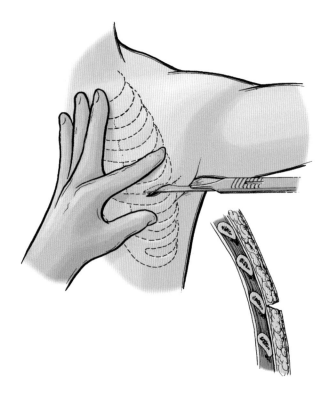

Figure 17.7 A transverse skin incision is made directly over the inferior aspect of the anesthetized rib down to the subcutaneous tissue. *(From Dumire SM, Paris PM:* Atlas of emergency procedures, *Philadelphia, 1994, Saunders.)*

11. Introduce the Kelly clamp through the incision, with the tips down, creating a tunnel through the subcutaneous tissue and muscle; use an opening and spreading maneuver; aim toward the superior aspect of the rib until the pleural space is reached (Fig. 17.8). **(Level E*)**	Facilitates insertion of the tube. Blunt dissection minimizes trauma to the neurovascular bundle.[3,12]	Additional lidocaine is infiltrated as needed. The direction of the tunnel created through the subcutaneous tissue and muscle determines the direction the chest tube takes after insertion. Be sure the clamp stays close to the ribs to avoid injury to the neurovascular bundle.
12. When the clamp is just over the superior portion of the rib, close the clamp and push it with steady pressure through the parietal pleura and into the pleural space, and then widen the hole in the pleural space by spreading the clamp (Fig. 17.9). **(Level E*)**	Ensures that the opening is large enough for the chest tube. Steady, even, controlled pressure provides control of the clamp once the pleura is perforated.[3,12]	This maneuver necessitates more pressure than might be anticipated. A lunging motion or use of the trocar, however, may cause a hole in the lung or injury to the liver or spleen.

*Level E: Multiple case reports, theory-based evidence from expert opinions, or peer-reviewed professional organizational standards without clinical studies to support recommendations.

Procedure continues on following page

Procedure	for Performing Pleural Chest Tube Placement—*Continued*	
Steps	Rationale	Special Considerations

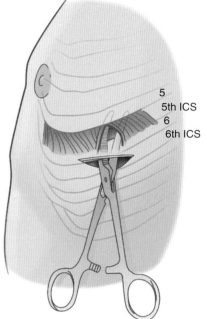

5
5th ICS
6
6th ICS

Figure 17.8   Blunt dissection is accomplished with forcing a closed clamp through the incision and using an opening-and-spreading maneuver to create a tunnel to the pleura. *ICS,* Intercostal space.

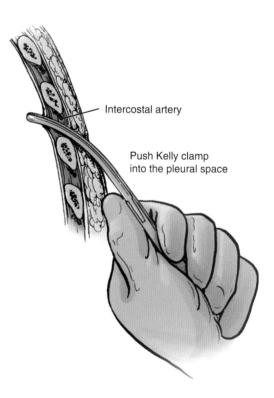

Intercostal artery

Push Kelly clamp
into the pleural space

Figure 17.9   Just over the superior portion of the rib, close the clamp and push with steady pressure into the pleura. *(From Dumire SM, Paris PM:* Atlas of emergency procedures, *Philadelphia, 1994, Saunders.)*

Procedure **for Performing Pleural Chest Tube Placement—*Continued***

Steps	Rationale	Special Considerations
13. Insert an index finger to dilate the tract and the hole in the pleura.	Relieves air or fluid accumulation when penetration of the space is made; ensures entry into the pleural space and not into a space inadvertently created between the parietal pleura and chest wall.[12]	Feel for lung tissue (the lung should expand and meet the finger on inspiration), diaphragm, or adhesions. Manually break up any clot, if found. If significant adhesions are unexpectedly encountered, abandon this site and select another one.
14. Insert the chest tube into the chest cavity with a curved Kelly clamp, holding the proximal end to guide the tip into the pleural space. Remove the clamp, and guide the tube in a rotating motion through the tract and into the space. The tube is advanced until the last hole is in the pleural space. Condensation of air or fluid in the tube should be noted.	The Kelly clamp provides stiffness to the chest tube, allowing for more control as it is inserted into the pleural space.	To drain air, aim the tube posteriorly and superiorly toward the apex of the lung; to drain fluid, aim the tube inferiorly and posteriorly. Do not allow any side holes of the tube to remain outside the thoracic cavity.
15. Connect the chest tube to the closed chest-drainage system (see Procedure 21, Closed Chest-Drainage System), and check for rise and fall (tidaling) of the H_2O column. An assistant applies the ordered amount of suction.	Ensures that the tube is properly positioned.	
16. Suture the tube to the chest wall. Wrap the free ends of the suture around the tube (similar to lacing a shoe). Tie the ends of the suture snugly around the top of the tube (Fig. 17.10).	Secures the position of the tube.[12] Sutures should be snug to prevent free air from passing into the subcutaneous tissue.	The type of stitch used depends on the preference of the provider; the goal is to prevent displacement of the chest tube.

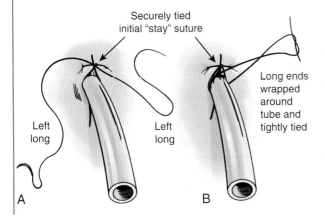

Figure 17.10 A "stay" suture is placed first next to the tube to close the skin incision. **A,** The knot is tied securely, and the ends, which subsequently are wrapped around the chest tube, are left long. **B,** The ends of the suture are wound twice around the tube, tightly enough to indent the tube slightly, and are tied securely. *(From Roberts JR, editor:* Roberts and Hedges' clinical procedures in emergency medicine, *ed 6, Philadelphia, 2014, Saunders.)*

UNIT 1

Patient Monitoring and Care —*Continued*

Steps	Rationale	Special Considerations
17. Apply an occlusive dressing. A. Dry slit drain sponges or 4 × 4 gauze pads are applied under and over top of the chest tube insertion site. **(Level B*)** B. Secure with a tape dressing. C. May consider a silicone foam dressing in place of a gauze and tape dressing. **(Level B*)**	Provides a cover for the wound, secures the dressing to the wound, and creates an airtight dressing.	Evidence supports the use of dry sterile dressings as an alternative to petroleum dressings due to a lower incidence of air leaks, wound infections, maceration of the skin around the chest tube, and loosening of sutures.[6,142] One study suggests that a silicone foam dressing may be used in place of gauze and tape dressings due to improved skin integrity and less pain at the insertion site and with dressing removal.[14]
18. Tape all connection points to the drainage system, or secure them with cable ties. **(Level E*)**	Creates an airtight system. Airtight connections prevent air leaks into the pleural space.[1,127]	Check that all tube drainage holes are in the pleural space.
19. Inferior to the dressing, secure the tube to the patient's skin with a commercial securing device or tape.	Functions as a strain relief to prevent tube and dressing dislodgment.	
20. Obtain a chest radiograph. **(Level E*)**	A chest radiograph confirms placement of the tube, expansion of the lung, and removal of fluid.[12]	Ensure that the distal drainage hole is within the pleural space. Document the result of the chest radiograph in the patient's record.
21. Dispose of equipment, and remove **PE**.		
22. **HH**		

*Level B: Well-designed, controlled studies with results that consistently support a specific action, intervention, or treatment.

*Level E: Multiple case reports, theory-based evidence from expert opinions, or peer-reviewed professional organizational standards without clinical studies to support recommendations.

Expected Outcomes

- Removal of air, fluid, or blood from the pleural space
- Relief of respiratory distress
- Reexpansion of the lung (validated with a chest radiograph)
- Restoration of negative pressure within the pleural space
- Successful delivery of solution or medication into the pleural space.

Unexpected Outcomes

- Hemorrhage or shock
- Increasing respiratory distress
- Infection
- Damage to the intercostal nerve that results in neuropathy or neuritis
- Incorrect tube placement
- Chest tube kinking, clogging, or dislodgment from the chest wall
- Subcutaneous emphysema
- Reexpansion pulmonary edema

Patient Monitoring and Care

Steps	Rationale	Reportable Conditions
		These conditions should be reported to the provider if they persist despite nursing interventions.
1. Assess cardiopulmonary and vital signs every 1–4 hours and as needed.	Provides baseline and ongoing assessment of the patient's condition. Abnormalities can indicate recurrence of the condition that necessitated chest tube insertion. Based on the patient's clinical condition or physician orders, vital signs may need to be checked more frequently.	• Tachypnea • Decreased or absent breath sounds • Hypoxemia • Tracheal deviation • Subcutaneous emphysema • Neck vein distention • Muffled heart tones • Tachycardia • Hypotension • Dysrhythmias • Fever
2. Monitor chest tube output every 1–4 hours, and record the amount and color.	Provides data for diagnosis. Higher drainage amounts require more frequent assessment. Based on the patient's clinical condition or physician orders, output may need to be checked more frequently.	• Bloody drainage greater than or equal to 200 mL/hour • Sudden cessation of drainage • Change in character of drainage
3. Assess for pain at the insertion site or for chest discomfort.	Pain interferes with adequate deep breathing. Pain at the insertion site, particularly with inspiration, may indicate improper tube placement.	• Continued pain despite pain interventions
4. Evaluate the chest drainage system for rise and fall (tidaling) and/or bubbling in the water-seal chamber. Check connections.[12] **(Level E*)**	The water level normally rises and falls with respiration until the lung is expanded. Bubbling immediately after insertion signifies that air is being removed from the pleural space; bubbling with exhalation and coughing is normal. Persistent bubbling indicates an air leak either in the patient's lung or in the chest drainage system.	• Absence of tidaling in the water-seal chamber • Persistent bubbling
5. Assess the insertion site and surrounding skin during dressing changes for impaired skin integrity, the presence of subcutaneous emphysema, or signs of infection or inflammation. **(Level B*)**	Skin integrity is altered during insertion, which can lead to infection. Research does not support daily dressing changes due to the increased risk of skin impairment, tube dislodgement, and reduced skin integrity.[14] Dressings should be changed if soiled, loose, and/or per institutional protocol.	• Fever • Redness around the insertion site • Purulent drainage • Subcutaneous emphysema

*Level B: Well-designed, controlled studies with results that consistently support a specific action, intervention, or treatment.
*Level E: Multiple case reports, theory-based evidence from expert opinions, or peer-reviewed professional organizational standards without clinical studies to support recommendations.

UNIT 1

Documentation

Documentation should include the following:
- Informed consent
- Patient and family education
- Reason for chest tube insertion
- Respiratory and vital sign assessment before, during, and after insertion
- Description of the procedure, including tube size, date and time of insertion, insertion site, and any complications associated with procedure
- Type and amount of drainage
- Presence of fluctuation and bubbling in the chest drainage system
- Amount of suction
- Patient's tolerance to the procedure
- Postinsertion chest radiograph results
- Unexpected outcomes
- Nursing interventions
- Pain assessment, interventions, and effectiveness

References and Additional Readings

For a complete list of references and additional readings for this procedure, scan this QR code with your smartphone, or visit https://www.elsevier.com/__data/assets/pdf_file/0005/1319792/Chapter0017.pdf

18 Chest Tube Placement (Assist)

Christine Slaughter

PURPOSE: Chest tubes are placed for the removal or drainage of air, blood, or fluid from the intrapleural space. They also are used to introduce sclerosing agents into the pleural space to prevent reaccumulation of fluid. The goals of placing a chest tube are to facilitate lung expansion and restore adequate gas exchange.[7]

PREREQUISITE NURSING KNOWLEDGE

- The thoracic cavity is a closed airspace in normal conditions. Any disruption results in the loss of negative pressure within the intrapleural space. Air or fluid that enters the space competes with the lung, resulting in collapse of the lung. Associated conditions are the result of disease, injury, surgery, or iatrogenic causes.
- Chest tubes are sterile flexible polyvinyl chloride (PVC) or silicone nonthrombogenic catheters approximately 20 inches (51 cm) long, varying in size from 8F to 40F. The size of the tube placed is determined by the indication and viscosity of the drainage.[9] The side of the chest tube usually has a radiopaque strip down the side to assist in visualization on chest radiographs.
- Indications for chest tube placement may include but are not limited to the following[10]:
  - ❖ Removal of an air collection in the pleural space:
    - ○ Pneumothorax
    - ○ Tension pneumothorax
    - ○ Hemopneumothorax
  - ❖ Removal of fluid collection or accumulation between the visceral and parietal pleura:
    - ○ Hemothorax
    - ○ Pleural effusion
    - ○ Chylothorax
    - ○ Empyema
  - ❖ Use as a conduit for the delivery of medication or fluid into the pleural space:
    - ○ Delivery of warmed fluid into the thoracic space as a method of internal warming of the core and circulating blood volume
    - ○ Instillation of anesthetic solutions, sclerosing agents, or fibrinolytic therapy
    - ○ Delivery of chemotherapeutic agents directly into the thoracic space
- Chest tubes inserted for traumatic hemopneumothorax or hemothorax (blood) should be large (36F to 40F). Medium tubes (24F to 36F) should be used for fluid accumulation (pleural effusions). Tubes inserted for pneumothorax (air) should be small (12F to 24F).[2,92]
- A pneumothorax may be classified as an *open, closed,* or *tension* pneumothorax.

- ❖ *Open pneumothorax:* The chest wall and the pleural space are penetrated, which allows air to enter the pleural space, as in a penetrating injury or trauma; a surgical incision in the thoracic cavity (i.e., thoracotomy); or a complication of surgical treatment (e.g., unintentional puncture during invasive procedures, such as thoracentesis or central venous catheter insertion).
- ❖ *Closed pneumothorax:* The pleural space is penetrated, but the chest wall is intact, which allows air to enter the pleural space from within the lung, as in spontaneous pneumothorax. A closed pneumothorax occurs without apparent injury and often is seen in individuals with chronic lung disorders (e.g., emphysema, cystic fibrosis, tuberculosis, necrotizing pneumonia) and in young, tall men who have a greater than normal height-to-width chest ratio; after blunt traumatic injury; or iatrogenically, occurring as a complication of medical treatment (e.g., intermittent positive-pressure breathing, mechanical ventilation with positive end-expiratory pressure, lung biopsy, bronchoscopy, central line insertion, pacemaker placement, lung biopsy, bronchoscopy, central line insertion, pacemaker placement).
- ❖ *Tension pneumothorax:* Air leaks into the pleural space through a tear in the lung and has no means to escape from the pleural cavity, creating a one-way valve effect. With each breath the patient takes, air accumulates and pressure within the pleural space increases, and the lung collapses. This condition causes the mediastinal structures (i.e., heart, great vessels, and trachea) to be compressed and shift to the opposite or unaffected side of the chest. Venous return and cardiac output are impeded, and collapse of the unaffected lung is possible. This life-threatening emergency requires prompt recognition and intervention.
- *Absolute contraindications:* Lung that is densely adherent to the chest wall throughout the hemithorax is an absolute contraindication to chest tube therapy.[8,105]
- *Relative contraindications:* Use of chest tubes in patients with multiple adhesions, giant blebs, or coagulopathies should be carefully considered; however, these relative contraindications are superseded by the need to reexpand the lung. When possible, any coagulopathy or platelet defect should be corrected before chest tube insertion. The differential diagnosis between a pneumothorax and bullous disease necessitates careful radiological assessment.[8]

- The tube size and insertion site selected for the chest tube are determined by the indication.[8,92] If draining air, the tube is placed near the apex of the lung (midclavicular second intercostal space); if draining fluid, the tube is placed near the base of the lung (midaxillary fifth or sixth intercostal space (Fig. 18.1).[7]
- Once the tube is in place, it should be sutured to the skin to prevent displacement, and an occlusive dressing should be applied. The chest tube also is connected to a chest-drainage system (see Procedure 21, Closed Chest-Drainage System) to remove air and fluid from the pleural space, which facilitates reexpansion of the collapsed lung. All connection points are secured with tape or zip ties (Parham-Martin bands) to ensure that the system remains air-tight.
- The water-seal chamber should bubble gently immediately on insertion of the chest tube and during expiration and with coughing. Continuous bubbling in this chamber indicates a leak within the patient or in the chest-drainage system. Fluctuations (tidaling) in the water level in the water-seal chamber of 5 to 10 cm, rising during inhalation and falling during expiration, should be observed with spontaneous respirations. If the patient is on mechanical ventilation, the pattern of fluctuation is just the opposite. Depending on the chest drainage system used, it may be necessary to disconnect suction temporarily to assess correctly for fluctuations in the water-seal chamber.[14]

EQUIPMENT

- Caps, masks, sterile gloves, gowns, drapes
- Protective eyewear (goggles)
- Antiseptic swab and/or solution: 2% chlorhexidine or povidone-iodine
- Local anesthetic: 1% or 2% lidocaine solution (with or without epinephrine)
  - 10-mL syringe with 20-gauge, 1½-inch needle
  - 5-mL syringe with 25-gauge, 1-inch needle

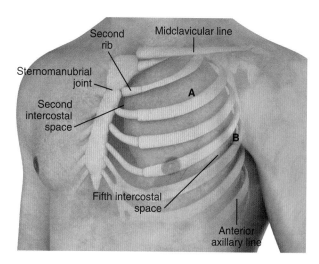

Figure 18.1 Entry sites for tube thoracostomy. The second intercostal space, the midclavicular line, is the preferred site for needle aspiration or catheter insertion (**A**). The fourth or fifth intercostal space, the midaxillary line, is the preferred site for a chest tube (**B**). (*From Margolis AM et al:* Roberts and Hedges' clinical procedures in emergency medicine and acute care, *ed 7, Philadelphia, 2019, Elsevier, pp 196–220.*)

- Tube thoracostomy tray
  - Sterile towels, 4 × 4 sterile gauze
  - Scalpel with No. 10 or 11 blade
  - Two Kelly clamps
  - Needle holder
  - Monofilament or silk suture material (No. 0 or 1-0)
  - Sterile basin or medicine cup
  - Suture scissors
  - Two hemostats
- Thoracotomy tubes (8F to 40F, as appropriate)
- Closed chest-drainage system
- Suction source
- Suction connector and connecting tubing (usually 6 feet for each tube)
- 1-inch adhesive tape or zip ties (Parham-Martin bands)
- Occlusive dressing materials
  - 4 × 4 gauze pads or slit drain sponges
  - Tape or a commercial securing device
- Additional equipment, to have available as needed, includes the following:
  - Ultrasound machine, ultrasound gel, and sterile probe cover

PATIENT AND FAMILY EDUCATION

- Assess the patient's and family's level of understanding about the condition and reason for the procedure if the clinical situation permits. ***Rationale:*** This assessment identifies the patient's and family's knowledge deficits concerning the patient's condition, the procedure, the expected benefits, and the potential risks. It also allows time for questions to clarify information and voice concerns. Explanations decrease patient anxiety and enhance cooperation.
- Explain the procedure if the clinical situation permits. If not, explain the procedure and reason for the chest tube insertion after it is completed. ***Rationale:*** This explanation enhances patient and family understanding and decreases anxiety.
- Explain that the patient's participation during the procedure is to remain as immobile as possible and to do relaxed breathing. ***Rationale:*** This explanation facilitates insertion of the chest tube and prevents complications during insertion.
- After the procedure, instruct the patient to sit in the semi-Fowler's position (unless contraindicated). ***Rationale:*** This position facilitates drainage, if present, from the pleural space by allowing air to rise and fluid to settle to be removed via the chest tube. This position also makes breathing easier.
- Instruct the patient to turn and change position every 2 hours. The patient may lie on the side with the chest tube but should keep the tubing free from kinks. ***Rationale:*** Turning and changing position prevent complications related to immobility and retained pulmonary secretions. Keeping the tube free from kinks maintains patency of the tube, facilitates drainage, and prevents the accumulation of pressure within the pleural space that interferes with lung reexpansion.
- Instruct the patient to cough and deep breathe, with splinting of the affected side. ***Rationale:*** Coughing and deep

breathing increase pressure within the pleural space, facilitating drainage, promoting lung reexpansion, and preventing respiratory complications associated with retained secretions. The application of firm pressure over the chest tube insertion site (i.e., splinting) may decrease pain and discomfort.

- Encourage active or passive range-of-motion exercises of the arm on the affected side. ***Rationale:*** The patient may limit movement of the arm on the affected side to decrease the discomfort at the insertion site, which may result in joint discomfort and potential joint contractures.
- Instruct the patient and family about activity as prescribed while maintaining the drainage system below the level of the chest. ***Rationale:*** This activity facilitates gravity drainage and prevents backflow and potential infectious contamination into the pleural space.
- Instruct the patient about the availability of prescribed analgesic medication and other pain-relief strategies. ***Rationale:*** Pain relief ensures comfort and facilitates coughing, deep breathing, positioning, range of motion, and recuperation.

PATIENT ASSESSMENT AND PREPARATION

Patient Assessment

- Assess for significant medical history or injury, including chronic lung disease, spontaneous pneumothorax, hemothorax, pulmonary disease, therapeutic procedures, lung surgery, and mechanism of injury. ***Rationale:*** Medical history or injury may provide the etiological basis for the occurrence of pneumothorax, empyema, pleural effusion, or chylothorax.
- Evaluate diagnostic test results (if the patient's condition does not necessitate immediate intervention), including chest radiograph, coagulation tests, and arterial blood gases. ***Rationale:*** Diagnostic testing confirms the presence of air or fluid in the pleural space, a collapsed lung, hypoxemia, and respiratory compromise.
- Assess baseline cardiopulmonary status for the following signs and symptoms that necessitate chest tube insertion.[5] ***Rationale:*** Accurate assessment of signs and symptoms allows for prompt recognition and treatment. Baseline assessment provides comparison data for evaluation of changes and outcomes of treatment.
  - ❖ Tachypnea
  - ❖ Decreased or absent breath sounds on affected side
  - ❖ Crackles adjacent to the affected area
  - ❖ Shortness of breath, dyspnea
  - ❖ Asymmetrical chest excursion with respirations
  - ❖ Cyanosis
  - ❖ Decreased oxygen saturation
  - ❖ Hyperresonance on the affected side (pneumothorax)
  - ❖ Subcutaneous emphysema (pneumothorax)
  - ❖ Dullness or flatness on the affected side (hemothorax, pleural effusion, empyema, chylothorax)
  - ❖ Sudden, sharp chest pain
  - ❖ Anxiety, restlessness, apprehension

- ❖ Tachycardia
- ❖ Hypotension
- ❖ Dysrhythmias
- ❖ Tracheal deviation to the unaffected side (tension pneumothorax)
- ❖ Neck vein distention (tension pneumothorax)
- ❖ Muffled heart sounds (tension pneumothorax)

Patient Preparation

- Verify the correct patient with two identifiers. ***Rationale:*** Before performing a procedure, the nurse should ensure the correct identification of the patient for the intended intervention.
- Ensure that the patient understands preprocedural teachings. Answer questions, and reinforce information as needed. ***Rationale:*** This communication evaluates and reinforces understanding of previously taught information.
- Obtain consent if circumstances allow. ***Rationale:*** Invasive procedures, unless performed with implied consent in a life-threatening situation, require written consent of the patient or significant other.
- Ensure that patient has a patent intravenous access. ***Rationale:*** This access provides a route for analgesics, sedation, and emergency medications.
- Consult with the practitioner for the appropriate-sized chest tube to be inserted. ***Rationale:*** Evacuation of air necessitates a smaller tube; evacuation of fluid necessitates a larger tube.
- If the patient has a pneumothorax, assist the patient to the lateral supine position; for a hemothorax, assist the patient to the semi-Fowler's position.[2,7,12] ***Rationale:*** This positioning enhances accessibility to the insertion site for positioning of the chest tube (Fig. 18.2).

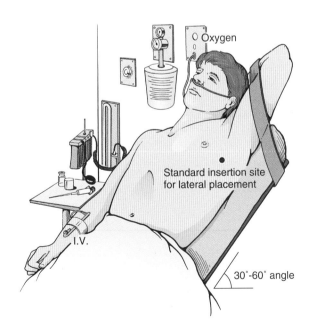

Figure 18.2 To insert a chest tube, position the patient semi-erect with the ipsilateral arm abducted as far as possible and preferably restrained. *(From Margolis AM et al: Roberts and Hedges' clinical procedures in emergency medicine and acute care, ed 7, Philadelphia, 2019, Elsevier, pp 196–220.)*

- Administer prescribed analgesics or sedatives as needed; follow institutional policy for procedural sedation. ***Rationale:*** Analgesics and sedatives reduce the discomfort and anxiety experienced and facilitate patient cooperation.

- Administer supplemental oxygen as needed. Monitor pulse oximeter or end-tidal carbon dioxide level. ***Rationale:*** Real-time assessment of the patient's respiratory status during the procedure is provided.

Procedure for Assisting With Pleural Chest Tube Placement

Steps	Rationale	Special Considerations
1. HH		
2. PE		
3. Open the chest tube insertion tray using sterile technique.	Reduces transmission of microorganisms.	
4. Assist with preparation of the equipment. A. Check that all equipment is present. B. Pour antiseptic solution into a basin or medicine cup with aseptic technique, or open the antiseptic swab packet and stand by. C. Open the chest tube package, and empty it onto the open sterile tray. D. Assist to prepare a syringe with lidocaine.	Facilitates insertion of the tube.	Ensure that the chest drainage system is also set up and ready for connection (see Procedure 21, Closed Chest-Drainage System).
5. Assist the physician or advanced practice nurse with preparation of the insertion site.	Assists in preparation of the area for insertion and proper tube placement.[12]	The insertion site for air removal is the midclavicular second intercostal space on the affected side. The insertion site for fluid removal is the fifth or sixth intercostal space, midaxillary line. The incision site is one rib below the insertion site (see Fig. 18.1).
6. Perform a preprocedural verification and time out, if nonemergent.	Ensures patient safety.	
7. After tube insertion, connect the chest tube to the closed chest-drainage system, and check for rise and fall (tidaling) of the H_2O column. Apply the ordered amount of suction.	Ensures that the tube is properly positioned.[4]	
8. Assist with suturing of the tube to the chest wall.	Secures the position of the tube.[5] Sutures should be snug to prevent free air from passing into the subcutaneous tissue.	The type of stitch used depends on the individual; the goal is to prevent displacement of the chest tube.
9. Apply an occlusive dressing. A. May use a slit drain sponge or 4 × 4 gauze under and over the top of the chest tube insertion site.[6,11,13] B. Secure with tape dressing. **(Level B*)**	Provides cover for the wound with the least damage to the surrounding skin.	Evidence does not support the use of petroleum gauze at the chest tube insertion site because of maceration of the skin around the chest tube and loosening of sutures.[6,13]

*Level B: Well-designed, controlled studies with results that consistently support a specific action, intervention, or treatment.

Procedure	for Assisting With Pleural Chest Tube Placement—*Continued*	
Steps	**Rationale**	**Special Considerations**
10. Tape all connection points to the drainage system, or secure with zip ties (Parham-Martin bands). **(Level E*)**	Creates an airtight system. Airtight connections prevent air leaks into the pleural space.[1,5]	Check that all tube drainage holes are in the pleural space.
11. Secure the tube below the dressing to the patient's skin with a commercial securing device or tape.	Functions as a strain relief to prevent tube and dressing dislodgement.	
12. Confirm tube placement with chest radiography. **(Level E*)**	A chest radiograph confirms tube placement, lung expansion, and fluid removal.[12]	Ensure that the distal drainage hole is within the pleural space. Document the result of the chest radiograph in the patient's record.
13. Dispose of used supplies, and remove PE		
14. HH		

*Level E: Multiple case reports, theory-based evidence from expert opinions, or peer-reviewed professional organizational standards without clinical studies to support recommendations.

Expected Outcomes

- Removal of air, fluid, or blood from the pleural space
- Relief of respiratory distress
- Reexpansion of the lung (validated with a chest radiograph)
- Restoration of negative pressure within the pleural space
- Successful delivery of solution or medication into the pleural space

Unexpected Outcomes

- Hemorrhage or shock
- Increasing respiratory distress
- Infection
- Damage to intercostal nerve that results in neuropathy or neuritis
- Incorrect tube placement
- Chest tube kinking, clogging, or dislodgment from chest wall
- Subcutaneous emphysema
- Reexpansion pulmonary edema

Patient Monitoring and Care

Steps	Rationale	Reportable Conditions
		These conditions should be reported to the provider if they persist despite nursing interventions.
1. Assess cardiopulmonary and vital signs every 1–4 hours and as needed.	Provides baseline and ongoing assessment of the patient's condition. Abnormalities can indicate recurrence of the condition that necessitated chest tube insertion. Based on the patient's clinical condition or physician orders, vital signs may need to be checked more frequently.	Tachypnea Decreased or absent breath sounds Hypoxemia Tracheal deviation Subcutaneous emphysema Neck vein distention Muffled heart sounds Tachycardia Hypotension Dysrhythmias Fever

Procedure continues on following page

Patient Monitoring and Care —*Continued*

Steps	Rationale	Reportable Conditions
2. Monitor chest tube output every 1–4 hours, and record the amount and color.	Provides data for diagnosis. Higher drainage amounts require more frequent assessment. Based on the patient's clinical condition or physician orders, output may need to be checked more frequently. Rapid removal of large amounts of fluid from the pleural space (>800 mL) may result in reexpansion pulmonary edema.[3,71]	Bloody drainage greater than or equal to 100 mL/hour Sudden cessation of drainage Change in character of drainage Sudden onset of coughing or worsening oxygenation (could indicate reexpansion pulmonary edema[7])
3. Assess for pain at the insertion site or for chest discomfort.	Pain interferes with adequate deep breathing. Pain at the insertion site, particularly with inspiration, may indicate improper tube placement.	Continued pain despite pain interventions If using opioids for analgesia, monitor for opioid-induced respiratory depression.[7]
4. Evaluate the chest-drainage system for rise and fall (tidaling) or bubbling in water-seal chamber. Check connections.	The water level normally rises and falls with respiration until the lung is expanded. Bubbling immediately after insertion signifies that air is being removed from the pleural space; bubbling with exhalation and coughing is normal. Persistent bubbling indicates an air leak either in the patient's lung or in the chest-drainage system.[3,49]	Absence of tidaling in water-seal chamber Persistent bubbling
5. Assess the insertion site and surrounding skin during dressing changes for presence of subcutaneous emphysema and signs of infection or inflammation.	Skin integrity is altered during insertion, which can lead to infection.[4,6,139] Studies do not support daily dressing changes because of the increased risk of skin impairment, tube dislodgement, and reduced skin integrity.[12]	Fever Redness around insertion site Purulent drainage Subcutaneous emphysema

Documentation

Documentation should include the following:
- Patient and family education
- Reason for chest tube insertion
- Respiratory and vital sign assessment before and after insertion
- Description of procedure, including tube size, date and time of insertion, insertion site, and any complications associated with the procedure
- Type and amount of drainage
- Presence of tidaling and bubbling
- Amount of suction
- Patient's tolerance of procedure
- Postinsertion chest radiograph results
- Unexpected outcomes
- Nursing interventions
- Pain assessment, interventions, and effectiveness

References and Additional Readings

For a complete list of references and additional readings for this procedure, scan this QR code with your smartphone, or visit https://www.elsevier.com/__data/assets/pdf_file/0006/1319793/Chapter0018.pdf

PROCEDURE

19 Chest Tube Removal (Perform)

Julie M. Waters

PURPOSE: Chest tube removal is performed to discontinue a chest tube when it is no longer needed for the removal or drainage of air, blood, or fluid from the intrapleural or mediastinal space.

PREREQUISITE NURSING KNOWLEDGE

- Chest tubes are placed in the pleural or mediastinal space to evacuate an abnormal collection of air, fluid, or both.
- For interpleural chest tubes, the air leak detector should bubble gently immediately on insertion of the chest tube during expiration and with coughing. Continuous bubbling in the air leak detector indicates a leak in the patient or the chest-drainage system. Fluctuations in the water level (also known as *tidaling*) in the water-seal chamber of 5 to 10 cm, rising during inhalation and falling during expiration, should be observed with spontaneous respirations. If the patient is on positive pressure mechanical ventilation, the pattern of fluctuation is just the opposite, with a rise during exhalation and a fall during inspiration. Any suction applied must be disconnected temporarily to assess correctly for fluctuations in the water-seal chamber.
- Flexible Silastic (Blake; Ethicon, Inc., Somerville, NJ) drains may be used in place of large-bore chest tubes in the mediastinal and pleural spaces after cardiac surgery. These tubes provide more efficient drainage and improved patient mobility with minimized tissue trauma and pain with removal.
- Chest radiographs are done periodically to determine whether the lung has reexpanded. Daily chest radiographs have been found not to be necessary while the tube is in place.[5] Reexpanded lungs, along with respiratory assessments that show improvement in the patient's respiratory status, are the basis for the decision to remove the chest tube.
- While the tubes are in place, patients may have related discomfort. Prompt removal of chest tubes encourages patients to increase ambulation and respiratory measures to improve lung expansion after surgery (e.g., coughing, deep breathing). However, removal of the chest tube may also be a painful procedure for the patient.[1,6]

AP This procedure should be performed only by clinicians who have demonstrated competence and are credentialed to perform it. In addition, the procedure must be within the scope of practice defined by their professional licensure, and in accordance with professional practice acts. Physicians, advanced practice nurses, and physician assistants may be credentialed to perform this procedure.

- The types of sutures used to secure chest tubes vary according to the preference of the physician, the physician assistant, or the advanced practice nurse. One common type is the horizontal mattress or purse-string suture, which is threaded around and through the wound edges in a U shape with the ends left unknotted until the chest tube is removed. Usually one or two anchor stitches accompany the purse-string suture (Fig. 19.1).
- A primary goal of chest tube removal is removal of tubes without introduction of air or contaminants into the pleural space.
- Available data indicate there is no consensus as to the rate of drainage that should be used as a threshold for tube removal and no evidence to suggest that it is unsafe to remove tubes that still have a relatively high rate of fluid drainage. Research has shown that, depending on the reason for the chest tube, volumes of 200 to 450 mL/day do not adversely affect length of stay or overall costs compared with lower threshold volumes, nor does the risk of pleural fluid reaccumulation increase.[4,8] However, some suggested guidelines include the following:
  - Drainage less than 200 to 400 mL over a 24-hour period. The presence of blood, purulent fluid, or chylous fluid are contraindications for chest tube removal.[4,7,9,11]
  - Another method, considering patient size for thoracic surgery patients, suggests chest drains can be removed when the 24-hour fluid output is ≤20% of whole-body lymphatic flow (i.e., about five times the patient's weight in kilograms).[5]
  - Chest tubes placed after cardiac surgery can be removed when drainage is less than 100 mL over the past 12 hours, no air leak is present, and no significant effusion is noted on chest x-ray. They are typically removed 24 to 48 hours after surgery.[2,5]
  - Lungs are reexpanded (as shown on chest radiographic results).
  - Respiratory status has improved (i.e., nonlabored respirations, equal bilateral breath sounds, absence of shortness of breath, decreased use of accessory muscles, symmetrical respiratory excursion, and respiratory rate less than 24 breaths/min).
  - For interpleural chest tubes, air leaks have resolved for at least 24 hours (the absence of continuous bubbling in the water-seal chamber or absence of air bubbles from right to left in the air leak detector), and the lung is fully reinflated on chest radiographic results.[11]

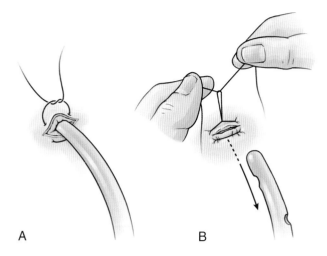

Figure 19.1 Purse-string suture. Removing the chest tube. **A,** First throw of a knot in the mattress suture. **B,** Removal of the chest tube and tying of the purse-string suture. *(From Leonar S, Nikaidoh H: Thoracentesis and chest tube insertion. In: Levin D, Morriss F, editors.* Essentials of Pediatric Intensive Care, *St Louis, 1990, Quality Medical Publishing.)*

❖ For chest tubes that have been placed for pneumothorax, the practice of clamping the tube for 4 to 6 hours to ensure that the air leak has resolved is controversial but still supported by some. This practice should only be performed with a provider's order. Clinically monitor the patient, and unclamp immediately if there are any signs of hemodynamic or respiratory distress. Consider obtaining a chest x-ray before removal.[4,7,11,12]

❖ Variable opinions exist regarding the removal of chest tubes for patients who are receiving mechanical ventilation. Some providers leave them in as long as the patient is on mechanical ventilation, while others maintain that removal should occur despite mechanical ventilation because of the risk of complications and continued pain, as soon as criteria for removal are met.[7,11]

EQUIPMENT

- Suture-removal set
- Antiseptic swabs (e.g., povidone-iodine, chlorhexidine gluconate)
- Plain or petrolatum gauze, as per hospital protocol
- Wide occlusive tape (2 inches)
- Elastic closure device, such as Steri-Strips (3M, St. Paul, MN)
- Dry 4 × 4 gauze sponges (two to four)
- Waterproof pad
- Personal protective equipment (goggles, sterile and non-sterile gloves, mask, gown)
  Additional equipment to have available as needed includes the following:
- Rubber-tipped Kelly clamps or disposable umbilical clamps
- Sterile scissors

PATIENT AND FAMILY EDUCATION

- Assess the patient's and family's level of understanding about the condition and rationale for the procedure. *Rationale:* This assessment identifies the patient's and family's knowledge deficits concerning the patient's condition, the procedure, the expected benefits, and the potential risks. It also allows time for questions to clarify information and voice concerns. Explanations decrease patient anxiety and enhance cooperation.
- Explain the procedure, reason for removal, and sensations to be expected. The most commonly reported sensations are pulling, pain or hurting, and burning.[1,6] *Rationale:* This explanation decreases patient anxiety and enhances cooperation.
- Explain the patient's role in assisting with removal. Explain that the patient should perform the Valsalva maneuver on the count of three. Have the patient practice the maneuver before the procedure. *Rationale:* This explanation elicits patient cooperation and facilitates removal, decreasing the risk of air entering the pleural space upon removal.
- Instruct the patient to turn and reposition every 2 hours after the chest tube has been removed. *Rationale:* This action prevents complications related to immobility and retained secretions.
- Instruct the patient to cough and breathe deeply after the chest tube has been removed, with splinting of the affected side or sternum (with mediastinal tubes). *Rationale:* This action prevents respiratory complications associated with retained secretions. The application of firm pressure over the insertion site (i.e., splinting) decreases pain and discomfort associated with coughing.
- Educate the patient about the availability of prescribed analgesic medication after the chest tube is removed. *Rationale:* Analgesics alleviate pain and facilitate coughing, deep breathing, and repositioning.[13]
- Instruct the patient and family to immediately report signs and symptoms of respiratory distress and/or infection. *Rationale:* Immediate reporting facilitates prompt intervention to treat a recurrent pneumothorax, accumulation of blood or fluid, or infection.

PATIENT ASSESSMENT AND PREPARATION

Patient Assessment

- Assess the patient's mental status and ability to follow directions. *Rationale:* Assessment verifies the patient's ability to cooperate with instructions during the procedure.
- Assess respiratory status. *Rationale:* Assessment of respiratory status verifies the patient's readiness for chest tube removal.
  ❖ Oxygen saturation within normal limits
  ❖ Nonlabored respirations
  ❖ Absence of shortness of breath
  ❖ Decreased use of accessory muscles
  ❖ Respiratory rate of less than 24 breaths/min
  ❖ Equal bilateral breath sounds

• Assess chest tube drainage amount and type.[9] **Rationale:** Assessment of drainage verifies patient readiness for chest tube removal. Thresholds are individualized depending on patient size, the indication for insertion, and provider discretion.

• For interpleural chest tubes, assess for minimal or no air leak in the air leak detector zone or indicator. **Rationale:** This assessment indicates whether the lung is reexpanded and whether an air leak is present.

• Evaluate chest radiographic results. **Rationale:** Lung reexpansion indicates that the need for a chest tube is resolved.

• Assess vital signs and (optional) arterial blood gases. **Rationale:** Vital sign assessment indicates whether the patient can tolerate chest tube removal.

• Assess laboratory results for clotting capability and medications that may affect clotting. **Rationale:** Thrombocytopenia, coagulopathy, or thrombolytic medications may precipitate excessive bleeding.

• Review the patient's medical record for allergies or sensitivity to antiseptics. **Rationale:** Patient allergies may require use of an alternative type of antiseptic of swab during the procedure.

Patient Preparation

• Verify the correct patient with two identifiers. **Rationale:** Before performing a procedure, the nurse should ensure the correct identification of the patient for the intended intervention.

• Ensure that the patient understands preprocedural teachings. Answer questions as they arise, and reinforce information as needed. **Rationale:** This communication evaluates and reinforces understanding of previously taught information. Anticipatory preparation may prepare patients for a better experience.

• Administer premedication of adequate analgesics at least 20 minutes before the procedure if indicated. Alternatively, subfascial lidocaine may be injected into the chest tube tract. In addition to opioids, adjunct methods shown to decrease pain during chest tube removal include slow deep-breathing relaxation exercises and application of cold packs.[10] **Rationale:** Intravenous 4-mg morphine 20 minutes before or 30-mg ketorolac 60 minutes before the procedure has been shown to provide substantial pain relief without excessive analgesia.[13] Pain medication, relaxation exercises, and application of cold reduces the discomfort and anxiety experienced, which facilitates patient cooperation.[1,6]

• Time the removal procedure to occur at peak analgesic effect. **Rationale:** This timing increases patient cooperation and decreases anxiety.[13]

• Place the patient in the semi-Fowler's position. Alternatively, place the patient on the unaffected side with the waterproof pad underneath the site. **Rationale:** This position enhances accessibility to the insertion site of the chest tube and protects the bed from drainage.

Procedure for Performing Chest Tube Removal

Steps	Rationale	Special Considerations
1. **HH**		
2. **PE**		
3. Open the sterile suture removal set, and prepare petrolatum or plain gauze dressing and two to four 4 × 4 gauze sponges, as per hospital protocol.	Aseptic technique is maintained to prevent contamination of the wound.	
4. Perform a preprocedure verification before chest tube removal.	Ensures patient safety.	If not removing all of the chest tubes at this time, ensure that they are correctly identified. Consider labeling in the presence of the ordering provider.
5. Discontinue suction from the chest-drainage system, and check for air leak in the air leak detector zone or indicator. Observe the air leak detector zone or indicator while the patient coughs.	Bubbling in the air leak detector is associated with an air leak. When an air leak is present, removal of the chest tube may cause development of a pneumothorax. Ensures that a recurrent pneumothorax has not occurred.	If an air leak is present, the tube should not be removed. Consult with the physician, physician assistant, or advanced practice nurse to determine the appropriate action.

Procedure continues on following page

Procedure for Performing Chest Tube Removal—*Continued*

Steps	Rationale	Special Considerations
6. Remove the existing dressing, and cleanse the area around the tubes with an antiseptic solution or swab. Determine the type of suture that secures each chest tube. Clip appropriately. If a purse-string suture is present, leave the long suture ends intact. (**Level D***)	Allows access to the chest tube at the skin level and prepares the sutures for removal.	Antiseptic swabs remove a broad spectrum of microbes quickly and provide high-level antimicrobial action for up to 6 hours after use.
7. Confirm that the tube is free from the suture and the tape.	Allows ease of removal and avoids tearing the skin.	
8. Hold the preferred gauze dressing with the nondominant hand near the chest tube insertion site.	Some institutions utilize petroleum gauze dressings for pleural insertion sites and 4 × 4 gauze pads for mediastinal insertions sites. Follow hospital policy.	Petroleum gauze on the chest tube site has not been demonstrated to decrease the risk of post-pull pneumothorax and also poses the theoretical risk of delayed wound healing.[7]
9. Instruct the patient to perform the Valsalva maneuver at either end inspiration or end expiration.[5,7] (**Level E***) Ask the patient to practice the planned technique.	The Valsalva maneuver is needed to provide positive pressure in the pleural cavity and decrease the incidence of an involuntary gasp by the patient when the tube is removed.[5,7]	An involuntary inhalation during chest tube removal may put the patient at risk for air entering the chest cavity.
A. End inspiration: Instruct the patient to take a deep breath and hold it while performing the Valsalva maneuver for each tube removed. If the patient is receiving ventilator support and is unable to follow instructions, remove the tube during peak inspiration.		Debate exists regarding the optimal timing of chest tube removal. As no method has shown to be superior, choose a consistent method when removing the tube.[3]
B. End expiration: Instruct the patient to forcibly exhale and perform the Valsalva maneuver at end expiration.		
C. If possible, patients may need to hold their breath until sutures are tied.	Avoids the influx of air.	
10. With the dominant hand, remove chest tubes rapidly, smoothly, and individually while the patient is performing the Valsalva maneuver or during peak inspiration if the patient is on a mechanical ventilator. Place the tube on the fluid-impermeable pad.	Prevents accidental entrance of air into the pleural space. Removal of pleural chest tubes should be accomplished rapidly with the simultaneous application of an occlusive dressing or closure with purse-string sutures to decrease the possibility of air from entering the pleural space.	*Some resistance is expected; however, if strong resistance is encountered and rapid removal of the tube is not possible, discontinue the procedure, and consult with the physician, physician's assistant, or advanced practice nurse immediately.* Resistance may indicate that the tube was inadvertently sutured during surgery or sternal closure.

*Level D: Peer-reviewed professional and organizational standards with the support of clinical study recommendations.

*Level E: Multiple case reports, theory-based evidence from expert opinions, or peer-reviewed professional organizational standards without clinical studies to support recommendations.

Procedure for Performing Chest Tube Removal—*Continued*

A. Hold sutures in the hand closer to the head of the patient, and apply mild pressure over the exit site with a folded 4 × 4 gauze pad.	Avoids influx of air.	
B. If the tube was "Y" connected to another tube, clamp the tube, and cut below the clamp to allow for easier manipulation when removing the remaining chest tubes.		Reconnect the other tube to the chest drainage system if it is not scheduled for removal at the same time.
11. If a purse-string suture is present, tie it off with a square knot (see Fig. 19,1). If no purse-string suture was used, the site may be closed with adhesive skin-closure strips.	Creates a firm closure of the chest tube site.	*Avoid pulling the suture too tight to prevent tissue necrosis at the site and to facilitate easier removal later.*
12. Secure the dressing with tape per hospital protocol.	Creates a firm closure of the chest tube site.	This action is easier with a second person to place the tape while holding pressure over the site.
13. Examine each chest tube to verify that the entire tube has been removed.	If portion of tube is not removed, surgical removal is necessary to remove it.	Consult with the physician, physician assistant, or advanced practice nurse immediately if a portion of the tube remains in the patient.
14. Assess the patient's condition after the procedure, and compare the results with the preprocedure assessment, as described previously.	Ensures stable respiratory status after the procedure.	Observe for warning signs of increased work of breathing, decreased oxygen saturation, increased restlessness, symptoms of chest discomfort, and diminished breath sounds on the affected side.
15. Obtain a chest radiograph (generally 1–4 hours after removal) only as clinically indicated.[14] (**Level B***)	Assesses that the lung has remained expanded.	Low incidence of complications. Recommended to perform a chest radiograph only if the patient is clinically deteriorating.[14]
16. Dispose of used supplies and equipment, and remove **PE**		
17. **HH**		

*Level B: Well-designed, controlled studies with results that consistently support a specific action, intervention, or treatment

Expected Outcomes
- Patient is comfortable and has no respiratory distress
- Lung remains expanded after chest tube removal
- Site remains free from bleeding, hematoma, or infection
- Patient is comfortable and has no respiratory distress

Unexpected Outcomes
- Pneumothorax
- Bleeding
- Skin necrosis
- Retained chest tube
- Infected chest tube insertion site

UNIT I

Patient Monitoring and Care

Steps	Rationale	Reportable Conditions
		These conditions should be reported to the provider if they persist despite nursing interventions.
1. Assess respiratory status, including oxygen saturation, work of breathing, breath sounds, and symptoms of chest discomfort. Obtain a chest radiograph if significant changes are found.	Diminished respiratory status could indicate a pneumothorax. Pneumothorax could be caused by removal of the chest tube before all of the air, fluid, or blood in the pleural space is drained, or it may recur after chest tube removal if air is introduced accidently into the pleural space through the chest tube tract.	• Decreased oxygen saturation on pulse oximetry • Increased work of breathing • Diminished breath sounds on the affected side • Increased restlessness and symptoms of chest discomfort • Persistent bleeding
2. Monitor the insertion site for bleeding. If bleeding is found, apply pressure, and place a tight occlusive dressing over the site, which may be removed after 48 hours.	Persistent bleeding from the insertion site could mean the chest tube was against a vein or a chest wall artery before removal.	
3. Monitor the suture site for signs of skin necrosis.	If the purse-string suture was pulled too tightly closed when the chest tube was removed, skin necrosis may be seen.	• Dark or inflamed skin with visible necrotic areas
4. Monitor the site for signs of infection.	Prolonged insertion of a chest tube increases the risk that the tract created by the chest tube may become infected, or infection may occur after removal of the chest tube if the opening created by the removal becomes contaminated.	• Purulent drainage • Increased body temperature • Inflammation • Tenderness • Warmth at site
5. Monitor the insertion area for development of subcutaneous emphysema.	Air may leak into the surrounding tissues and cause crepitus.	• Crepitus
6. Monitor for signs and symptoms of pericardial effusion or cardiac tamponade.	Removal of mediastinal chest tubes may cause increased bleeding into the pericardium. Pericardial bleeding may continue after chest tubes are removed.	• Distant heart tones • Decreased blood pressure, tachycardia • Pulsus paradoxus • Narrowed pulse pressure • Equalized pulmonary artery pressures
7. Follow institutional standards for assessing pain. Administer analgesia as prescribed.	Identifies the need for pain interventions.	• Continued pain despite pain interventions

Documentation

Documentation should include the following:
• Patient and family education
• Respiratory and vital signs assessments before and after the procedure
• Date and time of the procedure and who performed the procedure
• Amount, color, and consistency of any drainage
• Application of a sterile occlusive dressing
• Type of suture in place and what was done to it (cut and removed or tied)
• Patient's tolerance of the procedure
• Completion and results of the chest radiograph (if applicable)
• Specimens sent to the laboratory (if applicable)
• Unexpected outcomes
• Nursing interventions
• Pain assessment, interventions, and effectiveness

References and Additional Readings

For a complete list of references and additional readings for this procedure, scan this QR code with your smartphone, or visit https://www.elsevier.com/__data/assets/pdf_file/0007/1319794/Chapter0019.pdf

20 Chest Tube Removal (Assist)

Julie M. Waters

PURPOSE: Chest tube removal is performed to discontinue a chest tube when it is no longer needed for the removal or drainage of air, blood, or fluid from the intrapleural or mediastinal space.

PREREQUISITE NURSING KNOWLEDGE

- Chest tubes are placed in the pleural or mediastinal space to evacuate an abnormal collection of air, fluid, or both.
- For interpleural chest tubes, the air leak detector should bubble gently immediately on insertion of the chest tube during expiration and with coughing. Continuous bubbling in the air leak detector indicates a leak in the patient (from the lung to the pleural space) or the chest-drainage system. Fluctuations in the water level (also known as *tidaling*) in the water-seal chamber of 5 to 10 cm, rising during inhalation and falling during expiration, should be observed with spontaneous respirations. If the patient is on positive pressure mechanical ventilation, the pattern of fluctuation is just the opposite, with a rise during exhalation and a fall during inspiration. Any suction applied must be disconnected temporarily to assess correctly for fluctuations in the water-seal chamber.
- Flexible Silastic (Blake; Ethicon, Inc, Somerville, NJ) drains may be used in place of large-bore chest tubes in the mediastinal and pleural spaces after cardiac surgery. These tubes provide more efficient drainage and improved patient mobility with minimized tissue trauma and pain with removal.
- Chest radiographs are done periodically to determine whether the lung has reexpanded. Daily chest radiographs have been found to be unnecessary while the tube is in place.[5] Reexpanded lungs, along with respiratory assessments that show improvement in the patient's respiratory status as well as decreased drainage, are the basis for the decision to remove the chest tube.
- While the tubes are in place, patients may have related discomfort. Prompt removal of chest tubes encourages patients to increase ambulation and respiratory measures to improve lung expansion after surgery (e.g., coughing, deep breathing). However, removal of the chest tube may also be a painful procedure for the patient.[1,6]
- The types of sutures used to secure chest tubes vary according to the preference of the physician, the physician assistant, or the advanced practice nurse. One common type is the horizontal mattress or purse-string suture, which is threaded around and through the wound edges in a U shape with the ends left unknotted until the chest tube is removed. Usually, one or two anchor stitches accompany the purse-string suture (see Fig. 19.1).

- A primary goal of chest tube removal is removal of tubes without introduction of air or contaminants into the pleural space.
- Available data indicate that there is no consensus as to the rate of drainage that should be used as a threshold for tube removal and no evidence to suggest that it is unsafe to remove tubes that still have a relatively high rate of fluid drainage. Research has shown that, depending on the reason for the chest tube, volumes of 200 to 450 mL/day do not adversely affect length of stay or overall costs compared with lower threshold volumes, nor does the risk of increased pleural fluid reaccumulation.[4,8] However, some suggested guidelines include the following:
  - ❖ Drainage less than 200 to 400 mL over a 24-hour period. The presence of blood, purulent fluid, or chylous fluid are contraindications for chest tube removal.[4,7,9,11]
  - ❖ Another method considering patient size for thoracic surgery patients, suggests chest drains can be removed when the 24-hour fluid output is ≤20% of whole-body lymphatic flow (i.e., about 5 times the patient's weight in kilograms).[5]
  - ❖ Chest tubes placed after cardiac surgery can be removed when drainage is less than 100 mL over the past 12 hours, no air leak is present, and no significant effusion is noted on chest x-ray. They are typically removed 24 to 48 hours after surgery.[2,5]
  - ❖ Lungs are reexpanded (as shown on chest radiographic results).
  - ❖ Respiratory status has improved (i.e., nonlabored respirations, equal bilateral breath sounds, absence of shortness of breath, decreased use of accessory muscles, symmetrical respiratory excursion, and respiratory rate less than 24 breaths/min).
  - ❖ For interpleural chest tubes, air leaks have resolved for at least 24 hours (the absence of continuous bubbling in the water-seal chamber or absence of air bubbles from right to left in the air leak detector), and the lung is fully reinflated on chest radiographic results.[11]
  - ❖ For chest tubes that have been placed for pneumothorax, the practice of clamping the tube for 4 to 6 hours to ensure that the air leak has resolved is controversial but still supported by some. This practice should only be performed with a provider's order. Clinically monitor the patient, and unclamp immediately if there are any signs of hemodynamic or respiratory distress. Consider obtaining a chest radiograph before removal.[4,7,11,12]

❖ Variable opinions exist regarding the removal of chest tubes for patients who are receiving mechanical ventilation. Some providers leave them in as long as the patient is on mechanical ventilation, while others maintain that removal should occur because of the risk of complications and continued pain, as soon as criteria for removal are met.[7,11]

EQUIPMENT

- Suture-removal set
- Antiseptic swabs (e.g., povidone-iodine, chlorhexidine gluconate)
- Petrolatum gauze, as per hospital protocol
- Wide occlusive tape (2 inches)
- Elastic closure device, such as Steri-Strips (3M, St. Paul, MN)
- Dry 4 × 4 gauze sponges (two to four)
- Waterproof pad
- Personal protective equipment (goggles, sterile and non-sterile gloves, mask, gown)

Additional equipment to have available as needed includes the following:
- Rubber-tipped Kelly clamps or disposable umbilical clamps
- Sterile scissors

PATIENT AND FAMILY EDUCATION

- Assess the patient's and family's level of understanding about the condition and rationale for the procedure. ***Rationale:*** This assessment identifies the patient's and family's knowledge deficits concerning the patient's condition, the procedure, the expected benefits, and the potential risks. It also allows time for questions to clarify information and voice concerns. Explanations decrease patient anxiety and enhance cooperation.
- Explain the procedure, reason for removal, and sensations to be expected. The most commonly reported sensations are pulling, pain or hurting, and burning.[1,6] ***Rationale:*** This explanation prepares the patient and enhances cooperation.
- Explain the patient's role in assisting with removal. Explain that the patient should perform the Valsalva maneuver on the count of three. Have the patient practice the maneuver before the procedure. ***Rationale:*** This explanation elicits patient cooperation and facilitates removal.
- Instruct the patient to turn and reposition every 2 hours after the chest tube has been removed. ***Rationale:*** This action prevents complications related to immobility and retained secretions.
- Instruct the patient to cough and breathe deeply after the chest tube has been removed, with splinting of the affected side or sternum (with mediastinal tubes). ***Rationale:*** This action prevents respiratory complications associated with retained secretions. The application of firm pressure over the insertion site (i.e., splinting) decreases pain and discomfort associated with coughing.
- Educate the patient about the availability of prescribed analgesic medication after the chest tube is removed. ***Rationale:*** Analgesics alleviate pain and facilitate coughing, deep breathing, and repositioning.[13]

- Instruct the patient and family to immediately report signs and symptoms of respiratory distress and/or infection. ***Rationale:*** Immediate reporting facilitates prompt intervention to treat a recurrent pneumothorax, accumulation of blood or fluid, or infection.

PATIENT ASSESSMENT AND PREPARATION

Patient Assessment

- Assess the patient's mental status and ability to follow directions. ***Rationale:*** Assessment verifies the patient's ability to cooperate with instructions during the procedure.
- Assess respiratory status. ***Rationale:*** Assessment of respiratory status verifies the patient's readiness for chest tube removal.
  - ❖ Oxygen saturation within normal limits
  - ❖ Nonlabored respirations
  - ❖ Absence of shortness of breath
  - ❖ Decreased use of accessory muscles
  - ❖ Respiratory rate of less than 24 breaths/min
  - ❖ Equal bilateral breath sounds
- Assess chest tube drainage amount and type.[9] ***Rationale:*** Assessment of drainage verifies patient readiness for chest tube removal. Thresholds are individualized depending on patient size, the indication for insertion, and provider discretion.
- For interpleural chest tubes, assess for minimal or no air leak in the air leak detector zone or indicator. ***Rationale:*** This assessment indicates whether the lung is reexpanded and whether an air leak is present.
- Obtain chest radiographic results. ***Rationale:*** Lung reexpansion indicates that the need for a chest tube is resolved.
- Assess vital signs. ***Rationale:*** Vital sign assessment indicates whether the patient can tolerate chest tube removal.
- Assess laboratory results for clotting capability and medications that may affect clotting. ***Rationale:*** Thrombocytopenia, coagulopathy, or thrombolytic medications may precipitate excessive bleeding.
- Review the patient's medical record for allergies or sensitivity to antiseptics. ***Rationale:*** Patient allergies may require use of an alternative type of antiseptic of swab during the procedure.

Patient Preparation

- Verify the correct patient with two identifiers. ***Rationale:*** Before performing a procedure, the nurse should ensure the correct identification of the patient for the intended intervention.
- Ensure that the patient understands preprocedural teachings. Answer questions as they arise, and reinforce information as needed. ***Rationale:*** This communication evaluates and reinforces understanding of previously taught information. Anticipatory preparation may prepare patients for a better experience.
- Administer premedication of adequate analgesics at least 20 minutes before the procedure if indicated. Alternatively, subfascial lidocaine may be injected into the chest tube tract. In addition to opioids, adjunct methods shown

to decrease pain during chest tube removal include slow deep-breathing relaxation exercises and application of cold packs.[10] *Rationale:* Intravenous 4-mg morphine 20 minutes before or 30-mg ketorolac 60 minutes before the procedure has been shown to provide substantial pain relief without excessive analgesia.[13] Pain medication, relaxation exercises, and application of cold reduces the discomfort and anxiety experienced, which facilitates patient cooperation.[1,6]

- Time the removal procedure to occur at peak analgesic effect. Rationale: This timing increases patient cooperation and decreases anxiety.[13]
- Place the patient in the semi-Fowler's position. Alternatively, place the patient on the unaffected side with the waterproof pad underneath the site. *Rationale:* This position enhances accessibility to the insertion site of the chest tube and protects the bed from drainage.

Procedure | for Assisting with Chest Tube Removal

Steps	Rationale	Special Considerations
1. HH		
2. PE		
3. Assist with opening the sterile suture removal set and preparing petrolatum gauze dressing and two to four 4 × 4 gauze sponges, as per hospital protocol.	Aseptic technique is maintained to prevent contamination of the wound.	
4. Perform a preprocedure verification before chest tube removal.	Ensures patient safety.	If not removing all of the chest tubes at this time, ensure that they are correctly identified. Consider labeling in the presence of the ordering provider.
5. Assist with discontinuing suction from the chest-drainage system, and check for air leak in the air leak detector zone or indicator. Observe the air leak detector zone or indicator while the patient coughs.	Bubbling in the air leak detector is associated with an air leak. When an air leak is present, removal of the chest tube may cause development of a pneumothorax. Ensures that a recurrent pneumothorax has not occurred.	If an air leak is present, the tube should not be removed. Consult with the physician, physician assistant, or advanced practice nurse to determine the appropriate action.
6. Assist with removing the existing dressing, and cleanse the area around the tubes with an antiseptic solution or swab. (**Level D***)	Allows access to the chest tube at the skin level and prepares the sutures for removal.	Antiseptic swabs remove a broad spectrum of microbes quickly and provide high-level antimicrobial action for up to 6 hours after use.
7. Assist with covering the insertion sites with a dressing per hospital policy.	Some institutions utilize petroleum gauze dressings for pleural insertion sites and 4 × 4 gauze pads for mediastinal insertions sites.	Petroleum gauze on the chest tube site has not been demonstrated to decrease the risk of post-pull pneumothorax and also poses the theoretical risk of delayed wound healing.[7]
8. The tube is removed while the patient performs the Valsalva maneuver at either end inspiration or end expiration.[3,5,7] (**Level E***)	The Valsalva maneuver is needed to provide positive pressure in the pleural cavity and decrease the incidence of an involuntary gasp by the patient when the tube is removed.[3,5,7]	An involuntary inhalation during chest tube removal may put the patient at risk for air entering the chest cavity.
A. End inspiration: Instruct the patient to take a deep breath and hold it while performing the Valsalva maneuver for each tube removed. If the patient is receiving ventilator support and is unable to follow instructions, remove the tube during peak inspiration.	Removal of pleural chest tubes should be accomplished rapidly with the simultaneous application of an occlusive dressing or closure with purse-string sutures to decrease the possibility of air from entering the pleural space.	

*Level D: Peer-reviewed professional and organizational standards with the support of clinical study recommendations.
*Level E: Multiple case reports, theory-based evidence from expert opinions, or peer-reviewed professional organizational standards without clinical studies to support recommendations.

Procedure continues on following page

Procedure | for Assisting with Chest Tube Removal—*Continued*

Steps	Rationale	Special Considerations
B. End expiration: Instruct the patient to forcibly exhale and perform the Valsalva maneuver at end expiration.		
C. If possible, patients may need to hold their breath until sutures are tied.	Avoids the influx of air.	
9. Assist with securing the dressing with tape per hospital protocol.	Creates a firm closure of the chest tube site.	This action is easier with a second person to place the tape while holding pressure over the site.
10. Assess the patient's condition after the procedure, and compare the results with preprocedure assessment as noted previously.	Ensures stable respiratory status after the procedure.	Observe for warning signs of increased work of breathing, decreased oxygen saturation, increased restlessness, symptoms of chest discomfort, and diminished breath sounds on the affected side.
11. Ensure that a chest radiograph is obtained, if ordered (generally 1–4 hours after removal) only as clinically indicated.[14] **(Level B*)**	Assesses that the lung has remained expanded.	Low incidence of complication. Recommended to perform a chest radiograph only if the patient is clinically deteriorating.[14]
12. Dispose of used supplies and equipment, and remove **PE**		
13. **HH**		

*Level B: Well-designed, controlled studies with results that consistently support a specific action, intervention, or treatment.

Expected Outcomes

- Patient is comfortable and has no respiratory distress
- Lung remains expanded after chest tube removal
- Site remains free from bleeding, hematoma, or infection

Unexpected Outcomes

- Pneumothorax
- Bleeding
- Skin necrosis
- Retained chest tube
- Infected chest tube insertion site

Patient Monitoring and Care

Steps	Rationale	Reportable Conditions
		These conditions should be reported if they persist despite nursing interventions.
1. Assess respiratory status, including oxygen saturation, work of breathing, breath sounds, and symptoms of chest discomfort. Obtain a chest radiograph if significant changes are found.	Diminished respiratory status could indicate a pneumothorax. Pneumothorax could be caused by removal of the chest tube before all of the air, fluid, or blood in the pleural space had been drained, or it may recur after removal of the chest tube if air is introduced accidently into the pleural space through the chest tube tract.	- Decreased oxygen saturation on pulse oximetry - Increased work of breathing - Diminished breath sounds on the affected side - Increased restlessness and symptoms of chest discomfort
2. Monitor the insertion site for bleeding. If bleeding is found, apply pressure and place a tight occlusive dressing over the site, which may be removed after 48 hours.	Persistent bleeding from the insertion site could mean the chest tube was against a vein or chest wall artery before removal.	- Persistent bleeding

Patient Monitoring and Care —*Continued*

Steps	Rationale	Reportable Conditions
3. Monitor the suture site for signs of skin necrosis.	If the purse-string suture was pulled too tightly closed when chest tube was removed, skin necrosis may be seen.	• Dark or inflamed skin with visible necrotic areas
4. Monitor the site for signs of infection.	Prolonged insertion of a chest tube increases the risk that the tract created by the chest tube may become infected, or infection may occur after removal of the chest tube if the opening created by the removal becomes contaminated.	• Purulent drainage • Increased body temperature • Inflammation • Tenderness • Warmth at site
5. Monitor the insertion area for development of subcutaneous emphysema.	Air may leak into the surrounding tissues and cause crepitus.	• Crepitus
6. Monitor for signs and symptoms of pericardial effusion or cardiac tamponade.	Removal of mediastinal chest tubes may cause increased bleeding into the pericardium. Pericardial bleeding may continue after chest tubes are removed.	• Distant heart tones • Decreased blood pressure, tachycardia • Pulsus paradoxus • Narrowed pulse pressure • Equalized pulmonary artery pressures
7. Follow institutional standards for assessing pain. Administer analgesia as prescribed.	Identifies the need for pain interventions.	• Continued pain despite pain interventions

Documentation

Documentation should include the following:
- Patient and family education
- Respiratory and vital signs assessments before and after the procedure
- Date and time of the procedure and who performed the procedure
- Amount, color, and consistency of any drainage
- Application of a sterile occlusive dressing
- Patient's tolerance of the procedure
- Completion and results of the chest radiograph (if applicable)
- Specimens sent to the laboratory (if applicable)
- Unexpected outcomes
- Nursing interventions
- Pain assessment, interventions, and effectiveness

References and Additional Readings

For a complete list of references and additional readings for this procedure, scan this QR code with your smartphone, or visit https://www.elsevier.com/__data/assets/pdf_file/0008/1319795/Chapter0020.pdf

21 Closed Chest-Drainage System

Heidi Boddeker

PURPOSE Closed chest-drainage systems are used to facilitate the evacuation of fluid, blood, and air from the pleural space, the mediastinum, or both; to restore negative pressure to the pleural space; and to promote reexpansion of a collapsed lung.

PREREQUISITE NURSING KNOWLEDGE

- The clinical need for chest drainage arises whenever the negative pressure in the pleural cavity is disrupted by the presence of air and/or fluid, resulting in pulmonary compromise. The purpose of a chest-drainage system (CDS) is to evacuate the air and/or fluid from the chest cavity to reestablish normal intrathoracic pressure.
- Closed CDSs are integrated disposable systems (also known as *chest-drainage units*) that are modeled after the classic three-bottle CDS.
- Normal anatomy and physiology of the thorax:
  - ❖ Under usual conditions, normal intrapleural pressures measure approximately −4 cm H_2O during expiration, whereas pressure decreases to −8 cm H_2O at end inspiration.[2,3]
  - ❖ The mediastinum is within the musculoskeletal cage of the thorax and contains three subdivisions. The two lateral subdivisions hold the lungs. Between the lungs is the mediastinum, which contains the heart, the great vessels, parts of the trachea and esophagus, and other structures.
  - ❖ The lungs consist of the trachea and the bronchi, which divide into smaller branches until they reach the alveoli, known as the *air sacs.*
- Thoracic pathophysiology that requires a chest tube and CDS, which may occur spontaneously or as a result of trauma and/or surgery, is as follows:
  - ❖ Pneumothoraces (e.g., open, closed, and tension)
  - ❖ Hemothorax
  - ❖ Pleural effusions
  - ❖ Chylothorax
  - ❖ Empyema
  - ❖ Pericardial effusions, including cardiac tamponade
  - ❖ Bronchopleural fistula[14]
- CDSs include the following types:
  - ❖ Dry suction with a traditional water-seal, dry suction with a one-way valve, and wet suction with a traditional water-seal
  - ❖ Those that implement the use of gravity, suction, or both to restore negative pressure and remove air, fluid, and blood from the pleural space or the mediastinum

- Some CDSs use dry suction with a traditional water-seal and either a regulator or a restricted orifice mechanism. Although water is added to the water-seal chamber, water does not need to be added to the suction chamber. Instead, the suction source (usually a wall regulator) is increased until an indicator appears.
- Some CDSs are waterless, referred to as *dry-dry drains,* and have a one-way valve, which eliminates the need to fill any chambers (except an air-leak indicator zone, as needed). A valve opens on expiration and allows patient air to exit, and then it closes to prevent atmospheric air from entering during inspiration. This one-way valve feature allows the system to be used in the vertical or horizontal position without loss of the seal. These systems are safe if accidently tipped. The amount of suction delivered is regulated with an adjustable dial.
  - ❖ Advantages of dry suction are ease of setup; ease of application if higher, more precise levels of suction are needed; and a quiet system.
- CDSs may have some of the following components:
  - ❖ Tubing, which may or may not be latex free. See the manufacturer's guidelines for specific information
  - ❖ Collection chambers, which may be replaceable, allowing them to be removed when filled and replaced with a new collection chamber without changing the entire unit
  - ❖ Fluid-collection ports, which may be self-sealing ports or collection tubes for aspiration of drainage samples and removal of excess chamber fluid levels
  - ❖ A one-way mechanism created by a water-seal that permits air and fluid to be removed and prevents backflow into the chest
  - ❖ Accessories that may be used to convert systems to autotransfusion units
  - ❖ A digital or electronic component to quantify fluid drainage from the site, air leak if present, and intrathoracic pressures. This helps reduce variability in individual assessment of these findings.[1,8,11,14]
- Examples of CDSs include the Pleur-Evac, Thora-Klex, Argyle, Thopaz, Medela, and Atrium systems.
- CDSs contain the following chambers (Fig. 21.1):
  - ❖ The collection chamber, the largest of the three chambers, generally on the far-right side of the CDS, is the drainage reservoir. This is where drainage from the

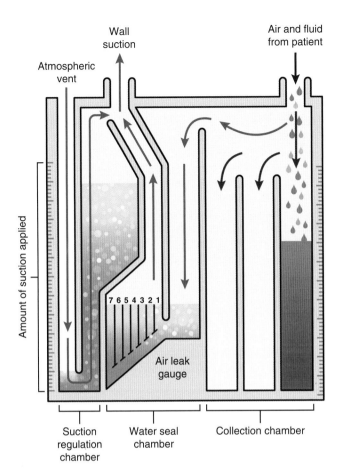

Figure 21.1 Chest drainage system. *(From Haas B, Nathens AB: (2015). Postoperative care including chest tube management. Injuries to the Chest Wall. https://doi.org/10.1007/978-3-319-18624-5_13).*

TABLE 21.1 Pressure Conversion Chart*

cm H$_2$O	mm Hg
20	15
25	18
30	22
35	26
40	30
45	33
50	37
60	44

*Approximate values.
Reprinted with permission of Atrium Medical Corporation, Hudson, NH.

pleural space accumulates. A window with calibrated markings is located on the exterior of the drainage collection for observation of the color, amount, and consistency of fluid.

❖ The suction-control chamber, generally on the far-left side of the CDS, is the suction chamber that regulates the amount of negative pressure applied to the system.

❖ The water-seal chamber, in traditional water-seal CDSs (wet systems), is usually the middle chamber and provides a one-way relief valve between the atmospheric pressure and the patient's negative intrapleural pressure.

❖ Positive-pressure relief valves are used to prevent a tension pneumothorax if the suction tubing becomes accidently occluded or if the suction source fails. In addition, automatic and manual pressure relief valves vent excessive negative pressure, such as may occur during deep inspiration or with milking of the chest tube.

• Suction guidelines include the following:

❖ When clinically indicated, the addition of a suction source can enhance drainage when large volumes of air or fluid must be evacuated.

❖ Current guidelines recommend that a water-seal alone is safe for most patients with a pneumothorax or

small air leak.[6,7,17] However, if the pneumothorax or air leak is large, expanding, or persistent, suction is recommended.[7]

❖ The most common amount of suction pressure ranges from −10 to −20 cm H$_2$O.[11,14,18] High suction levels may cause persistent pleural air leaks, air stealing, lung tissue entrapment, and reexpansion pulmonary edema.[18]

❖ There are differences in flow rates and in accuracy of delivered negative pressures noted in CDSs; however, they are not likely to be clinically important.[7]

❖ Some systems contain an exit vent from the water-seal chamber that ensures that the drainage unit remains vented when the suction device is off. Do not close or occlude the exit vent.[2,3] When using a CDS without an exit vent, the drainage systems should be disconnected from suction before they are turned off.[2,3]

❖ Some wall-mounted suction devices need control and pressure gauges to regulate and monitor for potential surges in suction levels.[2,3]

❖ If clinically appropriate, some wet suction with traditional water-seal drainage systems can provide suction levels greater than −25 cm H$_2$O. The suction-chamber vent holes can be occluded with nonporous tape or by replacing them with the manufacturer's special pronged vent plug and connecting directly to wall regulator suction. Suction levels must be converted from prescribed levels of cm H$_2$O suction to mm Hg of wall suction (Table 21.1).

• General guidelines in the proper care of the CDS include the following:

❖ Greater pressure within the chest than within the system is needed to maintain proper functioning of the closed system; this requirement is accomplished by keeping the drainage unit at least 1 foot below the chest tube insertion site and the tubing free from dependent loops and obstructions,[7,12,18] which prevents siphoning of the contents back into the pleural cavity.[7,12,18]

❖ Except for the exit vent, an airtight system is required to assist in maintaining negative pressure in the pleura and to prevent air entrapment in the pleural space.

❖ Tidaling, fluctuations that occur with inspiration and expiration, provides a continuous manometer of the pressure changes in the pleural space and indicates overall respiratory effort. Absence of fluctuations suggests obstruction of the drainage system from clots, contact with lung tissue, kinks, loss of subatmospheric pressure from fluid-filled dependent loops, or complete reexpansion of the lung.[2,3,10,12,18]

❖ In general, clamping of chest tubes is contraindicated. Clamping a chest tube in a patient with a pleural air leak may cause a tension pneumothorax. The few situations in which chest tubes may be clamped briefly (i.e., less than 1 minute) include locating the source of an air leak, replacing the CDS, and during chest tube removal.[11,14,18] Clamping in order to determine whether a patient is ready to have a chest tube discontinued is controversial and should only be performed with a provider order.[11,14,18]

❖ Stripping chest tubes or breaking the connection with the CDS to remove clots is not recommended.[5] Chest tubes that incorporate a guidewire-based clearance mechanism have been shown to reduce retained blood in patients following cardiac surgery.[8,13]

EQUIPMENT

Disposable Setup (Wet and Dry Systems)

- Disposable chest-drainage unit
- Gloves
- Suction source and regulator
- Connecting tubing
- 1-L bottle of sterile water or normal saline (for systems that use water)
- 50-mL irrigation syringe (if not supplied with unit) for systems that use water
- Tape (1 inch), one roll, or zip ties (e.g., Parham-Martin bands)

PATIENT AND FAMILY EDUCATION

- Explain the procedure, the indication for the chest tube insertion, and how the closed CDS works. **Rationale:** This communication identifies patient and family knowledge deficits about the patient's condition, procedure, expected benefits, and potential risks and allows time for questions to clarify information and to voice concerns. Explanations decrease patient anxiety and enhance cooperation.
- After chest tube insertion, instruct the patient to sit in the semi-Fowler's position (unless contraindicated). **Rationale:** Proper positioning facilitates drainage from the lung by allowing air to rise and fluid to settle, enhancing removal via the chest tube. This position also makes breathing easier.
- Instruct the patient to turn and reposition every 2 hours to facilitate drainage. The patient may lie on the side with the chest tube but should keep the tubing free from kinks. **Rationale:** Turning and positioning prevents complications related to immobility and retained secretions. Keeping the tubing free from kinks maintains patency of the tube, facilitates drainage, and prevents accumulation of pressure within the pleural space, which interferes with lung reexpansion.
- Instruct the patient to cough and deep breathe, with splinting of the affected side or sternum (if a mediastinal tube is

in place). **Rationale:** Coughing and deep breathing increase pressure within the pleural space, facilitating drainage, promoting lung reexpansion, and preventing respiratory complications associated with retained secretions. The application of firm pressure over the chest tube insertion site (e.g., splinting) may decrease pain and discomfort.

- Encourage active or passive range-of-motion exercises of the arm on the affected side. **Rationale:** The patient may limit the movement of the arm on the affected side to decrease the discomfort at the insertion site, which may result in joint discomfort and potential joint complications.
- Instruct the patient and family about activity as prescribed while maintaining the drainage system below the level of the chest. **Rationale:** The drainage system is maintained below the level of the chest to facilitate gravity drainage and to prevent backflow into the pleural space and potential infectious contamination into the pleural space.
- Instruct the patient and family about the availability of prescribed analgesic medication and other pain-relief strategies. **Rationale:** Pain relief ensures comfort; facilitates coughing, deep breathing, positioning, and range-of-motion exercises; and promotes healing.

PATIENT ASSESSMENT AND PREPARATION

Patient Assessment

- Assess significant medical history or injury, including chronic lung disease, spontaneous pneumothorax, pulmonary disease, therapeutic procedures, and mechanism of injury. **Rationale:** Medical history or injury may provide the etiological basis for the occurrence of pneumothorax, hemothorax, empyema, pleural effusion, or chylothorax.
- Assess the patient's baseline cardiopulmonary status (if the patient's condition does not necessitate immediate intervention). **Rationale:** Provides reference points for future assessments upon completion of the procedure.
- Assess baseline cardiopulmonary status, as follows:
  ❖ Vital signs (blood pressure, heart rate, respiratory rate)
  ❖ Shortness of breath or dyspnea
  ❖ Anxiety, restlessness, or apprehension
  ❖ Cyanosis
  ❖ Decreased oxygen saturation (e.g., pulse oximetry [SpO_2])
  ❖ Decreased or absent breath sounds on the affected side
  ❖ Crackles adjacent to the affected area
  ❖ Asymmetrical chest excursion with respirations
  ❖ Hyperresonance with percussion on the affected side (pneumothorax)
  ❖ Dullness or flatness with percussion on the affected side (hemothorax, pleural effusion, empyema, or chylothorax)
  ❖ Subcutaneous emphysema or crepitus (pneumothorax)
  ❖ Sudden sharp focal chest pain
  ❖ Tracheal deviation to the unaffected side (tension pneumothorax)
  ❖ Neck vein distention (tension pneumothorax, cardiac tamponade)
  ❖ Muffled heart sounds (cardiac tamponade)
  Rationale: Provides reference points for future tests upon completion of the procedure.

- Assess diagnostic tests (if the patient's condition does not necessitate immediate intervention):
  - ❖ Chest radiograph
  - ❖ Arterial blood gases

Patient Preparation

- Ensure that the patient understands the preprocedural teachings. Answer questions as they arise, and reinforce information as needed. *Rationale:* This communication evaluates and reinforces understanding of previously presented information.

- Verify the correct patient with two identifiers. *Rationale:* Before performing a procedure, the nurse should ensure the correct identification of the patient for the intended intervention.
- Administer prescribed analgesics or sedatives as needed. *Rationale:* Analgesics and sedatives reduce the discomfort and anxiety experienced, facilitating patient cooperation and improving outcomes.

Procedure	for Dry Suction Closed Chest-Drainage Systems	
Steps	**Rationale**	**Special Considerations**
1. HH		
2. PE		
3. Open sterile packages.	Maintains aseptic technique whenever changes are made to the system.	
4. Stabilize the unit. Some systems have a floor stand. For systems with an in-line connector, move the patient tube clamp down next to the in-line connector.	Keeping the clamp visible helps prevent inadvertent clamping.	Clamping of chest tubes can cause air trapped in the pleural space to accumulate and may cause tension pneumothorax.
5. *Dry suction with a traditional water-seal:* Remove the connector cap from the short tubing of the water-seal chamber and use the funnel provided or a 50-mL syringe to add sterile water or normal saline to the 2-cm level. Some systems provide prefilled sterile water containers. *Dry suction with a one-way valve:* Fill the air-leak monitor zone.	Depth of solution required to establish a water-seal; the water-seal permits air and fluid to be removed from the patient and prevents the backflow of air into the chest.[6,17,18]	Water-seal levels greater than 2 cm increase the work of breathing; levels less than 2 cm can expose the water-seal to air and increase the risk for pneumothorax.[3,18]
6. Hang the drainage unit from the bed frame, or place it on a floor stand. **(Level E*)**	Drainage unit must be kept below the level of the chest to promote gravity drainage and to prevent backflow of drainage into the pleural space, which interferes with lung expansion.[3,12,18]	Avoid hanging drainage unit from bed rails or other movable structures.
7. Connect the long tubing from the drainage collection chamber to the chest tube. **(Level C*)**	Creates the closed CDS; avoid dependent or fluid-filled loops.[3,12,18]	Avoid dependent or fluid-filled loops, which may create back pressure and decrease the effectiveness of suction.[3,12,18]
8. For gravity drainage, leave the suction-control chamber open to air. **(Level M*)**	Creates the exit vent for the escape of air.	*Clamping of chest tubes can cause air trapped in the pleural space to accumulate and may cause tension pneumothorax.*

*Level E: Multiple case reports, theory-based evidence from expert opinions, or peer-reviewed professional organizational standards without clinical studies to support recommendations.

*Level C: Qualitative studies, descriptive or correlational studies, integrative reviews, systematic reviews, or randomized controlled trials with inconsistent results.

*Level M: Manufacturer's recommendations only.

Procedure for Dry Suction Closed Chest-Drainage Systems—*Continued*

Steps	Rationale	Special Considerations
9. To initiate suction, connect the CDS to the suction source, and dial in the prescribed amount of suction (usually −10 to −20 cm H_2O); then increase the suction source until the indicator mark appears according to manufacturer's guidelines.	Activates suction.	Apply suction as per manufacturer's guidelines. For example, to apply −20 cm H_2O suction, use a minimum vacuum pressure of −80 mm Hg. Suction source vacuum should be >−80 mm Hg when multiple chest drains are used. For a suction level <−20 cm H_2O, any observed bellows expansion across the monitor window confirms adequate suction operation. To decrease suction, set the dial, confirm patient on suction, then depress the high-negativity vent, venting to the newer lower amount.
10. Tape all connection points in the CDS (see Fig. 17.3). A. One-inch tape is placed horizontally, extending over the connections (a portion of the connector may be left unobstructed by the tape).	Except for the exit vent, a secure and airtight system is required to avoid inadvertent disconnection that could cause air entrapment in the pleural space and decreased pleural negative pressure. This technique secures the connections but allows visualization of drainage in the connector.	Zip ties (Parham-Martin bands) may be used to secure connections instead of tape (see Fig. 17.4).
B. Reinforce the horizontal tape with tape placed vertically so that it encircles both ends of the connector.		
11. Dispose of soiled equipment and supplies and remove **PE**.		
12. **HH**		

Procedure for Wet Suction Closed Chest-Drainage Systems

Steps	Rationale	Special Considerations
1. **HH**		
2. **PE**		
3. Open sterile packages.	Maintains aseptic technique whenever changes are made to the system.	
4. Stabilize the unit. Some systems have a floor stand. For systems with an in-line connector, move the patient tube clamp down next to the in-line connector.	Keeping the clamp visible helps prevent inadvertent clamping.	Clamping of chest tubes can cause air trapped in the pleural space to accumulate and may cause tension pneumothorax.
5. Remove the connector cap from the short tubing of the water-seal chamber and use the funnel provided or a 50-mL syringe to add sterile water or normal saline to the 2-cm level.	Depth of solution required to establish a water-seal; the water-seal permits air and fluid to be removed from the chest and prevents backflow of air.[2,12,18]	Water-seal levels >2 cm increase the work of breathing; levels <2 cm can expose the water-seal to air and increase the risk for pneumothorax.[2,12,18]

Procedure continues on following page

Procedure for Wet Suction Closed Chest-Drainage Systems—*Continued*		
Steps	Rationale	Special Considerations
6. For gravity drainage, leave the short tubing from the suction control chamber open to air by turning stopcock to "open" or "on" position.	Creates the exit vent for the escape of air.	Clamping or occlusion of the exit vent can cause air to remain trapped in the pleural space, which may cause tension pneumothorax.
7. For suction drainage, fill the suction-control chamber with sterile water or normal saline to the prescribed level (usually −10 to −20 cm H_2O suction). Connect the short tubing from the suction-control chamber to the suction source.	Suction is regulated by the height of the solution level in this chamber.	Refill the solution level as necessary to the prescribed amount to replace solution lost through evaporation. Remove excess fluid as necessary via a self-sealing grommet.
8. Hang chest-drainage unit from bed frame or set it on a floor stand. **(Level E*)**	Drainage unit must be kept below the level of the chest to promote gravity drainage and to prevent backflow of drainage into the pleural space, which interferes with lung expansion.[2,12,18]	Avoid hanging the drainage unit from bed rails or other movable structures.
9. Connect the long tubing from the drainage collection chamber to the chest tube. **(Level C*)**	Creates the drainage-collection system; avoid dependent or fluid-filled loops.[7,12,18]	Dependent or fluid-filled loops may create back pressure and decrease the effectiveness of suction.[7,12,18]
10. Turn on the suction source, if prescribed, to elicit gentle constant bubbling. Leave stopcock between CDS and suction source fully open and adjust force of bubbling at suction source to decrease risk for pneumothorax.	Activates suction.	Some systems have a suction-control feature to maintain the desired suction level automatically despite fluctuations in the suction source. The stopcock should be kept fully in "open" or "on" position, and the force of bubbling should be adjusted at the suction source.
11. Tape all connection points in the CDS (see Fig. 17.3). A. Place 1-inch tape horizontally extending over the connections (a portion of the connector may be left unobstructed by the tape). B. Reinforce the horizontal tape with tape placed vertically so it encircles both ends of the connector.	Except for the exit vent, a secure and airtight system is required to avoid inadvertent disconnection that could cause air entrapment in the pleural space and decreased pleural negative pressure. This technique secures the connections but allows visualization of drainage in the connector.	Zip ties (Parham-Martin bands) may be used to secure connections instead of tape. (see Fig. 17.4)
12. Dispose of soiled equipment and supplies, and remove **PE**.		
13. **HH**		

*Level C: Qualitative studies, descriptive or correlational studies, integrative reviews, systematic reviews, or randomized controlled trials with inconsistent results.

*Level E: Multiple case reports, theory-based evidence from expert opinions, or peer-reviewed professional organizational standards without clinical studies to support recommendations.

UNIT I

Expected Outcomes

- Removal of air, fluid, or blood from the thoracic cavity
- Fluctuation or tidaling noted in the water-seal chamber (until lung is reexpanded)
- Relief of respiratory distress
- Reexpansion of the collapsed lung as validated with chest radiograph

Unexpected Outcomes

- Tension pneumothorax
- Hemorrhagic shock
- Absence of drainage and fluctuation or tidaling, or continuous bubbling in the water-seal chamber with continued respiratory distress
- No evidence of lung reexpansion
- Fever, purulent drainage, and redness around the insertion site or purulent drainage in the chest tube
- Respiratory distress (coughing, shortness of breath, decreased SaO_2, or chest pain or tightness)[12,18]

Patient Monitoring and Care

Steps	Rationale	Reportable Conditions
		These conditions should be reported to the provider if they persist despite nursing interventions.
1. Assess every 1–2 hours and with any change in patient condition or according to institutional protocol.	Provides baseline and ongoing assessment of the patient's condition.	• Tachypnea • Decreased or absent breath sounds • Hypoxemia • Tachycardia • Dysrhythmias • Hypotension • Muffled heart tones • Subcutaneous emphysema (crepitus) • Neck vein distention • Tracheal deviation • Fever • Absence of fluctuations in the water-seal chamber with respiratory distress
2. Monitor the amount and type of drainage by marking the drainage level on the outside of the drainage-collection chamber in hourly or shift increments (depending on the amount of drainage) or in time increments established by institutional policy or per practitioner orders. Monitor the amount and type of drainage.	Marking the container provides a reference point for future measurements. Volume loss can cause patients to become hypovolemic or can signal intrapulmonary bleeding. Drainage should decrease gradually and change from bloody to pink to straw-colored. Sudden flow of dark bloody drainage that occurs with position change is often old blood. Decreased or absent drainage associated with respiratory distress may indicate obstruction; decreased or absent drainage without respiratory distress may indicate lung reexpansion. Autotransfusion: if chest-drainage transfusion (autotransfusion) is being considered, please see Procedure 16, Autotransfusion.	• Drainage >100 mL/hour[7,12] or according to practitioner order • Sudden decrease or absence of drainage • Change in characteristics of drainage, such as unexpectedly bloody, cloudy, or milky • New onset of clots

Procedure continues on following page

Patient Monitoring and Care —*Continued*

Steps	Rationale	Reportable Conditions
3. Assess the patient and CDS for air leak. If a suction source has been added, momentarily turn the suction off, or pinch the suction tubing to accurately assess.[3,12,18] An air leak is present if air bubbles are observed in the water-seal chamber or going from right-to-left in the leak detector zone. When assessing the air-leak chamber, ask the patient to take deep breaths in and out. If you do not note an air leak, ask the patient to cough.[3,12,18] When the patient's pleural space is leaking air, intermittent bubbling is seen corresponding to respirations. If bubbling is continuous, suspect an air leak in the system. To locate the source, intermittently pinch the chest tube or drainage tubing for a moment (i.e., less than 1 minute), beginning at the insertion site and progressing to the chest-drainage unit.[3,12,18]	Assessing for air leak is one way to determine whether the patient is experiencing a pneumothorax. Bubbling when suction is initially turned on occurs with air displaced by fluid drainage in the collection chamber, loose connections in the system, or an air leak in the pleural space.[3,12,18] With a minor air leak, bubbling may occur only with coughing when airway pressures reach their peak.[3,12,18] An airtight system is required to help reestablish negative pressure in the pleural space. If bubbling in the water-seal chamber stops when the chest tube is occluded at the dressing site, the air leak is inside the patient's chest or under the dressing. If it is a new-onset air leak, reinforce the dressing, and notify the provider. If the bubbling stops when the drainage tubing is occluded along its length, the air leak is between the occlusion and the patient's chest; check to ensure that all connections are airtight.[3,12,18] If bubbling does not stop with occlusion, replace the CDS.	• New or increasing air leaks in the chest or around the chest tube insertion site • Chest tube drainage from a mediastinal tube does not normally cause bubbling in the water-seal chamber; if noted, it may indicate communication with the pleural space; notify the provider • Notify the provider of system knock-over and changing of the CDS (e.g., chest radiograph may be ordered).

4. Assess the chest tube and CDS patency on insertion, every 1–2 hours, and with a change in patient condition. Routine chest tube stripping or milking is not recommended.[3,12,18] For obstructed pleural tubes used in the treatment of recurrent effusions or retained hemothorax, a provider may order instillation of fibrinolytic medication to restore flow in the tube.[15,16]	Obstruction of drainage from the chest tube interferes with lung reexpansion or may cause cardiac tamponade. Stripping the entire length of the chest tube is contraindicated because it results in transient high negative pressures in the pleural space that could lead to lung entrapment.[3,12,18] No significant differences are reported in the amount of drainage when the tubing is milked as opposed to stripped.[3,12,18] Milking can cause excessive negativity. Use the high-negativity relief value to restore negativity to prescribed levels (see Step 8). Milking with a clamp on can result in a buildup of excessive thoracic pressure.	• Inability to establish patency
		• Excessive drainage
		• Signs and/or symptoms of increasing:
		  • Pneumothorax
		  • Cardiac tamponade
		  • Hemothorax

5. Maintain drainage tubing free from dependent loops (i.e., place the tube horizontally on the bed and down into the collection chamber, coiling the tubing on the bed). If a dependent loop cannot be avoided, lift and drain the tubing every 15 minutes.[3,12,18]	Drainage that accumulates in dependent loops obstructs chest drainage into the collecting system and increases pressure within the lung.[3,12,18] Allow enough length for patient movement.	• Loops or kinks that cannot be removed
6. Monitor fluid levels in the CDS chambers by briefly turning off the suction and refill (usually every 8 hours for the suction chamber and every 24 hours for the water-seal), or remove solution levels as necessary to the prescribed amount.	To maintain prescribed water-seal and suction levels and to prevent complications. Water-seal levels >2 cm increase the work of breathing; levels <2 cm expose the water-seal to air and increase the risk for pneumothorax.[6,17,18]	• Inability to maintain a water-seal or to keep suction at the prescribed level

Patient Monitoring and Care —*Continued*

Steps	Rationale	Reportable Conditions
7. Assess for CDS patency: note fluctuations or tidaling of fluid level in the water-seal chamber (disposable CDS) or the long straw of the water-seal bottle (bottle CDS) with respirations.[2,3,10,12,13,18] If a suction source has been added, momentarily turn the suction off, or pinch the suction tubing to accurately assess for fluctuations or tidaling.	Tidaling, fluid fluctuation up and down or back and forth, indicates effective communication between the pleural space and drainage system and provides an indication of lung expansion. Fluctuations or tidaling stops when the lung is reexpanded or when the tubing is obstructed by a kink, a fluid-filled loop, the patient lying on the tubing, or a clot or tissue at the distal end.[2,3,10,12,13,18] Suction must be turned off to accurately assess for tidaling.	• Absence of fluctuations or tidaling
8. Assess a CDS equipped with a float valve for increases in the patient's negative intrathoracic pressure. Inspect the water-seal chamber for increased levels (e.g., after milking the chest tube or when decreasing the amount of suction). Ensure that the CDS is operating on suction. Second, temporarily depress the filtered manual vent until the float valve releases and the water column lowers.	Changes in the patient's intrathoracic pressure are reflected by the height of the water in the water-seal column. Do not lower the water-seal column when suction is not operating or when the patient is on gravity drainage. Resume suction while performing this operation. If suction is not operative, or operating on gravity drainage, depressing the high-negative relief valve can reduce negative pressure within the collection chamber to zero (atmosphere), possibly resulting in a pneumothorax.	• Sustained increases in negative pressures
9. Assess the insertion site and surrounding skin for the presence of subcutaneous emphysema (crepitus) and signs of infection or inflammation daily and with each dressing change. Dressings should be changed when soiled, per institutional protocol, or when ordered by the practitioner. Routine petroleum dressings are not recommended.[9]	Crepitus may indicate chest tube obstruction or improper tube position. Skin integrity is altered during insertion and can lead to infection. Petroleum gauze dressing has been noted to cause skin maceration, potentiating the risk of infection.[9]	• New or increasing subcutaneous emphysema (crepitus) • Fever • Redness around the insertion site • Purulent drainage
10. Monitor the collection chamber for total amount of fluid. Change the CDS when approaching full or if system integrity is interrupted (i.e., cracked). Assess cardiopulmonary status and vital signs (including SpO_2) before and after the procedure. Prepare a new CDS according to manufacturer's instructions. Then, briefly (i.e., for less than 1 minute) cross-clamp the chest tube close to the patient's chest. Attach the new system, unclamp the chest tube, check connections, and assess the function of the drainage system.	When the patient has an air leak or pneumothorax, clamping of the chest tube may precipitate a tension pneumothorax because the air has no escape route and may accumulate in the pleural space.[11,14,18] Clamping of the chest tube should be as brief as possible.	• Respiratory distress noted during or after the procedure • Changes in breath sounds after the procedure • Nonfunctioning CDS

Procedure continues on following page

Patient Monitoring and Care —*Continued*

Steps	Rationale	Reportable Conditions
11. During gravity drainage, ambulation, or transport with gravity drainage, ensure that the CDS is upright, below the chest tube insertion site, and maintain the suction control stopcock in the "on" or "open" position. Utilize portable suction unless the provider has ordered that the patient can be ambulated or transported off suction. Do not clamp the chest tube during transport.[11,14,18]	The suction control stopcock should always remain in the "on" or "open" position. Do not clamp or cap the suction line. Leaving the port open allows air to exit and minimizes the possibility of tension pneumothorax.	• Notify the provider of inadvertent clamping or capping of the suction line • If the chest tube is accidently dislodged, apply a sterile dressing taped on three sides to allow air to escape.[4] Notify the provider immediately, and monitor the patient for increased respiratory distress or tension pneumothorax.
12. Follow institutional standards for assessing pain. Administer analgesia as prescribed.	Identifies need for pain interventions.	• Continued pain despite pain interventions.
13. Obtain a drainage specimen from some disposable CDSs. Cleanse the site with antiseptic solution, and use a syringe with a smaller (e.g., 20-gauge) needle to withdraw the specimen from the self-sealing diaphragm, or self-sealing drainage tubing, as available. Momentarily forming a dependent loop in the fluid collection tubing may be necessary to obtain a specimen.	Provides a specimen for analysis.	• Inability to obtain a specimen

*Level C: Qualitative studies, descriptive or correlational studies, integrative reviews, systematic reviews, or randomized controlled trials with inconsistent results.

*Level E: Multiple case reports, theory-based evidence from expert opinions, or peer-reviewed professional organizational standards without clinical studies to support recommendations.

Documentation

Documentation should include the following:
- Patient and family education
- Pain assessment, interventions, and effectiveness
- Cardiopulmonary and vital signs assessment
- Type of drainage system used
- Amount of suction, fluctuation or tidaling, type and amount of drainage
- Air leak: absence, presence, severity, resolution, and quantity (if a digital chest tube is used)
- Respiratory, thoracic, and vital sign assessment at baseline and with changes in therapy
- Intrathoracic pressure if a digital chest tube is used
- Chest tube dressing intact
- Completion and results of the postinsertion chest radiograph and any other ordered diagnostic tests
- Unexpected outcomes
- Nursing interventions
- Patient's tolerance of the therapy

References and Additional Readings

For a complete list of references and additional readings for this procedure, scan this QR code with your smartphone, or visit https://www.elsevier.com/__data/assets/pdf_file/0009/1319796/Chapter0021.pdf

22 Needle Thoracostomy [AP] (Perform)

Cynthia A. Goodrich

PURPOSE: Needle thoracostomy is performed to reduce a tension pneumothorax to a simple pneumothorax in a rapidly deteriorating patient. This temporary measure is quickly followed by insertion of a chest tube for more definitive management.

PREREQUISITE NURSING KNOWLEDGE

- Knowledge of anatomy and physiology of the pulmonary system.
- Under normal conditions, the thoracic cavity is a closed air space. Any disruption in its integrity will result in the loss of negative pressure within the intrapleural space. Air or fluid that enters the space competes with the lung, ultimately resulting in collapse of the lung. Pneumothorax may result from disease, trauma, surgery, or from iatrogenic causes such as central venous catheterization or mechanical ventilation.
- A pneumothorax is classified as an *open, closed,* or *tension* pneumothorax. In patients with tension pneumothorax, air leaks into the pleural space during inspiration through a tear in the lung, and with no means to escape from the pleural cavity during expiration, it creates a one-way valve effect. Air enters the pleural space during inspiration but is unable to escape during expiration. With each breath, air accumulates and pressure within the pleural space increases, ultimately resulting in collapse of the affected lung. Continued accumulation of air within the pleural space causes mediastinal structures (i.e., heart, great vessels, and trachea) to shift to the opposite or unaffected side of the chest. This impedes venous return and cardiac output, which may result in cardiopulmonary collapse and ultimately cardiac arrest.[2,7,8]
- A tension pneumothorax is a life-threatening condition that requires *immediate* intervention. It is a clinical diagnosis based on signs and symptoms, not a diagnostic diagnosis based on a chest x-ray. Accurate assessment of the following signs and symptoms allows for prompt recognition and treatment:
  - ❖ Tracheal deviation to the unaffected side
  - ❖ Jugular vein distention
  - ❖ Sudden, sharp chest pain
  - ❖ Decreased or absent breath sounds on the affected side
  - ❖ Asymmetrical chest excursion with respirations
  - ❖ Tachypnea, shortness of breath, dyspnea, increased work of breathing
  - ❖ Decreased oxygen saturation
  - ❖ Subcutaneous emphysema
  - ❖ Anxiety, restlessness, apprehension
  - ❖ Tachycardia
  - ❖ Hypotension
  - ❖ Dysrhythmias
  - ❖ Cyanosis
  - ❖ Decreased pulse oximetry readings
  - ❖ Pulseless electrical activity
- Needle thoracostomy is performed by placing a needle into the pleural space to remove air and reestablish negative pressure in patients who are rapidly deteriorating from a life-threatening tension pneumothorax (Fig. 22.1). Definitive treatment requires insertion of a chest tube as soon as possible after this temporary measure.[2]
- Sites for needle decompression include the second intercostal space, midclavicular line, or the fourth or fifth intercostal space (usually at the nipple level) just anterior to the midaxillary line.[2,3,5,8,9]
- Needle decompression success is influenced by chest wall thickness.[4] Current evidence suggests that an 8-cm needle will reach the pleural space more than 90% of the time, whereas a 5-cm needle will only reach the pleural space more than 50% of the time.[2] Insufficient needle length may lead to failed decompression of the pneumothorax.[4] The patient's body habitus should determine when a longer needle is required for effective decompression.[1,2,4,6]

EQUIPMENT

- Personal protective equipment including eye protection
- 14- to 16-gauge hollow needle or over-the-needle catheter at least 5 cm in length (5 cm for smaller adults, 8 cm for larger adults)[2]
- 10-cc syringe filled with 3 cc sterile saline (can be used to confirm entrance into the pleural space by observing for bubbling in the syringe)[2]
- Antiseptic solution
- 4 × 4 gauze dressing
- Tape
- Self-inflating manual resuscitation bag-valve-mask device
- Oxygen source and tubing

[AP] This procedure should be performed only by clinicians who have demonstrated competence and are credentialed to perform it. In addition, the procedure must be within the scope of practice defined by their professional licensure, and in accordance with professional practice acts. Physicians, advanced practice nurses, and physician assistants may be credentialed to perform this procedure.

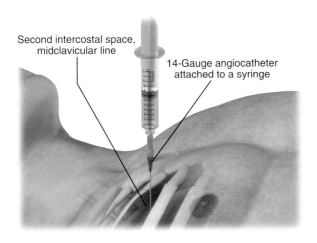

Second intercostal space, midclavicular line

14-Gauge angiocatheter attached to a syringe

Figure 22.1 Needle decompression. A large-bore needle or catheter-over-needle device is used to puncture the parietal pleura and establish the presence of blood or air in the pleural space. The needle can be placed anywhere in the pleural space, but is traditionally placed at the same sites used for tube thoracostomy: the anterior second intercostal space in the midclavicular line or the anterior axillary line in the fourth or fifth interspace. The needle is placed so it enters over the rib to avoid neurovascular injury. The needle is then withdrawn while leaving the catheter behind to create a simple open pneumothorax. The procedure can be performed either with or without the syringe attached to the catheter. This is only a temporary therapeutic maneuver for a tension pneumothorax, and a chest tube must also be inserted. *(From Margolis AM, Kirsch TD:* Roberts and Hedges' clinical procedures in emergency medicine and acute care, *ed 7, Philadelphia, 2019, Elsevier.)*

- Commercially available (Heimlich) flutter valve to attach to the needle or catheter, or, as an emergency alternative, a one-way valve may be created by using the following:
  - ❖ Scissors
  - ❖ Sterile glove (powder-free)
  - ❖ Small rubber band
  - ❖ Cut a finger off the glove, cut the very tip of the glove finger off, and attach it to the needle with the rubber band.[2]

PATIENT AND FAMILY EDUCATION

- If time permits, assess the patient's and family's level of understanding about the condition and rationale for the procedure. *Rationale:* This assessment identifies the patient's and family's knowledge deficits concerning the patient's condition, the procedure, the expected benefits, and the potential risks. It also allows time for questions to clarify information and voice concerns. Explanations decrease patient anxiety and enhance cooperation.
- Explain the procedure and the reason for the procedure if the clinical situation permits. If not, explain the procedure and reason for its implementation after it is completed. *Rationale:* This explanation enhances patient and family understanding and decreases anxiety.
- If indicated, explain the patient's role in assisting with needle thoracostomy. *Rationale:* Eliciting the patient's cooperation assists with insertion of a needle and flutter valve.

PATIENT ASSESSMENT AND PREPARATION

Patient Assessment

- Assess whether signs and symptoms are consistent with tension pneumothorax, as noted previously. *Rationale:* Accurate assessment of signs and symptoms allows for prompt recognition and treatment. Baseline assessment provides comparison data for evaluation of changes and outcomes of treatment. Tension pneumothorax is a life-threatening medical emergency that necessitates *immediate* intervention.
- If the situation allows, assess vital signs, including pulse oximetry. *Rationale:* Baseline assessment data provide information about the patient's condition and allows for comparison during and after the procedure.

Patient Preparation

- Verify the correct patient with two identifiers. *Rationale:* Before performing a procedure, the practitioner should ensure the correct identification of the patient for the intended intervention.
- Ensure that the patient and family understand the emergency nature of the procedure and preprocedural teachings, if appropriate. Answer questions as they arise, and reinforce information as needed. *Rationale:* This communication evaluates and reinforces understanding of previously taught information.
- Position the patient supine with the head of the bed flat. *Rationale:* This positioning allows for identification of landmarks for proper placement of the needle and flutter valve.
- Perform a preprocedural verification and time out, if non-emergent. *Rationale:* Ensures patient safety and improves communication.

Procedure	for Performing Needle Thoracostomy	
Steps	Rationale	Special Considerations
1. **HH**		
2. **PE**		Protective eyewear prevents exposure to secretions that may be expelled as the needle penetrates the pressurized pleural space.
3. Position supine with the head of the bed flat. Administer high-flow oxygen, and ventilate as needed.	Allows for oxygenation and ventilation before needle insertion.	
4. Prepare and assemble equipment for the procedure.	Ensures that all needed equipment is readily available.	Consider using a longer needle for patients with thicker chest walls.[1-4] (5 cm for smaller adults, 8 cm for larger adults).[2] (**Level D***) When using a longer needle, be aware of the risk of injury to underlying structures or complications such as pulmonary artery injury, hemothorax and cardiac tamponade.[4]
5. Locate the second intercostal space at the midclavicular line on the side of the suspected tension pneumothorax.	Identifies landmarks for needle thoracostomy.	An alternative site is the fourth or fifth intercostal space, just anterior to the midaxillary line.[2,3,5,8,9] It may be difficult to access this site in certain situations such as the transport environment or with trauma patients on a backboard.[2]
6. Prepare the skin with antiseptic solution using a circular motion.	Cleanses the area before needle insertion.	
7. Locate the upper margin of the third rib with several fingers. Insert the needle at a 90-degree angle into the second intercostal space at the midclavicular line (see Fig. 22.1), pointing the needle posterior but slightly upward and sliding it over the top of the third rib.[2,8]	Allows the proper placement of the needle into the pleural space. Inserting the needle above the third rib avoids damaging the nerve, artery, and vein that lie just beneath each rib.[2,8]	A 10-cc syringe filled with 3 cc of sterile saline may be attached to the needle. Bubbling in the syringe will be seen as air escapes from the pleural space.[2,8]
8. Puncture the parietal pleural space. Listen for an audible escape of air or bubbling in the syringe as the needle enters the pleural space. If a catheter-over-needle device is used, remove the needle.[2,8]	Although an audible rush of air indicates that needle decompression has been successful, a dramatic improvement in the patient's clinical condition is the best indicator of successful intervention.	This procedure may not be successful because of chest wall thickness, anatomical complications, or kinking of the catheter.[1,2,4,6] The clinician may need to repeat the procedure with a longer catheter to puncture the parietal pleura in patients with large, thick chests. Verify that the catheter is not kinked and that it is has been inserted into the proper anatomical location.
9. Attach a flutter valve to the needle or catheter, if not already attached.[2,8]	Allows air to escape the pleural space and prevents air from reentering.	The needle and flutter valve act as a one-way valve, preventing reentry of air into pleural space but allowing for escape of air during expiration (Fig. 22.2).

Procedure continues on following page

Procedure	**for Performing Needle Thoracostomy—***Continued*	
Steps	Rationale	Special Considerations
10. Apply a small dressing around the needle or catheter, and secure or suture it in place. 11. Prepare for immediate chest tube insertion (see Procedures 17 and 18). 12. Discard used supplies, and remove **PE**. 13. **HH**	Allows for temporary stabilization of the needle or catheter until a chest tube can be inserted. Provides definitive treatment of tension pneumothorax.	

Expected Outcomes

- Removal of air from the pleural space
- Reestablishment of negative intrapleural pressure
- Conversion of tension pneumothorax to simple pneumothorax
- Improved oxygenation and ventilation

Unexpected Outcomes

- Unresolved tension pneumothorax
- Resultant pneumothorax in a patient without tension pneumothorax
- Damage to nerves, veins, or arteries because of improper needle or catheter placement
- Local hematoma or cellulitis
- Pleural infection
- Unsuccessful placement of needle due to chest wall thickness, anatomical complications, or kinking of the catheter

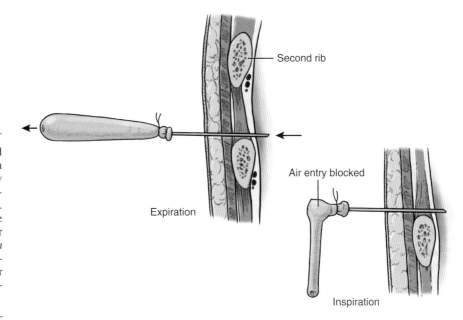

Figure 22.2 Use of a needle and a sterile finger cot or a finger from a sterile glove to fashion a one-way (flutter) valve for emergency evacuation of a tension pneumothorax. A small opening is made in the free end of the glove finger to allow air to escape during expiration. *(From Cosgriff JH: An atlas of diagnostic and therapeutic procedures for emergency personnel, Philadelphia, 1978, J.B. Lippincott.)*

Patient Monitoring and Care

Steps	Rationale	Reportable Conditions
		These conditions should be reported to the provider if they persist.
1. Assess vital signs.	Provides information regarding the patient's condition.	• Significant changes in the patient's vital signs
2. Stabilize the needle or catheter with a dressing until the chest tube is inserted.	Prevents movement and dislodgment of the needle or catheter. A chest tube should be inserted as soon as practical.	• Dislodged needle or catheter
3. Continuously monitor for signs and symptoms of tension pneumothorax.	Determines whether chest decompression has been successful and allows for early identification of new pneumothorax until a chest tube has been placed.	• Tracheal deviation to the unaffected side • Jugular vein distention • Sudden, sharp chest pain • Decreased or absent breath sounds on the affected side • Asymmetrical chest excursion with respirations • Tachypnea, shortness of breath, dyspnea, increased work of breathing • Decreased oxygen saturation • Subcutaneous emphysema • Anxiety, restlessness, apprehension • Tachycardia • Hypotension • Dysrhythmias • Cyanosis
4. Continuously monitor for catheter/needle occlusion due to clot formation at the catheter/needle tip.	Determines the need for repeated needle decompression and rapid insertion of a chest tube.	• Return of signs and symptoms of tension pneumothorax as listed previously
5. Follow institutional standards for assessing pain. Administer analgesia as prescribed.	Identifies the need for pain interventions.	• Continued pain despite pain interventions

Documentation

Documentation should include the following:
- Indications for needle thoracostomy
- Vital signs before and after insertion of the needle or catheter
- Location of the needle or catheter
- Size and length of the needle or catheter used
- Response after needle or catheter placement
- Occurrence of unexpected outcomes and related interventions
- Patient and family education
- Pain assessment, interventions, and effectiveness

References and Additional Readings

For a complete list of references and additional readings for this procedure, scan this QR code with your smartphone, or visit https://www.elsevier.com/__data/assets/pdf_file/0011/1319789/Chapter0022.pdf.

PROCEDURE

23 Thoracentesis (Perform) ![AP]

Kim Bowers

PURPOSE: Thoracentesis is performed to assist in the diagnosis and therapeutic management of patients with pleural effusions.

PREREQUISITE NURSING KNOWLEDGE

- Thoracentesis is performed with insertion of a needle or a catheter into the pleural space, which allows for removal of pleural fluid.
- Pleural effusions are defined as the accumulation of fluid in the pleural space that exceeds 10 mL and results from the overproduction of fluid or disruption in fluid reabsorption.[1]
- Thoracentesis is not used to verify the presence of pleural effusion. Diagnosis of pleural effusion is made via clinical examination, patient symptoms, and diagnostic techniques. A number of techniques can demonstrate pleural effusion with varying levels of sensitivity. Percussion requires a minimum of 300 to 400 mL for identification of a pleural effusion, whereas a standard chest radiography requires 200 to 300 mL. Lateral decubitus radiographs can be used to recognize smaller fluid amounts and highlight whether present fluid is free flowing. Ultrasound and computed tomography (CT) scan are more sensitive than chest radiographs in detecting very small effuisons.[1] Therefore initial diagnosis of pleural effusion may be optimized via imaging techniques such as chest radiographs, ultrasound scans, and CT scans combined with patient symptoms and clinical examination findings.
- Diagnostic thoracentesis is indicated for differential diagnosis in patients with pleural effusion of unknown etiology. A diagnostic thoracentesis may be repeated if initial results fail to yield a diagnosis.
- Therapeutic thoracentesis is indicated to relieve the symptoms (e.g., dyspnea, cough, hypoxemia, or chest pain) caused by a pleural effusion.
- Pleural effusions are classified as either *transudative* or *exudative* effusions.
- Samples of pleural fluid are analyzed and assist in distinguishing between exudative and transudative etiologies of effusion. Results of laboratory tests on pleural fluid alone do not establish a diagnosis; instead the laboratory results must be correlated with clinical findings and serum laboratory results.

![AP] This procedure should be performed only by clinicians who have demonstrated competence and are credentialed to perform it. In addition, the procedure must be within the scope of practice defined by their professional licensure, and in accordance with professional practice acts. Physicians, advanced practice nurses, and physician assistants may be credentialed to perform this procedure.

- Light's criteria should be used to distinguish between a pleural fluid exudate and transudate. To apply Light's criteria, the total protein and lactate dehydrogenase (LDH) should be measured in both blood and pleural fluid (Box 23.1).[6,8]
- Alternative diagnostic criteria also exist, including the two-test and three-test rule, which require one criterion to be met to define an exudate.[11]
  - ❖ Two test rule:
    - ○ Pleural fluid cholesterol is greater than 45 mg/dL
    - ○ Pleural fluid LDH greater than 0.45 times the upper limit of normal serum LDH
  - ❖ Three test rule:
    - ○ Pleural fluid protein is greater than 2.9 g/dL
    - ○ Pleural fluid cholesterol is greater than 45 mg/dL
    - ○ Pleural fluid LDH is greater than 0.45 times the upper limit of normal serum LDH
- Exudative effusions indicate a local etiology (e.g., pulmonary embolus, infection), whereas transudative effusions usually are associated with systemic etiologies (e.g., heart failure).[8]
- Relative contraindications for thoracentesis include the following:
  - ❖ Patient anatomy that hinders the practitioner from clearly identifying the appropriate landmarks
  - ❖ Patients actively undergoing anticoagulation therapy or with an uncorrectable coagulation disorder
  - ❖ Patients with severe hemodynamic compromise until stabilized
  - ❖ Patients with splenomegaly, elevated left hemidiaphragm, or left-sided pleural effusion
  - ❖ Patients with only one lung as a result of a previous pneumonectomy
  - ❖ Patients with active skin infection at the point of needle insertion (i.e., cellulitis or zoster)[5]
- Ultrasound-guided thoracentesis is thought to reduce complications.
- Complications commonly associated with thoracentesis include pneumothorax, hemopneumothorax, hemorrhage, hypotension, cough, pain, visceral injury, and reexpansion pulmonary edema.[4,5,7]
- The most common complications from pleural aspiration are pneumothorax, pain, hemothorax, and procedure failure.[10] The most serious complication is visceral injury.[4]
- Hypotension can occur as part of the vasovagal reaction, causing bradycardia, during or hours after the procedure. If it occurs during the procedure, cessation of the procedure and intravenous (IV) atropine may be necessary. If

BOX 23.1	Light's Criteria for Exudative Pleural Effusions (Applies If One or More Criteria Are Met)

EXUDATIVE CRITERIA

Ratio of pleural fluid protein to serum protein is >0.5.

Ratio of pleural fluid lactate dehydrogenase (LDH) to serum LDH is >0.6.

Pleural fluid LDH level is >$\frac{2}{3}$ of the upper limit of normal for serum LDH.

Modified from Porcel J, Light R: Diagnostic approach to pleural effusion in adults, *Am Fam Physician* 73(7):1211-1220, 2006.

hypotension occurs after the procedure, it is likely the result of fluid shifting from pleural effusion reaccumulation. In this situation, the patient is likely to respond to fluid resuscitation.[12]

- Development of cough generally initiates toward the end of the procedure and should result in procedure cessation.
- Reexpansion pulmonary edema is thought to occur from overdraining of fluid too quickly. The incidence is less than 1%, but asymptomatic radiologically apparent reperfusion pulmonary edema may be slightly more frequent.[4] The maximum volume of fluid that can be safely removed is uncertain because the volume removed does not clearly correlate with the onset of symptoms. Traditionally, to avoid this complication, discontinuation of fluid removal occurs with the onset of symptoms or when the total fluid removed reaches 1000 to 1500 mL.[4,7]
- If using continuous positive airway pressure, caution should be taken to avoid potential pneumothorax following aspiration if there is no pleural drain in place.[4] Patients receiving positive airway pressure can undergo thoracentesis with an ultrasound-guided incidence of less than 7% pneumothorax noted.[3,5]
- Baseline diagnostic study results (i.e., lateral decubitus chest radiograph, ultrasound imaging, CT scan, or MRI) should be reviewed before the procedure to identify the location and extent of pleural fluid accumulation.

EQUIPMENT

- Indelible marker
- Sterile drapes
- Sterile towels
- Adhesive bandage or adhesive strip
- Antiseptic solution
- Sterile 4 × 4 gauze pads
- Intervention medications (opioid, sedative, or hypnotic agents, local anesthetic 1% or 2% lidocaine)
- One small needle (25-gauge, ⅝-inch long)
- 5-mL syringe for local anesthetic
- Three large needles (20- to 22-gauge, 1½ to 2 inches long)
- Three-way stopcock
- Sterile 20-mL syringe
- Sterile 50-mL syringe
- Two chemistry blood tubes
- Hemostat or Kelly clamp
- Pulse oximetry equipment
- Side table

- Pillow or blanket to be placed on side table
- 14- and 16-gauge needle
- Thoracentesis kit
- Vacutainers or evacuated bottles (1 to 2 L) with pressure tubing

Additional equipment to have available as needed includes the following:

- Atropine, oxygen, thoracostomy supplies, advanced cardiac life-support equipment
- Ultrasound equipment as available and with a credentialed provider
- Two complete blood count tubes
- One anaerobic and one aerobic media bottle for culture and sensitivity
- Sterile tubes for fungal and tuberculosis cultures specimen tubes
- Commercially prepackaged thoracentesis kits, which are available in some institutions

PATIENT AND FAMILY EDUCATION

- Assess the patient's and family's level of understanding about the condition and rationale for the procedure. ***Rationale:*** This assessment identifies the patient's and family's knowledge deficits concerning the patient's condition, the procedure, the expected benefits, and the potential risks. It also allows time for questions to clarify information and voice concerns. Explanations decrease patient anxiety and enhance cooperation.
- Explain the procedure and the reason for the procedure if the clinical situation permits. If not, explain the procedure and reason for the thoracentesis after it is completed. ***Rationale:*** This explanation enhances patient and family understanding and decreases anxiety.
- Explain the patient's role in the thoracentesis. ***Rationale:*** This explanation increases patient compliance, facilitates needle and catheter insertion, and enhances fluid removal.

PATIENT ASSESSMENT AND PREPARATION

Patient Assessment

- Assess medical history of symptoms, occupational exposure, pleuritic chest pain, malignancy disease, heart failure, and medication usage. ***Rationale:*** Medical history may provide valuable clues to the cause of a patient's pleural effusion and the possible presence of any anticoagulation medications for underlying medical conditions. Knowledge of medication usage can indicate the need for anticoagulation reversal. In addition, an increasing number of medications are noted to contribute to exudative effusions. Visit http://www.pneumotox.com for more information.[2]
- Assess for signs and symptoms of pleural effusion. ***Rationale:*** Physical findings may suggest a pleural effusion.
  - ❖ Trachea deviated away from the affected side
  - ❖ Affected side dull to flat with percussion
  - ❖ Absent or decreased breath sounds

- ❖ Tactile fremitus
- ❖ Pleuritic chest pain
- ❖ Hypoxemia
- ❖ Tachypnea
- ❖ Dyspnea
- ❖ Cough, weight loss, night sweats, anorexia, and malaise may also occur with pleural infection or malignancy disease
- Assess chest radiograph or other imaging findings. Posterior-anterior chest radiographs should be performed in the assessment of all suspected pleural effusions.[6] *Rationale:* If at least half the hemidiaphragm is obliterated on erect anterior-posterior radiograph results, sufficient fluid is in the pleural space for a thoracentesis. Greater than 200 mL of fluid is considered abnormal in erect chest radiograph results.
- If a small amount of loculated fluid is noted, a lateral decubitus radiograph should be obtained. *Rationale:* Lateral decubitus radiographs assist with distinguishing between free-moving fluid and pleural thickening. Lateral radiographs show blunting of the costophrenic angle with 50 mL. If the pleural effusion is measured to be greater than 10 mm deep on a lateral decubitus radiograph, a diagnostic thoracentesis can be performed.[1]
- Anterior-posterior chest radiographs completed in the intensive care setting are typically completed in the supine position and are less sensitive in the identification of pleural effusions. In this setting, hazy opacification of one lung field or minor fissure thickening may be the only clues to the presence of a pleural effusion.[1] *Rationale:* In the supine position, pleural effusions tend to spread out across the posterior thoracic surface and are less evident on supine radiographs.
- Thoracic ultrasound guidance is strongly recommended for all pleural procedures for pleural fluid acquisition.[4,10] Marking of the site using thoracic ultrasound for subsequent remote aspiration is not recommended except for large pleural effusions.[4] *Rationale:* Ultrasound-guided pleural aspiration has been shown to increase the yield and reduce the risk of complications, particularly pneumothoraces and inadvertent organ puncture. Ultrasound detects pleural fluid septations with greater sensitivity than computed tomography.[6]
- CT scans with contrast should be performed for pleural enhancement before complete drainage of the fluid. *Rationale:* CT scans are useful in distinguishing malignant from benign pleural thickening. CT scan results may also be helpful when complicated pleural infection is present or if initial tube drainage is unsuccessful and surgery is to be considered.[6]

- Assess baseline vital signs, including pulse oximetry. *Rationale:* Baseline assessment data provide information about patient's cardiopulmonary status and allow for comparison during and after the procedure.
- Assess recent serum laboratory results, including the following. *Rationale:* These studies help determine whether the patient is at risk for bleeding. Although thoracentesis is considered to have a low risk of bleeding, an international normalized ratio of 2 or less is acceptable for invasive procedures.[4] Platelet transfusion is recommended for counts less than 50,000 mL. No consensus/recommendations exist for partial thromboplastin time and hematocrit thresholds. There is no evidence to support the use of bleeding times before minimally invasive procedures.[9]
  - ❖ Hematocrit
  - ❖ Platelet count
  - ❖ Prothrombin time/international normalized ratio
  - ❖ Partial thromboplastin time

Patient Preparation

- Verify the correct patient with two identifiers. *Rationale:* Before performing a procedure, the nurse should ensure the correct identification of the patient for the intended intervention.
- Ensure that the patient understands preprocedural teachings. Answer questions as they arise, and reinforce information as needed. *Rationale:* This communication evaluates and reinforces understanding of previously taught information.
- Obtain written informed consent for the procedure. *Rationale:* Invasive procedures, unless performed with implied consent in a life-threatening situation, require written consent of the patient or significant other.
- Consider medications for pain, sedation, or chemical paralysis, as indicated by the patient's condition. *Rationale:* Pain and sedation medications or chemical paralysis may be necessary to maximize positioning. If utilizing sedation or paralysis, ensure that airway adjuncts or definitive airways are secured before induction.
- Have atropine available. *Rationale:* Bradycardia, from a vasovagal reflex, can occur during thoracentesis.
- Initiate pulse oximetry monitoring. *Rationale:* Pulse oximetry provides a noninvasive means for monitoring oxygenation and heart rate at the bedside, which allows for prompt recognition and intervention should problems develop.
- Ensure patent intravenous access. *Rationale:* Provides IV access for both procedural and emergency medications, as necessary.

Procedure for Diagnostic and Therapeutic Thoracentesis

Steps	Rationale	Special Considerations
Diagnostic Thoracentesis 1. 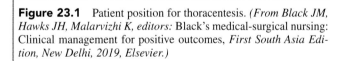 2. 3. Assemble equipment and review of available imaging.	Ensures that proper equipment is readily available throughout the procedure and in emergency situations. Review of imaging ensures that the proper side has been selected and provides anatomical guidance to the practitioner.[7]	Ultrasound guidance reduces complications associated with pleural procedures in the critical care setting, and its routine use is recommended.[4] **(Level D*)**
4. Position the patient for the procedure with an assistant standing in front of the patient. If the patient is alert and able, position the patient on the edge of the bed with feet supported on a stool and arms resting on a pillow on an elevated bedside table (Fig. 23.1). The patient may sit on a chair backward and rest arms on a pillow on the back of the chair. If the patient is unable to sit, position the patient in the lateral recumbent position on the unaffected side, with the back near the edge of the bed and the arm on the affected side above the head. Elevate the head of the bed to 30 or 45 degrees, as tolerated.	Positioning enhances ease of withdrawal of pleural fluid. Ensuring that the patient is comfortable increases the chance that the procedure will be successfully completed. Having the assistant in front of the patient ensures visualization of facial cues and enables the cessation of inadvertent patient movements that might interfere with the procedure.	

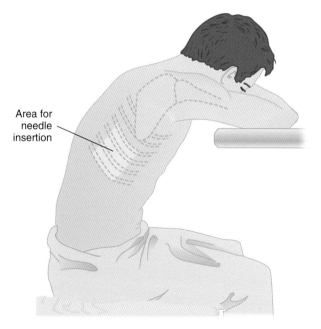

Area for needle insertion

Figure 23.1 Patient position for thoracentesis. *(From Black JM, Hawks JH, Malarvizhi K, editors:* Black's medical-surgical nursing: Clinical management for positive outcomes, *First South Asia Edition, New Delhi, 2019, Elsevier.)*

*Level D: Peer-reviewed professional and organizational standards with the support of clinical study recommendations

Procedure for Diagnostic and Therapeutic Thoracentesis—*Continued*

Steps	Rationale	Special Considerations
5. If not utilizing ultrasound, the following physical examination utilizing landmarks should be completed. Percuss the affected side posteriorly to determine the highest point of the pleural effusion. Effusion is generally noted using the following: one to two interspaces below the level at which breath sounds disappear on auscultation or become decreased, percussion becomes dull, or fremitus disappears. Identify the intercostal space below this point but above the ninth rib. Once the level is noted, a mark should be made 9–10 cm lateral to the spine moving toward the posterior axillary line.	Identifies the superior border of the pleural effusion and identifies and validates the planned site for thoracentesis. Palpation midway between the spine and posterior axillary line is a location where the ribs can generally be palpated. Accessing above the ninth rib minimizes potential injury to solid organs. Accessing 9–10 cm lateral to the spine below the eighth rib was noted to be associated with decreased cannulation of tortuous vessels and has been deemed the "safe zone."[4-6]	Use the posterior axillary line as the insertion point to avoid the spinal cord. If the space identified for insertion is below the eighth intercostal space (area is approximated at the posterior edge of the scapula), an ultrasound scan should be done to mark the fluid level and its relationship to the diaphragm, which helps identify a safe point of entry to avoid solid-organ damage. When able, ultrasound guidance should be utilized to identify effusion location.[4-6] **(Level D*)**
6. Apply PPE, while an assistant opens the necessary equipment onto a sterile field or opens the appropriate sterile tray with the equipment.	Reduces the transmission of microorganisms and body secretions during an invasive procedure.	
7. Have an assistant provide preprocedural medications.	Premedication with opioid, antianxiolytic, sedative, or hypnotic ensures patient comfort throughout the procedure.	
8. Perform a preprocedure verification and time out, if nonemergent.	Ensures patient safety.	
9. Sterilize a wide area surrounding the insertion site using 0.05% chlorhexidine or 10% povidone-iodine solution. Use concentric circles from the insertion site mark outward, and drape the area with a sterile drape.	Although the pleural space is efficient in clearing bacteria, aseptic technique minimizes skin contaminants, which reduces the risk of infection.[5]	
10. Anesthetize the skin with 1%–2% lidocaine (25-gauge, ⅝-inch needle) in the typical wheal fashion around the insertion site.	Increases patient comfort by anesthetizing the skin.	
11. With lidocaine, insert a 20- to 22-gauge, 1½- to 2-inch needle through the wheal. Advance the needle toward the rib, aspirating then injecting the lidocaine into the deep tissue. "Walk" the needle over the superior edge of the rib and periosteum of the underlying rib superiorly and laterally. The exact puncture site should be immediately above the superior aspect of a rib and, when possible, 8–10 cm lateral from the spine.[7]	Anesthetizes the work area for optimal patient comfort. Insertion above the rib minimizes manipulation or laceration of the vascular bundle located beneath the rib and the intercostal arteries (Fig. 23.2).[5,7] **(Level C*)**	Always aspirate before injecting to prevent lidocaine from entering a blood vessel or the pleural space. A longer needle may be needed in extremely obese patients.

*Level C: Qualitative studies, descriptive or correlational studies, integrative reviews, systematic reviews, or randomized controlled trials with inconsistent results
*Level D: Peer-reviewed professional and organizational standards with the support of clinical study recommendations

Procedure continues on following page

UNIT I

Procedure	for Diagnostic and Therapeutic Thoracentesis—*Continued*		
Steps	**Rationale**	**Special Considerations**	
12. After anesthetizing the periosteum of the underlying rib, gently advance the needle, and alternately aspirate and inject lidocaine until pleural fluid is obtained in the syringe.	In addition to anesthetizing the parietal pleura, utilizing this technique the pleural space is identified by pleural fluid aspirate in the syringe.[1,5] If air bubbles are noted, the lung tissue may have been violated, or air may have been introduced by the thoracentesis system. Withdraw the syringe to the tissue, and redirect. Withdrawal of the needle minimizes manipulation of lung tissue.		
13. When pleural fluid is obtained, place a sterile gloved finger on the needle at the point where the needle exits the skin. Withdraw the needle and syringe. For therapeutic thoracentesis, proceed to **Step 21.**	Approximates the length of insertion for the thoracentesis needle or catheter.		
14. Attach a three-way stopcock and 50-mL syringe to a 20- to 22-gauge, 1½- or 2-inch needle. Open the stopcock valve between the syringe and the needle.	The open stopcock valve allows for aspiration of pleural fluid during needle insertion and minimizes atmospheric air introduction.	Longer needles may be necessary in the obese patient.	

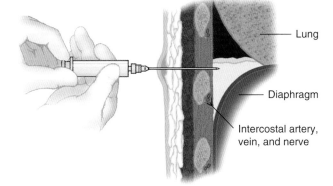

Figure 23.2 Ideal placement of needle insertion. *(From Kacmarek RM, Stoller JK, Heuer AJ, Egan's fundamentals of respiratory care, ed 12, St. Louis, MO, 2021, Elsevier.)*

Lung

Diaphragm

Intercostal artery, vein, and nerve

Steps	Rationale	Special Considerations
15. Insert the selected needle via the anesthetized tract, superior to the rib, and continually aspirate until pleural fluid is obtained, filling the 50-mL syringe. Fluid should be separated into three sterile containers for microbiology, biochemistry, and cytology analysis.	Inserting the needle superior to the rib avoids disruption of the vascular and lymph systems (see Fig. 23.2). The pleural fluid is used for laboratory testing for the differential diagnosis. A sample of 35–50 mL is needed for a diagnostic analysis of fluid. A change in patient position can be attempted to facilitate fluid drainage.	It is possible that no fluid is accessed (dry tap). If a dry tap occurs, the needle may be withdrawn and reinserted at a slightly different angle if the patient tolerated the initial "dry tap." A second tap warrants reevaluation with an ultrasound examination if not initially employed.[5] A larger-gauge needle may be needed for thick or loculated fluid, or the needle may have been inserted above or below the pleural fluid. When pleural fluid is aspirated, the needle may be stabilized with placing a hemostat or clamp on the needle at the skin site to keep the needle from advancing farther into the pleural space, preventing lung puncture. Note the appearance of the aspirated fluid because this may provide clues to the underlying etiology of the effusion. Straw-colored fluid is common and typical of transudates. Blood-stained fluid is suggestive of hemothorax, malignancy disease, pulmonary infarction, trauma, or postcoronary artery bypass surgery. Fluid turbidity suggests empyema or chylothorax, and food particles indicate esophageal rupture.
16. Fill the specimen tubes from the pleural fluid–filled syringe by turning the stopcock "off" to the patient and allowing the tubes to fill passively by vacuum or by depressing the syringe plunger (Fig. 23.3). Send the specimen tubes to the laboratory for appropriate analysis.	Analysis may aid in determining an etiology of the pleural effusion.	To interpret pleural fluid laboratory values utilizing Light's criteria, serum and pleural fluid chemistry laboratory values must be obtained (e.g., total protein and LDH). Initial laboratory testing may also include cytology, gram stain, culture, amylase, and glucose.[5]

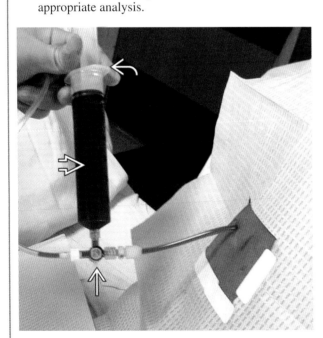

Figure 23.3 Attaching a catheter to a three-way stopcock and syringe. *(From Wible BC: Diagnostic imaging: Interventional procedures, ed 2, Salt Lake City, UT, 2018, Elsevier.)*

Procedure continues on following page

Procedure for Diagnostic and Therapeutic Thoracentesis—*Continued*

Steps	Rationale	Special Considerations
17. Evaluate patient response throughout the procedure.	Monitoring patient heart rate, pulse oximetry, and clinical response throughout the procedure enables prompt intervention or cessation of the procedure should complications arise.	
18. On completion of diagnostic thoracentesis, withdraw the needle. Apply pressure to the puncture site for a few minutes, and then apply an adhesive strip or adhesive bandage over the puncture site. Without concrete clinical indications, (i.e., withdraw of air, multiple needle passes, or clinical changes), a chest radiograph is not necessary after a routine thoracentesis.[5-7,10] (**Level C***)	If the patient is nonventilated and asymptomatic, only 1% of patients were noted to have a pneumothorax on a postthoracentesis chest radiograph.[5]	If air is aspirated during the procedure, multiple needle passes are required, or the patient develops signs of a pneumothorax, imaging should be ordered. Postthoracentesis chest radiography in mechanically ventilated patients remains controversial.[5]
19. Discard used supplies, and remove **PE**.		
20. **HH**		
Therapeutic Thoracentesis		
21. Once the insertion site is anesthetized, make a cut through the epidermis using the #11 blade scalpel in the thoracentesis kit.	The cut should be through the full thickness of the epidermis to ensure that the catheter does not become "hung up" on the skin surface, impeding its penetration.	
22. With the stopcock attached, the over-the-needle catheter is inserted into the skin while applying negative pressure to the syringe.	Over-the-needle catheters have stopcocks permanently affixed to the catheter and closed to the patient so when the needle is removed, there is no risk of pneumothorax from entrainment of air into the pleural space.	
23. When fluid is aspirated, the needle is inserted another 5 mm to ensure that both the needle and the catheter are positioned within the pleural fluid collection.		
24. The needle introducer is held stationary while the catheter is pushed forward over the needle until the catheter hub is against the skin. The needle is then removed (through the stopcock), and the catheter and stopcock remain in place.	Never pull the catheter back through the needle because the catheter may be cut or sheared by the needle tip.	

*Level C: Qualitative studies, descriptive or correlational studies, integrative reviews, systematic reviews, or randomized controlled trials with inconsistent results.

Procedure for Diagnostic and Therapeutic Thoracentesis—*Continued*		
Steps	**Rationale**	**Special Considerations**
25. Fill the 50-mL syringe with pleural fluid. Fill the specimen tubes from the pleural fluid–filled syringe by turning the stopcock "off" to the patient and allowing the tubes to fill passively by vacuum or by depressing the syringe plunger (see Fig. 23.3). Send the specimen tubes to the laboratory for appropriate analysis.	When changing syringes, be certain the stopcock is positioned such that air does not enter the pleural space. Analysis may aid in determining an etiology of the pleural effusion.	To interpret pleural fluid chemistry laboratory values, serum chemistry laboratory values also must be obtained (see the "Diagnostic Thoracentesis" section). Local anesthetics (i.e., lidocaine) are acidic; therefore care should be taken during pleural sampling to avoid contamination of the sample.[5]
26. Attach the vacutainer or evacuated bottles with tubing to the three-way stopcock. Open the valve to the vacutainer, and fill the vacutainer.	The vacutainer or evacuated bottles use negative pressure to withdraw pleural fluid from the pleural space, providing therapeutic relief. Reposition the catheter or patient, or both if drainage stops to determine whether fluid is still present.	The maximum volume of fluid that can be safely removed is uncertain because the volume removed does not clearly correlate with the onset of symptoms. Traditionally, to avoid this complication, discontinuation of fluid removal occurs with the onset of symptoms or when the total fluid removed reaches 1000–1500 mL.[4,7] **(Level E*)** The patient may feel the need to cough as the lung re-expands.
27. On completion of thoracentesis, remove the catheter. Apply pressure to the puncture site for a few minutes, and then apply an adhesive strip or adhesive bandage over the puncture site. **(Level C*)**	If the patient is nonventilated and asymptomatic, only 1% of patients were noted to have a pneumothorax on a postthoracentesis chest radiograph.[5]	If air is aspirated during the procedure, multiple needle passes are required, or if the patient develops signs of a pneumothorax, imaging should be ordered. Postthoracentesis chest radiography in mechanically ventilated patients remains controversial.[5]
28. Reposition the patient to optimize comfort.	The patient may desire to lie down after the procedure. Head of bed placement may vary if dyspnea, hypotension, or other symptoms re-present during procedure.	
29. Dispose of equipment, and remove **PE**.		
30. **HH**		

*Level C: Qualitative studies, descriptive or correlational studies, integrative reviews, systematic reviews, or randomized controlled trials with inconsistent results.
*Level E: Multiple case reports, theory-based evidence from expert opinions, or peer-reviewed professional organizational standards without clinical studies to support recommendations.

Expected Outcomes

- Patient is comfortable and has decreased respiratory distress
- Lung reexpansion occurs
- Site remains infection free
- Procedure aids in diagnosis of etiology of pleural effusion

Unexpected Outcomes

- Pneumothorax
- Vasovagal response
- Dyspnea
- Hypovolemia
- Hematoma
- Hemothorax
- Liver or splenic laceration
- Reexpansion pulmonary edema

Patient Monitoring and Care

Steps	Rationale	Reportable Conditions
		These conditions should be reported if they persist despite nursing interventions.
1. Monitor vital signs and cardiopulmonary status before and after thoracentesis and as needed.	Any change in vital signs may alert the practitioner of possible unexpected outcomes. Use of supplemental oxygen may be necessary.	• Tachypnea • Decreased or absent breath sounds on the affected side • Shortness of breath, dyspnea • Asymmetrical chest excursion with respirations • Decreased oxygen saturation • Subcutaneous emphysema • Sudden sharp chest pain • Anxiety, restlessness, apprehension • Tachycardia • Hypotension • Dysrhythmias • Tracheal deviation to the unaffected side • Neck vein distention • Muffled heart sounds
2. If indicated, obtain a postthoracentesis expiratory chest radiograph.[10] (**Level D***)	A chest radiograph is used to evaluate for lung reexpansion and evidence of a possible pneumothorax or hemothorax. If a pneumothorax or hemothorax is present, a chest tube may be necessary. Without concrete clinical indications, chest radiography is not necessary after a routine thoracentesis.[4,6,8]	• Pneumothorax • Expanding pleural effusion • Catheter migration
3. Follow institutional standards for assessing pain. Administer analgesia as prescribed.	Identifies need for pain interventions.	• Continued pain despite pain interventions

*Level D: Peer-reviewed professional and organizational standards with the support of clinical study recommendations.

Documentation

Documentation should include the following:
• Patient and family teaching
• Consent for procedure
• Patient positioning and monitoring devices
• Medication administration and patient response
• Patient tolerance, including procedural pain and instillation and response to pain medications
• Insertion of catheter or needle
• Catheter or needle size used
• Any difficulties in insertion
• Pleural fluid aspirate characteristics
• Total amount of pleural fluid aspirated
• Site assessment
• Intact catheter on withdrawal
• Occurrence of unexpected outcomes
• Post-thoracentesis radiograph acquisition and results, as needed/available
• Laboratory test ordered and results as available
• Interpretation of laboratory results
• Nursing interventions
• Pain assessment, interventions, and effectiveness

References and Additional Readings

For a complete list of references and additional readings for this procedure, scan this QR code with your smartphone, or visit https://www.elsevier.com/__data/assets/pdf_file/0011/1319798 /Chapter0023.pdf

24 Thoracentesis (Assist)

Kim Bowers

PURPOSE: Thoracentesis is performed to assist in the diagnosis and therapeutic management of patients with pleural effusions.

PREREQUISITE NURSING KNOWLEDGE

- Thoracentesis is performed with insertion of a needle or a catheter into the pleural space, which allows for removal of pleural fluid.
- Pleural effusions are defined as the accumulation of fluid in the pleural space that exceeds 10 mL and results from the overproduction of fluid or disruption in fluid reabsorption.[1]
- Diagnostic thoracentesis is indicated for differential diagnosis for patients with pleural effusion of unknown etiology. A diagnostic thoracentesis may be repeated if initial results fail to yield a diagnosis.
- Therapeutic thoracentesis is indicated to relieve the symptoms (e.g., dyspnea, cough, hypoxemia, or chest pain) caused by a pleural effusion.
- Samples of pleural fluid are analyzed and assist in distinguishing between exudative and transudative etiologies of effusion. Results of laboratory tests on pleural fluid alone do not establish a diagnosis; instead the laboratory results must be correlated with the clinical findings and serum laboratory results.
- Exudative effusions indicate a local etiology (e.g., pulmonary embolus, infection), whereas transudative effusions usually are associated with systemic etiologies (e.g., heart failure).
- Relative contraindications for thoracentesis include the following:
  - Patient anatomy that hinders the practitioner from clearly identifying the appropriate landmarks
  - Patients actively undergoing anticoagulation therapy or with an uncorrectable coagulation disorder
  - Patients with severe hemodynamic compromise until stabilized
  - Patients with splenomegaly, elevated left hemidiaphragm, or left-sided pleural effusion
  - Patients with only one lung as a result of a previous pneumonectomy
  - Patients with active skin infection at the point of needle insertion[5]
- Ultrasound-guided thoracentesis is thought to reduce complications.
- Complications commonly associated with thoracentesis include: pneumothorax, hemopneumothorax, hemorrhage, hypotension, cough, pain, visceral injury, and reexpansion pulmonary edema.[4,5,7]

- The most common complications from pleural aspiration are pneumothorax, pain, hemothorax, and procedure failure.[10] The most serious complication is visceral injury.[4]
- Hypotension can occur as part of the vasovagal reaction, causing bradycardia, during or hours after the procedure. If it occurs during the procedure, cessation of the procedure and intravenous (IV) atropine may be necessary. If hypotension occurs after the procedure, it is likely the result of fluid shifting from pleural effusion re-accumulation. In this situation, the patient is likely to respond to fluid resuscitation.[11]
- Development of cough generally initiates toward the end of the procedure and should result in procedure cessation.
- Reexpansion pulmonary edema is thought to occur from overdraining of fluid too quickly. The incidence is less than 1%, but asymptomatic radiological pulmonary edema may be slightly more frequent.[4] The maximum volume of fluid that can be safely removed is uncertain because the volume removed does not clearly correlate with the onset of symptoms. Traditionally, to avoid this complication, discontinuation of fluid removal occurs with the onset of symptoms or when the total fluid removed reaches 1000 to 1500 mL.[4,7]
- If using continuous positive airway pressure, caution should be taken to avoid potential pneumothorax following aspiration if there is no pleural drain in place.[5] Patients receiving positive airway pressure can undergo thoracentesis with an ultrasound-guided incidence of less than 7% pneumothorax noted.[3,5]

EQUIPMENT

- Indelible marker
- Sterile gloves
- Sterile drapes
- Sterile towels
- Adhesive bandage or adhesive strip
- Antiseptic solution
- Sterile 4 × 4 gauze pads
- Intervention medications (opioid, sedative, or hypnotic agents, local anesthetic 1% or 2% lidocaine)
- One small needle (25-gauge, ⅝-inch long)
- 5-mL syringe for local anesthetic
- Three large needles (20- to 22-gauge, 1½ to 2 inches long)
- Three-way stopcock
- Sterile 20-mL syringe
- Sterile 50-mL syringe

- Two chemistry blood tubes
- Hemostat or Kelly clamp
- Pulse oximetry equipment
- Side table
- Pillow or blanket to be placed on side table
- 14- and 16-gauge needle
- Thoracentesis kit: Safe T Plus Thora/Paracentesis Kit
- Vacutainers or evacuated bottles (1 to 2 L) with pressure tubing

Additional equipment to have available as needed includes the following:
- Atropine, oxygen, thoracostomy supplies, advanced cardiac life-support equipment
- Ultrasound equipment as available and with a credentialed provider
- Two complete blood count tubes
- One anaerobic and one aerobic media bottle for culture and sensitivity
- Sterile tubes for fungal and tuberculosis cultures specimen tubes
- Commercially prepackaged thoracentesis kits that are available in some institutions

PATIENT AND FAMILY EDUCATION

- Assess the patient's and family's level of understanding about the condition and rationale for the procedure. ***Rationale:*** This assessment identifies the patient's and family's knowledge deficits concerning the patient's condition, the procedure, the expected benefits, and the potential risks. It also allows time for questions to clarify information and voice concerns. Explanations decrease patient anxiety and enhance cooperation.
- Explain the procedure and the reason for the procedure if the clinical situation permits. If not, explain the procedure and reason for the thoracentesis after it is completed. ***Rationale:*** This explanation enhances patient and family understanding and decreases anxiety.
- Explain the patient's role in thoracentesis. ***Rationale:*** This explanation increases patient compliance, facilitates needle and catheter insertion, and enhances fluid removal.

PATIENT ASSESSMENT AND PREPARATION

Patient Assessment

- Assess medical history of symptoms, occupational exposure, pleuritic chest pain, malignancy disease, heart failure, and medication usage. ***Rationale:*** Medical history may provide valuable clues to the cause of a patient's pleural effusion and the possible presence of any anticoagulation medications for underlying medical conditions. Knowledge of medication usage can indicate the need for anticoagulation reversal. In addition, an increasing number of medications are noted to contribute to exudative effusions. Visit http://www.pneumotox.com for more information.[2]

- Assess for signs and symptoms of pleural effusion. ***Rationale:*** Physical findings may suggest a pleural effusion.
  - ❖ Trachea deviated away from the affected side
  - ❖ Affected side dull to flat with percussion
  - ❖ Absent or decreased breath sounds
  - ❖ Tactile fremitus
  - ❖ Pleuritic chest pain
  - ❖ Hypoxemia
  - ❖ Tachypnea
  - ❖ Dyspnea
  - ❖ Cough, weight loss, night sweats, anorexia, and malaise may also occur with pleural infection or malignancy disease
- Anterior-posterior chest radiographs completed in the intensive care setting are typically completed in the supine position and are less sensitive in the identification of pleural effusions. In this setting, hazy opacification of one lung field or minor fissure thickening may be the only clues to the presence of a pleural effusion.[1] ***Rationale:*** In the supine position, pleural effusions tend to spread out across the posterior thoracic surface and are less evident on supine radiographs.
- Assess baseline vital signs, including pulse oximetry. ***Rationale:*** Baseline assessment data provide information about patient status and allow for comparison during and after the procedure.
- Assess recent serum laboratory results, including the following. ***Rationale:*** These studies help determine whether the patient is at risk for bleeding. Although thoracentesis is considered to have a low risk of bleeding, an international normalized ratio of 2 or less is acceptable for invasive procedures.[4] Platelet transfusion is recommended for counts less than 50,000. No consensus/recommendations exist for partial thromboplastin time and hematocrit thresholds. There is no evidence to support the use of bleeding times before minimally invasive procedures.[9]
  - ❖ Hematocrit
  - ❖ Platelet count
  - ❖ Prothrombin time/international normalized ratio
  - ❖ Partial thromboplastin time

Patient Preparation

- Verify the correct patient with two identifiers. ***Rationale:*** Before performing a procedure, the nurse should ensure that a time out was completed to verify the correct identification of the patient for the intended intervention.
- Ensure that the patient understands the preprocedural teachings. Answer questions as they arise, and reinforce information. ***Rationale:*** This communication evaluates and reinforces understanding of previously taught information.
- Ensure that written informed consent for the procedure has been completed. ***Rationale:*** Invasive procedures, unless performed with implied consent in a life-threatening situation, require written consent of the patient or caregiver.
- Assist with patient positioning. Several alternative positions may be used, as follows. ***Rationale:*** Positioning enhances patient comfort and ease of pleural fluid withdraw.

- ❖ On the edge of the bed with legs supported and arms resting on a pillow on the elevated bedside table (see Fig. 23.1).
- ❖ Backwards on a chair with arms resting on a pillow over the chair back.
- If the patient is unable to sit, position the patient on the unaffected side, with the back near the edge of the bed and the arm on the affected side above the head. Elevate the head of the bed to 30 or 45 degrees, as tolerated. Position yourself or another member of the healthcare team in front of the patient. ***Rationale:*** This positioning enables visualization of facial cues and a close proximity to reassure or comfort the patient.

- Inquire about the need for sedation or paralysis. ***Rationale:*** For intubated patients, sedation or paralysis may be necessary to maximize positioning.
- Have atropine available. ***Rationale:*** Bradycardia, from a vasovagal reflex, is not uncommon during thoracentesis.
- Initiate pulse oximetry monitoring. ***Rationale:*** Pulse oximetry provides a noninvasive means for monitoring oxygenation and heart rate at the bedside, which allows for prompt recognition and intervention should problems develop.
- Ensure patent IV access. ***Rationale:*** Provides IV access for both procedural and emergency medications, as necessary.

Procedure for Assisting With Diagnostic and Therapeutic Thoracentesis

Steps	Rationale	Special Considerations
1. HH		
2. PE		
3. Assemble equipment and procedure tray.	Ensures that proper equipment is readily available throughout the procedure and in emergency situations.	
4. Assist with patient positioning.	Positioning that optimizes patient comfort aids in patient cooperation and completion of the procedure.	
5. Assume a position in front of the patient, and provide physical support for positioning, as necessary.	Positioning in front of the patient ensures visualization of facial cues and enables the cessation of inadvertent patient movements that might interfere with the procedure.	
6. As directed by physician or advanced practice provider, administer procedural medications.	Premedication with an opioid, antianxiolytic, sedative, or hypnotic ensures patient comfort throughout the procedure.	
7. Throughout procedure, assist with providing continuous monitoring of patient vital signs and response to the procedure and interventions.	The physician or advanced practice provider is focused on the technique required to obtain the fluid and may be delayed in noticing patient changes.	
8 As directed by the physician or advanced practice provider, assist with filling of the specimen tubes from the pleural fluid–filled syringe. Label it appropriately, and send the specimen tubes to the laboratory for appropriate analysis.	Analysis may aid in determining an etiology of the pleural effusion.	To interpret pleural fluid laboratory values, serum chemistry laboratory values must be obtained (e.g., pH, total protein, glucose, and lactate dehydrogenase).
9. As directed by physician or advanced practice provider, assist with attaching the vacutainer or evacuated bottles with tubing to the three-way stopcock.	The vacutainer or evacuated bottles use negative pressure to withdraw pleural fluid from the pleural space, providing therapeutic relief. Assist in repositioning the patient if drainage stops, as directed.	Evacuating more than 1000–1500 mL of pleural fluid at one time may cause hypovolemia, hypoxemia, or reexpansion pulmonary edema. The patient may feel the need to cough as the lung reexpands.

Procedure continues on following page

Procedure	for Assisting With Diagnostic and Therapeutic Thoracentesis—*Continued*	
Steps	**Rationale**	**Special Considerations**
10. On completion of thoracentesis, the physician or advanced practice provider may apply pressure to the puncture site for a few minutes. After pressure application has been completed, apply an adhesive bandage over the puncture site.		Without concrete clinical indications, a chest radiograph is not necessary after routine thoracentesis.
11. Reposition the patient to optimize comfort.	Patient may desire to lie down after procedure completion. Head-of-bed placement may vary if dyspnea, hypotension, or other symptoms are present during the procedure.	
12. Dispose of soiled supplies, and remove **PE**		
13. **HH**		

Expected Outcomes

- Patient is comfortable and has decreased respiratory distress
- Lung reexpansion occurs
- Site remains infection free
- Procedure aids in diagnosing of etiology of pleural effusion

Unexpected Outcomes

- Pneumothorax
- Vasovagal response
- Dyspnea
- Hypovolemia
- Hematoma
- Hemothorax
- Liver or splenic laceration
- Reexpansion pulmonary edema

Patient Monitoring and Care

Steps	Rationale	Reportable Conditions
1. Monitor vital signs and cardiopulmonary status before, during, and after thoracentesis.	Any change in vital signs may alert the practitioner of possible unexpected outcomes. Use of supplemental oxygen may be necessary.	*These conditions should be reported to the provider if they persist despite nursing interventions.* • Tachypnea • Decreased or absent breath sounds on the affected side • Shortness of breath, dyspnea • Asymmetrical chest excursion with respirations • Decreased oxygen saturation • Subcutaneous emphysema • Sudden sharp chest pain • Anxiety, restlessness, apprehension • Tachycardia • Hypotension • Dysrhythmias • Tracheal deviation to the unaffected side • Neck vein distention • Muffled heart sounds

Patient Monitoring and Care —*Continued*

Steps	Rationale	Reportable Conditions
2. If indicated, obtain a postthoracentesis expiratory chest radiograph.[10] (**Level D***)	A chest radiograph is used to evaluate for lung reexpansion and evidence of a possible pneumothorax or hemothorax. If a pneumothorax or hemothorax is present, a chest tube may be necessary. Without concrete clinical indications, a chest radiograph is not necessary after routine thoracentesis.[4,6,8]	• Pneumothorax • Catheter migration • Expanding pleural effusion
3. Follow institution standards for assessing pain. Administer analgesia as prescribed.	Identifies the need for pain interventions.	• Continued pain despite pain interventions

*Level D: Peer-reviewed professional and organizational standards with the support of clinical study recommendations.

Documentation

Documentation should include the following:
- Patient and family teaching
- Presence of completed consent for the procedure
- Adherence to Universal Protocol
- Patient positioning and monitoring devices
- Medication administration and patient response
- Patient tolerance, including procedural pain and instillation and response to pain medications
- Pleural fluid aspirate characteristics
- Total amount of pleural fluid aspirated
- Site assessment
- Occurrence of unexpected outcomes
- Postthoracentesis radiograph acquisition and results, as needed/available
- Laboratory tests ordered and results, as available
- Nursing interventions
- Pain assessment, interventions, and effectiveness

References and Additional Readings

For a complete list of references and additional readings for this procedure, scan this QR code with your smartphone, or visit https://www.elsevier.com/__data/assets/pdf_file/0012/1319799/Chapter0024.pdf

25 Bronchoscopy (Perform) AP

Chong Sherry Cheever

PURPOSE Bronchoscopy is an invasive procedure performed to assist in the diagnostic and therapeutic management of patients with abnormal respiratory function and/or abnormal radiographic findings.

PREREQUISITE NURSING KNOWLEDGE

- Bronchoscopy is performed by advancing a camera encased in a long tube through the oral cavity (or endotracheal tube), to the larynx, the bronchus, and to each section of the lung. This process allows for visualization of the lung and to obtain specimens to diagnose pulmonary illness.[9]
- Healthcare providers performing the procedure must have a knowledge of pulmonary physiology and the anatomy of each section of the lung (Fig. 25.1) as well as knowledge of how to operate bronchoscopy equipment.[1,2,5]
- A bronchoscope is a small-circumference tube that has three elements bundled within the tube: a fiberoptic camera, suction, and a small opening called a *C port* that is used for irrigation and to place assistive tools like a needle or protective brush (Fig. 25.2).[4]
- Chest x-ray or computed tomography (CT) of the chest should be performed before bronchoscopy to identify the segment of the lung that requires inspection or collection of a specimen.
- Bronchoscopy is indicated if imaging studies demonstrate abnormal findings such as consolidation, a foreign object, or a nodule.
- Bronchoscopy can be performed for diagnostic or therapeutic purposes. Indications for bronchoscopy include the following:
  - Removal of foreign objects that may have been aspirated
  - Pneumonia or infiltrates
  - Specimen collection (protected specimens without oral contamination may be obtained via bronchial lavage or a protected brush)
  - Pulmonary toileting (removal of thick secretions or mucous plugs using suction and saline lavage)
  - Assessment of patency and mechanical properties of the upper airway
  - Visual inspection to determine the degrees of toxic inhalation (smoke inhalation)
- Bronchoscopy may be performed in spontaneously breathing patients with procedural sedation or mechanically ventilated patients.
- Patients with severe chronic obstructive pulmonary disease (pulmonary function test with FEV <40% or Sao_2 <93% by arterial blood gas) should be considered for intubation before undergoing bronchoscopy.[4,12] These patients have a higher risk for hypoxia during the procedure and may also experience delayed recovery. They may be intubated for the procedure depending on the patient's risk factors.[2]
- Potential risks to bronchoscopy include hypoxemia from obstruction of airflow, cardiac arrhythmias or arrest secondary to hypoxia or vagus nerve stimulation, spontaneous pneumothorax caused by changes in intrathoracic pressure, bleeding secondary to accidental laceration or frail tissue, and unexpected anaphylactic reaction to the lubricant or anesthetic agent.
- Relative contraindications for bronchoscopy include the following:[3,4]
  - Recent (within 1 week) traumatic brain injury due to increasing intracranial pressure and hence herniation or ischemic stroke
  - Unstable angina or recent acute myocardial infarction (within 30 days)
  - Intubation requiring high positive end-expiratory pressure (PEEP >10 cm H_2O) or oxygen requirements (Fio_2 >0.60)[4]
  - Any hematological disorder, therapeutic anticoagulation, or coagulopathy (e.g., Factor V Leiden disorder or hemophilia).[4,7,12]
  - Known lung abscess: risk of purulent material flooding the airway
  - Recent (within 1 week) airway surgery (tonsil removal and adenoid removal)
  - Recent bleeding from Barret esophageal disease
  - Recent diagnosis of an airway nodule (e.g., vocal cord nodule caused by additional risk for airway obstruction or bleeding if dislodged during the procedure)[2]

AP This procedure should be performed only by clinicians who have demonstrated competence and are credentialed to perform it. In addition, the procedure must be within the scope of practice defined by their professional licensure, and in accordance with professional practice acts. Physicians, advanced practice nurses, and physician assistants may be credentialed to perform this procedure.

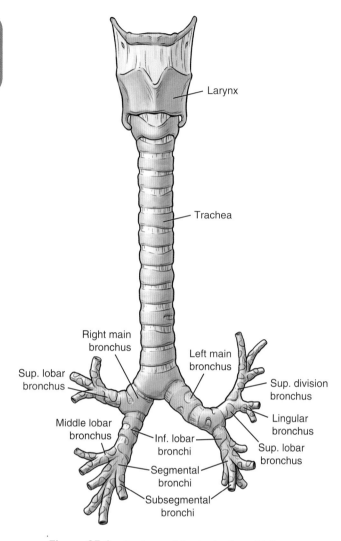

Figure 25.1   Anatomy of the tracheobronchial tree.

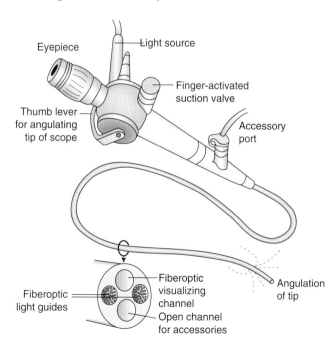

Figure 25.2   Components of a bronchoscope. (*From Pierce, LN. Management of the mechanically ventilated patient, ed 2, Philadelphia, 2007, Elsevier.*)

❖ Recent diagnosis of airway abscess in the vocal cords or trachea[5]

EQUIPMENT

- Bronchoscope
- Specimen containers (BAL specimen entrapment vial)
- Patient label(s) for specimen(s)
- Protective brush for specimen collection
- 500-mL bottle of sterile normal saline solution
- Water-soluble lubricant
- Local anesthetics (lidocaine jelly, 1% or 2% injectable lidocaine solution)
- Intubated patient: Endotracheal tube: connector for bronchoscopy (fiberoptic bronchoscope swivel adapter)
- Sterile 2 × 2 or 4 × 4 gauze sponges
- 25-cc or 50-cc syringe with lure connector end
- Wall suction or portable suction, container, and tubing
- Yankauer suction catheter (spontaneously breathing patients)
- Inline suction catheter (intubated patients)
- Medications (e.g., sedatives, nasal decongestant, glycopyrrolate) as prescribed by provider
- Oxygen source and tubing
- Resuscitation bag-valve-mask device
- Pulse oximeter
- Swivel adaptor for endotracheal tube (intubated patients)
- Bite block (nonintubated patients)

PATIENT AND FAMILY EDUCATION

- Assess patient's and family's level of understanding about the patient's condition and rationale for the procedure. Rationale: This assessment identifies the patient's and family's knowledge deficits concerning the patient's condition, the procedure, the expected benefits, and the potential risks. It also allows time for questions to clarify information and voice concerns. Explanations decrease patient anxiety and enhance cooperation.
- Explain the procedure and what the patient may experience if the clinical situation permits. Rationale: This explanation enhances patient and family understanding and decreases anxiety.

PATIENT ASSESSMENT AND PREPARATION

Patient Assessment

- Assess for significant medical history or surgery, including chronic lung disease, asthma, airway cancer, previous oral or tracheal surgery, bleeding disorders, splenectomy or known infections (tuberculosis, Hepatitis B or C, HIV). *Rationale:* Medical history or prior surgery may indicate the need for additional interventions before the procedure. Asthma patients require premedication with a bronchodilator before the procedure (10 to 30 minutes). Patients with active infection may require additional personal protective equipment or an isolation room.

Mallampati Classification

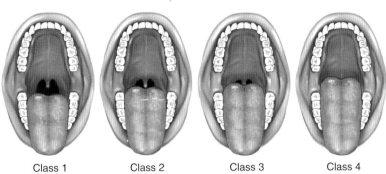

Class 1   Class 2   Class 3   Class 4

Class 1; soft palate, fauces, uvula, pillars
Class 2; soft palate, fauces, portion of uvula
Class 3; soft palate, base of uvula
Class 4; hard palate only

Figure 25.3   Mallampati classifications. *(From Fonseca R, Barber DH, Powers M, Frost D:* Oral and maxillofacial trauma, *ed 4, Philadelphia, 2013, Saunders.)*

- Assess for allergies. ***Rationale:*** Verifies that the patient is not allergic to lidocaine or lubricant used during procedure.
- Evaluate available imaging studies including chest radiography, CT, or ultrasound as available. ***Rationale:*** Imaging studies confirm the area of the lung that requires visualization or specimen collection during the bronchoscopy.
- Assess the patient's cardiovascular status, including heart rate, rhythm, blood pressure, and SpO_2. ***Rationale:*** Baseline assessment provides comparison data for evaluation of changes during the procedure. Sedation and hypoxemia may result in hypotension and dysrhythmias.
- Assess the stability of the patient's respiratory status, including recent arterial blood gases, oxygen requirements, and ventilator settings (if intubated). ***Rationale:*** Baseline assessment provides comparison data for evaluation of changes during the procedure. Procedural risk versus benefit should be considered in unstable patients.
- Review recent laboratory results, including platelets, hemoglobin, and international normalized ratio. ***Rationale:*** Bleeding risk is increased in thrombocytopenic patients and those taking anticoagulants.[10,12]
- Assess time of last oral intake. ***Rationale:*** Nothing by mouth for minimum of 4 hours, preferably 6 hours, to reduce the risk of aspiration during the procedure.[4,6]

Patient Preparation

- Obtain informed consent if circumstances allow. ***Rationale:*** Invasive procedures, unless performed with implied consent in a life-threatening situation, require written consent of the patient or significant other.

- Verify the correct patient with two identifiers. ***Rationale:*** Before performing a procedure, the nurse should ensure the correct identification of the patient for the intended intervention.
- Establish adequate monitoring of cardiopulmonary status, including pulse oximetry, ECG monitoring, and blood pressure. ***Rationale:*** Patients may experience hypoxemia and cardiovascular changes (hypotension, arrhythmias) during the procedure.
- Verify that the patient has a functional intravenous line. ***Rationale:*** Bronchoscopy requires administration of intravenous procedural sedation and may also require administration of emergency medications.
- Select the size and type of bronchoscope appropriate for the patient's condition. ***Rationale:*** In intubated patients, the internal diameter of the endotracheal tube or tracheostomy must be 2 mm larger than the bronchoscope so the scope does not cause complete occlusion of the ETT during the procedure. Disposable bronchoscopy tubes offer greater size selection: Small (5 to 6 mm), medium (6.5 to 7.5 mm), large (8 to 8.5 mm), and extra-large (9 mm).[3,5,10] For nonintubated patients, the Mallampati classification (Fig. 25.3) can be used to guide the provider in selecting bronchoscope size.[4,11]
- Confirm availability of staff to assist with the procedure. ***Rationale:*** The provider performing the bronchoscopy requires assistance in managing the airway and handing off specimens (usually a respiratory therapist) as well as a nurse to monitor the patient and administer prescribed medications.

Procedure for Diagnostic and Therapeutic Bronchoscopy		
Steps	**Rationale**	**Special Considerations**
1. 🔲		
2. 🔲 Don personal protective equipment: clean gown, gloves, eye goggle or face shield, mask (N-95 or respirator if warranted).		For patient with known or suspected infections (tuberculosis, COVID-19) all staff assisting with the procedure must wear PPE for an aerosol generating procedure (fit tested N-95 or respirators) to protect against airborne or and droplet exposure. Performing the procedure in an airborne isolation room is also preferred.[3,13] (**Level E***)
3. Confirm adequate personnel to assist with the procedure and clarify staff roles: • One to assist with equipment and airway management. • One to administer sedation and monitor the patient.	Communicate with assistants to ensure required supplies are available, including sedative agents and resuscitation equipment.	
4. Perform a preprocedure verification and time out, if nonemergent.	Ensures patient safety	Review imaging studies
5. Prepare and assemble the equipment for the procedure: • Ensure that suction equipment is in working order • Verify the correct size and type of bronchoscope • Check the fiberoptic light and camera on bronchoscope • For intubated patients, attach the fiberoptic bronchoscope swivel adapter; nonintubated patients will need a bite block.	All equipment and supplies needed to perform the procedure should be set up and in working order before beginning the bronchoscopy. Swivel connection is used to facilitate insertion of bronchoscope into the endotracheal tube. Bite block is used facilitate insertion of bronchoscope into oral airway.	Adjust camera settings as need-ed to obtain crisp clear picture. This may be done by focusing on a 4x4 gauze or a sterile towel.
6. Hold the scope, and verify the ability to manipulate components (Fig. 25.4): • Flex and release the thumb to move the leveler for up and down. • Tηε σecond digit will be used to press the suction button located at the opposite site of the leveler, the suction port on the lateral part of the scope, and any additional working ports, such as a retrieval line (see Fig. 25.4). • C port (located at the side of bronchoscopy) is used to administer saline flushes and to insert a covered brush to obtain a specimen (see Fig. 25.2).[4]	Practitioner should ensure proper function and ability to operate the scope before proceeding with procedure	Ensure fiberoptic is connected to monitor to verify you are able to see as scope enter into airway.

*Level E: Multiple case reports, theory-based evidence from expert opinions, or peer-reviewed professional organizational standards without clinical studies to support recommendations.

Procedure for Diagnostic and Therapeutic Bronchoscopy—*Continued*		
Steps	**Rationale**	**Special Considerations**

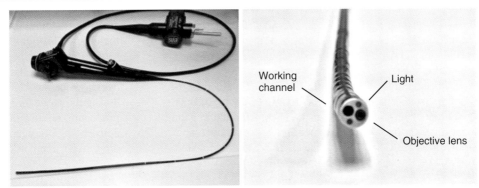

Figure 25.4 Handle of a scope with a lever. *(From Keszler M, Gautham KS:* Goldsmith's assisted ventilation of the neonate: An evidence-based approach to newborn respiratory care, *ed 7, Philadelphia, 2022, Elsevier.)*

Steps	Rationale	Special Considerations
7. Request administration of prescribed sedation appropriate for the patient's condition. • Intubated patients may receive sedation with propofol and fentanyl • Nonintubated patients receive moderate sedation with fentanyl and midazolam	Patients require some level of sedation to tolerate the discomfort of inserting the bronchoscope. Medications are titrated to achieve adequate sedation and analgesia without inducing significant hypotension or hypoxia	Vital signs and level of sedation must be monitored frequently during and after the procedure.
8. Preoxygenate the patient: • 100% Fio_2 administered via the ventilator for 1–2 minutes • Bag-valve-mask delivery for nonintubated patients	The scope will partially obstruct the airway decreasing the flow of oxygen. Preoxygenation can help prevent hypoxemia.	Nonvented patients should have their supplemental oxygen increased (for example, if stable on 2L consider increasing to 4L). If the patient is requiring high amounts of supplemental oxygen, bronchoscopy may be postponed or the patient may be intubated before performing the procedure.[2,8,9]
9. Apply local anesthetic before introducing the scope.[9] • Lidocaine 1% and 2% injectable lidocaine solution via direct administration or nebulizer • Nasal decongestant, topical solution • 2% lidocaine jelly	Local anesthetics applied to the back of the throat help prevent gag and cough.[1,5] (**Level D***)	
10. Slide the bronchoscopy tip to the mouthpiece (bite block) or ETT connector.		Ensured entire scope is well lubricated.
11. Proceed with advancing the bronchoscopy, examining each section of the lung segment (e.g., trachea, carina, right and left mainstem, right upper, middle, and lower lobes, left upper and middle lobes).	Visual inspection should be done on each section to explore and to confirm the area for specimen collection of mucus particle or secretion	If visualization of airway is poor due to phlegm or thick secretion, ask your assistant RT to lavage with specific amount of saline, 25–50 cc to side port.

*Level D: Peer-reviewed professional and organizational standards with the support of clinical study recommendations.

Procedure continues on following page

UNIT I

Procedure for Diagnostic and Therapeutic Bronchoscopy—*Continued*

Steps	Rationale	Special Considerations
12. Once visual inspection is complete, ask assisting staff to disconnect the suction from the bronchoscopy and connect the sterile specimen entrapment container.[5] If specimens are collected, ensure that staff label the container with the location (e.g., right upper lobe, carina) as specimens are obtained.	To clearly visualize the airway and obtain a clean specimen, lavage is performed. Instill 25cc or 50cc saline flush to side port or top of the bronchoscope. Bronchial washings can be obtained from large airways, or the tip of the scope can be positioned in a lung segment for bronchioalveolar lavage (BAL). Uncontaminated specimens for cytology or culture may be collected via C port, using a protected brush.	The patient should be monitored by an RN throughout the procedure, including vital signs, oxygen saturation and cardiac rhythm. If the patient oxygenation saturation decreases below 92% at any point during the procedure, stop the procedure, remove the scope and deliver 100% oxygen via ventilator or by bag valve mask bag.
13. After collecting the specimen, slowly withdraw the scope, inspecting each segment of the lung for any bleeding or phlegm that many need to be suctioned before removing the scope.	Check with assistant to ensure patient is oxygenating well.	Potential complications include scraping the inner lining of the airway or dislodging a nodule, resulting in bleeding. If this occurs, the procedure should be stopped, and the patient should be closely monitored. If desaturation or continued bleeding occurs the patient may require intubation.[3,8]
14. Have assisting staff remove the specimen cup, maintaining sterility, and verify that the specimen collection is adequate.		Ensure specimen is properly labeled with 2 patient identifiers and location that specimen was obtained.
15. Support the patient's postprocedure recovery: • Assess vital signs and oxygenation • Place the patient in the Fowler's position • Suction as needed 16. Discard used supplies, and remove ■■. 17. ■■	After the bronchoscope has been removed, the patient will have mild to moderate oral secretions related to recent removal of the scope	If procedure was abruptly stopped due to hypoxia, hypotension or cardiac arrhythmia, reassess until patient has stable vital signs and then proceed with procedure at Step 12.[10]

Expected Outcomes

- Patient is comfortable with adequate oxygenation and ventilation
- Specimens obtained to assist with clinical diagnoses

Unexpected Outcomes

- Increasing respiratory distress
- Hypoxemia
- Hemorrhage
- Pneumothorax
- Hypotension
- Aspiration

Patient Monitoring and Care

Steps	Rationale	Reportable Conditions
		These conditions should be reported to the provider if they persist despite nursing interventions.
1. Monitor respiratory status and vital signs before, during, and after bronchoscopy.	Changes may alert the practitioner of possible unexpected outcomes or the need for intervention. Use of supplemental oxygen or changes in ventilator settings may be necessary.	• Hypoxia • Shortness of breath, dyspnea, ventilator dyssynchrony • Dysrhythmias • Hypotension • Bleeding • Subcutaneous emphysema
2. Monitor level of consciousness and pain during and after administration of procedural sedation.	Changes may indicate a need for increasing or decreasing sedation or analgesia.	• Anxiety, restlessness • Oversedation • Increased pain
3. Obtain a chest radiograph.	Chest x-ray is performed following bronchoscopy to compare with the preprocedure x-rays and assess for any complications secondary to the procedure.[3,5,10] **(Level E*)**	

*Level E: Multiple case reports, theory-based evidence from expert opinions, or peer-reviewed professional organizational standards without clinical studies to support recommendations.

Documentation

Documentation should include the following:
- Consent for procedure
- Time out procedure
- Preprocedure and intraprocedure medications administered
- Patient's preprocedure airway status (intubated or natural airway and baseline oxygen apparatus)
- Airway grade: Mallampati classification
- The type and size of the scope
- Narrative of visual inspection of trachea, carina, right and left mainstem, and lung segments
- Specific locations of specimen collection and type of cultures sent
- Quantity and characteristics of specimen
- Amount of saline used for lavage
- Any complication event during the procedure
- Patient tolerance of the procedure, including vital signs, oxygenation, pain, and response to medications
- Postprocedure wakefulness
- Postprocedure airway and oxygenation support required
- Complications during the procedure
- Postprocedure imaging results

References and Additional Readings

For a complete list of references and additional readings for this procedure, scan this QR code with your smartphone, or visit https://www.elsevier.com/__data/assets/pdf_file/0004/1319800/Chapter0025.pdf

PROCEDURE

26 Bronchoscopy (Assist)

Chong Sherry Cheever

PURPOSE Bronchoscopy is an invasive procedure performed to assist in the diagnostic and therapeutic management of patients with abnormal respiratory function and/or abnormal radiographic findings.

PREREQUISITE NURSING KNOWLEDGE

- Bronchoscopy is performed by advancing a camera incased in a long tube through the oral cavity (or endotracheal tube), to the larynx, the bronchus, and to each section of the lung. This process allows for visualization of the lung and to obtain specimens to diagnose pulmonary illness.[9]
- A bronchoscope is a small circumference tube that has three elements bundled within the tube: a fiber-optic camera, suction, and a small opening called a C port that is used for irrigation and to place assistive tools like a needle or protective brush (Fig. 25.2A and B).[4]
- Chest x-ray or computed tomography (CT) of the chest is performed before bronchoscopy to identify the segment of the lung that requires inspection or lavage to obtain the specimen.
- Bronchoscopy is indicated if imaging studies demonstrate abnormal findings such as consolidation, a foreign object, or nodule.
- Bronchoscopy can be performed for diagnostic or therapeutic purposes. Indications for bronchoscopy include the following:
  - ❖ Removal of foreign objects that may have been aspirated
  - ❖ Pneumonia or infiltrates
  - ❖ Specimen collection (protected specimens without oral contamination may be obtained via bronchial lavage or a protected brush)
  - ❖ Pulmonary toileting (removal of thick secretions or mucous plugs using suction and saline lavage)
  - ❖ Assessment of patency and mechanical properties of the upper airway
  - ❖ Visual inspection to determine the degrees of toxic inhalation (smoke inhalation)
- Bronchoscopy may be performed in spontaneously breathing patients with procedural sedation or in mechanically ventilated patients.
- Potential risks to bronchoscopy include hypoxemia from obstruction of airflow, cardiac arrhythmias or arrest secondary to hypoxia or vagus nerve stimulation, spontaneous pneumothorax caused by changes in intrathoracic pressure, bleeding secondary to accidental laceration or frail tissue, and unexpected anaphylactic reaction to the lubricant or anesthetic agent.

- Relative contraindications for bronchoscopy include the following[3,4]:
  - ❖ Recent (within 1 week) traumatic brain injury due to risk for increasing intracranial pressure and hence herniation or ischemic stroke
  - ❖ Unstable angina or recent acute myocardial infarction (within 30 days)
  - ❖ Intubated patients requiring high positive end-expiratory pressure (PEEP >10 cm H_2O) or oxygen requirements (Fio_2 >0.60)[4]
  - ❖ Any hematological disorder, therapeutic anticoagulation, or coagulopathy (e.g., Factor V Leidan disorder or hemophilia)[4,7,11]
  - ❖ Known lung abscess: risk of purulent material flooding the airway
  - ❖ Recent (within 1 week) airway surgery (tonsil removal and adenoid removal)
  - ❖ Recent bleeding from Barret's esophageal disease
  - ❖ Recent diagnosis of an airway nodule, such as vocal cord nodule (due to additional risk for airway obstruction or bleeding if dislodged during the procedure)[2]
  - ❖ Recent diagnosis of airway abscess in the vocal cords or trachea[5]

EQUIPMENT

- Bronchoscope
- Specimen containers (BAL specimen entrapment vial)
- Patient label(s) for specimen(s)
- Protective brush for specimen collection
- 500-mL bottle of sterile normal saline
- Water-soluble lubricant
- Local anesthetics (lidocaine jelly, 1% or 2% injectable lidocaine solution)
- Intubated patient: Endotracheal tube connector for bronchoscopy (fiber-optic bronchoscope swivel adapter)
- Sterile 2 × 2 or 4 × 4 gauze sponges
- 25-cc or 500-cc syringe with lure connector end
- Wall suction or portable suction, container and tubing
- Yankauer suction catheter (spontaneously breathing patients)
- Inline suction catheter (intubated patients)
- Medications (e.g., sedatives, nasal decongestant, glycopyrrolate) as prescribed by the provider
- Oxygen source and tubing
- Resuscitation bag-valve-mask device
- Swivel adaptor for endotracheal tube (intubated patients)
- Bite block (nonintubated patients)

PATIENT AND FAMILY EDUCATION

- Assess patient's and family's level of understanding about their condition and rationale for the procedure. *Rationale:* This assessment identifies the patient's and family's knowledge deficits concerning the patient's condition, the procedure, the expected benefits, and the potential risks. It also allows time for questions to clarify information and voice concerns. Explanations decrease patient anxiety and enhance cooperation.
- Explain the procedure and what the patient may experience if the clinical situation permits. If not, explain the procedure and reason for the bronchoscopy after it is completed. *Rationale:* This explanation enhances patient and family understanding and decreases anxiety.

PATIENT ASSESSMENT AND PREPARATION

Patient Assessment

- Assess for significant medical history or surgery, including chronic lung disease, asthma, airway cancer, previous oral or tracheal surgery, bleeding disorders, splenectomy or known infections (tuberculosis, hepatitis B or C, HIV). *Rationale:* Medical history or prior surgery may indicate the need for additional interventions before the procedure. Asthma patients require premedication with a bronchodilator before the procedure (10 to 30 minutes). Patients with active infection may require additional personal protective equipment or an isolation room.
- Assess for allergies. *Rationale:* Verifies that the patient is not allergic to lidocaine or lubricant used during the procedure.
- Ensure that imaging studies including chest radiography, CT scan, or ultrasound as available are accessible for review. *Rationale:* Imaging studies confirm the area of the lung that requires visualization or specimen collection during the bronchoscopy.
- Assess the patient's cardiovascular status, including heart rate, rhythm, and blood pressure. *Rationale:* Baseline assessment provides comparison data for evaluation of changes during the procedure. Sedation and hypoxemia may result in hypotension and dysrhythmias.

- Assess the stability of the patient's respiratory status, including pulse oximetry readings, recent arterial blood gases, oxygen requirements, and ventilator settings (if intubated). *Rationale:* Baseline assessment provides comparison data for evaluation of changes during the procedure. Procedural risk versus benefit should be considered in unstable patients.
- Review recent laboratory tests including platelets, hemoglobin, and INR. *Rationale:* Bleeding risk is increased in thrombocytopenic patients and those taking anticoagulants.[10,12]
- Assess the time of last oral intake. *Rationale:* Patients should have nothing by mouth for a minimum of 4 hours, preferably 6 hours, to reduce risk of aspiration during the procedure.[4,6]

PATIENT PREPARATION

- Ensure that written informed consent for the procedure has been completed if circumstances allow. *Rationale:* Invasive procedures, unless performed with implied consent in a life-threatening situation, require written consent of the patient or family member.
- Verify the correct patient with two identifiers. *Rationale:* Before performing a procedure, the nurse should ensure the correct identification of the patient for the intended intervention.
- Establish adequate monitoring of cardiopulmonary status, including pulse oximetry, ECG monitoring, and blood pressure. *Rationale:* Patients may experience hypoxemia and cardiovascular changes (hypotension, arrhythmias) during the procedure.
- Verify that the patient has a functional intravenous line. *Rationale:* Bronchoscopy requires administration of intravenous procedural sedation and may also require administration of emergency medications.
- Confirm availability of staff to assist with the procedure. *Rationale:* The provider performing the bronchoscopy requires assistance in managing the airway and handing off specimens (usually a respiratory therapist) as well as a nurse to monitor the patient and administer prescribed medications.

Procedure	**for Diagnostic and Therapeutic Bronchoscopy**		
Steps	Rationale	Special Considerations
1. **HH**		
2. **PE** Don personal protective equipment: clean gown, gloves, eye goggles or face shield, mask (N-95 or respirator if warranted)		For patients with known or suspected infections (tuberculosis, COVID-19), all staff assisting with the procedure must wear PPE for an aerosol-generating procedure (fit-tested N-95 or respirators) to protect against airborne and droplet exposure. Performing the procedure in an airborne isolation room is also preferred.[3,12] **(Level E*)**

*Level E: Multiple case reports, theory-based evidence from expert opinions, or peer-reviewed professional organizational standards without clinical studies to support recommendations.

Procedure | for Diagnostic and Therapeutic Bronchoscopy—*Continued*

Steps	Rationale	Special Considerations
3. Perform a preprocedure verification and time out, if nonemergent.	Ensures patient safety.	
4. Prepare and assemble equipment for the procedure: A. Ensure that suction equipment is in working order. B. For intubated patients, attach the fiber-optic bronchoscope swivel adapter; nonintubated patients will need a bite block.	All equipment and supplies needed to perform the procedure should be set up and in working order before beginning the bronchoscopy. The swivel connection is used to facilitate insertion of the bronchoscope into the endotracheal tube. The bite block is used facilitate insertion of the bronchoscope into the oral airway.	The provider will confirm that the fiber-optic light and camera on the bronchoscope are working correctly.
5. Administer procedural sedation as ordered by the physician or advanced practice provider. A. Nonintubated patients receive moderate sedation. B. Intubated patients may receive deeper sedation.	Premedication with an opioid, antianxiolytic, sedative, or hypnotic ensures patient comfort throughout the procedure. Medications are titrated to achieve adequate sedation and analgesia without inducing significant hypotension or hypoxia.	Local anesthetics (1% or 2% injectable lidocaine solution or 2% lidocaine jelly) may be applied to the back of the patient's throat to help prevent gag and cough.[1,5] **(Level D*)**
6. Assist with preoxygenating the patient: A. 100% Fio_2 administered via the ventilator for 1–2 minutes. B. Bag-valve-mask delivery for nonintubated patients	The scope will partially obstruct the airway, decreasing the flow of oxygen. Preoxygenation can help prevent hypoxemia.	Nonintubated patients should be placed on supplemental oxygen. If the patient is requiring high levels of oxygen before the procedure, bronchoscopy may be postponed, or the patient may be intubated before performing the procedure.[2,8,9]
7. Throughout the procedure, assist with providing continuous monitoring of patient vital signs and response to the procedure and interventions.	The physician or advanced practice provider is focused on the technique required to obtain the fluid and may be delayed in noticing patient changes.	If the patient oxygenation saturation decreases below 92% at any point during the procedure, notify the provider so they can stop the procedure, remove the scope, and deliver 100% oxygen via ventilator or by bag-valve-mask device.
8. As directed by the physician or advanced practice provider, assist with hand-off of specimens obtained through the bronchoscope. Label them with two patient identifiers and the location where the specimen was obtained (e.g., carina, right upper lobe), and send it to the laboratory for appropriate analysis.	Analysis may aid in determining an etiology for pulmonary disease or other pathology.	Verify the order for microbiology or sputum culture; also note any specific information requested by the provider, such as collection with a protective brush, if warranted.
9. After the provider removes the bronchoscope, assist with removing the bite block or swivel adaptor (on intubated patients), and suction the patient as needed.	After the bronchoscope has been removed, the patient will have mild to moderate oral secretions related to recent removal of the scope.	

*Level D: Peer-reviewed professional and organizational standards with the support of clinical study recommendations.

Procedure continues on following page

Procedure for Diagnostic and Therapeutic Bronchoscopy—*Continued*

Steps	Rationale	Special Considerations

10. Support the patient's postprocedure recovery.
  A. Assess vital signs and oxygenation.
  B. Place the patient in the Fowler's position per direction of the provider.
11. Discard used supplies, and remove 🔲PE.
12. 🔲HH
	Hypoxia, hypotension, or difficulty ventilating the patient may indicate potential complications related to the procedure or sedation.	Patients may experience complications after bronchoscopy such as migration of a mucous plug, bleeding from a dislodged nodule, or a pneumothorax.

Expected Outcomes

- Patient is comfortable with adequate oxygenation and ventilation
- Specimens are obtained to assist with clinical diagnoses

Unexpected Outcomes

- Increasing respiratory distress
- Hypoxemia
- Hemorrhage
- Pneumothorax
- Hypotension
- Aspiration

Patient Monitoring and Care

Steps	Rationale	Reportable Conditions
		These conditions should be reported to the provider if they persist despite nursing interventions.
1. Monitor respiratory status and vital signs before, during, and after bronchoscopy.	Changes may alert the practitioner of possible unexpected outcomes or the need for intervention. Use of supplemental oxygen or changes in ventilator settings may be necessary.	- Hypoxia - Shortness of breath, dyspnea - Dysrhythmias - Hypotension
2. Monitor level of consciousness and pain during and after administration of procedural sedation.	Changes may indicate a need for increasing or decreasing sedation or analgesia.	- Anxiety, restlessness - Oversedation - Increased pain
3. Obtain a chest radiograph as directed by the physician or advanced practice provider.	Chest x-ray is performed following bronchoscopy to verify aeration and success of the procedure.[3,5,10] **(Level E*)**	

*Level E: Multiple case reports, theory-based evidence from expert opinions, or peer-reviewed professional organizational standards without clinical studies to support recommendations.

Documentation

Documentation should include the following:
- Patient and family teaching
- Completed consent for the procedure
- Patient's airway status pre- and postprocedure (intubated or not)
- Medication administration and patient response
- Postbronchoscopy radiograph acquisition and results as available
- Laboratory tests ordered and results as available
- Patient tolerance of the procedure, including vital signs, oxygenation, pain, and response to medications
- Wakefulness postprocedure
- Airway and oxygenation support required postprocedure
- Occurrence of unexpected outcomes

UNIT I

References and Additional Readings

For a complete list of references and additional readings for this procedure, scan this QR code with your smartphone, or visit https://www.elsevier.com/__data/assets/pdf_file/0005/1319801/Chapter0026.pdf.

PROCEDURE

27

Invasive Mechanical Ventilation (Through an Artificial Airway): Volume and Pressure Modes

John J. Gallagher

PURPOSE Initiation and maintenance of positive-pressure ventilation (PPV) through an artificial airway are accomplished to maintain or improve oxygenation and ventilation and to provide respiratory muscle rest. Selection of volume or pressure modes is dependent on the available evidence, clinical goals, availability of modes, and practitioner preference.

PREREQUISITE NURSING KNOWLEDGE

- Indications for the initiation of mechanical ventilation include the following:
  - Apnea (e.g., neuromuscular or cardiopulmonary collapse)
  - Acute ventilatory failure, which is generally defined as a pH less than or equal to 7.25 with an arterial partial pressure of carbon dioxide ($Paco_2$) greater than or equal to 50 mm Hg
  - Impending ventilatory failure (serial decrement of arterial blood gas values or progressive increase in signs and symptoms of increased work of breathing)
  - Severe hypoxemia: an arterial partial pressure of oxygen (Pao_2) less than or equal to 50 mm Hg on room air indicates a critical level of oxygen in the blood. Although oxygen-delivery devices may be used before intubation, the refractory nature of the shunt (perfusion without ventilation) may necessitate that positive pressure be applied to reexpand closed alveoli. Restoration of functional residual capacity (FRC; lung volume that remains at the end of a passive exhalation) is the goal.
  - Respiratory muscle fatigue: the muscles of respiration can become fatigued if they are made to contract repetitively at high workloads. Fatigue occurs when muscle energy stores become depleted. Weakness, hypermetabolic states, and chronic lung disease are examples of conditions in which patients are especially prone to fatigue. When fatigue occurs, the muscles no longer contract optimally, and hypercarbia results. To rest the muscles, patients are typically required to get 12 to 24 hours of rest. Respiratory muscle rest requires that the workload of the muscles (or muscle loading) be offset so mitochondrial energy stores can be repleted. Respiratory work and rest vary with different modes and the application of the same. In general, when hypercarbia is present, mechanical ventilation is necessary

to relieve the work of breathing. Muscle unloading is accomplished differently and depends on patient-ventilator interaction and the mode.

- Ventilators are categorized as either negative or positive pressure. Although negative-pressure ventilation (i.e., the iron lung) was used extensively in the 1940s, introduction of the cuffed endotracheal tube resulted in the dominance of PPV in clinical practice during the second half of the 20th century. Although sporadic interest in negative-pressure ventilation continues, the cumbersome nature of the ventilators and the lack of airway protection associated with this form of ventilation preclude a serious resurgence of this mode of ventilation.[32,72]
  - PPV: positive-pressure modes of ventilation have traditionally been categorized into volume and pressure. However, with the advent of microprocessor technology, sophisticated iterations of traditional volume and pressure modes of ventilation have evolved. Many of the modes have names that are different from traditional volume and pressure modes, but they are similar in many characteristics. Little data exist to show that the newer modes improve outcomes. A wide variety of modes described in this procedure are actually a combination of volume and pressure but for ease of learning are classified into specific categories.[16,17,32,72]
  - Volume ventilation has traditionally been the most popular form of PPV, largely because tidal volume (Vt) and minute ventilation (MV) are ensured, which is an essential goal in the patient with acute illness. With volume ventilation, a predetermined Vt is delivered with each breath regardless of resistance and compliance. Vt is stable from breath to breath, but airway pressure may vary. The gas flow-rate pattern of volume ventilation is generally constant from the beginning to the end of the breath (square wave). In modern ventilators, this can be changed to accelerating, decelerating, or even sine patterns. To rest the respiratory muscles with volume

ventilation, the ventilator rate must be increased until spontaneous respiratory effort ceases. When spontaneous effort is present, such as with initiation of an assist/control (A/C) breath, respiratory muscle work continues throughout the breath.[17,32,80]

❖ With traditional *pressure ventilation*, the practitioner selects the desired pressure level, and the Vt is determined by the selected pressure level, airway resistance, and lung compliance.[1,64] This characteristic is important to note when caring for a patient with an unstable condition on a pressure mode of ventilation. Careful attention to Vt is necessary to prevent inadvertent hyperventilation or hypoventilation. To ensure respiratory muscle rest on pressure-support ventilation (PSV), the workload must be offset with appropriate adjustment of the pressure-support level. To accomplish this adjustment, the pressure-support level is increased to lower the spontaneous respiratory rate (RR) to less than or equal to 20 breaths/min and to attain a Vt of 6 to 10 mL/kg of predicted body weight (PBW).

❖ Pressure ventilation provides for an augmented inspiration (pressure is maintained throughout inspiration). The flow pattern (speed of the gas) is described as *decelerating;* that is, gas-flow delivery is high at the beginning of the breath and tapers off toward the end of the breath. This pattern contrasts with volume ventilation in which the flow rate is typically more consistent during inspiration (i.e., the same at the beginning of the breath as at the end of the breath). The decelerating flow pattern associated with pressure ventilation is thought to provide better gas distribution and more efficient ventilation.

❖ Increasingly, sophisticated ventilator technology has resulted in the development of volume-assured pressure modes of ventilation. These pressure modes of ventilation are designed in such a way that the minimum desired tidal volume be can be achieved on a breath-to-breath basis. These are called *adaptive pressure control* or *dual-control pressure modes.* The more desirable decelerating flow pattern may be provided and plateau pressures controlled, with more consistent Vt and MV.

❖ Additional modes of ventilation have been promoted for use in patients with acute respiratory distress syndrome (ARDS), including high-frequency oscillation ventilation (HFOV), airway pressure-release ventilation (APRV), and other ventilator-specific modes, such as biphasic, adaptive support ventilation (ASV), and proportional assist ventilation (PAV). Although some data exist that suggest the modes may be beneficial in patients with ARDS, to date no change in mortality rate has been noted, although positive trends have been demonstrated in some variables of interest such as oxygenation.[17,20,27,28,29,32,37,54,55,59,60,63,66,68,75,76]

• Summary descriptions of modes, mode parameters, and ventilator alarms are provided within this procedure and in Boxes 27.1 and 27.2 and Table 27.1.

• Complications of PPV include volume-pressure trauma, hemodynamic changes, and pulmonary barotrauma.
   ❖ Volume-pressure trauma, in contrast with barotrauma (or air-leak disease), was first described in animals with

---

| BOX 27.1 | **Traditional Modes of Mechanical Ventilation (on All Ventilators)** |

VOLUME MODES

Control Ventilation (CV) or Controlled Mandatory Ventilation (CMV)
Description: With this mode, the ventilator provides all of the patient's minute ventilation. The clinician sets the rate, Vt, inspiratory time, and PEEP. Generally, this term is used to describe situations in which the patient is chemically relaxed or is paralyzed from a spinal cord or neuromuscular disease and is unable to initiate spontaneous breaths. This mode does not exist as a standard mode on modern ventilators. Patients on assist/control (A/C) mode who are unable to trigger the machine are essentially in CMV.

Assist/Control (A/C) Ventilation
Description: This option requires that a rate, Vt, inspiratory time, and PEEP be set for the patient. The ventilator sensitivity also is set, and when the patient initiates a spontaneous breath, a full-volume breath is delivered.

Synchronized Intermittent Mandatory Ventilation (SIMV)
Description: This mode requires that the rate, Vt, inspiratory time, sensitivity, and PEEP are set by the clinician. In between mandatory breaths, patients can spontaneously breathe at their own rates and Vt. With SIMV, the ventilator synchronizes the mandatory breaths with the patient's own breaths.

PRESSURE MODES

Pressure Support Ventilation (PSV)
Description: This mode provides augmented inspiration to a patient who is spontaneously breathing. With pressure support (PS), the clinician selects an IPL, PEEP, and sensitivity. When the patient initiates a breath, a high flow of gas is delivered to the preselected pressure level, and pressure is maintained throughout inspiration. The patient determines the parameters of Vt, rate, and inspiratory time.

Pressure-Controlled (PC) and Pressure-Controlled Inverse Ratio Ventilation (PC/IRV)
Description: This mode may provide pressure-limited ventilation (PC) alone or combined with an inverse ratio of inspiration to expiration (PC/IRV). The clinician selects the pressure level, rate, inspiratory time (1:1, 2:1, 3:1, 4:1), and PEEP level. With prolonged inspiratory times, auto-PEEP may result. The auto-PEEP may be a desirable outcome of the inverse ratios. In PC without IRV, conventional inspiratory times are used, and rate, pressure level, and PEEP are selected.

Positive End-Expiratory Pressure (PEEP) and Continuous Positive Airway Pressure (CPAP)
Description: This ventilatory option creates positive pressure at end exhalation. PEEP restores functional residual capacity. The term *PEEP* is used when end-expiratory pressure is provided during ventilator positive pressure breaths.

---

stiff noncompliant lungs who were ventilated with traditional lung volumes (range, 10 to 12 mL/kg PBW). The investigators noted that the large volumes translated into high plateau pressures (also known as *static, distending,* or *alveolar* pressure) and subsequent acute lung injury. The lung injury was described as a loss of alveolar integrity (i.e., alveolar fractures) and movement of fluids and proteins into the alveolar space. Plateau pressures of 30 cm H_2O or more for greater than 48 to 72 hours were associated with the injury.

<table>
<tr><td>

BOX 27.2   **Ventilator Alarms**

DISCONNECT ALARMS (LOW-PRESSURE OR LOW-VOLUME ALARMS)

When disconnection occurs, the clinician must be immediately notified. Generally, this alarm is a continuous one and is triggered when a preselected IPL or minute ventilation is not sensed. With circuit leaks, this same alarm may be activated even though the patient may still be receiving a portion of the preset breath. Physical assessment, digital displays, and manometers are helpful in troubleshooting the cause of the alarms.

PRESSURE ALARMS

High-pressure alarms are set to ensure notification of pressures that exceed the selected threshold. These alarms are usually set 10–15 cm H_2O above the usual peak inspiratory pressure (PIP). Some causes for alarm activation (generally an intermittent alarm) include secretions, condensation in the tubing, biting on the endotracheal tubing, increased resistance (i.e., bronchospasm), decreased compliance (e.g., pulmonary edema, pneumothorax), and tubing compression. When this alarm is triggered, the breath delivery is halted and the remaining tidal volume to be delivered by the machine is not delivered. This will then often result in the occurrence of a low-volume alarm.

Low-pressure alarms are used to sense disconnection, circuit leaks, and changing compliance and resistance. They are generally set 5–10 cm H_2O below the usual PIP or 1–2 cm H_2O below the PEEP level or both.

Minute ventilation alarms may be used to sense disconnection or changes in breathing pattern (rate and volume). Generally, low-minute ventilation and high-minute ventilation alarms are set (usually 5–10 L/min above and below usual minute ventilation). When stand-alone pressure support ventilation (PSV) is in use, this alarm may be the only audible alarm available on some ventilators.

Fio_2 alarms are provided on most new ventilators and are set 5–10 mm Hg above and below the selected Fio_2 level.

Alarm silence or pause options are built in by ventilator manufacturers so clinicians can temporarily silence alarms for short periods (i.e., 20 seconds) because alarms must stay activated at all times. The ventilators reset the alarms automatically.

Alarms provide important protection for patients on ventilation. However, inappropriate threshold settings decrease usefulness. When threshold gradients are set too narrowly, alarms occur needlessly and frequently. Conversely, alarms that are set too loosely (wide gradients) do not allow for accurate and timely assessments.

</td></tr>
</table>

- Studies in humans followed the recognition that a large Vt may be associated with lung injury. The ARDS Network conducted a randomized controlled trial of adult patients with ARDS that compared low–lung-volume ventilation (6 mL/kg) with more traditional volumes (i.e., 12 mL/kg). The results showed that the lower-volume ventilation resulted in a lower mortality rate.[1] As a result, current recommendations are to limit volumes (and lower pressures) in patients with stiff lungs. With pressure ventilation, pressure is limited by definition; however, until additional evidence emerges on the efficacy of controlling pressures versus volumes in ARDS, a goal should be to ensure a Vt in the 4 to 8 mL/kg range.[3,5,7,10,11,12,18,24,30,33,34,57,58] Another lung-protective strategy is that of "recruitment" and the prevention of "derecruitment." Investigators showed that stiff noncompliant lungs were at risk of trauma from the repetitive opening associated with tidal breaths. The application of higher levels of positive end-expiratory pressure (PEEP) was associated with better recruitment and resulted in improved mortality rates.[22,33,36,44,78]

- The extent of hemodynamic changes associated with PPV depends on the level of applied positive pressure, the duration of positive pressure during different phases of the breathing cycle, the amount of pressure transmitted to the vascular structures, the patient's intravascular volume, and the adequacy of hemodynamic compensatory mechanisms. PPV can reduce venous return, shift the intraventricular septum to the left, and increase right-ventricular afterload as a result of increased pulmonary vascular resistance. The hemodynamic effects of PPV may be prevented or corrected by optimizing filling pressures to accommodate the PPV-induced changes in intrathoracic pressures; minimizing the peak pressure, plateau pressure, and PEEP; and optimizing the inspiratory-to-expiratory (I:E) ratio.[19,45,46,53,64,65]

- Pulmonary barotrauma (i.e., air-leak disease) is damage to the lung from extrapulmonary air that may result from changes in intrathoracic pressures during PPV. Barotrauma is manifested by pneumothorax, pneumomediastinum, pneumopericardium, pneumoperitoneum, and

TABLE 27.1   **Volume and Pressure Modes and Corresponding Ventilator Parameters**

Mode Name and Description	Main Parameters	Comments
Assist Control (A/C)	Vt Rate Inspiratory time (Ti) Sensitivity Fio_2 PEEP	Generally considered a full support mode. Must switch to another mode or method for weaning.
Synchronized Mandatory Ventilation (SIMV)	Vt Rate Ti Sensitivity Fio_2 PEEP	Originally used as a weaning mode; however, work of breathing is high at low SIMV rates. Often used in conjunction with PSV.

Continued

UNIT I

TABLE 27.1   Volume and Pressure Modes and Corresponding Ventilator Parameters—cont'd

Mode Name and Description	Main Parameters	Comments
Pressure Support Ventilation (PSV)	PS level Sensitivity Fio_2 PEEP	Often pressure is arbitrarily selected (e.g., 10–20 cm H_2O) and then adjusted up or down to attain the desired tidal volume. Some use the plateau pressure if transitioning from volume ventilation as a starting point.
Pressure-Controlled Ventilation (PCV)	Inspiratory pressure limit (IPL) Rate Ti Sensitivity Fio_2 PEEP	Variants of PCV include Volume-Assured Pressure Options and some other modes such as Airway Pressure Release Ventilation and Bilevel Ventilation.
Pressure Controlled–Inverse Ratio Ventilation	As for PCV, but an inverse inspiratory : expiratory (I:E) ratio is attained by lengthening the Ti. Inverse ratios include 1:1, 2:1, 3:1, and 4:1.	Some ventilators allow for the I:E ratio to be selected.
Bilevel Positive Airway Pressure (Bilevel or BiPAP)	$Pressure_{HIGH}$ (P_{HIGH}) $Pressure_{LOW}$ (P_{LOW}) T_{HIGH} (similar to I time in PC) T_{LOW} (similar to E time in PC) Or set ratio T_{HIGH}/T_{LOW} ratio Rate Fio_2	Similar in many ways to PC in that an inspiratory pressure (P_{HIGH}) and PEEP (P_{LOW}) are set. However, unlike PC, the patient may take spontaneous breaths as well. If additional support is desired for patient-initiated breathing, pressure support in bilevel mode may be selected as well. Attention to Vt is important because the patient can augment Vt significantly with supported spontaneous breaths.
Airway Pressure Release Ventilation (APRV)	$Pressure_{HIGH}$ (P_{HIGH}): high CPAP level $Pressure_{LOW}$ (P_{LOW}) is generally 0–5 cm H_2O $Time_{HIGH}$ (T_{HIGH}) $Time_{LOW}$ (T_{LOW}) Fio_2	APRV is a form of biphasic ventilation with a very short expiratory time. Generally, the CPAP level is adjusted to ensure adequate oxygenation while the rate of the releases are increased or decreased to meet ventilation goals. Vt is variably dependent on the CPAP level, compliance and resistance of the patient, and patient spontaneous effort.
Dual Control or Volume-Assured Pressure Modes (1–5 listed here)	These modes provide pressure breaths with a minimum tidal volume assurance.	These modes are ventilator specific. Although the similarities are greater than the differences, they are called different names. Often the names suggest that the mode is a volume mode, yet a decelerating flow pattern (associated with pressure ventilation) is always provided.
Volume Support (VS)	Vt Sensitivity Fio_2 PEEP	The pressure level is automatically adjusted to attain the desired Vt. If control of pressure is desired, it must be carefully monitored.
Pressure-Regulated Control (PRVC)	Rate and Ti are set in addition to those set for VS.	As with VS. The difference is that this is a control mode. Spontaneous breaths, however, may also occur.
Volume Control Plus (VC+)	Rate and Ti are set in addition to those set for VS.	This is a mode option listed in the category called Volume Ventilation Plus. To access this mode, the user selects the SIMV or A/C (both control modes) and then selects VC+. For some clinicians, this is confusing because it appears that the patient is on two different modes versus VC+.
Adaptive Support Ventilation (ASV)	Body weight %MinVol (minute volume), high pressure limit	Once basic settings are selected, ASV is started and %MinVol is adjusted if indicated. Spontaneous breathing is automatically encouraged, and when the inspiratory pressure (Pinsp) is consistently 0 and the rate is 0, extubation may be considered.
Proportional Assist Ventilation (PAV)	Proportional Pressure Support (PPS): PEEP, Fio_2, percent volume assist and flow assist Proportional Assist Plus: PAV+: PEEP, Fio_2, percent support	Depending on the ventilator, the amount of assist that is provided is determined by the clinician, and different parameters are selected to do so. Default percent support numbers are recommended, but the clinician must determine the timing of reductions of same.
Automatic Tube Compensation (ATC)	Endotracheal tube internal diameter Percent compensation	This is not a mode but rather a pressure option to offset the work associated with tube resistance. It can be combined with other modes or used alone as in a CPAP weaning trial.

subcutaneous emphysema. The risk of barotrauma in a patient receiving PPV is increased with preexisting lung lesions (e.g., localized infections, blebs), high inflation pressures (i.e., large Vt, PEEP, main-stem bronchus intubation, patient-ventilator asynchrony), and invasive thoracic procedures (e.g., subclavian catheter insertion, bronchoscopy, thoracentesis). Barotrauma from PPV may be prevented by controlling peak and plateau pressures, optimizing PEEP, preventing auto-PEEP, ensuring patient-ventilator synchrony, and ensuring proper artificial airway position.[23,40,61,79]

- ❖ Auto-PEEP is a common complication of mechanical ventilation and can result in hemodynamic compromise and even death. Because increased intrathoracic pressures are transmitted to the adjacent capillaries, venous return is decreased, and the effect can be profound. Auto-PEEP and dynamic hyperinflation should be assumed in the patient on ventilation with acute severe asthma whose condition is hemodynamically compromised, and a brief cessation of mechanical ventilation or decrease in rate and shortening of inspiratory time should be accomplished.[2,19,23,40,52,61,79] Auto-PEEP is caused by inadequate expiratory time relative to the patient's lung condition. Auto-PEEP is often seen in patients with prolonged inspiratory times, short expiratory times, high minute ventilation requirements, bronchospasm, low elastic recoil (lung elastance), mucus hypersecretion, increased bronchial wall thickness, airway closure or collapse, and mechanical factors (e.g., water in the ventilator circuit, pinched ventilator tubing). Correcting these factors reduces auto-PEEP. In some cases in which auto-PEEP cannot be eliminated, adding set PEEP to the level of auto-PEEP results in a decreased inspiratory trigger threshold and thus improvement of patient triggering.[2,19,23,40,52,61,79]

- Ventilator-associated complications include ventilator-associated pneumonia (VAP) and ventilator associated conditions (pneumonia, pulmonary edema, atelectasis, acute respiratory distress syndrome).
  - ❖ VAP occurs after 3 days of mechanical ventilation and accounts for one-third of all healthcare-associated infections and between 50% and 83% of infections patients with MV.[9,42,70,73]
  - ❖ Modifiable risk factors to the aspiration of colonized organisms in the patient on ventilation include interventions such as proper endotracheal tube cuff inflation (secretions that collect above the cuff of the endotracheal or tracheostomy tube and leak past the cuff into the lungs), use of continuous-aspiration subglottic suctioning (CASS) tubes, decreased ventilator tubing changes, use of heat and moisture exchangers (HMEs), stringent hand washing, backrest elevation (BRE) of greater than 30 degrees, and when possible the use of noninvasive ventilation (especially in patients with immunocompromise).[13,14,21,31,48,50,51]
  - ❖ Other interventions with a lower level of evidence supporting their use include oral care techniques such as mouth care and oral decontamination with agents such as chlorhexidine or oral antibiotics. Of interest, gastric residual volumes have not been found to be consistently

---

BOX 27.3 Top Modifiable Ventilator-Associated Pneumonia Prevention Interventions

- Backrest elevation (>30–45 degrees)
- Continuous aspiration of subglottic secretions tubes
- Limit/interrupt sedation (spontaneous awakening trial)
- Spontaneous awakening trial (SAT)
- Spontaneous breathing trial (SBT)
- Assess readiness to extubate daily
- Noninvasive ventilation when possible
- Early mobility
- No routine ventilator circuit change
- Hand washing and aseptic technique

Modified from Klompas M, Branson R, Eichenwald E, et al: Strategies to prevent ventilator-associated pneumonia in acute care hospitals: 2014 update. *Infect Control Hosp Epidemiol* 35(S2): S133-S154, 2014; Society of Critical Care Medicine: ICU Liberation. https://www.sccm.org/ICULiberation/Home; American Association of Critical Care Nurses. AACN Practice Alert. *Ventilator associated pneumonia in adults.* https://www.aacn.org/~/media/aacn-website/clincial-resources/practice-alerts/preventingvapinadults2017.pdf/

associated with VAP.[49,62,81] Box 27.3 lists the top recommendations of authoritative professional organizations for the prevention of VAP.

EQUIPMENT

- Endotracheal or tracheostomy tube
- Electrocardiogram and pulse oximetry
- Supplemental oxygen source
- Manual self-inflating resuscitation bag-valve-mask device (with PEEP valve adjusted to patient baseline level)
- Appropriate-sized resuscitation face mask
- Ventilator
- Suction equipment

PATIENT AND FAMILY EDUCATION

- Explain the procedure and the reasons for PPV to the patient and family. ***Rationale:*** Communication and explanations for therapy are important needs of patients and families.
- Discuss the potential sensations the patient will experience, such as relief of dyspnea, lung inflation, noise of ventilator operation, and alarm sounds. ***Rationale:*** Knowledge of anticipated sensory experiences reduces anxiety and stress.
- Encourage the patient to relax. ***Rationale:*** This encouragement promotes general relaxation, oxygenation, and ventilation.
- Explain that the patient will be unable to speak. Establish a method of communication in conjunction with the patient and family before initiating mechanical ventilation, if necessary. ***Rationale:*** Ensuring the patient's ability to communicate is important to alleviate anxiety.
- Teach the family how to perform desired and appropriate activities of direct patient care, such as pharyngeal suction with the tonsil-tip suction device, range-of-motion

exercises, and reconnection to ventilator if inadvertent disconnection occurs. Demonstrate use of the call bell. *Rationale:* Family members have identified the need and desire to help in the patient's care.

- Explain to the patient and family the importance of not touching the ventilator controls, including silencing and resetting alarms. *Rationale:* Families may become familiar with the ventilator over time and, in a desire to help, reset or silence an alarm without an understanding of the cause/underlying problem.

- Provide the patient and family with information on the critical nature of the patient's dependence on PPV. *Rationale:* Knowledge of the prognosis, probable outcome, or chance for recovery is cited as an important need of patients and families.

- Offer the opportunity for the patient and family to ask questions about PPV. *Rationale:* Asking questions and having questions answered honestly are cited consistently as the most important need of patients and families.

PATIENT ASSESSMENT AND PREPARATION

Patient Assessment

- Assess for signs and symptoms of acute ventilatory failure and fatigue. *Rationale:* Ventilatory failure indicates the need for initiation of PPV. While PPV is being considered and assembled, support ventilation via a self-inflating manual resuscitation bag-valve-mask device, if necessary.
  - ❖ Increasing arterial carbon dioxide tension
  - ❖ Chest-abdominal dyssynchrony
  - ❖ Shallow or irregular respirations
  - ❖ Tachypnea, bradypnea, or dyspnea
  - ❖ Decreased mental status
  - ❖ Restlessness, confusion, or lethargy
  - ❖ Increasing or decreasing arterial blood pressure
  - ❖ Tachycardia
  - ❖ Atrial or ventricular dysrhythmias
- Determine arterial pH and carbon dioxide tension. *Rationale:* Acute ventilatory failure is confirmed by an uncompensated respiratory acidosis. Ventilatory failure is an indication for PPV.
- Assess for signs and symptoms of inadequate oxygenation. *Rationale:* Hypoxemia may indicate the need for PPV. While PPV is being considered and assembled, provide 100% oxygen via a manual resuscitation bag-valve-mask device or an oxygen delivery device such as a nonrebreather mask.
  - ❖ Decreasing arterial oxygen tension

- ❖ Tachypnea
- ❖ Dyspnea
- ❖ Central cyanosis
- ❖ Alterations in level of consciousness
- ❖ Restlessness
- ❖ Confusion
- ❖ Agitation
- ❖ Tachycardia
- ❖ Bradycardia
- ❖ Dysrhythmias
- ❖ Intercostal and suprasternal retractions
- ❖ Increasing or decreasing arterial blood pressure
- ❖ Adventitious breath sounds
- ❖ Decreasing urine output
- ❖ Metabolic acidosis
- Determine PaO_2 or arterial oxygen saturation (SaO_2). *Rationale:* Hypoxemia is confirmed by a PaO_2 <60 mm Hg or SaO_2 less than 90% on supplemental oxygen. Hypoxemia may indicate the need for PPV.
- Assess for signs and symptoms of inadequate breathing patterns. *Rationale:* Respiratory distress is an indication for PPV.
  - ❖ Dyspnea
  - ❖ Chest-abdominal dyssynchrony
  - ❖ Rapid-shallow breathing pattern
  - ❖ Irregular respirations
  - ❖ Intercostal or suprasternal retractions
  - ❖ Inability to say a whole sentence

Patient Preparation

- Verify the correct patient with two identifiers. *Rationale:* Before performing a procedure, the nurse should ensure the correct identification of the patient for the intended intervention.
- Perform a preprocedural verification and time out, if nonemergent. *Rationale:* Ensures patient safety.
- If the patient is not in distress, ensure that the patient understands the preprocedural teachings. Answer questions as they arise and reinforce information as needed. *Rationale:* This communication evaluates and reinforces understanding of previously taught information.
- Premedicate as needed. *Rationale:* Administration of sedatives, narcotics, or muscle relaxants may be necessary to provide adequate oxygenation and ventilation in some patients.
- Ensure that the patient is positioned properly for optimum ventilation. *Rationale:* Elevating the head of the bed at least 30 degrees enhances diaphragmatic excursion, decreases intrathoracic pressure, and helps prevent aspiration and VAP.

Procedure for Invasive Mechanical Ventilation (Through an Artificial Airway): Volume and Pressure Modes

Steps	Rationale	Special Considerations
1. **HH**		
2. **PE**		
Volume-Control Modes		
3. Select mode (see Box 27.1 and Table 27.1). The three traditional volume modes and mode settings are control mechanical ventilation (CMV), assist/control (A/C), and synchronized intermittent mandatory ventilation (SIMV).	Mode selection varies depending on the clinical goal and clinician preference. Traditional volume modes that may provide total ventilatory support include control, SIMV, and A/C. Other modes may also provide complete support depending on the settings. Remember that the goal is to offset the patient's work of breathing. See subsequent description of other modes and their applications.	SIMV is often used in conjunction with PSV (to overcome circuit resistance and to decrease the work of breathing associated with spontaneous effort). The use of SIMV plus PSV has been associated with prolonged weaning times. If respiratory muscle rest is the goal with SIMV plus PSV, the level of PSV should be high enough to provide a Vt of 6–12 mL/kg and to maintain a total rate (IMV plus PSV breaths) of ≤20 breaths/min.[15,40,68]
A. CMV: The intent of control ventilation is to ensure the Vt and rate (fx). As with all modes of ventilation, the patient is never completely "locked out" and can breathe between the control breaths, which is ensured by setting the sensitivity or flow triggers **(see Step 8)**. However, should control over ventilation be desired, sedation and often paralytic agents are provided to ensure the goal.		
B. A/C: Ventilation ensures that a control rate and Vt are set. Patient-initiated (assist) breaths are delivered at the predetermined volume selected for the control breaths.		
C. SIMV: With this mode, a rate (fx) and Vt are set and are delivered in synchrony with the patient's respiratory effort. Between mandatory breaths, the patient may initiate breaths at a patient-determined volume and rate.		
4. Set Vt <10 mL/kg PBW. In patients with ARDS, Vt should be set at 4–6 mL/kg PBW. **(Level B*)**	Vt is selected in conjunction with fx to attain an MV 5–10 L/min with a $Paco_2$ 35–45 mm Hg. Large Vt values (12 mL/kg) have been associated with lung injury in patients with ARDS.[1,3,5,7,10,11,12,18,24,30,33,34,57,58]	When lower Vt values are used to reduce lung injury, patients may need sedation and potentially paralytic agents if they are dyssynchronous with the ventilator. Hypercarbia is an expected outcome of low Vt values. Permissive hypercapnia is generally well tolerated in patients if the pH is reduced gradually (over 24–48 hours); A pH around 7.2 is cited as an end point if tolerated.[6,25,52] Occasionally, bicarbonate infusions are used to keep the pH within an acceptable range. However, this temporizing maneuver may result in a higher $Paco_2$ because bicarbonate is metabolized into CO_2 and H_2O. Permissive hypercapnia should not be attempted in patients with elevated intracranial pressure or those with myocardial ischemia, myocardial injury, or dysrhythmias. Patients who are allowed to become hypercarbic may need sedation and often paralytic agents to control ventilation.

*Level B: Well-designed, controlled studies with results that consistently support a specific action, intervention, or treatment.

Procedure continues on following page

Procedure	**for Invasive Mechanical Ventilation (Through an Artificial Airway): Volume and Pressure Modes—*Continued***

Steps	Rationale	Special Considerations
5. Select RR (frequency) between 10 and 20 breaths/min.	Vt and rate are selected to maintain an acceptable $Paco_2$ with an MV between 5 and 10 L/min. Generally, once Vt is selected, the rate is the parameter adjusted to attain a desired $Paco_2$; the rate selected depends on whether the clinical goal is to rest or work the respiratory muscles.	When low Vts are used, as in ARDS, a higher rate may be necessary to maintain pH and $Paco_2$ at acceptable levels because smaller Vt provides less-efficient ventilation; the result is higher CO_2 and lower pH.[6,25,52]
6. For I:E times, select inspiratory time (this parameter name is different, depending on the ventilator). Examples of parameter names include percent inspiratory time, inspiratory time, flow rate, and peak flow. 1.1.1 I:E ratios are usually 1:2 or 1:3. A typical inspiratory time for an adult is in the range of 0.75–1.2 second.	Inspiratory flow refers to the speed with which Vt is delivered during inspiration. Increasing the flow rate shortens the inspiratory time. Conversely, slowing the flow rate lengthens the inspiratory time.	Generally, flow rates of approximately 50 L/min are used initially and adjusted to provide an inspiratory time that synchronizes with patient effort. Short inspiratory times and long expiratory times are necessary in patients with obstructive lung diseases (e.g., emphysema, asthma). In contrast, patients with restrictive diseases, such as ARDS, have noncompliant lungs. Longer inspiratory times enhance recruitment and prevent derecruitment.[12,55,64]
7. Adjust flow as necessary to attain patient ventilator synchrony.	Achieves the desired I:E ratio and comfortable breathing patterns.	
8. Set the sensitivity (trigger sensitivity). Most ventilators have pressure-sensing sensitivity mechanisms that trigger a machine breath, which means that the patient must generate a decrease in the system pressure with an inspiratory effort. When the ventilator senses the drop in pressure, gas flow (or a breath) is delivered. If a pressure trigger is used, sensitivity is set between −1 and −2 cm H_2O pressure.	The more negative the number, the less sensitive the ventilator is to patient effort, which increases the patient respiratory workload and may lead to dyssynchrony.	When auto-PEEP is present, the patient must generate a negative pressure equal to the set sensitivity plus the level of auto-PEEP. Auto-PEEP is common in patients with asthma, chronic obstructive pulmonary disease, and high RRs and minute ventilation. This additional work may fatigue the patient. Patient ventilator dyssynchrony is likely.[2,19,23,40,52,61,79]
9. If the ventilator has a flow-triggering option, select the flow trigger in L/min. The smaller the number, the more sensitive the ventilator. Flow triggering is set in conjunction with a base flow (flow in L/min that is provided between ventilator breaths). Flow rate is monitored in the expiratory limb of the ventilator. When flow is disrupted during a spontaneous breath, a decrease in flow downstream is sensed; additional flow or a breath is delivered.	Flow triggering has been associated with faster ventilator response times and less work of breathing than pressure triggering.	

Procedure	for Invasive Mechanical Ventilation (Through an Artificial Airway): Volume and Pressure Modes—*Continued*		
Steps	**Rationale**	**Special Considerations**	
10. Set Fio$_2$ to 0.60–1.0 (60%–100%), if Pao$_2$ is unknown. A. Adjust Fio$_2$ downward as tolerated by monitoring Sao$_2$ and arterial blood gas values.	Initiation of PPV with maximal oxygen concentration avoids hypoxemia while optimal ventilator settings are being determined and evaluated. In addition, it permits measurement of the percentage of venous admixture (shunt), which provides an estimate of the severity of the gas-exchange abnormality.	The goal is an Fio$_2$ ≤0.5; high levels of Fio$_2$ result in increased risk of oxygen toxicity, absorption atelectasis, and reduction of surfactant synthesis.[41,43]	
11. Select PEEP or continuous positive airway pressure (CPAP) level. Initial setting is often 5 cm H$_2$O. A. PEEP may be adjusted as needed after evaluation of tolerance (e.g., Sao$_2$, Pao$_2$, physical assessment). PEEP levels are increased to restore lung functional residual capacity (FRC) and allow for reduction of FiO$_2$ to safe levels (i.e., ≤0.5) to decrease the risk of oxygen toxicity.	A PEEP level of 5 cm H$_2$O is considered physiological (essentially the amount of pressure at end exhalation normally provided by the glottis). Higher levels of PEEP may be used to prevent alveolar collapse during the expiratory phase of the ventilator breath in atelectasis or ARDS.	High levels of PEEP ≥10 cm H$_2$O should rarely be interrupted because reestablishment of FRC (and Pao$_2$) may take hours. Prevention of this derecruitment in the patient with ARDS is especially important. Super-PEEP levels (i.e., ≥20 cm H$_2$O) may be necessary in patients with noncompliant lungs (e.g., patients with ARDS) to prevent lung injury. The repetitive opening and closing of stiff alveoli is thought to result in alveolar damage; to this end, the use of high PEEP levels to maintain alveolar distention and to prevent injury during PPV is considered a protective lung strategy.[12,30,58] In general, when high PEEP levels are used, Vt values are lower than normal and subsequent hypercarbia may be anticipated. Use of muscle relaxants, sedatives, and narcotics is often necessary to prevent patient spontaneous breathing.	
B. Continuous positive airway pressure (CPAP) is often referred to as *PEEP* without the positive pressure breaths. CPAP is a spontaneous breathing mode that provides continuous pressure throughout the ventilator cycle. It is commonly used as a mode for spontaneous-breathing trials (SBT).	Patients who are spontaneously breathing may not require delivery of ventilator breaths but may require positive pressure applied to the airways and alveoli to prevent collapse or obstruction during exhalation.	Generally, the pressure levels of CPAP are relatively low but vary with individual patient conditions. A traditional application of CPAP is for obstructive sleep apnea (OSA) through a noninvasive mask or prongs. When used for OSA, the mode provides a pneumatic splint to the airways to prevent obstruction during sleep.	
Pressure Modes (Invasive)			
1. Select mode: PSV, pressure-controlled/inverse ratio ventilation (PC/IRV), volume-assured pressure support option, Biphasic, APRV, ASV, PAV, automatic tube compensation (ATC), or HFO.	Mode selection depends on clinical goals, mode availability (these vary widely with different ventilators), and clinician preference. To date, no mode has emerged as superior. Modes include those designed for spontaneous breathing and those for control or partial control of ventilation.[32]	Many new modes that use microprocessor technology are available on specific ventilators. Although many are similar to traditional modes, others are not. Parameter names also vary. Refer to the specific ventilator operating manuals and websites for details not contained in this procedure.	

Procedure continues on following page

Procedure for Invasive Mechanical Ventilation (Through an Artificial Airway): Volume and Pressure Modes—*Continued*

Steps	Rationale	Special Considerations
2. PSV augments spontaneous respirations with a clinician-selected pressure level. Adjust the PSV level to attain a Vt <10 mL/kg PBW with a spontaneous RR ≤20 breaths/min (if respiratory muscle rest is desired; this is called *PSVmax*). Decrease PSV level during weaning trials as tolerated by the patient. Tolerance criteria for trials may be predetermined by protocols or on an individual basis. Often during trials, Vt values can be lower (i.e., 5–8 mL/kg) and RR higher (i.e., 25–30 breaths/min) than when rest is the goal. However, these parameters are always evaluated in conjunction with other signs and symptoms of fatigue and intolerance. **(Level B*)**	The pressure level in conjunction with compliance and resistance determines delivered Vt.	PSV sometimes is used between IMV breaths to offset the work of breathing associated with artificial airways and circuits during spontaneous breathing. PSV generally is considered a weaning mode of ventilation, which necessitates stability of patient condition. PSV may be used in patients with less stable conditions provided that close attention is given to changes in Vt and RR. High levels of PSV may provide respiratory muscle unloading.
A. Set sensitivity (as with volume ventilation).	The less sensitive the ventilator is to patient effort, the more the patient respiratory workload increases, which may lead to dyssynchrony.	
B. Set Fio$_2$ (as with volume ventilation).	Initiation of PPV with maximal oxygen concentration avoids hypoxemia while optimal ventilator settings are being determined and evaluated. In addition, it permits measurement of the percentage of venous admixture (shunt), which provides an estimate of the severity of the gas-exchange abnormality.	
C. Set PEEP (as with volume ventilation).	A PEEP level of 5 cm H$_2$O is considered physiological (essentially the amount of pressure at end exhalation normally provided by the glottis). Higher levels of PEEP may be used to prevent alveolar collapse during the expiratory phase of the ventilator breath in atelectasis or ARDS.	

*Level B: Well-designed, controlled studies with results that consistently support a specific action, intervention, or treatment.

Procedure	for Invasive Mechanical Ventilation (Through an Artificial Airway): Volume and Pressure Modes—*Continued*	
Steps	**Rationale**	**Special Considerations**
3. PC/IRV is a control mode of ventilation. With this mode, an inspiratory pressure level (IPL) is selected; the rate and inspiratory time are selected as well. They were originally used to manage patients with ARDS in whom the goal was to limit the pressure level. In addition, the decelerating flow pattern of the modes was considered desirable. PC/IRV was used to enhance lung recruitment by prolonging inspiration. Expiration was shortened, thereby decreasing the potential for derecruitment.[4,32,64]	Absolute pressure level is the sum of the IPL and PEEP.	If the clinical goal is to ensure a plateau pressure of ≤30 cm H_2O, the IPL may be lowered gradually over 24–48 hours to prevent sudden changes in $Paco_2$ and pH.[4,64]
A. Select IPL. With this pressure mode, the inspiratory pressure setting is often identified as IPL versus PS level of PSV.	Rate and IPL determine MV.	
B. Select the rate.	IPL and rate are selected to maintain an acceptable $Paco_2$ with an MV between 5 and 10 L/min. Generally, once IPL is selected, rate is the parameter adjusted to attain a desired $Paco_2$; the rate selected depends on whether or not the clinical goal is to rest or work the respiratory muscles.	When low Vts are desired, as in ARDS, a higher rate may be necessary to maintain pH and $Paco_2$ at acceptable levels because smaller Vts provide less-efficient ventilation; the result is higher CO_2 and lower pH.[25,52]
C. Select the inspiratory time or inverse I:E ratio (ventilators vary).	I:E ratios are set at 1:1, 2:1, 3:1, or 4:1 by selecting the appropriate inspiratory time. Ratios are adjusted upward to recruit collapsed alveoli and improve shunt and oxygenation. Blood pressure may be adversely affected. Rate is usually relatively high (e.g., 20–25 breaths/min).	Generally, clinicians start with 1:1 ratios and increase as necessary to improve oxygenation. A limiting factor related to prolonged inspiratory times is hemodynamic compromise and hypotension, which is generally why the use of ratios >2:1 rarely is seen clinically. Auto-PEEP is common and may be a desired outcome of PC/IRV.[23,79]
D. Select the PEEP level. When transitioning from volume ventilation to PC/IRV, the PEEP initially is maintained at the level used previously until the effect of the IRV is assessed. **(Level C*)**	Because IRV may result in auto-PEEP, evaluation of the total amount of PEEP present is important. This can be measured through the performance of an expiratory hold maneuver on the ventilator.	Auto-PEEP generated by IRV is expected and helpful in expanding collapsed alveoli.

*Level C: Qualitative studies, descriptive or correlational studies, integrative reviews, systematic reviews, or randomized controlled trials with inconsistent results.

Procedure continues on following page

Procedure   for Invasive Mechanical Ventilation (Through an Artificial Airway): Volume and Pressure Modes—*Continued*

Steps	Rationale	Special Considerations
E. Set Fio_2 to 0.60–1.0 (60%–100%) if Pao_2 is unknown. Adjust Fio_2 downward as tolerated by monitoring SaO_2 and arterial blood gas values.	Initiation of PPV with maximal oxygen concentration avoids hypoxemia while optimal ventilator settings are being determined and evaluated. In addition, it permits measurement of the percentage of venous admixture (shunt), which provides an estimate of the severity of the gas-exchange abnormality.	The goal is an Fio_2 ≤0.5; high levels of Fio_2 result in increased risk of oxygen toxicity, absorption atelectasis, and reduction of surfactant synthesis.[41,43]
F. Set the sensitivity (as with volume ventilation). **(Level B*)**	The goal of PC/IRV is to improve oxygenation and allow for reduction of Fio_2 to ≤0.5.[41,43] This is done in conjunction with the addition of PEEP. Always set sensitivity so the patient can get a breath if needed.	If controlled ventilation is the goal, chemical relaxation may be necessary in conjunction with sedatives and narcotics. Patient tolerance of IRV (i.e., the prolonged inspiratory times) is unlikely without such interventions. Remember that IRV may result in auto-PEEP (which may be a desirable outcome of the mode). Regardless, auto-PEEP should be anticipated and measured regularly.
4. Dual-control pressure mode options are pressure modes that ensure a minimum set tidal volume. The breath delivery varies with the specific mode. For dual-control pressure-support options, parameter selection (i.e., pressure, volume, rate) is specific to the ventilator; however, selection of desired (or guaranteed) Vt is required. Some ventilators also require selection of the pressure level. Spontaneous breathing modes and controlled modes are available.[16,17,32] **(Level C*)** A. For volume-guaranteed pressure options, please see the specific ventilator manual for the parameter setting. **(Level M*)** B. PEEP, Fio_2, and sensitivity are set as per volume ventilation as are rate and inspiratory time if the mode is a control mode. However, the desired Vt must be selected as well.	Specific names vary depending on ventilator manufacturer. Examples include Pressure Augmentation (Carefusion, San Diego, CA) and Volume Support and Pressure Regulated Volume Control (Maquet, Wayne, NJ); similar modes are available on other manufacturers' ventilators.	Few studies have been accomplished that show the superiority of these modes. In addition, many modes are available only on specific ventilators. These modes are complex; concurrent use of pressure, flow, and volume waveform displays may be necessary to assess the modes accurately. These modes will deliver the set minimum tidal volume within the set IPL, but depending on patient effort, larger tidal volumes may be generated by the patient. If consistent control of tidal volume is desired, volume control ventilation should be used. Refer to specific ventilator operating manuals or websites for additional information (see Table 27.1 for volume-guaranteed pressure options).

*Level B: Well-designed, controlled studies with results that consistently support a specific action, intervention, or treatment.

*Level C: Qualitative studies, descriptive or correlational studies, integrative reviews, systematic reviews, or randomized controlled trials with inconsistent results.

*Level M: Manufacturer's recommendations only.

Procedure	for Invasive Mechanical Ventilation (Through an Artificial Airway): Volume and Pressure Modes—*Continued*	
Steps	**Rationale**	**Special Considerations**
5. Biphasic and APRV ventilation are relatively new modes that appear on selected ventilators. Used most commonly for patients with ARDS, the modes use relatively high levels of pressure to recruit the lung (restore FRC). APRV is a type of biphasic ventilation with a very short expiratory (release) time.[12,32,59,71] **(Level C*)**	Although the modes appear to be safe and effective, randomized controlled trials are not available. One advantage to these modes is that they do not require that the patient be heavily sedated or paralyzed. Spontaneous breathing is expected. Generally, the patient's breathing pattern is rapid.	Few studies have been accomplished that show the superiority of these modes. These ventilatory modes require a steep learning curve on the part of the physician, advanced practice nurse, and other healthcare professionals who care for these patients; as with most new forms of ventilation, education of staff should occur before the mode is used. Although the appeal of APRV and biphasic ventilation is in part because the patient may breathe spontaneously, it is unclear whether the associated workload is advantageous. Additionally, large spontaneous tidal volumes may result in injurious overdistention of alveoli.
A. With APRV, a high level of CPAP is selected, and brief expiratory "releases" are provided at set intervals (similar to setting RR); the releases are very brief (≤1.5 seconds).	The high level of CPAP helps "recruit" the lung. Alveolar filling and emptying time constants in the ARDS lung vary; the brief expiratory releases provided with APRV allow for more uniform emptying throughout the lung and ultimately improved gas distribution. An additional benefit of periodic airway pressure releases is that they may decrease the potential negative effect of the high CPAP level on venous return. At the high CPAP level, patients may take spontaneous breaths at the rate they determine.[12,29,32]	On some machines, the formal mode name APRV may not be used. It may be incorporated under "Biphasic ventilation."
B. With the Biphasic mode, two different levels of PEEP are selected and are called *high-PEEP* and *low PEEP*. This is really an iteration of traditional PC ventilation. A rate is set, and the cycles look similar to PC or PC/IRV ventilation (depending on the I:E ratio). The major difference is that flow is available to the patient for spontaneous breathing at both pressure levels. In addition, pressure support (PS) may be added to assist in decreasing the work associated with spontaneous breathing.[12,32] **(Level E*)**	The theoretical advantage of this mode over traditional PC/IRV is that the mode may fully support lung recruitment while still allowing for spontaneous breathing at the two pressure levels.[12,32] In contrast with traditional PC/IRV, the patient receives additional flow adequate to meet inspiratory demands throughout the ventilatory cycle. Deterioration with spontaneous effort is less likely; as a result, heavy sedation and paralytics may be avoided.	The APRV mode as described previously may be achieved in ventilators with biphasic modes. Biphasic modes have many trade names (BiVent, BiLevel, BiPAP, DuoPap). The APRV settings are achieved on each type of ventilator in a slightly different manner. Refer to the specific ventilator manual for parameter settings.

*Level C: Qualitative studies, descriptive or correlational studies, integrative reviews, systematic reviews, or randomized controlled trials with inconsistent results.
*Level E: Multiple case reports, theory-based evidence from expert opinions, or peer-reviewed professional organizational standards without clinical studies to support recommendations.

Procedure continues on following page

Procedure	**for Invasive Mechanical Ventilation (Through an Artificial Airway): Volume and Pressure Modes—*Continued***	
Steps	Rationale	Special Considerations
C. For APRV and biphasic mode options, please see the specific ventilator manual for parameter settings. (**Level M***)	Manufacturers have different names for parameters settings. Although there are similarities among the ventilator models, it is important to be familiar with the ventilators used at your practice area.	

D. Specific APRV settings:
  i. Pressure high (P_{HIGH}), which is the high-PEEP level. This may be set at the measured plateau pressure to start.
  ii. Pressure low (P_{LOW}), which is the low-PEEP level, is generally set at 0 cm H_2O.
  iii. Time high (T_{HIGH}): 4–6 seconds.
  iv. Time low (T_{LOW}): 0.4–0.8 seconds (keep <1.5 seconds). Rate is determined by the combined inspiratory (T_{HIGH}) expiratory time (T_{LOW}).[12,32,59,71]
	The combination of the inspiratory pressure (P_{HIGH}) and inspiratory time (T_{HIGH}) determine the machine-delivered tidal volume. The expiratory time (T_{LOW}) determines the duration of exhalation. In APRV, the expiratory time is very short (usually <1.0 second). Therefore, the P_{LOW} is set at 0 cm H_2O, because there is insufficient time for the alveoli to collapse before the next breath.	Patients on APRV should be transported on the ventilator to avoid alveolar derecruitment associated with disconnection from the ventilator circuit. This can occur when the patient is transitioned to a bag-valve-mask device for transport. If the patient must be disconnected from the ventilator, the endotracheal tube may be clamped during the inspiratory phase before circuit disconnection to reduce the chance of alveolar derecruitment.

E. Specific Biphasic settings:
  i. Pressure high (P_{HIGH}).
  Set to achieve the desired tidal volume for the patient
  ii. Pressure low (P_{LOW}). Set to attain the best PEEP
  iii. Rate: 8–10
  iv. Inspiratory time (T_{HIGH}): 1.5 seconds or set T_{HIGH}/T_{LOW} ratio (I:E ratio)
  v. FiO_2.
F. FiO_2 and sensitivity are set as outlined in **Steps 8 and 9** under "Volume-Control Modes."
	The combination of the inspiratory pressure (P_{HIGH}) and inspiratory time (T_{HIGH}) determines the machine-delivered tidal volume. The expiratory time (T_{LOW}) determines the duration of exhalation. In biphasic (non-APRV), the I:E ratio is usually set at conventional ratios (1:2 or 1:3).
	
	See **Steps 8 and 9.**	

6. Adaptive Support Ventilation: This mode is referred to by the ventilator manufacturer as *intelligent ventilation* and is designed to assess lung mechanics on a breath-to-breath basis (controlled loop ventilation) for spontaneous and control settings. It achieves an optimal Vt by automatically adjusting mandatory respiratory fx and inspiratory pressure. Built into the mode are algorithms that are "lung protective." The protective strategies are designed to minimize auto-PEEP and prevent apnea, tachypnea, excessive dead space, and excessively large breaths.[26,32,47] (**Level C***) Parameters to set include PBW, minute volume (%MinVol), and high pressure limit in addition to Fio_2. (**Level M***)	The working concept with this mode is that the patient will breathe at fx and Vt that minimize elastic and resistive loads. In all modes, the opportunity for spontaneous breathing is promoted (the user does not have to switch back and forth from one mode to another to encourage spontaneous breathing because this is automatically done). Thus the interactions required by the clinician are few.	The higher the %MinVol, the higher the level of support provided to the patient.

*Level M: Manufacturer's recommendations only.
*Level C: Qualitative studies, descriptive or correlational studies, integrative reviews, systematic reviews, or randomized controlled trials with inconsistent results.

Procedure	for Invasive Mechanical Ventilation (Through an Artificial Airway): Volume and Pressure Modes—*Continued*	
Steps	**Rationale**	**Special Considerations**
7. PAV: The concept with this pressure mode is to prevent fatiguing workloads while still allowing the patient to breathe spontaneously. Current PAV modes take measurements throughout the inspiratory cycle and automatically adjust the pressure, flow, and volume proportionally to offset the resistance and elastance of the system with each inspiration (patient and circuit). Different names for the modes are provided by specific manufacturers, and parameters that require adjustment vary somewhat among ventilators.[8,32,69] **(Level M*)** Parameter settings include PEEP, Fio_2, percent volume assist, and percent flow assist.	PAV may provide a more physiological breathing pattern. These modes recognize that patient effort reflects work and demand and base the adjustments accordingly. The percent of assist is adjusted to a higher percent if less work is desired and a lower percent if more work is necessary.[8,32,69]	Few studies have been accomplished that show the superiority of this mode. In addition, many modes are available on specific ventilators.
8. ATC is a ventilatory adjunct rather than a mode and is available on many current ventilators. It is designed to overcome the work of breathing imposed by the artificial airway. Parameters include type of airway (endotracheal tube or tracheostomy tube), internal diameter size of the airway, and the desired percent of compensation.[32,74] **(Level C*)**	ATC adjusts the pressure (proportional to tube resistance) needed to provide a variable fast inspiratory flow during spontaneous breathing.	ATC is increased during inspiration and lowered during expiration, thus decreasing the work of breathing as a result of tube resistance. In some patients, the use of ATC has resulted in auto-PEEP.[32,75]
9. High-frequency oscillation ventilation (HFOV) differs significantly from conventional ventilator modes or mode options. HFOV does not require bulk movement of volume in and out of the lungs; rather, a bias flow of gases is provided, and an oscillator disperses the gases throughout the lung in what has been called augmented dispersion at high frequencies.[29,35,56] **(Level C*)** The parameters for HFOV are different from conventional ventilation and are outlined in the following.	The method achieves oscillation of the lung around a constant airway pressure (essentially opening the lung and keeping it open).[29,35,56]	Studies to date have not shown the superiority of this mode over traditional modes in adults with ARDS. The mode is safe if appropriately applied by those with experience in its use; however, it is not easily understood by clinicians. Especially of concern is the fact that patients on the mode often need sedation and neuromuscular blockade.
A. Bias flow: flow in L/min (usual range, 40–50 L/min)	The bias flow combined with the oscillatory activity (extremely rapid pulses in a back-and-forth motion) results in the constant infusion of fresh gases and evacuation of old gases.	

*Level M: Manufacturer's recommendations only.
*Level C: Qualitative studies, descriptive or correlational studies, integrative reviews, systematic reviews, or randomized controlled trials with inconsistent results.

Procedure continues on following page

Procedure	for Invasive Mechanical Ventilation (Through an Artificial Airway): Volume and Pressure Modes—*Continued*	
Steps	Rationale	Special Considerations
B. Oscillatory frequency (fx): in Hz (usual range, 3–6 Hz)[29,35,56]	Increases in frequency in HFOV actually reduce CO_2 elimination because there is less time for CO_2 to be removed from the lungs between the oscillatory breaths. This is different from conventional ventilation in which an increase in rate may reduce CO_2.	1 Hz is equivalent to 60 breaths.
C. Mean airway pressure: generally slightly greater than conventional ventilation initially		
D. ΔP: Change in pressure or pressure amplitude (generally adjusted to achieve chest wall vibration)	ΔP and fx are adjusted to achieve $Paco_2$ within a target range.	
E. Fio_2 level and PEEP level: as in conventional ventilation (generally PEEP is >10)		
F. Percent inspiratory time: controls the percentage of time the oscillator spends in the inspiratory phase; a starting place is 33%		
10. Discard used supplies, and remove 🔲 PE		
11. 🔲 HH		

Humidity

1. Humidity is essential to prevent the drying effect of the gases provided by the ventilator.	Inspired gases may be humidified with the use of standard humidifiers. Many institutions use disposable HMEs in place of conventional humidifiers.	HMEs are popular because they decrease the risk of infection and are inexpensive. The heat and moisture exchanger filter (HMEF) is a version of heat moisture exchanger that includes bacterial and viral filtration properties.
2. For conventional humidifiers, ensure that the humidifier has adequate fluid (sterile distilled water) and that the thermostat setting is adjusted according to manufacturer's recommendations. **(Level M*)**	Gases generally are humidified before entering the artificial airway. Temperature is measured at the patient's airway; temperatures between 35°C and 37°C (95°F and 98°F) are considered optimal.	Cool circuits may be tolerated well in patients without secretions. In patients with thick or tenacious secretions, attention to inspired temperature is important to prevent mucus plugging; circuit temperatures may need to be closer to body temperature (37°C vs. 35°C) in these cases.
3. HMEs are placed between the airway and the ventilator circuit.	The moisture in warmed exhaled gases passes through the vast surface area of the HME and condenses. With inspiration, dry gases pass through the HME and become humidified. The use of HMEs has been associated with decreased incidence of ventilator-associated pneumonias in patients on ventilation.[38,77] **(Level B*)**	

*Level M: Manufacturer's recommendations only.
*Level B: Well-designed, controlled studies with results that consistently support a specific action, intervention, or treatment.

Procedure	for Invasive Mechanical Ventilation (Through an Artificial Airway): Volume and Pressure Modes—*Continued*		
Steps	**Rationale**	**Special Considerations**
A. Change HMEs per manufacturer's instructions. **(Level M*)**	The longer the HME is in line, the more efficient the humidification; however, inspiratory resistance increases over time. HMEs are often changed every 2–3 days (refer to manufacturer's instructions).	In patients undergoing weaning, the additional resistive load added by these humidifiers may preclude their use.[38]
B. Do not use if secretions are copious or bloody.	Obstruction is possible, and HMEs are not indicated in these conditions.	
4. Discard used supplies, and remove PE.		
5. HH		

*Level M: Manufacturer's recommendations only.

Expected Outcomes

- Maintenance of adequate pH and $Paco_2$
- Maintenance of adequate Pao_2
- Maintenance of adequate breathing pattern
- Respiratory muscle rest

Unexpected Outcomes

- Abnormal pH, $Paco_2$, and Pao_2
- Hemodynamic instability
- Pulmonary barotrauma
- Inadvertent extubation
- Malpositioned endotracheal tube
- Nosocomial lung infection
- Acid-base disturbance
- Respiratory muscle fatigue

Patient Monitoring and Care

Steps	Rationale	Reportable Conditions
		These conditions should be reported to the provider if they persist despite nursing interventions.
1. Ensure activation of all alarms during each shift (see Box 27.2).	Ensures patient safety.	• Continued activation of alarms
2. Check for secure stabilization and maintenance of the endotracheal or tracheostomy tube.	Reduces the risk of inadvertent extubation or decannulation.	• Unplanned extubation or decannulation
3. Monitor the in-line thermometer to maintain inspired gas temperature (in the range 35°C–37°C [95°F–98°F]).	Reduces the risk of thermal injury from overheated inspired gas and the risk of poor humidity from underheated inspired gas.	• Dislodgment of airway • Temperature <35°C or >37°C
4. Keep ventilator tubing clear of condensation. Drain any condensation in the ventilator tubing toward condensation-collection reservoirs on the expiratory limb of the circuit (clean to dirty). Avoid draining condensation back toward the patient (dirty to clean).	Reduces the risk of respiratory infection by decreasing inhalation of contaminated water droplets.	• Continued condensation

Procedure continues on following page

Patient Monitoring and Care —*Continued*

Steps	Rationale	Reportable Conditions
5. Ensure availability of a self-inflating manual resuscitation bag-valve-mask device attached to supplemental oxygen at the head of the bed. Attach or adjust the PEEP valve if the patient is on >5 cm H_2O of PEEP.	Provides capability for immediate delivering of ventilation and oxygenation to relieve acute respiratory distress caused by hypoxemia or acidosis.	• Inability to oxygenate or ventilate
6. Check the ventilator for baseline Fio_2, peak inspiratory pressure (PIP), Vt, fx, and alarm activation with initial assessment and after removal of the ventilator from the patient for suctioning, bagging, or draining the ventilator tubing.	Ensures that prescribed ventilator parameters are used (e.g., 100% oxygen used for suctioning is not inadvertently delivered after the suctioning procedure), provides diagnostic data to evaluate interventions (e.g., PIP is reduced after suctioning or bagging), and ensures that the monitoring and warning functions of the ventilator are functional (i.e., alarms).	• Fio_2, PIP, Vt, or fx settings different from prescribed
7. Explore any changes in peak inspiratory pressure >4 cm H_2O or decreased (sustained) Vt on PSV. Immediately explore the cause of high-pressure alarms.	Acute changes in PIP or Vt may indicate mechanical malfunction, such as tubing disconnection, cuff or connector leaks, tubing or airway kinks, or changes in resistance and compliance. Always consider the possibility of tension pneumothorax or dynamic hyperinflation.	• Unexplained high-pressure alarms
8. Place a bite-block between the teeth if the patient is biting on the oral endotracheal tube.	An oral airway serves the same purpose but may not be tolerated as well as the bite-block because it may induce gagging.	• Biting on tube
9. Evaluate patient-ventilator dyssynchrony by manually ventilating the patient with a self-inflating manual resuscitation bag-valve-mask device.	By taking the patient off the ventilator for manual ventilation, synchrony may be accomplished more quickly than on the ventilator. This intervention may reduce the risk of barotrauma and cardiovascular depression. If the patient breathes in synchrony with bagging, consider changes in ventilatory parameters. If the patient does not breathe synchronously with bagging, explore the differential diagnoses of problems distal to the airway. Respiratory care practitioner, nurse practitioner, or physician consultation may be necessary.	• Patient-ventilator dyssynchrony
10. Assess for signs of atelectasis.	May occur because of hypoventilation as well as mucous plugging of bronchioles. Early detection of atelectasis indicates the need for alteration to promote resolution (tidal volume adjustment, recruitment maneuver, PEEP adjustment).	• Localized changes in auscultation (increased or bronchial breath sounds) • Localized dullness to percussion • Increased breathing effort • Tracheal deviation toward the side of abnormal findings • Increased peak and plateau pressures • Decreased compliance • Decreased Pao_2 or Sao_2 (with constant ventilator parameters) • Localized consolidation ("whiteout," opacity) on chest radiograph

Patient Monitoring and Care —*Continued*

Steps	Rationale	Reportable Conditions
11. Assess for signs and symptoms of pulmonary barotrauma (i.e., pneumothorax).	Early detection of pneumothorax is essential to minimize progression to obstructive shock and death. Tension pneumothorax requires immediate emergency decompression with a large-bore needle (i.e., 14-gauge) into the second or third intercostal space, midclavicular line on the affected side, followed by immediate chest tube placement.	• Acute, increasing, or severe dyspnea • Restlessness • Agitation • Localized changes in auscultation (decreased or absent breath sounds) on the affected side • Localized hyperresonance or tympany to percussion on the affected side • Elevated chest on the affected side • Increased breathing effort • Tracheal deviation away from the side of abnormal findings • Increased peak and plateau pressures • Decreased lung compliance • Decreased Pao_2 or Sao_2 • Subcutaneous emphysema • Localized increased lucency with absent lung markings on chest radiograph. • Hypotension
12. Assess for signs that are consistent with ARDS.	Ventilatory management should focus on ensuring that lung-protective strategies are in place so additional injury does not ensue. This includes Vt of 6 mL/kg (4 mL/kg to 8 mL/kg) and lung recruitment with PEEP.	• Acute, increasing, or severe dyspnea • Restlessness • Agitation • Generalized crackles, especially in the dependent portions of the lung • Refractory hypoxemia • Increased peak and plateau pressures • Decreased lung compliance • Decreased Pao_2 or Sao_2 • Bilateral diffuse lung opacity on chest radiograph or computer axial tomography (CAT) scan of the chest • $Pao_2 : Fio_2 < 200$ • A noncardiac etiology for the pulmonary edema
13. Monitor for signs and symptoms of acute respiratory distress, hypoxemia, hypercarbia, and fatigue.	Respiratory distress indicates the need for changes in PPV. While troubleshooting the difficulties, support ventilation via a manual self-inflating resuscitation bag if necessary.	• Chest-abdominal dyssynchrony • Shallow or irregular respirations • Tachypnea, bradypnea, or dyspnea • Decreased mental status • Restlessness, confusion, lethargy • Increasing or decreasing arterial blood pressure • Tachycardia • Atrial or ventricular dysrhythmias • Significant changes in arterial pH, Pao_2, $Paco_2$, or Sao_2

Procedure continues on following page

Patient Monitoring and Care —*Continued*

Steps	Rationale	Reportable Conditions
14. Assess for signs and symptoms of a malpositioned endotracheal tube.	Early detection and correction of a malpositioned endotracheal tube can prevent inadvertent extubation, atelectasis, barotrauma, and problems with gas exchange.	• Dyspnea • Restlessness or agitation • Unilateral decreased or absent breath sounds • Unilateral dullness to percussion • Increased breathing effort • Asymmetrical chest expansion • Increased PIP • Changes in endotracheal tube depth • Radiographic evidence of malposition.
15. Assess for signs and symptoms of inadvertent extubation.	Inadvertent extubation is sometimes obvious (e.g., the endotracheal tube is in the patient's hand). Often, the tip of the endotracheal tube is in the hypopharynx or in the esophagus; however, an inadvertent extubation may not be immediately apparent. Reintubation may be necessary, although some patients may not need reintubation. If reintubation is necessary, ventilation and oxygenation are assisted with a manual self-inflating resuscitation bag-valve-mask device and face mask.	• Decreased Sao_2 • Vocalization • Activated ventilator alarms • Low pressure • Low minute ventilation • Inability to deliver preset pressure • Decreased or absent breath sounds • Gastric distention • Changes in endotracheal tube depth • Signs and symptoms of inadequate ventilation, oxygenation, and breathing pattern
16. Evaluate the patient's need for long-term mechanical ventilation.	This evaluation allows the nurse to anticipate patient and family needs for the patient's discharge to an extended-care facility, rehabilitation center, or home on PPV.	• Spontaneous breathing trial failure • Inability to wean from the ventilator
17. Observe for hemodynamic changes associated with increased Vt, PEEP/CPAP, or recruitment maneuver.	PPV can cause decreased venous return and increase right ventricular afterload because of the increase in intrathoracic pressure. This mechanism often manifests immediately after initiation of mechanical ventilation and with increases in Vt, PEEP or CPAP levels and manual hyperinflation techniques. Cardiovascular depression associated with manual or periodic ventilator hyperinflation is immediately reversible with cessation of hyperinflation. Decreases in blood pressure with PPV also may be seen with hypovolemia. Always consider the potential for pneumothorax with acute changes.	• Decreased blood pressure • Change in heart rate (increase or decrease of >10% of baseline) • Weak peripheral pulses, pulsus paradoxus, or decreased pulse pressure • Decreased cardiac output • Decreased mixed venous oxygen tension • Increased arteriovenous oxygen difference

Documentation

Documentation should include the following:
- Depth of endotracheal tube at the teeth or gums
- Reason for initiation of PPV
- Date and time ventilatory assistance was instituted
- Ventilator settings, including the following: Fio_2, mode of ventilation, Vt or IPL, respiratory frequency (total and mandatory), PEEP level, I:E ratio or inspiratory time, PIP, dynamic compliance, and static compliance
- Humidifier change maintenance
- Arterial blood gas results
- Sao_2 readings
- Patient responses to PPV (including the patient's indication of level of comfort and respiratory symptoms)
- Respiratory assessment findings
- Assessment of pain, interventions, and response to intervention
- Vital signs and hemodynamic values
- Degree of backrest elevation
- Nursing interventions
- Unexpected outcomes

References and Additional Readings

For a complete list of references and additional readings for this procedure, scan this QR code with your smartphone, or visit https://www.elsevier.com/__data/assets/pdf_file/0006/1319802/Chapter0027.pdf

28 Noninvasive Ventilation

Christine Slaughter

PURPOSE: Noninvasive ventilation (NIV) is delivery of ventilatory support without placement of an artificial airway (an oral or nasal endotracheal tube or tracheostomy); ventilatory support is provided through a specialized nasal cannula, nasal mask, nasal pillows, full face mask, or helmet mask. NIV is used to prevent airway obstruction during sleep, to maintain or improve ventilation and/or oxygenation, and to provide respiratory muscle rest in patients in whom invasive mechanical ventilation is not possible, acceptable, or desired.

PREREQUISITE NURSING KNOWLEDGE

- An understanding of the terminology used to describe different methods of delivering NIV:
  - Continuous positive airway pressure (CPAP) is the provision of positive airway pressure throughout inspiration and expiration.
  - Bilevel positive airway pressure (BiPAP) is the administration of two levels of airway pressure: one during inspiration and another during expiration. BiPAP is a proprietary name of Philips Respironics (Murrysville, PA), but for the purposes of this procedure, the acronym *BiPAP* indicates bilevel positive airway pressure.
  - High-flow nasal cannula (HFNC) oxygen therapy delivers heated and humidified oxygen and air via specialized nasal prongs with a maximum flow of 60 L/min and at a prescribed inspired oxygen concentration, both of which can be independently titrated for hypoxemic respiratory failure.
- Although invasive mechanical ventilation delivered through an artificial airway has been the principal support strategy for patients with impaired ventilation and oxygenation in critical care since the early 1970s, Sullivan and colleagues[50] introduced the use of CPAP delivered through a nasal mask to patients with obstructive sleep apnea in 1981 and to patients with acquired muscle weakness and muscular dystrophy in 1987.[14]
- The use of NIV has become common and is often a first-line support. Ugurlu and colleagues[52] determined that nearly 40% of patients who required ventilator support initially received NIV; most common diagnoses managed with NIV were acute exacerbation of chronic obstructive pulmonary disease (COPD) and cardiogenic pulmonary edema (CPE). Nearly three-fourths of these patients were successful users of NIV, and the mortality rate of those who received NIV was nearly one-half that of patients who were ventilated invasively. The use of NIV has also been shown to reduce intubation rates and hospital mortality in patients with acute hypoxemic nonhypercapnic respiratory failure excluding COPD and CPE.[61]

- Lin and colleagues[26] identified a reduction in the likelihood of postextubation respiratory failure, a decrease in the likelihood of reintubation, and a reduction in the likelihood of intensive care unit (ICU) and hospital mortality compared with standard therapy. Chandra and colleagues[10] reported a 400% increase in the use of NIV for patients with an acute exacerbation of COPD over the decade from 1998 to 2008, and a subsequent reduction in invasive ventilation. In 2017, the American College of Chest Physicians and the American Thoracic Society published a clinical practice guideline that strongly recommended the use of preventive NIV in high-risk patients ventilated for more than 24 hours immediately after extubation.[39]
- The use of NIV maintains upper-airway protective reflexes and the ability to speak and swallow and avoids complications associated with intubation and invasive ventilation such as airway trauma, barotrauma, ventilation-induced acute lung injury, and hospital-acquired ventilator-associated pneumonia.[31] Complications associated with NIV include airway dryness, nasal congestion, gastric insufflation, facial erythema, nasal/sinus/ear pain, minor air leaks, major air leaks, claustrophobia, carbon dioxide (CO_2) rebreathing, nasal skin lesions, and general discomfort.[9]
- Patient predictors of potential failure of NIV before application of NIV include established severe acute respiratory distress syndrome, reduced level of consciousness, shock of any etiology, Glasgow coma score less than 11, Acute Physiology and Chronic Health Evaluation (APACHE) II severity of illness score higher than 29, profuse secretions, tachypnea (>35 breaths/min), pH less than 7.25, hypotension (systolic blood pressure <90 mm Hg), age older than 40 years, edentulism, severe agitation, and asynchronous breathing.[18,31] Predictors observed after initiation of NIV include major air leaks, poor tolerance, and ventilatory asynchrony. After 1 hour of ventilation, continued tachypnea, lack of improvement in oxygenation, hypercarbia, acidosis, and evident fatigue predicts failure of NIV.[18,28]

- The use of HFNC, which delivers heated and humidified oxygen and air, may provide an alternative to conventional oxygen therapy and NIV in patients postextubation, especially when the risk of reintubation is caused by hypoxemic respiratory failure.[20] HFNC provides a reduction in anatomical dead space, a positive end-expiratory pressure (PEEP) effect, a constant fraction of inspired oxygen (FiO_2), along with high level of humidity to aid in patient comfort.[37] Because the inspiratory flow of patients experiencing respiratory failure varies widely and may exceed 100 L/min, HFNC exceeds traditional oxygen delivery devices, which are limited to 15 L/min.[37]

Indications for Noninvasive Ventilation

- *Obstructive sleep apnea.* Obstructive sleep apnea (OSA) is characterized by repeated episodes of upper-airway collapse during sleep with subsequent oxyhemoglobin desaturation, hypoxemia, and recurrent sleep arousal. OSA can cause fragmented sleep, daytime fatigue, systemic inflammation, overactivation of the sympathetic nervous system, and endothelial dysfunction.[3] Exaggerated fluctuations in intrathoracic pressure, blood pressure, and cardiac rhythm are also seen in patients with OSA.[3] Long-term consequences of OSA include hypertension,[62] atherosclerosis and cardiovascular disease,[7] cognitive dysfunction, decreased quality of life, depression,[1] and premature all-cause mortality.[30,33] Although CPAP is highly effective as a pneumatic splint to the upper airway, investigators have reported poor adherence, with nonadherence rates of 46% to 83%.[36,57]

- *Obesity hypoventilation syndrome*: Obesity hypoventilation syndrome (OHS), along with sleep-disordered breathing, are the most common pulmonary complications related to obesity class III.[46] OHS is defined as a combination of obesity (body mass index of ≥ 30 kg/m^2) and daytime hypercapnia ($PaCO_2 > 45$ mm Hg) that is not secondary to other known causes of hypoventilation, where patients may present with acute hypercapnic respiratory failure that requires immediate intervention with NIV or invasive ventilation.[32,46] The goals of treatment for OHS using NIV are to improve alveolar ventilation and gas exchange and to maintain a patent airway.[46] Patients with OHS experiencing acute hypercapnic respiratory failure can be effectively treated with NIV using similar protocols developed for COPD.[8]

- *Acute exacerbation of COPD.* Bilevel NIV is recommended in the care of acute respiratory failure, which leads to respiratory acidosis (pH <7.35) resulting from an acute exacerbation of COPD.[42,32] The use of NIV to manage patients with acute exacerbation of COPD has been associated with a reduction in hospital-acquired pneumonia, a decrease in hospital length of stay, a reduction in medical costs, and reductions in mortality in patients with low, moderate, and high comorbidity burdens compared with patients managed with invasive ventilation.[27] Predictors of those patients who failed NIV included weak cough, high severity of illness (APACHE II >19), and malnutrition as indicated by total protein less than 5.8 mg; those with one or more of these risk factors had an increased risk of NIV failure.[15,28,47]

- *Acute cardiogenic pulmonary edema (ACPE).* Respiratory failure related to ACPE is caused by a decrease in respiratory compliance and high capillary pressures that flood the alveoli.[43] The use of NIV reduces left ventricular filling pressures by decreasing systemic venous return and left ventricular afterload.[4] Bilevel NIV and CPAP were demonstrated to reduce the need for intubation and respiratory distress in patients with acute cardiogenic pulmonary edema, particularly those with edema subsequent to myocardial ischemia or infarction.[19]

- *Asthma.* There is theoretical support for the use of NIV in the management of acute asthma; however, there currently are few data to support its use. Small trials have described improvements in dyspnea, respiratory rate, and airflow, which were attributed to the use of positive airway pressure and improved dispersal of inhaled bronchodilators.[40,43,48]

- *Pneumonia.* The use of NIV in acute hypoxemic nonhypercapnic respiratory failure associated with community-acquired and hospital-acquired pneumonia has shown improved survival to hospital discharge in patients who have a noncardiopulmonary comorbidity.[43,49,53] Patients who failed NIV initially and were subsequently intubated experienced high in-hospital mortality.[43] HFNC has emerged as an effective therapy for mild to moderate hypoxemic respiratory failure compared with CPAP/BiPAP because of improved patient tolerance and reduction in dead space.[29,37,43] HFNC has recently been used to support patients with moderate to severe acute hypoxemic respiratory failure associated with COVID-19.[12] Observational studies have shown decreased rates of intubation in patients with COVID infection, although mortality outcomes have varied.[13,56] Ease of setup has allowed for initiation of treatment outside intensive care units, providing additional resources during the pandemic.

- *Weaning from mechanical ventilation/postextubation respiratory failure.* The use of preventive NIV to facilitate weaning of patients with hypercapnic respiratory failure who received invasive mechanical ventilation for greater than 24 hours was associated with a significant decrease in mortality, reduction in ventilator-associated pneumonia, shorter hospital and ICU length of stay, and shorter duration of invasive mechanical ventilation.[5,43,44] Patients at high risk for extubation failure include those with hypercapnia, COPD, CHF, or other serious morbidities.[39] NIV should be applied immediately after extubation, and the combined use of HFNC and CPAP/BiPAP may further improve gas exchange and work of breathing, thereby reducing reintubation.[39,51] In patients with low risk for reintubation (<65 years of age, CHF not the indication for intubation, APACHE II score <12 on day of extubation, BMI <30, ventilated less than 7 days, no airway patency issues, and able to manage secretions), HFNC was found to have lower reintubation rates compared with conventional oxygen therapy.[17,29]

- *Postoperative acute respiratory failure.* Patients undergoing thoracic or abdominal surgery are at risk for postoperative acute respiratory failure resulting from anesthesia, pain, and the surgery itself.[21,43] The negative effects of postoperative acute respiratory failure may include decreased lung volumes, hypoxemia, and atelectasis, which in turn may lead to intubation.[21,43] The use of NIV improves gas exchange, improves lung aeration, decreases the work of breathing, and reduces the amount of atelectasis during the immediate postoperative period.[21,43] The use of NIV was associated with reduced rates of intubation, mortality, and hospital-acquired infections compared with conventional oxygen therapy.[63] Zayed found that HFNC also reduced intubation rates and hospital-acquired infections when compared with standard oxygen therapy; there were no significant differences between CPAP/BiPAP and HFNC in postoperative respiratory failure.[63]
- *Thoracic trauma.* There is evidence to support the effective use of NIV in patients with rib fractures, pulmonary contusions, pneumothorax, hemothorax, and flail chest.[23] The use of NIV showed a reduction in mortality, decreased risk for intubation, decreased ICU length of stay, improved oxygenation, reduced risk for nosocomial pneumonia, and reduced respiratory rate in patients with adequate pain control and hypoxemia that is not severe.[11,43]
- *Palliative care and do-not-intubate orders.* Because of the increasing number of patients who are in palliative care or have designated that they do not wish to be intubated, NIV may prove effective in relieving breathlessness and dyspnea.[23,37,43] Patients may benefit from the use of NIV when they do not wish to be intubated but desire treatment of a reversible process or seek symptom management when survival is not the goal.[43] The use of NIV may allow treatment outside the ICU and may reduce the amount of morphine administered to allow for less sedation and better cognitive function for end-stage patients with COPD, cancer, and neuromuscular disorders.[16,23,29,36,41,59]
- *Neuromuscular disorders.* The use of NIV with neuromuscular disorders such as Duchenne muscular dystrophy and amyotrophic lateral sclerosis increased minute ventilation, reduced respiratory rate, reduced hypoxemia time, decreased energy expenditure, and prolonged survival.[23,35,55]

Contraindications for Noninvasive Ventilation
Absolute Contraindications*
- Respiratory arrest, apnea
- Uncontrolled vomiting
- Absence of upper-airway reflexes
- Pneumothorax (untreated)
- Acute, copious upper gastrointestinal bleeding
- Recent gastric, laryngeal, or esophageal surgery

---

*Absolute contraindications for HFNC are lacking because of sufficient evidence; therefore careful consideration should be utilized in the application of HFNC in patients for whom NIV is contraindicated.[37,38]

- Facial and/or airway trauma or significant burns or deformity precluding proper mask fit unless a helmet is used
- Total upper airway obstruction

Relative Contraindications
- Medically unstable—hypotension, cardiac dysrhythmias, need for vasopressors
- Severe hypoxia and or hypercapnia, PaO_2/FiO_2 ratio of less than 200 mm Hg
- Agitated or uncooperative with fitting and wearing the interface
- Excessive secretions
- Impaired swallow reflex
- Cardiac ischemia

Noninvasive Ventilation Interfaces
An interface is a device that connects the positive pressure source (ventilator) to the patient airway. NIV interfaces can be categorized as a *nasal interface* or *facial interface* (Fig. 28.1).[18,31]
- *Nasal interfaces* are most commonly used in patients with chronic conditions such as OSA.[23,31] Nasal interfaces include nasal pillows and nasal masks. Nasal interfaces permit speech and feeding; unfortunately, these interfaces are also associated with greater resistance to gas flow and the potential for considerable leak of gas from the mouth.[58] Thus nasal interfaces are of minimal use during critical illness.[23]
- *Facial interfaces* are the most common in critical care clinical practice and include oronasal masks, face masks, and full face masks.[23,31] These interfaces vary in size and the area of the face covered and are particularly useful for patients who are mouth breathers. An oronasal and traditional face mask covers the mouth and nose, whereas a total face mask covers the mouth, nose, and eyes. These interfaces are associated with nasal congestion, skin breakdown, nasal and mouth dryness, and claustrophobia and are less useful in patients who are vomiting.[23,31] Total face masks may be better tolerated and induce fewer adverse effects, especially in patients with a do-not-resuscitate order.[23,25]
- The *high-flow nasal cannula* uses a wide-bore nasal cannula. The HFNC prongs are lighter and more tolerable than other NIV interfaces. The device utilizes an oxygen and air blender, heat, and humidification and provides fixed flow rates up to 60 L/minute[29,31,38] (Fig. 28.2). HFNC is better tolerated than other NIV interfaces because of a better balance of oxygenation and patient comfort; oronasal masks are more prone to skin breakdown, which leads to treatment interruptions and discontinuation of therapy.[38]

Modes of Noninvasive Ventilation
- *CPAP* elevates the pressures above atmospheric pressure and provides the same fixed positive pressure during both the inspiratory and expiratory cycles.[23,45] As a result of increased intrathoracic pressure, collapsed alveoli are recruited, functional residual capacity is increased, lung compliance is optimized, and the work of breathing is

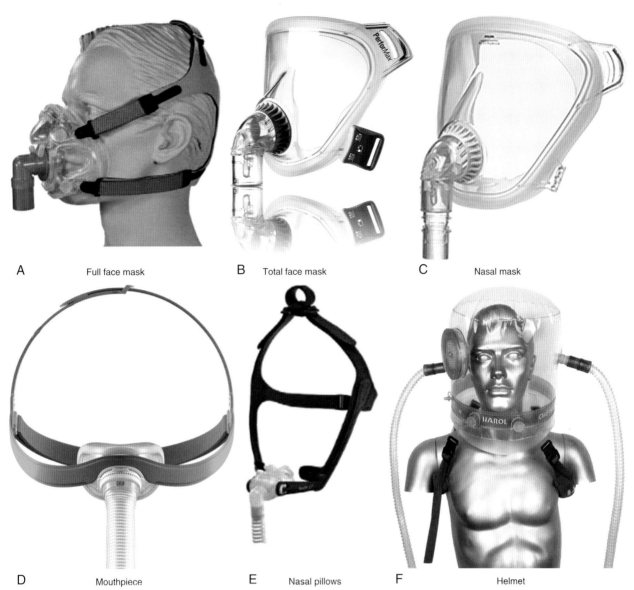

A Full face mask   B Total face mask   C Nasal mask

D Mouthpiece   E Nasal pillows   F Helmet

Figure 28.1 Different types of interfaces. **A,** Full face mask; **B,** Total face mask; **C,** Nasal mask; **D,** Mouthpiece; **E,** Nasal pillows; **F,** Helmet. *(A image reproduced with permission from Hans-Rudolph, Inc. C Courtesy of Philips RS North America LLC. All rights reserved. D image reproduced with permission from Fisher & Paykel Healthcare. E Courtesy of © ResMed. All rights reserved. F Image reproduced with permission from Harol Srl.)*

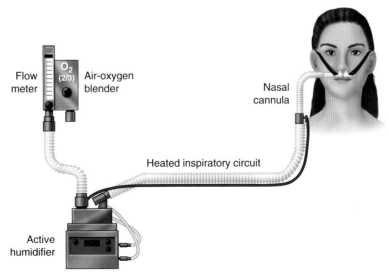

Flow meter   O₂ (2/3)   Air-oxygen blender   Nasal cannula

Heated inspiratory circuit

Active humidifier

Figure 28.2 High-flow nasal cannula interface.

TABLE 28.1	Mechanisms and Benefits of High Flow Nasal Cannula Oxygen
Mechanism	**Physiological and Clinical Benefit**
Small, pliable nasal prongs	• Enhanced patient comfort
Heat and humidification	• Facilitates removal of airway secretions • Avoids airway desiccation and epithelial injury • Decreased work of breathing • Enhances patient comfort
Washout of nasopharyngeal deadspace	• Improved ventilation and oxygen delivery
Positive end-expiratory (PEEP) effect	• Unload auto-PEEP (if present) • Decrease work of breathing • Enhance oxygenation
High nasal flow rate	• Reliable delivery of fraction of inspired oxygen (Fio_2) • Improved breathing pattern (e.g., increased tidal volume, decreased respiratory rate)

From UptoDate. https://www.uptodate.com/contents/image?imageKey=PULM%2F115105.

lessened.[31] Of note, there is no inspiratory muscle unloading with CPAP; thus tidal volume is dependent on respiratory muscles.[18,45]

• *Noninvasive bilevel positive airway pressure* provides two levels of pressure, an inspiratory positive airway pressure (IPAP), which may also be referred to as *pressure support*, and an expiratory positive airway pressure (EPAP) or positive end expiratory pressure (PEEP). IPAP and EPAP can be independently adjusted.[23] If the respiratory rate is fixed, the greater the difference between EPAP and IPAP, the greater the minute ventilation and decreased partial pressure of oxygen (Pao_2).[23] Bilevel NIV augments tidal volume, thus improving gas exchange, and allows the unloading of the respiratory muscles.[18,45] Bilevel ventilation is commonly used in acute-care patients.[31]

• *High-flow nasal cannula* is an open circuit that does not push or pull gases but provides warmed, humidified oxygen at fixed flow rates up to 60 L/min.[29,31,37,38] Mechanisms and benefits of HFNC are described in Table 28.1. Like CPAP, a high-flow nasal cannula does not provide inspiratory support.[31]

EQUIPMENT FOR CONTINUOUS POSITIVE AIRWAY PRESSURE OR BILEVEL NONINVASIVE VENTILATION

• Noninvasive interface (see Fig. 28.1)
• CPAP or BiPAP ventilator
• Electrocardiographic monitor
• Pulse oximeter—stand-alone or monitor module

• End-tidal carbon dioxide ($Etco_2$) capnography cannula and module or stand-alone module (may be used in conjunction with facial interfaces)
• Self-inflating manual resuscitation bag-valve-mask device
• Oxygen source and tubing
• Suction equipment
• Personal protective equipment (gloves, mask, goggles, gown, as appropriate)
• Humidification equipment as required

Additional equipment to have available depending on patient need includes the following:
• Medications, as indicated
• Intubation equipment and endotracheal tubes
• Equipment for needle thoracostomy or tube thoracostomy

EQUIPMENT FOR HIGH-FLOW NASAL CANNULA

• High-flow oxygen flow meter with attached muffler
• Air-oxygen blender
• Oxygen and air hose with quick-connects
• Specialized nasal cannula
• Heated inspiratory circuit
• Active humidifier
• Sterile water bag
• Temperature probes and heater wire adapter
• Electrocardiographic monitor
• Pulse oximeter—stand-alone or monitor module
• Self-inflating manual resuscitation bag-valve-mask device
• Suction equipment
• Personal protective equipment (gloves, mask, goggles, gown, as appropriate)

Additional equipment to have available depending on patient need includes the following:
• Medications, as indicated
• Intubation equipment and endotracheal tubes
• Equipment for needle thoracostomy or tube thoracostomy

PATIENT AND FAMILY EDUCATION

• If time permits, assess the patient's and family's level of understanding about the condition and rationale for the procedure. **Rationale:** This assessment identifies knowledge deficits about the patient's condition, the procedure, the expected benefits, and the potential risks. The nurse should provide sufficient time for questions to clarify information and for the patient and family to voice concerns. Explanations decrease patient anxiety and enhance cooperation.
• Explain the procedure and the reason for the procedure before and during the institution of NIV. Reinforce the information as required by the patient's condition. **Rationale:** This explanation enhances patient and family understanding, decreases anxiety, and increases cooperation.
• Provide details about the potential sensations associated with CPAP/BiPAP NIV (dyspnea, claustrophobia, lung inflation, noise, alarms). **Rationale:** Clear, complete

explanations reduces anxiety, fear, and distress and may improve patient tolerance.

- Promote relaxation in the patient. Techniques such as distraction may be useful. ***Rationale:*** Relaxation and cooperation promote optimal delivery of positive pressure gas flow, improve ventilation and oxygenation, and reduce the work of breathing.

- Establish a method of communication in conjunction with the patient and family before initiation of NIV. Explain that the patient will be able to speak, but this should be minimized to optimize the therapy. ***Rationale:*** The ability to communicate needs, symptoms, and feelings is vital to effective patient care and will reduce anxiety and fear.

- Instruct the patient and family about how to use the call system to obtain assistance and how to perform selected activities to improve patient comfort. This includes how to remove the mask if nausea and vomiting occur. ***Rationale:*** This supports autonomy of the patient and family; includes the family in caregiving, which is an identified need; and reduces anxiety of the patient and family members. Air insufflation may produce gastric distension, nausea, and vomiting with potential for pulmonary aspiration.

- Explain that the patient will not be permitted oral intake during CPAP/BiPAP NIV. ***Rationale:*** Reduces the risk for pulmonary aspiration.

- Offer information about the goals of NIV for the patient and frequent reports about progress. ***Rationale:*** Information about care, goals, and probable outcome is a stated need of patients and family members.

- Provide the opportunity for questions during NIV. ***Rationale:*** Family members state that the ability to ask questions and receive honest understandable answers is their most important need.

PATIENT ASSESSMENT AND PREPARATION

Patient Assessment

- Evaluate for signs and symptoms of respiratory muscle fatigue and impending acute ventilatory failure. These include increasing arterial partial pressure of carbon dioxide ($Paco_2$) and end-tidal carbon dioxide ($Etco_2$), chest wall-abdominal dyssynchrony, shallow or irregular respirations, tachypnea, bradypnea, dyspnea, reduced level of consciousness, confusion, lethargy, restlessness, change in arterial blood pressure (increase or decrease), tachycardia, and cardiac dysrhythmias. ***Rationale:*** Early detection of inadequate ventilation permits the clinician to intervene and improve ventilation with a noninvasive method or rapidly institute intubation and invasive mechanical ventilation.

- Evaluate the patient for signs and symptoms of inadequate oxygenation. These include decreased oxygen saturation by pulse oximetry (Spo_2), Pao_2 ≤60 mm Hg, tachypnea, dyspnea, central cyanosis, restlessness, confusion, decreased level of consciousness, agitation, tachycardia, bradycardia, cardiac dysrhythmias, intercostal and suprasternal retractions, alteration in arterial blood pressure (increased or decreased), adventitious breath sounds, reduced urine output, and acidosis. ***Rationale:*** Early detection of hypoxemia permits the clinician to intervene and institute additional supports to maintain adequate tissue oxygenation.

- Evaluate ventilation with measurement of $Paco_2$ and pH or $Etco_2$/capnography. Hypercarbia and respiratory acidosis indicate inadequate ventilation. ***Rationale:*** $Paco_2$ is the best indicator of adequacy of ventilation. Early detection of inadequate ventilation permits the clinician to intervene and improve ventilation with the noninvasive method or rapidly institute intubation and invasive mechanical ventilation.

Patient Preparation

- Verify the correct patient with two identifiers. ***Rationale:*** Ensures correct identification of the appropriate patient for the procedure.

- Evaluate patient understanding of the information provided. Answer questions, and reinforce information as needed. ***Rationale:*** Determines patient understanding, reinforces information, and reduces anxiety of the patient and family.

- Premedicate the patient as needed. ***Rationale:*** Cautious use of low-dose narcotics, sedatives, or anxiolytics may be required to improve patient tolerance, reduce anxiety, and promote optimal ventilation. Medication should not reduce the level of consciousness or central ventilatory drive.

Procedure	for Noninvasive Ventilation (Continuous Positive Airway Pressure and Bilevel Ventilation)	
Steps	**Rationale**	**Special Considerations**
1. **HH**		
2. **PE**		
3. Assemble and prepare equipment.	Readies equipment for the procedure.	
4. Select a noninvasive interface for use with NIV (see Fig. 28.1).[24,26,54,58] **(Level C*)**	Interface device fit is essential to efficacy. The interface should be carefully selected with attention to patient preference, face and nose size, facial deformities, skin integrity, presence of nasal or oral gastric tubes, and availability.	Not all interfaces may be available. The presence of a nasal or oral gastric tube does not preclude NIV. Most of the ventilators have leak compensation built into the system. However, a large leak may make patient-initiated cycling more difficult. Obtunded patients and patients with excessive secretions are not good choices.[31] **(Level E*)** Full face mask ventilation should be used cautiously. The patient should be able to remove the interface quickly if nausea and vomiting are imminent; otherwise, the potential for aspiration is high.
5. A chin strap may be used with a nasal mask to prevent excessive leaks through the mouth.	Optimal mask fit is vital so the patient receives adequate support.	
CPAP		
1. Select mode: CPAP.[3,6,11,24,26,27,60] **(Level A*)**	Prepares the ventilator to deliver CPAP.	This mode may be labeled CPAP or another vendor-specific name. Refer to the specific ventilator manufacturer's information for specific names of the mode.
2. Select desired CPAP level.	Establishes the initial pressures settings, which may be adjusted as needed.	Selection of a CPAP level of 3–5 cm H_2O or less is adequate to initiate.[31] **(Level D*)** Increase as needed to attain goal (e.g., relief of dyspnea, improved oxygenation, and comfortable breathing pattern). Begin by holding the mask in place, initiate with 1 cm H_2O pressure, and increase slowly to improve tolerance.
3. Select desired FiO_2 level.	Establishes the initial oxygen setting, which may be adjusted as needed.	There are limitations to the absolute amount of oxygen that may be bled into the system. Follow manufacturer's directions. A majority of ventilators that deliver CPAP provide a full range of FiO_2 from room air to 1.0. Oxygen may also be delivered by an oxygen flow meter in L/min, whereby oxygen is bled into the ventilator at the patient interface, or into the patient circuit. Begin with the current patient FiO_2, and increase as indicated. Monitoring of arterial oxygen saturation allows for adjustment as needed. If adequate oxygenation is not attained by adjusting oxygen to manufacturer specifications, a traditional ventilator may be used to supply CPAP using a noninvasive interface.[31] **(Level D*)**
4. Discard used supplies, and remove **PE**		
5. **HH**		

*Level C: Qualitative studies, descriptive or correlational studies, integrative reviews, systematic reviews, or randomized controlled trials with inconsistent results.

*Level E: Multiple case reports, theory-based evidence from expert opinions, or peer-reviewed professional organizational standards without clinical studies to support recommendations.

*Level A: Meta-analysis of quantitative studies or metasynthesis of qualitative studies with results that consistently support a specific action, intervention, or treatment (including systematic review of randomized controlled trials).

*Level D: Peer-reviewed professional and organizational standards with the support of clinical study recommendations.

Procedure continues on following page

Procedure	for Noninvasive Ventilation (Continuous Positive Airway Pressure and Bilevel Ventilation)—*Continued*		
Steps	**Rationale**	**Special Considerations**	

BiPAP or Bilevel

Steps	Rationale	Special Considerations
1. Select levels of support. Bilevel provides two levels of support: IPAP and EPAP.[6,11,43,26,27] (**Level A***) Depending on the ventilator, the two levels may have different names. For example, one vendor refers to pressure support ventilation as *IPAP* and positive end-expiratory pressure (PEEP) as *EPAP*.	Establishes inspiratory and expiratory pressure levels of support.	Selections of the levels of support are arbitrary, but in general start low and adjust upward. The concepts related to use of pressure support and PEEP are described in Procedure 27 for invasive mechanical ventilation. Refer to the specific ventilator manufacturer's information for specific names of the modes. Initiation at low levels is reasonable (i.e., pressure support of 5 cm H_2O and PEEP of 3 cm H_2O); slowly increase levels as tolerated to attain a comfortable respiratory rate and pattern and acceptable arterial blood gas values.
2. Select the bilevel options (dependent on ventilator manufacturer), which include the following: A. A spontaneous mode whereby the patient initiates all breaths (similar to "stand-alone" mode). B. A spontaneous-timed option, which is similar to pressure support with a backup rate (some vendors call this *assist-control*). C. Control mode. In contrast with the spontaneous and spontaneous-timed modes, the control mode requires that a control rate and inspiratory time be selected.	Establishes desired bilevel modes.	The selection of the specific BiPAP option is dependent on patient condition and the goals of therapy. If leaks around the interface prevent patient cycling, consider a spontaneous timed option or a control option. Settings on specific ventilators vary. However, concepts related to the settings are the same as with invasive ventilation (see Procedure 27, Invasive Mechanical Ventilation [Through an Artificial Airway]: Volume and Pressure Modes).
3. Adjust Fio_2 by means of an oxygen source (oxygen tubing connected to a flow meter) that is connected into the mask or in the inspiratory line at the junction of the ventilator and ventilator interface.	Establishes desired Fio_2 level.	Each ventilator has specifications that dictate the maximal flows allowed. Ventilator function may be adversely affected if the manufacturer's recommendations are not followed. Delivery of high levels of Fio_2 is not possible. For patients with a high Fio_2 requirement, BiPAP may not be a good option because the degree of intrapulmonary shunt may require high inspiratory and expiratory pressures that will not be tolerated.[18,24,31,52] (**Level C***) Consider the use of a traditional ventilator for NIV.[31] With use of a traditional ventilator, pressure support may not be the best mode to use because cycling may be impeded by mask leaks. The assist-control mode or a volume guaranteed-pressure mode may be used as an alternative[31] (exceptions exist and are ventilator specific) (see Procedure 27, Invasive Mechanical Ventilation [Through an Artificial Airway]: Volume and Pressure Modes).
4. Discard used supplies, and remove **PE**.		
5. **HH**		

High-Flow Nasal Cannula

Steps	Rationale	Special Considerations
1. **HH**		
2. **PE**		
3. Assemble and prepare equipment.	Readies equipment for the procedure.	

*Level A: Meta-analysis of quantitative studies or metasynthesis of qualitative studies with results that consistently support a specific action, intervention, or treatment (including systematic review of randomized controlled trials).

*Level C: Qualitative studies, descriptive or correlational studies, integrative reviews, systematic reviews, or randomized controlled trials with inconsistent results.

UNIT I

Procedure	for Noninvasive Ventilation (Continuous Positive Airway Pressure and Bilevel Ventilation)—*Continued*	
Steps	**Rationale**	**Special Considerations**
4. Select a wide-bore nasal cannula that fits snugly into the nares and is held in place with a head strap.[29]	Interface device fit is essential to prevent entrapment of room air around the cannula. Manufacturers have a maximum flow rate for each cannula size corresponding to the size and age of the patient.[29]	
5. Place the device on the patient, and ensure proper fit	The device should not be too tight. Straps for HFNC should be placed at the crown of the head. Use clothing clips and/or neck straps. Nasal prongs should be placed inside the nose.	Device placement at the crown of the head reduces skin injury to the ears. Clothing clips and neck straps help alleviate pulling of the device. Nasal prongs should not be pressed against the nose or against the outer edges of the nare.
6. Adjust liter flow and Fio_2		Adjust the liter flow and Fio_2 based on patient response (work of breathing, Spo_2)
7. Inspect for secretions or membrane swelling	Secretions and/or membrane swelling may alter the original fit of the cannula in the patient's nares	Inspect for device-related skin injury inside the nares.
8. Discard used supplies, and remove **PE**.		
9. **HH**		

Expected Outcomes

- Maintenance of pH (7.35 to 7.45) and $Paco_2$ (35 to 45 mm Hg); goal arterial blood gases should be individualized, particularly for patients with chronic hypercapnia and some degree of hypoxemia with obstructive lung disease.
- Maintenance of adequate Pao_2 (80 to 100 mm Hg); individualize goal for those with COPD or at higher altitudes.
- Regular ventilation with adequate minute volume
- Respiratory muscle rest
- Intact skin under interface

Unexpected Outcomes

- Failure of the NIV to improve pH, $Paco_2$, and Pao_2
- Hemodynamic instability
- Pulmonary barotrauma
- Respiratory muscle fatigue
- Skin breakdown under interface
- Aspiration
- Claustrophobia and panic

Patient Monitoring and Care

Steps	Rationale	Reportable Conditions
		These conditions should be reported to the provider if they persist despite nursing interventions.
1. Activate available alarms with high and low limits. Use reasonable alarm values (high pressure at 10 cm H_2O above patient peak, low exhaled volume/flow at least 2 L/min, low rate 8–10 breaths/min.[6,24] **(Level C*)**	Alerts clinicians of monitored values outside of high and low limits. Limits should be individualized and determined based on ventilator settings and patient condition. Ensures patient safety.	• Continued activation of alarms despite interventions to improve ventilation, intolerance, inadequate airway clearance, and excessive work of breathing

*Level C: Qualitative studies, descriptive or correlational studies, integrative reviews, systematic reviews, or randomized controlled trials with inconsistent results.

Procedure continues on following page

Patient Monitoring and Care —*Continued*

Steps	Rationale	Reportable Conditions
2. Evaluate regularly for stabilization and maintenance of the interface.[3,11] (**Level A***)	Ensures delivery of adequate positive pressure flow with minimal to no leaks. Reduces risk of inadvertent mask removal and subsequent inadequate ventilation.	• Inability to rapidly stabilize interface and maintain adequate ventilation • Uncontrolled agitation and panic that results in poor stabilization of interface • Inspired gas temperature <35°C or >37°C
3. Monitor the in-line thermometer to maintain inspired gas temperature when humidification is added to the circuit (in the range 35°C–37°C [95°F–98°F]; only applies to some devices).[18,31,60] (**Level E***, **M***)	Reduces risk of thermal inhalation injury from overheated inspired gas and risk of poor humidity from underheated inspired gas.	
4. Keep the interface and circuit clear of secretions and condensation when humidification is used.[18,31] (**Level M***)	Reduces risk of respiratory infection by decreasing inhalation of contaminated water droplets and secretions.	• Excessive secretions
5. Ensure availability of a manual self-inflating resuscitation bag with supplemental oxygen at the head of the bed. Attach or adjust the PEEP valve if the patient is receiving more than 5 cm H_2O CPAP.	Ensures that there will be immediate delivery of ventilation and oxygenation to relieve acute respiratory distress caused by hypoxemia or acidosis if needed.	
6. Regularly monitor the device for baseline settings and alarm activation with initial assessment and after removal and reapplication of NIV.	Ensures that prescribed device settings are delivered.	• Settings different from those prescribed
7. Evaluate alarms to determine the cause and correct issues. When capability is available, alarms should be integrated into the central system.	Multiple reasons for alarms exist and may indicate mask or tubing disconnection, kinks in the tubing, or serious changes in patient condition. Always consider the possibility of tension pneumothorax. Maintain equipment for emergency needle decompression of tension pneumothorax near the patient.	• Unexplained high or low pressure, exhaled volume, and rate alarms
8. Change patient position as often as possible but at least every 2 hours. Rotating beds may be helpful. Elevating the head of the bed may improve functional residual capacity.	Frequent position changes are indicated to reduce the potential for atelectasis and pneumonia caused by secretion stasis. Promotes airway clearance.	

*Level A: Meta-analysis of quantitative studies or metasynthesis of qualitative studies with results that consistently support a specific action, intervention, or treatment (including systematic review of randomized controlled trials).

*Level E: Multiple case reports, theory-based evidence from expert opinions, or peer-reviewed professional organizational standards without clinical studies to support recommendations.

*Level M: Manufacturer's recommendations only.

Patient Monitoring and Care —*Continued*

Steps	Rationale	Reportable Conditions
9. Evaluate patient-ventilator synchrony with CPAP/BiPAP.	There may be asynchrony of the trigger, flow, or cycle.[31] **(Level C*)** Trigger asynchrony is demonstrated by ineffective ventilatory efforts and auto-triggering; adjustment of pressure support and reduction of leaks should rectify. Flow asynchrony is demonstrated by inadequate flow time for patient demand; adjustment to a higher flow cycle will address this. Cycle asynchrony is demonstrated by asynchrony of the device and the patient inspiratory time; alteration of cycle time should address this issue. Notify the physician and respiratory care practitioner, and assess the patient frequently with any changes in settings to ensure resolution of asynchrony.	• Dyspnea • Chest-abdominal asynchrony • Rapid-shallow breathing pattern • Irregular, ineffective ventilation • Intercostal or suprasternal retractions
10. Observe for hemodynamic changes associated with increased inspiratory and expiratory pressures.	Hemodynamic changes may indicate functional changes in circulating volume caused by positive intrathoracic pressure. Always consider the potential for pneumothorax with acute changes. Equipment used for rapid release of tension pneumothorax should be in close proximity (i.e., 14-gauge needle; see Procedure 22, Needle Thoracostomy). Chest tube insertion equipment should be readily available.	• Hypotension • Heart rate increase or decrease of >10% of baseline value with worsening hemodynamic state • Decreased cardiac output
11. Monitor for signs and symptoms of acute respiratory distress, hypoxemia, hypercarbia, and respiratory muscle fatigue.	Respiratory distress indicates the need for changes in device settings or need for intubation and invasive ventilation. While troubleshooting, support ventilation via a self-inflating manual resuscitation bag-valve-mask device, if indicated (see Procedure 29, Manual Self-Inflating Resuscitation Bag-Valve-Mask Device).	• Hypercarbia • Chest-abdominal asynchrony • Shallow or irregular ventilation • Tachypnea, bradypnea, or dyspnea • Reduced level of consciousness • Restlessness, confusion, lethargy • Increase in pulmonary artery occlusion pressure • Decreased mixed venous oxygen saturation • Tachycardia • Atrial or ventricular dysrhythmias • Acidosis, hypoxemia, hypercarbia

*Level C: Qualitative studies, descriptive or correlational studies, integrative reviews, systematic reviews, or randomized controlled trials with inconsistent results.

Procedure continues on following page

Patient Monitoring and Care —*Continued*

Steps	Rationale	Reportable Conditions
12. Evaluate the patient regularly for signs and symptoms of pulmonary barotrauma (i.e., pneumothorax).	Early detection of pneumothorax is essential to minimize progression and adverse effects. Tension pneumothorax requires immediate emergency decompression with a large-bore needle (i.e., 14-gauge) into the second intercostal space or midclavicular line on the affected side (see Procedure 22, Needle Thoracostomy) or immediate chest tube placement (see Procedure 17, Chest Tube Placement).	• Acute, increasing, or severe dyspnea • Restlessness • Agitation • Decreased or absent breath sounds on the affected side • Localized hyperresonance or tympany to percussion on the affected side • Elevated chest on the affected side • Increased breathing effort • Tracheal deviation away from the side of abnormal findings • Increased peak and plateau airway pressures • Decreased compliance • Decreased Pao_2 and Sao_2 • Subcutaneous emphysema • Localized increased lucency with absent lung markings on chest radiograph
13. Assess skin under the interface every 1–2 hours for skin breakdown.[31] **(Level E*)**	The pressure of the tightly fitting interface may cause skin breakdown.	• Skin breakdown under the interface
14. Implement regular oral care for patients on HFNC and other NIV patients who are stable enough to tolerate temporary removal of the mask interface. Brush the teeth, tongue, and gums at least twice a day with a soft toothbrush, and moisturize the lips and oral mucosa every 2–4 hours.[2] **(Level E*)**	Tooth brushing removes dental plaque to prevent oral colonization, and moisturizing reduces inflammation. Oral care decreases the risk of hospital-acquired pneumonia and improves patient comfort.[22,34]	• Hypoxemia associated with mask removal

*Level E: Multiple case reports, theory-based evidence from expert opinions, or peer-reviewed professional organizational standards without clinical studies to support recommendations.

Documentation

Documentation should include the following:
• Patient and family education
• Date and time ventilatory assistance was instituted
• Ventilator settings, including the following: type of interface used, Fio_2, mode of ventilation, pressure levels (inspiratory and expiratory), respiratory frequency (total and mandatory if set)
• Arterial blood gas results
• Spo_2 measurements and/or $Etco_2$ measurements
• Reason for initiating NIV
• Patient responses to NIV including respiratory symptoms and patient-reported comfort level
• Hemodynamic values that are available
• Standard vital signs
• Respiratory assessments
• Skin assessments under interface
• Unexpected outcomes
• Nursing interventions

UNIT I

References and Additional Readings

For a complete list of references and additional readings for this procedure, scan this QR code with your smartphone, or visit https://www.elsevier.com/__data/assets/pdf_file/0007/1319803/Chapter0028.pdf

PROCEDURE

29 Manual Self-Inflating Resuscitation Bag-Valve-Mask Device

Kim Wigen-Dewey

PURPOSE: The use of a manual self-inflating resuscitation bag, otherwise known as *bagging,* is an essential skill for all levels of providers. It is used to deliver positive pressure ventilation when ventilations are either inadequate or absent. Using a bag-valve-mask device is a challenging skill to perform and requires practice to become proficient.

PREREQUISITE NURSING KNOWLEDGE

- The self-inflating bag consists of an air and oxygen inlet, reservoir bag, expiratory valve, and pressure release valve (Fig. 29.1). Positive end-expiratory pressure (PEEP) can also be added by using an external PEEP valve.
- Bagging is an essential skill utilized in many emergency situations.
  - ❖ Cardiac arrest
  - ❖ General anesthesia/neuromuscular blockade
  - ❖ Altered level of consciousness
  - ❖ To assess the patency of airway devices such as an endotracheal tube
  - ❖ To assist patients in respiratory distress
  - ❖ To provide oxygenation and ventilation before and after airway suctioning
  - ❖ To provide oxygenation and ventilation during patient transport
  - ❖ To evaluate issues with the patient's ventilation versus issues with the ventilator
- Bagging should result in chest movement and auscultatory evidence of bilateral air entry.
- Some factors that may make mask ventilation of bagging more difficult include facial hair or injuries, obesity, age (older than 55 years), having a history of snoring, or having no teeth.[4]
- In patients without an artificial airway in place, effective bagging requires an unobstructed airway, slight head and neck extension (i.e., the same technique used for mouth-to-mouth ventilation), and placement of a face mask over the nose and mouth (Fig. 29.2). An exception to this technique is with known or suspected cervical spine injury, in which the patient's airway is opened with the jaw thrust (without neck hyperextension) (Fig. 29.3). Bagging is most effective when performed with two people: one person to secure the mask and ensure head and neck placement, and another person to ventilate using the bag-valve-mask device[4] (Fig. 29.4).
- In patients with artificial airways, such as endotracheal or nasotracheal tubes or tracheostomies, the nurse must understand the components of artificial airways and their relationship to the upper-airway anatomy.
- When signs and symptoms of respiratory distress are noted in a patient on mechanical ventilation and troubleshooting the ventilator does not immediately resolve the issue, the patient should be bagged using 100% oxygen. Disconnect the ventilator from the patient's endotracheal or tracheostomy tube, and connect the bag-valve-mask device.
- The rate and depth of manually delivered breaths should be monitored.
  - ❖ Large volumes or pressure, or an increased rate of manually delivered breaths, may cause morbidity from hyperinflation, stomach insufflation, and/or hemodynamic changes.[3]
  - ❖ The lungs may not have complete deflation at end expiration if the manual ventilation rate or bagging rate is too fast, thus promoting dynamic hyperinflation. Hyperinflation occurs when exhalation time is inadequate, which results in auto-PEEP.
  - ❖ Auto-PEEP increases intrathoracic pressures and may decrease venous return; this may result in hypotension. It may also cause significant barotrauma and increase the possibility of pneumothorax or tension pneumothorax. A rapid solution to auto-PEEP with hemodynamic or respiratory compromise is a brief disconnection from the bag to allow passive deflation and a decrease in intrathoracic pressures. This should result in improved hemodynamics. With resumption of bagging, providing a longer exhalation time (smaller tidal volumes with a lower respiratory rate) will help minimize auto-PEEP.

EQUIPMENT

- Manual self-inflating resuscitation bag and mask of appropriate size
- Appropriate-sized airway adjuncts in the nonintubated patient
  - ❖ Oral pharyngeal airway (patient without cough or gag)
  - ❖ Nasopharyngeal airway and water-soluble lubricant

267

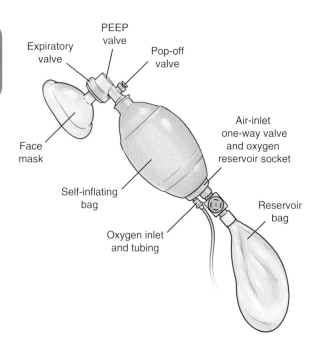

Figure 29.1   Components of a self-inflating manual resuscitation bag.

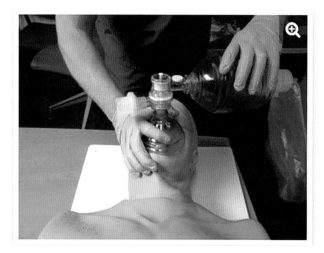

Figure 29.2   One-person technique. One person is holding the face mask while using a self-inflating manual resuscitation bag. *(From Davies JD, Costa BK, Asciutto AJ: Approaches to manual ventilation.* Respir Care *59[6]:810–822; discussion 822–824, 2014.)*

- Oxygen source and regulator
- Large-bore suction
- Personal protective equipment (PPE)
  - ❖ Eye protection
  - ❖ Face mask/face shield
  - ❖ Gloves
  - ❖ Gown

Additional equipment to have available as needed includes the following:
- PEEP valve, if required
- McGill forceps of various sizes
- High-efficiency particulate-absorbing (HEPA) filter

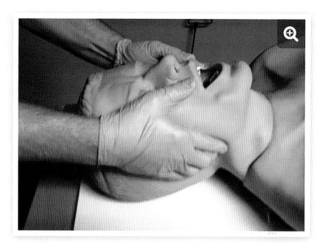

Figure 29.3   Jaw thrust. *(From Davies JD, Costa BK, Asciutto AJ: Approaches to manual ventilation.* Respir Care *59[6]:810–822; discussion 822–824, 2014.)*

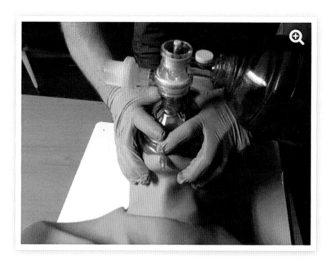

Figure 29.4   Two-person technique. One person is holding the face mask with two hands, and another person provides ventilations. *(From Davies JD, Costa BK, Asciutto AJ: Approaches to manual ventilation.* Respir Care *59[6]:810–822; discussion 822–824, 2014.)*

PATIENT AND FAMILY EDUCATION

- If time permits, assess the patient's and family's level of understanding about the condition and rationale for the procedure. ***Rationale:*** This assessment identifies the patient's and family's knowledge deficits concerning the patient's condition, the procedure, the expected benefits, and the potential risks. It also allows time for questions to clarify information and voice concerns. Explanations decrease patient anxiety and enhance cooperation.
- Explain the procedure and the reason for the procedure if the clinical situation permits. If not, explain the procedure after it is completed. ***Rationale:*** This explanation enhances patient and family understanding and decreases anxiety.
- If the patient is currently on a ventilator, inform the patient if possible and the family if present that the patient will be

disconnected from the ventilator and bagging will be performed. Describe the reason (e.g., ventilator malfunction, suctioning, patient comfort, the need for patient transport) for bagging. Explain that if the patient is in respiratory distress, bagging must be done immediately. **Rationale:** Information about the patient's therapy is an important need of the patient and family members. Dyspnea is uncomfortable and frightening. It leads to anxiety, fear, and distrust. Failure to diagnose promptly and alleviate the cause of respiratory distress puts the patient at risk for further decompensation.
- Discuss the sensory experience associated with bagging. **Rationale:** Knowledge of anticipated sensory experiences decreases anxiety and distress.
- Instruct the patient to communicate discomfort with breathing during bagging, if possible. **Rationale:** The bagging technique can be altered to produce a more comfortable breathing pattern by working with the patient's spontaneous respiratory efforts.
- Offer the opportunity for the patient if possible and the family to ask questions about bagging. **Rationale:** The ability to ask questions and have questions answered honestly is cited consistently as the most important need of patients and families.

PATIENT ASSESSMENT AND PREPARATION

Patient Assessment

- Verify the correct patient with two identifiers if possible. **Rationale:** Before performing a procedure, the nurse should ensure the correct identification of the patient for the intended intervention, though completing this in patients in severe distress should *not* delay intervention.

- Assess for signs of respiratory distress, including mental status changes; respiratory rate, rhythm, and quality; breath sounds; heart rhythm and rate; hypoxemia or hypoxia; hypertension or hypotension; or diaphoresis. **Rationale:** Any acute change in patient status may indicate that bagging is necessary.
- If present, assess for a sudden increase or decrease in end-tidal carbon dioxide ($EtCO_2$) readings. **Rationale:** Any acute change in patient status may indicate that bagging is necessary.
- Assess the patency of the patient's airway. **Rationale:** This establishes if there are any obstructions of the patient's airway and the patency of the patient's ability to maintain an open airway. Suction as necessary with a large-bore suction device, or utilize McGill forceps to remove larger foreign bodies. If *no* protective airway reflexes are present, consider inserting an oropharyngeal airway or nasopharyngeal airway.
- Use ventilator alarms if the patient is receiving mechanical ventilation, including low- or high-pressure or apnea alarms. **Rationale:** Any acute change in patient status may indicate that bagging is necessary. Rapid response with 100% fraction of inspired oxygen (FiO_2) protects the patient and allows for rapid evaluation of airway resistance, placement, and function of the artificial airway if one is in place.
- If present, ensure proper placement and function of any artificial airway. **Rationale:** The positioning and patency of the airway must be ensured.

Patient Preparation

- Ensure that the patient understands preprocedural teachings if possible. Answer questions as they arise, and reinforce information as needed. **Rationale:** This communication evaluates and reinforces understanding of previously taught information.

Procedure	for Manual Self-Inflating Resuscitation Bag	
Steps	Rationale	Special Considerations
Using the Manual Self-Inflating Bag-Valve-Mask Device in Patients without an Advanced Airway		
1. HH 2. PE 3. Attach the bag to an oxygen source, and open the oxygen source to a minimum of 15 L/min. 4. If the patient is spontaneously breathing, place the mask over the patient's face, covering the nose and mouth, and attempt to assist with spontaneous respirations.	A minimum amount of oxygen is required to provide a high FiO_2, usually >15 L/min flow. Avoid delivering a ventilation when the patient exhales. Working with the patient's spontaneous respirations will minimize patient discomfort.	If a reservoir bag is present, it must be fully inflated to provide a high concentration of oxygen. Use the thumb and index fingers of the nondominant hand over the top of the mask to provide downward pressure on mask. Place the third, fourth, and fifth fingers around the mandible to lift the mandible toward the mask rather than pushing the mask toward the face (see Fig. 29.2). Avoid placing the fingers beneath the mandible on the soft tissue because this may worsen airway obstruction. Fingers/pressure should be placed on the mandible itself.

Procedure continues on following page

Procedure for Manual Self-Inflating Resuscitation Bag—*Continued*

Steps	Rationale	Special Considerations
5. If the patient is *not* breathing spontaneously, open the airway using either the head-tilt/chin-lift or jaw-thrust maneuver.	Opening the airway allows the patient either to attempt self-ventilation or to be bagged.	Jaw thrust (see Fig. 29.3) if cervical spine trauma is suspected. If the patient is unable to maintain an airway, consider inserting an oropharyngeal airway or nasopharyngeal airway.
6. After obtaining an adequate seal with the mask, slowly compress the bag over 1 second, with sufficient volume to allow chest rise (500–600 mL). Ventilate at approximately 10–12 breaths/min (1 breath every 5–6 seconds).[1]	Compressing the bag too fast may result in gastric insufflation, emesis, and the possibility of breath stacking (dynamic hyperinflation).	If adequate mask seal cannot be obtained and ventilations are inadequate with a single provider, utilize a two-person technique with one provider maintaining a mask seal while the other ventilates the patient by compressing the bag-valve mask[1] (see Fig. 29.4). Obtaining an adequate mask seal with a single provider is frequently difficult. If bagging the patient is difficult, look for causes of high airway resistance (e.g., obstructed airway) or low lung compliance (e.g., bronchospasm, mucus plugging, pulmonary edema, pneumonia, acute lung injury, or pneumothorax).
7. Assess chest rise and fall with each ventilation, and listen for bilateral breath sounds with each bag compression. Is the chest rising? Do you still have an adequate seal with the mask?	Confirms the effectiveness of the bagging.	If ventilations are not effective, be prepared to intervene by assessing the mask size and/or adjusting hand placement to obtain a better seal or repositioning the patient's head. Call for assistance, and prepare for intubation or another rescue airway-device placement.
8. When assistance arrives, discard used supplies and **PE**.		

9. **HH**

Using the Manual Self-Inflating Bag-Valve-Mask Device in Patients With an Advanced Airway (i.e., Endotracheal Tube, Tracheostomy, Laryngeal Mask Airway, or King Airway)

Steps	Rationale	Special Considerations
1. **HH**		
2. **PE**		
3. Attach the bag to an oxygen source, and open the oxygen source to a minimum of 15 L/min.	A minimum amount of oxygen is required to provide a high FiO_2, usually >15 L/min flow.	Attach a PEEP valve if the patient is on a ventilator with a PEEP of 5 cm H_2O or more; adjust the PEEP level to that of the ventilator settings.
4. Silence the ventilator alarms.	Eliminates the ventilator alarms when the circuit is disconnected.	
5. Disconnect the patient from the ventilator.	Allows for attachment of the bag-valve-mask device.	Suspend ventilator breaths while disconnected.
6. Connect the bag to an artificial airway.	Allows for manual ventilation.	

Procedure for Manual Self-Inflating Resuscitation Bag—*Continued*		
Steps	Rationale	Special Considerations
7. Slowly compress the bag over 1 second at approximately 10–12 breaths/min (1 breath every 5–6 seconds).[1]	Compressing the bag too fast may result in breath stacking (dynamic hyperinflation).	If bagging the patient is difficult, look for causes of high airway resistance (e.g., obstructed airway, misplaced artificial airway) or low lung compliance (e.g., bronchospasm, mucus plugging, pulmonary edema, pneumonia, acute lung injury, or pneumothorax).
8. Observe the patient's breathing pattern and rate, and attempt to synchronize manual breaths with the patient's spontaneous effort.	Helps ensure adequate ventilation and oxygenation.	A higher manual rate may be required initially because larger breaths are more difficult to provide with manual ventilation compared with breaths provided by the ventilator.
9. If the patient is awake and alert, encourage the patient to relax and breathe with the manual breaths that are provided.	Provides synchrony between patient breaths and manual breaths.	
10. Gradually adjust the rate of manual breaths to a rate that meets the patient's demand.	Reestablishes synchrony.	A return to higher ventilator support settings may be necessary after bagging.
11. Ascertain whether the patient is comfortable with the manual breaths.	Promotes comfort.	
12. Assess the ease or difficulty with which the bag is compressed.	Difficulty in bag compression may identify presence of a pneumothorax or pulmonary emboli.	
13. If signs and symptoms of distress are resolved, reconnect the patient to the ventilator.	Indicates that respiratory distress is relieved.	Reassess the patient once the patient is placed back on the ventilator.
14. If the patient's distress is not eliminated with bagging, consider the following steps: A. Hyperoxygenate and suctioning. B. Assess for the presence of bilateral breath sounds and symmetrical chest expansion. C. Assess the ease (or difficulty) with which the bag can be compressed. D. Assess anxiety and discomfort as potential causes of dyspnea.	Indicates that respiratory distress cannot be relieved with bagging. Further assessment is needed. Suctioning provides information related to the presence of secretions or airway obstruction. By auscultating the lungs during bagging, essential information related to tube placement (e.g., migration to right mainstem or displaced) or patient status (e.g., bronchospasm, pulmonary edema) may be obtained. Asymmetrical chest expansion may be the result of a displaced artificial airway, pneumothorax, or obstruction. A change in ease of bag compression provides gross data about increasing (improved) or decreasing (deteriorating) lung compliance. Although psychological reasons for respiratory distress are possible, rule out physiological causes first.	In some situations, such as pulmonary embolus, no distinct physical assessment findings may be immediately evident. Support the patient until appropriate interventions are accomplished. The use of anxiolytics, analgesics, or both may be appropriate to decrease anxiety and pain. However, a thorough evaluation of the cause of distress must be undertaken both before and after administration.

Procedure continues on following page

Procedure   **for Manual Self-Inflating Resuscitation Bag—*Continued***

Steps	Rationale	Special Considerations
15. Return the patient to the ventilator when respiratory distress is relieved.	Returns the patient to baseline.	
16. Reactivate and check ventilator alarms and settings.	Safety precautions. Alerts staff to actual or potential life-threatening problems.	
17. Observe breathing pattern, patient ventilator synchrony, peak inspiratory pressure (volume ventilation), and tidal volume and respiratory frequency (patient initiated).		
18. Check that the call system is within patient's reach, if appropriate.		
19. Discard used supplies, and remove **PE**.		
20. **HH**		

Maintenance Ventilation During Patient Transport in Patients With an Advanced Airway

Portable ventilators are highly recommended for use during transport instead of manual bagging.[5] (**Level E***) If a transport ventilator is not available, bagging may be required. Procedures may vary depending on institutional standards.

Steps	Rationale	Special Considerations
1. **HH**		
2. **PE**		
3. Obtain an appropriate-sized bag and mask.	Ensures that appropriate equipment is available during the transport.	An appropriate-sized mask must accompany the patient in the event of inadvertent removal of the invasive airway.
4. Attach the bag to an oxygen source, and open the oxygen source to a minimum of 15 L/min.	A minimum amount of oxygen is required to provide a high Fio_2, usually >15 L/min flow.	Attach a PEEP valve if the patient is on a ventilator with a PEEP of 5 cm H_2O or more, and adjust the bag's PEEP level to that of the ventilator settings.
5. Confirm airway placement and the patient's tolerance to the ventilator and settings.	Establishes patency of the airway and ventilator's settings.	
6. Silence the ventilator alarms.	Eliminates the ventilator alarm when the circuit is disconnected.	
7. Disconnect the patient from the ventilator.	Allows for attachment of the bag-valve-mask device.	
8. Connect the bag-valve-mask device, and bag the patient with Fio_2 of 1.0 at an approximate rate depth and pattern as ventilator breaths.	Maintains a ventilation pattern like that being provided by the ventilator.	1.0 Fio_2 is typically used during patient transports. Adjust the liter flow of oxygen to maintain the patient's arterial blood oxygen saturation (Sao_2) at the desired level. If bagging the patient is difficult, look for causes of high airway resistance (e.g., obstructed airway, misplaced artificial airway) or low lung compliance (e.g., bronchospasm, mucus plugging, pulmonary edema, pneumonia, acute lung injury, or pneumothorax).

Procedure	for Manual Self-Inflating Resuscitation Bag—*Continued*	
Steps	**Rationale**	**Special Considerations**
9. Attach the continuous $Etco_2$ monitor.	$Etco_2$ monitoring continuously monitors airway placement and the adequacy of ventilations.	$Etco_2$ monitoring is recommended and an essential part of monitoring during patient transport to ensure continued airway patency and adequate ventilations.[2,5] **(Level E*)**
10. Frequently reassess the patient to ensure that the patient is comfortable with the bagging technique.	Promotes patient comfort.	Frequent reassessment is vital to patient comfort and safety. Adjustments may be needed to maintain patient comfort with manual ventilation.
11. Reattach the patient's advanced airway to the ventilator when the transport is completed.	Reestablishes mechanical ventilation.	
12. Discard used supplies, and remove 🅷🅷.		
13. 🅿🅴		

Level E: Multiple case reports, theory-based evidence from expert opinions, or peer-reviewed professional organizational standards without clinical studies to support recommendations.

Expected Outcomes

- Maintenance of adequate oxygenation and ventilation
- Resolution of respiratory distress if present

Unexpected Outcomes

- Hemodynamic instability from dynamic hyperinflation
- Pulmonary barotrauma (e.g., pneumothorax)
- Inability to restore adequate ventilation and oxygenation with bagging
- Inadvertent extubation during bagging
- Equipment failure and inability to bag

Patient Monitoring and Care

Steps	**Rationale**	**Reportable Conditions**
		These conditions should be reported to the provider if they persist despite nursing interventions.
1. Evaluate trends or sudden changes in lung compliance, airway resistance, or the patient's condition.	Impairment of the patient's lung function or airway may be identified by changes in the patient's condition or the ability to bag the patient.	• Difficulty bagging (stiff) • No observable chest wall movement • Agitation • Diaphoresis • Hypertension or hypotension • Tachycardia or bradycardia • Dyssynchronous breathing
2. Observe for signs and symptoms of synchrony with the bagging, including adequate chest rise and fall.	Proper technique results in a comfortable synchronous breathing pattern.	
3. Monitor Spo_2 and $Etco_2$ values and trends.	Spo_2 and $Etco_2$ provide information regarding the adequacy of oxygenation and ventilation.	• Decrease in Spo_2 >10% • Increase in $Etco_2$ >10%

UNIT I

Additional Considerations

Certain medical interventions such as bag-valve-mask ventilations may create localized aerosol generation that can allow airborne transmission of viruses. Appropriate PPE and HEPA filtration to filter expired air are currently recommended if aerosol generation is a concern (see Fig. 29.5). Additionally, follow all national and international recommendations for precautions regarding any updated practice updates.

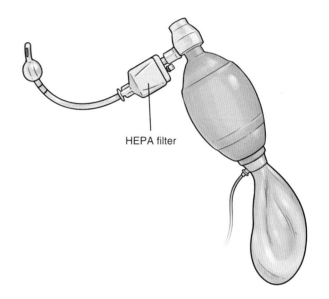

HEPA filter

Figure 29.5   Use of a HEPA filter with a manual resuscitation bag.

References and Additional Readings

For a complete list of references and additional readings for this procedure, scan this QR code with your smartphone, or visit https://www.elsevier.com/__data/assets/pdf_file/0008/1319804/Chapter0029.pdf

30 Weaning Mechanical Ventilation

Stephen Hopkins

PURPOSE: Weaning from mechanical ventilation is a process whereby the work of breathing is transferred from the ventilator to the individual. Once patients are able maintain adequate gas exchange with spontaneous breathing, they can be liberated from mechanical support.

PREREQUISITE NURSING KNOWLEDGE

- Invasive mechanical ventilation is a life-saving therapy but is also associated with complications, including barotrauma, hemodynamic compromise, ventilator-associated pneumonia, and generalized muscle weakness.[7,27] Once the condition that led to the need for ventilatory support has been adequately addressed, the process for liberating the patient from the ventilator should be initiated. However, premature ventilator removal also carries risks, including the potential for airway obstruction, hypoxemia, pulmonary aspiration, respiratory muscle failure, and respiratory arrest.[42] Thus clinicians seek the ideal point in the patient's clinical course to initiate weaning.
- Current guidelines recommend that all patients who require mechanical ventilation for 24 hours or more should be screened daily for readiness to wean with a standardized liberation protocol.[14] These systematic assessments have been shown to reduce time on the ventilator and improve patient outcomes.[4,5] The ABCDEF bundle is a protocolized approach to optimizing ICU patient care including weaning that has been well studied (Box 30.1).[39] The bundle incorporates spontaneous awakening trial (SAT) safety screens and spontaneous breathing trial (SBT) safety screening in a protocolized approach to weaning (Fig. 30.1).[1,9]
- Factors that affect weaning include respiratory and cardiovascular function, nutritional status, laboratory results (blood pH, hemoglobin, electrolytes), and psychological and neurological stability.[5,25]
- Excessive or prolonged use of sedation has been shown to increase the duration of mechanical ventilation.[8] Daily interruptions in sedation (spontaneous awakening trials) to allow for assessment of continued need and dosage of sedatives have been implemented in many critical care units.[32] Recent practice guidelines for the management of pain and sedation in critically ill patients suggest using light sedation in mechanically ventilated patients.[12]
- Prolonged immobility can lead to deconditioning, which can affect respiratory muscle strength. Clinical practice guidelines for liberation from mechanical ventilation include a recommendation that ventilated patients

| BOX 30.1 | ABCDEF Bundle and Components |

Requires a coordinated effort between the healthcare team

A–Assess, Prevent, and Manage Pain

B–Both Spontaneous Awakening Trials (SAT) and Spontaneous Breathing Trials (SBT)

- Spontaneous Awakening Trial
  - Daily assessment of SAT safety screen to turn off continuous sedation
  - Daily SAT (sedation interruption or light targeted level of sedation)
- Spontaneous Breathing Trial
  - Daily assessment of SBT safety screen
  - Daily SBT

C–Choice of Analgesia and Sedation

- Assessment of pain and sedation using validated tools
  - Sedation: Richmond Agitation Sedation Scale (RASS) or Sedation Agitation Scale (SAS)
  - Pain: Numeric Rating Scale (NRS), or Behavioral Pain Scale (BPS), or Critical Care Pain Observation Tool (CPOT)

D–Delirium: Assess, Prevent, and Manage

- Routine assessment of delirium using either validated tool
  - Confusion Assessment Method for the ICU (CAM-ICU)
  - Intensive Care Delirium Screening Checklist (ICDSC)

E–Early Mobility and Exercise

- Daily assessment of mobility readiness and activity
  - Early Mobility Protocol/Mobility Program

F–Family Engagement and Empowerment

- Patient and family centered care

From Society of Critical Care Medicine. ICU liberation bundle (A–F). Available at https://www.sccm.org/Clinical-Resources/ICULiberation-Home/ABCDEF-Bundles. Retrieved August 20, 2021.

receive rehabilitation directed toward early mobilization as tolerated.[17]
- The use of weaning protocols directed by registered nurses, respiratory therapists, or computer-driven protocols has demonstrated significant reductions in ventilator hours, intensive care days, and hospital length of stay compared with usual care.[4,6,21,37] Although there are variations in protocols based on institution or clinician preference, most involve a stepwise approach to implementing

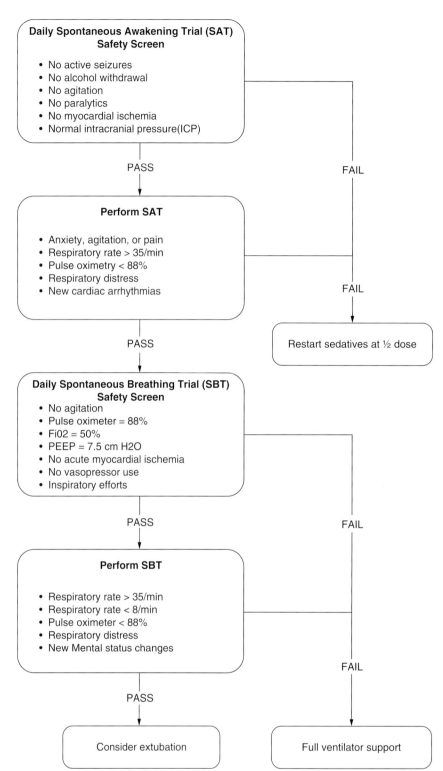

Figure 30.1 Spontaneous awakening trial (SAT) and spontaneous breathing trial (SBT). *(Data from Society of Critical Care Medicine. Implementing the B element of the ABCDEF bundle. Available at https://www.sccm.org/Clinical-Resources/ICULiberation-Home/ABCDEF-Bundles Retrieved June 30, 2021.)*

weaning. Protocols typically include clinical parameters that indicate readiness to wean, the method of weaning that should be used, and criteria used to evaluate success or failure.[4,42]

Evaluation of Weaning Readiness

- A number of parameters have been studied as predictors for identifying which patients are ready to successfully wean from mechanical ventilation. Traditional parameters focused on the respiratory muscle strength, gas exchange, and breathing pattern. Some of these are described in Box 30.1. One of the most commonly used indices in clinical practice is the rapid shallow breathing index (RSBI).[3,29] This index is the ratio of the breathing frequency divided by the spontaneously generated tidal volume over 1 minute. An RSBI <105 breaths/min/L is considered an indicator for weaning readiness.[38] Although this parameter can be a positive predictor for weaning success, it may also rule out patients who could be successfully weaned.[16]

- Nonrespiratory parameters have also been investigated for their impact on predicting weaning success, including as brain natriuretic peptide (BNP)[11,33] and heart rate variability[20,23] but have not been routinely used in clinical practice.[3] To date, none of the predictors of readiness to wean are sufficiently sensitive and specific in all populations, which limits their clinical utility. These parameters may play a role in selected high-risk patient populations who require prolonged mechanical ventilation.[29]

- Readiness to wean is most often determined by assessment of the patient based on a defined set of clinical criteria. Positive screening typically includes evidence of the following[26,34]:
  - ❖ Improvement in the condition that caused respiratory failure
  - ❖ Adequate oxygenation (with low PEEP and Fio_2 requirements)
  - ❖ Hemodynamic stability (on minimal vasopressors, no significant arrhythmias)
  - ❖ Ability to initiate breaths
  - ❖ Awake and able to tolerate minimal sedation

Weaning Methods

- Weaning requires that the patient assume responsibility for breathing, but there are different strategies for reducing ventilatory support.[7] In the past, support was withdrawn gradually, either by decreasing the rate of breaths or the level of pressure provided by the ventilator. This has now been replaced in many protocols by rapid transition to a period of spontaneous breathing, once the patient has met safety criteria.[7,32]

- Well-established evidence-based guidelines support the use of SBTs for 30 to 120 minutes to evaluate individual ability to sustain independent spontaneous ventilation.[7,31,35] Trials of spontaneous ventilation consist of cessation of mechanical ventilation and administration of supplemental humidified oxygen, often accompanied by some level of support (such as pressure support [PS] or automatic tube compensation) to overcome the resistance imposed by the endotracheal tube.[6] Methods used to perform a spontaneous breathing trial include the following:
  - ❖ *T-piece* trial provides administration of supplemental oxygen through tubing connected directly to the endotracheal tube. This method provides no inspiratory or expiratory support and requires the patient to overcome endotracheal tube resistance but may more closely mimic the work of breathing following extubation.[38] A recent meta-analysis found comparable rates for successful extubation with SBTs performed with T-piece or PS ventilation.[30]

- ❖ *Continuous positive airway pressure (CPAP)* trial delivers positive airway pressure throughout the ventilatory cycle during spontaneous breathing. Positive pressure applied at end-expiration in particular increases functional residual capacity and improves pulmonary compliance, oxygenation, and ventilation-perfusion match. Since CPAP offers minimal inspiratory support, this may be combined with automatic tube compensation (ATC), a setting within the ventilator that applies pressure to compensate for flow resistance of the endotracheal tube.[6,18]

- ❖ *PS* provides pressure during inspiration to overcome the work of breathing imposed by breathing through an endotracheal tube. This method permits the patient to trigger inspiration and control respiratory rate, depth, length, and flow during each spontaneous breath, with augmentation of tidal volume supported by a preset inspiratory pressure. Several investigators have concluded that PS weaning was associated with greater weaning success compared with T-piece weaning, particularly in patients who required simple weaning.[28] Current guidelines recommend that SBTs be conducted with inspiratory pressure augmentation of 5 to 8 cm H_2O.[14]

- ❖ *Automated weaning systems* use a closed-loop circuit to adjust ventilator settings in response to continuous monitoring and interpretation of data from the patient (end-tidal CO_2 concentration, respiratory rate, and tidal volume).[22] A systematic review of 21 trials concluded that these systems may reduce weaning and ventilation duration but indicated that more trials were needed.[36]

- Some evidence supports noninvasive ventilation (NIV) as a strategy for ventilator weaning in certain patient populations. This method differs in that it facilitates removal of the endotracheal tube before a patient has demonstrated criteria for successful weaning. Studies demonstrate successful weaning outcomes with a decrease in ventilator-associated events due to a shorter overall time with invasive ventilation.[35,41] The use of NIV as a weaning strategy may be most beneficial in patients with COPD.[41]

Evaluation of Weaning

- During weaning, patients are carefully monitored to ensure that they can tolerate the increased work of spontaneous breathing. Criteria for a successful SBT include acceptable physiological parameters (heart rate, blood pressure, respiratory rate, oxygen saturation) and no evidence of patient distress (diaphoresis, increased work of breathing, agitation).

- Failure of the spontaneous breathing trial is identified by tachypnea, a rapid shallow breathing pattern, decrease in oxygen saturation, changes in heart rate and/or blood pressure by >20% from baseline values, increased in work of breathing, and alteration in level of consciousness.[42] If the patient is unable to tolerate weaning, ventilator support is resumed while further assessment is performed for potential contributing factors. Reassessment for weaning is performed in 24 hours or at a time specified by the protocol.

- Weaning outcomes have been classified based on duration and difficulty of weaning. Patients who require simple weaning are those who are successful on the initial attempt;

difficult weaning requires at least three spontaneous breathing trials and as long as 7 days to achieve a successful transition. Those who require prolonged weaning need more than three spontaneous breathing trials and longer than 7 days to achieve successful independent ventilation.[15,24] Typically, a majority of patients (approximately 70%) require simple ventilator weaning; difficult weaning is required by approximately 20% and prolonged weaning by 10%.[24]

EQUIPMENT

- Standardized weaning protocol approved for your facility
- Personal protective equipment (i.e., gloves, mask, goggles, gown)
- Force meter/aneroid pressure manometer—typically a component of the mechanical ventilator
- Spirometer to measure volumes—typically a component of the mechanical ventilator
- Equipment for endotracheal suctioning
  Additional equipment to have available as needed includes the following:
- Self-inflating manual resuscitation bag-valve-mask device connected to an oxygen source as needed
- Oxygen flow meter connected to an oxygen source with heated aerosol humidifier with in-line thermometer and water trap for T-piece weaning or tracheostomy collar as appropriate for those using this method of weaning

PATIENT AND FAMILY EDUCATION

- Assess the patient's and family's level of understanding about the condition and rationale for the procedure. ***Rationale:*** Assessment identifies the patient and family knowledge deficits about the patient's condition, the procedure, the expected benefits, and the potential risks. The clinician should permit time for questions to clarify information and voice concerns. Explanations decrease patient anxiety and enhance cooperation.
- Explain the procedure and the reason for the procedure before and during the procedure. Reinforce information frequently. ***Rationale:*** Explanation enhances patient and family understanding and decreases anxiety.
- Maintain the clear and frequent transmission of information about patient progress, change in status, and prognosis with the patient and family members. ***Rationale:*** Establishes an open trusting relationship and encourages a realistic perception of the situation and patient prognosis.
- Describe the potential sensations (dyspnea, increased airway resistance, increased ventilatory effort, palpitations) that the patient may experience during evaluation and spontaneous breathing trials, and explain the importance of cooperation and maximal effort. Explain that prolonged ventilation may require muscle conditioning and produce more sensations associated with distress. ***Rationale:*** A clear understanding of expected sensations reduces anxiety and improves understanding and cooperation.
- Provide reassurance during the procedure; ensure continuous presence of qualified, experienced clinician(s).

Rationale: May reduce anxiety, promote patient cooperation, and improve and enhance effort.
- Explain how the patient will be monitored and evaluated for tolerance of spontaneous breathing, and assure the patient and family that mechanical ventilation will be reinstituted should the patient demonstrate intolerance. ***Rationale:*** Provides assurance to the patient and family that clinicians will protect the patient from harm during the procedure.

PATIENT ASSESSMENT AND PREPARATION

Patient Assessment

- Evaluate the patient for improvement or reversal of conditions that induced the need for mechanical ventilation in the individual, and address those before implementing weaning. Considerations include correction of the underlying cause of the respiratory failure, improvement in mental status, cardiovascular stability, adequate neuromuscular function, and sufficient ventilatory drive. These factors should be effectively managed before the initiation of weaning. ***Rationale:*** Adequate attention to all factors that influence the ability to ventilate spontaneously improves the likelihood of successful weaning from ventilation.
- Evaluate the patient for objective and subjective measures indicating readiness to wean as specified in the weaning protocol. Objective measures include oxygenation (Pao_2, Spo_2) and ventilation ($Paco_2$, end-tidal CO_2), acidosis (arterial pH), respiratory function (inspiratory effort, rate, tidal volume), volume of secretions, level of consciousness, stable blood pressure and heart rate, no new cardiac dysrhythmias, and normal temperature. Subjective indicators include self-reported dyspnea, sensation of excessive work of breathing, anxiety, and fatigue. ***Rationale:*** Premature weaning can put the patient at risk for adverse outcomes. Weaning should not begin until patient meets specified screening criteria to ensure patient safety.
- Evaluate the level of patient responsiveness and degree of sedation for patients receiving intermittent or continuous sedation infusion using a reliable and valid instrument like the Richmond Agitation-Sedation scale.[2,12] Assess the patient for delirium with a reliable and valid instrument like the Confusion Assessment Method for the Intensive Care Unit (CAM-ICU)[12,32] because the presence of delirium has previously been hypothesized to be associated with the use of sedation and mechanical ventilation, and this combination may trigger weaning failure.[2,10,40] ***Rationale:*** Adequate cognitive function supports the ability of the patient to cooperate and participate in the procedure and increases the likelihood of success.

Patient Preparation

- Verify the correct patient with two identifiers. ***Rationale:*** Ensures correct identification of the appropriate patient for the procedure.

- Negative inspiratory pressure (NIP) ≤ -20 to -30 cm H_2O
- Spontaneous tidal volume (Vt) >5 mL/kg
- Vital capacity (VC) >10-15 mL/kg
- Fraction of inspired oxygen (Fio_2) ≤40%-50%
- Pao_2/Fio_2 > 150-200 mm Hg
- Positive end-expiratory pressure (PEEP) ≤5-8 cm H_2O
- Minute ventilation (V_E) <10 L/min
- Rapid Shallow Breathing Index (RSBI) <105 breaths/min/L

Modified from Kacmarek RM, Stoller JK, Heuer AJ. (Eds). *Egan's Fundamentals of Respiratory Care.* 12th ed. St. Louis: Elsevier, 2019.

- Review the procedure and expected sensations with the patient and family; answer questions as they arise. Reinforce the importance of patient relaxation, cooperation, and maximal effort. **Rationale:** Determines patient understanding, reinforces information, and reduces anxiety of the patient and family.
- Position the patient for comfort and physiological support of ventilation; consider the use of a position elevated 45 degrees, as this supports optimal respiratory muscle function. **Rationale:** Investigators found that a 45-degree elevation reduced work of breathing and intrinsic positive end-expiratory pressure level compared with supine and sitting positions.[13]
- Initiate titration/reduction or cessation of sedation (sedation interruption, sedation vacation) following hospital protocol. **Rationale:** Sedative agents can alter mental status and suppress respiratory drive, thus impeding weaning. Minimal sedation optimizes the ability of the patient to understand the procedure, understand the sensations detected during weaning, and cooperate, thereby increasing the likelihood of success.

Procedure	for Ventilator Weaning	
Steps	**Rationale**	**Special Considerations**
Evaluation of Readiness 1. **HH** 2. **PE** 3. Assemble and prepare equipment and supplies.	Prepares equipment for the procedure.	Refer to institutional policy regarding the role of nursing in measuring ventilator parameters. These measures may be the responsibility of respiratory therapy.
4. Use the spirometer as indicated in the facility protocol to evaluate specific indicators if they are to be measured before a weaning trial.	The spirometer in the ventilator may be used to measure spontaneous Vt and V_E and VC (Box 30.2).	Ensure that there is minimal leak around the endotracheal tube cuff because this will give inaccurate measures of volumes measured through the tube. Provide the patient with rest periods on the ventilator between measurements.
5. Request that the patient breathe normally for 1 minute; the spirometer in the ventilator may be used to determine values required by your facility protocol.	The ventilator may measure the V_E, the total volume exhaled in 1 minute. Spontaneous Vt is also measured breath to breath or determined by dividing the 1-minute total exhaled volume by the measured respiratory rate.	Evaluate patient status, and discontinue evaluation if intolerance is detected (e.g., Spo_2 <90%, tachypnea, bradypnea, agitation, diaphoresis, tachycardia).
6. Calculate the RSBI if this is a required component of your facility protocol. This parameter is obtained by dividing the measured spontaneous Vt by the respiratory rate (f/Vt) over 1 minute.	An RSBI value <105 breaths/min/L is generally considered an indication of weaning readiness.	

Procedure continues on following page

Procedure for Ventilator Weaning—*Continued*

Steps	Rationale	Special Considerations
7. Measure the VC if this is a component of your facility protocol. For a VC measure, instruct the patient to exhale and then inhale as deeply as possible (maximal inspiration), followed by an exhalation of all the gas possible (maximal expiration).	VC measurement requires patient cooperation and effort. This measure is typically repeated at least three times and the average value used.	Most often used with patients who have a neuromuscular disorder.
8. When indicated by your facility protocol, measure the negative inspiratory force. Instruct the patient to maximally inhale. Determine the maximal pressure generated during the inspiratory effort over a 20-second period.	This measure is typically repeated at least three times, and either the best effort is achieved or the average value used. This measure can be effort independent in patients who are unable to cooperate. Threshold −20 to −30 cm H_2O pressure (a greater negative value is desirable).	Some ventilators will permit this measure to be made while the patient is connected to the ventilator. The patient will be unable to ventilate normally during this measure and may become anxious. Prior explanation should reduce this anxiety. Abort the measure with signs of excessive anxiety and intolerance.
9. Evaluate patient condition; return to mechanical ventilation using previous settings *or* initiate a spontaneous breathing trial based on facility weaning protocol.	Patient measures that indicate adequate ventilatory drive, respiratory muscle strength, and endurance lead to initiating a spontaneous breathing trial in most protocols.	A spontaneous breathing trial in those deemed ready to wean may be supported with PS, CPAP, or ATC to reduce the effect of the endotracheal tube on flow.
10. Discard used supplies, and remove **PE**.		
11. **HH**		

Ensure that the patient has passed a spontaneous awakening trial and met safety criteria for readiness to wean before proceeding with the spontaneous breathing trial.

Spontaneous Breathing Trial With T-Piece or Tracheostomy Collar

1. **HH**		
2. **PE**		
3. Position the patient for optimal respiratory muscle function and comfort.	Elevating the head of the bed 45 degrees provides optimal support of respiratory muscle function.[13]	
4. Remove the patient from the ventilator, and connect the endotracheal tube or tracheostomy to a humidified, heated oxygen source with the same Fio_2 as the patient received via the ventilator unless otherwise prescribed. The recommended time for spontaneous breathing trials is 30–120 minutes, driven by patient tolerance.[19,31] **(Level B*)**	The endotracheal tube or tracheostomy removes the upper-airway mechanisms that warm and humidify the inhaled gas.	Monitor respiratory frequency, breathing pattern, heart rate, cardiac rhythm, Sao_2, and general appearance of the patient continuously during the trial. General appearance includes skin color and temperature, presence of mottling or cyanosis, perceived anxiety, degree of subjective work of breathing, and patient report of tolerance.
5. Monitor the patient closely during the trial. Provide coaching, encouragement, and information to the patient and family during the trial. Celebrate successes, and provide encouragement for those who are not tolerant of the trial.	The patient and family require frequent accurate information about status and care. Frequent encouragement and reminders that spontaneous breathing will have different sensation from mechanical ventilation may increase tolerance of the trial.	Abort the trial if patient intolerance develops.
6. At the end of the trial time, return the patient to the mechanical ventilator at the previous settings.	Report the measures obtained before the trial as well as the length and tolerance of the trial to the care team.	As many as 70% of patients require simple weaning most commonly with spontaneous breathing trials and can be extubated after the initial weaning trial.

*Level B: Well-designed, controlled studies with results that consistently support a specific action, intervention, or treatment.

Procedure   for Ventilator Weaning—*Continued*

Steps	Rationale	Special Considerations
7. Discard used supplies, and remove .		
8. [HH]		

Spontaneous Breathing Trial Supported With CPAP or PS

Steps	Rationale	Special Considerations
1. [HH]		
2. [PE]		
3. Position the patient for optimal respiratory muscle function and comfort.	Elevating the head of the bed 45 degrees provides optimal support of respiratory muscle function.[13]	
4. Set the ventilator to the prescribed level of CPAP or PS and spontaneous ventilation. Typical levels of CPAP are 5–8 cm H_2O; PS is recommended at 5–8 cm H_2O in current guidelines.[12] (*Level D)	The patient will remain connected to the ventilator, but all ventilation will be patient-initiated/spontaneous. CPAP will maintain a positive pressure throughout the ventilatory cycle; PS will provide inspiratory gas with the set level of inspiratory support. The initial PS level should attain a spontaneous respiratory rate of ≤20 breaths/min with the absence of accessory muscle use, and a Vt of 6–10 mL/kg ideal body weight.	Monitor respiratory frequency, breathing pattern, heart rate, cardiac rhythm, SaO_2, and general appearance of the patient during the trial. Use caution with high levels of PS because patients who have obstructive lung disease may develop alveolar overdistension and air trapping.
5. Monitor the patient closely during the trial. Provide coaching, encouragement, and information to the patient and family during the trial. Celebrate successes, and provide encouragement for those who do not tolerate the trial.	The patient and family require frequent accurate information about status and care. Frequent encouragement and reminders that spontaneous breathing with these modes will have different sensations from mechanical ventilation may increase tolerance of the trial.	Abort the trial if patient intolerance develops. This type of weaning increases endurance of respiratory muscles as levels of support are decreased. Full ventilatory support should be provided at night to promote rest, especially early in the weaning process. If the endotracheal or tracheostomy cuff is insufficiently inflated, the PS cycle-off mechanism may not activate (i.e., the ventilator cycles off when it senses that flow is one-fourth the original flow). If this decrement of flow is not recognized, the result is an inappropriately long inspiratory time.
6. Depending on the facility protocol, the CPAP or PS level may be titrated downward until a lower limit is reached and tolerated by the patient. In patients who have difficult or require prolonged weaning, a gradual reduction in support may be performed with an automatic ventilator system or with use of a nurse, physician, or respiratory therapist–driven protocol.	Report the measures obtained before the trial, the length and tolerance of the trial, and the titration of CPAP or PS to the care team.	
7. Discard used supplies, and remove [PE].		
8. [HH]		

*Level D: Peer-reviewed professional and organizational standards with the support of clinical study recommendations.

Procedure continues on following page

UNIT I

Expected Outcomes

- Identification of the appropriate time for ventilator weaning
- Effective transition from mechanical to spontaneous independent ventilation without complication
- Ability to sustain adequate independent ventilation for more than 48 hours

Unexpected Outcomes

- Cardiac or respiratory distress or arrest during trial
- Cardiac dysrhythmias that influence hemodynamic state during weaning
- Pulmonary aspiration
- Ventilator-associated pneumonia
- Respiratory muscle fatigue/failure
- Hypoxemia and/or hypercapnia with acidosis
- Dyspnea, anxiety and agitation
- Unsuccessful, demoralizing weaning trials

Patient Monitoring and Care

Steps	Rationale	Reportable Conditions
		These conditions should be reported to the provider if they persist despite nursing interventions.
1. Evaluate patient responses to ventilation and weaning systematically. Be vigilant for deviations from a homeostatic condition.	Premature spontaneous breathing trials are associated with poorer patient outcomes.	Abort the trial with signs of patient intolerance to prevent complications and subsequently poorer outcomes. Signs and symptoms include anxiety; agitation; tachypnea or bradypnea; thoracic abdominal asynchrony; worsening dyspnea; altered level of consciousness; decreased Pao_2, Spo_2, or Sao_2; increased end-tidal CO_2 or $Paco_2$; tachycardia or bradycardia; cardiac dysrhythmias; and/or change in blood pressure or heart rate more than 20% from baseline.

Documentation

Documentation should include the following:
- Patient and family education provided before and during ventilator weaning
- Individualized goals set by the multidisciplinary team and patient for weaning
- Method and procedures used for weaning
- Preweaning measures of readiness for a spontaneous breathing trial per facility protocol
- Patient physiological and psychological responses to the weaning trial
- Duration of the trial and measured criteria per protocol at the end of the trial time
- Titration of support level, decreases in support level timing, and tolerance of titration
- Complications and unexpected outcomes
- Notification of the multidisciplinary team
- Extubation and subsequent status

References and Additional Readings

For a complete list of references and additional readings for this procedure, scan this QR code with your smartphone, or visit https://www.elsevier.com/__data/assets/pdf_file/0009/1319805/Chapter0030.pdf

PROCEDURE

31 Automated External Defibrillation

Kiersten Henry

PURPOSE: An automated external defibrillator (AED) is an electronic medical device that, by using a computerized detection system, analyzes cardiac rhythms, distinguishes between rhythms that require defibrillation and rhythms that do not, and delivers a series of preprogrammed electrical shocks. The AED is designed to allow early defibrillation by healthcare providers and laypersons who have minimal or no training in rhythm recognition or manual defibrillation.

PREREQUISITE NURSING KNOWLEDGE

- *Defibrillation* is the therapeutic use of an electrical shock that temporarily stops or stuns an irregularly beating heart and allows the spontaneously repolarizing pacemaking cells within the heart to recover and resume more normal electrical activity. Ventricular fibrillation (VF) and pulseless ventricular tachycardia (VT) are the only two rhythms recognized as shockable by an AED (Fig. 31.1).
- Time is the major determining factor in the success rates of defibrillation. In out-of-hospital cardiac arrests, for every minute defibrillation is delayed, the chance of success decreases by 7% to 10%. When used in conjunction with effective cardiopulmonary resuscitation (CPR), the decrease in the likelihood of success is more gradual and averages 3% to 4% per minute. Effective CPR increases the amount of time in which defibrillation may be effective.[3,11]
- Although defibrillation is the definitive treatment for VF and pulseless VT, the use of the AED is not a stand-alone

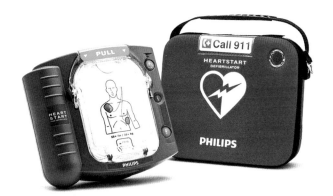

Figure 31.1 Automated external defibrillator device. (*Courtesy of Royal Philips.*)

skill; it is used in conjunction with CPR. CPR should be started as soon as the patient is found to be pulseless and not stopped until the AED has been turned on, the pads have been attached, and the machine is prompting the provider to "stand clear" or "don't touch the patient."[1,2] Immediate postshock CPR starting with compressions has been documented to lead to increased return of spontaneous circulation and increased cerebral survival,[1,3] which is why time is not taken to check for a rhythm or pulse after defibrillation.
- Ventricular fibrillation depletes the cardiac energy stores of adenosine triphosphate (ATP) more rapidly than a normal rhythm. The longer the heart goes without circulation, the more depleted its energy stores. In a heart with depleted energy stores, defibrillation is more likely to result in asystole because no fuel remains to support spontaneous depolarization or myocardial contraction. Effective CPR can supply the needed oxygen and energy substrates to the heart cells and allow them to return to a perfusing rhythm.[1,7]
- Three stages of VF are seen in cardiac arrest. The first phase is the electrical phase. During this phase, which is considered the first 4 to 5 minutes of VF, defibrillation is most likely to be effective, and the sooner the shock can be delivered, the more likely it is to work. During the next 5 to 10 minutes after VF occurs, the hemodynamic or circulatory phase, a brief period of CPR may "prime the pump" and provide oxygen to the myocardial cells, improving the effectiveness of the defibrillation. The metabolic phase starts 10 minutes after VF. During this phase, the cardiac cells have experienced global ischemia and energy depletion if no CPR has been initiated. CPR before defibrillation is more likely to be successful and needs to be used in conjunction with advanced cardiac life support (ACLS) therapies.[1,7]
- The AED is attached to the patient with adhesive electrode pads. Through these pads, the rhythm is analyzed and a

shock delivered, if indicated. If the AED recognizes VF or VT, visual and/or verbal prompts guide the operator to deliver a shock to the patient. The AED, not the operator, makes the decision about whether the rhythm is appropriate for defibrillation.

- The chance of the AED shocking inappropriately is minimal. There is a higher incidence of inappropriate shocks with manual defibrillation than with AED.[8,9] The AED should be applied only to unresponsive, nonbreathing, pulseless patients. To keep artifact interference to a minimum, the patient should not be touched or moved during the analysis time.
- The mnemonic "PAAD" makes it easy for the rescuer to remember the steps of operation of the AED: *P* for Power on, *A* for Attach the pads, *A* for clear to Analyze, and *D* for clear to Defibrillate.
- Although AEDs are simple to use, healthcare personnel should be familiar with and technically competent in the use of AEDs.
- Never use pediatric pads on an adult or large child because the reduced energy levels delivered by these electrodes may not be effective for treatment of VF.[6]
- The use of AEDs in prehospital settings has increased the success of defibrillation. The goal for in-hospital cardiac arrest is rapid CPR and defibrillation followed by medications and airway interventions.[3] Placement of AED units in unmonitored patient units and in public use areas of a hospital decreases the time to defibrillation. The largest study of in-hospital cardiac arrest found overall survival to discharge to be 15%.[2,10] AEDs are also needed in freestanding or ambulatory care settings. The majority of in-hospital cardiac arrests do not involve VT/VF and therefore are not indications for defibrillation.[4,10] High-quality CPR and rapid initiation of ACLS should remain a focus for in-hospital cardiac arrest.
- Many manual defibrillators have analysis capability that allows a tiered response (i.e., individuals with different skill levels can use the same defibrillator).
- Most AEDs in use in emergency response systems (EMS) or in the hospital have a method of recording the event in the form of rhythm strip printouts, audio and event recording devices, data cards, or computer chips that can print an event summary.
- AEDs may or may not have monitor screens. AEDs with screens may allow the provider with rhythm recognition skills to override the AED's analysis and recommendations.
- An important safety issue an AED operator must address is the possibility of inadvertently shocking a bystander or other provider at the scene. The operator must clear the patient verbally and visibly by looking at the patient from head to toe before and during the discharge of energy to the patient.
- All defibrillation programs need to include training for the potential operators. Training should include psychomotor skills, troubleshooting, equipment maintenance, and interfacing with ACLS providers. Healthcare providers and laypersons have the responsibility to be familiar with the machine they will use.
- When a resuscitation team (e.g., 911 responders, code team, ACLS providers) arrives, the team assumes responsibility for monitoring and treating the patient.

EQUIPMENT

- AED
- Nonsterile gloves
- Barrier device or airway management equipment (bag-valve-mask device with oxygen)
- Hand towel
- At least two sets of adult defibrillation pads and potentially one set of child defibrillation pads

Additional equipment to have available as needed includes the following:

- Trauma shears (with ability to cut through clothing)
- Clippers or scissors
- Extra electrocardiographic (ECG) paper
- Cardiac backboard

PATIENT AND FAMILY EDUCATION

- AEDs are used in emergency situations with limited or no time to educate the family about the equipment or the procedure. If family is present in the room during the arrest, a staff member should be assigned to keep the family informed of the procedures taking place and to offer support. *Rationale:* Information provides education and support.[5]
- After a sudden cardiac event, a patient may be discharged from an institution with an implanted cardioverter defibrillator (see Procedure 42, Implantable Cardioverter-Defibrillator: Post-Insertion Care) or a wearable cardioverter defibrillator (see Procedure 36, External Wearable Cardioverter-Defibrillator). In these situations, patient and family education is essential and should include information regarding performing CPR. *Rationale:* Education prepares the family for potential future procedures and emergencies.

PATIENT ASSESSMENT AND PREPARATION

Patient Assessment

- Establish that the patient is unresponsive, has absent or abnormal breathing, and is pulseless. *Rationale:* AEDs are indicated for the treatment of patients in cardiac arrest.
- Ensure that the patient does not have a Do Not Resuscitate (DNR) order indicating that CPR and defibrillation should not be performed. Gathering this information should not delay delivery of care. *Rationale:* Honors previously determined patient wishes.

Patient Preparation

- Remove clothing from the patient's chest, and ensure that the skin is dry where the AED electrodes will be placed. *Rationale:* This action prepares the patient for placement of the AED electrodes and minimizes the risk of electrical burns.
- Call for or obtain the AED; activate emergency response procedures for your setting. *Rationale:* Ensures the availability of the AED and additional emergency personnel.

Procedure	for Automated External Defibrillation	
Steps	Rationale	Special Considerations
1. HH		
2. PE		
3. Assess the patient. Perform CPR until the AED is available, turned on, attached to the patient, and prompts you to clear the patient. (If another provider is not nearby, it is reasonable for the healthcare provider to leave the patient and quickly obtain the AED.)	CPR helps keep the patient in a shockable rhythm longer, increasing the chance that defibrillation will be effective.	Place a backboard under the patient who is in bed.
4. The person in charge of the AED should: A. Open the AED. B. Press the "on" button. C. Proceed with the next steps as instructed by the AED.	When the AED is on, the prompts tell you what to do.	Some AEDs automatically turn on when they are opened. CPR should continue during the next few steps.
5. Attach the electrode pads to the patient's bare, dry chest:	Moisture under the pads can decrease the effectiveness of the contact of the electrode pads. Ensure that appropriate-sized pads are used.	Patients 1–8 years of age may use pediatric or adult pads; adult patients must use adult-sized pads.[2]
A. Place one pad below the right clavicle to the right of the sternum and the other to the left of the left nipple or slightly lower than the nipple line with the center of the electrode pad on the midaxillary line. The electrode pads have pictures that indicate where to place them (Fig. 31.2).	This placement ensures that the heart is between the two electrode pads, maximizing the current flow through the heart.	Placing an electrode pad on the sternum decreases effectiveness. Bone blocks some of the energy. Even with proper placement, only 4%–25% of the delivered current actually passes through the heart, so proper pad placement is crucial.[1] Polarity of the electrode pads is interchangeable for defibrillation purposes. However, if ECG monitoring is being done, the QRS complex is inverted if the positive and negative pads are reversed.

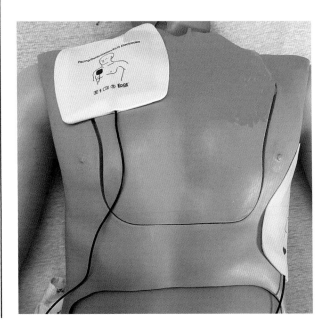

Figure 31.2 Automated external defibrillator pad placement. Place one pad below the right clavicle to the right of the sternum and the other to the left of the left nipple or slightly lower than the nipple line with the center of the electrode pad on the midaxillary line.

Procedure continues on following page

UNIT II

Procedure	for Automated External Defibrillation—*Continued*	
Steps	Rationale	Special Considerations
B. An alternative electrode pad position is anterior-posterior placement, where one pad is anterior over the left apex and the other is posterior behind the heart in the infrascapular location (Fig. 31.3).	This placement also ensures that the heart is between the two electrode pads.	Ensure that the electrode pads are directly above and below each other.
6. Connect the cables from the electrode pads to the AED.	Prepares equipment.	
7. Place the electrode pads firmly to eliminate air pockets and to form a complete seal. Excessive hair on the chest may prevent adequate adhesion of the electrodes. Apply additional pressure to the pads, and if the seal remains inadequate, remove the initial set of pads briskly and apply a second set.[2]	The AED uses the electrode pads to monitor and to shock. Good contact must be ensured to defibrillate most effectively; air pockets under the electrode can cause electrical sparks and skin burns.[1,2]	
A. Do not place the electrode pads over any medication or monitoring patches. Remove any medication pads from the chest, and wipe the chest clean.	Defibrillating over medication patches can cause burns and block the transfer of energy from the electrode pad to the heart.[1,2]	

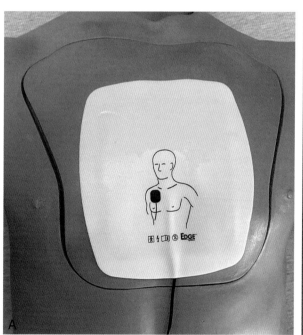
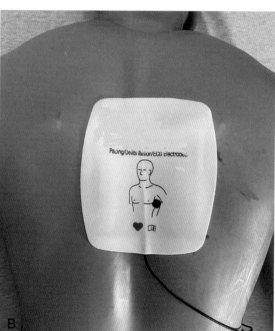

Figure 31.3   Anterior/posterior placement of automated external defibrillator pads. **A,** Place the anterior pad over the left apex. **B,** Place the posterior pad on the back over the infrascapular location.

Procedure for Automated External Defibrillation—*Continued*

Steps	Rationale	Special Considerations
B. For the patient with an implantable cardioverter defibrillator (ICD) or pacemaker, keep the electrode pads a minimum of 1 inch from the device generator. When possible for these patients, anterior-posterior placement is preferred. Other acceptable placement options are on the lateral chest wall on the right and left sides (biaxillary) or placement of the left pad in the standard apical position and the other pad on the right or left upper back.	Placement of electrode pads directly over an implanted device can divert energy away from the heart and can damage the device.[1,2]	Electrode pads should be placed a minimum of 1 inch from pacemaker and ICD generators if possible. The ICD or pacemaker should be checked for possible damage to the device after defibrillation. Try to place the pads without interrupting CPR. Pad placement should not delay defibrillation.[1,2]
8. Once the electrode pads are in place and plugged in, most AEDs sense an electrical pattern and tell the operator to make sure no one is touching the patient ("stand clear" or "don't touch the patient").	The machine needs to analyze the rhythm to determine whether defibrillation is needed; therefore touching the patient or doing CPR may give the machine a false message or delay the ability of the AED to analyze the rhythm.	CPR must be stopped at this point. No one should be touching the patient when the AED is analyzing.
9. Wait for the AED to analyze the patient's rhythm: A. If a shock is advised, clear the patient visually and verbally.	The AED has determined that the rhythm is either VF or VT; defibrillation is needed. Maintain safety for everyone around the patient. Anyone touching the patient or any conductive apparatus that is in contact with the patient (e.g., stretcher frame, intubation stylet) when the energy is discharged receives some of that shock. Free-flowing oxygen (such as disconnected ventilator tubing) should be directed away from the defibrillator pads.	Use a mnemonic such as "I'm clear, you're clear, we're all clear," and look at the patient while talking to ensure that no one is touching the patient. Another mnemonic is "Shocking on three. One, I am clear. Two, you are clear. Three, we are all clear. Shocking now."
B. If no shock is advised, restart CPR.	If the patient is not in a shockable rhythm and was pulseless, the only treatment is CPR until the ACLS team arrives.	
10. Push the shock button or buttons if shock advised, as prompted while looking at the patient.	Delivering the shock quickly is the best way to convert the fatal rhythm. Most AEDs discharge the energy into the machine if the shock button is not pushed within a preset time frame, usually about 10–15 seconds.	The energy levels for AEDs are preset to an energy level recommended by the manufacturer. Some AEDs are fully automatic and deliver a shock if needed without user interaction. In this case, the AED warns the user to stand clear before delivering the shock.

Procedure continues on following page

UNIT II

UNIT II

Procedure	for Automated External Defibrillation—*Continued*

Steps	Rationale	Special Considerations
11. Immediately restart CPR, beginning with compressions. Continue CPR for 2 minutes, approximately five cycles of 30 compressions to 2 breaths. If an advanced airway has been achieved, an asynchronous breath should be delivered 10 times/min.[3] **(Level D*)**	Providing immediate postshock compressions increases the probability of return of spontaneous circulation.[1,2,3]	Change compressors every 2 minutes to ensure effectiveness of the CPR. Performing chest compressions is tiring, and effectiveness decreases after 2 minutes.[1]
12. After 2 minutes, the AED prompts the healthcare providers or laypersons to "stand clear" or "don't touch the patient" to allow it to analyze the rhythm, determining whether the rhythm remains shockable.	Checks to see whether the initial shock was effective or whether the patient needs to be defibrillated again.	Ensure that no one touches the patient during the analysis. A good time to change compressors is during the analysis pause.
13. **Repeat steps 9A and 10** if prompted to shock again.	If the patient remains in a shockable rhythm, CPR and defibrillation are most likely to be effective in return of spontaneous circulation.	Be sure to clear the patient for analysis and shocking.
14. If you receive a "no shock advised" message, resume CPR beginning with compressions until the ACLS team arrives and the rhythm can be checked, or the patient begins to move.[2]	Continues emergency intervention.	If a change occurs in the patient's condition, check a pulse. If a pulse is found, check for adequate breathing. If adequate breathing is not found and the patient has a pulse, provide rescue breaths at a rate of 1 breath every 5–6 seconds with a bag-valve-mask device and oxygen if available.
15. Once the patient has a pulse, obtain vital signs and assess level of consciousness.	Determines the patient's response to CPR and use of the AED.	
16. Transfer the patient to a critical care unit.	Continues assessment and medical intervention.	
17. Ensure that the AED is cleaned and electrodes are replaced.	Prepares emergency equipment for future use.	
18. Discard **PE** any used supplies in an appropriate receptacle.	Reduces the transmission of microorganisms; standard precautions.	
19. **HH**		

*Level D: Peer-reviewed professional and organizational standards with the support of clinical study recommendations.

Expected Outcomes	Unexpected Outcomes
• Restoration of perfusing rhythm • Restoration of spontaneous respirations • Transfer to a critical care unit for postresuscitation care	• Operator or bystander shocked • Skin burns • Pain • Unsuccessful resuscitation; death

Patient Monitoring and Care

Steps	Rationale	Reportable Conditions
		These conditions should be reported to the provider if they persist despite nursing interventions.
1. Monitor vital signs at least every 15 minutes until stable.	Determines hemodynamic stability.	• Abnormal vital signs • Dysrhythmias
2. Monitor ECG rate and rhythm.	A patient with VF or pulseless VT is at risk for additional dysrhythmias.	• Dysrhythmias
3. Administer antidysrhythmic and vasopressor medications as prescribed.	Antidysrhythmic medications may prevent the risk of additional dysrhythmias. Vasopressors may be required to maintain adequate blood pressure in patients who are hypotensive postarrest.	• Dysrhythmias • Hypotension
4. Follow institutional standards for assessing pain. Administer analgesia as prescribed.	Identifies need for pain interventions.	• Continued pain despite pain interventions
5. Initiate induced hypothermia (targeted temperature management) postarrest if prescribed.	Reduces the incidence of hypoxic brain injury after cardiac arrest.	

Documentation

Documentation should include the following:
• Type of arrest (witnessed or not witnessed)
• Time from patient collapse to first shock (only if witnessed)
• CPR information (including start and stop times)
• CPR performed before AED application: yes/no
• Time of application of AED
• Time of first shock
• Number of times patient was defibrillated and shock dosage
• Preshock and postshock rhythms
• Any complications
• Assessment after resuscitation (if applicable)
• Pain assessment, interventions, and effectiveness
• Unexpected outcomes
• Nursing interventions
• Patient and family education

References and Additional Readings

For a complete list of references and additional readings for this procedure, scan this QR code with your smartphone, or visit https://www.elsevier.com/__data/assets/pdf_file/0010/1319806/Chapter0031.pdf

UNIT II

PROCEDURE

32 Cardioversion

Cynthia Hambach

PURPOSE: Electrical cardioversion is the therapy of choice for terminating hemodynamically unstable tachydysrhythmias such as supraventricular tachycardia, atrial fibrillation, atrial flutter, and monomorphic ventricular tachycardia with a pulse. It also may be used to convert hemodynamically stable atrial fibrillation or atrial flutter to normal sinus rhythm.

PREREQUISITE NURSING KNOWLEDGE

- Understanding of the anatomy and physiology of the cardiovascular system, principles of cardiac conduction, basic dysrhythmia interpretation, and electrical safety.
- Basic and advanced cardiac life support knowledge and skills.
- Clinical and technical competence in the use of the defibrillator.
- Synchronized cardioversion is recommended for termination of dysrhythmias that result from a reentrant circuit, which include unstable supraventricular tachycardia, atrial fibrillation, atrial flutter, and unstable monomorphic ventricular tachycardia with a pulse.[3,4,7,9]
- Elective cardioversion also may be used in patients with hemodynamically stable ventricular or supraventricular tachydysrhythmias that are unresponsive to medication therapy.[3]
- The electrical current delivered with cardioversion depolarizes the myocardial tissue involved in the reentrant circuit. This depolarization renders the tissue refractory; thus it is no longer able to initiate or sustain reentry. A countershock synchronized to the QRS complex allows for the electrical current to be delivered outside the heart's vulnerable period in which a shock can precipitate ventricular fibrillation. This synchronization occurs a few milliseconds after the highest part of the R wave but before the vulnerable period associated with the T wave.[3,4,7,9]
- Cardioversion should be considered emergently in patients with persistent tachydysrhythmia that is causing the following unstable symptoms: hypotension, acutely altered mental status, signs of shock, ischemic chest discomfort, and/or acute heart failure.[4,7,9]
- Elective cardioversion may be used to convert hemodynamically stable atrial fibrillation or atrial flutter to a normal sinus rhythm. When used to convert atrial fibrillation or atrial flutter, anticoagulation therapy may be required for at least 3 weeks before cardioversion and for a varying duration postcardioversion to decrease the risk of thromboembolism. The duration of postcardioversion anticoagulation is dependent of the thromboembolic risk profile and bleeding risk profile.[2]

- Anticoagulation therapy may not be necessary if atrial fibrillation or atrial flutter has been present for less than 48 hours, depending on thromboembolic risk.[2]
- A physician, advanced practice nurse, or other healthcare professional may choose to perform a transesophageal echocardiogram (TEE) to exclude the possibility of an atrial thrombus before cardioversion for patients at high risk for thromboembolism (see Chapter 72). The patient is immediately placed on an anticoagulant, and the cardioversion is performed once anticoagulation is achieved.[2]
- If time and clinical condition permit, the patient should be given a combination of analgesia and sedation to minimize discomfort.[4,8,9]
- Defibrillators deliver energy or current in waveform patterns. Delivered energy levels may differ among the various defibrillators and waveforms. Various types of monophasic waveforms are used in older defibrillators. Biphasic waveforms have been designed more recently and are used currently in implantable cardioverter defibrillators (ICDs), automated external defibrillators, and manual defibrillators sold at the present time.[3,7]
  - ❖ Monophasic waveforms deliver energy in one direction. The energy travels through the heart from one pad or paddle to the other.[3]
  - ❖ Biphasic waveforms deliver energy in two directions. The energy travels through the heart in a positive direction and then reverses itself and flows back through the heart in a negative direction.[3]
  - ❖ Because of their increased success in terminating dysrhythmias, defibrillators with biphasic waveforms are preferred for the treatment of atrial and ventricular dysrhythmias.[6,7]
- When performing synchronized cardioversion, follow the manufacturer's energy recommendations per the specific device used.[3,7,9]

EQUIPMENT

- Defibrillator/monitor with electrocardiogram (ECG) oscilloscope/recorder capable of delivering a synchronized shock
- ECG cable with leads and electrodes
- Self-adhesive defibrillation pads or conductive gel, paste, or prepackaged gelled conduction pads to be used with defibrillator paddles

290

- Intravenous sedative and/or analgesic pharmacological agents as prescribed
- Bag-valve-mask device with mask and oxygen delivery
- Flow meter for oxygen administration, oxygen source
- Emergency suction and intubation equipment
- Blood pressure–monitoring equipment
- Pulse oximeter
- Intravenous infusion pumps
- Code cart with ACLS medications, intubation tray, and cardiac backboard for CPR
- Personal protective equipment as needed
- Emergency transcutaneous pacing equipment

PATIENT AND FAMILY EDUCATION

- Assess patient and family understanding of the etiology of the dysrhythmia. *Rationale:* This assessment determines the patient and family understanding of the condition and additional educational needs.
- Explain the procedure to the patient and family. *Rationale:* This explanation decreases anxiety and promotes patient cooperation.
- Discuss the use of sedative and analgesic pharmacology agents. *Rationale:* This discussion will help alleviate the patient's fear and anxiety about receiving an electrical shock.
- Explain the signs and symptoms of hemodynamic compromise associated with the preexisting cardiac dysrhythmias to the patient and family. *Rationale:* This explanation enables the patient and family to recognize when the patient needs to notify the nurse or physician.
- Evaluate and discuss with the patient the need for long-term pharmacological support. *Rationale:* This discussion allows the nurse to anticipate educational needs of the patient and family regarding specific discharge medications.
- Assess and discuss with the patient the need for lifestyle changes. *Rationale:* The underlying pathophysiology may necessitate alterations in the patient's current lifestyle and require a plan for behavioral changes.

PATIENT ASSESSMENT AND PREPARATION

Patient Assessment

- Assess the patient's ECG results for tachydysrhythmias, including paroxysmal supraventricular tachycardia, atrial fibrillation, atrial flutter, and monomorphic ventricular tachycardia with a pulse, which could require synchronized cardioversion. *Rationale:* Tachydysrhythmias may precipitate deterioration of hemodynamic stability.[4,7,9]
- Assess the patient's vital signs and any associated symptoms of hemodynamic compromise with each significant change in ECG rate and rhythm. *Rationale:* Deterioration of vital signs or the presence of associated symptoms indicates hemodynamic compromise that could become life threatening.[4,7,9]

- Assess for the presence or absence of peripheral pulses and the patient's level of consciousness. *Rationale:* This baseline determination assists in the detection of cardioversion-induced peripheral embolization.[1]
- Obtain the patient's serum potassium, magnesium, digoxin levels (if taking this medication), international normalized ratio (INR) if on warfarin, and arterial blood gas results. *Rationale:* Electrolyte imbalances, acid-base disturbances, and digitalis toxicity contribute significantly to electrical instability and may potentiate postconversion dysrhythmias.[1] Hypokalemia should be corrected to prevent postconversion dysrhythmias. Although cardioversion is considered a safe practice in patients taking digitalis glycosides, the medication may be discontinued on the day of cardioversion. Elective cardioversion is contraindicated in patients with a dysrhythmia associated with digoxin toxicity.[1]

Patient Preparation

- Verify the correct patient with two identifiers. *Rationale:* Before performing a procedure, the nurse should ensure the correct identification of the patient for the intended intervention.
- Ensure that the patient and family understand the pre-procedural teaching. Answer questions as they arise, and reinforce information as needed. *Rationale:* This communication evaluates and reinforces understanding of previously taught information.
- Ensure that informed consent is obtained. *Rationale:* Informed consent protects the rights of the patient and makes competent decision making possible for the patient; however, in emergency circumstances, time may not allow the consent form to be signed.
- Perform a preprocedure verification and time out if nonemergent. *Rationale:* Ensures patient safety.
- Obtain a 12-lead ECG. *Rationale:* Provides baseline data and verifies for elective procedures that the indication for cardioversion exists/remains.
- Give the patient nothing by mouth per institutional policy. *Rationale:* Decreases the risk of aspiration.
- Establish a patent intravenous access. *Rationale:* Medication administration may be necessary.[3,4,9]
- Assist the patient to the supine position. *Rationale:* Supine positioning provides the best access for procedure initiation, intervention, and management of possible adverse effects.
- Remove transdermal medication patches from the patient's chest and wipe the area clean, or ensure that the defibrillator pad or paddle does not touch the patch. *Rationale:* Transdermal medication patches may block the transfer of energy from the pad or paddle to the patient and produce a chest burn when the pad or paddle is placed over it.[3]
- Ensure that the patient is in a dry environment, and dry the patient's chest if it is wet. *Rationale:* Water is a conductor of electricity. If the patient and rescuer are in contact with water, the rescuer may receive a shock, or the patient may receive a skin burn. Also, if the patient's chest is wet, the current may travel from one pad across the water to the other, resulting in a decreased amount of energy to the myocardium.[3]

- If the patient has a hairy chest, self-adhesive defibrillation pads may stick to the patient's hair instead of the skin. Apply pressure to the pads to ensure contact. If this does not work and it is an emergency, briskly remove the pads to remove hair, and reapply a new set of pads. Hair may also be clipped if time is available. *Rationale:* This action allows the electrodes to adhere to the chest.[3]
- Remove loose-fitting dentures, partial plates, or other mouth prostheses. *Rationale:* Removal decreases the risk of airway obstruction during the procedure. Evaluate each individual situation (e.g., dentures may facilitate a tighter seal for airway management).

- Preoxygenate the patient as prescribed and appropriate to the condition. *Rationale:* This will optimize oxygen delivery until the patient is stabilized.[4,9]
- If time and clinical condition allow, consider administration of sedation and analgesia as prescribed. *Rationale:* These medications provide amnesia and decrease anxiety and pain during the procedure.[4,7-9]
- Maintain a patent airway with oxygenation throughout the procedure. *Rationale:* Respiratory depression and hypoventilation can occur after administration of sedatives and analgesics.[8]

Procedure for Cardioversion

Steps	Rationale	Special Considerations
1. **HH**		
2. **PE**		
3. Connect the patient to the monitoring lead wires on the defibrillator.	The R wave must be sensed by the defibrillator to achieve synchronization for cardioversion.[3,4,9]	
4. Select a monitor lead that displays an R wave of sufficient amplitude to activate the synchronization mode of the defibrillator. In most models, synchronization is achieved when the monitoring lead produces a tall R wave. (**Level M***)	Synchronized cardioversion must sense the R wave to deliver the current outside the heart's vulnerable period.[3,4,9] Lead II generally produces a large R wave.	
5. Place the defibrillator in the synchronization mode. Ensure that the patient's QRS complexes appear with a marker to signify correct synchronization of the defibrillator with the patient's ECG rhythm (Fig. 32.1). To confirm that the synchronization has been achieved, observe for visual flashing on the screen, or listen for auditory beeps. If necessary, adjust the R-wave gain until the synchronization marker appears on each R wave. (**Level D***)	Synchronization prevents the random delivery of an electrical charge, which may cause ventricular fibrillation.[3,4,7,9]	
6. If the defibrillator is unable to distinguish between the peak of the QRS complex and the peak of the T wave, as in polymorphic ventricular tachycardia, proceed with unsynchronized defibrillation (see Procedure 33, Defibrillation [External]).	Avoids a delay or failure of shock delivery in the synchronized mode.[3,4,9]	

*Level M: Manufacturer's recommendations only.
*Level D: Peer-reviewed professional and organizational standards with the support of clinical study recommendations.

Procedure for Cardioversion—*Continued*

Steps	Rationale	Special Considerations

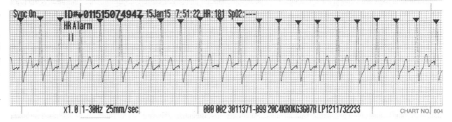

Figure 32.1 R-wave synchronization. Note the synchronization marker above each R wave. *(Courtesy Drexel University Center for Interdisciplinary Clinical Simulation and Practice.)*

Steps	Rationale	Special Considerations
7. Apply self-adhesive defibrillation pads, or prepare defibrillation paddles with the proper conductive agent. **(Level D*)**	Reduces transthoracic resistance, enhancing electrical conduction through subcutaneous tissue.[3,7,9] Minimizes erythema from the electrical current.	Self-adhesive defibrillation pads connected directly to the defibrillator have been found to be as effective as paddles.[3,7,9] Advantages of hands-free defibrillation pads are safety and convenience of use. These pads can be used for monitoring, and they allow for rapid delivery of a shock if necessary. For that reason, they are recommended for routine use instead of standard paddles.[3,7,9] Prepackaged gelled conductive pads are available for placement in the area of each paddle.[3] Gel pads should be replaced if they appear to be drying out or as per manufacturer recommendations. Conductive gel should be evenly dispersed on the defibrillator paddles and should adequately cover the surface. Be careful not to smear gel between paddles because current may follow an alternate pathway over the chest wall and avoid the heart. It may also cause a potential for a spark, causing a fire hazard. For that reason, gel pads are preferred.[3]
8. Follow these steps for pad or paddle placement: A. Place one pad or paddle at the heart's apex, just to the left of the nipple at the midaxillary line. Place the other pad or paddle just below the right clavicle to the right of the sternum (Fig. 32.2). B. In women, the apex pad or paddle is placed at the fifth to sixth intercostal space with the center of the pad or paddle at the midaxillary line.	Cardioversion is achieved by passing an electrical current through the cardiac muscle mass to restore a single source of impulse generation; this pathway maximizes current flow through the myocardium.[3] Placement over a woman's breast should be avoided to reduce transthoracic resistance.	Most pads or paddles are 8–12 cm in diameter.[3,7] Avoid placing pads or paddles over lead wires or implanted devices (ports, pacemakers, ICD).[3]

*Level D: Peer-reviewed professional and organizational standards with the support of clinical study recommendations.

UNIT II

Procedure continues on following page

UNIT II

Procedure for Cardioversion—*Continued*

Steps	Rationale	Special Considerations

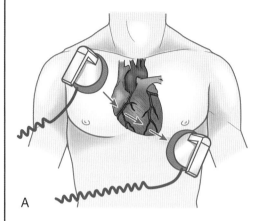

A

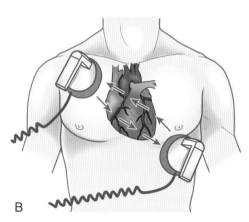

B

Figure 32.2   Paddle placement and current flow in (**A**) monophasic defibrillation and (**B**) biphasic defibrillation. *(From Harding M, Kwong J, Roberts D, et al.: Medical-surgical nursing: Assessment and management of clinical problems, ed 11, St Louis, 2019, Elsevier.)*

Steps	Rationale	Special Considerations

C. Anterior-posterior placement may also be used.
  i. Self-adhesive defibrillation pads are used for this approach.
  ii. The anterior pad is placed in the anterior left precordial area, and the posterior pad is placed posteriorly behind the heart in the right or left infrascapular area (Fig. 32.3).
  iii. An alternative approach is to place the anterior pad in the right infraclavicular area and the posterior pad in the left infrascapular position.
	All methods of pad or paddle placement are effective.[3,7]	

D. In a patient with a permanent pacemaker, do not place pads or paddles directly over the pulse generator.	Cardioversion over an implanted pacemaker may impair passage of current to the patient and may cause the device to malfunction or become damaged.[3]	Do not place the pad or paddle over the pulse generator and lead wire.[3] Anterior-posterior placement is also suggested.[3] The pacemaker should be assessed after any electrical countershock. Standby emergency pacing equipment should be available should pacemaker failure occur.

Procedure for Cardioversion—*Continued*

Steps	Rationale	Special Considerations

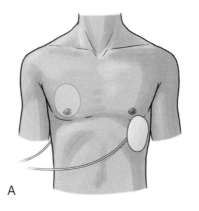 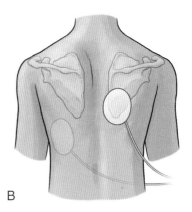

Figure 32.3 Anterior-posterior placement of self-adhesive defibrillation pads. **A,** Anterior pad placed over the left precordium. **B,** Posterior pad placed under the right scapula.

A   B

Steps	Rationale	Special Considerations
E. Pad or paddle placement in the patient with an ICD is the same as standard pad or paddle placement for cardioversion (see Fig. 32.2). Pads or paddles should not be placed over the device. **(Level D*)**	Cardioversion over an ICD may impair passage of current to the patient and cause the device to malfunction or become damaged.[3]	Do not place the pad or paddle over the pulse generator and lead wire.[3] Anterior-posterior placement is also suggested.[3] The ICD should be checked after external countershock. If the ICD is delivering anti-tachycardic pacing or shocks to the patient, wait 30–60 seconds before cardioverting the patient with the manual defibrillator.[3]
9. Ensure that the defibrillator cables are positioned to allow for adequate access to the patient.	Allows cardioversion to occur without excessive tension on the cables.	
10. Turn on the ECG recorder for a continuous printout.	Establishes a visual recording of the patient's current ECG status and response to intervention. Provides a permanent record of the patient's response to intervention.	
11. Charge the defibrillator as prescribed or in accordance with the manufacturer's energy recommendations per the specific device used. **(Level D*)**	The defibrillator is charged with the lowest energy level necessary to convert the tachydysrhythmia.[3,9]	
12. Disconnect the oxygen source during actual cardioversion.	Decreases the risk of combustion in the presence of electrical current.[3]	Arcing of electrical current in the presence of oxygen could precipitate an explosion and subsequent fire hazard.[3]
13. State "clear, shocking," and visually verify that everyone is clear of contact with the patient, bed, and equipment.	Maintains safety to caregivers because electrical current can be conducted from the patient to another individual if contact occurs.	State the warning firmly, using a forceful voice and look at the patient while talking to ensure that no one is touching or is in contact with the patient.[9] When using hands-free cardioversion, take special care to clear other personnel from patient contact because they do not have the visual cue of the paddles being placed on the patient's chest.

*Level D: Peer-reviewed professional and organizational standards with the support of clinical study recommendations.

Procedure continues on following page

UNIT II

Procedure   for Cardioversion—*Continued*

Steps	Rationale	Special Considerations
14. Verify that the defibrillator is still in the synchronization mode and that the patient's QRS complexes appear with a marker to signify correct synchronization of the defibrillator with the patient's ECG rhythm (see Fig. 32.1). **(Level D*)**	Synchronization prevents the random delivery of an electrical charge, which may potentiate ventricular fibrillation.[3,7,9]	
15. When using self-adhesive hands-free defibrillation pads, depress and hold the discharge button on the defibrillator to deliver the charge.	Depolarizes the cardiac muscle.[3,9] In the synchronized mode, a delay occurs before the charge is released, which allows the sensing mechanism to detect the QRS complex.	
16. If using handheld paddles, apply pressure to each paddle against the chest wall, depress both buttons on the paddles simultaneously, and then hold until the defibrillator fires.	Firm paddle pressure decreases transthoracic resistance, thus improving the flow of electrical current across the axis of the heart.[3]	This application of pressure is not necessary for defibrillator models with hands-free and automatic transthoracic impedance sensing/correction options built in.
17. Observe the monitor for conversion of the tachydysrhythmia, and assess the patient's carotid pulse. If a pulse is palpated, assess the patient's vital signs and level of consciousness.	Simultaneous depolarization of the myocardial muscle cells should reestablish a single source of impulse generation.[3,9]	If unsuccessful in converting the rhythm, proceed with repeated energy recommendations per the specific device used.[9] Ensure that the defibrillator is still in the synchronization mode; many defibrillators revert back to the unsynchronized mode after cardioversion. Ventricular fibrillation may develop after cardioversion. If so, deactivate the synchronizer and follow the procedure for defibrillation (see Procedure 33, Defibrillation [External]).[3,9]
18. Clean the defibrillator and remove any gel from the paddles.	Conductive gel accumulated on the defibrillator paddles impedes surface contact and increases transthoracic resistance.	
19. If self-adhesive defibrillation pads were used, evaluate the placement and integrity of the pads. In the case of elective cardioversion, remove the pads while the patient still sedated/anesthetized postprocedure, if possible, to minimize pain.	Self-adhesive defibrillation pads may crimp, crack, or fold with loss of adhesiveness.	Loss of adhesive integrity in self-adhesive defibrillation pads may occur in restless or diaphoretic patients. Pads should be left on the patient per manufacturer recommendations.
20. Remove PPE and discard used supplies in appropriate receptacle.	Reduces the transmission of microorganisms; standard precautions.	
21. 🖐		

*Level M: Manufacturer's recommendations only.

Expected Outcomes

- Reestablishment of sinus rhythm
- Hemodynamic stability

Unexpected Outcomes

- Continued tachydysrhythmias/unsuccessful cardioversion
- Ventricular fibrillation that progresses to cardiopulmonary arrest
- Bradycardia
- Asystole
- Pulmonary edema
- Systemic embolization
- Respiratory complications
- Hypotension
- Pacemaker or ICD dysfunction
- Skin burns
- Pain

Patient Monitoring and Care

Steps	Rationale	Reportable Conditions
		These conditions should be reported to the provider if they persist despite nursing interventions.
1. Evaluate neurological status before and after cardioversion. Reorient the patient as needed to person, place, and time.	An altered level of consciousness may occur after hemodynamically unstable dysrhythmias.[5,9] Cerebral or systemic emboli may develop as a postprocedural complication.[1]	• Change in level of consciousness • Sensory or motor changes
2. Monitor pulmonary status before and after cardioversion.	Hemodynamically unstable tachydysrhythmias may cause respiratory complications.[4,9] Respiratory depression and hypoventilation can occur after administration of sedatives and analgesics.[8]	• Dyspnea • Crackles • Rhonchi • Slow shallow respirations • Decrease in oxygen saturation as measured with pulse oximetry
3. Monitor cardiovascular status (blood pressure, heart rate, and rhythm) before and after cardioversion.	Dysrhythmias may develop after cardioversion.[5,9]	• Hypotension • Supraventricular dysrhythmias • Ventricular dysrhythmias • Bradycardia • Asystole
4. Prepare for administration of intravenous antidysrhythmic medications as prescribed.	Dysrhythmias may develop after cardioversion.[5,9]	• Supraventricular dysrhythmias • Ventricular dysrhythmias • Bradycardia • Asystole
5. Assess for burns.	Erythema at electrode sites may be seen from local hyperemia in the current pathway. Skin burns may be minimized with use of gel pads or placement of appropriate paste or gel on the paddles. Local cold application to the electrode site after cardioversion may decrease the incidence and severity of burns and pain at the site.[10]	• Skin burns
6. Follow institutional standards for assessing pain. Administer analgesia as prescribed.	Identifies the need for pain interventions.	• Continued pain despite pain interventions

Procedure continues on following page

Documentation

Documentation should include the following:
- Patient and family education
- Signed informed consent
- Universal protocol requirements, if nonemergent
- Neurological, pulmonary, and cardiovascular assessment before and after cardioversion
- Interventions to prepare the patient for cardioversion, including anticoagulation or TEE
- The joules used and the number of cardioversion attempts made
- Pain assessment, interventions, and effectiveness
- Printout of the ECG tracing depicting the cardiac rhythm before and after cardioversion (before and after each attempt if more than one attempt is used) or medication administration (e.g., antidysrhythmics, analgesics, sedatives)
- Condition of the skin of the chest wall
- Unexpected outcomes and nursing interventions
- Serum electrolytes, digoxin level, and coagulation laboratory results

References and Additional Readings

For a complete list of references and additional readings for this procedure, scan this QR code with your smartphone, or visit https://www.elsevier.com/__data/assets/pdf_file/0011/1319807/Chapter0032.pdf.

33 Defibrillation (External)

Cynthia Hambach

PURPOSE: External defibrillation is performed to eradicate life-threatening ventricular fibrillation or pulseless ventricular tachycardia. The goal for defibrillation is to terminate lethal dysrhythmias and to restore a perfusing rhythm. Coordinated cardiac electrical and mechanical pumping action results in restored cardiac output, tissue perfusion, and oxygenation.

PREREQUISITE NURSING KNOWLEDGE

- Anatomy and physiology of the cardiovascular system, principles of cardiac conduction, basic dysrhythmia interpretation, and electrical safety.
- Basic and advanced cardiac life support (ACLS) knowledge and skills.
- Clinical and technical competence in the use of a defibrillator.
- Recognition of ventricular fibrillation and pulseless ventricular tachycardia (VT) as lethal dysrhythmias.
- Early emergent defibrillation is the treatment of choice to restore normal electrical activity and coordinated contractile activity within the heart.[1,2,3]
- Recognition that the chances of successful defibrillation decrease as the length of time the ventricular tachycardia or fibrillation continues.[1,2,3]
- The electrical current delivered with defibrillation depolarizes the myocardium, terminating all electrical activity and allowing the heart's intrinsic pacemaker to resume electrical activity within the heart.[9] Defibrillator pads or paddles placed over the patient's chest wall surface in the anterior-apex or anterior-posterior position maximize the current flow through the myocardium.[1,2]
- Defibrillators deliver energy or current in waveform patterns. Delivered energy levels may differ among different defibrillators and waveforms. Various types of monophasic waveforms are used in older defibrillators. Biphasic waveforms have been designed more recently and are used currently in implantable cardioverter defibrillators (ICDs), automated external defibrillators, and manual defibrillators sold at the present time.[1]
- Monophasic waveforms deliver energy in one direction. The energy travels through the heart from one pad or paddle to the other.[1]
- Biphasic waveforms deliver energy in two directions. The energy travels through the heart in a positive direction and then reverses itself and flows back through the heart in a negative direction. Investigators in both in-hospital and out-of-hospital studies concluded that lower energy biphasic waveform shocks had equal or higher success rates for eradicating ventricular fibrillation than monophasic defibrillators.[1,2] Because of their increased

success in terminating dysrhythmias, defibrillators with biphasic waveforms are preferred for the treatment of atrial and ventricular dysrhythmias.[2,4] More research is needed to determine a specific recommendation for the optimal energy level for biphasic waveform defibrillation. Biphasic energy recommendations are device specific, using a variety of waveforms that are effective in terminating fatal dysrhythmias. When using biphasic defibrillators, the American Heart Association (AHA) recommends using the amount of energy specified by the manufacturer (120 to 200 J). If operators are unaware of the effective biphasic dose, they should use the maximal amount specified on the defibrillator for the first and all subsequent shocks.[2,3]

EQUIPMENT

- Personal protective equipment if needed depending on patient diagnosis
- Code cart with backboard/ACLS drugs and intubation equipment
- Defibrillator with electrocardiogram (ECG) oscilloscope/ recorder
- ECG cable with leads and electrodes
- Self-adhesive defibrillation pads or conductive gel, paste, or prepackaged gelled conduction pads to be used with defibrillator paddles
- Bag-valve-mask device with oxygen delivery
- Flow meter for oxygen administration, oxygen source
- Emergency suction
- Blood pressure monitoring equipment
- Pulse oximeter
- End-tidal carbon dioxide ($ETco_2$) monitoring equipment
- Intravenous infusion pumps
  Additional equipment to have available as needed includes the following:
- Emergency transcutaneous pacing equipment

PATIENT AND FAMILY EDUCATION

- Teaching may need to be performed after the procedure. *Rationale:* If emergent defibrillation is performed in the face of hemodynamic collapse, education may be impossible until after the procedure has been performed.

- Assess patient and family understanding of the etiology of the dysrhythmia. *Rationale:* This assessment determines the patient's and family's understanding of the condition and guides additional educational needs.
- Explain the procedure to the patient and family. *Rationale:* This explanation decreases anxiety and promotes understanding.
- Explain to the patient and family the signs and symptoms of hemodynamic compromise associated with preexisting cardiac dysrhythmias. *Rationale:* This explanation enables the patient and the family to recognize when to contact the nurse or physician.
- Evaluate and discuss with the patient the need for long-term pharmacological support. *Rationale:* This evaluation and discussion allow the nurse to anticipate the educational needs of the patient and family regarding specific discharge medications.
- Assess and discuss with the patient the need for lifestyle changes. *Rationale:* Underlying pathophysiology may necessitate alterations in the patient's current lifestyle and require a plan for behavioral changes.
- Assess and discuss with the patient the need as applicable for an ICD. *Rationale:* Life-threatening dysrhythmias may persist after initial defibrillation and pharmacological interventions.[5]
- Assess and discuss with the patient and family the need as applicable for an emergency communication system such as calling emergency medical services if the patient develops symptoms of hemodynamic compromise. *Rationale:* People with recurrent life-threatening dysrhythmias are at risk for cardiac arrest.[5]

PATIENT ASSESSMENT AND PREPARATION

Patient Assessment

- Assess the ECG monitor for ventricular fibrillation or ventricular tachycardia. *Rationale:* Both dysrhythmias can cause cardiac arrest.[2,3,5]
- Assess pulse. *Rationale*: Pulse is absent in the presence of ventricular fibrillation because of the loss of cardiac output.[9] If there is no pulse, initiate chest compressions while awaiting the defibrillator.

Patient Preparation

- Verify the correct patient with two identifiers. *Rationale:* Before performing a procedure, the nurse should ensure the correct identification of the patient for the intended intervention.
- If the family is present during the procedure, a staff member should be assigned, if possible, to provide support and keep the family informed. A member of pastoral care may also be called upon to provide support. *Rationale:* By relaying information and answering questions, a staff member and/or a pastoral care team member may provide support to ease family members' anxiety during the procedure.[10]
- Place the patient bed flat, and lower the side rails. *Rationale:* This prepares the environment for the procedure. the
- Remove transdermal medication patches from the patient's chest and wipe the area clean, or ensure that the defibrillator pad or paddle does not touch the patch. *Rationale:* Transdermal medication patches may block the transfer of energy from the pad or paddle to the patient and produce a chest burn when the pad or paddle is placed over it.[1]
- Ensure that the patient is in a dry environment, and dry the patient's chest if it is wet. *Rationale*: Water is a conductor of electricity. If the patient and rescuer are in contact with water, the rescuer may receive a shock, or the patient may receive a skin burn. Also, if the patient's chest is wet, the current may travel from one pad or paddle across the water to the other, resulting in a decreased amount of energy to the myocardium.[1]
- If the patient has a hairy chest, self-adhesive defibrillation pads may stick to the patient's hair instead of the skin. Apply pressure to pads to ensure contact. If this does not work, remove the pads briskly to remove hair, and replace with a new set of pads. *Rationale:* This action allows the electrodes to adhere to the chest.[1]
- Initiate basic life support (BLS) if immediate defibrillation is not available, and ensure that cardiopulmonary resuscitation continues with minimal interruption between defibrillation attempts and during charging of the defibrillator. *Rationale:* Basic life support maintains cardiac output to diminish irreversible organ and tissue damage.[2,5]
- Oxygenate the patient with a bag-valve-mask device and 100% oxygen. *Rationale:* This will optimize oxygen delivery until the patient is stabilized.[2,4,8,9] Use of bag-valve-mask ventilation is more effective with two rescuers.[3,5]
- Place the defibrillator in the defibrillation mode. *Rationale:* The defibrillation mode must be set to disperse the electrical charge randomly because the synchronization mode does not fire in the absence of a QRS complex.[1,3]

Procedure for Defibrillation (External)

Steps	Rationale	Special Considerations
1. 🔲 2. PPE 3. Apply self-adhesive defibrillation pads, or prepare defibrillation paddles with the proper conductive agent. **(Level D*)**	Reduces transthoracic resistance, thus enhancing electrical conduction through subcutaneous tissue.[1,2,3] Minimizes erythema from the electrical current.	Self-adhesive defibrillation pads connected directly to the defibrillator have been found to be as effective as paddles. Advantages of hands-free defibrillation pads are safety and convenience of use. Self-adhesive defibrillation pads decrease the risk of arcing, they can be used for monitoring, and they allow for fast delivery of a shock if necessary. For those reasons, the pads are recommended for routine use instead of standard paddles.[2,3] Prepackaged gelled conductive pads are available for placement in the area of the defibrillation paddles.[1] Gel pads should be replaced if they appear to be drying out or as per manufacturer recommendations. Conductive gel should be evenly dispersed on the defibrillator paddles and should adequately cover the surface. Be careful not to smear gel between paddles because current may follow an alternate pathway over the chest wall and avoid the heart. It may also cause a potential for a spark, causing a fire hazard. For this reason, gel pads are preferred.[1]
4. Ensure that the defibrillator cables are positioned to allow for adequate access to the patient.	Allows defibrillation to occur without excessive tension on cables.	
5. Turn on the ECG recorder for a continuous printout.	Establishes a visual recording of the patient's current ECG, verifies response to intervention, and provides a permanent record of the response to defibrillation.	
6. Follow these steps for pad or paddle placement: A. Place one pad or paddle at the heart's apex, just to the left of the nipple at the midaxillary line. Place the other pad or paddle below the right clavicle to the right of the sternum (see Fig. 32.2). B. In female patients, the apex pad or paddle is placed at the fifth to sixth intercostal space with the center of the pad or paddle at the midaxillary line.	Defibrillation is achieved by passing an electrical current through the cardiac muscle mass to restore a single source of impulse generation. This pathway maximizes current flow through the myocardium.[1] Placement over a female patient's breast should be avoided to reduce transthoracic resistance.	Most pads or paddles range from 8–12 cm in diameter.[2] Avoid placing pads or paddles over lead wires or implanted devices (ports, pacemakers, ICD).[1]

*Level D: Peer-reviewed professional and organizational standards with the support of clinical study recommendations.

Procedure continues on following page

Procedure for Defibrillation (External)—*Continued*

Steps	Rationale	Special Considerations
C. Anterior-posterior placement may also be used. i. Self-adhesive defibrillation pads are used for this approach. ii. The anterior pad is placed in the anterior left precordial area, and the posterior pad is placed posteriorly behind the heart in the right or left infrascapular area (see Fig. 32.3). iii. An alternative approach is to place the anterior pad in the right infraclavicular area and the posterior pad in the left infrascapular position.	All methods of pad placement are effective.[2]	
D. If the patient has a permanent pacemaker, do not place pads or paddles directly over the pulse generator.	Defibrillation over an implanted pacemaker may impair the passage of current to the patient and may cause the device to malfunction or become damaged.[1]	Do not place the pad or paddle over the pulse generator and lead wire.[1] Anterior-posterior placement is also suggested.[1] The pacemaker should be assessed after any electrical countershock. Standby emergency pacing equipment should be available in case the patient's permanent pacemaker does not function appropriately.
E. Pad or paddle placement in the patient with an ICD is the same as standard placement for defibrillation (see Fig. 32.2). Pads or paddles should not be placed over the device. **(Level D*)**	Defibrillation over an implanted ICD may impair the passage of current to the patient and cause the device to malfunction or become damaged.[1]	Do not place the pad or paddle over the pulse generator and lead wire.[1] Anterior-posterior placement is also suggested.[1] The ICD should be checked after external countershock. If the ICD is delivering antitachycardic pacing or shocks to the patient, wait until the ICD has finished delivering the pacing/shock algorithm (watch for pacing/shock activity on the ECG), and then defibrillate.[1]
7. Ensure that the mode dial is on defibrillation. Charge the defibrillator as prescribed or in accordance with AHA recommendations. **(Level D*)**	The defibrillator is charged with the lowest energy level needed to convert ventricular fibrillation or pulseless ventricular tachycardia.[1]	AHA monophasic energy recommendations for adults are for a 360-J shock.[1,2,3] When using biphasic defibrillators, the AHA recommends using the amount of energy specified by the manufacturer (120–200 J). If operators are unaware of the effective biphasic dose, they should use the maximal amount specified on the defibrillator for the first shock and all subsequent shocks.[2,3,4]
8. Disconnect the oxygen source during actual defibrillation.	Decreases the risk of combustion in the presence of electrical current.[1]	Arcing of electrical current in the presence of oxygen could precipitate an explosion and subsequent fire hazard.[1]

*Level D: Peer-reviewed professional and organizational standards with the support of clinical study recommendations.

Procedure	for Defibrillation (External)—*Continued*		
Steps	**Rationale**	**Special Considerations**	
9. State "clear, shocking," and visually verify that all personnel are clear of contact with the patient, bed, and equipment.	Maximizes safety to self and caregivers because electrical current can be conducted from the patient to another person if contact occurs.	State the warning firmly, using a forceful voice, and look at the patient while talking to ensure that no one is touching or is in contact with the patient.[3] With use of a hands-free defibrillation, take special care to clear other personnel from patient contact because they do not have the visual cue of the paddles being placed on the patient's chest.	
10. Verify that the patient is still in ventricular fibrillation or pulseless ventricular tachycardia.	Ensures that defibrillation is necessary.		
11. When using self-adhesive hands-free defibrillation pads, depress the discharge button on the defibrillator to deliver the charge. In the defibrillation mode, an immediate release of the electrical charge occurs.	Depolarizes the cardiac muscle.[3]		
12. If using handheld paddles, apply pressure to each paddle against the chest wall, depress both buttons on the paddles simultaneously, and then hold until the defibrillator fires. Ensure that paddles do not come in contact with ECG leads.	Firm paddle pressure decreases transthoracic resistance, thus improving the flow of electrical current across the axis of the heart.	This application of pressure is not necessary for defibrillator models with hands-free and automatic transthoracic impedance sensing/correction options built in.	
13. Immediately administer 2 minutes of CPR. (**Level D***)	CPR is needed for 2 minutes to provide some coronary and cerebral perfusion until adequate heart function resumes.[1,2,3] Studies have reported increased return of spontaneous circulation with shorter pauses in CPR for shock.[2,3]		
14. Observe the monitor for conversion of the dysrhythmia. If a stable rhythm is noted, assess for the presence of a carotid pulse. If a pulse is palpated, assess vital signs and level of consciousness.	Simultaneous depolarization of the myocardial muscle cells should reestablish a single source of impulse generation.[3]	If using $ETco_2$ monitoring, observe for a capnography waveform that indicates return of spontaneous circulation (ROSC).[3,5]	
15. If the patient is still in ventricular fibrillation or pulseless VT, continue CPR for 2 minutes, immediately charge the paddles to 360 J (monophasic) or a device-specific value (escalating; biphasic), and then **repeat Steps 8–14. (Level D***)	Immediate action increases the chance of successful subsequent depolarization of cardiac muscle.[1]	A vasopressive medication such as epinephrine may be given during CPR to improve cardiac output and blood pressure.[2,3,4,7] This recommendation is based on a significant difference in 30-day survival, survival to hospital discharge, and short-term outcomes of return to spontaneous circulation and survival to hospital admission.[7]	

*Level D: Peer-reviewed professional and organizational standards with the support of clinical study recommendations.

Procedure continues on following page

Procedure for Defibrillation (External)—*Continued*

Steps	Rationale	Special Considerations
16. If the second attempt is unsuccessful, continue CPR for 2 minutes, immediately charge the paddles to 360 J (monophasic) or a device-specific value (escalating; biphasic), and **repeat Steps 8–14. (Level D*)**	Immediate action increases the chance of successful subsequent depolarization of cardiac muscle.[1]	An antidysrhythmic medication such as amiodarone or lidocaine may be given during CPR to assist in terminating the dysrhythmia. There is no evidence that the use of an antidysrhythmic medication will increase long-term survival or survival with a positive neurological outcome after cardiac arrest.[2,3,4,8]
17. If the third attempt is unsuccessful, continue with ACLS. **(Level D*)**	Actions necessary to maintain the delivery of oxygenated blood to vital organs.[2,8,9]	BLS must be continued throughout resuscitation.[2,3,5] If the defibrillator is charged and defibrillation is not needed, turn the mode dial to monitor to safely remove the charge.
18. Observe the monitor for conversion of the dysrhythmia. If a stable rhythm is noted, assess for the presence of a carotid pulse. If a pulse is palpated, assess vital signs and level of consciousness.	Determines patient response to defibrillation.	
19. Transfer the patient to a critical care unit (if not there already).	Continues assessment and medical intervention.[3]	
20. After the emergency has ended, clean the defibrillator and remove the gel.	Prepares emergency equipment for future use.	
21. If the self-adhesive defibrillation pads were used, evaluate the placement and integrity of the pads.	Self-adhesive defibrillation pads may crimp, crack, or fold with loss of adhesiveness.	Loss of adhesive integrity in self-adhesive defibrillator pads can occur in restless or diaphoretic patients. Pads should be left on the patient per manufacturer recommendations.
22. Remove PPE, and discard used supplies in an appropriate receptacle.	Reduces transmission of microorganisms; standard precautions.	
23. 🅷🅷		

*Level D: Peer-reviewed professional and organizational standards with the support of clinical study recommendations.

Expected Outcomes

- Reestablishment of a perfusing rhythm such as sinus rhythm
- Hemodynamic stability

Unexpected Outcomes

- Continued ventricular fibrillation
- Continued cardiopulmonary arrest
- Asystole
- Myocardial infarction (MI)
- Respiratory complications
- Cerebral anoxia and brain injury/death
- Systemic embolization
- Hypotension
- Pacemaker or ICD dysfunction
- Skin burns
- Pain

Patient Monitoring and Care

Steps	Rationale	Reportable Conditions
		These conditions should be reported to the provider if they persist despite nursing interventions.
1. Evaluate neurological status before and after defibrillation. Reorient the patient as necessary to person, place, and time.	Altered level of consciousness may occur after cardiac arrest.[2,3,9]	• Change in level of consciousness
2. If the patient's neurological status is decreased (unable to follow verbal commands), prepare for procedures to achieve targeted temperature management (see Chapter 125). Maintain the patient's temperature between 32°C and 36°C for 24 hours. Follow institutional standards.	Therapeutic hypothermia has been shown to improve neurological recovery for patients post–cardiac arrest.[3,5,8,9]	• Core temperature < 32°C or >36°C during treatment protocol
3. Monitor the patient's airway and pulmonary status after defibrillation.	The goal is to support cardiac and pulmonary function to optimize tissue perfusion to vital organs, especially the brain.[2,3,9]	• Change in respirations • Change in breath sounds • Decreased oxygen saturation as measured with pulse oximetry • Abnormal arterial blood gas results
4. Prepare for insertion of an advanced airway if the patient remains unconscious or unresponsive, and administer 10 breaths/min to achieve a $Paco_2$ of 35–45 mm Hg. Mechanical ventilatory support may be necessary.	Hyperventilation of the patient should be avoided as it may cause adverse hemodynamic effects secondary to increased thoracic pressure. It may also decrease $Paco_2$ leading to decreased cerebral blood flow.[9,10]	• Abnormal $Paco_2$ results
5. Administer sedation and analgesia in mechanically ventilated patients as prescribed.	Intubation and mechanical ventilation as well as CPR and defibrillation can cause the patient pain and anxiety.[3]	• Continued pain or anxiety despite interventions
6. Administer oxygen therapy as prescribed.	The goal is to administer enough oxygen to maintain oxygen saturation (Sao_2) 92%–98% and to avoid oxygen toxicity.[2,3,5,9]	• Sao_2 < 92%
7. Monitor vital signs immediately after defibrillation and at least every 15 minutes until stable.	Vital signs should stabilize after achieving a normal heart rate and rhythm.	• Hypotension • Hypertension • Tachycardia • Bradycardia
8. Administer intravenous fluids followed by vasopressive medications to support cardiac output and maintain normal blood pressure as prescribed.	The goal is a systolic blood pressure ≥90 mm Hg or mean arterial pressure ≥65 mm Hg.[3,5,8,9]	• Hypotension • Hypertension
9. Continue to monitor the ECG after defibrillation.	Postdefibrillation dysrhythmias may occur. Administration of antidysrhythmic medications may be prescribed.[4,5]	• Dysrhythmias
10. Monitor electrolyte levels.	Abnormal electrolyte levels may have contributed to the development of ventricular dysrhythmias.[2,3,8]	• Abnormal electrolyte results

Procedure continues on following page

UNIT II

Patient Monitoring and Care —*Continued*

Steps	Rationale	Reportable Conditions
11. Obtain a 12-lead ECG, and prepare for emergent coronary angiography if warranted.	Cardiac arrest may be caused by acute coronary syndrome.[2,3,9]	• ECG changes
12. Assess for burns.	Erythema at electrode sites may be seen from local hyperemia in the current pathway.[11] Skin burns may be minimized with use of gel pads or placement of appropriate paste or gel on the paddles. Local cold application to the electrode site after defibrillation may decrease the incidence and severity of burns and pain at the site.[11]	• Skin burns
13. Consider other possible causes for ventricular fibrillation or pulseless ventricular tachycardia.	Interventions may be aimed at correcting the underlying pathophysiology and preventing the recurrence of lethal dysrhythmias.[2,3]	
14. Closely monitor neurological status.	The goal is to return patients to their pre–cardiac arrest neurological function.[2,3]	• Changes in level of consciousness • Changes in neurological examination

Documentation

Documentation should include the following:
- Neurological, pulmonary, and cardiovascular assessments before and after defibrillation
- Interventions to prepare the patient for defibrillation
- The joules (J) used and the number of defibrillation attempts made
- Medications administered during resuscitation
- Printout of ECG tracings that depict the cardiac rhythm before and after defibrillation
- Pain assessment, interventions, and effectiveness
- Patient response to defibrillation
- Condition of skin of the chest wall
- Unexpected outcomes and nursing interventions
- Team members present during resuscitation efforts
- Patient and family education

References and Additional Readings

For a complete list of references and additional readings for this procedure, scan this QR code with your smartphone, or visit https://www.elsevier.com/__data/assets/pdf_file/0003/1319808/Chapter0033.pdf

34 Emergent Open Sternotomy (Perform) and Defibrillation (Internal) (Perform)

Alice Chan and Marion E. McRae

PURPOSE Emergent open sternotomy is performed for a patient after cardiac surgery to identify and eliminate areas of persistent hemorrhage, relieve pericardial tamponade, and provide access for open cardiac massage and internal defibrillation.

PREREQUISITE NURSING KNOWLEDGE

- Knowledge of anatomy and physiology of the cardiovascular system, principles of cardiac conduction, dysrhythmia interpretation, and electrical safety are necessary.
- Advanced cardiac life support knowledge and skills are needed.
- Understanding the signs and symptoms of cardiac tamponade is necessary.
- Cardiac arrest after cardiac surgery occurs in about 0.7% to 8% of patients.[14] Ventricular fibrillation is the cause of arrest in 25% to 50% of cases.[14]
- Clinical competence in the use of the defibrillator is needed.
- Knowledge of internal paddle placement and energy requirements for internal defibrillation is needed.
- Emergent open sternotomy is performed for patients who have undergone a median sternotomy.
- If open chest resuscitation with internal defibrillation is attempted in cardiac arrest, it should be performed within the first 5 minutes after arrest for the most favorable outcomes.[14-15]
- Emergent open sternotomy is indicated for exsanguinating hemorrhage or cardiac tamponade with imminent cardiac arrest.[7]
  - ❖ The goal of mediastinal exploration for persistent hemorrhage is to stop the bleeding and retain circulating blood volume. The requirement for homologous blood transfusion and incidence of wound infection associated with an undrained mediastinal hematoma may be decreased.[2]
  - ❖ The goal of mediastinal exploration for cardiac tamponade is to relieve the pressure on the ventricles during diastole. The decreased pressure allows the ventricles to fill during diastole, which should increase contractility, stroke volume, and cardiac output to improve systemic perfusion.[2]
- Knowledge and skills related to aseptic and sterile technique, surgical instrumentation, sternal opening, sternal exploration, sternal closure, and suturing are needed.[11]
- Paralytic agents may be a necessary adjunct to sedation and analgesia to improve oxygenation, diminish muscle activity, and enhance visualization.
- Evidence shows that practicing open sternotomy skills with simulation can reduce the time to chest reopening, reduce resternotomy complications by 50%,[14] and increase survival to discharge.[8]

EQUIPMENT

- Antiseptic solution (e.g., 2% chlorhexidine gluconate skin preparation)
- Head cover, masks, eye protection, sterile gown, sterile gloves, sterile drapes
- Emergency resternotomy set (Fig. 34.1). A small resternotomy set containing the following items is recommended[14]:
  - ❖ Wire cutter
  - ❖ Rib spreader
  - ❖ Kelly clamps
  - ❖ Disposable scalpel
  - ❖ Drape
  - ❖ Nonvented Yankauer suction
  - ❖ Sterile suction tubing
- Electrocautery equipment: generator, cautery, electrical dispersing pad (e.g., grounding pad)
- Suction containers, tubing, regulator, and suction source
- Radiopaque gauze or other surgical sponge materials

UNIT II

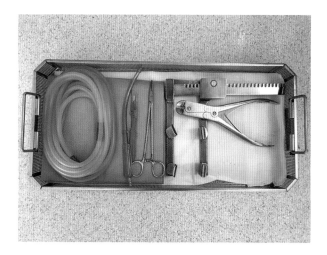

Figure 34.1 Emergency resternotomy set containing *(left to right)* sterile suction tubing, Yankauer suction (nonvented), disposable scalpel with blade, Kelly clamps, sternal retractor, and wire cutters.

- Polypropylene (Prolene) suture (cutting needle) and other suture material according to preference
- Clip applicator and clips
- Syringes: 3 mL, 5 mL, 10 mL, and 20 mL
- Disposable 10, 11, and 15 scalpels
- Sternal wires or bands
- Sterile stapler or sutures
- Sterile dressing supplies
- Emergency medication and resuscitation equipment, including internal defibrillation paddles and external defibrillation pads or paddles
- Prescribed analgesia or sedation
  Additional equipment to have available as needed includes the following:
- Prescribed blood products and intravenous solutions
- Warm saline solution with or without an antibiotic, as prescribed
- Chest tubes and chest tube drainage system
- Epicardial wires
- Intraaortic balloon catheter and pump console or other mechanical assist device
- Peripheral nerve stimulator (used if paralytic agents are administered)
- Sterile staple remover

PATIENT AND FAMILY EDUCATION

- Teaching may not be provided until after the procedure. *Rationale:* When an emergent sternotomy and internal defibrillation is performed for rapid hemodynamic collapse, education for the patient and family may not be possible before the procedure.
- Explain the reason that the open sternotomy procedure and defibrillation, if used, was performed and its outcome or anticipated outcome. *Rationale:* This explanation provides information and encourages the patient and family to ask questions and clarify details about the patient and procedure.

PATIENT ASSESSMENT AND PREPARATION

Patient Assessment

- Assess hemodynamic and neurological status. *Rationale:* This assessment identifies baseline data that may indicate the need for emergent open sternotomy and provides comparison data.
- Assess for dysrhythmias, especially ventricular ectopy. *Rationale:* Ventricular dysrhythmias may precede ventricular tachycardia and ventricular fibrillation.
- Assess vital signs when dysrhythmias occur. *Rationale:* This assessment provides data about the patient's response to dysrhythmias.
- Assess the patient's medical history, specifically for coagulation disorders, renal disease with coexistent uremia, and functional status of the right and left ventricle. *Rationale:* Baseline data are obtained.
- Assess current laboratory data, specifically complete blood cell count, platelet count, international normalized ratio, activated partial thromboplastin time, fibrinogen, and electrolytes. *Rationale:* Near-normal baseline coagulation study results decrease the likelihood of coagulopathy as a possible cause for ongoing hemorrhage. Abnormal electrolytes may lead to dysrhythmias.
- Assess for signs and symptoms of cardiac tamponade. *Rationale:* The presence of some or all of these signs and symptoms helps the physician, advanced practice nurse, or other healthcare professional determine whether the emergent open sternotomy is indicated:
  - ❖ Sudden decrease or cessation in chest tube drainage
  - ❖ Hypotension (mean arterial blood pressure <60 mm Hg)
  - ❖ Altered mental status
  - ❖ Apical heart rate greater than 110 beats/min
  - ❖ Narrowing of pulse pressure
  - ❖ Distended neck veins
  - ❖ Distant heart sounds
  - ❖ Equalization of intracardiac pressures, including right atrial, pulmonary artery diastolic, and pulmonary artery occlusion pressures
  - ❖ Decreased cardiac output and cardiac index
  - ❖ Pulsus paradoxus
- Assess for excessive chest tube drainage. *Rationale:* Severity of bleeding assists with the determination of the need for emergent mediastinal exploration. Follow institutional guidelines regarding determination of the timing of mediastinal exploration. One recommendation for timing the procedure is when chest tube drainage continues at equal to or greater than 3 mL/kg/hour for at least 3 hours.[3,5]

Patient Preparation

- Verify the correct patient with two identifiers. *Rationale:* Before performing a procedure, the nurse should ensure the correct identification of the patient for the intended intervention.
- Ensure that the patient and family understand the procedural teaching (if time is available). Answer questions as they arise, and reinforce information as needed.

Rationale: Understanding of the information provided is evaluated and reinforced.

- Obtain informed consent (may not be possible if the procedure is an emergency). *Rationale:* Informed consent protects the rights of the patient and ensures a competent decision for the patient and family.
- Perform a preprocedure verification and time out, if nonemergent. *Rationale:* Ensures patient safety.
- Ensure that the patient's airway is protected and that supplemental oxygen is delivered, if needed. *Rationale:* The probability that the patient's ventilatory needs will be met is enhanced.
- Position the patient in the supine position with the head of the bed flat. *Rationale:* This position ensures visualization of the chest and enhances hemodynamic stability.
- Remove all metallic objects from the patient's skin. *Rationale:* Metallic objects are conductors of electrical current and may cause burns.
- Prescribe and ensure that an analgesic and/or sedative are administered. *Rationale:* Promotes patient comfort.

Procedure | for Performing Emergent Open Sternotomy

Steps	Rationale	Special Considerations
1. HH		
2. PE		
3. Ensure that the nurse has applied an electrical dispersing pad (i.e., grounding pad) to the patient's dry skin over a large well perfused muscle mass. **(Level M*)**	Electrocautery is used to terminate capillary oozing or bleeding.	Grounding is essential to avoid burning the patient and possible electrical shock to healthcare providers. Electrocautery may not be immediately available in the critical care setting; follow institutional standards.
4. Ensure that the nurse has a new sterile suction system set up.	Suction within the mediastinum is necessary during the procedure.	
5. Either have the nurse remove the sternal dressing and cleanse the chest with an antiseptic solution (e.g., 2% chlorhexidine gluconate solution), or perform the procedure yourself. If performing the procedure yourself, remove gloves when cleansing is completed, and wash hands.	Inhibits microorganism transmission.	Prepare the skin beginning at the incision line, extending outward to include the area from the chin to the mid-abdomen (caudal to the umbilicus) and to include the area outward to one anterior axillary line and then outward to the opposite anterior axillary line. Prevent the solution from running off the surgical site, dripping, pooling, and soaking fabric and the patient's hair. Ensure that alcohol-based preparation agents do not wet the patient's hair or bedding or pool in skin folds or the umbilicus because this increases the risk of fire (nonflammable preparations eliminate the risk of fire).[1]

6. Don personal protective equipment and sterile equipment:
  i. Surgical head cover, mask, and eye protection
  ii. Perform hand antisepsis/hand scrub
  iii. Sterile gown and sterile gloves
	Minimizes microorganisms, thereby preventing infection.[1,10]	All personnel in the room must don caps and masks.

*Level M: Manufacturer's recommendations only.

Procedure continues on following page

Procedure	for Performing Emergent Open Sternotomy—*Continued*	
Steps	**Rationale**	**Special Considerations**
7. Ask the nurse or person assisting to open the sternotomy tray and place necessary items on the sterile field.	Prepares equipment.	
8. Fully drape the patient with exposure of only the surgical site.[1,10] **(Level D*)**	A large sterile field minimizes the risk of infection and provides space to maintain asepsis of instruments and supplies during the procedure.[1,10]	
9. Hand off the distal end of the electrocautery cable (active electrode) to the nurse or assisting healthcare provider for connection to the electrocautery machine (if used).	Cautery is used to stop bleeding from small vessels.	
10. Open the incision down to the sternum with the staple remover or scalpel, exposing the sternal wires or bands.	Ensures visualization of the sternal wires or bands.	Remove staples with a staple remover; cut sutures and tissue with a scalpel.
11. Cut the sternal wires (or bands) from the top to the bottom of the sternum with the wire cutter, or untwist the wires with the heavy needle holder or Kelly clamps.	Provides access to the mediastinum. The sternal wires fatigue and break when untwisted.	Use care when removing the sternal wires to minimize damage to the heart, underlying equipment (e.g., epicardial pacing wires, chest tubes), and coronary artery bypass grafts and to avoid injury to the healthcare provider.
12. Gently separate the sternum with your hands.	Caution must be taken to separate the sternum gently because the heart, bypass grafts, and pacing wires rest just under the sternal bone.	
13. Place the sternal retractor under the sternal bone. Slowly crank it open while feeling along the edge of the retractor blades and observing the mediastinal cavity and heart for anything caught in the retractor.	Exposes the heart and mediastinum.	Sternal retractor blades can trap and tear bypass grafts and pacing wires if caught and pulled apart when the retractor is cranked open.
14. For bleeding, apply pressure with a finger over any bleeding site, and suction the remainder of the chest, evacuating any clots.	Pressure on the bleeding site may minimize blood loss.	Resuscitate with intravenous fluids, inotropic medications, and blood products as necessary.
15. Control and ligate bleeding sites, enhance sternal retraction, and provide suctioning and electrocautery as needed.	May eliminate the need for further exploration. Assists with better visualization of the surgical field.	Determine whether the patient needs to be transferred to the operating room for further surgical intervention.
16. If pulseless ventricular tachycardia or ventricular fibrillation occurs, internal defibrillation is needed.	Emergency intervention is needed.	The nurse or additional assistive personnel obtain the defibrillator and the internal defibrillation paddles (Fig. 34.2).

*Level D: Peer-reviewed professional and organizational standards with the support of clinical study recommendations.

Procedure for Performing Emergent Open Sternotomy—*Continued*		
Steps	Rationale	Special Considerations

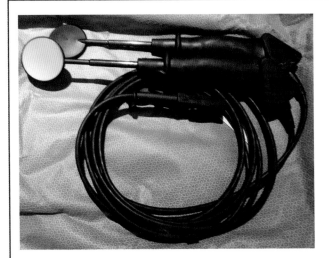

Figure 34.2 Internal defibrillation paddles.

Steps	Rationale	Special Considerations
17. Have the nurse open and place internal paddles on the sterile field. Hand off the connection cable to be attached to the defibrillator. If the internal paddles are two-part paddles, connect the defibrillation paddles to the handles (usually via a screw mechanism).	Prepares the internal paddles for use.	
18. Request that the nurse set the defibrillator to the desired energy (usually 20 J for biphasic shocks)[15,9] **(Level E*)**	Although 5 J can defibrillate the heart, use of 10 to 20 J optimizes more rapid defibrillation and fewer shocks[13]	Refer to the defibrillator manufacturer's operation guidelines for specific recommendations, and follow institutional guidelines.
19. Ask the nurse to charge the defibrillator. Place one paddle over the right atrium or right ventricle; place the other paddle over the apex of the heart (Fig. 34.3).	This will aid in depolarizing the entire myocardium.	
20. State "all clear," and visually verify that all personnel are clear of contact with the patient, bed, and equipment.	Electrical current can be conducted from the patient to another person if contact occurs with the patient, bed, or other equipment.	
21. Simultaneously depress and hold the buttons on each paddle until the defibrillator discharges if the paddles are equipped with defibrillation buttons. If the paddles are not equipped with defibrillation buttons, ask the nurse to activate the shock button on the defibrillator. **(Level M*)**	In the defibrillation mode, an immediate release of the electrical charge depolarizes cardiac muscle. Simultaneous depolarization of the myocardium may result in simultaneous repolarization of enough myocardium to reestablish a single cardiac impulse.	
22. Assess the patient's response to defibrillation (heart rate and rhythm, blood pressure, level of consciousness).	Determines whether additional interventions may be needed.	

*Level E: Multiple case reports, theory-based evidence from expert opinions or peer-reviewed professional organizational standards without clinical studies to support recommendations.
*Level M: Manufacturer's recommendations only.

Procedure continues on following page

Procedure | for Performing Emergent Open Sternotomy—*Continued*

Steps	Rationale	Special Considerations

Figure 34.3 Paddle placement for internal defibrillation. *(From Kinkade S, Lohrman JE: Critical care nursing procedures: a team approach, Philadelphia, 1990, BC Decker.)*

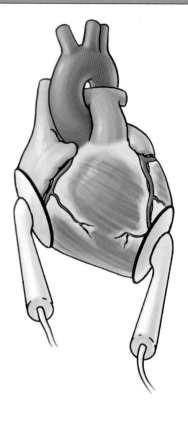

23. If the first defibrillation is not successful, perform additional defibrillations as needed.

    Continues emergency treatment.

24. Open chest compressions may be initiated if needed:
    i. Place one hand around the surface of the apex of the heart toward the posterior aspect of the heart with the palm up and fingers straight.
    ii. Avoid lifting the apex of the heart.
    iii. Avoid any grafts or other structures on the heart such as epicardial pacemaker leads.
    iv. Place the palm of the other hand on the anterior surface of the heart keeping the fingers straight.
    v. Squeeze the heart between your two hands at 100–120 compressions per minute.[14] **(Level D*)**
    vi. Aim for an SBP of >60 mm Hg via arterial line[14] with compressions. **(Level D*)**

    Open-chest cardiac compression may be initiated if internal defibrillation is not successful. Internal cardiac massage is superior to external cardiac massage.[6]

    Do not press your fingers into the epicardial surface of the heart as tears can occur in thin or weak areas of tissue. Do not lift the apex of the heart as posterior ventricular rupture can occur,[6] especially if there are prosthetic atrioventricular valve prostheses in situ.

*Level D: Peer-reviewed professional and organizational standards with the support of clinical study recommendations.

Procedure	**for Performing Emergent Open Sternotomy—*Continued***	
Steps	Rationale	Special Considerations
25. If defibrillation is successful, obtain vital signs, and assess the patient.	Aids in determining whether additional interventions are needed.	Provide additional supportive therapies such as antiarrhythmic drugs, epicardial pacing, and/or vasoactive agents.
26. Insert chest tubes and/or epicardial pacing wires if needed.	Chest tubes and epicardial pacing wires can be displaced during sternal retraction or mediastinal exploration.	
27. Warm saline solution with or without an antibiotic may be used to flush the chest cavity before closing the incision.	May decrease the incidence of infection.	Determine whether additional antibiotic coverage is needed.
28. Assist with placement of mechanical assist devices if needed.	Cardiac tamponade may conceal right or left ventricular dysfunction; mechanical assistance may be necessary to improve cardiac output.	
29. Assist with patient transport to the operating room if necessary.	The patient may need further exploration; surgical repair of coronary artery bypass grafts, cardiac valves, or the myocardium; or insertion of an assist device (e.g., intra-aortic balloon pump, ventricular assist device).	Ensure that the patient's chest is covered with sterile drapes or with a dressing during transportation.

30. If the patient does not need to return to the operating room, reinsert sternal wires as follows:
  i. Grasp the sternal wire with the needle holder.
  ii. From under the sternum, push one end of the wire up between two ribs at the sternal border.
  iii. Repeat step B with the other end of the wire on the opposite side of the sternum (same intercostal space).
  iv. Pull the sternum together with the wire, and twist the edges of the wires together with the needle holder.
  v. Cut off the excess wire, and bend the twisted edges flat against the sternum.
  vi. Repeat with additional wires every two to three ribs until the sternum is closed.
	Ensures sternal closure.	Caution must be taken not to penetrate the heart, pericostal vessels, lungs, or bypass grafts with the sternal wires.
		Multiple wiring techniques can be used for sternal wound closure; the advanced practice nurse or physician performing the procedure may use an alternate method or use sternal bands to close the sternum.

31. Close the skin closure according to preference (staples or sutures).	Promotes wound healing.	The patient's chest may be left open and covered with a sterile occlusive dressing if severe tissue swelling or ventricular dysfunction exists.

Procedure continues on following page

UNIT II

Procedure   for Performing Emergent Open Sternotomy—*Continued*

Steps	Rationale	Special Considerations
32. Apply an occlusive dressing to the sternal incision, epicardial pacing wires, and chest tube sites.	Dressings provide a physical barrier to external sources of contamination and cushion from physical contact and trauma; they absorb drainage and help maintain a moist environment at body temperature to enhance wound healing.	
33. Dispose of sharps per facility standards.[11]	Minimizes the risk of sharps injury.	A chest radiograph may be prescribed to rule out the presence of any retained surgical sponges, needles, or instruments.
34. Discard used supplies in appropriate receptacles **PE**.	Reduces the transmission of microorganisms and body secretions; standard precautions.	
35. **HH**		
36. Remove and package instruments for cleaning and sterilization.	Prepares for another emergency.	

Expected Outcomes

- Resolution of the condition that necessitated the emergent open sternotomy
- Resolution of cardiac dysrhythmias
- Increased cardiac output/hemodynamic stability
- Increased tissue perfusion, including cerebral, renal, and peripheral perfusion
- Minimal chest tube drainage
- Decreased need for blood transfusions

Unexpected Outcomes

- Severe right or left ventricular dysfunction
- Continued dysrhythmias, bleeding, or coagulation disorders
- Myocardial, aortic, coronary artery, or coronary artery bypass graft perforation
- Pneumothorax
- Pain
- Surgical infection
- Death

Patient Monitoring and Care

Steps	Rationale	Reportable Conditions
		These conditions should be reported to the provider if they persist despite nursing interventions.
1. Perform cardiovascular, hemodynamic, and peripheral vascular assessments every 15–30 minutes as patient status requires (including vital signs, pulmonary artery pressure, cardiac index, level of consciousness, and urine output).	Determines hemodynamic stability and volume status; recurrent tamponade or dysrhythmias may develop during and after sternotomy. Determines the adequacy of cerebral perfusion; hemodynamic instability can lead to cerebral anoxia. Determines adequate perfusion to the kidneys.	• Mean arterial blood pressure <60 mm Hg • Abnormal changes in heart rate and rhythm • Decrease in cardiac index • Abnormal pulmonary artery pressures • Urine output <0.5 mL/kg/hour • Equalizing pulmonary artery pressures • Change in level of consciousness • Impaired level of consciousness
2. If the patient's neurological condition is compromised after a chest procedure with cardiac arrest (e.g., comatose), consider therapeutic hypothermia at 32°–36°C for at least 24 hours[14] **(Level D*)**	The benefit of therapeutic hypothermia in cardiac arrest after cardiac surgery is unknown, with only case reports.[12] However, there is a strength of evidence in other populations; therefore it should be considered. Hypothermia can impair coagulation, which is a concern if the patient is bleeding.	

*Level D: Peer-reviewed professional and organizational standards with the support of clinical study recommendations.

Patient Monitoring and Care —*Continued*

Steps	Rationale	Reportable Conditions
3. Assess heart and lung sounds every 2 hours and as needed.	Abnormal heart and lung sounds may indicate the need for additional treatment.	• Distant heart sounds • Abnormal lung sounds
4. Monitor coagulation, hematologic, and electrolyte laboratory blood study results.	Coagulation and hematological profiles provide data that indicate the risk of bleeding and indicate the need for additional treatment. Electrolyte studies provide data regarding the risk for dysrhythmias and decreased contractility.	• Abnormal hemoglobin and hematocrit, activated partial thromboplastin time, international normalized ratio, platelets, fibrinogen, calcium, magnesium, or potassium
5. Closely monitor chest tube drainage.	Determines functioning of the chest tube drainage system and the amount of chest drainage.	• Cessation of chest tube drainage • Increased chest tube drainage • Clots in the chest tube drainage system
6. Provide orders for a 12-lead electrocardiogram (ECG), and interpret the ECG.	Assess for myocardial ischemia/infarction	• ECG abnormalities
7. Assess pain, and prescribe analgesia as needed.	Identifies the need for pain interventions.	• Continued pain despite pain interventions

Documentation

Documentation should include the following:
- Patient and family education
- Signed informed consent, if nonemergent
- Universal protocol requirement, if nonemergent
- Pain assessment, interventions, and effectiveness
- Indications for the procedure and the procedure performed
- Amount of blood collected from chest suctioning; estimated blood loss
- Patient therapies and response, including hemodynamic parameters, antiarrhythmic agents, inotropic or vasopressor agents, analgesia, sedation, ventilation, and neurological status
- Additional interventions
- Unexpected outcomes

References and Additional Readings

For a complete list of references and additional readings for this procedure, scan this QR code with your smartphone, or visit https://www.elsevier.com/__data/assets/pdf_file/0004/1319809/Chapter0034.pdf

35 Emergent Open Sternotomy and Internal Defibrillation (Assist)

Alice Chan and Marion E. McRae

PURPOSE: Emergent open sternotomy is performed for a patient after cardiac surgery to identify and eliminate areas of persistent hemorrhage, relieve pericardial tamponade, and provide access for open cardiac massage and internal defibrillation.

The purpose of internal defibrillation is to deliver electrical current directly to the epicardial surface of the heart when a shockable rhythm is present.

PREREQUISITE NURSING KNOWLEDGE

- Knowledge of the anatomy and physiology of the cardiovascular system, principles of cardiac conduction, dysrhythmia interpretation, and electrical safety is necessary.
- Advanced cardiac life support knowledge and skills are needed.
- Understanding the signs and symptoms of cardiac tamponade is necessary.
- Clinical competence in the use of the defibrillator is needed.
- Knowledge of energy requirements for internal defibrillation is needed.
- Emergency open sternotomy is performed for patients who have undergone a median sternotomy.
- Emergent open sternotomy is indicated for exsanguinating hemorrhage or cardiac tamponade with imminent cardiac arrest.[6,7]
  - ❖ The goal of mediastinal exploration for persistent hemorrhage is to stop the bleeding and retain circulating blood volume. The requirement for homologous blood transfusion and incidence of wound infection associated with an undrained mediastinal hematoma may be decreased.[2]
  - ❖ The goal of mediastinal exploration for cardiac tamponade is to relieve pressure on the ventricles during diastole. The decreased pressure allows the ventricles to fill during diastole, which should increase contractility, stroke volume, and cardiac output to improve systemic perfusion.
- Cardiac arrest after cardiac surgery occurs in about 0.7% to 8% of patients.[13] Ventricular fibrillation is the cause of arrest in 25% to 50% of cases.[13]
- If open-chest resuscitation with internal defibrillation is attempted in cardiac arrest, it should be performed within the first 5 minutes after cardiac arrest for the most favorable outcomes.[13]

- Internal defibrillation may be necessary if life-threatening dysrhythmias occur.
- Knowledge and skills related to aseptic and sterile technique are needed.
- Paralytic agents may be a necessary adjunct to sedation and analgesia to improve oxygenation, diminish muscle activity, and enhance visualization.
- Evidence shows that practicing open sternotomy skills with simulation can reduce the time to chest reopening,[4] reduce resternotomy complications by 50%,[13] and increase survival to discharge.[8]

EQUIPMENT

- Antiseptic solution (e.g., 2% chlorhexidine gluconate skin preparation)
- Head cover, masks, eye protection, sterile gown, sterile gloves, sterile drapes
- Emergency resternotomy set (see Fig. 34.1). A small resternotomy set containing the following items is recommended[13]:
  - ❖ Wire cutter
  - ❖ Rib spreader
  - ❖ Kelly clamps
  - ❖ Disposable scalpel
  - ❖ Drape
  - ❖ Nonvented Yankauer suction
- Electrocautery equipment: generator, cautery, electrical dispersing pad (e.g., grounding pad)
- Suction containers, tubing, regulator, and suction source
- Radiopaque gauze or other surgical sponge materials
- Polypropylene (Prolene) suture (cutting needle), other suture material as requested
- Clip applicator and clips
- Syringes: 3 mL, 5 mL, 10 mL, and 20 mL
- Disposable scalpel: 10, 11, and 15 scalpels
- Sternal wires or bands
- Sterile stapler or sutures
- Sterile dressing supplies
- Emergency medication and resuscitation equipment
- Defibrillator

- Sterile internal paddles (ensure compatibility with the defibrillator). Adult internal paddles are usually 5 to 7.5 cm in diameter (see Fig. 34.2)

Additional equipment to have available as needed includes the following:

- Prescribed analgesia and sedation
- Blood products and intravenous solutions as prescribed
- Warm saline solution with or without an antibiotic, as prescribed
- Chest tubes and chest tube drainage system
- Epicardial wires
- Intraaortic balloon catheter and pump console or other mechanical assist device
- Peripheral nerve stimulator (used if paralytic agents are administered)
- Sterile staple remover

PATIENT AND FAMILY EDUCATION

- Teaching may not be provided until after the procedure. *Rationale:* When emergent sternotomy and internal defibrillation are performed for rapid hemodynamic collapse, education for the patient and family may not be possible before the procedure.
- Explain the reason why the open sternotomy procedure/internal defibrillation was performed. *Rationale:* This explanation provides information and encourages the patient and family to ask questions and clarify details about the patient and procedure.

PATIENT ASSESSMENT AND PREPARATION

Patient Assessment

- Assess hemodynamic and neurological status. *Rationale:* This assessment identifies baseline data that may indicate the need for emergent open sternotomy and provides comparison data.
- Assess for dysrhythmias, especially ventricular ectopy. *Rationale:* Ventricular dysrhythmias may precede ventricular tachycardia and ventricular fibrillation.
- Assess vital signs when dysrhythmias occur. *Rationale:* This assessment provides data about the patient's response to dysrhythmias.
- Assess for pulseless ventricular tachycardia or ventricular fibrillation. *Rationale:* This assessment determines the need for resuscitation, which includes internal cardiac defibrillation. If immediate intervention is not initiated, return of circulation may not be possible.
- Assess current laboratory data, specifically complete blood cell count, platelet count, international normalized ratio, activated partial thromboplastin time, and fibrinogen. Abnormal electrolytes may lead to dysrhythmias. *Rationale:* Near-normal baseline coagulation study results decrease the likelihood of coagulopathy as a possible cause for ongoing hemorrhage.

- Assess for signs and symptoms of cardiac tamponade. *Rationale:* The presence of some or all of these signs and symptoms assists the healthcare team to decide whether an emergent open sternotomy is necessary:
  - ❖ Sudden decrease or cessation in chest tube drainage
  - ❖ Hypotension (mean arterial blood pressure <60 mm Hg)
  - ❖ Altered mental status
  - ❖ Apical heart rate greater than 110 beats/min
  - ❖ Narrowing of pulse pressure
  - ❖ Distended neck veins
  - ❖ Distant heart sounds
  - ❖ Equalization of intracardiac pressures, including right atrial, pulmonary artery diastolic, and pulmonary artery occlusion pressures
  - ❖ Decreased cardiac output and cardiac index
  - ❖ Pulsus paradoxus
- Assess for excessive chest tube drainage. *Rationale:* The presence of bleeding assists with determination of the need for mediastinal exploration. Follow institutional guidelines regarding determination of the timing of mediastinal exploration. One recommendation for timing the procedure is when chest tube drainage continues at equal to or greater than 3 mL/kg/hour for at least 3 hours.[3,5]

Patient Preparation

- Verify the correct patient with two identifiers. *Rationale:* Before performing a procedure, the nurse should ensure the correct identification of the patient for the intended intervention.
- Ensure that the patient and family understand the procedural teaching (if time is available). Answer questions as they arise, and reinforce information as needed. *Rationale:* Comprehension of the information provided is evaluated and reinforced.
- Ensure that informed consent was obtained (may not be possible if the procedure is an emergency). *Rationale:* Informed consent protects the rights of the patient and ensures a competent decision for the patient and family.
- Perform a preprocedure verification and time out, if nonemergent. *Rationale:* Ensures patient safety.
- Ensure that the patient's airway is protected (reintubate if necessary) and that supplemental oxygen is delivered, if needed. *Rationale:* Ensures adequate ventilation and oxygenation.
- Position the patient in the supine position with the head of the bed flat. *Rationale:* This position ensures visualization of the chest and enhances hemodynamic stability.
- Remove all metallic objects from the patient's skin. *Rationale:* Metallic objects are conductors of electrical current and may cause burns.
- Administer analgesia and sedation as prescribed. *Rationale:* Promotes patient comfort.

UNIT II

Procedure | for Assisting With Emergent Open Sternotomy

Steps	Rationale	Special Considerations
1. Assist as needed with calling the patient's physician and operative team.	The physician can reassess the need for further surgical intervention. The operative team may be needed to assist at the bedside or to prepare the operating room if further exploration is needed.	Follow institutional standards.
2. 🅷🅷		
3. 🅿🅴		

4. Assist with preparation of the electrocautery device for possible use:
  i. Apply the electrical dispersing pad (i.e., grounding pad) to the patient's dry skin over a large well-perfused muscle.
  ii. Attach the grounding cable to the electrocautery device. **(Level M*)**
	Electrocautery may be used to terminate capillary bleeding.	Grounding is essential to avoid burning the patient and possible electrical shock to healthcare providers.
		Electrocautery may not be immediately available in the critical care setting; follow institutional standards.

5. Set up a new sterile suction system.	Suction within the mediastinum is necessary during the procedure.	
6. Assist if needed with removing the sternal dressing.	Prepares for the procedure.	
7. Assist if needed with cleansing the patient's chest with an antiseptic solution (e.g., 2% chlorhexidine gluconate solution).[1]	Inhibits microorganism transmission.	The skin is cleansed beginning at the incision line, extending outward to include the area from the chin to the mid-abdomen (caudal to the umbilicus) and to include the area outward to one anterior axillary line and then outward to the opposite anterior axillary line. Minimize solution from running off of the surgical site. Ensure that alcohol-based preparation agents do not wet the patient's hair or bedding or pool in skin folds or the umbilicus because this increases the risk of fire.[1]

8. If needed, assist the physician, advanced practice nurse, or other healthcare provider performing the procedure with:
  A. Donning surgical head cover, mask, and eye protection.
  B. Donning sterile gown and sterile gloves.
	Prevents infection.	All personnel in the room must don head covers and masks.

9. Assist with opening the sternotomy tray on a clean, dry surface. Keep a count of any instruments/needles/ sponges placed on the sterile field.	Prepares equipment.	

*Level M: Manufacturer's recommendations only.

Procedure continues on following page

Procedure for Assisting With Emergent Open Sternotomy—*Continued*

Steps	Rationale	Special Considerations
10. As needed, assist with fully draping the patient with exposure of only the surgical site.[1,10] **(Level D*)**	A large sterile field minimizes the risk of infection and provides space to maintain asepsis of instruments and supplies during the procedure.	Allows good view of the incision.
11. As needed, assist with setting up the electrocautery system (e.g., adjusting the settings).	Cautery is used to stop bleeding from small vessels.	The connection must be handed off the sterile field to the nonsterile staff to connect to the machine.
12. As needed, assist with providing supplies and with removing sharp objects (e.g., cut wires) from the surgical field.	Assists with the procedure and ensures that removed wires are safely discarded.	
13. Assist with suctioning as needed.	Clears blood from the field.	
14. If pulseless ventricular tachycardia or ventricular fibrillation occurs, assist with obtaining a defibrillator and sterile internal paddles.	Provides emergent intervention.	
15. Open and place internal paddles on the sterile field. The individual performing the procedure will hand off the connection cable to be attached to the defibrillator.	Prepares the internal paddles for use.	
16. Set the defibrillator to the requested joules (usually 20 J for biphasic shocks[9,14] **(Level E*)**	Although 5 J can defibrillate the heart, use of 10 to 20 J optimizes more rapid defibrillation and fewer shocks.[12]	Refer to the defibrillator manufacturer's operation guidelines for specific recommendations, and follow institution guidelines.
17. Charge the defibrillator when requested to do so. If the defibrillator paddles do not have defibrillation buttons, discharge the defibrillator when requested to do so after ensuring that all personnel are clear of contact with the patient, bed, and equipment. **(Level M*)**	Defibrillation releases the electrical charge to depolarize cardiac muscle. Simultaneous depolarization of the myocardium may result in simultaneous repolarization of enough myocardium to reestablish a single cardiac impulse.	
18. Assess the patient's response to defibrillation (heart rate and rhythm, blood pressure, level of consciousness).	Determines whether additional interventions may be needed.	
19. If the first defibrillation is not successful, perform additional defibrillations as needed.	Continues emergency treatment.	
20. If internal cardiac compressions are needed, monitor the blood pressure response, aiming for a systolic blood pressure of >60 mm Hg via an arterial line.[13] **(Level D*)**	Ensures perfusion of major organs.	
21. If resuscitation is successful, obtain vital signs, and assess the patient.	Aids in determining whether additional interventions are needed.	Provide additional supportive therapies as needed. Vasoactive agents, antiarrhythmic agent, and other therapies may be needed.

*Level D: Peer-reviewed professional and organizational standards with the support of clinical study recommendations.
*Level E: Multiple case reports, theory-based evidence from expert opinions, or peer-reviewed professional organization standards without clinical studies to support recommendations.
*Level M: Manufacturer's recommendations only.

Procedure for Assisting With Emergent Open Sternotomy—*Continued*		
Steps	Rationale	Special Considerations
22. Prepare the chest tube drainage system and pacemaker to be connected after placement of chest tubes or epicardial pacing wires.	Epicardial pacing wires and chest tubes can be displaced during sternal retraction.	
23. Assist as needed with obtaining or preparing warm saline solution with or without an antibiotic for irrigation of the chest cavity.	May decrease the incidence of infection.	
24. Prepare equipment for placement of mechanical assist devices if needed.	Cardiac tamponade can conceal right or left ventricular dysfunction; mechanical assistance may be necessary to improve cardiac output.	
25. Assist with transporting the patient to the operating room if necessary.	The patient may need further exploration or surgical repair of coronary artery bypass grafts, cardiac valves, the myocardium, or placement of an assist device (e.g., intraaortic balloon pump, ventricular assist device).	Ensure that the patient's chest is covered with sterile drapes or with a dressing during transportation.
26. If the patient does not return to the operating room, assist the healthcare provider performing the procedure by providing supplies for reinsertion of the sternal wires.	Ensures sternal closure.	
27. Provide supplies for tissue and skin closure.	Ensures closure of the sternal incision.	
28. Assist with or apply an occlusive dressing to the sternal incision, epicardial pacing wires, and chest tube sites after the procedure is completed. Assist with counting instruments/needles/sponges to ensure that none are left behind in the chest.	Dressings provide a physical barrier to external sources of contamination; they absorb drainage and maintain a dry environment to enhance wound healing.	The patient's chest may be left open and covered with a sterile and occlusive surgical dressing if severe ventricular dysfunction occurs. A chest radiograph may be ordered to rule out the presence of any retained surgical sponges, needles, or instruments.
29. Discard used supplies, and remove and discard **PE**	Reduces the transmission of microorganisms and body fluids; standard precautions.	
30. Assist, if needed, with gathering used instruments for sterilization.	Prepares equipment for future use.	Ensure that the open chest tray and internal paddles are restocked to prepare for another emergency.
31. **HH**		

Expected Outcomes

- Resolution of the condition that necessitated the emergent open sternotomy
- Increased cardiac output/hemodynamic stability
- Increased tissue perfusion, including cerebral, renal, and peripheral perfusion
- Minimal chest tube drainage
- Decreased need for blood transfusions

Unexpected Outcomes

- Severe right or left ventricular dysfunction
- Continued dysrhythmias, bleeding, or coagulation disorders
- Myocardial, aortic, coronary artery, or coronary artery bypass graft perforation
- Pneumothorax
- Pain
- Surgical site infection
- Death

Procedure continues on following page

Patient Monitoring and Care

Steps	Rationale	Reportable Conditions
		These conditions should be reported to the provider if they persist despite nursing interventions.
1. Perform cardiovascular, hemodynamic, capnographic, and peripheral vascular assessments every 15–30 minutes as patient status requires (including vital signs, pulmonary artery pressure, cardiac index, level of consciousness, and urine output).	Determines hemodynamic stability and volume status; recurrent tamponade or dysrhythmias may develop during and after sternotomy. Determines the adequacy of cerebral perfusion; hemodynamic instability can lead to cerebral anoxia. Determines perfusion to the kidneys.	• Mean arterial blood pressure <60 mm Hg • Abnormal changes in heart rate and rhythm • Decrease in cardiac index • Abnormal pulmonary artery pressure • Urine output <0.5 mL/kg/hour • Equalizing pulmonary artery pressure • Change in level of consciousness • Impaired level of consciousness
2. If the patient's neurological condition is compromised after a chest procedure with cardiac arrest (e.g., comatose), consider therapeutic hypothermia at 32°–36°C for at least 24 hours[14] **(Level D*)**	The benefit of therapeutic hypothermia in cardiac arrest after cardiac surgery is unknown with only case reports.[11] However, there is a strength of evidence in other populations; therefore it should be considered. Hypothermia can impair coagulation, which is a concern if a patient is bleeding.	
3. Assess heart and lung sounds every 2 hours and as needed.	Abnormal heart and lung sounds may indicate the need for additional treatment.	• Distant heart sounds • Abnormal lung sounds
4. Monitor coagulation, hematologic, and electrolyte laboratory blood study results as prescribed.	Coagulation and hematological profiles provide data that indicate the risk of bleeding and indicate the need for additional treatment. Electrolyte studies provide data regarding the risk for dysrhythmias and decreased contractility.	• Abnormal hemoglobin and hematocrit, activated partial thromboplastin time, international normalized ratio, platelets, fibrinogen, calcium, magnesium, or potassium levels
5. Obtain and interpret a 12-lead electrocardiogram (ECG).	Assesses for myocardial ischemia/infarction	• ECG abnormalities
6. Monitor chest tube drainage.	Determines functioning of the chest tube drainage system and the amount of chest drainage.	• Cessation of chest tube drainage • Increased chest tube drainage • Clots in chest tube drainage system
7. Follow institutional standards for assessing pain. Administer analgesia as prescribed.	Identifies the need for pain interventions.	• Continued pain despite pain interventions

*Level D: Peer-reviewed professional and organizational standards with the support of clinical study recommendations.

UNIT II

Documentation

Documentation should include the following:
- Patient and family education
- Signed informed consent, if nonemergent
- Universal protocol requirement, if nonemergent
- Pain assessment, interventions, and effectiveness
- Indications for the procedure and the procedure performed
- Amount of blood collected from chest suctioning; estimated blood loss
- Patient therapies and response, including hemodynamic values, antiarrhythmic agents, inotropic or vasopressor agents, ventilation, and neurological status
- Additional interventions
- Unexpected outcomes

References and Additional Readings

For a complete list of references and additional readings for this procedure, scan this QR code with your smartphone, or visit https://www.elsevier.com/__data/assets/pdf_file/0005/1319810/Chapter0035.pdf

PROCEDURE

36 External Wearable Cardioverter-Defibrillator

Kiersten Henry

PURPOSE: The external wearable cardioverter-defibrillator (WCD) is a temporary device that is used to prevent sudden cardiac death from malignant ventricular arrhythmias. The WCD continuously monitors a patient's heart rate and rhythm and attempts to convert ventricular tachycardia (VT) or ventricular fibrillation (VF) via defibrillation.

PREREQUISITE NURSING KNOWLEDGE

- Knowledge of the anatomy and physiology of the cardiovascular system, principles of cardiac conduction, and basic arrhythmia interpretation.
- Knowledge of basic functioning of the WCD and patient response to WCD therapy.
- Knowledge of the principles of defibrillation threshold, antiarrhythmia medications, alteration in electrolytes, and effect on the defibrillation threshold.
- Basic life support (BLS) and advanced cardiac life support (ACLS) knowledge and skills.
- The WCD may be utilized as bridge therapy to the implantable cardioverter-defibrillator (ICD).
- The WCD is different from an automated external defibrillator (AED) because it requires no bystander assistance.
- The WCD currently commercially available in the United States is the Zoll LifeVest. The Zoll LifeVest is a wearable cardioverter defibrillator (WCD), which is currently available in the United States and several countries worldwide. The LifeVest is worn by the patient underneath his or her clothes. The purpose of the vest is to sense life-threatening ventricular arrhythmias and defibrillate as appropriate.[6]
- The vest contains four nonadhesive electrodes that continuously monitor the cardiac rhythm. Three defibrillator pads release gel just before defibrillation to protect the skin from burns and decrease electrical impedence.[6]
- The WCD monitor and batteries are worn in a holster around the waist or in a bag over their shoulder (Fig. 36.1).
- Patients are advised to change the rechargeable battery daily. Batteries need approximately 1 to 2 hours to recharge on the charging unit.
- If the WCD senses VF or VT, it can deliver a series of up to five defibrillations. The energy delivered is selected by the provider when the device is ordered. The LifeVest can deliver up to 150 J per defibrillation. The heart rate threshold for defibrillation is also determined by the ordering provider.[4,6]
- When a shockable ventricular rhythm is detected, the vest begins a series of audible warnings and physical vibrations to alert the patient and bystanders. The warnings continue for at least 25 seconds, allowing the patient to deactivate the device if the detected arrhythmia is

actually interference due to electronic devices or motion artifact. The patient can deactivate the WCD by pushing a button located on the battery pack. If defibrillation is indicated, the device will audibly warn bystanders to stand clear.[4,6,8]
- Audible alerts with the ZOLL LifeVest include the following[8]:
  - Gong followed by no verbal message (signaling the patient to check for instruction on the device screen) or followed by "Treatment has been given, call your doctor." This indicates that therapy has been given and the patient is being monitored.
  - Two-tone alarm followed by "If patient is not responsive, call for help. Perform CPR." These means the ZOLL LifeVest is not sensing a shockable rhythm, has delivered the maximum number of therapies, or cannot detect the electrocardiogram (ECG).
  - Two-tone alarm accompanied by "Press response buttons to delay treatment" or "Bystanders do not interfere." A shock will be delivered within 25 to 60 seconds unless the patient deactivates the device. Bystanders should stand clear until defibrillation is completed as they can be shocked if the patient is touched during defibrillation. The siren alert will stop when it is safe to contact the patient to evaluate for return of circulation.
  - The presence of blue gel on the patient's chest indicates that a defibrillation has likely been delivered.
- The WCD monitors patient rhythm and stores data about vest utilization. This information is transmitted electronically to the manufacturing company, which provides clinical information to the prescribing provider.
- Indications for the WCD include any situation in which a patient is at risk for sudden cardiac death but is not eligible for an ICD. Delays in ICD eligibility are related to the fact that a patient may regain left ventricular function with optimal medical therapy, reducing the risk of sudden cardiac death.[1,3-5,7]
  - Patients who may require ICD implantation but are within the guideline-directed waiting period include[1,3-5]:
    - Patients within 40 days of a myocardial infarction who did not undergo coronary intervention
    - Patients within 90 days of a myocardial infarction who underwent percutaneous coronary intervention or coronary artery bypass grafting

323

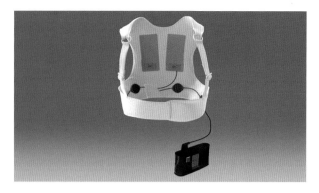

Figure 36.1   LifeVest wearable cardioverter-defibrillator. *(Courtesy ZOLL Medical, Pittsburgh, PA.)*

○ Patients with cardiomyopathy who have not been on maximum tolerated guideline-directed medical therapy for at least 90 days
○ Patients awaiting cardiac transplantation
○ Patients with ICD indications when the patient's condition prohibits ICD implantation

- A meta-analysis of WCD trials found a 95.5% rate of successful conversion from VT/VF in patients who received appropriate shock therapy from their WCD. Inappropriate shocks (for artifact or rhythms other than VT/VF) occurred in <1% of patients. This is a rate lower than that seen with implanted cardioverter-defibrillators, likely because of the ability of WCD patients to abort defibrillation if they are awake when the alert cycle begins.[3]
- Studies of WCD patients show higher survival rates after discharge from coronary artery bypass grafting or percutaneous coronary intervention than patients discharged without a WCD. Patient discontinuation rates average 14%, with WCD patients wearing their device an average of 19 to 23 hours per day.[3,4]
- If a patient meets eligibility criteria for an ICD, the ICD is preferable to the WCD.[1]
- For patients presenting to the hospital wearing a WCD, refer to facility-specific protocols regarding management of the device, including communication to all team members regarding safety precautions with WCD use. Some facilities require that the device be removed during hospitalization, whereas others encourage patients to wear it at all times. If hospital policy requires removal of the WCD, the patient should be on telemetry monitoring at all times.

EQUIPMENT

- LifeVest garment
- Sensing electrodes
- Defibrillator pads
- Battery pack with waist holster
- Extra battery pack
- Charging/transmission station
- Cardiac monitor
- Nonsterile gloves
  Additional equipment, to have available as needed, includes the following:
- Emergency medications
- Cardiac board
- Resuscitation equipment

PATIENT AND FAMILY EDUCATION

- Assess learning needs, readiness to learn, and factors that influence or impede learning. ***Rationale:*** This assessment allows the nurse to individualize teaching in a meaningful manner.
- Assess patient and family understanding of WCD therapy and the reason for its use. ***Rationale:*** This assessment provides information regarding knowledge level and the necessity of additional teaching.
- Provide information about the normal conduction system, such as the structure of the conduction system, the source of the heartbeat, the normal and abnormal heart rhythms, the symptoms of abnormal heart rhythms, and the potentially life-threatening nature of VT and VF. ***Rationale:*** Understanding the conduction system and dangerous arrhythmias assists the patient and family in recognizing the seriousness of the patient's condition and the need for WCD therapy.
- Provide information about WCD therapy, including the indication for the WCD, device operation, location of the device, types of therapy given by the device, risks and benefits of the device, and follow-up. This will occur in conjunction with the provider who ordered the device and the WCD company representative, who provides fitting of the device and patient education. ***Rationale:*** Understanding WCD functioning assists the patient and family in developing realistic perceptions of WCD therapy.
- Reinforce with the patient and family the importance of wearing the vest at all times (including during sleep), except when showering or bathing. Another responsible adult should be present during showering or bathing to obtain help in the event of a life-threatening arrhythmia. The device is not waterproof but should be worn at all other times. ***Rationale:*** Understanding the importance of compliance with wearing the vest will help decrease the risk of sudden cardiac death.
- Reinforce with the patient and family that only the patient should press the button to cancel defibrillation if the device begins alert. If the patient is not coherent to abort the defibrillation, it is likely indicated. If defibrillation occurs, family members should be educated to stand clear of the patient and immediately call 911. ***Rationale:*** Understanding that the device is likely functioning appropriately if defibrillating an unconscious patient will help limit the likelihood of inappropriate deactivation by bystanders or the risk of bystander injury caused by electrical shock.

PATIENT ASSESSMENT AND PREPARATION

Patient Assessment

- In conjunction with the physician, advanced practice nurse, and other healthcare professionals, assess the patient for orientation and mental capacity to manage the WCD. ***Rationale:*** Patients who cannot exercise compliance with the WCD or deactivate the device before inappropriate defibrillation are not candidates for WCD therapy.[6]

- Monitor and document the cardiac rhythm per unit protocol during hospitalization. *Rationale:* This will allow real-time assessment of any arrhythmias that occur in the WCD patient and early diagnosis of lethal arrhythmias during hospitalization.

Patient Preparation

- Verify the correct patient with two identifiers. *Rationale:* Before performing a procedure, the nurse should ensure the correct identification of the patient for the intended intervention.

- Ensure that the patient and family understand preprocedural teaching. Answer questions as they arise, and reinforce information as needed. *Rationale:* Understanding of previously taught information is evaluated and reinforced.
- Consent for monitoring and using the device is obtained from the patient by the WCD product representative. *Rationale:* Placement of the WCD is not an invasive procedure. The patient is consenting to the company monitoring vest utilization and therapy.

Procedure	for External Wearable Cardioverter-Defibrillator		
Steps	**Rationale**	**Special Considerations**	
1. **HH**			
2. **PE**			
3. Assist the WCD product representative as needed in determining the appropriate vest size for the patient.[2]	There are different vest sizes. Utilization of the appropriate-size vest will increase compliance as well as increase cardiac monitoring accuracy.		
4. Assist with placing the WCD on the patient if needed.	Provides assistance and begins therapy.		
5. The patient should wear the device as prescribed.	This provides an opportunity for the patient to get comfortable with the fit of the device and how it operates.	The patient should demonstrate an understanding of WCD placement, the rationale for wearing the device, and appropriate utilization of the device.	
6. Continue cardiac monitoring even though the patient is wearing the WCD.	Monitors for changes in heart rate and rhythm.	The WCD does not protect against arrest from bradyarrhythmias/ pulseless electrical activity/ asystole.	
7. If the device indicates that defibrillation is indicated:[8]			
A. Assess and stay with the patient. Do not touch the patient.	A bystander can be shocked during defibrillation with the WCD.		
B. Wait for the device to function. Do not touch the patient until the audible alert stops or the device advises bystanders "If patient is unresponsive, call for help. Perform CPR." (**Level M***)	The audible alerts will indicate which phase of the process the WCD is in (monitoring or preparing to defibrillate).	Observe the heart rate and rhythm on the cardiac monitor.	
C. If the device successfully converts a life-threatening arrhythmia:	Determines the patient's response to the therapy.		
i. Assess the patient's level of consciousness.			
ii. Assess the patient's vital signs and heart rhythm.			
D. If the device is not successful in converting a life-threatening arrhythmia:		CPR can be interpreted by the device as ventricular arrhythmia.	

*Level M: Manufacturer's recommendations only.

Procedure continues on following page

UNIT II

Procedure for External Wearable Cardioverter-Defibrillator—*Continued*

Steps	Rationale	Special Considerations
i. Remove the WCD battery and/or vest after defibrillation attempts are complete.	Disconnecting the battery will deactivate the defibrillator. If anterior/posterior placement of defibrillator pads is required, the vest should be removed.	The battery should be removed or disconnected before initiation of CPR to avoid inappropriate defibrillation. When removing the WCD, if cutting the cloth vest off is required, make every attempt to avoid cutting through the ECG leads. This allows the device to be utilized by the patient at a later time.
ii. Initiate BLS and ACLS.	Provides emergency interventions.	Patients may progress to pulseless electrical activity/asystole, which the device will not treat.
8. After successful or unsuccessful treatment, contact the WCD product representative to download the device information.	The device download can be helpful in determining rhythm type (if not captured on a hospital-based monitor).	The device will store pre- and posttherapy ECG strips. This information can also be obtained from the cardiac monitoring system.
9. Discard used supplies and personal protective equipment in appropriate receptacles.	Reduces the transmission of microorganisms and body secretions; standard precautions.	
10. 🅷🅷		
11. Obtain an additional WCD vest and defibrillator pads from the company representative.	Provides equipment needed for ongoing therapy.	

Expected Outcomes

- WCD detects life-threatening VT or VF.
- WCD delivers appropriate defibrillation.
- Patient deactivates the WCD if audible/physical warnings begin and the patient is conscious.
- Emergency treatment is provided if the patient receives defibrillation from the WCD.

Unexpected Outcomes

- WCD delivers inappropriate defibrillation.
- WCD fails to detect VF/VT.
- Patient is noncompliant with wearing of the WCD.
- Staff/bystander injury occurs.

Patient Monitoring and Care

Steps	Rationale	Reportable Conditions
		These conditions should be reported to the provider if they persist despite nursing interventions.
1. Continuous cardiac monitoring.	Detects arrhythmias.	• Abnormal heart rate • Arrhythmias
2. Assess the patient's response to WCD defibrillation, including anxiety, cardiac rate and rhythm, level of consciousness, and vital signs.	Determines patient status after defibrillation.	• Anxiety • Abnormal heart rate • Arrhythmias • Hypotension • WCD therapy • Defibrillation • WCD malfunction • Hemodynamic instability • Neurological changes
3. Follow institutional standards for assessing pain. Administer analgesia as prescribed.	Identifies the need for pain interventions.	• Continued pain despite pain interventions

Documentation

Documentation should include the following:
- WCD settings
- Patient and family education
- Patient's return demonstration of device placement and utilization
- All rhythm-strip recordings
- Pain
- Patient response to WCD therapy
- Anxiety assessment, interventions, and effectiveness
- Occurrence of any unexpected outcomes
- Additional interventions

UNIT II

References and Additional Readings

For a complete list of references and additional readings for this procedure, scan this QR code with your smartphone, or visit https://www.elsevier.com/__data/assets/pdf_file/0006/1319811/Chapter0036.pdf

PROCEDURE

37 Pericardiocentesis (Perform) 🅰🅿

Brandi L. Holcomb

PURPOSE: Pericardiocentesis is the removal of excess fluid from the pericardial sac for identification of the etiology of pericardial effusion by fluid analysis (diagnostic pericardiocentesis) and/or prevention or treatment of cardiac tamponade (therapeutic pericardiocentesis).

PREREQUISITE NURSING KNOWLEDGE

- Advanced cardiac life support (ACLS) knowledge and skills.
- Knowledge and skills related to sterile technique
- Clinical and technical competence in the performance of pericardiocentesis
- Knowledge of cardiovascular anatomy and physiology
- The pericardial space normally contains 20 to 50 mL of fluid.
- Pericardial fluid has electrolyte and protein profiles similar to plasma.
- Pericardial effusion is generally defined as the accumulation of fluid within the pericardial sac that exceeds the stretch capacity of the pericardium, generally more than 50 to 100 mL.[8]
- The space within the pericardial sac is finite; however, initially large increases in intrapericardial volume result in relatively small changes in intrapericardial pressure. If fluid continues to accumulate and increases intrapericardial pressures above the filling pressures of the right heart, right-ventricular diastolic filling is compromised, resulting in cardiac tamponade.[6]
- Intrapericardial fluid accumulation can be acute or chronic and therefore varies in presentation of symptoms. Acute effusions are usually a rapid collection of fluid occurring over minutes to hours and may result in hemodynamic compromise with volumes of less than 250 mL.[7] Chronically developing effusions occurring over days to weeks allow for hypertrophy and distention of the fibrous pericardial membrane. Patients with chronic effusions may accumulate greater than or equal to 2000 mL of fluid before exhibiting symptoms of hemodynamic compromise. Pericardiocentesis is recommended for cardiac tamponade to relieve symptoms and establish a diagnosis of malignant or bacterial pericardial effusion utilizing cytology.[1]
- Symptoms of cardiac tamponade are nonspecific, so the diagnosis relies on clinical suspicion and associated signs and symptoms. Acute pericardial effusions are usually a result of trauma, myocardial infarction, cardiac surgery, or iatrogenic injury, whereas chronic effusions can result from conditions such as bacterial or viral pericarditis, cancer, autoimmune disorders, uremia, and so on.[3] With a decrease in cardiac output, the patient may present with the classic symptoms of cardiac tamponade including Beck's triad: hypotension, distant heart sounds, and jugular venous distension. Other common signs and symptoms include dyspnea, tachycardia, chest pain, pulsus paradoxus, pallor, diaphoresis, hypotension, impaired cerebral and renal function, and decreased ECG voltage.[5]
- The amount of fluid in the pericardium is best evaluated through a two-dimensional echocardiogram, electrocardiography (ECG), and clinical findings. Chest x-rays may not be diagnostically significant in patients with acute traumatic tamponade.[7] Chest radiographs are nonspecific and may suggest a pericardial effusion with identification of an enlarged cardiac silhouette.[6] Electrographic markers of pericardial effusion include widespread ST segment elevation, PR depression (elevation may be seen in lead aVR), and low voltage.
- Pericardiocentesis is performed therapeutically to relieve tamponade or to diagnose the etiology of the effusion. An acute tamponade resulting in hemodynamic instability necessitates an emergency procedure. Blind pericardiocentesis should be performed only in extreme emergency situations.[8]
- Pericardiocentesis is recommended for cardiac tamponade to relieve symptoms and establish etiology of a pericardial effusion if there is suspicion of either bacterial or neoplastic etiology.[1]
- Pericardiocentesis is usually performed via a subxiphoid approach.
- Two-dimensional echocardiography or ultrasound to assist in guiding the needle during pericardiocentesis is strongly recommended.[3,7,8]

- This procedure may also be performed with fluoroscopy in a cardiac catheterization or interventional radiology suite.
- Urgent or emergent chest exploration is necessary in the face of cardiac injury, rapid reaccumulation of pericardial fluid, or ineffective drainage of the pericardium.
- There are no absolute contraindications to pericardiocentesis in the setting of life-threatening hemodynamic instability. Relative contraindications include uncorrected coagulopathy in the hemodynamically stable patient.[7] Prior thoracic surgery, pacemaker placement, artificial heart valves, or other cardiac devices may limit the ultrasound field of vision as a result of surgical adhesions. If ultrasound identification of effusion is compromised, then direct visualization utilizing a surgical approach is recomended.[7]
- Cardiac output is generally improved after pericardiocentesis.

EQUIPMENT

- Pericardiocentesis tray (or thoracentesis tray)
- 16-gauge or 18-gauge, 3-inch cardiac needle or catheter over the needle
- Antiseptic skin preparation solution (e.g., 2% chlorhexidine-based preparation)
- Two packs of 4 × 4 gauze sponges
- No. 11 knife blade with handle (scalpel)
- Sterile 50-mL to 60-mL, 10-mL, 5-mL, and 3-mL syringes
- Sterile drapes and towels
- Masks, goggles or face shields, surgical head covers, sterile gowns, and gloves
- Two three-way stopcocks
- 1% lidocaine (injectable)
- 10-mL syringe with 25-gauge needle
- Culture bottles and specimen tubes for fluid analysis
- 2-inch and 3-inch tape
  Additional equipment to have available as needed includes the following:
- Emergency cart (defibrillator, emergency respiratory equipment, emergency cardiac medications, and temporary pacemaker)
- Two-dimensional echocardiography equipment
- 12-lead ECG machine
- Sterile marker
- Echocardiogram contrast medium
- Suture supplies
- Scissors
- If continuous drainage is necessary:
  - ❖ J guidewire, 0.035 diameter
  - ❖ Vessel dilator, 7F
  - ❖ Pigtail catheter, 7F
  - ❖ Tubing and drainage bag or bottle
  - ❖ Three-way stopcock and nonvented caps

PATIENT AND FAMILY EDUCATION

- Explain to the patient and family the reason necessitating the pericardiocentesis (e.g., relief of pressure on the heart); describe the procedure in detail including risks, benefits, alternatives, expected outcomes, and potential complications. *Rationale:* Communication of pertinent information helps the patient and family understand the procedure

and the potential risks and benefits, subsequently reducing anxiety and apprehension.[2]
- Teach the patient and family about the signs and symptoms of pericardial effusion (e.g., dyspnea, dull ache or pressure within the chest, dysphagia, cough, tachypnea, hoarseness, hiccups, or nausea).[5,6] *Rationale:* Early recognition of signs and symptoms of recurrent pericardial effusion may prompt detection of a potentially life-threatening problem.

PATIENT ASSESSMENT AND PREPARATION

Patient Assessment

- Elicit the patient's history of the present illness and mechanism of injury (if applicable), past medical history, and current medications and/or medical therapies from the patient or reliable source. *Rationale:* A thorough history is necessary to determine the patient's baseline health status and to identify potential risk factors. The nurse-patient interaction provides an opportunity for the nurse to establish a therapeutic relationship focused on the patient.[3]
- Assess the patient's neurological status, heart rate, cardiac rhythm, heart sounds (S_1, S_2, rubs, murmurs), pulmonary artery pressures if PA catheter is in situ, central venous pressure (noninvasive or invasive), blood pressure, mean arterial pressure (MAP), oxygen saturation via pulse oximetry (SpO_2), and respiratory status. *Rationale:* This provides baseline data.
- Evaluate current laboratory values to include a complete blood cell count, electrolytes, and coagulation profile. *Rationale:* Review of these data is essential to identify the potential risk of cardiac dysrhythmias or abnormal bleeding. If the international normalized ratio, partial thromboplastin time, or both are elevated, reversing the level of anticoagulation therapy should be considered before performing the procedure. It may be prudent to defer the procedure until the blood levels indicate a reduction in bleeding risk.[7]

Patient Preparation

- Confirm that the patient and family understand preprocedural teaching by having them verbalize understanding. Clarify key points by reinforcing important information and answer all questions. *Rationale:* Preprocedural communication provides a framework of patient expectations, enhances cooperation, and reduces anxiety.[2]
- Verify the correct patient with two identifiers. *Rationale:* The provider should always ensure the correct identification of the patient for the intended intervention for patient safety.
- Obtain informed consent by providing specific and relevant information about the procedure. Implied consent may be assumed if emergent life-saving intervention is necessary. *Rationale:* Informed consent is based on the autonomous right of the patient and facilitates a competent decision for the patient and the family.[2]
- Perform a preprocedural verification and time out, if nonemergent. *Rationale:* Ensures patient safety.

- Coordinate the procedure with the echocardiogram technician or ultrasonographer to assist with the two-dimensional echocardiogram or ultrasound examination if this approach is being used. **Rationale:** Echocardiogram- or ultrasound-directed pericardiocentesis allows for more precise localization of the effusion and is associated with higher success rates and lower complication rates.[6,7,8]

- If nonemergent, prescribe and ensure that an analgesic and/or sedative is administered. **Rationale:** Analgesia and sedation reduce anxiety and promote comfort and cooperation.
- Apply the limb leads, and connect the leads to the cardiac bedside monitoring system or to the 12-lead ECG machine. **Rationale:** The ECG is monitored during and after the procedure for changes that may indicate cardiac injury.

Procedure	for Performing Pericardiocentesis AP		
Steps	**Rationale**		**Special Considerations**
1. HH			
2. PE			Consider putting a mask on the patient during the actual procedure if the patient is not intubated (in a contained system), especially if the patient has methicillin-resistant *Staphylococcus aureus* (MRSA)–positive results or if MRSA status is unknown at the time of the procedure.
3. Prepare the pericardiocentesis tray and supplies with aseptic technique.	Reduces the potential for infection.		
4. Position the patient in the supine position with the head of the bed elevated 30–45 degrees as the patient's condition allows.	Facilitates patient comfort, decreases work of breathing, and permits fluid to pool on the inferior surface of the heart, aiding fluid aspiration.		
5. Cleanse the skin with antiseptic solution (e.g., 2% chlorhexidine-based preparation), and perform HH. HH	Minimizes the potential for infection.		Clipping the hair may be necessary before applying antiseptic solution.
6. If two-dimensional echocardiogram or ultrasound is being used, skip to **Step 14.**			
7. Using maximal barrier precautions, fully drape the patient with exposure of only the surgical site, and apply a mask, goggles or face shield, surgical cap, sterile gown, and sterile gloves.[3]	Minimizes the risk of infection; maintains aseptic and sterile precautions.		
8. Attach a three-way stopcock to a 3-inch cardiac needle, and attach it to a 50-mL or 60-mL syringe.	Provides the mechanism to aspirate fluid.		
9. If time and patient condition permit, inject the access site with 2–3 mL 1% lidocaine using a 10-mL syringe and a 25-gauge needle, raising a wheal. If unable to perform this step, attach a syringe with 1% lidocaine to one side of the stopcock to inject analgesia during the access procedure.	Reduces patient discomfort.		Local infiltration of analgesia reduces patient discomfort. Alternatively, as the needle is introduced, the physician, advanced practice nurse, or other healthcare professional may insert a small amount of 1% lidocaine to add analgesic effect.
10. Continuously monitor the bedside ECG, vital signs, SpO₂, and pulmonary artery pressures and central venous pressure, if a pulmonary artery and/or central venous catheter is present, during needle aspiration and fluid withdrawal.[3,5,6]	Determines patient response during the procedure.		A 12-lead ECG machine can also be used for cardiac monitoring.

Procedure for Performing Pericardiocentesis AP—*Continued*

Steps	Rationale	Special Considerations
11. Subxiphoid approach to pericardiocentesis (Fig. 37.1): A. A 16- or 18-gauge needle is slowly inserted into the left xiphocostal angle perpendicular to the skin 3–4 mm below the left costal margin. Slowly advance the needle under the xiphoid toward the left shoulder while maintaining negative pressure on the syringe (aspirating). B. After the needle is advanced to the inner aspect of the rib cage, the needle's hub is depressed while the needle points toward the patient's left shoulder. The needle is slowly advanced 5–10 mm until fluid is aspirated. You may feel a distinct "give" when the needle penetrates the pericardium. Successful removal of fluid confirms needle position.	Minimizes the risk of cardiac injury; angles >45 degrees may lacerate the liver or stomach.	The movement of the heart usually defibrinates blood in the pericardial space so it cannot clot.[9] Clotting usually indicates penetration of the heart chamber and blood obtained from within a ventricle or atrium.[6] If clotting occurs with the fluid obtained, withdraw the needle. If no fluid is aspirated, withdraw the needle completely, and redirect it working from the patient's left to right.
12. When the needle position is confirmed, obtain the fluid samples, and remove the needle. No more than 50–150 mL of pericardial fluid should be removed at one time.[6,7] **(Level E*)** Sterile specimens should be collected and sent to the laboratory for analysis.[1] If continuous drainage is needed, go to **Step 19.**	Removes the pericardial fluid for analysis.	Samples of pericardial fluid should be sent for appropriate biochemical, cytological, bacteriological, and immunological analysis to assist in the diagnosis and cause of the effusion. The first sample is usually reserved for microbiological studies.[1] These samples should be collected by the performing provider.
13. Label the specimen, and send the specimen to the laboratory.	Prepares the sample for analysis.	Label it with the patient's name and date of birth. Time and date the sample.

When Two-Dimensional Echocardiogram or Ultrasound Is Used

14. Perform a two-dimensional echocardiogram or ultrasound to determine the location and size of the effusion.	Two-dimensional echocardiogram or ultrasound can help identify the location and size of the pericardial effusion.	
15. Determine the ideal entry site and needle trajectory for the pericardiocentesis.	The ideal entry site is the point where the effusion is closest to the transducer and fluid accumulation is maximal.[5,7,8]	A straight trajectory that best avoids vital structures, including the liver, myocardium, and lung, should be chosen. The internal mammary artery also should be avoided.[7-8,9]
16. Mark the skin with a sterile marker.	May aid with the procedure.	
17. Return to **Step 7**, and follow the procedural steps.		

*Level E: Multiple case reports, theory-based evidence from expert opinions, or peer-reviewed professional organizational standards without clinical studies to support recommendations.

Procedure continues on following page

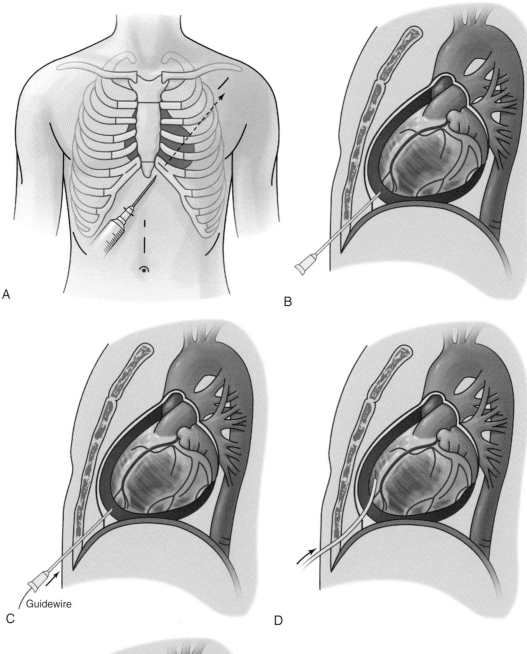

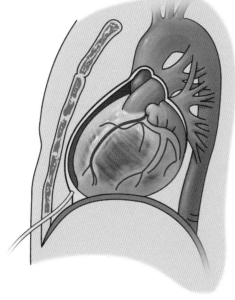

Figure 37.1   The subxiphoid approach to catheter placement into the pericordial space. **A,** A short needle (16 gauge or 18 gauge) is inserted into the left xiphocostal angle perpendicular to the skin and 3 to 4 mm below the left costal margin. **B,** After the needle is advanced to the inner aspect of the rib cage, the needle's hub is depressed so the needle points toward the patient's left shoulder. The needle is then cautiously advanced about 5 to 10 mm until fluid is reached. The fingers may sense a distinct "give" when the needle penetrates the parietal pericardium. Successful removal of fluid confirms the needle's position. **C,** The syringe is then disconnected from the needle, and the flexible tip of the guidewire is advanced into the pericardial space. The needle is withdrawn and replaced with a soft multihole pigtail catheter (6F to 8F) with use of the Seldinger technique. **D,** After dilation of the needle tract, the catheter is advanced over the guidewire into the pericardial space. **E,** Once the catheter is properly positioned, aspiration of fluid should result in rapid improvement in blood pressure and cardiac output, a decrease in atrial and pericardial pressures, and a decrease in the degree of any paradoxical pulse. Electrical alternans, if present, also decreases or disappears. *(From Spodick DH: The technique of pericardiocentesis.* J Crit Ill *2:91, 1987.)*

Procedure	**for Performing Pericardiocentesis AP—*Continued***	
Steps	Rationale	Special Considerations
18. If bloody fluid is aspirated, a few milliliters of echo contrast medium can be infused to confirm position.[7,8] A. Echocardiogenic saline can be prepared by using two 5-mL syringes attached to a three-way stopcock (one filled with sterile normal saline and one with air). B. Agitate the saline between the two syringes, and inject into the sheath. The agitated saline should appear as an echogenic stream.[9] C. When the fluid is determined to be pericardial, return to **Step 12.**	If the contrast material appears in the pericardial space, the procedure can be continued. If the contrast material disappears, the needle may be in one of the heart chambers and must be withdrawn and repositioned.	Two-dimensional echocardiogram or ultrasound assists in determining the position of the needle. Echo contrast is agitated saline solution that is injected via the side port of the stopcock.[7]
When Continuous Drainage Is Desired		
19. When the needle tip position is confirmed to be within the pericardial space, insert the flexible tip of the guidewire through the needle into the pericardial space, and then remove the needle, leaving the guidewire in place. The guidewire is passed so it wraps around the heart within the pericardial space.[7,8]	A soft guidewire minimizes the risk of cardiac injury and allows for the passage of the guidewire and placement within the pericardial space.	
20. A multiholed pigtail or 8 raight soft catheter is passed over the guidewire using the Seldinger technique[6] (see Fig. 37.1).	A flexible-tipped soft catheter with multiple holes in the tip is used to facilitate drainage of the effusion. Use of a soft-tipped catheter reduces the chances of causing myocardial injury and dysrhythmias during the procedure.[2]	Either a pigtail catheter or a straight catheter with multiple holes can be used for better drainage.
21. Remove the guidewire, and connect the end of the catheter to the three-way stopcock and the drainage collection bag.[6,7,8]	Maintains asepsis; allows for continual drainage of the effusion.	If the effusion is small, remove the catheter when the fluid is drained.
22. If an indwelling catheter is placed to continuously drain a large pericardial effusion, attach the catheter to the sterile bag or bottle using aseptic technique	Facilitates fluid drainage; minimizes the potential for infection.	
23. If an indwelling catheter is to remain in place, secure the catheter by suturing the cathcter securely to the patient's chest wall.	Prevents dislodging or accidental removal.	
24. Cleanse the area around the catheter with an antiseptic solution, and apply an occlusive sterile dressing.[4]	May reduce the risk of infection.	
25. Continue bedside ECG monitoring, and discontinue the 12-lead ECG if used.	Allows monitoring of cardiac rate and rhythm.	
26. Dispose of sharps **PE** and used supplies in appropriate receptacles.	Reduces the transmission of microorganisms; standard precautions.	
27. **HH**		
28. If an indwelling catheter is placed, consider prescribing antibiotics.	May reduce the risk of infection.	

Expected Outcomes

- Fluid removed from the pericardial sac
- Relief of pain, dyspnea, or other symptoms that indicated the need for the procedure
- Improved cardiac output
- Patient's blood pressure, venous pressure, heart sounds, pulse pressure, and cardiac rhythm within normal limits

Unexpected Outcomes

- Injury to the myocardium, coronary arteries, lungs, large blood vessels or abdominal viscera
- Hemodynamic instability resulting in any of the following:
  - Hypotension or low cardiac output
  - Increase in pulmonary artery pressure or venous pressure
  - Sustained cardiac dysrhythmias
  - Excessive bleeding
- ECG changes:
  - ST-segment depression
  - PR-segment elevation
- Cardiac tamponade
- Pain
- Dyspnea

Patient Monitoring and Care

Steps	Rationale	Reportable Conditions
		These conditions should be reported to the provider if they persist despite nursing interventions.
1. Continuously monitor the ECG; assess the pulmonary artery pressure (PA) if a PA catheter is in situ, venous pressure, blood pressure, SpO$_2$, and neurological status during and frequently after the procedure until stable (if available, continuously monitor cardiac index and systemic vascular resistance).	Assess for early recognition of possible postprocedure complications including tamponade, cardiac injury, or hemodynamic instability.	• Increasing venous pressure • Decreasing arterial pressure • Change in level of consciousness • Pulsus paradoxus • Equalizing PA pressures • Decreased cardiac index • Abnormal systemic vascular resistance
2. Treat dysrhythmias if they occur.	Dysrhythmias may lead to cardiac decompensation.	• Persistent dysrhythmias despite appropriate intervention
3. Auscultate heart and lung sounds immediately before and after the procedure.	Muffled or distant heart sounds may indicate fluid reaccumulation. Decreased or absent breath sounds may indicate pneumothorax or hemothorax.	• Asymmetrical breath sounds • Dyspnea • Tachypnea • Decreased SpO$_2$ • Distant or faint heart sounds
4. Obtain a portable chest radiograph immediately after the procedure.	Assesses for pneumothorax and hemothorax.	• Pneumothorax • Hemothorax
5. Obtain a two-dimensional echocardiogram within several hours after the procedure.	Determines the effectiveness of the pericardial drainage.	• Pericardial effusion
6. Monitor the pericardiocentesis site for bleeding frequently after the procedure is completed until the patient's condition is stable and then every 4 hours for 24 hours. If an indwelling catheter is present, continue to monitor the site every 4 hours until the catheter is removed.	Assesses for postprocedural hemostasis and possible drainage.	• Bleeding or hematoma at the insertion site. • Drainage at the insertion site, erythema, fever, or foul odor.

Patient Monitoring and Care —*Continued*

Steps	Rationale	Reportable Conditions
7. Monitor hemoglobin, hematocrit, and coagulation studies every 8 hours after the procedure for 24 hours or as indicated.	Assesses for potential of effusion recurrence or bleeding at the site.	• Bleeding or hematoma at the insertion site • Decrease in hemoglobin or hematocrit values • Changes in coagulation study results
8. Assess for pericardiocentesis site every day.	Determines the presence of infection.	• Erythema • Edema • Purulent drainage • Foul odor • Temperature >100.5°F (>38°C)
9. Prescribe site care: A. Cleanse the area surrounding the pericardial catheter with an antiseptic solution (e.g., 2% chlorhexidine-based preparation). B. Apply a dry sterile gauze or transparent dressing with the date and time of the dressing change. Follow institutional standards. **(Level E*)**	May reduce infection. The U.S. Centers for Disease Control and Prevention (CDC) does not have a specific recommendation for care of pericardial catheters or site care. The CDC recommends replacing intravascular catheter dressings when the dressing becomes damp, loosened, or soiled or when inspection of the site is necessary.[4]	
10. Evaluate the size of the effusion within 24 hours of indwelling catheter placement with use of a two-dimensional echocardiogram.	Records how effective drainage was and whether the need for the indwelling catheter continues to exist.	• Increased size of the effusion
11. Should the indwelling catheter be left in the pericardial space, a collection bag is connected by a stopcock to the indwelling catheter. Using sterile technique, heparinized saline (2–3 mL) should be instilled following each drainage attempt.[1]	Facilitates pleural fluid drainage by gravity or alternatively drained manually to avoid recurrence of pleural effusion. Maintains a patent catheter. Minimizes the potential for infection.	• Continued drainage >25 mL/24 hours • Color or consistency of fluid changes
12. Remove the indwelling catheter using aseptic technique when no longer needed.		
13. Be prepared for emergent chest exploration if sudden deterioration in the patient's condition occurs.	Deterioration in the patient's hemodynamic status may indicate an increasing effusion and the need for immediate surgical intervention.	• Decreased blood pressure • Presence of dysrhythmias • Increased venous pressure • Change in mental or respiratory status • Diaphoresis • Distant heart sounds
14. Provide emotional support to the patient throughout the procedure.	Minimizes apprehension and anxiety.	
15. Keep the patient and family informed about the patient's condition. Be available to answer the patient's and family's questions, and facilitate meeting their needs as appropriate.	The unknown increases the anxiety and apprehension of the patient and family.	
16. Assess for pain, and prescribe analgesia as needed.	Identifies the need for pain interventions.	• Continued pain despite pain interventions

*Level E: Multiple case reports, theory-based evidence from expert opinions, or peer-reviewed professional organizational standards without clinical studies to support recommendation.

Documentation

Documentation should include the following:
- Specific preprocedural instructions and the patient's and family's satisfactory understanding
- Universal protocol requirement, if nonemergent
- Legally signed consent form
- Pre- and postprocedural level of consciousness; blood pressure; venous pressures; pulmonary arterial pressures; cardiac index, cardiac output, systemic vascular resistance, if available; heart sounds and cardiac rhythm; respiratory status and pulse oximetry reading
- Pre- and postprocedural hemoglobin, hematocrit, and coagulation results, if performed
- Medications administered with dosage and times noted
- Placement of an indwelling catheter (if used) to include total length, diameter, and length from skin to hub
- Removal of the indwelling catheter, if used
- Assessment of pericardiocentesis fluid
- Amount and consistency of postprocedural drainage
- Occurrence of unexpected outcomes
- Pain assessment, interventions, and effectiveness
- Pre- and postprocedural evaluation and location of effusion with two-dimensional echocardiogram, if used
- ECG rhythm strips
- Emergency interventions performed if necessary
- Specimens sent to the laboratory

References and Additional Readings

For a complete list of references and additional readings for this procedure, scan this QR code with your smartphone, or visit https://www.elsevier.com/__data/assets/pdf_file/0007/1319812/Chapter0037.pdf

38 Pericardiocentesis (Assist)

Brandi L. Holcomb

PURPOSE: Pericardiocentesis is the removal of excess fluid from the pericardial sac for the diagnosis and management of acute and chronic pericardial effusions. It can be palliative for symptom management and lifesaving in the case of cardiac tamponade.

PREREQUISITE NURSING KNOWLEDGE

- Advanced cardiac life support (ACLS) knowledge and skills.
- Knowledge and skills related to aseptic technique.
- Knowledge of hematology and coagulation laboratory values
- Knowledge of cardiovascular anatomy and physiology.
- The pericardial space normally contains 20 to 50 mL of clear, serous fluid.
- Pericardial fluid has electrolyte and protein profiles similar to plasma and acts as a lubricant between the pericardium and the heart.
- Pericardial effusion is defined as the abnormal accumulation of fluid within the pericardial sac that exceeds the stretch capacity of the pericardium, generally more than 50 to 100 mL.[7]
- The space within the pericardial sac is finite; initially large increases in intrapericardial volume result in relatively small changes in intrapericardial pressure. If fluid continues to accumulate and increases intrapericardial pressures above the filling pressures of the right heart, right-ventricular diastolic filling is compromised, resulting in cardiac tamponade.[5]
- Intrapericardial fluid accumulation can be acute or chronic and therefore varies in presentation of symptoms. Acute effusions are usually a rapid collection of fluid occurring over minutes to hours and may result in hemodynamic compromise with volumes less than 250 mL.[6] Chronic effusions develop over days to weeks allowing for hypertrophy and distention of the fibrous pericardial membrane. Patients with chronic effusions may accumulate greater than or equal to 2000 mL of fluid before exhibiting symptoms of hemodynamic compromise.[6]
- Classic symptoms of cardiac tamponade include Beck's triad: hypotension, distant heart sounds, and jugular venous distension. Other common signs and symptoms include dyspnea, tachycardia, chest pain, pulsus paradoxus, pallor, diaphoresis, hypotension, impaired cerebral and renal function, and decreased ECG voltage.[5]
- Acute pericardial effusions can occur from trauma, myocardial infarction, cardiac surgery, aortic aneurysm rupture, or iatrogenic injury, whereas chronic effusions can result from conditions such as bacterial or viral pericarditis, cancer, autoimmune disorders, uremia, congestive heart failure, and infection.[2] Pericardial effusions may also be idiopathic.
- The amount of fluid in the pericardium is best evaluated by a two-dimensional echocardiogram. Chest radiographs are nonspecific and may suggest a pericardial effusion with identification of an enlarged cardiac silhouette.[6] Electrographic markers of pericardial effusion include widespread ST segment elevation, PR depression (elevation may be seen in lead aVR), and low voltage.
- Pericardiocentesis is performed therapeutically to relieve tamponade or to diagnose the etiology of the effusion. Acute tamponade resulting in hemodynamic instability necessitates an emergency procedure. Blind pericardiocentesis should only be performed in emergency situations.[7]
- The patient should be under continuous cardiac monitoring during the procedure. Pericardiocentesis is usually performed via a subxiphoid approach. Alternative sites include subcostal or parasternal approaches.
- Two-dimensional echocardiography or ultrasound to assist in guiding the needle to the safest entry site and needle trajectory during pericardiocentesis is strongly recommended.[2,6,8,9]
- This procedure may also be performed with fluoroscopy in a cardiac catheterization or interventional radiology suite.
- When reaccumulation of pericardial fluid is expected, a pericardial drain may be placed to facilitate continuous or serial drainage. Urgent or emergent chest exploration is necessary in the face of cardiac injury, rapid reaccumulation of pericardial fluid, or ineffective drainage of the pericardium.[1]
- Pericardiocentesis is contraindicated in the setting of aortic dissection or post–myocardial infarction free wall rupture. Relative contraindications include coagulopathy, prior thoracic surgery or pacemaker placement in which adhesions may have formed, artificial heart valves or other cardiac devices, or inability to directly visualize the effusion using ultrasound during the procedure.[6]
- The effect of pericardiocentesis is typically immediate. Drainage of even a small amount of fluid can decrease intrapericardial pressures and restore cardiac output.

EQUIPMENT

- Echocardiography machine with cardiac probe, sterile probe cover, and echo gel

- Pericardiocentesis tray (or thoracentesis tray)
- 16-gauge or 18-gauge, 3-inch cardiac needle or catheter over the needle
- Antiseptic skin preparation solution (e.g., 2% chlorhexidine-based preparation)
- Two packs of 4 × 4 gauze sponges
- No. 11 knife blade with handle (scalpel)
- Sterile 50-mL to 60-mL, 10-mL, 5-mL, and 3-mL syringes
- Sterile drapes and towels
- Masks, goggles or face shields, surgical head covers, sterile gowns, and gloves
- Two three-way stopcocks
- 1% lidocaine (injectable)
- 10-mL syringe with 25-gauge needle
- Culture bottles and specimen tubes for fluid analysis
- 2-inch and 3-inch tape

Additional equipment to have available as needed includes the following:

- Emergency cart (defibrillator, emergency respiratory equipment, emergency cardiac medications, and temporary pacemaker)
- 12-lead ECG machine
- Sterile marker
- Echocardiogram contrast medium
- Suture supplies
- Scissors
- If continuous drainage is necessary:
  - ❖ J guidewire, 0.035 diameter
  - ❖ Vessel dilator, 7F
  - ❖ Pigtail catheter, 7F
  - ❖ Tubing and drainage bag or bottle
  - ❖ Three-way stopcock and nonvented caps

PATIENT AND FAMILY EDUCATION

- Explain to the patient and family the reason necessitating the pericardiocentesis (e.g., relief of pressure on the heart). *Rationale:* Communication of pertinent information helps the patient and family understand the procedure, make an informed decision to proceed, and may reduce anxiety and apprehension.[2]
- Teach the patient and family about the signs and symptoms of pericardial effusion (e.g., dyspnea, dull ache or pressure within the chest, dysphagia, cough, tachypnea, hoarseness, hiccups, and/or nausea).[5,6] *Rationale:* Recognition of signs and symptoms of recurrent pericardial effusion may prompt early detection of a potentially life-threatening problem.

PATIENT ASSESSMENT AND PREPARATION

Patient Assessment

- Obtain a complete history of present illness including mechanism of injury (if applicable), past medical history,

and current medications and/or medical therapies from the patient or a reliable source. *Rationale:* A thorough history is necessary to determine the patient's baseline health status and to identify potential risk factors. The nurse-patient interaction provides an opportunity for the nurse to establish a therapeutic relationship focused on the patient.[2]

- Assess the patient's neurological status, heart rate, blood pressure, cardiac rhythm, heart sounds (S_1, S_2, rubs, murmurs), central venous pressure (noninvasive or invasive), mean arterial pressure, oxygen saturation via pulse oximetry (SpO_2), and respiratory status. If a pulmonary artery catheter is in situ, assess pulmonary artery pressures. *Rationale:* Provides baseline data.
- Evaluate current laboratory values to include a complete blood cell count, electrolytes, and coagulation profile. *Rationale:* Review of these data is essential to identify the potential risk of cardiac dysrhythmias or abnormal bleeding. If the international normalized ratio (INR) or partial thromboplastin time (PTT) or both are elevated, reversing anticoagulation therapy should be considered before performing the procedure. If the patient is hemodynamically stable, it may be prudent to defer the procedure until blood levels indicate a reduction in bleeding risk.[6]

Patient Preparation

- Confirm that the patient and family understand preprocedural teaching by having them verbalize understanding. Clarify key points by reinforcing important information, and answer all questions. *Rationale:* Preprocedural communication provides a framework of patient expectations, enhances cooperation, and reduces anxiety.[2]
- Verify that the patient is the correct patient using two identifiers. *Rationale:* The nurse should always ensure correct identification of the patient for the intended intervention for patient safety.
- Ensure that informed consent is obtained. Implied consent may be assumed if emergent life-saving intervention is necessary. *Rationale:* Informed consent is based on the autonomous right of the patient and facilitates a competent decision for the patient and family.[2]
- If nonemergent, assist as needed with a preprocedural verification and time out. *Rationale:* Ensures patient safety.
- Assist with coordinating the procedure with the echocardiogram technician or ultrasonographer to assist with the two-dimensional echocardiogram or ultrasound examination if this approach is being used. *Rationale:* Echocardiogram- or ultrasound-directed pericardiocentesis allows for more precise localization of the effusion and is associated with higher success rates and lower complication rates.[5-7]
- Administer analgesics or sedatives as prescribed. *Rationale:* Analgesia and sedation reduce anxiety and promote patient comfort and cooperation.
- Continue cardiac monitoring, or initiate bedside cardiac monitoring. *Rationale:* The ECG is monitored during and after the procedure for changes that may indicate cardiac injury.

Procedure	for Assisting With Pericardiocentesis		
Steps		Rationale	Special Considerations
1. **HH**			
2. **PE**			Consider putting a mask on the patient during the actual procedure if the patient is not intubated (in a contained system), especially if the patient has methicillin-resistant *Staphylococcus aureus* (MRSA)-positive results on nasal swab or MRSA status is unknown
3. Using aseptic technique, assist as needed with opening the pericardiocentesis tray and supplies.		Prepares for the procedure.	
4. If tolerated, position the patient in the supine position with the head of the bed elevated 30–45 degrees.		Facilitates patient comfort, decreases work of breathing, and permits fluid to pool on the inferior surface of the heart, aiding fluid aspiration.	Rotating the patient slightly to the left may enhance ease of imaging and fluid drainage.
5. Assist the physician, advance practice nurse, or healthcare provider performing the procedure with cleansing the patient's skin with antiseptic solution (e.g., 2% chlorhexidine-based preparation), and perform **HH**		Minimizes the potential for infection.	Clipping hair from the area may be necessary before applying the antiseptic solution.
6. If two-dimensional echocardiogram or ultrasound is being used, **skip to Step 14.**			
7. Assist as needed with applying personal protective equipment and sterile equipment (e.g., masks, head covers, sterile gowns, sterile gloves), and if needed assist with fully draping the patient with exposure of only the surgical site.		Protects the provider and maintains aseptic and sterile technique.	
8. Assist if needed with providing a three-way stopcock, 3-inch cardiac needle, and 50-mL or 60-mL syringe.		Provides needed supplies.	
9. Assist if needed with preparing for a local injection (e.g., 10-mL syringe with 1% lidocaine and a 25-gauge needle).		Reduces patient discomfort.	As the needle is introduced, the physician, advanced practice nurse, or other healthcare professional may insert a small amount of 1% lidocaine to add analgesic effect.
10. Continuously monitor the bedside ECG, vital signs, Spo$_2$, pulmonary artery pressures, and central venous pressure (if pulmonary artery catheter present) during needle aspiration and fluid withdrawal.[3,5,6]		Determines the patient's response during the procedure.	
11. Continuously monitor the patient as the physician, advanced practice nurse, or other healthcare professional slowly inserts the needle.		Continues to determine patient response during the procedure.	The movement of the heart usually defibrinates blood in the pericardial space so it cannot clot. Clotting usually indicates penetration of the heart chamber and blood obtained from within a ventricle or atrium.[1,3]

Procedure continues on following page

Procedure for Assisting With Pericardiocentesis—*Continued*		
Steps	Rationale	Special Considerations
12. Assist if needed with obtaining pericardial fluid samples. If continuous drainage is used, **go to step 17.**	Provides diagnosis of the organism involved in pericardial effusion.	Samples of pericardial fluid should be sent for appropriate biochemical, cytologic, bacteriologic, and immunological analysis to assist in the diagnosis of the cause of the effusion. The first sample is usually reserved for microbiological studies.[1] These samples should be collected by the performing provider.
13. Assist if needed with labeling the specimens, and send the specimens to the laboratory.	Prepares the samples for analysis.	Label with the patient's name and date of birth. Time and date the sample.
When Two-Dimensional Echocardiogram or Ultrasound Is Used		
14. Assist the physician, advanced practice nurse, or other healthcare professional and the echocardiogram/ultrasound technician as needed.	Provides assistance.	Assist if needed with marking the skin with a sterile marker.
15. **Return to Step 7** and proceed.		
16. If bloody fluid is aspirated, be prepared to assist the physician, advanced practice nurse, or other healthcare professional in infusing a few milliliters of echo contrast medium into the space where the needle is to confirm position.[6,7] If requested, prepare echocardiogenic saline with aseptic technique by: A. Opening two sterile 5-mL syringes and a three-way stopcock onto the sterile field for the provider to assemble (one filled with air and one with 5 mL sterile normal saline). B. Inverting the sterile saline vial so the performing provider can accurately aspirate saline into sterile syringe. The physician, advanced practice nurse, or other healthcare professional will perform the procedure. When this is determined to be pericardial fluid, **return to step 12.**	Provides assistance.	Sterile technique is utilized to decrease the risk of sample contamination and infection. Bloody aspirate may indicate myocardial puncture or hemorrhagic pericardial effusion. Chronic effusions usually contain serous or serosanguineous fluid while acute effusions from trauma or arterial perforations are frankly bloody. Echo contrast or agitated saline can be viewed on the echocardiogram. If the needle is in a cardiac chamber, then the contrast/bubbles will be seen in the right ventricular cavity and rapidly disperse with the next right ventricular ejection.
When Continuous Drainage Is Desired		
17. Assist the physician, advanced practice nurse, or other healthcare professional if needed as they remove the needle and insert a soft floppy-tipped guidewire through the needle or sheath. The guidewire is passed so it wraps around the heart within the pericardial space. A multiholed pigtail or straight soft catheter is passed over the guidewire to facilitate drainage of the effusion.[6,7]	Provides assistance. Fluid volume and characteristics can provide important clinical information to help manage the patient.	Can be viewed on echocardiographic and/or fluoroscopic imaging.

Procedure | for Assisting With Pericardiocentesis—*Continued*

Steps	Rationale	Special Considerations
18. Assist the physician, advanced practice nurse, or other healthcare professional with removing the guidewire and connecting the end of the catheter to the three-way stopcock and the drainage collection bag.[5-7] Assist with evaluation and documentation of fluid aspirate.	Maintains asepsis; allows for continual drainage of the effusion.[1]	
19. If an indwelling catheter is placed to continuously drain a pericardial effusion, assist the physician, advanced practice nurse, or other healthcare professional with attaching the sterile end or the catheter to the bag or bottle with aseptic technique.	Facilitates fluid drainage and maintenance; minimizes the potential for infection.	Pericardial fluid should intermittently be aspirated every 4–6 hours as this ensures catheter drainage. Sterile saline may be used to flush the catheter after drainage; this will ensure patency.[8]
20. If an indwelling catheter is in place, assist the physician, advanced practice nurse, or other healthcare professional if needed by providing suture supplies.	Prevents dislodging or accidental discontinuation of the drainage catheter.	
21. Assist if needed with cleansing the area around the catheter with antiseptic solution, and apply an occlusive sterile dressing.[3]	May reduce the risk of infection.	
22. Continue bedside ECG monitoring, and discontinue the 12-lead ECG if used.	Allows monitoring of cardiac rate and rhythm.	
23. Dispose of **PE** and used supplies in appropriate receptacles.	Reduces the transmission of microorganisms; Standard Precautions.	
24. **HH**		
25. Administer antibiotics as prescribed.	May reduce the risk of infection.	

Expected Outcomes

- Fluid removed from the pericardial sac.
- Diagnostic pericardial fluid samples sent to the laboratory if indicated.
- Relief of pain, dyspnea, or other symptoms necessitating the procedure.
- Improved cardiac output.
- Patient's blood pressure, venous pressure, heart sounds, pulmonary artery pressures, and cardiac rhythm within normal limits

Unexpected Outcomes

- Injury to the myocardium, coronary arteries, lungs, large blood vessels, or abdominal viscera
- Hemodynamic instability resulting in any of the following:
  - Hypotension or low cardiac output
  - Increase in pulmonary artery pressure or venous pressure
  - Sustained cardiac dysrhythmias
  - Excessive bleeding
- ECG changes
  - ST-segment depression
  - PR-segment elevation
  - Cardiac tamponade
- Pain
- Dyspnea

UNIT 2

Patient Monitoring and Care

Steps	Rationale	Reportable Conditions
		These conditions should be reported to the provider if they persist despite nursing interventions.
1. Continuously monitor and assess the patient's ECG pulmonary artery (PA) pressures if a PA catheter is in situ, venous pressure, blood pressure, SpO_2, and neurological status during and frequently after the procedure until stable (if available, continuously monitor cardiac index and systemic vascular resistance).	Assess for early recognition of possible postprocedure complications including cardiac tamponade, cardiac injury, or hemodynamic instability.	• Increasing venous pressure • Decreasing arterial pressure • Change in level of consciousness • Pulsus paradoxus • Equalizing PA pressures • Decreased cardiac index • Decreased systemic vascular resistance
2. Treat dysrhythmias as prescribed.	Dysrhythmias may lead to cardiac decompensation.	• Persistent dysrhythmias despite appropriate intervention • New-onset dysrhythmia
3. Auscultate heart and lung sounds immediately before and after the procedure.	Muffled or distant heart sounds may indicate fluid reaccumulation. Decreased or absent breath sounds may indicate pneumothorax or hemothorax.	• Distant or faint heart sounds • Asymmetrical or absent breath sounds • Dyspnea • Tachypnea • Decreased SpO_2
4. Ensure that a portable chest radiograph is obtained immediately after the procedure as prescribed.	Assesses for pneumothorax and hemothorax.	• Pneumothorax • Hemothorax
5. Ensure that a two-dimensional echocardiogram is obtained within several hours after the procedure as ordered and after removal of catheter/drain (if placed post procedure).	Confirms absence of fluid reaccumulation.	• Pericardial effusion reaccumulation
6. Monitor the pericardiocentesis site for bleeding frequently after the procedure is completed until the patient's condition is stable and then every 4 hours for 24 hours. If an indwelling catheter is present, continue to monitor the site every 4 hours until the catheter has been removed.	Assesses for postprocedural hemostasis and drainage or signs of infection.	• Bleeding or hematoma at the site • Drainage at the insertion site, erythema, fever, or foul odor
7. Monitor hemoglobin, hematocrit, and coagulation levels as ordered (e.g., every 8 hours after the procedure for 24 hours and then as indicated).	Assesses for effusion recurrence or bleeding at the site.	• Decrease in hemoglobin or hematocrit • Changes in coagulation study results

Patient Monitoring and Care *—Continued*		
Steps	**Rationale**	**Reportable Conditions**
8. Assess the pericardiocentesis site every day.	Determines the presence of infection.	• Erythema • Edema • Purulent drainage • Foul odor • Temperature >100.5°F (>38°C) • Signs and symptoms of infection
9. Perform site care as ordered or according to institutional standards: 　A. Ensure that the catheter/ drain is appropriately sutured/ secured. 　B. Assess and document the amount and type of drainage. 　C. Cleanse the area surrounding the pericardial catheter with an antiseptic solution (e.g., 2% chlorhexidine-based preparation). 　D. Apply a dry sterile gauze or transparent dressing with the date and time of the dressing change. Follow institutional standards. **(Level E*)**	Reduces infection. The Centers for Disease Control and Prevention (CDC) does not have a specific recommendation for care of pericardial catheters or site care. The CDC recommends replacing intravascular catheter dressings when the dressing becomes damp, loosened, or soiled or when inspection of the site is necessary.[4]	• Dislodgement of catheter/drain • Evidence of infection
10. Should the indwelling catheter be left in the pericardial space, a collection bag is connected by a stopcock to the indwelling catheter. Using sterile technique, heparinized saline (2–3 mL) should be instilled following each drainage attempt.[1] 11. Remove the indwelling catheter using aseptic technique when no longer needed. 12. Be prepared for chest exploration if the patient's status deteriorates.	Facilitates pleural fluid drainage by gravity or alternatively drained manually to avoid recurrence of pleural effusion. Maintains a patent catheter. Minimizes the potential for infection. Deterioration in the patient's hemodynamic status may indicate an increasing effusion and the need for immediate surgical intervention.	• Decreased blood pressure • Dysrhythmias • Increased venous pressure • Change in mental or respiratory status • Diaphoresis • Distant or faint heart sounds
13. Provide emotional support to the patient throughout and after the procedure.	Minimizes apprehension and anxiety.	
14. Keep the patient and family informed about the patient's condition. Be available to answer their questions and facilitate meeting their needs as appropriate.	The unknown increases the anxiety and apprehension of the patient and family.	
15. Follow institutional standards for assessing pain. Administer analgesia as needed.	Identifies the need for pain interventions.	• Continued pain despite pain interventions

*Level E: Multiple case reports, theory-based evidence from expert opinions, or peer-reviewed professional organizational standards without clinical studies to support recommendations.

Documentation

Documentation should include the following:
- Specific preprocedural instruction and patient's and family's satisfactory understanding of the procedure
- Legally signed informed consent
- Universal protocol requirement, if nonemergent
- Pre- and postprocedure level of consciousness; blood pressure; ECG findings, venous pressure; pulmonary arterial pressure; cardiac index, cardiac output, and systemic vascular resistance, if available; heart sounds and cardiac rhythm; respiratory status and pulse oximetry reading
- Preprocedure and postprocedure hemoglobin, hematocrit, and coagulation results, if performed
- Medications administered
- Assessment of pericardiocentesis fluid volume and characteristics
- Placement of indwelling catheter and/or drain if applicable
- Removal of indwelling catheter if used
- Occurrence of unexpected outcomes
- Pain assessment, interventions, and effectiveness
- Emergency interventions necessary
- Specimens sent to the laboratory

References and Additional Readings

For a complete list of references and additional readings for this procedure, scan this QR code with your smartphone, or visit https://www.elsevier.com/__data/assets/pdf_file/0008/1319813/Chapter0038.pdf.

PROCEDURE

39

Atrial Electrogram

Marion E. McRae

PURPOSE: An atrial electrogram (AEG) is obtained to determine the presence of atrial activity in a dysrhythmia or to identify the relationship between atrial and ventricular depolarizations.

PREREQUISITE NURSING KNOWLEDGE

- Anatomy and physiology of the cardiovascular system, principles of cardiac conduction, and basic dysrhythmia interpretation.
- Principles of general electrical safety applied with use the of epicardial pacing wires. Gloves should always be worn when handling pacing electrodes to prevent microshock because even small amounts of electrical current can cause serious dysrhythmias if transmitted to the heart.[1,8,10-11]
- Advanced cardiac life support knowledge and skills.
- AEG is a method of recording electrical activity that originates from the atria using temporary atrial epicardial wires placed during cardiac surgery. Standard electrocardiogram (ECG) monitoring records electrical events from the heart with electrodes located on the surface of the patient's body, which is a considerable distance from the myocardium. One limitation of ECG monitoring may be its inability to detect P waves effectively.
- AEGs detect electrical events directly from the atria, which provides a greatly enhanced tracing of atrial activity. This enhanced tracing allows for the determination of atrial activity, comparison of atrial events with ventricular events, and determination of the relationship between the two.
- The American Heart Association Practice Standards for Electrocardiographic Monitoring in Hospital Settings recommend recording an AEG whenever tachycardia of unknown origin develops in a patient after cardiac surgery.[2]
- Indications for AEG are as follows[2]:
  - When atrial activity is not clearly detected on ECG monitoring
  - For determining the relationship between atrial and ventricular activity including heart blocks
  - For differentiating wide-complex rhythms (i.e., ventricular tachycardia and supraventricular tachycardia with aberrant ventricular conduction)
  - For differentiating narrow-complex supraventricular tachycardias (i.e., sinus tachycardia, atrial tachycardia, paroxysmal supraventricular tachycardia, atrial flutter, atrial fibrillation with relatively regular ventricular rate intervals, or junctional tachycardia)
- AEGs can be performed with multichannel telemetry or a bedside ECG monitor that allows for simultaneous display

of the AEG along with the surface ECG.[3-5] The AtriAmp device (Atrility Medical, Madison, WI) allows recording of a unipolar AEG as well as allowing intermittent or continuous atrial pacing.[9] A 12-lead ECG machine also can be used to obtain an AEG, but this method is not preferred as it does not allow continuous AEG recording and increases requirements for equipment disinfection.

- Accurate identification of the epicardial atrial pacing wire or wires is important.
- The two types of AEGs that can be obtained from epicardial pacing wires are unipolar and bipolar.
  - A unipolar electrogram identifies electrical activity between one atrial epicardial wire and a surface ECG electrode. The unipolar AEG detects atrial and ventricular activity and the relationship between the two. If there is only one atrial electrode or an atrial and a ground electrode, one can only record a unipolar AEG.
  - A bipolar electrogram detects electrical activity between the two atrial epicardial wires. The bipolar AEG predominantly detects atrial activity because both electrodes are attached to the atria (atrial activity generally appears larger than on a unipolar AEG).
- Atrial electrograms increase the accuracy of nurses' diagnoses of cardiac arrhythmias.[4,7] However, they remain underused in clinical practice.[5]
- An AEG cannot be performed if the patient is dependent on atrial pacing for hemodynamic stability because at least one atrial pacing wire must be disconnected from the pacemaker to perform the AEG, resulting in a loss of atrial pacing unless the AtriAmp device is used.

EQUIPMENT

- Nonsterile gloves
- Temporary atrial epicardial pacing wires placed during cardiac surgery
- Multichannel ECG monitor and recorder (ensure that biomedical safety standards are met and that the machine is safe for use with epicardial wires)
- Sterile dressings and materials needed for site care, including antiseptic solution

  Additional equipment to have available as needed includes the following:
- ECG electrodes

- ECG lead with alligator clips
- Insulating material for epicardial pacing wires (e.g., built-in insulators on some epicardial wires, finger cots, needle caps, glove, ear plug)
- An AtriAmp device (optional)

PATIENT AND FAMILY EDUCATION

- Provide information about the normal conduction system, normal and abnormal heart rhythms, and symptoms of abnormal heart rhythms. *Rationale:* This information helps the patient and family understand the patient's condition and encourages the patient and family to ask questions.
- Provide information about the AEG, the reason for the AEG, and an explanation of the equipment. *Rationale:* This communication may decrease patient anxiety and help the patient and family understand the procedure, why it is needed, and how it will help the patient.
- Explain the patient's expected participation during the procedure, including the need to lie still to avoid artifact on the AEG. *Rationale:* This explanation encourages patient assistance.

PATIENT ASSESSMENT AND PREPARATION

Patient Assessment

- Assess the patient's cardiac rhythm for the presence of atrial activity in more than one lead from the multichannel ECG monitor. *Rationale:* This assessment determines the presence or absence of P waves and the potential need for an AEG.
- Assess the patient's cardiac rhythm for the relationship between atrial and ventricular activity. *Rationale:* This assessment determines the relationship between P waves and QRS complexes and the potential need for an AEG.
- Assess for dysrhythmias. *Rationale:* This assessment determines the patient's baseline cardiac rhythm.
- Assess the patient's hemodynamic status (e.g., systolic, diastolic, and mean arterial pressure; level of consciousness; dizziness; dyspnea; nausea; vomiting; cool or clammy skin; and chest pain). *Rationale:* This determines the patient's hemodynamic status and need for immediate intervention.

Patient Preparation

- Verify the correct patient with two identifiers. *Rationale:* Before performing a procedure, the nurse should ensure the correct identification of the patient for the intended intervention.
- Ensure that the patient understands the preprocedure teaching. Answer questions as they arise, and reinforce information as needed. *Rationale:* This communication evaluates and reinforces understanding of previously taught information.
- Expose the patient's chest, and identify the epicardial pacing wires. *Rationale:* This action provides access to the atrial pacing wires.

Procedure	for Atrial Electrogram	
Steps	**Rationale**	**Special Considerations**
1. **HH**		
2. **PE**		Epicardial wires are a direct source of electrical conduction to the myocardium. Use of gloves prevents microshocks with handling of epicardial wires that could cause arrhythmias.[2,8,10,11]
3. Touch a large metal object such as the patient's bed before touching the wires.[8] (**Level E***)	Prevents microshock that can cause arrythmias.[7]	Any static electricity is discharged before touching the pacing wires.
4. Expose and identify the atrial epicardial pacing wires.	Differentiation of the atrial from the ventricular wires is important to ensure that the appropriate epicardial wires are used.	Typically the atrial wires exit the chest to the right of the patient's sternum, and the ventricular wires exit to the left of the patient's sternum (Fig. 39.1).
5. Ensure that you are not using a ground wire (one only sutured to the chest wall and not on the surface of the heart).[4]	Using a ground wire will record only a surface ECG, not an AEG.	

*Level E: Multiple case reports, theory-based evidence from expert opinions, or peer-reviewed professional organizational standards without clinical studies to support recommendations.

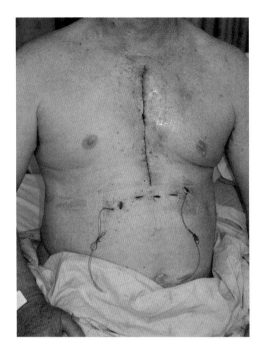

Figure 39.1 Atrial wires exit the chest to the right of the patient's sternum. Ventricular wires exit the chest to the left of the patient's sternum.

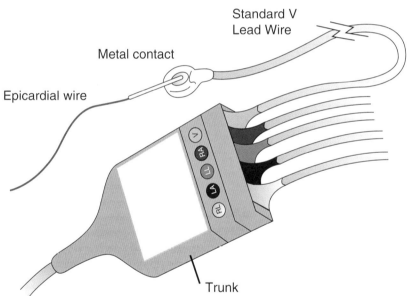

Standard V
Lead Wire

Metal contact

Epicardial wire

Trunk

ECG Bedside Monitor Cable

Figure 39.2 The tip of atrial epicardial wire in direct contact with the metal on the end of the V lead wire. *(Drawing courtesy Paul W. Schiffmacher, Thomas Jefferson University, Philadelphia.)*

Procedure for Atrial Electrogram—*Continued*		
Steps	Rationale	Special Considerations
Obtaining a Unipolar AEG with Multichannel Telemetry or Bedside ECG Monitor: Lead V		
1. Detach the precordial V lead from the precordial V lead electrode on the patient's chest.	Prepares equipment.	Determine that the ECG monitoring system meets all safety requirements.
2. Place the tip of one of the atrial epicardial wires in direct contact with: A. The metal on the end of the V lead (Fig. 39.2). **(Level D*)**	Electrical activity is transmitted from the epicardial wire to the ECG monitoring system.	A lead wire with alligator clips at both ends also can be used to connect the epicardial pacing wire to the monitor lead.

*Level D: Peer-reviewed professional and organizational standards with the support of clinical study recommendations.

Procedure continues on following page

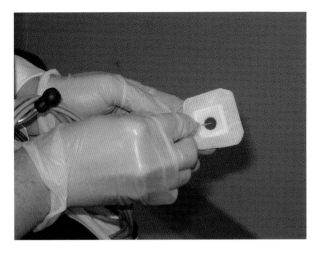

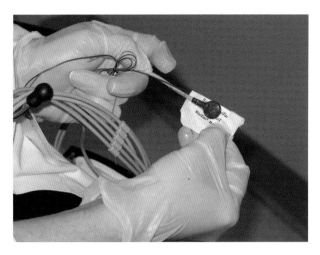

Figure 39.3 The tip of the atrial epicardial wire in direct contact with the conductive gel on the adhesive side of the electrode.

Figure 39.4 An electrode wrapped around the tip of the atrial epicardial wires.

Procedure   for Atrial Electrogram—*Continued*

Steps	Rationale	Special Considerations
or B. The conductive gel on the adhesive side of the electrode is attached to the V lead electrode (Fig. 39.3).[3-5]	Electrical activity is transmitted from the epicardial wire to the ECG monitoring system.	The electrode can be wrapped around the atrial wire if continuous monitoring of the AEG is indicated to diagnose an unknown intermittent rhythm (Fig. 39.4).[3]
3. Select lead V on the ECG monitor and a surface ECG lead (I, II, III, augmented vector foot [avF], augmented vector right [avR], or augmented vector left [avL]).	Use of the precordial V lead allows for the detection of atrial electrical activity between the precordial V lead and an indifferent limb lead in a unipolar configuration.	
4. Record a dual-channel continuous strip.	Displays the AEG simultaneously with a surface ECG lead.	Label the precordial V lead on the ECG strip as the AEG.

5. Analyze the AEG strip, and compare the surface ECG:
  A. Vertically line up the QRS complexes on the ECG strip with the ventricular deflections on the AEG (Fig. 39.5).
  B. All other spikes should be atrial activity either being initiated in the atrium or being conducted retrograde to the atrium (Fig. 39.6).
	Identifies P waves and QRS complexes and determines the relationship between the P waves and the QRS complexes.	Multiple atrial spikes will exist between ventricular spikes if the atrial rate is greater than the ventricular rate (e.g., atrial flutter, atrial fibrillation, second- or third-degree atrioventricular block).

Obtaining a Unipolar AEG With Multichannel Telemetry or Bedside ECG Monitor: Lead I

1. Detach the right arm (RA) lead from the electrode on the patient's chest.	Prepares equipment.	Determine that the ECG bedside monitoring system meets all safety requirements.

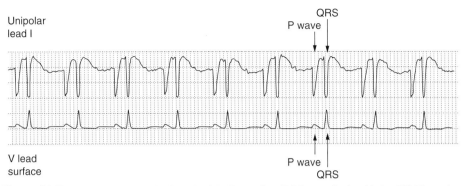

Figure 39.5 Unipolar AEG strip from lead I. The surface ECG was obtained in lead V. The unipolar AEG was obtained in lead I. The atrial activity is magnified in lead I.

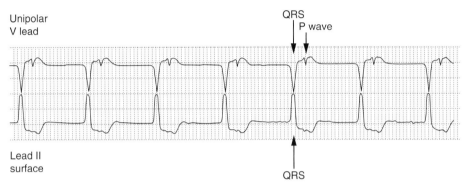

Figure 39.6 Unipolar AEG strip from lead V. The surface ECG was obtained in lead II. On the basis of the surface ECG, the rhythm appears to be junctional with no evidence of P waves or atrial activity. The unipolar AEG shows retrograde P waves that follow the QRS complex, confirming the junctional rhythm interpretation.

Procedure for Atrial Electrogram—*Continued*		
Steps	**Rationale**	**Special Considerations**
2. Place the tip of one of the atrial epicardial wires in direct contact with: A. The metal on the end of the RA lead.[2] **(Level D*)** *or*	Electrical activity is transmitted from the epicardial wire to the ECG monitoring system.	A lead wire with alligator clips at both ends also can be used to connect the epicardial pacing wire to the monitor.
B. The conductive gel on the adhesive side of the electrode is attached to the RA lead (see Fig. 39.3).[3]	Electrical activity is transmitted from the epicardial wire to the ECG monitoring system.	The electrode can be wrapped around the atrial wire if continued monitoring is indicated to diagnose an unknown intermittent rhythm (see Fig. 39.4).[3]
3. Select lead I and a surface ECG lead on the ECG monitor.	Lead I detects electrical activity between the right arm (RA) and the left arm (LA) limb lead. Because the atrial pacing wire is in contact with the RA lead, lead I detects the electrical activity between the atrial wire and the surface LA limb lead.	Label lead I on the ECG strip as the AEG.

*Level D: Peer-reviewed professional and organizational standards with the support of clinical study recommendations.

Procedure continues on following page

Procedure for Atrial Electrogram—*Continued*		
Steps	Rationale	Special Considerations
4. Record a dual-channel strip.	Displays the AEG simultaneously with a surface ECG lead.	A dual-channel recorder permits comparison of the surface ECG with the AEG.
5. Analyze the AEG strip and compare the surface ECG with the AEG (see Fig. 39.5). A. Vertically line up the QRS complexes on the ECG strip with the ventricular deflections on the AEG. B. All other spikes should be atrial activity either being initiated in the atrium or being conducted retrograde to the atrium (see Fig. 39.6).	Identifies P waves and QRS complexes and determines the relationship between the P waves and the QRS complexes.	
Obtaining a Bipolar AEG With Multichannel Telemetry or Bedside ECG Monitor		
1. Detach the RA and LA leads from the electrodes on the patient.	Two atrial pacing wires are used when obtaining a bipolar AEG.	Determine that the ECG monitoring system meets all safety requirements.
2. Atrial pacing wires: A. Place the tip of one atrial epicardial pacing wire to the metal on the end of the RA lead, and place the tip of the other atrial epicardial pacing wire to the metal on the end of the LA lead.	Connection to the limb leads of the ECG monitor allows for the detection and recording of atrial electrical activity.	A lead wire with alligator clips at both ends also can be used to connect the epicardial pacing wires to the monitor leads.
or		
B. Place the tip of one atrial epicardial pacing wire to the conductive gel on the adhesive side of the electrode of the RA lead, and place the tip of the other atrial epicardial pacing wire to the conductive gel on the adhesive side of the electrode of the LA lead (see Fig. 39.3).	Electrical activity is transmitted from the epicardial wire to the ECG monitoring system.	The electrodes can be wrapped around the atrial wires if continued monitoring is indicated to diagnose an unknown intermittent rhythm (see Fig. 39.4).[3]
3. Select lead I on the bedside ECG monitor.	Lead I detects electrical activity between the RA limb lead and the LA limb lead. Because the atrial pacing wires are in contact with the RA lead and the LA lead, lead I detects the electrical activity between the two atrial wires and therefore records an AEG.	Bipolar tracings magnify atrial activity and minimize ventricular activity.
4. Record a dual-channel strip of lead I and another surface lead.	Displays the AEG simultaneously with a surface ECG.	Label lead I on the ECG strip as the bipolar AEG.
5. Analyze the AEG strip (Fig. 39.7).	Identifies P waves and QRS complexes; determines the relationship between the P waves and the QRS complexes.	

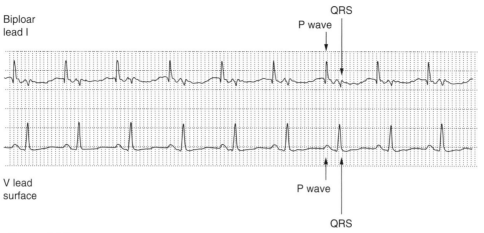

Figure 39.7 Bipolar AEG strip from lead I. The surface ECG was obtained in lead V. The bipolar AEG was obtained in lead I. The atrial activity is magnified in lead I. Also note how small the ventricular activity is in lead I.

Procedure for Atrial Electrogram—*Continued*		
Steps	Rationale	Special Considerations
Obtaining an AEG (Unipolar) Using an AtriAmp Device (Fig. 39.8A)[9]		
1. Place one atrial epicardial pacing wire into the negative port on the AtriAmp device by pushing the button beside the negative port and inserting the wire in the port.		Specific pacing cables are supplied for various pacemaker brands.
2. Place a second atrial epicardial pacing wire or a ground wire into the positive port on the AtriAmp device by pressing the button beside the positive port on the Atriamp device and inserting the wire into the port (see Fig. 39.8B).		
3. Connect the precordial V lead or V1 monitor lead to the V port at the top of the AtriAmp device (see Fig 39.8C).		
4. Connect the supplied atrial pacing cable into the pacing cable port at the top of the device and the other end into the temporary pacemaker generator if intermittent or continuous atrial pacing is needed (Fig. 39.8D).		
5. Set the bedside monitor to display a limb lead and a precordial V lead or precordial lead V1 simultaneously. The precordial V or monitor V1 lead will be the AEG. **(Level M*)**		
After the AEG Is Obtained		
1. Disconnect the atrial epicardial wires from the lead electrode.	Disconnects the wires from the bedside monitoring system.	
2. Reconnect or ensure that the ECG leads are connected to the electrodes on the patient.	Establishes continuous ECG monitoring.	

*Level M: Manufacturer's recommendations only.

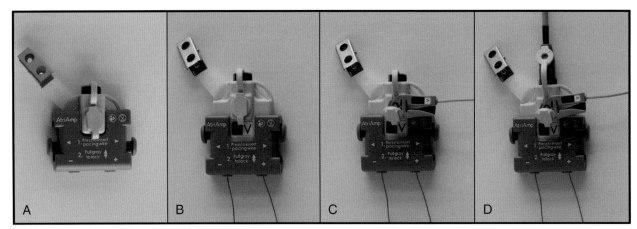

Figure 39.8 A, The AtriAmp device. **B,** Insertion of atrial pacing wire into the negative port on the device. Insertion of a second atrial wire or a ground wire into the positive port on the device. **C,** Precordial V lead or V1 bedside monitor lead connected to a V port on top of the device. **D,** Atrial pacing cable connected to the top of the device for intermittent or continuous atrial pacing using the supplied cable. *(Courtesy Atrility Medical, Madison, WI.)*

Procedure   for Atrial Electrogram—*Continued*

Steps	Rationale	Special Considerations
3. Apply a dry sterile dressing to the epicardial wire exit sites if this was removed to access the atrial epicardial wires.	Reduces the transmission of microorganisms; standard precautions.	Follow institutional guidelines for site care.
4. Place the uninsulated portion of the epicardial wires in an insulated material (e.g., built-in insulators on some wires, finger cot, needle cap, needle barrel, glove, ear plug).[10-11] **(Level E*)**	Prevents microshock.	
5. Remove gloves, and discard used supplies in the appropriate receptacle.	Reduces the transmission of microorganisms; standard precautions.	
6. 🏥		

*Level E: Multiple case reports, theory-based evidence from expert opinions, or peer-reviewed professional organizational standards without clinical studies to support recommendations.

Expected Outcomes
- Atrial activity is identified
- The relationship between atrial and ventricular activity is determined

Unexpected Outcomes
- Hemodynamically significant dysrhythmias
- Dysrhythmias in which atrial activity is unclear or the relationship between atrial and ventricular activity is unclear
- Microshocks that cause dysrhythmias

Patient Monitoring and Care

Steps	Rationale	Reportable Conditions
		These conditions should be reported to the provider if they persist despite nursing interventions.
1. Evaluate the AEG for the presence of atrial activity and its relationship to ventricular activity. Compare it with the surface ECG for interpretation.	AEG determines the presence or absence of atrial activity.	• Inability to identify atrial activity (junctional rhythm) • Inability to determine the relationship between the atrial and ventricular activity
2. Monitor the ECG rhythm for changes.	The underlying dysrhythmia may change during the AEG.	• Altered hemodynamic status caused by a change in ECG rhythm
3. Monitor vital signs and level of consciousness during the AEG and as needed.	Ensures adequate tissue perfusion.	• Hemodynamic instability • Change in level of consciousness
4. Assess and treat dysrhythmias identified by the AEG and ECG. An AEG can increase the diagnostic accuracy of arrhythmias.[4,7] (**Level C***)	Identifies dysrhythmias that need intervention.	• Return of rhythm stability • Change in cardiac rate or rhythm
5. Site care should be as follows: A. Cleanse the area surrounding the epicardial pacing wires with an antiseptic solution (e.g., 2% chlorhexidine-based preparation). (**Level D***)	May reduce infection. There are no specific recommendations for epicardial pacing wire site care.[7]	• Any signs or symptoms of infection
B. Apply a dry, sterile dressing with the date and time of the dressing change. Follow institutional standards for frequency and type of dressing. (**Level D***)	There are no specific recommendations for epicardial pacing wire dressing care. The Centers for Disease Control and Prevention recommends replacing gauze dressings every 2 days and transparent dressings at least every 7 days.[6] Dressings should be replaced when they become damp, loosened, or soiled or when inspection of the site is necessary.[6] Wet materials increase the likelihood of microshock as electrical current travels more effectively through fluid.	
C. Protect the exposed uninsulated portion of the epicardial pacing wires in an insulated environment according to institutional standards (e.g., built-in insulators on some epicardial wires, finger cot, glove, plastic needle cap, needle barrel, ear plug).[3,10,11](**Level E***)	Prevents microshocks and potentially lethal dysrhythmias.	• Dysrhythmias • Hemodynamic instability • Microshocks

*Level C: Qualitative studies, descriptive or correlational studies, integrative reviews, systematic reviews, or randomized controlled trials with inconsistent results.
*Level M: Manufacturer's recommendations only.
*Level D: Peer-reviewed professional and organizational standards with the support of clinical study recommendations.
*Level E: Multiple case reports, theory-based evidence from expert opinions, or peer-reviewed professional organizational standards without clinical studies to support recommendations.

UNIT 2

UNIT 2

Documentation

Documentation should include the following:
- Patient and family education
- Date and time of AEG tracing with interpretation
- Treatment undertaken for arrhythmias present
- Hemodynamic status and level of consciousness
- Patient tolerance of the procedure
- Occurrence of unexpected outcome

References and Additional Readings

For a complete list of references and additional readings for this procedure, scan this QR code with your smartphone, or visit https://www.elsevier.com/__data/assets/pdf_file/0009/1319814/Chapter0039.pdf.

Additional Reading

Reade MC. Temporary epicardial pacing after cardiac surgery: a practical review: part 2: selection of epicardial pacing modes and troubleshooting. *Anaesthesia*. 2007;62:364–373.

PROCEDURE 40

Atrial Overdrive Pacing AP (Perform)

Eliza Ajero Granflor

PURPOSE: The purpose of atrial overdrive pacing is to attempt to restore sinus rhythm in the setting of reentrant atrial dysrhythmias, especially atrial flutter, by intermittently pacing at a rate faster than the intrinsic atrial tachycardia so the sinus node can resume heart rate control. Several randomized trials have also demonstrated reduced rates of postoperative atrial fibrillation with preventive atrial pacing.[8] Sinus rhythm enhances cardiac output by allowing atrial contraction to contribute to ventricular filling.

PREREQUISITE NURSING KNOWLEDGE

- Knowledge of the anatomy and physiology of the cardiovascular system, principles of cardiac conduction, as well as basic and advanced dysrhythmia interpretation.
- Supraventricular dysrhythmias (e.g., right-sided atrial flutter, reentrant atrial tachycardia, atrioventricular [AV] nodal reentry tachycardia [AVNRT], atrioventricular reentrant tachycardia [AVRT] that use an accessory pathway, such as Wolff-Parkinson-White [WPW] syndrome) sometimes can be terminated by overdrive atrial pacing.[1,2]
- Atrial fibrillation occasionally terminates with overdrive atrial pacing, but this is not a reliable therapy for this rhythm. Many contemporary permanent pacemakers have arrhythmia response algorithms that include antitachycardia pacing (ATP); however, research has not yet shown that continuous atrial overdrive pacing prevents progression to permanent atrial fibrillation or reduces other major adverse cardiac events.[4]
- Knowledge of modes of cardiac pacing function and patient response to pacemaker therapy.
- Principles of general electrical safety with use of temporary invasive pacing.
- Gloves always should be worn when handling pacemaker electrodes to prevent microshock because even small amounts of electrical current can cause serious dysrhythmias if they are transmitted to the heart.[5,9]
- Clinical and technical competence related to the use of a temporary atrial pacemaker pulse generator and the rapid atrial pacing feature (Fig. 40.1).
- Advanced cardiac life support knowledge and skills are necessary.
- In the acute care setting, overdrive atrial pacing is performed most commonly with epicardial atrial pacing wires placed during cardiac surgery. A transvenous atrial pacing lead with an active fixation tip to help keep the lead in the atrium also can be used.
- Overdrive atrial pacing involves the delivery of short bursts of rapid pacing stimuli through an epicardial atrial pacing wire or a transvenous lead in the atrium. The physician or advanced practice nurse determines the duration and rate of the burst.
    - ❖ One approach to overdrive pacing is to atrial pace the heart with 20 milliamperes (mA) at a rate 20% to 30% faster than the intrinsic atrial rate for 30 seconds, then abruptly stop pacing. An alternate approach is to initiate atrial pacing at a rate 20 beats/min faster than

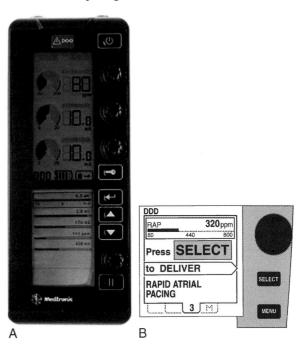

A   B

Figure 40.1 **A,** Temporary dual-chamber pulse generator with overdrive atrial pacing capability (Images used with permission from Medtronic, plc © 2022.). **B,** Enlargement of the lower screen on the pacemaker showing rapid atrial pacing controls. *(Images used with permission from Medtronic, plc © 2022.)*

AP This procedure should be performed only by clinicians who have demonstrated competence and are credentialed to perform it. In addition, the procedure must be within the scope of practice defined by their professional licensure, and in accordance with professional practice acts. Physicians, advanced practice nurses, and physician assistants may be credentialed to perform this procedure.

355

the intrinsic atrial rate; if 1:1 capture does not occur after 30 seconds, the paced rate can be increased by 20 beats/min; repeat every 30 seconds until 1:1 capture is achieved. Continue pacing until the heart rate decreases from AV block (e.g., 2:1, 3:1) or 1 to 2 minutes of 1:1 pacing have occurred, and then stop pacing.[7]

- ❖ Successive bursts usually are performed at gradually increasing rates (maximal capability of the pulse generator for overdrive atrial pacing is 800 pulses/min) and may be delivered for up to 2 minutes.[7]
- The atrial pacing wire or atrial pacing lead must be accurately identified with initiation of overdrive pacing because pacing the ventricle at rapid rates may induce ventricular tachycardia or ventricular fibrillation.
- Rapid atrial pacing may result in degeneration of the atrial rhythm to atrial fibrillation with a rapid ventricular response. This pacemaker-induced atrial fibrillation usually does not sustain itself for more than a few minutes before it converts to normal sinus rhythm.[7]
- If an accessory pathway is present, rapid atrial pacing can result in conduction to the ventricles over the accessory pathway, leading to ventricular fibrillation.
- Overdrive suppression of the sinus node may result in periods of bradycardia, asystole, junctional or ventricular escape rhythms, or polymorphic ventricular tachycardia.
- Conversion of an atrial tachydysrhythmia can result in dislodgment of atrial thrombus and embolization of clots to the pulmonary or systemic circulation.

EQUIPMENT

- Nonsterile gloves
- External pulse generator (pacemaker box) capable of rapid atrial pacing
- Pacing cable (connects the pulse generator to the patient's pacemaker leads)
- Cardiac monitor and recorder
- Electrocardiogram (ECG) electrodes
- Double alligator clip or wire with connector pins (if needed to create a ground wire)
- Materials for epicardial pacing wire site care
  - ❖ Antiseptic pads or swab sticks (e.g., 2% chlorhexidine-based preparation)
  - ❖ Gauze pads
  - ❖ Tape
- Insulating material for epicardial pacing wires or transvenous pacing electrode connector pins (e.g., finger cot, needle cap, needle barrel, glove, ear plug)
- Blood pressure monitoring system

Additional equipment to have available as needed includes the following:

- Defibrillator
- Emergency medications
- Airway management equipment
- Standard pulse generator or transcutaneous pacemaker and equipment
- Subcutaneous needle for a ground wire

PATIENT AND FAMILY EDUCATION

- Explain the procedure and its purpose to the patient and family. ***Rationale:*** This explanation may decrease patient and family anxiety and promote cooperation with the procedure.
- Reassure the patient that atrial pacing usually cannot be felt and that any sensation most likely will be a "fluttering" feeling in the chest. ***Rationale:*** This reassurance prepares the patient and may decrease the patient's anxiety.

PATIENT ASSESSMENT AND PREPARATION

Patient Assessment

- Identify the patient's ECG rhythm. Verify ECG intervals as well as atrial and ventricular rates. ***Rationale:*** This assessment determines baseline cardiac conduction.
- Assess the patient's vital signs and hemodynamic parameters. ***Rationale:*** This assessment determines the patient's stability and ability to tolerate the procedure.
- Assess for signs and symptoms that might be caused by the dysrhythmia (e.g., shortness of breath, dizziness, nausea, chest pain, signs of poor peripheral perfusion). ***Rationale:*** This determines the patient's response to the dysrhythmia.
- Assess the patency of the intravenous access. ***Rationale:*** Intravenous access is needed for possible administration of fluids and medications.
- Note any medications that might have an effect on the patient's cardiac rhythm or hemodynamic parameters (e.g., beta blockers, calcium channel blockers, antidysrhythmics, or digoxin). ***Rationale:*** Knowledge of medication therapy can alert healthcare providers to potential cardiac rhythms (e.g., bradycardia or atrioventricular block) after termination of the atrial dysrhythmia.
- Verify the patient's coagulation laboratory results. ***Rationale:*** Therapeutic coagulation levels may decrease the risk of embolization.[1,3]

Patient Preparation

- Verify the correct patient with two identifiers. ***Rationale:*** Before performing a procedure, the nurse should ensure the correct identification of the patient for the intended intervention.
- Obtain informed consent (may not be possible in an emergency). ***Rationale:*** Informed consent protects the rights of the patient who is a competent decision maker.
- Ensure that the patient and family understand preprocedural teaching. Answer questions as they arise, and educate as needed. ***Rationale:*** This communication evaluates and reinforces understanding of previously taught information.
- Perform a preprocedure verification and time out, if nonemergent. ***Rationale:*** This ensures patient safety.
- Initiate continuous bedside cardiac monitoring (if not already in place). ***Rationale:*** The patient's cardiac rate and

rhythm must be visible at the bedside during the procedure to determine atrial capture during pacing and to evaluate the response of the patient's cardiac rate and rhythm after pacing.
• Obtain a 12-lead ECG as needed. ***Rationale:*** The ECG may aid in determining the patient's baseline cardiac rhythm.

• Assist the patient to the supine position. ***Rationale:*** This position facilitates access to the epicardial pacemaker wires or the transvenous atrial pacing lead wire.
• Obtain the patient's blood pressure via a blood pressure cuff or arterial line. ***Rationale:*** This aids in assessment of the patient's baseline blood pressure and hemodynamic response to rapid atrial pacing.

Procedure   **for Performing Atrial Overdrive Pacing**

Visit https://www.youtube.com/watch?v=zLHRQFFaAzw for a short video on how to perform atrial overdrive pacing along with rhythm before and after atrial overdrive pacing with a dual-chamber temporary pacemaker.

Steps	Rationale	Special Considerations
1. **HH**		
2. **PE**		Gloves protect the patient from microshock while the pacemaker wires are being handled.[5,9]
3. Attach the connecting (pacing) cable to the external pulse generator, ensuring that the positive (+) pole of the cable is connected to the (+) terminal of the pulse generator and the negative (−) pole of the cable is connected to the (−) terminal.	The connecting cable provides extra length so the pulse generator does not have to be placed on the patient's chest or abdomen.	
4. For epicardial atrial pacing: A. Expose the atrial epicardial pacing wires.	The atrial epicardial wires usually exit the chest to the right of the patient's sternum (see Fig. 39.1).	The atrial epicardial pacing wires can be verified by performing an atrial electrogram (see Procedure 39, Atrial Electrogram).
B. Connect an atrial epicardial pacing wire to the negative terminal of the connecting cable.	The pacing current is delivered through the negative terminal of the pulse generator; an epicardial pacing wire on the atrium must be connected to the negative terminal for the atrium to receive pacing impulses.	
C. Connect a second epicardial pacing wire or a ground wire to the positive terminal of the connecting cable.	The pacing circuit is completed as energy reaches the positive electrode.	If only one atrial pacing wire is present, additional options for a ground wire include an ECG monitoring electrode on the chest near the epicardial pacing wire exit site or a subcutaneous needle in the tissue on the chest. The positive terminal of the connecting cable is connected to the metal snap of the monitoring electrode or the subcutaneous needle hub with a double alligator clip.
5. For transvenous atrial pacing: A. Identify the proximal and the distal electrode connector pins on the external portion of the atrial pacing lead.	The pacing stimulus travels from the pulse generator to the negative terminal, and energy returns to the pulse generator via the positive terminal.	

Procedure continues on following page

UNIT II

Procedure	for Performing Atrial Overdrive Pacing—*Continued*	
Steps	**Rationale**	**Special Considerations**
B. Connect the distal (negative) electrode connector pin to the negative terminal of the connecting cable.	Energy from the pulse generator is directed to the distal electrode in contact with the atrium.	
C. Connect the proximal (positive) electrode connecting pin to the positive terminal of the connecting cable.	The pacing circuit is completed as energy reaches the positive electrode.	
6. Set the rate and the milliampere (mA/output) controls on the pulse generator.	The settings are based on the characteristics of the patient's dysrhythmia and the threshold needed for atrial capture.	
7. Initiate atrial overdrive pacing. Pace the atrium for a brief period of 30 seconds to 2 minutes, and then abruptly terminate pacing (Figs. 40.2 and 40.3).	Short bursts of pacing stimuli at a rapid rate are intended to create refractory tissue in the atrium and interrupt the reentry circuit responsible for the tachydysrhythmia.	Bursts can be repeated at faster rates and for longer intervals until the dysrhythmia terminates or changes.
A. Pace the heart with 20 mA at a rate 20%–30% faster than the intrinsic atrial rate for 30 seconds, and then stop pacing.		Refer to the manufacturer's recommendations in the pulse generator's technical manual for instructions on how to initiate rapid atrial pacing.

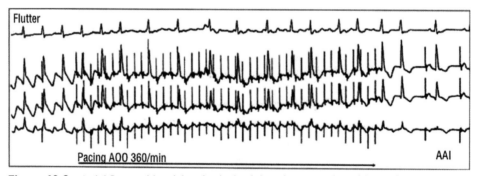

Figure 40.2   Atrial flutter with atrial pacing in the right atrium *(Panel A)* with entrainment achieved at the *asterisk*. Cessation of rapid atrial pacing led to conversion to sinus rhythm *(Panel B)*. *(From Cosio FG, Pastor A, Nunez, A, Magalhaes AP, Awamieh P. Atrial flutter: an update.* Revista Espanola de Cardiologia. *2006;59(8):822.)*

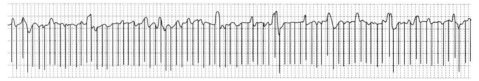

Figure 40.3   Rhythm strip showing rapid atrial pacing in an attempt to terminate atrial flutter.

UNIT II

Procedure for Performing Atrial Overdrive Pacing—*Continued*		
Steps	Rationale	Special Considerations
B. An alternate approach is to initiate atrial pacing at a rate 20 beats/min faster than the intrinsic atrial rate; if 1:1 capture does not occur after 30 seconds, increase the paced rate by 20 beats/min; repeat every 30 seconds until 1:1 capture is achieved. Continue pacing until the heart rate decreases from AV block (e.g., 2:1, 3:1) or 1–2 minutes of 1:1 pacing have occurred, and then stop pacing.[9] (**Level E***)		On termination of the dysrhythmia, the sinus node may be suppressed for a period, resulting in bradycardia, asystole, junctional or ventricular escape rhythms, or ventricular tachycardia. Initiation of temporary atrial, ventricular, or transcutaneous pacing may be necessary until normal sinus function returns.
Perform a 12-lead ECG to verify the rhythm after overdrive pacing. When atrial pacing is completed, disconnect the connecting cable from the epicardial pacing wires or from the transvenous pacing electrode connector pins.	Removes the rapid atrial pacemaker.	Standard pacemaker therapy can be initiated if necessary.
9. Apply a sterile occlusive dressing to the pacemaker site if not already in place.	May reduce the incidence of infection.	
10. Protect the exposed pacemaker electrode connector pins or epicardial pacemaker wires with an insulating material (e.g., finger cot, needle cap, needle barrel, glove, ear plug).[5,9] (**Level E***)	Prevents microshock, which can result in symptomatic dysrhythmias.	
11. Secure the pacing wires or connector pins.	Prevents accidental dislodgment.	
12. Label each epicardial pacemaker wire or dressing to identify atrial and ventricular pacing wires.	Aids in identification of the epicardial pacemaker wires.	
13. Remove gloves, and discard used supplies in appropriate receptacles.	Reduces the transmission of microorganisms; standard precautions.	
14. 🖐️		

*Level E: Multiple case reports, theory-based evidence from expert opinions, or peer-reviewed professional organizational standards without clinical studies to support recommendations.

Expected Outcomes

- Return to normal sinus rhythm
- Stable or improved hemodynamic status

Unexpected Outcomes

- Continuation of tachydysrhythmia
- Conversion to atrial fibrillation
- Prolonged period of bradycardia or asystole after termination of tachydysrhythmia
- Rapid conduction of atrial paced impulses to the ventricle through an accessory pathway, resulting in ventricular tachycardia or ventricular fibrillation
- Emergence of a slow junctional or ventricular escape rhythm or ventricular tachycardia after termination of the tachydysrhythmia
- Microshock that results in ventricular tachycardia or fibrillation
- Pain

Procedure continues on following page

Patient Monitoring and Care

Steps	Rationale	Reportable Conditions
		These conditions should be reported to the provider if they persist despite nursing interventions.
1. Monitor the patient's cardiac rhythm continuously at the bedside during the procedure and after the procedure.	Allows for immediate recognition of rhythm changes or return of the initial tachydysrhythmia.	• Heart rate or rhythm changes • Return of initial tachydysrhythmia • Any significant or hemodynamically unstable dysrhythmia • Need for additional temporary pacing to maintain adequate heart rate after conversion of the tachydysrhythmia
2. Monitor the patient's vital signs before initiating overdrive pacing, every 5–10 minutes during attempts to overdrive pace, with any significant heart rate or rhythm change during the procedure, and on termination of the procedure. If the patient's condition is not hemodynamically stable after the procedure, monitor vital signs every 5–10 minutes until stable. Monitor vital signs per institutional standards if the patient's condition is stable after the procedure.	Changes in vital signs may indicate significant change in the patient's condition. Blood pressure often improves with cessation of the tachydysrhythmia or restoration of normal sinus rhythm; blood pressure may deteriorate if the ventricular rate accelerates because of overdrive pacing. If the patient is receiving antidysrhythmic medications, changes in vital signs may indicate an adverse medication reaction.	• Abnormal heart rate or rhythm • Hypotension
3. Replace gauze dressings every 2 days and transparent dressings at least every 7 days.[6] Cleanse the site with an antiseptic solution (e.g., 2% chlorhexidine-based solution). Follow institutional standards. **(Level D*)**	Although guidelines specific to epicardial wires and transvenous pacemaker sites do not exist, the U.S. Centers for Disease Control and Prevention (CDC) recommend replacing dressings on intravascular catheters when the dressing becomes damp, loosened, or soiled or when inspection of the site is necessary.[6]	• Redness or exudate around the site • Increased white blood cell count, increased band neutrophil values • Elevated temperature
4. Monitor the patient's response to antidysrhythmic medications.	Antidysrhythmic medications may be necessary to prevent recurrence of the initial tachydysrhythmia or to control the ventricular rate.[7]	• Prolonged QT interval • Rhythm changes
5. Follow institutional standards for assessing pain. Administer analgesia as prescribed.	Identifies the need for pain interventions.	• Continued pain despite pain interventions

*Level D: Peer-reviewed professional and organizational standards with the support of clinical study recommendations.

Documentation

Documentation should include the following:

- Signed informed consent, if nonemergent
- Universal protocol requirements, if nonemergent
- Patient and family education provided and an evaluation of their understanding of the procedure
- Rhythm strip documenting initial cardiac rate and rhythm
- Initial vital signs
- Pacemaker settings for each attempt of overdrive pacing: rate, mA, duration
- Rhythm strip documenting each overdrive pacing burst
- Number of pacing attempts
- Patient's response to the procedure (e.g., anxiety, pain)
- Pain assessment, interventions, and effectiveness
- Postprocedure rhythm strip
- Postprocedure vital signs
- Any medications given during procedure
- Any unexpected outcomes
- Additional interventions

References and Additional Readings

For a complete list of references and additional readings for this procedure, scan this QR code with your smartphone, or visit https://www.elsevier.com/__data/assets/pdf_file/0010/1319815/Chapter0040.pdf.

41 Temporary Epicardial Pacing AP Wire Removal

Marion E. McRae

PURPOSE: Temporary epicardial pacing wires are inserted into the epicardium during cardiac surgery and are removed when pacing therapy is no longer needed.

PREREQUISITE NURSING KNOWLEDGE

- Knowledge of cardiovascular anatomy and physiology is necessary.
- Knowledge of where the atrial, ventricular, and ground wires exit on the chest is necessary.
- Temporary epicardial pacing wires can be unipolar wires (Fig. 41.1) or bipolar wires (Fig. 41.2).
- Knowledge of the function of epicardial pacing wires is necessary.
- Advanced cardiac life support knowledge and skills are needed.
- Principles of general electrical safety must be applied with use of temporary epicardial pacemaker wires.[21]
- Gloves always should be worn when handling epicardial pacemaker electrodes to prevent microshock because even small amounts of electrical current can cause serious dysrhythmias if they are transmitted to the heart.[1,26]
- Knowledge of cardiac dysrhythmias and treatment of life-threatening dysrhythmias is necessary.
- Relative contraindications to epicardial pacing wire removal include abnormal coagulation study results (elevated international normalized ratio [INR], partial thromboplastin time [PTT], heparin level, or heparin anti-Xa level), very low platelet counts, presence of dysrhythmias that necessitate pacing, and compromised hemodynamic status.[7,8,21] Acceptable levels for INR, PTT, heparin level, anti-Xa level, and platelet counts before epicardial pacing wire removal are determined by institutional policy. Low-dose aspirin therapy is not a contraindication to epicardial pacing wire removal. Direct oral anticoagulants (DOACs) pose a bleeding risk and should be held for at least 24 hours (or longer with reduced renal function) before pacing wire removal per institutional policy.[6]

AP This procedure should be performed only by clinicians who have demonstrated competence and are credentialed to perform it. In addition, the procedure must be within the scope of practice defined by their professional licensure, and in accordance with professional practice acts. Physicians, advanced practice nurses, and physician assistants may be credentialed to perform this procedure.

- Knowledge of the signs and symptoms of cardiac tamponade is needed (e.g., hemodynamic instability, dyspnea, muffled heart sounds, diaphoresis with cool skin, equalizing pulmonary artery pressures, jugular venous distention, pulsus paradoxus, narrowed pulse pressure, orthopnea, altered level of consciousness or mental status).[20,28]
- Epicardial pacing wires should not be cut but should be removed unless excessive force is needed to remove them (3% to 4% of wires are cut and left in situ as a result of extreme resistance on removal[31]). Retained epicardial pacing wires can cause long-term problems. The wires can eventually protrude through the skin, cause local infection or infective endocarditis,[10] or migrate within the heart[32] and outside the heart. There are documented cases of pacing wires being found in the jaw,[17] breast,[13] carotid artery,[15] diaphragm,[2] and colon[29] causing paracardiac masses[16] resulting in serious tissue and organ injury. If there is difficulty pulling an epicardial pacing wire because of resistance, an anterior and lateral chest x-ray may identify if the wire is trapped under a sternal wire or wrapped around anatomical structures.
- Although it is not recommended, if cut epicardial pacemaker wires are left in situ, the patient must be educated about the warning signs to look for (e.g., redness, pain, drainage, fever) and to identify that the wires are in situ before magnetic resonance image (MRI) scanning. Although MRI scanning with retained epicardial wires may be safe at 1.5 Tesla,[5,19,24,25,31] institutions may have their own policies about this. The concern with higher magnetic field strength is heating of the wires and cardiac damage. If problems develop with retained wires, they will need to be surgically removed.
- Complications have been reported to occur in less than 1% of patients having temporary epicardial pacing wires removed.[3,9,11,18,20,22]

EQUIPMENT

- Nonsterile gloves
- Antiseptic solution (e.g., 2% chlorhexidine-based solution)
- Suture removal kit
- Sterile gauze
- Tape

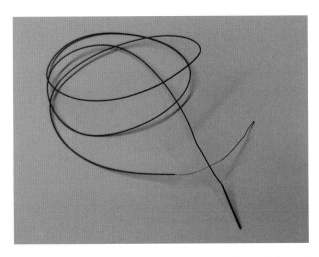

Figure 41.1 Unipolar pacemaker wire. One electrode is on the heart *(uninsulated section, upper right),* and one pin is connected to the temporary pacemaker cable *(bottom right).*

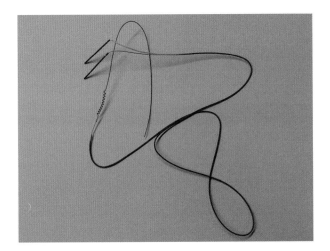

Figure 41.2 Bipolar pacemaker wire. Two electrodes (straight and coiled, uninsulated section of the wire) split into two pins to connect to the temporary pacemaker cable.

Additional equipment to have available as needed includes the following:
- Emergency equipment including resuscitation cart and sternotomy tray (see Procedure 35: Emergent Open Sternotomy (Assist) and Defibrillation (Internal) Assist)
- Temporary transcutaneous or transvenous pacing equipment

PATIENT AND FAMILY EDUCATION

- Assess patient and family readiness to learn and identify factors that affect learning. *Rationale:* This assessment allows the nurse to individualize teaching.
- Provide information about the epicardial pacing wires, the reason for their removal, and an explanation of the procedure. *Rationale:* This information helps the patient and family understand the procedure and why it is needed and may decrease anxiety.
- Explain the patient's expected participation during and after the procedure. *Rationale:* Encourages patient participation in the treatment plan and may decrease anxiety.

- Explain that the patient may feel pain and a burning or pulling sensation during the procedure.[23,27] *Rationale:* This explanation prepares the patient for the procedure.

PATIENT ASSESSMENT AND PREPARATION

Patient Assessment

- Assess the patient's baseline cardiovascular, hemodynamic, and peripheral vascular status. *Rationale:* This assessment provides data that can be used for comparison with postremoval assessment data and hemodynamic values.
- Assess the patient's current laboratory data, including electrolyte and coagulation study results. *Rationale:* This assessment identifies laboratory abnormalities. Baseline coagulation studies (INR [if on warfarin], PTT or heparin levels [if on heparin], anti-Xa levels [if on low-molecular-weight heparin]) and platelet counts are helpful in determining the patient's risk for bleeding.[8] Electrolyte abnormalities such as hypokalemia, hyperkalemia, or hypomagnesemia may increase cardiac irritability.
- Ensure that the patient is not fully anticoagulated and/ or that the platelet count is not very low. Based on the half-life of heparin (1.5 hours),[14] discontinue a heparin infusion 2 to 4 hours before pacemaker wire removal and begin the heparin infusion 1 hour after pacemaker removal as long as there is no apparent bleeding.[8,14] Remove pacemaker wires at the nadir of low-molecular-weight heparin doses, or hold for several hours when the next dose is due. Ensure that the INR is less than 1.5 to 2 before removing pacemaker wires if the patient is on warfarin.[8,21] Ensure DOACs have been discontinued at least 24 hours (longer with reduced renal function)[6] per institutional policy. When possible, remove the epicardial pacing wires before beginning anticoagulants. Ensure that the platelet count is greater than 50,000. Always check institutional policy for guidelines about acceptable laboratory values or periods to hold medications before epicardial pacemaker wire removal. *Rationale:* Bleeding is more likely to occur if the patient is anticoagulated or the platelet count is low.

Patient Preparation

- Verify the correct patient with two identifiers. *Rationale:* Before performing a procedure, the nurse should ensure the correct identification of the patient for the intended intervention.
- Ensure that the patient and family understand preprocedural teaching. Answer questions as they arise, and reinforce information as needed. *Rationale:* Evaluates and reinforces understanding of previously taught information.
- Remove epicardial pacing wires at least the day before discharge (approximately 24 hours or longer).[21] *Rationale:* Removal at this time provides time for observation for potential complications.
- Remove epicardial pacing wires at a time of the day when access to echocardiography and surgical services is immediately available. *Rationale:* Cardiac tamponade is an emergency that must be dealt with rapidly.

UNIT II

• Administer prescribed analgesic medication before removing the epicardial pacing wires.[23,27] ***Rationale:*** Analgesics may minimize discomfort during epicardial pacing wire removal. Patients report pain and a burning or pulling sensation during the procedure.[23,27]

• Determine the patency of an intravenous (IV) catheter. ***Rationale:*** A patent IV is necessary should emergency fluids, blood, or medications be needed.

• Ensure that patient has electrocardiographic (ECG) monitoring. ***Rationale:*** ECG monitoring provides assessment for the presence of potential dysrhythmias during epicardial wire removal.[4]

Procedure	**for Epicardial Pacing Wire Removal**	
Steps	Rationale	Special Considerations
1. 🄷🄷		
2. 🄿🄴		Gloves minimize the possibility of microshock when in contact with the epicardial pacing wires.[1,26]
3. Assist the patient into the supine position with the head of the bed raised 30 degrees.	This position provides the best access during the procedure.	Epicardial pacing wires are removed with the patient lying in bed.
4. Touch a large metal object such as the patient bed before touching the wires to ensure that any static electricity is discharged.[1,26] **(Level E*)**	Static electricity could be conducted to the pacemaker wires resulting in microshock.	
5. Remove the dressing and tape over the epicardial wires. Identify each wire so you are clear whether it is an atrial wire, a ground wire, or a ventricular wire (see Fig. 41.3 for the usual location of atrial and ventricular wires).	Exposes the epicardial wire exit sites.	

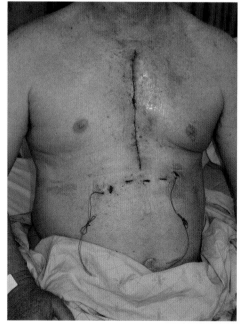

Figure 41.3 Temporary epicardial wires on the right side of the patient's chest are generally atrial wires. Wires exiting the left side of the patient's chest are generally ventricular wires.

Procedure continues on following page

Procedure for Epicardial Pacing Wire Removal—*Continued*

Steps	Rationale	Special Considerations
6. Cleanse each of the epicardial pacing wire exit sites with an antiseptic solution (e.g., 2% chlorhexidine solution).	May reduce the risk of infection.	Cleanse at least a 3-inch area around each of the exit sites.
7. Untie or cut the suture knot of each of the epicardial pacing wires at the skin.	Prepares for epicardial pacing wire removal.	
8. Obtain an ECG strip, and observe the patient's ECG monitor while removing epicardial wires.	Ensures you have documented the preprocedure rhythm. Dysrhythmias may occur during epicardial wire removal, particularly ventricular ectopy.[4]	
9. Remove each epicardial atrial pacing wire and then right ventricular epicardial pacing wires by pulling with steady, slow, gentle tension. There may also be epicardial wires on the left ventricle for right atrial–left ventricular or biventricular pacing that require removal.[12] Ground pacing wires are anchored only in the skin and are removed similar to skin sutures.	Steady, slow, gentle tension uncoils the pacing lead from the epicardial surface of the heart. Removing the atrial wires first allows ventricular pacing if hemodynamic instability occurs.	Follow institutional standards. If slow, steady, gentle tension does not remove the wires, discontinue the procedure and notify the surgeon. Wires can become trapped in adhesions.
10. Inspect each epicardial pacing wire to ensure that each wire is intact and to assess for the presence of tissue on the tip of the wires.[10] (**Level E***)	Ensures that each epicardial wire extracted is completely intact.	If bleeding occurs at the epicardial pacing wire site, apply direct pressure until bleeding stops. If tissue is noted on the epicardial wire(s), observe the patient for hemodynamic instability. Notify the physician if tissue is noted on the epicardial wire(s) and if bleeding or oozing continues.
11. Apply a sterile dressing over the epicardial exit sites.	Decreases the risk of infection until the exit sites heal. Contains drainage from the site.	
12. Remove **PE**, and discard used supplies in an appropriate receptacle.	Reduces the transmission of microorganisms and body secretions; standard precautions.	
13. **HH**		

*Level E: Multiple case reports, theory-based evidence from expert opinions, or peer-reviewed professional organizational standards without clinical studies to support recommendations.

Expected Outcomes

- Removal of the epicardial pacing wires
- Stable cardiac rate and rhythm
- Stable vital signs

Unexpected Outcomes

- Dysrhythmias
- Hemodynamic instability
- Pain
- Hemorrhage
- Cardiac tamponade
- Hematoma
- Infection
- Coronary graft laceration[22]

UNIT II

Patient Monitoring and Care

Steps	Rationale	Reportable Conditions
		These conditions should be reported to the provider if they occur.
1. Ask the patient to let you know if any pain, changes in breathing, sweating, or lightheadedness occur. (**Level C***)	These signs and symptoms have been found to correlate with cardiac tamponade after pacemaker wire removal.[20] Dyspnea has a sensitivity of 87%–89% for cardiac tamponade[28] and was the most common symptom reported by patients with cardiac tamponade.[20]	• Dyspnea • Bleeding • Palpitations • Diaphoresis • Chest pressure • Presyncope
2. After the epicardial wires are removed, monitor vital signs frequently for at least 2 hours. Follow institutional standards. (**Level C***)	Determines the patient's hemodynamic status. Abrupt hypotension can occur within 4 hours of pacemaker wire removal although in some cases it can also be delayed if tamponade occurs more slowly.[20]	• Abnormal vital signs
3. Continue ECG monitoring for at least 24 hours after removal of epicardial pacing wires.[21] (**Level E***)	Provides assessment of possible dysrhythmias.	• Dysrhythmias • ECG changes
4. Follow institutional standards regarding activity limitations after epicardial pacing wire removal.	There is little evidence that activity limitation after removal of pacemaker wires prevents complications.[30]	
5. When obtaining vital signs, assess for signs and symptoms of cardiac tamponade. If cardiac tamponade is suspected, a stat echocardiogram or use of a handheld echocardiographic device should be obtained to ascertain the presence of cardiac tamponade. If tamponade has occurred, notify the surgeon immediately, and prepare to assist with plans to surgically or interventionally drain the pericardial effusion.	Early detection is important because cardiac tamponade is a potentially fatal complication.	• Hypotension and tachycardia • Pulsus paradoxus • Beck's triad (jugular venous distention, hypotension, and muffled heart sounds) • Presyncope • Altered level of consciousness • Orthopnea
6. Follow institutional standards for assessing pain. Administer analgesia as prescribed.	Identifies the need for pain interventions.	• Continued pain despite pain interventions

*Level C: Qualitative studies, descriptive or correlational studies, integrative reviews, systematic reviews, or randomized controlled trials with inconsistent results.

*Level E: Multiple case reports, theory-based evidence from expert opinions, or peer-reviewed professional organizational standards without clinical studies to support recommendations.

Documentation

Documentation should include the following:
- Patient and family education
- Removal of epicardial pacing wires
- Patient tolerance of the procedure
- Pain assessment, interventions, and effectiveness
- Site assessment
- Vital signs and ECG strip
- Occurrence of unexpected outcomes and interventions

References and Additional Readings

For a complete list of references and additional readings for this procedure, scan this QR code with your smartphone, or visit https://www.elsevier.com/__data/assets/pdf_ file/0011/1319816/Chapter0041.pdf

PROCEDURE

42 Implantable Cardioverter-Defibrillator: Post-Insertion Care

Kiersten Henry

PURPOSE: The implantable cardioverter-defibrillator (ICD) is a device that is used to prevent sudden cardiac death from malignant ventricular dysrhythmias. The ICD continuously monitors a patient's rhythm and attempts to convert ventricular tachycardia or ventricular fibrillation via antitachycardia pacing, defibrillation, or some combination of these. Electric cardioversion for arrhythmias may be delivered manually through the ICD by a healthcare provider if deemed appropriate for atrial or ventricular arrhythmias that do not trigger automatic therapies from the ICD. The ICD has the capability for backup bradycardia pacing.

PREREQUISITE NURSING KNOWLEDGE

- Knowledge of the anatomy and physiology of the cardio-vascular system, principles of cardiac conduction, and basic dysrhythmia interpretation.
- Knowledge of basic functioning of ICDs and patient response to ICD therapy.
- Knowledge of principles of defibrillation threshold, anti-dysrhythmia medications, alteration in electrolytes, and effect on the defibrillation threshold.
- Advanced cardiac life support (ACLS) knowledge and skills.
- Clinical and technical competence related to use of the external defibrillator.
- Indications for ICD implantation, based on the 2012 Update of the American College of Cardiology (ACC)/American Heart Association (AHA)/Heart Rhythm Society (HRS) guidelines[6,12] Class I:
  - ❖ Indicated in survivors of cardiac arrest because of ventricular fibrillation (VF) or sustained unstable ventricular tachycardia (VT)
  - ❖ Patients with structural heart disease and sustained VT (hemodynamically stable or unstable)
  - ❖ Patients with syncope of undetermined origin with hemodynamically significant VT or VF at electrophysiology study (EPS)
  - ❖ Patients with nonischemic dilated cardiomyopathy (DCM) with left ventricular ejection fraction (LVEF) less than or equal to 35%, New York Heart Association (NYHA) functional class II or III
  - ❖ Patients with LVEF less than 35% because of prior myocardial infarction (MI; more than 40 days after MI), NYHA class II or III; or LVEF less than 30%, NYHA functional class I
  - ❖ Patients with nonsustained VT as a result of prior MI, LVEF less than 40%, with inducible VF or sustained VT at EPS

- Class IIa: Reasonable for:
  - ❖ Patients with unexplained syncope, significant left ventricular (LV) dysfunction, nonischemic dilated cardiomyopathy
  - ❖ Patients with sustained VT with normal or near-normal ventricular function
  - ❖ Patients with hypertrophic cardiomyopathy (HCM) or arrhythmogenic right ventricular dysplasia (ARVD) and with one or more major risk factors for sudden cardiac death (SCD). Patients with long QT syndrome who are having syncope or VT while receiving beta blockers
  - ❖ Patients who are not hospitalized and awaiting transplantation who are at high risk for sudden cardiac death (e.g., left ventricular ejection fraction <35%, on home inotropic therapy)
  - ❖ Patients with Brugada syndrome, with either syncope or with documented VT, that has not resulted in cardiac arrest
  - ❖ Patients with catecholaminergic polymorphic VT with syncope or documented sustained VT on beta blocker therapy
  - ❖ Patients with cardiac sarcoidosis, giant cell myocarditis, or Chagas disease
- Class IIb: May be considered in:
  - ❖ Patients with nonischemic cardiomyopathy with LVEF less than or equal to 35%, NYHA functional class I
  - ❖ Patients with long QT syndrome and risk factors for SCD
  - ❖ Patients with syncope and advanced structural heart disease in whom thorough invasive and noninvasive investigations have failed to define a cause
  - ❖ Patients with familial cardiomyopathy associated with SCD
  - ❖ Patients with LV noncompaction
- Class III: Not indicated in:
  - ❖ Patients without a clinical expectation of survival for at least 1 year (with reasonable functional status), even if other implantation criteria are met

- Patients with refractory VT or VF
- Patients with significant psychiatric illness that may affect device implantation or the patient's ability to follow up
- Patients who have NYHA class IV heart failure that is refractory to drug therapy and are not candidates for transplantation or cardiac resynchronization therapy
- Patients with syncope of undetermined cause and no evidence of inducible ventricular tachyarrhythmias or structural heart disease
- Patients with VF/VT that can be treated with catheter or surgical ablation
- Patients with ventricular dysrhythmias due to a reversible disorder (such as electrolyte imbalance or medications) without evidence of structural heart disease.

- Indications for subcutaneous ICD implantation, based on the 2017 guideline for management of patients with ventricular arrhythmias and the prevention of sudden cardiac death from the American Heart Association (AHA)/American College of Cardiology (ACC)/Heart Rhythm Society (HRS)[1]:
  - Class I: Indicated in patients who meet criteria for an ICD with inadequate vascular access or high risk for infection. These patients must not have an anticipated need for pacing for bradycardia or termination of VT
  - Class IIa: Indicated in patients who meet indication for ICD and do not have an anticipated need for pacing to treat bradycardia or terminate VT
  - Class III: Contraindicated in: patients with an indication for bradycardia pacing or cardiac resynchronization therapy or for whom antitachycardia pacing is required.

- A specific time period of guideline-driven medical therapy must be initiated before implantation of an ICD. The indication for implantation determines the necessary waiting period:
  - Patients with any cardiomyopathy not on optimal medical therapy must be reassessed for eligibility after 3 months.
  - Patients who are post-MI or post–ischemic cardiomyopathy and are revascularized with percutaneous coronary intervention or coronary artery bypass must be reassessed for eligibility after 3 months.
  - Patients who are post-MI without revascularization must be reassessed for eligibility after 40 days.
  - Patients with any cardiomyopathy who have been on guideline-directed medical therapy for the required interval can be referred for ICD implantation.[1]
- The ICD system is composed of a pulse generator and a lead system. The pulse generator is titanium and contains the capacitors, circuitry, and a lithium battery (Fig. 42.1).
- Battery longevity may be greater than 5 years, depending on the number of times therapies are delivered and the frequency of pacing.[25] The pulse generator is typically located in a pectoral subcutaneous pocket.
- The leads are insulated wires that sense the patient's intrinsic rhythm and can pace or deliver therapies (see Fig. 42.1). Leads are classified as atrial or ventricular, endocardial (transvenous) or epicardial (myocardial), unipolar or

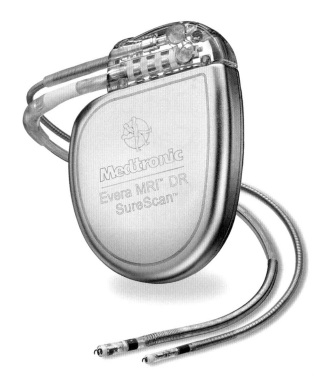

Figure 42.1 ICD and transvenous lead system. *(Images used with permission from Medtronic, plc © 2022.)*

bipolar, and active or passive fixation. The lead systems may be single, double (dual), or multiple (biventricular).
- Leads may be attached to the heart via active or passive fixation. Active fixation leads use a screw, barb, or hook at the tip that is embedded into the myocardium to ensure stability of the lead. Passive fixation leads (which are infrequently used) use tines or fins at the tip that allow the lead to attach to trabeculae of the myocardium.
- Most leads are endocardial (transvenous) leads and are inserted transvenously through the subclavian, cephalic, or axillary veins.
- Epicardial leads are less common but are used in special circumstances. Epicardial pacing leads may be placed on the outside of the left ventricle to provide biventricular pacing when coronary sinus placement of the LV lead has been unsuccessful. Epicardial leads may be placed during cardiac surgery.
- All leads have a cathode (negative pole) and an anode (positive pole). A unipolar lead uses one conductor wire, with a distal electrode as the cathode and the metal can as the anode. This configuration produces a large electrical circuit and a large pacing artifact on electrocardiography (ECG). Because of the large area covered, this configuration is susceptible to stimulation of chest muscles and also to electromagnetic interference. A bipolar lead uses two electrodes on the distal end of the lead to form the circuit. The cathode is located at the distal tip, and the anode is located several millimeters proximal to the tip. Because of the closer circuitry, a smaller pacing artifact is seen on ECG.
- All ICDs function as pacemakers. Some ICDs are also biventricular pacemakers if they have leads in the right and left ventricles. Cardiac resynchronization therapy (CRT)

paces the right and left ventricles together to establish synchrony in an effort to improve LV function.[21] Biventricular pacing must be as close to 100% as possible for the greatest benefit. Biventricular pacing leads are placed in the right atrium, the right ventricle, and an epicardial vein on the surface of the left ventricle accessed through the coronary sinus. Patients must be on guideline-directed medical therapy before placement of a device for CRT. Indications for biventricular pacing, based on the 2012 Update of the American College of Cardiology (ACC)/ American Heart Association (AHA)/ Heart Rhythm Society (HRS) guidelines[12]:

❖ Class I: Indicated in:
  ○ Patients with LVEF less than or equal to 35%, left bundle branch block (LBBB) with a QRS duration greater than or equal to 150 ms, NYHA class II to IV symptoms, and sinus rhythm
❖ Class IIa: May be useful in:
  ○ Patients with LVEF less than or equal to 35%, LBBB with a QRS duration 120 to 149 ms or non-LBBB pattern with QRS duration greater than or equal to 150 ms, NYHA class II to IV symptoms, and sinus rhythm
  ○ Patients with ejection fraction less than or equal to 35% who require ventricular pacing for other reasons
  ○ Patients with ejection fraction less than or equal to 35% who are undergoing new or replacement device placement and are expected to have ventricular pacing greater than 40% of the time
❖ Class IIb: May be considered in:
  ○ Patients with ischemic cardiomyopathy, LVEF less than or equal to 30%, LBBB with a QRS greater than or equal to 150 ms, NYHA class I symptoms, and sinus rhythm
  ○ Patients with LVEF of less than or equal to 35%, a non-LBBB pattern with QRS 120 to 149 ms, NYHA class III/IV symptoms, and sinus rhythm
  ○ Patients with LVEF of less than or equal to 35%, a non-LBBB pattern with QRS greater than or equal to 150 ms, NYHA class II symptoms, and sinus rhythm
❖ Class III: Not indicated in:
  ○ Patients with a non-LBBB pattern and QRS duration less than 150 ms who have NYHA class I/II symptoms
  ○ Patients whose expected survival with good functional capacity is less than 1 year

• The ICD detects tachydysrhythmias, delivers antitachycardia pacing (ATP) or electrical therapy (shock), and provides bradycardia pacing. ATP attempts to convert monomorphic VT by pacing at a rate faster than the VT rate, thereby terminating the dysrhythmia. ATP is a painless way of treating VT, sometimes avoiding shock therapy altogether. The PainFree II trial demonstrated that compared with shocks, empirical ATP for fast VT was highly effective, was equally safe, and improved quality of life.[24] Defibrillation is not synchronized and is generally used to convert ventricular dysrhythmias.[10]

• The ICD therapies may be programmed from one to three zones based on detected heart rate sensed by the ventricular lead. The device may be programmed to differentiate between supraventricular tachycardia (SVT) and VF/VT using certain parameters such as onset of the tachyarrhythmia, stability, or regularity of the rhythm and QRS morphology to avoid inappropriate shocks for supraventricular tachycardia. Tachycardia detection windows that require a certain number of sensed consecutive ventricular beats before tachyarrhythmia therapies are initiated are also programmed (e.g., 30 of 40 beats) to avoid unnecessary shocks because some rhythms will spontaneously terminate. Additional zones based on heart rates (201 to 250 and >250) allow for more aggressive management of tachyarrhythmias. Zones may be programmed for sequential therapies of ATP followed by electrical defibrillation if ATP is unsuccessful. Programming of multiple zones helps reduce inappropriate defibrillator shocks.[13,20,30]

• A defibrillator code was developed in 1993 by the North American Society of Pacing and Electrophysiology and the British Pacing and Electrophysiology Group to describe the capabilities and operation of ICDs. The defibrillator code is patterned after the pacemaker code; however, it has some important differences (Table 42.1).[5] The defibrillator code offers less information about the ICD's antibradycardia pacing function but more specific information about the shock functions.

• A magnet (Fig. 42.2A) applied over an ICD disables the device therapies of ATP and electrical /defibrillation but does not affect pacemaker function. The magnet is used during procedures that may cause electromagnetic interference (EMI). EMI from cautery devices, for example, may be improperly sensed as a tachydysrhythmia, possibly leading to inappropriate device shock. In most models, removal of the magnet restores normal ICD function. Some models, however, do not resume previous settings once the magnet is removed.[4] If a device programmer (see

TABLE 42.1 NASPE/BPEG Defibrillator Code

Position I	Position II	Position III	Position IV
Shock Chamber	Antitachycardia Pacing Chamber	Tachycardia Detection	Antibradycardia Pacing Chamber
O = none	O = none	E = electrogram	O = none
A = atrium	A = atrium	H = hemodynamic	A = atrium
V = ventricle	V = ventricle		V = ventricle
D = dual (A + V)	D = dual (A + V)		D = dual (A + V)

NASPE/BPEG, North American Society of Pacing and Electrophysiology/British Pacing and Electrophysiology Group.
From Bernstein AD, et al: The NASPE/BPEG defibrillator code (NBD code). *Pacing Clin Electrophysiol,* 16, 1776, 1993.

Fig. 42.2B) and trained personnel are available, device tachydysrhythmia detection and therapies can be disabled through the programmer for the duration of the procedure.

- Emotional adjustments vary with each patient and family. Patients may experience depression, anxiety, fear, and anger. Some patients view the device as an activity restriction, and others see it as a life-saving device that allows normal life to resume. Preimplantation psychological variables, such as degree of optimism or pessimism, and an anxious personality style may place patients at a higher risk for difficulty adjusting to the ICD.[22] Support groups may serve a vital role for ICD recipients who are anxious and for patients who may need additional support. Education interventions with patients and family members help reduce psychosocial distress. Delivery of shock is shown to increase the risk of posttraumatic stress disorder in patients with ICDs.[18,22]

- The option of ICD deactivation should be discussed before the device is implanted.[28] Early discussions of device deactivation facilitate later discussions and are an important part of shared decision making and the informed consent process.[7,17,29]

For patients with a contraindication to a transvenous implanted cardioverter-defibrillator, including patients with complex vascular anatomy or high risk for infection, the subcutaneous-implanted cardioverter defibrillator (S-ICD) is a therapeutic option. The S-ICD, implanted in the left axillary area, provides defibrillation but not pacing therapies.[15]

EQUIPMENT

- ECG monitor and recorder
- ECG electrodes
  Additional equipment to have available as needed includes the following:
- ICD programmer (commonly obtained from the electrophysiology department or specific manufacturer)
- Magnet (doughnut or bar type)
- 12-lead ECG machine
- Analgesia and sedation as prescribed
- Emergency medications and resuscitation equipment
- Antidysrhythmia medications as prescribed

PATIENT AND FAMILY EDUCATION

- Assess learning needs, readiness to learn, and factors that influence learning. *Rationale:* This assessment allows the nurse to individualize teaching in a meaningful manner.
- Assess patient and family understanding of ICD therapy and the reason for its use. *Rationale:* This assessment provides information regarding knowledge level and necessity of additional teaching.
- Provide information about the normal conduction system, such as structure of the conduction system, source of the heartbeat, normal and abnormal heart rhythms, symptoms of abnormal heart rhythms, and the potentially life-threatening nature of VT and VF. *Rationale:* Understanding of the conduction system and dangerous dysrhythmias assists the patient and family in recognizing the seriousness of the patient's condition and the need for ICD therapy.

- Provide information about ICD therapy, including the reason for the ICD, device operation, location of the device, types of therapy given by the device, risks and benefits of the device, and follow-up. *Rationale:* Understanding of ICD functioning assists the patient and family in developing realistic perceptions of ICD therapy.

- Discuss postimplant incision care, including inspection of the incision and pocket. The incision is kept dry for several days after the procedure. *Rationale:* The nurse or physician needs to know whether any of the following

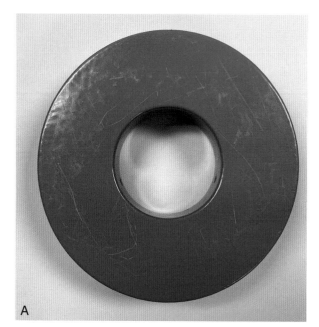

A

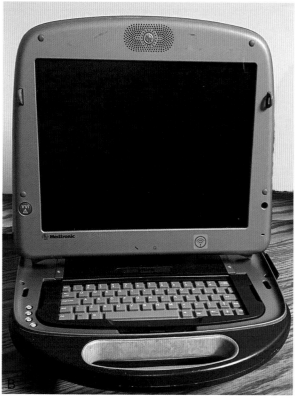

B

Figure 42.2 A, ICD magnet. **B,** ICD device programmer *(Source: Author.)*

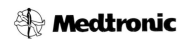

Medtronic **Quick Look**

Device: En Trust Serial Number: Date of Interrogation: **-Feb-2007 16:08:52**

Patient: Physician:

				Measured on:
1	**Device Status (Implanted: 13-Jun-2006)**			
	Battery Voltage (ERI=2.61 V)	3.17 V		24-Feb-2007
	Last Full Energy Charge	7.9 sec		13-Dec-2006
2		**Atrial(5076)**	**RV**	
	Pacing Impedance	488 ohms	504 ohms	24-Feb-2007
	Defibrillation Impedance		RV=76 ohms	24-Feb-2007
	Programmed Amplitude/Pulse Width	3 V / 0.4 ms	3 V / 0.4 ms	
3	Measured P/R Wave	3 mV	20 mV	24-Feb-2007
	Programmed Sensitivity	0.3 mV	0.45 mV	

4	**Parameter Summary**					
	Mode AAI<=>DDD	Lower Rate	60 bpm	Paced AV	180 ms
	Mode Switch 171 bpm	Upper Track	130 bpm	Sensed AV	150 ms
		Upper Sensor	130 bpm		

5	**Detection**		**Rates**	**Therapies**
	AT/AF	Monitor	>171 bpm	All Rx Off
	VF	On	>200 bpm	ATP During Charging, 25J, 35J × 5
	FVT	OFF		All Rx Off
	VT	On	171-200 bpm	Burst(3), Ramp(3), 20J, 35J × 3

Enhancements On: AF/All, Sinus Tach

	Clinical Status	**Since 24-Oct-2006**
6	**Treated**	
	VF	0
	FVT (Off)	
	VT	1
	AT/AF (Monitor)	
7	**Monitored**	
	VT (Off)	
	VT-NS (>4 beats, >171 bpm)	3
	SVT: VT/VF Rx Withheld	0
	AT/AF	1
	Time in AT/AF	<0.1 hr/day (<0.1%)
	Longest AT/AF	2 hours
	Functional	**Last Week**
	Patient Activity	0.9 hr/day

Cardiac Compass Trends (Jun-2006 to Feb-2007)

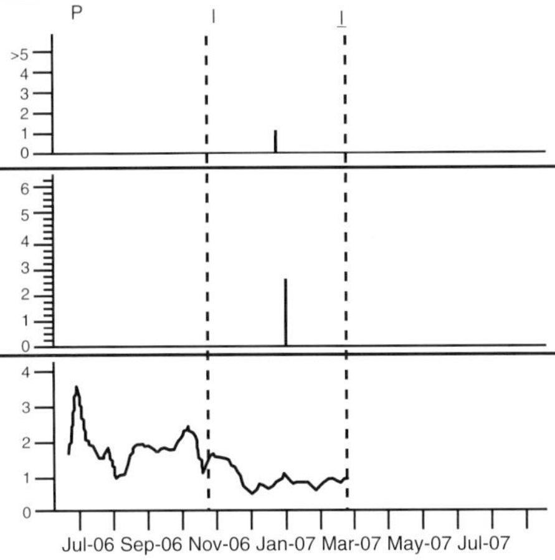
Treated VT/VF (#/day)
AT/AF (hr/day)
Patient Activity (hr/day)
Jul-06 Sep-06 Nov-06 Jan-07 Mar-07 May-07 Jul-07

9	**Therapy Summary**	**VT/VF**	**AT/AF**
	Pace-Terminated Episodes	1 of 1	0
	Shock-Terminated Episodes	0	0
	Total Shocks	0	0
	Aborted Charges	0	0

Pacing	**(% of Time Since 24-Oct-2006)**	8
AS-VS	44.5%	
AS-VP	<0.1%	
AP-VS	55.4%	
AP-VP	<0.1%	
MVP	On	

10	**OBSERVATIONS (1)**
	Patient Activity less than 2 hr/day for 17 weeks.

Medtronic CareLink Network Confidential Patient Information 02-May-2007 16:27:07

Copyright © 2001-2005 Medtronic, Inc Page 1

Figure 42.3 Printout from an ICD interrogation.

signs or symptoms of infection appear: redness, edema, warmth, drainage, and/or fever.

- Discuss postoperative activity. For the first 4 to 6 weeks after implant: (1) no lifting of the arm on the side of the ICD above the shoulder or extending the arm to back (including activities such as swimming, golfing, and bowling); (2) no lifting of items heavier than 10 lb.; and (3) no excessive pushing, pulling, or twisting. *Rationale:* The activity restrictions help prevent new leads from dislodgment.

- Provide patients with an identification card (temporary cards are usually given to patients at the time of implant, and permanent cards are sent to patients by the manufacturer several weeks later). Encourage the patient to wear Medic Alert identification and to carry the identification card at all times. *Rationale:* This identification ensures that appropriate information is available to anyone caring for the patient.

- If patients are prescribed antidysrhythmic medication, stress the importance of continuing the medication. *Rationale:* Antidysrhythmic medications suppress dysrhythmias and may limit potential ICD shocks.

- Discuss the need for patients to keep a current list of medications in their wallets. *Rationale:* The patient or other family members should be prepared to provide necessary information to healthcare providers in an emergency situation.

- Encourage family members to learn community CPR. *Rationale:* Family members may be more prepared for an emergency situation (e.g., if the ICD does not convert a life-threatening rhythm or the ICD malfunctions).

- Educate patients and families about what to do for a device shock. The shock varies in intensity from mild to severe pain. If patients have received an isolated shock and are asymptomatic afterward, they should call their healthcare provider to determine further action (usually an appointment for device interrogation). If patients have received multiple shocks in a short period (within minutes to hours) or if they have had one shock and do not feel well, they should activate the emergency medical services (EMS) system by calling 911 to seek emergency evaluation at an emergency department.[9] *Rationale:* Repeated shocks may indicate conditions that necessitate prompt treatment, such as electrolyte imbalance or ischemia. They may also indicate malfunction of the device sensing, which may occur with lead fracture.

- Inform patients to call their healthcare provider if they hear an audible tone emitted from the device. An audible tone may indicate battery depletion or signal device parameter alerts (such as lead impedance out of normal range). Some devices use vibratory alerts in place of audible tones to signal an alert condition. *Rationale:* The ICD should be interrogated to determine the reason for the tone and to ensure safe device function.

- Inform patients and families that family members are not harmed if they touch the patient when a shock is delivered. *Rationale:* This information prepares the patient and family and may decrease anxiety.

- Driving restrictions vary from state to state and among physicians. Each patient should discuss plans for long trips and driving restrictions with the physician. Current guidelines prohibit anyone with an ICD from obtaining a commercial driver's license.[26] *Rationale:* These restrictions are intended to prevent motor vehicle accidents from sudden loss of consciousness while driving.

- Educate patients and families that the terms *elective replacement indicated* (ERI) and *end of life* (EOL) are used to describe the status of the battery. At ERI, the battery is able to function for approximately another 2 to 3 months. A generator change is performed as soon as possible during this period. At EOL, the generator must be changed promptly. *Rationale:* This teaching prepares patients and families for generator changes, alleviates misunderstanding, and may decrease anxiety.

- Inform patients and family members about follow-up device checks or *interrogations*. Stress the importance of keeping these appointments. Devices are checked every 3 to 6 months (but may be more frequent if any issues arise that necessitate monitoring). Many follow-up checks are now done remotely through Internet-based systems. A transmitter device is mailed to the patient from the device manufacturer.[23] *Rationale:* Routine interrogation maintains optimal functioning of the ICD and alerts providers of dysrhythmias or device issues.

- Inform the patient and family of potential sources of EMI to the ICD. In the hospital, EMI includes magnetic resonance imaging, diathermy, computed tomography, lithotripsy, electrocautery, radiation therapy, and nerve stimulators. Outside the hospital, these include handheld wands used by airport security, arc welders, large transformers or motors, antitheft devices at stores or libraries, cellular phones less than 6 inches away from the pulse generator, the antenna of an operating citizen's band or ham radio, improperly grounded electrical equipment, and handheld tools less than 12 inches away from the pulse generator or any strong magnetic fields. Cellular phones should be positioned on the opposite side of device.[3] *Rationale:* EMI can result in inappropriate ICD sensing and therapies.

- Explore the patient's feelings about having an ICD. Provide education to the patient and family about the device implantation. *Rationale:* Acknowledging these stressors may alleviate the most common psychological disturbances after ICD implantation, which include stress, anxiety, depression, and fear.[14,18]

- Inform patients to notify their provider if the device begins to wear through the skin or the device site becomes reddened, warm, painful, or has discharge. *Rationale:* These signs and symptoms identify problems (e.g., infection) that need additional medical care.

PATIENT ASSESSMENT AND PREPARATION

Patient Assessment

- Assess the patient's cardiac rate and rhythm. *Rationale:* This assessment establishes baseline data.

- Presurgical instructions usually include maintaining nothing by mouth (NPO) for at least 8 hours before the procedure and obtaining complete blood cell count (CBC), chemistries, prothrombin time (PT), and partial thromboplastin time (PTT) for baseline data. *Rationale:* All of these actions ensure patient safety to prevent complications such as excessive bleeding and aspiration.

- For patients prescribed oral anticoagulation, review with the provider who will be implanting the device whether the anticoagulation medication should be continued. Warfarin may be continued if the international normalized ratio is therapeutic but less than 3. Direct oral anticoagulants should be held before implantation and resumed per the implanting provider. The duration of holding direct oral anticoagulants is determined by renal function and should be discussed with the implanting provider before cessation of therapy. *Rationale:* Historically, warfarin was held for several days before the implant procedure with heparin as a bridge to surgery. Recent research shows a lower incidence of bleeding with continuation of warfarin rather than bridging with heparin. The rapid onset of action with direct oral anticoagulants allows resumption after surgery with minimal interruption in therapy.[2]
- Assess the patency of the patient's intravenous access. IV access is usually requested in the left arm because the preferred site of implantation is left pectoral. *Rationale:* Intravenous access should be ensured for administration of prescribed medications.
- Administer antibiotics as prescribed. *Rationale:* Antibiotics are administered to reduce infection from skin microorganisms such as *Staphylococcus aureus* (cause of early infection) and *Staphylococcus epidermidis* (cause of later infection).[16]
- Identify the manufacturer of the ICD and how it is programmed. *Rationale:* Interrogation of the device provides important information: battery voltage and impedance,

charge time, dysrhythmias detected by device (logbook) and any therapies given (ATP or shock), pacing and sensing thresholds, and impedances for all leads, percent of pacing and sensing in each chamber, and review of programmed parameters.[23,27] Interrogation usually also reveals device and lead information (models and serial numbers), implant date, and implanting physician information. See Figure 42.3 for an example of an ICD interrogation report.

Patient Preparation

- Verify the correct patient with two identifiers. *Rationale:* Before performing a procedure, the nurse should ensure the correct identification of the patient for the intended intervention.
- Ensure that the patient and family understand the preprocedural teaching. Answer questions as they arise, and reinforce information as needed. *Rationale:* Understanding of previously taught information is evaluated and reinforced.
- Ensure that informed consent has been obtained (before ICD insertion). *Rationale:* Informed consent protects the rights of the patient and makes a competent decision possible for the patient.
- Ensure appropriate laboratory tests have been obtained to assess anticoagulation (if applicable) and renal function. *Rationale:* Ensures patient safety and decreases the risk of postprocedure bleeding and contrast-induced nephropathy.
- Perform a preprocedure verification and time out (before ICD insertion). *Rationale:* Ensures patient safety.
- Provide analgesia or sedatives as prescribed and needed. *Rationale:* Analgesia and sedatives promote comfort and may decrease anxiety.

Procedure	**for Implantable Cardioverter-Defibrillator**	
Steps	Rationale	Special Considerations
Preimplantation		
1. 🔲		
2. 🔲		
3. Cleanse the skin for application of the ECG electrodes with cleansing pads or soap and water.	Proper skin preparation is essential to maintain appropriate skin-to-electrode contact.	Clipping of chest hair may be necessary to ensure good skin contact with the electrodes.
4. Attach the ECG leads to the electrodes, place the electrodes on the patient's chest, and record the ECG.	Assesses cardiac rhythm.	
Postimplantation Monitoring and Care		
		These conditions should be reported to the provider if they persist despite nursing interventions.
1. Monitor the ECG continuously.	Detects dysrhythmias.	• Dysrhythmias
2. Ensure completion of postinsertion chest x-ray per institution protocol.	Detects pneumothorax, a potential complication of ICD insertion.	• Pneumothorax • Lead placement (check for threshold or impedance changes)

Procedure continues on following page

UNIT II

Procedure for Implantable Cardioverter-Defibrillator—*Continued*

Steps	Rationale	Special Considerations
3. Monitor the ICD for antitachycardia pacing and defibrillation.	Detects functioning of the ICD.	• Atrial dysrhythmias • Ventricular dysrhythmias • Conduction abnormalities • ICD therapy • Defibrillation • ICD malfunction
4. Assess the patient's response to ICD defibrillation, including cardiac rate and rhythm, level of consciousness, and vital signs.	Determines patient status and necessity for additional treatment.	• Cardiac rate and rhythm before and after defibrillation • Level of consciousness • Vital signs
5. Follow institutional standards for assessing pain. Administer analgesia as prescribed.	Identifies the need for pain interventions.	• Continued pain despite pain interventions
6. Monitor for signs and symptoms of infection.	Placement of an invasive device may result in infection.	• Redness • Edema • Drainage • Increased white blood cell count • Increased temperature
7. Monitor for signs of bleeding and hematoma at the ICD insertion site.	Placement of an invasive device may result in untoward bleeding.	• Bleeding at incision site • Edema around ICD site

Management of the Patient With an ICD

Steps	Rationale	Special Considerations
1. If the patient experiences VT or VF: A. Assess and stay with the patient.	Ensures patient safety and provides an opportunity to assess the patient's response to the dysrhythmia.	Run a continuous ECG strip of the dysrhythmia from the bedside monitor if possible; record a 12-lead ECG if possible.
B. Wait for the device to function: antitachycardia pacing or shock therapy.	The ICD requires a brief period (8–30 seconds) to assess the VT or VF and to initiate therapy.	Note: The device may not detect VT/VF if the rate of the VT is below the programmed detection rate.[30]
C. If the dysrhythmia continues, wait for the ICD to recharge and shock again, or deliver antitachycardia pacing if indicated.	The ICD reassesses the cardiac rhythm, recharges, and shocks again as preprogrammed.	
D. If the ICD has been functioning as preprogrammed and still does not convert the dysrhythmia, initiate BLS and ACLS.	Provides emergency care.	Assess the patient's response to VT; the patient's condition may be hemodynamically stable or unstable. Notify the provider immediately, and prepare emergency equipment.
E. Apply defibrillation electrodes (patches) or paddles in one of the two following ways: i. Place one electrode or paddle at the heart's apex just to the left of the nipple in the midaxillary line (fifth to sixth intercostal space), and place the other electrode or paddle just below the right clavicle to the right of the sternum.	The electrical current passes through the cardiac muscle.	Defibrillator paddles and defibrillation electrodes should not be placed over medication patches or the ICD generator. The paddles and electrodes should be a minimum of 2 inches away from the generator when external shocks are delivered.

or

Procedure | for Implantable Cardioverter-Defibrillator—*Continued*

Steps	Rationale	Special Considerations
ii. Apply anterior-posterior defibrillation electrodes or paddles. The anterior electrode or paddle is placed in the anterior left precordial area, and the posterior electrode or paddle is placed posteriorly behind the heart in the left infrascapular area.	The electrical current passes through the cardiac muscle.	
F. If the ICD does not convert VT/ VF and the patient's condition is hemodynamically unstable, externally defibrillate the patient according to ACLS guidelines (see Procedure 33, Defibrillation [External]).	Provides emergency treatment.	ICDs have preprogrammed pacing capability; cardiac pacing is initiated by the ICD if the result of defibrillation is bradycardia or asystole. If external defibrillation is needed, the ICD should be interrogated to assess for potential damage to the device.
ICD Deactivation 1. Prepare for deactivation of the ICD: A. Review the provider prescription. B. Obtain supplies including ICD magnet or device programmer (see Fig. 42.2)	The ICD may need to be deactivated if it is defibrillating a cardiac rhythm that is not VT or VF, such as atrial fibrillation with a rapid ventricular response. The device also can be temporarily deactivated during surgical procedures in which EMI may interfere with appropriate device function. The ICD may be deactivated if therapy is no longer effective or needed or is not desired.[7,28]	If the device is functioning inappropriately, deactivation may be necessary to prevent harm to the patient. The following circumstances may necessitate ICD deactivation: • Lead dislodgment • Lead migration • Lead fracture • Inappropriate identification of the rhythm • Inappropriate defibrillation threshold Consider connecting the patient to an external defibrillator as indicated and desired.
2. ▦ 3. ▦		
4. Determine who will deactivate the ICD. This may include a physician, nurse, advance practice nurse, or other healthcare professional.	The ICD may be deprogrammed by personnel trained in use of the ICD programmer. Ensures that the device is deprogrammed as prescribed.	Follow institutional standards regarding personnel who can deactivate the ICD with use of the programmer.

Procedure continues on following page

Procedure   for Implantable Cardioverter-Defibrillator—*Continued*

Steps	Rationale	Special Considerations
5. If the ICD programmer is unavailable, a magnet may be used to deactivate the device: A. Place a bar or doughnut magnet over the ICD generator. B. Follow the manufacturer's guidelines regarding removing the magnet or taping the magnet in place. **(Level M*)**	The deactivation response to a magnet varies among manufacturers. Some ICDs are deactivated when the magnet is placed on the skin above the generator, and then the magnet can be removed. Other ICDs are deactivated only when the magnet remains on the skin over the generator.	Follow institutional standards regarding personnel who can deactivate the ICD with a magnet. A magnet applied over an ICD disables the device therapies of ATP and electrical cardioversion/defibrillation, but it does not turn off pacemaker function. The magnet may initiate asynchronous pacing. If information about a patient's ICD model and magnet features is unknown or is not clear, contact the personnel responsible for ICDs at your institution, or contact the manufacturer to determine this information. Some ICDs emit a synchronous tone that occurs with each R wave when the device is activated and a constant tone when the ICD is deactivated. Knowledge of which manufacturers have this ability and whether the feature is turned on is important; not all devices emit a synchronous tone.[8,19]
6. Remove gloves, discard used supplies, and ensure that equipment is cleaned.	Reduces the transmission of microorganisms; standard precautions.	
7. **HH**		
ICD Reactivation		
1. **HH**		
2. **PE**		
3. Determine who will reactivate the ICD if a device programmer was utilized to turn off the VT/VF therapy. This may include a physician, nurse, advance practice nurse, or other healthcare professional trained in the management of ICDs.	The ICD may be reprogrammed by personnel trained in use of the ICD programmer. Ensures that the device is reprogrammed as prescribed.	Follow institutional standards regarding personnel who can reactivate the ICD with use of the programmer.
A. If a bar or doughnut magnet is over the ICD generator, remove the magnet. B. If a bar or doughnut magnet is not over the ICD generator, place one there, and then remove the magnet. **(Level M*)**	When the magnet is removed, most ICDs automatically reactivate.	Follow the manufacturer's recommendations regarding magnet features. Some ICDs (Boston Scientific ICDs only) emit a synchronous tone that occurs with each R wave with magnet application for 60 seconds unless this feature has been turned off. Knowledge of which manufacturers have this ability and whether the feature is turned on is important; not all devices emit a synchronous tone.
5. Remove gloves, discard used supplies, and ensure that equipment is cleaned.	Reduces the transmission of microorganisms; standard precautions.	
6. **HH**		

*Level M: Manufacturer's recommendations only.

Expected Outcomes	Unexpected Outcomes
• ICD detects life-threatening VT or VF • ICD delivers appropriate therapy, including antitachycardia pacing and defibrillation as necessary • Cardiac rhythm is converted to a hemodynamically stable rhythm • ICD provides bradycardia pacing as needed	• Failure of the ICD to detect VT or VF • Failure of the ICD to convert life-threatening dysrhythmia despite appropriate therapy and defibrillation attempts • Failure of the backup pacing system to pace if bradycardia or asystole is the result of defibrillation • Inappropriate therapies: antitachycardia or shock • Infection at the ICD pulse generator site, leads, or myocardium • Lead fracture or migration • Pulse generator migration • Pulse generator pocket hematoma • Loosened set screw in device header (this screw holds the lead circuitry in place in the device header); loose set screws usually manifest as improper device function and occur generally immediately after implant • Air embolism • Venous thrombosis • Cardiac tamponade • Skin erosion • Pneumothorax • Frozen shoulder on operative side • Twiddler's syndrome (manipulation of the device in the device pocket by a patient, either intentionally or unintentionally, which may lead to dislodgement)

UNIT II

Documentation

Documentation should include the following:
• Presenting rhythm and underlying rhythm
• Device interrogation information: battery voltage and charge time, dysrhythmias detected by device and any therapies given, status of leads, programmed parameters
• Patient and family education[7]
• Adjustment to device settings
• All rhythm strip recordings
• Patient response to ICD therapy
• Pain assessment, interventions, and effectiveness
• Anxiety assessment, interventions, and effectiveness
• Occurrence of any unexpected outcomes
• Additional interventions

References and Additional Readings

For a complete list of references and additional readings for this procedure, scan this QR code with your smartphone, or visit https://www.elsevier.com/__data/assets/pdf_file/0003/1319817/Chapter0042.pdf.

43 Permanent Pacemaker (Assessing Function)

Mary Leier

PURPOSE The purpose of permanent pacing is to electrically stimulate myocardial contraction and to restore and maintain an appropriate heart rate, rhythm, or ventricular synchrony when a chronic conduction or impulse-formation disturbance exists in the cardiac conduction system. Assessment of the permanent pacemaker is important in maintaining proper function.

PREREQUISITE NURSING KNOWLEDGE

• Knowledge of the normal anatomy and physiology of the cardiovascular system, cardiac conduction, and basic dysrhythmia interpretation is necessary.
• Knowledge of pacemaker function and patient response to pacemaker therapy is needed.
• Advanced cardiac life support (ACLS) knowledge and skills are needed.
• Permanent pacing is indicated for the following clinical conditions.[10]
   ❖ Symptomatic sinus node dysfunction
   ❖ Acquired atrioventricular (AV) block in adults
   ❖ Chronic bifascicular and trifascicular block
   ❖ AV block associated with acute myocardial infarction
   ❖ Hypersensitive carotid sinus and neurocardiogenic syncope
   ❖ Specific conditions related to cardiac transplantation, neuromuscular diseases, sleep apnea syndromes, or infiltrative and inflammatory diseases such as cardiac sarcoidosis
   ❖ Prevention and termination of supraventricular tachycardia via pacing
   ❖ Hypertrophic cardiomyopathy with sinus node dysfunction or AV block
   ❖ Certain congenital heart defects
   ❖ Certain cases of left-ventricular dysfunction, to restore ventricular synchrony (cardiac resynchronization therapy [CRT]).[3,5]
• Relative contraindications to permanent pacemakers include the following:
   ❖ Active infection (e.g., endocarditis, positive blood culture results)
   ❖ Bleeding with abnormal coagulation laboratory results
• Components of the traditional transvenous pacemaker are the pulse generator and the leads. The pulse generator weighs less than 1 ounce and is typically implanted subcutaneously or submuscularly in a pocket created either above or below the pectoral muscle. The outer casing is made of titanium and contains the electronic components and the battery (Fig. 43.1). The typical battery life is 10

to 12 years and is dependent on variables such as output values, impedance, and the percentage of pacing. Transvenous pacing leads may be positioned in the right atrium, the right ventricle, a cardiac vein supplying the left ventricle on the His bundle (before it branches to the left and right ventricle) in the right atrium against the septal wall, and/or at the left bundle trunk or its proximal fascicles depending on the type of pacing needed. Alternatively, epicardial leads can be considered in patients with increased risk for infection, those whose vasculature cannot accommodate additional leads, or those with single-ventricle anatomy.
• In leadless pacemakers, the entire pacing system is a self-contained generator and electrode system that is implanted

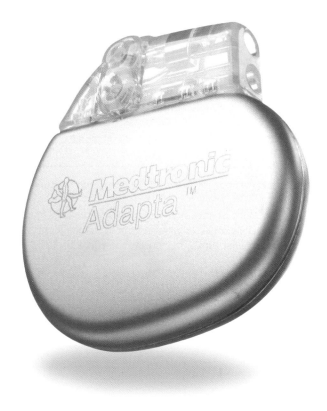

Figure 43.1 Permanent pacemaker pulse generator. (*Courtesy Medtronic, Inc., Minneapolis, MN.*)

directly into the right ventricle. The leadless pacing system weighs 1.75 g and has a volume of 0.8 cc. The typical battery life is 8 to 13 years and is dependent on the same variables as the traditional pacemaker battery. The outer casing of the leadless device is also titanium, and the device is anchored into the right ventricle using four Nitinol tines (equal parts nickel and titanium) that splay outward and grab the endocardial tissue of the RV apex, allowing for optimal electrode/tissue interface and stable low thresholds (Fig. 43.2).[14]

- Most modern pacing leads utilize a bipolar system with the positive and negative electrode at the distal tip of the pacing wire. A bipolar lead can be converted to a unipolar system by making the pacemaker case the positive pole. Some older leads only have unipolar capability. Unipolar pacing involves a relatively large electrical circuit. The distal tip of the pacing lead is the negative electrode and

is in contact with the myocardium. The positive electrode encompasses the metallic pacemaker case, located in the soft tissue. Energy is delivered from the negative electrode in contact with the myocardium. The pacing lead has a second positive electrode that is located within 1 cm of the negative electrode. Energy is delivered from the negative electrode to the positive electrode, causing myocardial depolarization. The ECG tracing may show small spikes, or the spikes may not be visible on a surface ECG.

- Basic principles of cardiac pacing include sensing, pulse generation, capture, and impedance (see Table 43.1 for definitions).
- Depending on the type of pacemaker, the pacemaker lead may be placed in the atrium, the right ventricle, the left ventricle, along the bundle of His, or at the left bundle trunk or its proximal fascicles. A leadless pacemaker will not have any leads. A standard code exists to describe

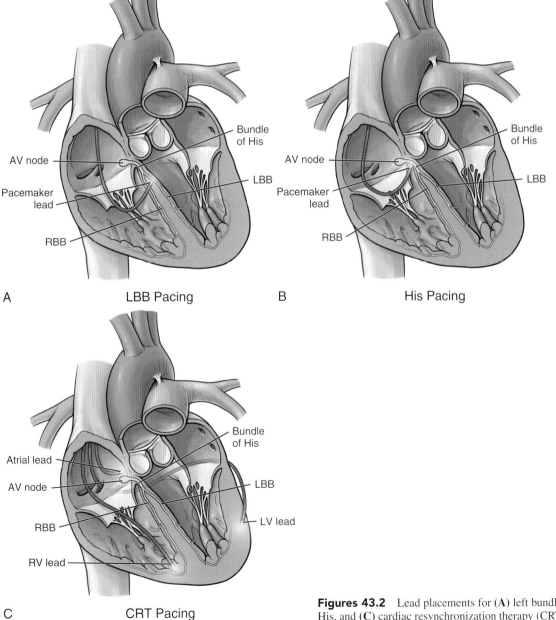

Figures 43.2 Lead placements for (**A**) left bundle branch (LBB), (**B**) His, and (**C**) cardiac resynchronization therapy (CRT) pacing leads.

TABLE 43.1	Pertinent Definitions Related to Pacemakers
Sensing	Ability of the pacemaker to detect intrinsic myocardial electrical activity. The pacemaker is either inhibited from delivering a stimulus or initiates an electrical impulse based on the programmed response.
Pulse generation	Occurs when the pacemaker produces a programmed electrical current for a programmed duration. This energy travels through the transvenous lead wires to the myocardium. In a leadless pacemaker, the entire pacing system is a self-contained generator and electrode system that is implanted into the right ventricle, allowing for pulse generation through direct contact between the generator and the myocardium. The electrical impulse is seen as a line or spike on the ECG recording (pacemaker spikes are shown in Fig. 43.8).
Capture	Successful stimulation of the myocardium by the pacemaker impulse that results in depolarization. Two settings are used to ensure capture: amplitude and pulse width as evidenced on the ECG by a pacemaker spike/stimulus followed by either an atrial or ventricular complex, depending on the chambers being paced (see Fig. 43.8).
Lead impedance	Opposition to flow of electrical current by the leads, electrodes, the electrode-myocardial interface, and body tissues.[12] It is measured in ohms (normally between 200 and 1200 ohms). A lead insulation break can cause impedance to fall below 200 ohms. A lead fracture can cause impedance to exceed 2000 ohms.
Failure of pulse generation	The pacemaker does not discharge a pacing stimulus to the myocardium at its programmed time. This is evidenced by the absence of a pacemaker spike on the ECG where expected (see Fig. 43.10).
Failure to sense	The pacemaker has either detected extraneous signals that mimic intrinsic cardiac activity (oversensing) or has not accurately identified intrinsic activity (undersensing). Oversensing is recognized on the ECG by pauses where paced beats were expected and prolongation of the interval between paced beats (see Fig. 43.11). Oversensing leads to underpacing. Undersensing is recognized on the ECG by inappropriate pacemaker spikes relative to the intrinsic electrical activity (pacemaker spikes occurring where they are not needed) and shortened distances between paced beats (see Fig. 43.12). Undersensing leads to overpacing. Spikes may appear during the QRS complex as part of normal pacemaker function seen with fusion and pseudofusion beats.
Failure to capture	Pacemaker has delivered a pacing stimulus that was unable to initiate depolarization and contraction of the myocardium. Evidenced on the ECG by pacemaker spikes that are not followed by a P wave for atrial pacing or spikes not followed by a QRS complex for ventricular pacing (see Fig. 43.13).
Hysteresis	Rate hysteresis is a pacemaker setting that is designed to allow for longer periods of intrinsic rhythm by temporarily allowing both atrial and ventricular intrinsic and paced rates to fall below the lower rate limit/set base rate of pacemaker.

TABLE 43.2	Revised NASPE/BPEG Generic Code for Antibradycardia Pacing			
I	II	III	IV	V
Chambers Paced	Chambers Sensed	Response to Sensing	Rate Modulation	Multisite Pacing
O = None	O = None	O = None	O = None	O = None
A = Atrium	A = Atrium	T = Triggered	R = Rate modulation	A = Atrium
V = Ventricle	V = Ventricle	I = Inhibited		V = Ventricle
D = Dual (A + V)	D = Dual (A + V)	D = Dual (T + I)		D = Dual (A + V)
S = Single (A or V)*	S + Single (A or V)*			

*Manufacturer's designation only. *NASPE,* North American Society of Pacing and Electrophysiology; *BPEG,* British Pacing and Electrophysiology Group.
From Bernstein AD, Daubert JC, Fletcher RD, et al: The revised NASPE/BPEG generic code for antibradycardia, adaptive-rate, and multisite pacing, *Pacing Clin Electrophysiol* 25(2):261, 2002.

pacemakers (Table 43.2).[2] The nurse must know the programmed mode with the pacemaker code to determine whether the device is functioning appropriately. See Table 43.3 for a review of different programmed modes for pacemakers.

- Dual-chamber pacemakers contain pacing leads that are fixed in the right atrium and the right ventricle. Pacing and sensing occur in both chambers when programmed in DDD or DDI modes. Pacing is inhibited by sensed atrial or ventricular activity. Sensed or paced atrial activity triggers a ventricular paced response in the absence of intrinsic ventricular activity within a programmed AV interval.
- In a leadless pacemaker system, the pacing capsule is fixed to the right ventricle (Fig. 43.4). In first-generation

leadless pacemakers, only ventricular sensing and pacing are capable, allowing for VVI, VVIR, and VOO modes.[14] In second-generation leadless pacemakers, the capability of atrial sensing was added, allowing for VVI, VVIR, VOO, VDD, and VDI modes.[17] In these devices, pacing is inhibited by sensed ventricular activity. In the VDD leadless pacing device, the capability of atrial sensing triggers the ventricular response in the absence of intrinsic ventricular activity within the programmed AV interval. Atrial sensing is enabled by an accelerometer to detect blood flow through the tricuspid valve, indicating mechanical atrial contractions.[17]

- Biventricular pacemaker systems (Figs. 43.2C and 43.5) contain three leads: one in the right atrium, one in the right

TABLE 43.3	Programmed Pacing Modes
Pacemaker Code	**Pacemaker Response**
AOO	Atrial pacing; no sensing; asynchronous mode → paces in atria at a fixed, preprogrammed rate.
AAI	Atrial pacing, atrial sensing and inhibition; intrinsic P waves inhibit atrial pacing; if no sensed atrial events → paces in atria at a preprogrammed rate.
AAIR	Atrial pacing; atrial sensing; intrinsic P waves inhibit atrial pacing; if no sensed atrial events → paces in atria; rate response to patient's activity.
VOO	Ventricular pacing; no sensing; asynchronous mode → paces in ventricle at a fixed, preprogrammed rate.
VVI	Ventricular pacing: ventricular sensing; intrinsic QRS inhibits ventricular pacing; if no sensed events → paces in ventricle at a preprogrammed rate.
VVIR	Ventricular pacing: ventricular sensing; intrinsic QRS inhibits ventricular pacing; if no sensed events → paces in ventricle; rate response to patient's activity.
VDI	Ventricular pacing: atrial and ventricular sensing; intrinsic QRS inhibits ventricular pacing; if no sensed events, device will pace the ventricle at a preprogrammed rate.
VDD	Ventricular pacing: atrial and ventricular sensing.
DOO	Atrial and ventricular pacing: no sensing; asynchronous mode → paces in atria and ventricles at a fixed, preprogrammed rate.
DDI	Atrial and ventricular pacing; atria and ventricular sensing; no tracking of atria: sensed atrial events inhibit atrial pacing/do not trigger a ventricular pacing pulse; sensed atrial events with absent ventricular event inhibit atrial pacing but do pace ventricle at preprogrammed rate; if both atrial and ventricular events absent → AV sequential pacing results at a preprogrammed rate.
DDIR	Atrial and ventricular pacing; atrial and ventricular sensing; no tracking of atria (as described previously in DDI); AV sequential rate modulation.
DDD	Atrial and ventricular pacing; atrial and ventricular sensing; intrinsic P wave and intrinsic QRS can inhibit pacing; intrinsic P wave can trigger a paced QRS (tracks the atrium). May see four possible combinations in DDD mode: 1, atrial sensed/ventricular sensed; 2, atrial sensed/ventricular paced; 3, atrial paced/ventricular sensed; 4, atrial paced/ventricular paced.
DDDR	Atrial and ventricular pacing; atrial and ventricular sensing; tracks the atrium: intrinsic P wave and intrinsic QRS can inhibit pacing, intrinsic P wave can trigger a paced QRS; AV sequential rate modulation.

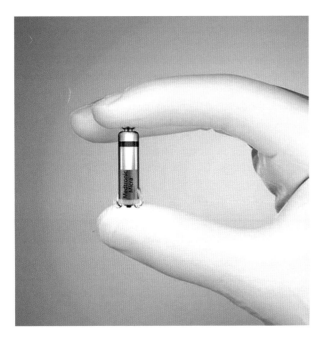

Figure 43.3 Leadless pacemaker. *(Courtesy Medtronic, Inc., Minneapolis, MN.)*

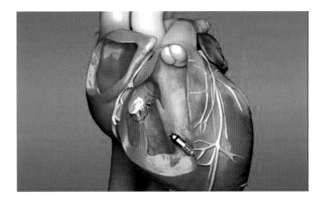

Figure 43.4 Placement of leadless pacemaker in the right ventricle. *(Courtesy Medtronic, Inc., Minneapolis, MN.)*

ventricle, and one on the surface of the left ventricle (cannulated through the coronary sinus vessel) that provides simultaneous pacing of the right and left ventricles for cardiac resynchronization therapy (Fig. 43.5). Epicardial leads can also be utilized if needed in this system.

- His bundle pacing systems (Fig. 43.2B) contain two leads; one in the right atrium and a second lead fixed along the His bundle, before branching down the left and right bundles, at the right atrial wall along the septum (Fig. 43.6). The His pacing lead paces the His bundle to produce normal physiological ventricular activation of the His-Purkinje system, helping synchronize right and left ventricular contraction (Fig. 43.7). This can provide an alternative site for pacing in patients who meet CRT indications to tighten QRS duration in left bundle branch block or in patients with heart block in whom long-term right ventricular pacing will be inevitable.[13] Because of placement in the septum to target the His-Purkinje system,

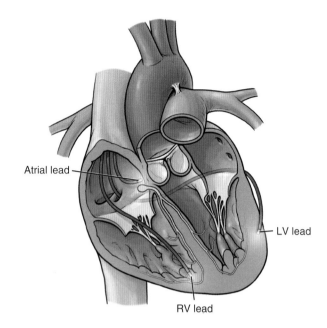

Figure 43.5   Biventricular pacemaker (cardiac resynchronization therapy). *(Courtesy Medtronic, Inc, Minneapolis, MN.)*

His bundle pacing often requires higher pacing thresholds and can lead to quicker depletion of battery life.[6]

- Left bundle branch pacing (LBBP) (Fig. 43.2A) is an alternative method to His bundle pacing and the three-lead bi-ventricular system to achieve synchrony of left ventricular contraction in patients with infranodal atrioventricular block and left bundle branch block. In LBBP, there are two leads: the atrial lead and the ventricular lead. The ventricular lead is advanced transseptally, past the His-Purkinje conduction system, targeting the proximal left bundle branches that run through the LV septum to form a wider target for lead placement and LV stimulation. LBBP offers lower pacing thresholds and therefore increased battery longevity when compared with His bundle pacing.[6]
- Some pacemaker systems also include an implantable cardioverter-defibrillator, using a defibrillator lead placed in the RV. This lead allows for pacing as well as defibrillation if needed (see Procedure 42).
- Some pacemakers can be programmed to switch modes (e.g., DDD mode to DDI mode) to avoid pacing at the upper rate in patients who experience intermittent atrial dysrhythmias in which rapid atrial rates are generated.
- Certain pacemakers can be programmed with pacing therapies for atrial dysrhythmias. This programming is called *antitachycardia pacing,* in which the device paces the atrium faster than a patient's rate in an attempt to convert the atrial arrhythmia.
- Rate-responsive pacemakers include a sensor and are designed to mimic normal changes in heart rate based on the patient's physiological needs. Most commonly, the sensor reacts to motion and vibration through respirations and can initiate an appropriate change in the pacing rate, depending on metabolic activity. In the VDD leadless pacemaker system, the accelerometer detects atrial contractions via flow through the tricuspid valve using the device's built-in three-axis accelerometer and triggers the ventricular rate accordingly. These patients have a set pacemaker rate range, which can be adjusted based on their baseline activity level.
- Inappropriate pacemaker function includes failure of pulse generation, failure to sense, and failure to capture (see Table 43.1 for definitions).[13]
- Electromagnetic interference (EMI) may interfere with pacemaker function and includes electrocautery, cardioversion and defibrillation, magnetic resonance imaging, diathermy, and transcutaneous nerve stimulation. Patients with pacemakers with MRI conditional labeling on the leads and the generator can undergo MRIs as necessary.[7] Patients with MRI nonconditional devices can also undergo MRI if there are no fractured, epicardial, or abandoned leads; the MRI is the best test for the condition; there is an institutional protocol, and a designated responsible MR physician, electrophysiologist, or a trained advanced practice provider supervises the imaging[7] **(Level B*).** Other outside causes of EMI include welding equipment less than 24 inches from the device, electrical motors, chainsaws, battery-powered cordless power tools and drills less than 12 inches from the device, magnetic mattresses and chairs, and airport wands for security checks. Household appliances such as microwave ovens rarely cause EMI. Cell phones may cause EMI and should be used on the ear opposite the device. The cell phone should be carried on the opposite side of the body, with at least 6 inches maintained between the cell phone and the device.[10,13] Patients who are pacemaker-dependent may experience dizziness, lightheadedness, near-syncope, or syncope if EMI inhibits proper sensing and therefore inhibits pacing.
- A pacemaker programmer appropriate for the pacemaker make and model is required for a device check or *interrogation.* Note that some situations may require notification of the device manufacturer to obtain the proper interrogation equipment (the device programmer). Manufacturer information can be found on the patient's pacemaker identification card and via chest radiography.
- A pacemaker remote monitor allows for patient devices to transmit from an outside location (e.g., home) either using analog telephone lines or a cellular wireless data network to a central storage repository that is available via a secure dedicated website for the provider to retrieve and review.[16]

EQUIPMENT

- ECG monitor and recorder with paper
- ECG cable and electrodes

Additional equipment to have available as needed includes the following:

- Pacemaker magnet
- Pacemaker programmer appropriate for the pacemaker manufacturer and model

PATIENT AND FAMILY EDUCATION

- Assess learning needs, readiness to learn, and factors that influence learning. *Rationale:* This assessment allows the nurse to individualize teaching in a meaningful manner.

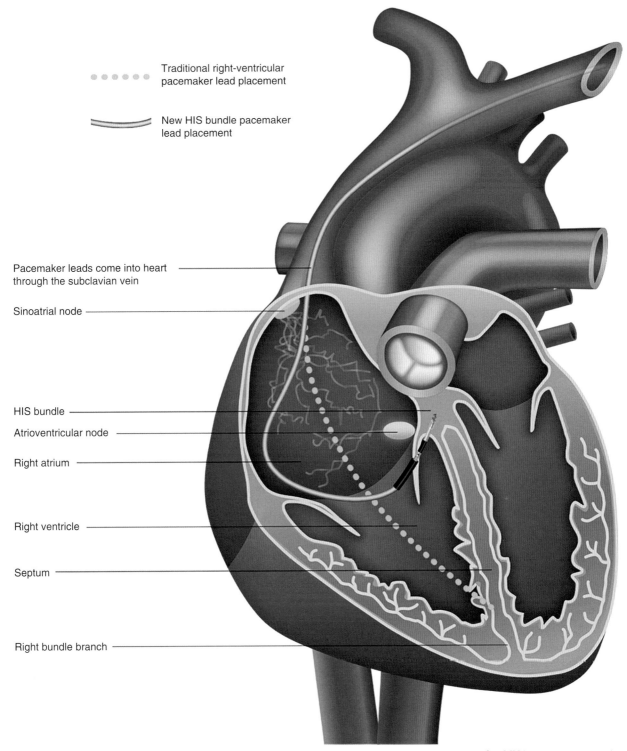

Figure 43.6 His bundle lead placement. *(Courtesy Medtronic, Inc., Minneapolis, MN.)*

- Provide information about the normal conduction system, such as structure of the conduction system, source of heartbeat, normal and abnormal heart rhythms, and symptoms of abnormal heart rhythms. Patients with cardiomyopathy and heart failure need further information about ventricular dyssynchrony. *Rationale:* Understanding of the normal conduction system and pumping function assists the patient and family in recognizing the need for permanent pacemaker therapy.

- Provide information about permanent pacing, including the indications for pacing; explanation of the equipment; what to expect during permanent pacing; precautions and restrictions in activities of daily living; signs and symptoms of complications; instructions on when to call the physician, advanced practice nurse, or pacemaker clinic; and information on expected follow-up. *Rationale:* Understanding of pacemaker functioning and expectations after discharge assists the patient and family in developing

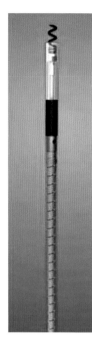

Figure 43.7 His bundle pacing lead. *(Courtesy Medtronic, Inc., Minneapolis, MN.)*

realistic perceptions of permanent pacing therapy. Information may improve compliance with restrictions and promote effective lifestyle management after discharge.

- Provide information about required device follow-up, including in-clinic evaluation, or remote monitoring. *Rationale:* Periodic pacemaker checks are essential for routine device monitoring and evaluation of changes in patient condition related to the pacemaker. Current guidelines recommend the following minimum frequency of routine device checks: within 72 hours of device implant (in person) then 2 to 12 weeks after implantation (in person), followed by every 3 to 12 months (in person or remote), annually, and then every 1 to 3 months at signs of battery depletion (in person or remote). For VDD leadless devices, the first interrogation is recommended to be performed within 1 hour of implantation to ensure appropriate atrial sensing **(Level M*).** Devices may be checked more frequently as needed (e.g., if a change occurs in symptoms, antiarrhythmic medications, or heart failure therapies).[10,13] Pacemakers and defibrillators are commonly followed by electrophysiologists or cardiologists via remote monitoring. This allows for independence from scheduled appointments, early detection for arrhythmia based on provider-selected criteria, immediate detection of device malfunction, lead integrity breaches, and battery voltage elective replacement indicator status **(Level B*).** Remote monitoring also allows for symptomatic patients to initiate transmissions, enabling the provider to correlate possible arrhythmia with reported symptoms.[16] Device setting changes cannot be made remotely and can only be made in person using the device programmer.
- Always instruct patients to carry their device identification card. Patients receive identification cards from the manufacturer at the time of implant. These cards identify the indication for pacing and the model of pacemaker generator and leads used. Also encourage patients to wear Medic Alert information. *Rationale:* This instruction ensures that appropriate identifying information is available to other healthcare providers, if needed.

PATIENT ASSESSMENT AND PREPARATION

Patient Assessment

- Identify the manufacturer of the pacemaker. This information may be found on the patient's identification card. If no card is available, the manufacturer of the device may be identified on chest radiography. Additionally, device type can be identified by evaluation of the magnet rate, as each device manufacturer has a unique magnet rate. The Medtronic pacemaker magnet rate is 85 beats/min at the beginning of life and 65 beats/min when it reaches elective replacement interval. The Boston Scientific magnet rate is 100 beats/min, Biotronik is 90 beats/min in the first 6 beats of magnet evaluation, and St. Jude Medical devices is about 100 beats/min and 85 beats/min once ERI is reached. *Rationale:* Identification of the manufacturer ensures that the correct programmer is used to review the programmed pacemaker parameters.
- Identify the reason for permanent pacemaker support. *Rationale:* Knowledge of the clinical indication (e.g., complete heart block) provides the nurse with baseline data such as pacemaker dependency, when evaluating pacemaker function and patient response.
- Determine the patient's pacemaker history: date of insertion; last battery change; most recent pacemaker check; any problems with the pacemaker or pacemaker site; and any unexpected symptoms such as dizziness, chest pain, shortness of breath, palpitations, or activity intolerance. *Rationale:* The pacemaker history provides information useful for determining any problems that may occur.
- Identify the programmed mode of the pacemaker. *Rationale:* Knowledge of how the pacemaker is intended to respond is necessary to detect appropriate and inappropriate function.
- Assess the patient's ECG for appropriate pacemaker function. *Rationale:* Evidence of inappropriate function determines the need for further testing.[18]

- Assess the patient's hemodynamic response to the paced rhythm. ***Rationale:*** The patient's hemodynamic response indicates how effective the pacemaker is in maintaining an adequate cardiac output in response to the patient's physiological needs. Evidence of inadequate cardiac output may be exhibited as decreased level of consciousness, fatigue, dizziness, shortness of breath, pallor, diaphoresis, chest pain, or hypotension.
- Patients with new biventricular pacemakers should also be assessed for signs and symptoms of dehydration. ***Rationale:*** Patients on long-term diuretics may have increased diuresis after pacemaker implantation due to improved circulation and hemodynamics.[3]
- Evaluate the patient for diaphragmatic stimulation. Phrenic nerve stimulation can occur in patients with traditional cardiac resynchronization devices because of the proximity of the phrenic nerve to the pericardial veins, which can expose the nerve to stimulation by the left ventricular lead. This is commonly described by affected patients as an uncomfortable pulsation with certain position changes, such as left-sided lying.

Patient Preparation

- Verify the correct patient with two identifiers. ***Rationale:*** Before performing a procedure, the nurse should ensure the correct identification of the patient for the intended intervention.
- Ensure that the patient and family understand teaching. Answer questions as they arise, and reinforce information as needed. ***Rationale:*** This communication evaluates and reinforces understanding of previously taught information.
- Pacemaker interrogation may be performed with the patient either sitting or in the supine position. ***Rationale:*** This position prepares the patient for pacemaker interrogation.

Procedure	for Assessing Function of a Permanent Pacemaker		
Steps	**Rationale**	**Special Considerations**
1. 🅷🅷		Assess the patient's pacemaker pocket incision site for any new signs of redness, swelling, or erosion.
2. 🅿🅴		
3. Prepare skin by cleansing with soap and water before application of ECG electrodes.	Proper skin preparation is essential to maintain appropriate skin-to-electrode contact.	
4. Attach the ECG leads to the electrodes, and place the electrodes on the patient's chest (see Procedure 49).	Attaching the leads to the electrodes first and then placing the electrodes on the chest produces less discomfort.	
5. Record an ECG rhythm strip.	Allows for evaluation of the patient's intrinsic rhythm and aids in assessment of pacemaker function.	
6. Follow institutional standards for recording a rhythm strip with a magnet placed over the pacemaker. **(Level M*)**		
A. Place the pacemaker magnet on top of the pacemaker generator.	A magnet placed over the pacemaker causes the pacemaker to pace at the preprogrammed parameters.	Follow institutional standards to ensure that a nurse can use the pacemaker magnet.
B. Record the ECG rhythm strip.	This is needed to assess the rhythm and for documentation.	
C. Remove the magnet.	After the magnet is removed, the ECG rhythm represents the patient's current status (intrinsic rhythm, paced rhythm, or a combination).	
D. Assess the ECG rhythm.	Can help determine the patient's inherent rhythm.	May not be useful if the patient is pacer dependent (No ventricular signal/no R wave).
7. Inspect the ECG rhythm strip for pacemaker spikes, and evaluate for evidence of failure to sense or failure to capture (Figs. 43.8 to 43.14).	Determines whether the pacemaker is functioning adequately and assesses electrical activity of the atria and ventricles.	Depending on the type of lead and programming, pacemaker spikes may be difficult to detect on the surface ECG.

*Level M: Manufacturer's recommendations only.

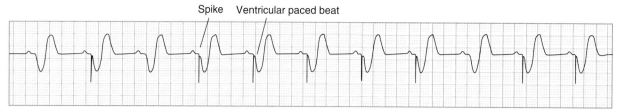

Figure 43.8   DDD pacing, normal operation: atrial activity sensed, ventricle paced.

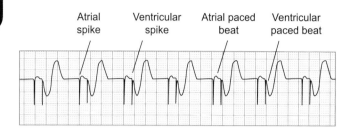

Figure 43.9   Dual-chamber DDD pacing, normal operation: atrial paced, ventricle paced.

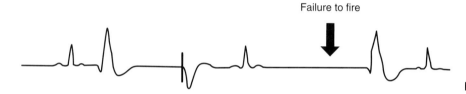

Figure 43.10   Failure of pulse generation.

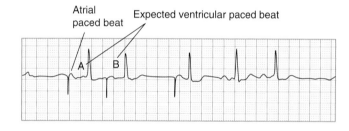

Figure 43.11   Ventricular oversensing and possibly ventricular pulse-generation failure. Ventricular spike expected at 150 ms. Ventricular spike and corresponding ventricular depolarization did not occur at points A and B. Also, atrial timing reset by oversensed ventricular activity resulted in erratic atrial pacing (suspicious for fracture of ventricular lead).

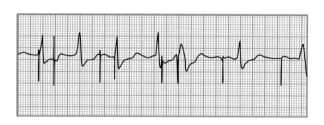

Figure 43.12   Ventricular undersensing. Pacemaker appears to be firing asynchronously. The third and sixth ventricular complexes represent concurrent intrinsic ventricular depolarization overlaid by inappropriate pacemaker fire.

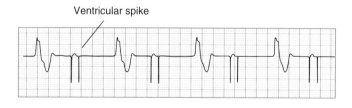

Figure 43.13   DDD system with failure to capture or sense ventricular activity. All ventricular spikes show absence of corresponding ventricular depolarization. There is no timing circuit reset by intrinsic ventricular complexes.

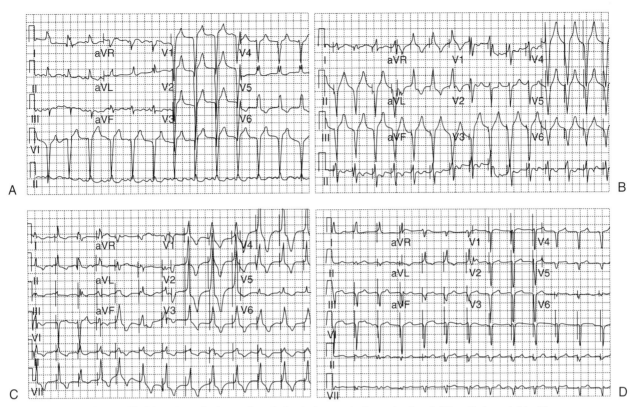

Figure 43.14 Biventricular pacing. **A,** Intrinsic ventricular activation (left bundle branch block). **B,** Right-ventricular pacing. **C,** Left-ventricular pacing. **D,** Biventricular pacing. *(From Ellenbogen KA, Wood MA:* Cardiac pacing and ICDs, *ed 5, Oxford, 2008, Blackwell Publishing, 1095.)*

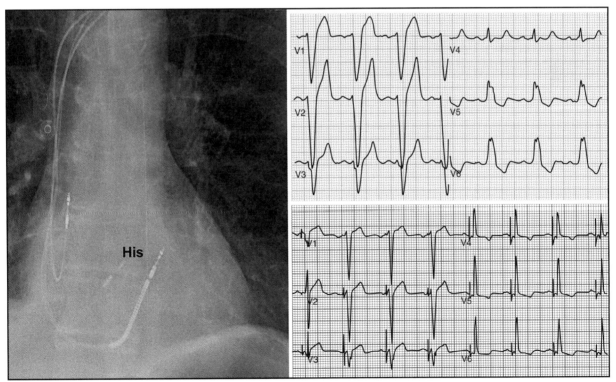

Figure 43.15 His bundle ICD system seen on chest x-ray showing placement of leads *(left).* His bundle pacing capture *(bottom right)* versus noncapture *(top right),* demonstrated on ECG. *(From Ajijola OA, Upadhyay GA, Macias C, Shivkumar K, Tung R: Permanent His-bundle pacing for cardiac resynchronization therapy: Initial feasibility study in lieu of left ventricular lead.* Heart Rhythm *14[9]:1353–1361, 2017.)*

UNIT II

Procedure for Assessing Function of a Permanent Pacemaker—*Continued*

Steps	Rationale	Special Considerations
A. Identify atrial activity. Is the pacemaker programmed to detect atrial activity? Was the atrial activity sensed? What is the pacemaker programmed to do when atrial activity is sensed? If the pacemaker is programmed to trigger ventricular pacing with sensed atrial activity, is a ventricular-paced complex seen at the programmed AV interval? If not, did an intrinsic QRS complex occur before the programmed AV interval? In VDD leadless pacemakers, the manual atrial mechanical test is a press-and-hold test that allows for assessment and adjustment of atrial sensing markers. ECG, accelerometer waveform, markers, and marker intervals from the live waveform are collected to determine the best accelerometer vector to use to provide the most accurate AV synchrony. **(Level M*)**	Determines the presence of atrial activity in response to the pacemaker settings.	Different AV intervals may be programmed for sensed and paced events. In VDD leadless pacemakers, consider having the patient perform activity such as walking in the clinic hallway, walking stairs, or marching in place to help assess accelerometer wave form, marking intervals during times of increased heart rate to allow for optimal sensing parameters during activity and rest. **(Level M*)**
B. If no intrinsic atrial activity is present, determine whether the pacemaker is programmed to pace the atrium. If atrial pacing should be occurring, determine the lower rate limit at which the pacemaker stimulates atrial activity. Evaluate whether the pacemaker is firing at this rate.		If atrial pacing is occurring below the set rate, consider that a sleep rate or hysteresis may be on. If atrial pacing is occurring above the set rate, consider that rate response, rate drop response, or atrial preferred pacing may be turned on. If a pacemaker spike is present but evidence of atrial capture is not present, attempt to assess the presence of atrial contraction as follows: 1. Looking for the *"a"* wave in the central venous pressure (or right-atrial pressure) waveform (if available). 2. Changing the ECG lead. 3. Listening to the heart sounds (S_1 becomes softer in the absence of atrial contraction because left-ventricular contractility affects the loudness of S_1).[13,19] 4. Examine a 12-lead ECG tracing, which may show pacemaker spikes not seen on a monitor strip.
C. Identify ventricular activity. Is the pacemaker programmed to detect intrinsic activity? Is it sensed appropriately? What is the pacemaker programmed to do when ventricular activity is sensed? Does inhibition of ventricular pacing occur?	Determines the presence of ventricular activity in response to the pacemaker settings.	Failure of ventricular capture, or ventricular undersensing can be a life-threatening situation.

*Level M: Manufacturer's recommendations only.

Procedure for Assessing Function of a Permanent Pacemaker—*Continued*

Steps	Rationale	Special Considerations
D. If no intrinsic ventricular activity is found, determine whether the pacemaker is programmed to pace the ventricles. If pacing should occur, identify the lower rate limit, and determine whether ventricular pacing spikes are occurring at this rate. If ventricular pacing spikes are occurring at intervals that are longer than the lower rate limit, evaluate for oversensing of unwanted signals. If ventricular pacing spikes are occurring at intervals that are shorter than the lower rate limit, is the pacemaker in a rate-responsive mode? Is hidden atrial activity triggering a ventricular output? Is atrial oversensing found? Determine whether each ventricular pacing spike is followed by a QRS complex. If the pacemaker has an upper rate limit, determine whether the patient is being paced appropriately when this limit is reached.	Determines the presence of ventricular activity in response to the pacemaker settings.	If ventricular activity is not present as expected, determine whether other pacemaker features are enabled, such as programming to minimize ventricular pacing or programmed change in base rate caused by atrial dysrhythmia, rate response, sleep rate, or hysteresis.
E. If antitachycardia pacing is programmed, determine whether the tachycardia detection criterion has been met and whether the pacemaker intervened appropriately.	Determines appropriate pacemaker function.	
F. If the patient has a biventricular pacemaker, His bundle pacing lead, or LBBP for CRT purposes, verify that the ventricles are consistently paced.[3,5,6,18]	The purpose of biventricular, his bundle, or LBB pacing is to pace both ventricles simultaneously to restore ventricular synchrony. If the patient is not consistently being paced in the ventricles, the system is not working properly, and there likely is a burden of ectopy (PACs/PVCs) or atrial arrhythmia present.[1,3,8]	Detailed interrogation of function is needed because a surface ECG rhythm strip does not provide enough information to assess proper function adequately. Fig. 43.14 illustrates various aspects of biventricular pacing. With biventricular, His bundle, or LBB pacing, the loss of capture may be seen only by a change in the patient's condition or a change in the QRS width or appearance (see Fig. 43.15)[4,5,13,18] and must be reported to the supervising physician.

Procedure continues on following page

UNIT II

Procedure　for Assessing Function of a Permanent Pacemaker—*Continued*

Steps	Rationale	Special Considerations
8. Perform a check of the pacemaker using the manufacturer's programmer (only done by trained personnel), when available and as prescribed: 　A. Place the wand attached to the programmer over the patient's pacemaker. 　B. Perform testing of sensing, capture thresholds, and lead impedances. **(Level M*)**	Determines appropriate pacemaker function. The wand retrieves and transmits the programmed information. Allows for determination of pacemaker function, programmed parameters, dysrhythmias, and alerts.	• Follow institutional standards regarding training required before use of the pacemaker programmer. Some devices have a wireless connection to the programmer and a wand is not used. Pacemaker device check with the programmer provides the following information:[13,16,19] 　• Battery voltage (and impedance) 　• Magnet rate (varies by manufacturer) 　• Pacing and sensing thresholds for leads placed in the atrium and right ventricle and pacing threshold for leads stimulating the left ventricle 　• Pacing lead impedance for all leads 　• Dysrhythmias detected by the device (e.g., mode switches, high ventricular rate episodes) 　• Percentage of pacing in each chamber 　• Review of programmed parameters 　• Review of any "safety" or automatic device alerts 　• Review of hemodynamic measurements or recordings of any other programmed parameters (e.g., heart rate variability, activity level), depending on the type of device
C. Determine whether the pacemaker needs to be reprogrammed.	Ensures proper programming.	
9. Assess the patient's vital signs, symptoms, and hemodynamic response.	The patient may have the electrical activity of pacing without the associated mechanical activity of cardiac contraction (e.g., pulseless electrical activity).	
10. If inappropriate pacemaker function is detected, notify the physician or advanced practice nurse immediately, and implement basic life support and advanced cardiac life support as needed.	Inappropriate pacemaker function may compromise cardiac output and necessitate immediate adjustment of settings or replacement of malfunctioning components.	
11. Remove gloves; clean the ECG leads, programmer, and wand; and discard used supplies in an appropriate receptacle. **HH**	Reduces the transmission of microorganisms; standard precautions.	

*Level M: Manufacturer's recommendations only.

UNIT II

Expected Outcomes

- Appropriate pacemaker functioning based on programmed parameters
- Improvement or resolution of bradycardia-induced symptoms (adequate systemic tissue perfusion and cardiac output as evidenced by the patient being alert, oriented, and normotensive, with no dizziness, shortness of breath, chest discomfort, or lightheadedness).
- Minimal discomfort with new implant; no discomfort with preexisting implant
- No signs or symptoms of fluid, infection, or erosion at the pocket incision site.
- Patient understanding of interrogation results and recommended setting changes.

Unexpected Outcomes

- Failure to sense (e.g., oversensing, undersensing) or failure to capture; failure to sense or capture in the immediate postimplant period may indicate lead dislodgment.
- Lead perforation of the myocardium may occur within the first 24 hours of implant; signs and symptoms may include intermittent failure of pacing or sensing, distant heart sounds, pericardial rub, and in extreme cases hemodynamic instability.
- Diaphragmatic stimulation may occur if high-voltage outputs are needed to pace the ventricles.
- Hematoma
- Wound infection
- Upper extremity venous thrombus
- Device or lead recall
- Lead fracture
- Lead insulation breech
- Ongoing site discomfort
- Extra cardiac stimulation other than the phrenic nerve
- Frozen shoulder due to postoperative arm limitations
- Anxiety or lack of coping due to a new health condition

Patient Monitoring and Care

Steps	Rationale	Reportable Conditions
		These conditions should be reported to the provider if they persist despite nursing interventions.
1. Monitor the ECG continuously.	Determines whether the patient's cardiac rate and rhythm are consistent with the programmed pacemaker parameters.	• Failure of the pacemaker to perform as programmed • Oversensing • Undersensing • Failure to capture
2. Monitor the patient's vital signs and hemodynamic status.	Determines the patient's response to pacemaker therapy.	• Abnormal vital signs or symptoms • Hemodynamic instability
3. Assess the pacemaker pocket in the acute postimplant phase.	Determines healing and the presence of fluid.	• Bleeding at incision, hematoma. • Edema around pacemaker site • Increased pain at incision site
4. Assess the upper extremity on the side of the implanted device in the acute postimplant phase.	Determines patent vasculature supplying the upper extremity and the presence of a thrombus.	• Swelling or tenderness to palpation of the upper extremity
5. Assess for signs and symptoms of infection.	Identifies infection.	• Redness • Edema • Drainage • Elevated white blood cell count • Elevated temperature • Increased pain or tenderness at the pacemaker site • Night sweats or chills
6. Follow institutional standards for assessing pain. Administer analgesia as prescribed.	Identifies the need for pain interventions.	• Continued pain despite pain interventions

Documentation

Documentation should include the following:

- Indication for implanting device, date of implant (generator and leads), and device type
- Patient education and evaluation of patient and family understanding
- Programmed parameters
- ECG rhythm strip recordings
- Underlying rhythm
- Evaluation of pacemaker function
- Battery longevity
- Physical assessment, including vital signs and hemodynamic response
- Evaluation of device incision site and surrounding skin
- Unexpected outcomes
- Interventions needed and evaluation of interventions
- Pain assessment, interventions, and effectiveness
- Recommended follow-up care and scheduling

References and Additional Readings

For a complete list of references and additional readings for this procedure, scan this QR code with your smartphone, or visit https://www.elsevier.com/__data/assets/pdf_file/0004/1319818/Chapter0043.pdf

PROCEDURE

44

Temporary Transcutaneous (External) Pacing

Valerie Spotts, Nikki J. Taylor, and Jennifer Pesenecker

PURPOSE Transcutaneous or external pacing stimulates myocardial depolarization through the chest wall. External pacing is used as a temporary measure when normal cardiac conduction fails to produce myocardial contraction and the patient experiences hemodynamic instability.

PREREQUISITE NURSING KNOWLEDGE

- Cardiac anatomy and physiology.
- Cardiac monitoring (see Procedure 49).
- Dysrhythmia interpretation.
- Temporary pacemaker function and expected patient responses to pacemaker therapy.
- Clinical and technical competence in the use of the external pacing equipment (Fig. 44.1).
- Indications for transcutaneous pacing are as follows[1-4]:
  - ❖ Symptomatic bradycardia unresponsive to medications
  - ❖ In standby mode for the following rhythms in the acute myocardial infarction setting[4,5]:
  - ❖ Symptomatic sinus node dysfunction
  - ❖ Mobitz type II second-degree heart block
  - ❖ Third-degree heart block
- Newly acquired left, right, or alternating bundle-branch block or bifascicular block
- Temporary transvenous pacing is indicated when prolonged pacing.
- Contraindications for transcutaneous pacing are as follows[2,6,7]:
  - ❖ Severe hypothermia
  - ❖ Asystole (as presenting rhythm)
- Pacing is contraindicated in severe hypothermia because cold ventricles are more prone to ventricular fibrillation and are more resistant to defibrillation.[6]
- External cardiac pacing is a temporary method of stimulating ventricular myocardial depolarization through the chest wall via two large pacing electrodes (patches). The electrodes are placed on the anterior and posterior chest wall (Figs. 44.2 and 44.3) or anterior and lateral chest wall (Fig. 44.4) and are attached by a cable to an external pulse generator. The external pulse generator delivers energy (milliamps) to the myocardium based on the set pacing rate, output, and sensitivity. Some models of external pulse generators are combined with an external defibrillator, and the electrodes of these models may be used for pacing and defibrillation. Some external pulse generators need the ECG leads attached to view the rhythm.

- *Sensitivity* refers to the ability of the pacemaker to detect intrinsic myocardial activity.
- In the nondemand or asynchronous mode, pacing occurs at the set rate regardless of the patient's intrinsic rate. In the demand or synchronous mode, the pacemaker senses intrinsic myocardial activity and paces when the intrinsic cardiac rate is lower than the set rate on the external pulse generator.
- *Pacing* occurs when the external pulse generator delivers enough energy through the pacing electrodes to the myocardium, which is known as *pacemaker firing* and is represented as a spike on the electrocardiograph (ECG) tracing.
- *Electrical capture* occurs when the pacemaker delivers enough energy to the myocardium so depolarization occurs. Capture is seen on the ECG with a pacemaker spike followed by a ventricular complex. The ventricular complex occurs after the pacemaker spike, and the QRS is wide (greater than 0.11 seconds), with the initial and terminal deflections in opposite directions. In Figure 44.5, paced complexes have a downward QRS negative following the pacer spike, and the T wave is in the opposite direction. *Mechanical capture* occurs when a paced QRS complex results in a palpable pulse.
- *Standby pacing* is when the pacing electrodes are applied in anticipation of possible use but pacing is not needed at the time.

EQUIPMENT

- Nonsterile gloves
- Blood pressure monitoring equipment
- External pulse generator
- Pacing cable
- Pacemaker electrodes (patches)
- ECG electrodes
- ECG monitor
- ECG cable
  Additional equipment to have available as needed includes the following:
- Emergency cart
- Medications including sedatives and analgesics
- Scissors
- Transvenous pacing equipment

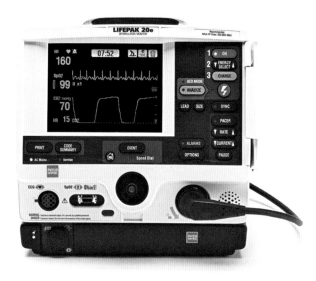

Figure 44.1   The LIFEPAK 20E provides defibrillation, monitoring, and external pacing. *(Reproduced with permission of Stryker.)*

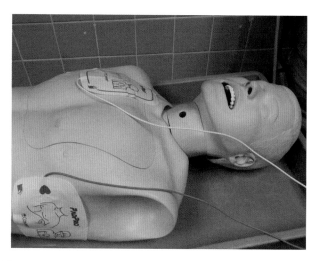

Figure 44.4   Location of anterior-lateral pacing electrodes. *(Courtesy Valerie Spotts.)*

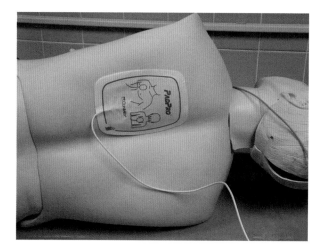

Figure 44.2   Location of the posterior (back) pacing electrode. *(Courtesy Valerie Spotts.)*

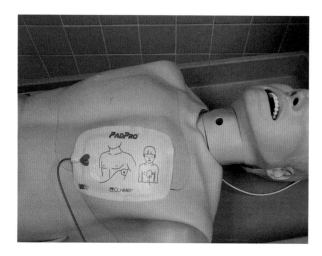

Figure 44.3   Location of the anterior (front) pacing electrode. *(Courtesy Valerie Spotts.)*

PATIENT AND FAMILY EDUCATION

- Assess learning needs, readiness to learn, and factors that influence learning. *Rationale:* This assessment reveals the patient's and family's knowledge so teaching can be individualized to be meaningful to the patient and family.
- Discuss basic facts about the normal conduction system, the reason external cardiac pacing is indicated, and what happens to the patient when pacing occurs. *Rationale:* This discussion assists the patient and family in recognizing the need for external pacing and what to expect when pacing occurs.
- Discuss discomfort experienced with transcutaneous pacing and interventions to alleviate it. *Rationale:* This discussion provides the patient with an opportunity to validate perceptions. It gives the patient and family knowledge that interventions are used to minimize the level of discomfort.
- If indicated, inform the patient and family of the possibility of the need for transvenous or permanent pacing support. *Rationale:* This information prepares the patient and family for the possibility of additional therapy. If permanent pacing is necessary, the patient and family need further instruction about possible lifestyle modifications, follow-up visits, and information about the pacemaker to be implanted.

PATIENT ASSESSMENT AND PREPARATION

Patient Assessment

- Assess the patient's cardiac rate and rhythm for the presence of dysrhythmias that indicate the need for external cardiac pacing. *Rationale:* Recognition of a dysrhythmia is the first step in determining the need for external cardiac pacing or placing the external pacemaker on standby.

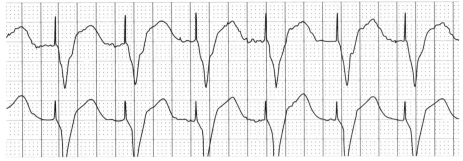

Figure 44.5   Electrocardiograph tracing of external pacing. *(Courtesy Valerie Spotts.)*

- Determine the patient's hemodynamic response to the dysrhythmia, such as the presence or absence of a pulse; presence of hypotension; altered level of consciousness; dizziness; shortness of breath; nausea and vomiting; cool, clammy, diaphoretic skin; or the development of chest pain. ***Rationale:*** The decision to initiate pacing depends on the effect of the dysrhythmia on the patient's cardiac output.

Patient Preparation

- Verify the correct patient with two identifiers. ***Rationale:*** Before performing a procedure, the nurse should ensure the correct identification of the patient for the intended intervention.

- Ensure that the patient and family understand preprocedural teaching. Answer questions as they arise, and reinforce information as needed. ***Rationale:*** This communication evaluates and reinforces understanding of previously taught information.
- Maintain bedside ECG monitoring. ***Rationale:*** External pacing units do not provide central monitoring or dysrhythmia detection.
- Establish or ensure patency of intravenous access. ***Rationale:*** Medication administration may be necessary.
- Assist the patient to the supine position, and expose the patient's torso while maintaining modesty. ***Rationale:*** This positioning prepares for electrode (patch) placement.

Procedure	**for Temporary Transcutaneous (External) Pacing**	
Steps	Rationale	Special Considerations
1. **HH**		
2. **PE**		
3. Administer sedative or analgesic medications as prescribed. **(Level D*)**	Decreases discomfort associated with external cardiac pacing.[2,3,6]	Not indicated for patients who are unconscious with hemodynamically unstable conditions. Not indicated for standby because pacing may not be needed.
4. Turn on the pulse generator and monitor. **(Level M*)**	Provides the power source.	Many devices work on battery or alternating current (AC) power.
5. Prepare the skin on the patient's chest and back by washing with nonemollient soap and water. **(Level B*)**	Removal of skin oils, lotion, and moisture improves electrode adherence and maximizes delivery of energy through the chest wall.	Optional step in an emergency. Dry thoroughly. Trim body hair with scissors, if necessary. Avoid use of flammable liquids to prepare the skin (e.g., alcohol, benzoin) because of the increased potential for burns.[2,6,7] Avoid shaving the chest hair because the presence of nicks in the skin under the pacing electrodes can increase patient discomfort. Remove any medication patches applied to the chest area.
6. Apply the ECG electrodes to the ECG leads.	Prepares the equipment.	

*Level B: Well-designed controlled studies with results that consistently support a specific action, intervention, or treatment.
*Level M: Manufacturer's recommendations only.

Procedure continues on following page

Procedure	for Temporary Transcutaneous (External) Pacing—*Continued*	
Steps	Rationale	Special Considerations
7. Connect the ECG cable to the monitor inlet of the pulse generator. **(Level M*)**	Prepares the equipment.	Follow the manufacturer's recommendations. Attachment of the ECG electrodes to the ECG leads and the ECG cable to the pacemaker monitor is optional for some manufacturers in an emergency. If the ECG leads are not placed, the pacemaker may function in the asynchronous mode. The pacemaker may not function unless both the ECG monitoring connection and the pacing electrode connection are both connected to the pacemaker.
8. Apply the ECG electrodes to the patient (see Procedure 49).	Displays the patient's intrinsic rhythm on the monitor.	
9. Adjust the ECG lead and size to the maximum R wave size. Look for an indicator that the pacemaker is sensing the QRS complexes on the intrinsic rhythm, usually seen as a marker above each native QRS complex.	Detection of the intrinsic rhythm is necessary for the demand mode of pacing.	Lead II usually provides the most prominent R wave.
10. Apply the back (posterior, positive) pacing electrode between the spine and left scapula at the level of the heart (see Fig. 44.2).	Placement of the pacing electrodes in the recommended anatomical location enhances the potential for successful pacing.	Avoid placing the pacing electrodes over bone because this increases the level of energy needed to pace, increases patient discomfort, and increases the possibility of noncapture.
11. Apply the front (anterior, negative) pacing electrode at the left, fourth intercostal space, midclavicular line (see Fig. 44.3). **(Level M*)**	Placement of the pacing electrodes in the recommended anatomical locations enhances the potential for successful pacing.	For women, adjust the position of the pacing electrode below and lateral to breast tissue to ensure optimal adherence. Avoid placement of the pacing electrodes over the bedside monitor ECG electrodes and permanently placed devices, such as implantable cardioverter-defibrillators or permanent pacemakers.
12. If the patient's condition is hemodynamically unstable, the back (posterior) electrode may be placed over the patient's right sternal area at the second or third intercostal space. The front (anterior) electrode is maintained at the apex (fourth or fifth intercostal space, midclavicular line (see Fig. 44.4).	Facilitates ease of electrode placement for emergent pacing.	Pacing may be less effective with this method of electrode placement.[1,6]
13. Connect the pacing electrodes to the pacemaker cable, and connect the pacemaker cable to the external pulse generator. **(Level M*)**	Necessary for the delivery of electrical energy.	

*Level M: Manufacturer's recommendations only.

Procedure for Temporary Transcutaneous (External) Pacing—*Continued*

Steps	Rationale	Special Considerations
14. Set the pacemaker rate, level of energy (output, mA) (Fig. 44.6).	Each patient needs different pacemaker settings to provide safe and effective external pacing.	Follow institutional standards regarding who can initiate external cardiac pacing. The demand mode is used as long as the ECG leads are attached to the pacemaker monitor.
A. Set the demand or the synchronous mode.	The demand mode is used to prevent competition from the patient's intrinsic rhythm.	In the asynchronous mode, the pacemaker fires regardless of the intrinsic rhythm and rate.
B. Set the rate.	Pacing should be at a rate that maintains adequate cardiac output but does not induce ischemia.	The pacemaker may have a default setting (e.g., 80 beats/min) that can be adjusted as needed.

C. Set the mA.
  i. Slowly increase the mA setting (output) until capture is present.
  ii. Set the mA slightly higher than the capture threshold (an additional 2 mA).[6,8]
	Use the lowest amount of energy that consistently results in myocardial capture and contraction to minimize discomfort.[8]	The pacemaker may have a default setting that can be adjusted as needed, or the pacemaker may turn on at 0 mA and will need to be increased for pacing to occur. The average adult usually can be paced with a current of 40–70 mA.

Procedure continues on following page

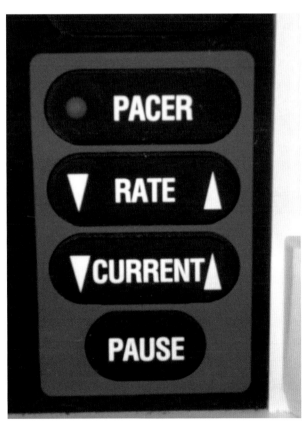

Figure 44.6 Controls for external pacemaker settings. *(Courtesy Valerie Spotts.)*

Patient Monitoring and Care —*Continued*

Steps	Rationale	Special Considerations
15. When the pacemaker fires, observe that each pacemaker spike is followed by a wide ventricular complex and a T wave in the opposite deflection of the QRS (see Fig. 44.5).	Identifies appropriate functioning of the pacemaker.	If a pacemaker spike occurs and is not followed by a ventricular complex, slowly increase the energy (mA) level. Artifact from skeletal muscle twitching may make an ECG tracing difficult to interpret. Skeletal muscle twitching occurs at lower mA settings, before capture of the myocardium.[1,7,8] Confirm mechanical capture by assessing pulse or intraarterial waveform.
16. Palpate the patient's pulse (e.g., femoral pulse, right brachial pulse, radial pulse).	Ensures adequate blood flow with paced complexes.	The carotid pulses usually are not palpated because the electrical stimulation from the pacemaker may mimic a pulse.[2,7,8]
17. Evaluate the patient's vital signs and hemodynamic response to pacing.	The patient's hemodynamic response should improve with pacing if symptoms were related to bradycardia.[1,8]	If symptoms do not improve with pacing, assess for other causes such as electrolyte abnormalities.
18. Remove **PE**, and discard used supplies in appropriate receptacles.	Reduces the transmission of microorganisms; standard precautions.	
19. **HH**		

Expected Outcomes

- Adequate systemic tissue perfusion and cardiac output as evidenced by blood pressure greater than 90 mm Hg systolic (or resolution of hypotension), return to baseline mental status, absence of dizziness or syncope, absence of shortness of breath, absence of nausea and vomiting, and absence of ischemic chest pain
- Stable cardiac rate and rhythm
- Appropriate sensing, pacing, and capture present

Unexpected Outcomes

- Failure of the pacemaker to sense the patient's underlying rhythm with the possibility of R-on-T phenomenon (initiation of ventricular tachydysrhythmias as a result of an improperly timed spike on the T wave)
- Failure of the pacemaker to capture the myocardium
- Failure of the pacemaker to pace
- Discomfort, including skin burns from the delivery of high levels of energy through the chest wall, painful sensations, and skeletal muscle twitching

Patient Monitoring and Care

Steps	Rationale	Reportable Conditions
		These conditions should be reported to the provider if they persist despite nursing interventions.
1. Monitor vital signs every 15 minutes until stable, and then hourly or more frequently as needed. (**Level E***)	Ensures adequate tissue perfusion with paced beats. Adjustments in the pacing rate may need to be made based on vital signs. Continuous assessment is needed because pacing thresholds may change, and response to the pacemaker settings can change over time.	- Change in vital signs - Hemodynamic instability

*Level E: Multiple case reports, theory-based evidence from expert opinions, or peer-reviewed professional organizational standards without clinical studies to support recommendations.

Patient Monitoring and Care *—Continued*

Steps	Rationale	Reportable Conditions
2. Continue to monitor the patient's cardiac rate and rhythm through the central monitoring system. The pacing spike may obscure or mimic the QRS complex, making ventricular capture difficult to see.[2,7,9] Select a lead that minimizes the size of the pacing spike and maximizes the QRS complex.[2,7] Set the pacemaker option on the central monitoring system.	Provides an alarm system. Of note, if ECG leads are disconnected from the pacemaker monitor, pacing reverts to asynchronous, which could compete with the native rhythm.	• Changes in capture or sensing • Dysrhythmias

3. Monitor level of comfort and sedation level:
  A. Assess the patient's level of comfort and sedation level following institutional standards.
  B. Administer the prescribed analgesic and sedative medications as needed.
  C. Adjust the level of energy to the lowest level for capture.
  D. Evaluate the patient's response to interventions.
	The external delivery of energy through the chest wall may cause varying degrees of discomfort.[1,2,4,7]	• Continued pain despite interventions to alleviate pain
		• Patient intolerance of the prescribed medications (e.g., nausea, hypotension, decreased respirations)

4. Obtain an ECG recording strip to document pacing function on initiation of pacing, every 4–8 hours, and as needed or according to institutional standards.	Documents cardiac rate, rhythm, and pacemaker activity.	• Dysrhythmias • Failure to capture • Failure to pace
5. Obtain blood samples for laboratory analysis as prescribed.	Acidosis and electrolyte abnormalities need to be corrected for an effective response to pacing.	• Electrolyte abnormalities • Acidosis
6. Evaluate pacemaker function (capturing and sensing) with any change in patient condition or vital signs. If changes to capturing or sensing occurs, assess the position of the electrode pads.	Ensures continued functioning of the pacemaker.	• Inability to maintain appropriate sensing and capture • Changes in patient condition that affect appropriate pacemaker function

7. Monitor the patient's cardiac rate and rhythm for resolution of the dysrhythmia that necessitates pacemaker intervention.
  A. This monitoring may necessitate turning the pacemaker off, if prescribed, to assess the patient's underlying rate and rhythm. Do not turn the pacemaker off if the patient is 100% paced.
  B. When assessing the patient's intrinsic rate and rhythm, reduce the pacing rate slowly.
	Determines whether the dysrhythmia has subsided. Some devices have the ability to reduce the percentage of pacing to allow assessment of the underlying rhythm. A sudden cessation of pacing can lead to asystole because the intrinsic rate and rhythm may be suppressed by continuous pacing.[2,6,7]	• Worsening of baseline cardiac rate and rhythm (e.g., change from symptomatic second-degree heart block to complete heart block)

Procedure continues on following page

UNIT II

Patient Monitoring and Care —*Continued*

Steps	Rationale	Reportable Conditions
8. Check the adherence of the pacing electrodes to the skin at least every 4 hours. If pacing is not occurring, assess the skin integrity under the pacing electrodes. 9. Change the electrodes at least every 24 hours or after 8 hours of continuous pacing.[2,7] (**Level M***) Prepare for an alternate method of pacing if pacing need continues.	Changes in skin integrity caused by burns or skin breaks significantly alter the patient's level of comfort and expose the patient to possible infection. Pacing electrodes should not be used once they have been out of the package for 24 hours.[2,6,7]	• Changes in skin integrity • Burns

*Level M: Manufacturer's recommendations only.

Documentation

Documentation should include the following:
- Patient and family education
- Patient preparation
- Date and time external cardiac pacing is initiated
- Description of events that warranted intervention
- Vital signs and physical assessment before and after external cardiac pacing
- ECG recordings before and after pacing
- Pain assessment, interventions, and effectiveness
- Medications administered
- Pacing rate, mode, mA
- Percentage of the time the patient is paced if in the demand mode
- Status of skin integrity when the pacing electrodes are changed
- Interventions to secure an alternate and less painful method of pacing if the need continues
- Unexpected outcomes
- Additional interventions

References and Additional Readings

For a complete list of references and additional readings for this procedure, scan this QR code with your smartphone, or visit https://www.elsevier.com/__data/assets/pdf_file/0005/1319819/Chapter0044.pdf.

45 Temporary Transvenous AP Pacemaker Insertion (Perform)

Nikki J. Taylor

PURPOSE The purpose of temporary cardiac pacing is to ensure or restore an adequate heart rate and rhythm. A transvenous pacemaker is inserted as a temporary measure when the normal conduction system of the heart fails to produce or conduct an electrical impulse, resulting in hemodynamic decompensation.

PREREQUISITE NURSING KNOWLEDGE

- Knowledge of the anatomy and physiology of the cardiovascular system, principles of cardiac conduction, as well as basic and advanced dysrhythmia interpretation.
- Temporary pacemaker function and expected patient responses to pacemaker therapy.
- Clinical and technical competence in central line insertion, temporary transvenous pacemaker insertion, and suturing.
- Principles of sterile technique.
- Clinical and technical competence related to the use of temporary pacemakers.
- Competence in chest radiograph interpretation.
- Advanced cardiac life support (ACLS) knowledge and skills.
- Application of principles of general electrical safety with the use of temporary invasive pacing.
- Gloves always should be worn when handling pacemaker electrodes to prevent microshock because even small amounts of electrical current can cause serious dysrhythmias if they are transmitted to the heart.[9]
- Knowledge of the care of the patient with central venous catheters (see Procedures 74, Central Venous Catheter Insertion [Perform], and 75, Central Venous Catheter Insertion [Assist], Nursing Care and Removal)
- The insertion of a temporary transvenous pacemaker is performed in emergency and elective clinical situations. Temporary transvenous pacing may be used for the following:
  - ❖ Stimulate the myocardium to contract in the absence of an intrinsic rhythm
  - ❖ Establish adequate cardiac output and blood pressure
  - ❖ Ensure tissue perfusion to vital organs
  - ❖ Reduce the possibility of ventricular dysrhythmias in the presence of bradycardia

  - ❖ Supplement an inadequate rhythm, such as when transient decreases in heart rate occur (e.g., chronotropic incompetence in shock)
  - ❖ Allow the administration of medications that may cause a rhythm or conduction abnormalities (e.g., beta blockers).
- Temporary transvenous pacing is indicated for the following:
  - ❖ Symptomatic third-degree atrioventricular (AV) block
  - ❖ Symptomatic Type II AV block
  - ❖ Dysrhythmias that may occur in the setting of an acute myocardial infarction (e.g., symptomatic bradycardia, complete heart block, new bundle-branch block with transient complete heart block, alternating bundle-branch block)
  - ❖ Sinus node dysfunction (e.g., symptomatic bradyarrhythmias, treatment of bradycardia-tachycardia syndromes, sick sinus syndrome)
  - ❖ Ventricular standstill or cardiac arrest
  - ❖ Long QT syndrome with ventricular dysrhythmias
  - ❖ Medication toxicity or adverse side effects of a medication
  - ❖ Postoperative cardiac surgery in the absence of working temporary epicardial pacemaker wires
  - ❖ Prophylaxis with cardiac diagnostic, interventional procedures or surgical procedures
  - ❖ Chronotropic incompetence in the setting of cardiogenic shock
  - ❖ Malfunction/infection of a permanent cardiac pacemaker
- When temporary transvenous pacing is used, the pulse generator is attached externally to one or more pacing leads that are inserted through a vein into the right atrium and/or right ventricle.
- Veins used for the insertion of a transvenous pacing lead wire include the subclavian, femoral, brachial, internal jugular, or external jugular vein.
- Single-chamber ventricular pacing is the most appropriate method in an emergency because the goal is to establish a heart rate as quickly as possible.
- The transvenous pacing lead is an insulated wire with one or two electrodes at the tip of the wire (Fig. 45.1).

AP This procedure should be performed only by clinicians who have demonstrated competence and are credentialed to perform it. In addition, the procedure must be within the scope of practice defined by their professional licensure, and in accordance with professional practice acts. Physicians, advanced practice nurses, and physician assistants may be credentialed to perform this procedure.

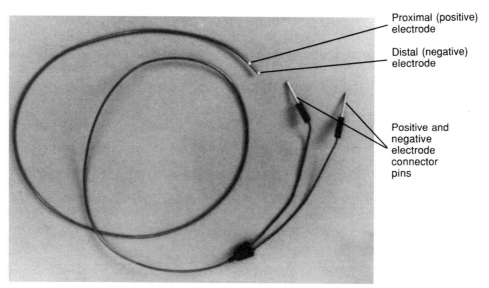

Figure 45.1   Bipolar lead wire.

- The pacing lead can be a hard-tipped or a balloon-tipped pacing catheter that is placed in direct contact with the endocardium. Most temporary leads are bipolar with the distal tip electrode (seen as a metal ring) separated from the proximal electrode by 1 to 2 cm of pacing catheter (also seen as a metal ring; see Figs. 45.1 and 46.1).
- Basic principles of cardiac pacing include sensing, pacing, and capture.
  - ❖ *Sensing* refers to the ability of the pacemaker device to detect intrinsic myocardial electrical activity. Sensing occurs if the pulse generator is in the synchronous or demand mode. The pacemaker either is inhibited from delivering a stimulus or initiates an electrical impulse in response to a sensed event.
  - ❖ *Pacing* occurs when the temporary pulse generator is activated and the programmed level of energy travels from the pulse generator through the temporary pacing lead wire to the endocardium. This is known as *pacemaker firing* and is exhibited as a vertical line or spike on the electrocardiogram (ECG) recording.
  - ❖ *Capture* refers to the successful conduction of the pacemaker impulse through the myocardium, resulting in depolarization. Capture is evidenced on the ECG by a pacemaker spike followed by either an atrial or a ventricular complex, depending on the chamber being paced. The healthcare provider can assess whether the electrical depolarization resulted in mechanical activity by observing pressure waveforms for evidence of contraction (right or left atrial, pulmonary artery, or arterial) or by palpating a pulse.
- Pulse generators can be used for single-chamber pacing with one set of terminals at the top of the pulse generator, into which the pacing wires are inserted (via a connecting cable). A dual-chamber pacemaker requires two sets of terminals, one each for the atrial and ventricular wires (see Fig. 46.6).
- The temporary pulse generator houses the controls and the energy source for pacing. Different models of pacemakers use either dials or touchpads to adjust the following settings (see Figs. 46.5 to 46.6):

  - ❖ Pacing rate adjusts the number of pacing stimuli delivered per minute.
  - ❖ Pacing output determines the amount of energy delivered to the endocardium in milliamperes (mA). Dual-chamber pacing requires that mA are set for both the atria and the ventricle.
  - ❖ AV interval on a dual-chamber pacemaker controls the amount of time between atrial and ventricular stimulation (electronic PR interval).
  - ❖ Sensitivity determines the size of the intrinsic activity in millivolts (mV) that will be detected by the generator.
- The ability of the pacemaker to detect the patient's intrinsic rhythm is determined by the pacing mode. In an asynchronous mode, the pacemaker functions as a fixed-rate pacemaker and is not able to sense any of the patient's inherent cardiac electrical activity. In a synchronous mode, the pacemaker is able to sense the patient's inherent cardiac electrical activity.
- The ability of the pacemaker to depolarize the myocardium depends on many variables: position of the electrode and degree of contact with viable endocardial tissue; level of energy delivered through the pacing wire; presence of hypoxia, acidosis, or electrolyte imbalances; fibrosis around the tip of the catheter; and concomitant medication therapy.[8]
- All electrical equipment in the patient's room must be properly grounded to prevent interference from occurring (this may be seen as a 60-cycle interference on the ECG).
- Exposed pacing leads should be insulated when not in use to prevent microshock.

EQUIPMENT

- Antiseptic skin preparation solution (e.g., 2% chlorhexidine-based solution)
- Sterile drapes, gloves and gowns, and towels
- Masks, head cover, goggles, or face shields
- Pacing catheter (flexible or rigid with or without balloon) and insertion tray
- Pulse generator
- Appropriate batteries for the pulse generator

- Connecting cables
- Alligator clips or wires with connecting pins
- ECG monitor and recorder
- Supplies for dressing at the insertion site

Additional equipment to have available as needed includes the following:

- Local anesthetic
- Percutaneous introducer needle or 14-gauge needle
- Introducer sheath with dilator
- Guidewire (per physician or advanced practice nurse choice)
- Suture, syringes, needles, and scalpel
- Emergency equipment (e.g., automated external defibrillator [AED], defibrillator)
- Portable ultrasound scan equipment with sterile probe sheath and gel
- Fluoroscopy
- Lead aprons or shields
- 12-lead ECG machine

PATIENT AND FAMILY EDUCATION

- Assess learning needs, readiness to learn, and factors that influence learning. *Rationale:* This assessment enables teaching to be individualized in a manner that is meaningful to the patient and family.
- Discuss basic facts about the normal conduction system, such as structure and function of the conduction system, normal and abnormal heart rhythms, and symptoms and significance of abnormal heart rhythms. *Rationale:* The patient and family should understand the conduction system, why the procedure is necessary, and what potential risks and benefits are associated with this invasive procedure.
- Provide a basic description of the temporary transvenous pacemaker insertion procedure. *Rationale:* The patient and family should be informed of the invasive nature of the procedure and any risks associated with the procedure. An understanding of the procedure may reduce anxiety associated with the procedure.
- Describe the precautions and restrictions required while the temporary pacemaker is in place, such as limitation of movement, avoiding handling the pacemaker or touching exposed portions of the electrodes, and situations in which the nurse should be notified (e.g., if the dressing becomes damp, if the patient experiences dizziness). Patients with femoral temporary pacemakers will most likely be placed on bed rest with limited motion in the limb that the pacemaker was placed. *Rationale:* Understanding potential limitations may improve the patient's cooperation with restrictions and precautions.

PATIENT ASSESSMENT AND PREPARATION

Patient Assessment

- Assess the patient's cardiac rhythm for the presence of the dysrhythmia that necessitates the initiation of temporary

cardiac pacing. *Rationale:* This assessment determines the need for invasive cardiac pacing.

- Assess the patient's hemodynamic response to the dysrhythmia. Rhythm disturbances may reduce cardiac output significantly, with detrimental effects on perfusion of vital organs. *Rationale:* This assessment determines the urgency of the procedure. It may indicate the need for temporizing measures (e.g., vasopressors or transcutaneous pacing [see Procedure 44, Temporary Transcutaneous (External) Pacing]).
- Review current medications. *Rationale:* Medications may be implicated as a cause of the dysrhythmia that led to the need for pacemaker therapy, or medications may need to be held as a result of concomitant effect. Other medications, such as antidysrhythmics, may alter the pacing threshold. Review of medications could also determine whether reversal agents could be used as an alternative to pacemaker therapy.
- Review the patient's current laboratory study results, including chemistry, electrolyte profile, arterial blood gases, coagulation profile, platelet count, and cardioactive serum medication levels. *Rationale:* This review assists in determining whether inserting the pacemaker was precipitated by metabolic disturbances or medication toxicity and establishes the pacing milieu. The review provides the healthcare provider with information regarding the risk for abnormal bleeding during or after the procedure is performed.

Patient Preparation

- Verify the correct patient with two identifiers. *Rationale:* Before performing a procedure, the nurse should ensure the correct identification of the patient for the intended intervention.
- Ensure that the patient and family understand the preprocedural teaching. Answer questions as they arise, and reinforce information as needed. *Rationale:* Evaluates and reinforces understanding of previously taught information.
- Obtain informed consent. *Rationale:* Informed consent protects the rights of the patient and makes a competent decision possible for the patient; however, in emergency circumstances, time may not allow a consent form to be signed.
- Perform a "time-out" procedure to confirm the correct patient, site and procedure, if nonemergent. *Rationale:* This ensures patient safety.
- Connect the patient to a 5-lead monitoring system or to a 12-lead ECG machine. *Rationale:* This monitoring facilitates placement of the balloon-tipped catheter by indicating the position of the catheter during placement. Also, it allows for monitoring of the patient's cardiac rhythm during the procedure.
- Prescribe and ensure that pain medication and/or sedation is administered. *Rationale:* Medication may be indicated depending on the patient's level of anxiety and pain. Sedation or pain medication may not be possible if the patient's condition is hemodynamically unstable.

Procedure for Performing Temporary Transvenous Pacemaker Insertion

Steps	Rationale	Special Considerations
1. 🅷🅷		
2. 🅿🅴		
3. Connect the patient to the bedside monitoring system, and monitor the ECG continuously (see Procedure 49, Electrocardiographic Leads and Cardiac Monitoring).	Monitors the patient's intrinsic heart rate and rhythm during and after the procedure to evaluate for adequate rate and pacemaker function.	If the monitoring system is not a 5-lead system, also connect the patient to the 12-lead ECG machine (see Procedure 49, Electrocardiographic Leads and Cardiac Monitoring).
4. Dispose of used supplies, and wash hands.	Minimizes the risk of infection.	
5. Check the placement of the central venous access with chest radiography before beginning the procedure.	Central venous access is needed as the transvenous pacing catheter is passed through the central venous system.	If central venous access is needed, refer to Procedures 74 (Central Venous Catheter Insertion [Perform]) and 75 (Central Venous Catheter Insertion [Assist], Nursing Care and Removal). A modified pulmonary artery catheter may be used with dedicated arterial and ventricular ports while still allowing routine thermodilution hemodynamic monitoring.[2,91]
6. Assess functioning of the temporary pacemaker, check the battery life indicator to see the battery (or batteries) level, and insert a new battery into the pulse generator before beginning therapy if needed or according to institutional policy. (**Level M***)	Ensures a functional pacemaker pulse generator.	Different ways to assess battery function depend on the model and manufacturer; check the manufacturer's recommendations for specific instructions.
7. Attach the connecting cable to the pulse generator, connecting the "positive" on the cable to the "positive" on the pulse generator and the "negative" on the cable to the "negative" on the pulse generator.	Prepares the pacing system; the pacing stimulus travels from the pulse generator to the negative terminal, and energy returns to the pulse generator via the positive terminal.	Some lead wires are labeled "distal" and "proximal"; distal connects to negative, and proximal connects to positive. Some lead wires do not have "negative" and "positive" marked on them. Polarity is established when the wires are placed in the connecting cable. Two connecting cables are needed with both atrial and ventricular pacing.
8. All personnel performing and assisting with the procedure should wash hands and apply 🅿🅴 and sterile equipment (e.g., masks, head covers, goggles or face shields, sterile gowns, and gloves).	Minimizes the risk of infection and maintains standard and sterile precautions.	Gloves should be worn whenever the pacing electrodes are handled to prevent microshock. If fluoroscopy will be used, all personnel must be shielded from the radiation with lead aprons under the sterile gowns or be positioned behind lead shields. A lead sheet or apron should also be placed below the patient's waist.
9. Cleanse the site with antiseptic solution (e.g., 2% chlorhexidine-based preparation).	Minimizes the risk of infection.	
10. Drape the site with the sterile drapes.	Provides a sterile field and reduces the transmission of microorganisms.	A full drape will minimize the patient's risk for infection.
11. Insert the balloon-tipped pacing catheter through the introducer, and slowly advance the pacing lead, using one of the following insertion techniques:	The transvenous pacing catheter is threaded through the central venous system, using one of four methods to confirm proper placement.	For transvenous, ventricular pacing, the negative pacing electrode is positioned in the endocardium (at the apex) of the right ventricle.

*Level M: Manufacturer's recommendations only.

Procedure for Performing Temporary Transvenous Pacemaker Insertion—*Continued*		
Steps	Rationale	Special Considerations
A. Blind technique: 　i. Continue advancing the pacing lead.	This technique can be used to quickly achieve pacing in unstable patients.	If premature ventricular contractions or runs of ventricular tachycardia occur, deflate the balloon and slightly withdraw the catheter.
ii. The balloon can be inflated when the tip of the pacing lead is in the vena cava, approximately at the 20 cm marking.	The balloon allows blood flow to facilitate catheter advancement.	Once capture is identified on ECG, mechanical contraction should be confirmed with palpation of a pulse.
iii. As the catheter advances, pacemaker spikes will be seen on the ECG monitor. When the catheter enters the right ventricle and makes contact with the right ventricular wall, a left bundle branch will be seen after every pacemaker spike indicating capture.		
B. Ultrasound-guided technique increases first pass success and decreases hematoma/complication rate. **(Level E*)**: 　i. Obtain ultrasound equipment. 　ii. Continue advancing the pacing lead. 　iii. The balloon can be inflated when the tip of the pacing lead can be visualized in the vena cava. 　iv. Advance the pacing lead to the desired intracardiac position guided by ultrasound.	Transcutaneous ultrasound scan visualization of the pacing lead as it is passed through the central venous system may ensure quicker and more accurate placement of the pacing electrode within the endocardium of the right ventricle.[2,4,10,11]	
C. Fluoroscopy-guided technique: 　i. Obtain fluoroscopy equipment. 　ii. Continue advancing the pacing lead. 　iii. The balloon can be inflated when the tip of the pacing lead can be visualized in the vena cava. 　iv. Advance the pacing catheter to the desired intracardiac position guided by fluoroscopy.	Fluoroscopy may be needed to permit direct visualization of the pacing electrode.[2,11]	If fluoroscopy is used, all personnel must be shielded from the radiation with lead aprons or be positioned behind lead shields. A lead sheet or apron should also be placed below the patient's waist. The provider operating the fluoroscopy should have a fluoroscopy license per state and/or according to institutional guidelines.

*Level E: Multiple case reports, theory-based evidence from expert opinions, or peer-reviewed professional organizational standards without clinical studies to support recommendations.

Procedure continues on following page

Procedure	for Performing Temporary Transvenous Pacemaker Insertion—*Continued*	
Steps	Rationale	Special Considerations

D. ECG-guided technique:
  i. The V lead of a 5-lead system can be used.
  ii. Alternatively, a 12-lead ECG machine can be used.
  iii. Connect the patient to the limb leads of the 12-lead ECG machine if this method is used.
  iv. Attach the V lead of the ECG monitoring system or the 12-lead ECG machine to the negative electrode connector pin (distal pin) of the pacing lead wire.
  v. An alligator clip or a wire with connector pins can be used if needed (see Fig. 45.2).
  vi. Set the monitoring system to record the V lead continuously.
  vii. Continue advancing the pacing lead.
  viii. The balloon can be inflated when the tip of the pacing lead is in the vena cava, approximately at the 20-cm marking.
  ix. Advance the pacing lead, and observe the ECG for ST segment elevation in the V lead (Fig. 45.3).
  x. Observe for a left bundle-branch block pattern and left-axis deviation that usually can be identified (Fig. 45.4).
	When an ECG is obtained directly from the pacing electrode, proper positioning of the catheter tip is verified by visualization of the ST-segment elevation indicating catheter contact with the endocardium.[4,5,114]	As a result of temporary pacing catheter transmission of impulses from within the right ventricle, conduction of the impulse throughout the ventricles occurs via cellular conduction of the impulse rather than transmission down the bundle branches.

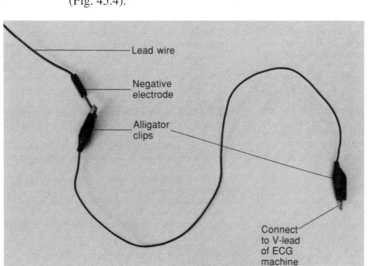

Figure 45.2   Alligator clips. *ECG,* Electrocardiogram.

Procedure   **for Performing Temporary Transvenous Pacemaker Insertion—*Continued***

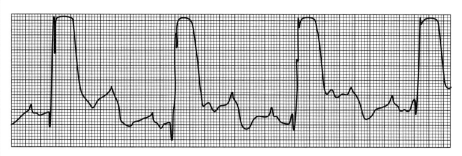

Figure 45.3 Electrocardiogram rhythm recorded in the right ventricle; elevated ST segments when the pacing electrode is wedged against the endocardial wall of the right ventricle. *(From Meltzer LE, Pinneo R, Kitchell JR: Intensive coronary care, ed 4, Bowie, MD, 1983, Robert J. Brady Co.)*

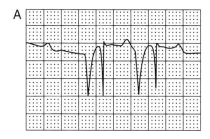

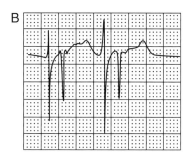

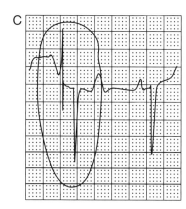

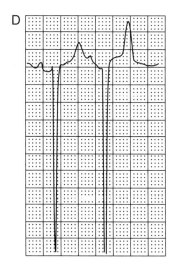

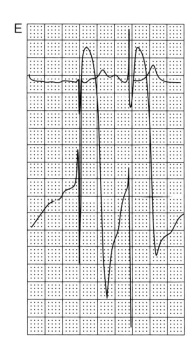

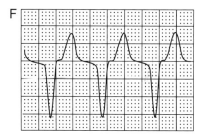

Figure 45.4 ECG recordings during transvenous pacemaker placement. A. High right atrium, B. Mid to low right atrium, C. Low right atrium to tricuspid annulus D. Right ventricle, E. Contact with right ventricular endocardium, and F. Surface ECG demonstrating pacemaker capture. *(Courtesy of Joyce W. Wald, DO.)*

Procedure continues on following page

Procedure	for Performing Temporary Transvenous Pacemaker Insertion—*Continued*	
Steps	Rationale	Special Considerations

12. After the electrodes are properly positioned:
  A. Deflate the balloon.
  B. Connect the pacing lead external electrode pins to the pulse generator via the connecting cables.
  C. Ensure that the positive and negative electrodes are connected to the respective positive and negative terminals on the pulse generator via the connecting cables.
	Energy from the pulse generator is directed to the negative electrode in contact with the ventricle. The pacing circuit is completed as energy reaches the positive electrode.
	The lead wires must be connected securely to the pacemaker to ensure appropriate sensing and capture and to prevent inadvertent disconnection.
		A bridging connecting cable is recommended for use between the pacing lead and the pulse generator.

13. Set the pacemaker settings and initiate pacing (see Procedure 46, Temporary Transvenous and Epicardial Pacing).	Initiates pacemaker therapy.	
14. Suture the pacing lead in place.	Minimizes the risk of dislodgment.	
15. Apply a sterile occlusive dressing over the site.	Minimizes the risk of infection.	
16. Secure the pacemaker equipment such as strapping the pulse generator to the patient's torso or securing the pulse generator in a carrying device.	The pulse generator should be protected from falling or becoming inadvertently detached by patient movement. Disconnection or tension on the pacing electrodes may lead to pacemaker malfunction.	Pinning the generator to the patient's sheets or pillow is not recommended because the pacing lead may be inadvertently disconnected if the patient moves, sits up, or gets out of bed.
17. Remove **PE**, and discard used supplies in appropriate receptacles.	Reduces the transmission of microorganisms; standard precautions.	
18. **HH**		
19. Obtain a chest radiograph.	In the absence of fluoroscopy, a chest radiograph is essential to detect potential complications associated with insertion and to visualize lead position.	

Expected Outcomes

- Paced rhythm on ECG consistent with parameters set on the pacemaker, as evidenced by appropriate heart rate, proper sensing, and proper capture
- Patient exhibits hemodynamic stability, as evidenced by systolic blood pressure greater than 90 mm Hg, mean arterial blood pressure greater than 60 mm Hg, alert and oriented condition, and no syncope or ischemia
- Pacemaker leads securely connected to the pulse generator

Unexpected Outcomes

- Inability to achieve proper placement of the pacing catheter
- Failure of the pacemaker to sense, causing competition between the pacemaker-initiated impulses and the patient's intrinsic cardiac rhythm
- Failure of the pacemaker to capture the myocardium
- Pacemaker oversensing that causes the pacemaker to be inappropriately inhibited
- Stimulation of the diaphragm that causes hiccupping, possibly related to pacing the phrenic nerve, perforation, wire dislodgment, or excessively high pacemaker mA setting
- Phlebitis, thrombosis, embolism, or catheter-related blood stream infections
- Ventricular dysrhythmias
- Arterial puncture, pseudoaneurysm, arteriovenous fistula, hematoma, pneumothorax, hemothorax, pneumomediastinum, or the development of subcutaneous emphysema from the insertion procedure[12]
- Myocardial perforation, cardiac tamponade, or postpericardiotomy syndrome from the insertion procedure and electrode placement
- Air embolism
- Lead dislodgment
- Pain

Patient Monitoring and Care

Steps	Rationale	Reportable Conditions
		These conditions should be reported if they persist despite nursing interventions.
1. Monitor vital signs and hemodynamic response to pacing following institutional standards and as often as the patient's condition warrants.	The goal of cardiac pacing is to improve cardiac output by increasing heart rate or by overriding life-threatening dysrhythmias.	• Change in vital signs associated with signs and symptoms of hemodynamic deterioration
2. Evaluate the ECG for the presence of the paced rhythm or resolution of the initiating dysrhythmia.	Proper pacemaker functioning is assessed by observing the ECG for pacemaker activity consistent with the set parameters.	• Dysrhythmias • Inability to obtain capture • Oversensing • Undersensing
3. Follow institutional standards for assessing pain. Prescribe analgesia.	Promotes comfort.	• Continual hiccups (may indicate wire perforation or phrenic nerve stimulation) • Continued pain despite pain interventions
4. Check and document the sensitivity and pacing threshold at least every 24 hours. The pacemaker settings may be set slightly above the pacing threshold and slightly below the sensing threshold for safety.	Ensures proper pacemaker functioning. Prevents loss of sensing and capture.	• Problems with sensitivity or threshold

Procedure continues on following page

Patient Monitoring and Care—*Continued*

Steps	Rationale	Reportable Conditions
The threshold may be checked by physicians or advanced practice nurses in patients at high risk or per institutional policy (e.g., if pacemaker dependent).	Prevents unnecessarily high levels of energy delivery to the myocardium.	
Follow institutional standards.	Threshold may be checked more frequently if the patient's condition changes or pacemaker function is questioned.	
5. Replace gauze dressings every 2 days and transparent dressings at least every 7 days or per institutional standards.[9] Cleanse the site with an antiseptic solution (e.g., 2% chlorhexidine-based preparation). Follow institutional standards. **(Level D*)**	Although guidelines specific to pacing leads do not exist, the U.S. Centers for Disease Control and Prevention (CDC) recommend replacing dressings on intravascular catheters when the dressing becomes damp, loosened, or soiled or when inspection of the site is necessary.[1]	• Increased temperature • Increased white blood cell count • Purulent drainage at the insertion site • Warmth, redness, discoloration, or pain at the site
6. Monitor for other complications.	Early recognition leads to prompt treatment.	• Embolus • Thrombosis • Perforation of the myocardium • Pneumothorax • Hemothorax • Phlebitis
7. Monitor electrolyte levels.	Electrolyte imbalances may precipitate dysrhythmias.	• Abnormal electrolyte values
8. Ensure that all pacemaker connections are secure.	Maintenance of tight connections is necessary to ensure proper sensing, ensure impulse conduction, and minimize the risk of microshock conduction to the heart.	• Inability to maintain tight connections with available equipment, jeopardizing pacing therapy

*Level D: Peer-reviewed professional and organizational standards with the support of clinical study recommendations.

Documentation

Documentation should include the following:
• Description of the events that warranted intervention
• Patient and family education and response to education
• Signed informed consent form
• Universal protocol requirements, if nonemergent
• Date and time of insertion
• Date and time of initiation of pacing
• Type of pacing wire inserted and location of insertion
• Pacemaker settings: mode, rate, output, sensitivity setting, threshold measurements, and whether pacemaker is on or off. These settings should be documented on insertion and at least per shift or per institutional standards.
• ECG monitoring strip recording before and after pacemaker insertion, with interpretation
• Vital signs and hemodynamic parameters before, during, and after the procedure
• Proper placement confirmed with chest radiography or fluoroscopy
• Patient response to the procedure
• Complications and interventions
• Occurrence of unexpected outcomes and interventions taken
• Pain assessment, interventions, and patient response to medication
• Date and time pacing was discontinued
• Adjustment to monitoring system to ensure detection of paced rhythms
• ICD coding

References and Additional Readings

For a complete list of references and additional readings for this procedure, scan this QR code with your smartphone, or visit https://www.elsevier.com/__data/assets/pdf_file/0006/1319820/Chapter0045.pdf

UNIT II

46 Temporary Transvenous and Epicardial Pacing

Valerie Spotts, Nikki J. Taylor, and Jennifer Pesenecker

PURPOSE The purpose of temporary cardiac pacing is to ensure or restore an adequate heart rate and rhythm. Transvenous and epicardial pacing are initiated as temporary measures when failure of the normal conduction system of the heart to produce an electrical impulse results in hemodynamic decompensation.

PREREQUISITE NURSING KNOWLEDGE

- Normal anatomy and physiology of the cardiovascular system, principles of cardiac conduction, and basic dysrhythmia interpretation.
- Understanding of temporary pacemakers to evaluate pacemaker function and the patient's response to pacemaker therapy.
- Clinical and technical competence related to the use of temporary pacemakers.
- Advanced Cardiac Life Support (ACLS) knowledge and skills.
- Basic principles of hemodynamic monitoring in the assessment of the efficacy of temporary pacing therapy.
- Pulmonary artery (PA) catheter function and its use relative to hemodynamic monitoring with use of a PA catheter with pacing function (see Procedure 59, Pulmonary Artery Catheter Insertion (Assist) and Pressure Monitoring).
- Care of patients with a central venous catheter (see Procedure 75, Central Venous Catheter Insertion [Assist], Nursing Care and Removal).
- Understanding of application of the principles of general electrical safety with the use of temporary invasive pacing methods. Gloves always should be worn when handling electrodes to prevent microshock. In addition, the exposed proximal ends of the pacing wires should be insulated when not in use to prevent microshock.[10,14]
- The insertion of a temporary pacemaker is performed in emergent and elective clinical situations.
- Temporary pacing may be used to stimulate the myocardium to contract in the absence of an intrinsic rhythm, establish an adequate cardiac output and blood pressure to ensure tissue perfusion to vital organs, reduce the possibility of ventricular dysrhythmias in the presence of bradycardia, supplement an inadequate rhythm with transient decreases in heart rate (e.g., chronotropic incompetence in shock), or allow the administration of medications (e.g., beta blockers) to treat ischemia or tachydysrhythmias in the presence of conduction system dysfunction or bradycardia.

- Temporary invasive pacing is indicated for the following[1,5,9,11-13]:
  - ❖ Symptomatic third-degree atrioventricular (AV) block
  - ❖ Symptomatic second-degree heart block
  - ❖ Dysrhythmias that complicate acute myocardial infarction
  - ❖ Symptomatic bradycardia or bradysrhythmia
  - ❖ New bundle-branch block with transient complete heart block
  - ❖ Alternating bundle-branch block
  - ❖ Symptomatic sinus node dysfunction
  - ❖ Treatment of bradycardia-tachycardia syndrome (sick sinus syndrome)
  - ❖ Ventricular standstill or cardiac arrest
  - ❖ Long QT syndrome with ventricular dysrhythmia
  - ❖ Brugada syndrome
  - ❖ Medication toxicity (e.g., digoxin) or adverse effects of a medication
  - ❖ Postoperative cardiac surgery
  - ❖ Low cardiac output states
  - ❖ Electrolyte abnormalities (e.g., hyperkalemia)
  - ❖ Prophylaxis with cardiac diagnostic, interventional, or surgical procedures
  - ❖ Chronotropic incompetence in the setting of cardiogenic shock
  - ❖ During the perioperative period during a surgical or other procedural intervention[13]
- The three primary methods of invasive temporary pacing are transvenous endocardial pacing, pacing via a PA catheter, and epicardial pacing.
- Transvenous pacing:
  - ❖ In temporary transvenous pacing, the pulse generator is externally attached to a pacing lead that is inserted through a vein into the right atrium or ventricle.
  - ❖ Veins used for insertion of the pacing lead are the subclavian, femoral, brachial, internal jugular, or external jugular veins.
  - ❖ Single-chamber ventricular pacing is the most common method-used in an emergency because the goal is to establish a heart rate as quickly as possible.

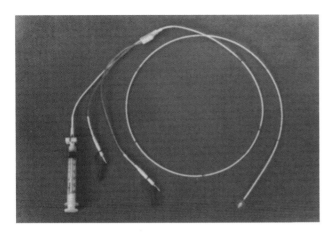

Figure 46.1 Balloon-tipped bipolar lead wire for transvenous pacing.

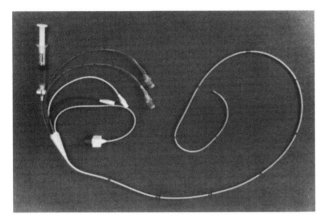

Figure 46.2 Pulmonary artery catheter with atrial and ventricular pacing lumens.

❖ Temporary atrial or dual-chamber pacing can be initiated if the patient needs atrial contraction for improvement in hemodynamics.
❖ The pacing lead is an insulated wire with one or two electrodes at the tip of the wire (see Fig. 45.1)
❖ The pacing lead can be a hard-tipped or balloon-tipped pacing catheter that is placed in direct contact with the endocardium (Fig. 46.1). Most temporary leads are bipolar, with the distal tip electrode separated from the proximal ring by 1 to 2 cm (see Fig. 45.1).
❖ An external temporary pulse generator is connected to the transvenous pacing wire via a bridging or connecting cable.
• Pacing via a PA catheter:
❖ Temporary atrial or ventricular pacing via a thermodilution PA catheter can be done with combination catheters that are specifically designed for temporary pacing.
❖ PA pacing catheters feature atrial and ventricular ports for the introduction of the pacing lead wires (Fig. 46.2).
❖ Use of a PA catheter combines the capabilities of PA pressure monitoring, thermodilution cardiac output measurement, fluid infusion, mixed venous oxygen sampling, and temporary pacing.

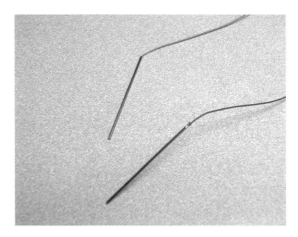

Figure 46.3 Epicardial wires.

❖ One limitation of these multifunction catheters is that the simultaneous measurement of pulmonary artery occlusion pressure (PAOP) and pacing is usually not possible. Balloon inflation can cause repositioning of the pacing electrode with catheter movement; measurement of the PAOP may cause pacing to become intermittent.[8]
• Temporary epicardial pacing:
❖ Temporary epicardial pacing is a method of stimulating the myocardium through the use of polytetrafluoroethylene (PTFE)-coated, unipolar or bipolar stainless steel wires that are sutured loosely to the epicardium after cardiac surgery (Fig. 46.3).
❖ The epicardial wires may be attached to the right atrium for atrial pacing, the right ventricle for ventricular pacing, or both for AV pacing.
❖ Each pacing wire is brought through the chest wall before the chest is closed.
❖ Epicardial wires can be placed in a unipolar or bipolar configuration. Bipolar configuration is more common. With bipolar placement, both leads are connected to the myocardium, and both are able to function as negative poles. Unipolar placement has one lead on the myocardium (negative) and another lead placed on the chest wall (positive). This positive lead is sometimes referred to as a *ground* or *skin* lead.
❖ Typically, the atrial wires are located on the right of the sternum, and the ventricular wires exit to the left of the sternum (Fig. 46.4).
❖ If a minimally invasive surgery was performed, the pacing wires may be in different locations; discuss and label the pacing wires so it is clear which wires are atrial and which are ventricular.
❖ An external temporary pulse generator (Figs. 46.5 to 46.6) is connected to the epicardial pacing wires via a bridging or connecting cable (Fig. 46.7).
❖ Atrial and ventricular thresholds for epicardial wires increase by the fourth postoperative day.[9]
• Basic principles of cardiac pacing include sensing, pacing, and capture.
❖ *Sensing* refers to the ability of the pacemaker device to detect intrinsic myocardial electrical activity. Sensing

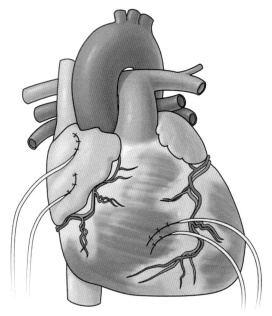

Two atrial wires   Two ventricular wires

Figure 46.4 Location of atrial and ventricular epicardial lead wires.

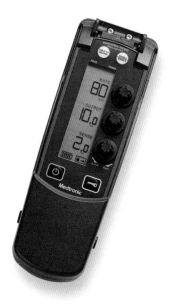

Figure 46.5 Single-chamber temporary pulse generator, Model 53401. *(Images used with permission from Medtronic, plc © 2022.)*

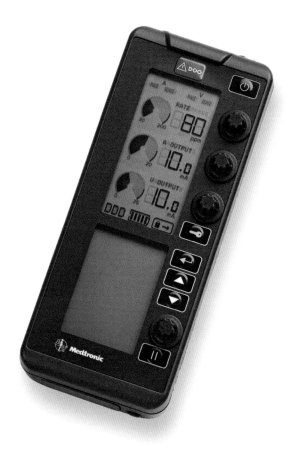

Figure 46.6 Dual-chamber temporary pulse generator, model 5392. *(Images used with permission from Medtronic, plc © 2022.)*

occurs if the pulse generator is in the synchronous or demand mode. The pacemaker either is inhibited from delivering a stimulus or initiates an electrical impulse.
- ❖ *Pacing* occurs when the temporary pulse generator is activated, and the requisite level of energy travels from the pulse generator through the temporary wires to the myocardium. This is known as *pacemaker firing* and is represented as a line or spike on the electrocardiogram (ECG) recording.

- ❖ *Electrical capture* refers to the successful stimulation of the myocardium by the pacemaker, resulting in depolarization. Capture is evidenced on the ECG as an atrial or ventricular complex following the pacemaker spike, depending on the chamber being paced. Mechanical capture is evidenced by generation of a pulse.
- Temporary pulse generator:
  - ❖ The temporary pulse generator houses the controls and energy source for pacing.
  - ❖ Some pulse generators are for single-chamber pacing only and have one set of terminals at the top of the pulse generator into which the pacing wires are inserted (via a connecting cable; Fig. 46.9).
- A dual-chamber pacemaker requires two sets of terminals for the atrial and ventricular wires (see Figs. 46.6 and 46.8). A dual-chamber pacemaker can be used for single-chamber pacing, but settings for the chamber that is not being paced should be programmed to "off" to avoid signal interference.[5,6]
- Different models of pacemakers use either dials or touch pads to change the settings.
  - ❖ The pacing rate is determined by the rate dial or touchpad.
  - ❖ The AV interval dial or pad on a dual-chamber pacemaker controls the amount of time between atrial and ventricular stimulation (electronic PR interval).

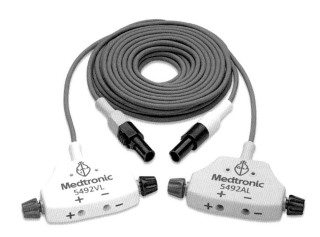

Figure 46.7 Connecting cables. *(Images used with permission from Medtronic, plc © 2022.)*

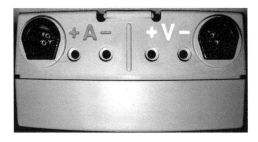

Figure 46.8 Pulse generator terminals to connect cables from atrial and ventricular leads. *(Images used with permission from Medtronic, plc © 2022.)*

❖ The energy delivered to the myocardium is determined by setting the output (milliampere [mA]) dial or pad on the pulse generator.

❖ Dual-chamber pacing requires that mA be set for the atria and the ventricle.

• The ability of the pacemaker to detect the patient's intrinsic rhythm is determined by the pacing mode and sensitivity setting. In the asynchronous mode, the pacemaker functions as a fixed-rate pacemaker and is not able to sense any of the patient's inherent cardiac activity. In the synchronous mode, the pacemaker is able to sense the patient's inherent cardiac activity.

• The ability of the pacemaker to depolarize the myocardium depends on many variables: the position of the electrodes and degree of contact with viable myocardial tissue; the level of energy delivered through the pacing wire; the presence of hypoxia, acidosis, or electrolyte imbalances; fibrosis around the tip of the catheter; and concomitant medication therapy.[13,18]

EQUIPMENT

• Antiseptic solution (e.g., 2% chlorhexidine-based preparation)
• Nonsterile gloves
• Pacing lead wires
• Pulse generator
• Battery/batteries for pulse generator (usually 9 V or AA)

• Connecting cables
• ECG monitoring equipment
• Dressing supplies

Additional equipment to have available as needed includes the following:

• Central venous catheter insertion supplies (see Procedure 74, Central Venous Catheter Insertion [Perform])
• Alligator clips or wire with connector pins
• Suture, needles, syringes
• Emergency equipment
• Fluoroscopy
• Limited bedside echocardiogram using a phased array probe
• Lead aprons or shields
• Multiple-pressure transducer system, with use of PA catheter (see Procedure 59, Pulmonary Artery Catheter Insertion (Assist) and Pressure Monitoring)
• 12-lead ECG machine
• Local anesthetic
• Sterile drapes, towels, masks, goggles or face shields, gowns, caps
• Insulating material for epicardial wires (e.g., finger cots, glove, needle caps, ear plug)

PATIENT AND FAMILY EDUCATION

• Assess learning needs, readiness to learn, and factors that influence learning. *Rationale:* This assessment enables teaching to be individualized in a manner that is meaningful to the patient and family.

• Discuss basic information about the normal conduction system, such as structure and function of the conduction system, normal and abnormal heart rhythms, signs, symptoms, and the significance of abnormal heart rhythms. *Rationale:* The patient and family should understand the conduction system and why the procedure is necessary.

• Provide a basic description of the temporary pacemaker insertion procedure. *Rationale:* The patient and family should be informed of the invasive nature of the procedure and any risks associated with it. An understanding of the procedure may reduce anxiety.

• Describe the precautions and restrictions required while the temporary pacemaker is in place, such as limitation of movement, avoidance of handling the pacemaker or touching exposed portions of the electrodes, and when to notify the nurse (e.g., if the dressing becomes wet, if the patient experiences dizziness). *Rationale:* Understanding limitations may improve patient cooperation with restrictions and precautions. The patient and family also will alert nurses to potential problems.

PATIENT ASSESSMENT AND PREPARATION

Patient Assessment

• Assess the patient's baseline cardiac rhythm for the presence of the dysrhythmia that necessitates temporary cardiac pacing. *Rationale:* This assessment determines the need for invasive cardiac pacing.

- Assess the patient's hemodynamic response to dysrhythmia. Rhythm disturbances may reduce cardiac output significantly with detrimental effects on perfusion to vital organs. *Rationale:* This assessment determines the urgency of the procedure. It may indicate the need for temporizing measures, such as vasopressors or transcutaneous pacing.
- Review the patient's current medications. *Rationale:* Medications may be a cause of the dysrhythmia that led to the need for pacemaker therapy, or medications may need to be held because of concomitant effect. Other medications, such as antidysrhythmics, may alter the pacing threshold.
- Review the patient's current laboratory study results, including chemistry or electrolyte profile, arterial blood gases, and/or cardioactive medication levels. *Rationale:* This review assists in determining whether the need for pacing was precipitated by metabolic disturbances or medication toxicity and establishes the pacing milieu.

Patient Preparation

- Verify the correct patient with two identifiers. *Rationale:* Before performing a procedure, the nurse should ensure the correct identification of the patient for the intended intervention.
- Ensure that the patient and family understand the preprocedural teaching. Answer questions as they arise, and reinforce information as needed. *Rationale:* This communication evaluates and reinforces understanding of previously taught information.
- Confirm that informed consent has been obtained. *Rationale:* Informed consent protects the rights of the patient and makes a competent decision possible for the patient; however, in emergency circumstances, time may not allow the consent form to be signed.
- Perform a preprocedure verification and time out, if nonemergent. *Rationale:* Ensures patient safety.

Procedure for Temporary Transvenous and Epicardial Pacing

Steps	Rationale	Special Considerations
Initiating Temporary Pacing		
1. 🅷🅷		
2. 🅿🅴		
3. Connect the patient to the bedside monitoring system, and monitor the ECG continuously (see Procedure 49, Electrocardiographic Leads and Cardiac Monitoring).	Monitors the patient's intrinsic rhythm and the patient's rhythm during and after the procedure to evaluate for adequate pacemaker function.	Skin preparations may be needed to remove oils to improve impulse transmission.
4. Assess pacemaker functioning, and insert a new battery into the pulse generator before beginning therapy. **(Level M*)** If the pacemaker has a battery indicator and there is sufficient power, it may not be necessary to insert a new battery.	Ensures a functional pacemaker pulse generator.	Different ways to assess battery function depend on the model and manufacturer; check the manufacturer's recommendations for specific instructions.
5. Prepare the pacing system: A. Ensure that the pulse generator is turned off. B. Attach the connecting cable to the pulse generator. C. The atrial cable connects into the socket labeled "A." D. The ventricular cable connects into the socket labeled "V."	Prepares equipment; the pacing stimulus travels from the pulse generator to the negative terminal, and energy returns to the pulse generator via the positive terminal.	Connecting cables are specific to either transvenous or epicardial wires. Some lead wires are labeled distal and proximal; distal connects to negative, and proximal connects to positive. Some lead wires may not have "negative" and "positive" marked on them. Polarity is established when the wires are placed in the connecting cable. Two connecting cables are needed with both atrial and ventricular pacing.

*Level M: Manufacturer's recommendations only.

Procedure for Temporary Transvenous and Epicardial Pacing—*Continued*		
Steps	Rationale	Special Considerations

Assisting With Initiation of Temporary Transvenous Pacing

Steps	Rationale	Special Considerations
1. Follow **Steps 1 to 5** in Initiating Temporary Pacing.		
2. If a central venous catheter is not in place, assist as needed with catheter insertion (see Procedures 74, Central Venous Catheter Insertion [Perform], and 75, Central Venous Catheter Insertion [Assist], Nursing Care and Removal).	A central line is needed for transvenous pacing.	An introducer sheath is used that fits the pacemaker wire that is being inserted.
3. Assist as needed with insertion of the transvenous pacing lead wire.	Provides needed assistance.	
4. All personnel performing and assisting with the procedure should apply PE and sterile equipment (e.g., masks, head covers, goggles or face shields, sterile gowns, and sterile gloves).[2,8]	Minimizes the risk of infection, maintains sterility, and maintains standard and sterile precautions.	
5. Assist as needed with cleansing the insertion site with antiseptic solution (e.g., 2% chlorhexidine-based preparation).	Minimizes the risk of infection.	Gloves should be worn whenever handling the pacing electrodes to prevent microshock.[2,10,14]
6. Assist as needed with draping the insertion site.	Provides a sterile field and reduces the transmission of microorganisms.	
7. Assist as needed as the pacing lead is passed through the introducer.	Facilitates the insertion process.	If a balloon-tipped pacing lead is used, balloon inflation occurs when the tip of the pacing lead is in the vena cava. The air-filled balloon allows the blood flow to carry the catheter tip into the desired position in the right ventricle.
8. Assist with verifying the position of the transvenous pacing lead wire:	For transvenous, ventricular pacing, the negative pacing electrode is positioned in the endocardium (at the apex) of the right ventricle.	
A. Ultrasound scan	Transcutaneous ultrasound may be used to assist with insertion of the pacing electrode.	
B. Fluoroscopy	Fluoroscopy may be used to assist with visualization of the pacing electrode.	If fluoroscopy is used, all personnel must be shielded from the radiation with lead aprons or be positioned behind lead shields.
C. Chest radiography	X-ray may be used to confirm placement of the pacing electrode.	

Procedure continues on following page

UNIT II

Procedure for Temporary Transvenous and Epicardial Pacing—*Continued*		
Steps	**Rationale**	**Special Considerations**

D. Bedside monitoring system or 12-lead ECG machine
   i. Connect the patient to the limb leads.
   ii. Attach the V lead of the ECG monitoring system or the 12-lead ECG machine to the negative electrode connector pin (distal pin) of the pacing lead wire (an alligator clip or wire with connector pins may be needed (see Fig. 45.1).
   iii. Set the monitoring system to record the V lead continuously.
   iv. Observe the ECG for ST-segment elevation in the V lead recording.
   v. Observe for a left bundle-branch block pattern and left-axis deviation that usually can be identified.
	The ECG is derived directly from the pacing electrode, and the position of the catheter tip is verified by the internal electrical recording, which shows ST-segment elevation when in contact with the myocardium.	Determine that the ECG monitoring system meets all safety requirements. As a result of the temporary pacing catheter transmission of impulses from within the right ventricle, conduction of the impulse throughout the ventricles occurs via cellular conduction of the impulse rather than transmission down the bundle branches.

9. After the pacing lead wire is properly positioned:
   A. Connect the external electrode pins to the pulse generator via the connecting cables.
   B. Ensure that the positive and negative electrode connector pins are connected to the respective positive and negative terminals on the pulse generator (see Fig. 46.8) via the connecting cables (Fig. 46.9).
   C. Ensure that all connections are secure.
	Energy from the pulse generator is directed to the negative electrode in contact with the ventricle. The pacing circuit is completed as energy reaches the positive electrode. The lead wires must be connected securely to the pacemaker to ensure appropriate sensing and capture and to prevent inadvertent disconnection.	A connecting cable is recommended for use between the pacing wires and the pulse generator. Some lead wires are labeled distal and proximal; distal connects to negative, and proximal connects to positive. Some lead wires may not have "negative" and "positive" marked on them. Polarity is established when the wires are placed in the connecting cable.

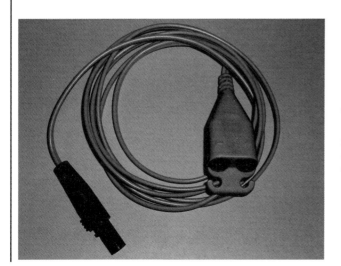

Figure 46.9 Transvenous cable that connects to transvenous pacemaker leads with shrouded pins. *(Courtesy Medtronic, Inc., Minneapolis, MN.)*

Procedure for Temporary Transvenous and Epicardial Pacing—*Continued*		
Steps	Rationale	Special Considerations

10. For AV demand pacing, when an atrial lead is placed in addition to a ventricular lead:
  A. Connect the atrial electrodes to the atrial terminals via the connecting cable.
  B. Connect the ventricular electrodes to the ventricular terminals via the connecting cable.
  C. The connecting cable(s) should already be connected to the pulse generator for each chamber that is being paced (see Fig. 46.9).
	Ensures that the atrial electrodes are connected correctly to the pulse generator. Ensures that the ventricular electrodes are connected correctly to the pulse generator. The pacing stimulus travels from the pulse generator to the negative terminal, and energy returns to the pulse generator via the positive terminal.	Transvenous temporary atrial leads may be placed short term for procedures and then removed.

Assisting With Initiating Temporary Pacing via a Pulmonary Artery Catheter		
1. Follow **Steps 1 to 5** in "Initiating Temporary Pacing."	Prepares equipment.	
2. Assist the provider with insertion of the PA catheter (see Procedure 58, Pulmonary Artery Catheter Insertion [Perform]).	Provides assistance as needed.	Pacing electrodes may be inserted at the time of PA catheter insertion, or they may be inserted at a later time, when temporary pacing is needed because of a change in the patient's condition.
3. Obtain the appropriate pacing lead for insertion.	Only probes specifically manufactured for use with the PA catheter should be used; check the manufacturer's recommendations for specific instructions.	Continuous monitoring of the right-ventricular pressure waveform via the pacing lumen is recommended before insertion of the electrode to ensure correct placement of the right ventricular port 1–2 cm distal to the tricuspid valve.
4. Assist as needed with insertion of the pacing lead wire.	Close monitoring of the ECG during insertion of the pacing lead is necessary to detect dysrhythmias.	Follow specific manufacturer's instructions regarding pacing lead insertion and securing the pacing lead in place within the catheter lumen.[11,14]

5. After the pacing lead wire is properly positioned:
  A. Connect the positive and negative electrode connector pins to the pulse generator via the connecting cable.
  B. Ensure that the positive and negative electrodes are connected to the respective positive and negative terminals on the pulse generator via the connecting cables.
  C. Ensure that all connections are secure.
	Energy from the pulse generator is directed to the negative electrode.
	The pacing circuit is completed as energy reaches the positive electrode. The pacing electrode must be securely connected to the pulse generator to ensure appropriate sensing and capture and to prevent inadvertent disconnection.
		Gloves should be worn whenever handling the pacing electrodes to prevent microshock.

6. Check institutional policy, or obtain specific provider prescription regarding not wedging the PA catheter.	Intermittent capture has been noted during the wedging procedure as a result of movement of the electrode with catheter migration into the wedge position.	Usually, the PA catheter is not wedged during pacing therapy.

Procedure continues on following page

UNIT II

Procedure for Temporary Transvenous and Epicardial Pacing—*Continued*		
Steps	Rationale	Special Considerations
Epicardial Pacing		
1. Follow **Steps 1 to 5** in "Initiating Temporary Pacing."		
2. Expose the epicardial pacing wires (see Fig. 46.3), and identify the chamber of origin (see Fig. 46.4). A. Epicardial wires that exit to the right of the sternum are atrial in origin. B. Epicardial wires that exit to the left of the sternum are ventricular in origin.	Identifies the correct chamber for pacing.	Gloves should be worn when handling the epicardial wires to prevent microshock.
3. Set up the system: A. Connect the epicardial wires to the pulse generator via the connecting cables (see **Step 4**). B. Ensure that the positive and negative electrodes are connected to the respective positive and negative terminals on the pulse generator via the connecting cables. C. Ensure that all connections are secure.	Energy from the pulse generator is directed to the negative electrode in contact with the myocardium. The pacing circuit is completed as energy reaches the positive electrode. The epicardial wires must be connected securely to the pacemaker to ensure appropriate sensing and capture and to prevent inadvertent disconnection.	
4. Determine which type of pacing will be initiated: A. Unipolar pacing B. Bipolar pacing	In a unipolar pacing system, only one epicardial pacing electrode is in contact with the chamber being paced (the negative electrode). The positive, or indifferent (ground), electrode may be an ECG electrode patch, may be an epicardial wire sewn to the subcutaneous tissue of the chest wall, or may be a subcutaneous needle inserted into the chest wall. In a bipolar pacing system, two epicardial pacing electrodes are in direct contact with the myocardial tissue of the chamber being paced.	With unipolar pacing (one electrode in contact with the heart), the epicardial wire must be the negative electrode, and the ECG patch, skin wire, or subcutaneous needle is the positive electrode. With AV demand pacing, both atrial epicardial wires are connected to the atrium (via the connecting cable), and the ventricular epicardial wires are connected to the terminal labeled "ventricle" (via the connecting cable).
All Methods of Temporary Pacing		
1. Determine the mode of pacing desired.	The pacing mode chosen should be the one that best achieves the goal of pacing therapy. Possibilities include atrial, ventricular, or AV asynchronous (fixed rate) pacing or atrial, ventricular, or AV synchronous (demand) pacing.	Asynchronous pacing in the presence of an intrinsic rhythm may result in an R-on-T phenomenon, leading to a lethal dysrhythmia, and should be used only in the absence of an intrinsic rhythm.[5,6,8,13]

Procedure	for Temporary Transvenous and Epicardial Pacing—*Continued*		
Steps	**Rationale**	**Special Considerations**	
2. Set the pacemaker mode, pacemaker rate, and level of energy (output or mA) as prescribed or as determined by sensitivity and stimulation threshold testing (see **Steps 3, 4, and 5**).	Prepares pacemaker equipment.	Follow institutional standards regarding whether critical care nurses can set the pacemaker mode and energy level, and test the sensitivity and stimulation threshold levels. The demand or the synchronous mode is recommended to avoid competition between the pacemaker-initiated beats and the patient's intrinsic rhythm. Output is set to ensure capture of the myocardium. In AV pacing, separate output settings are used to ensure capture of the atrium and the ventricle.	
3. Depending on the pulse generator, turn all settings to the lowest level, and then turn on the pulse generator. **(Level M*)**	Prepares the equipment.	Follow the manufacturer's recommendations. Settings cannot be adjusted on some pulse generators until after the pulse generator is turned on. Other pulse generators turn on at default settings, after a self-test, and the settings can be adjusted at that time.	
4. Determine the sensitivity threshold (for each chamber as appropriate). Set the rate for 10 beats/min below the patient's intrinsic rate.[1,6,7] **(Level M*)**	Sensitivity threshold is the level at which intrinsic myocardial activity is recognized by the sensing electrodes. Setting the pacemaker rate lower than the intrinsic rate avoids competition between the pacemaker and the patient's intrinsic rhythm. For demand pacing, the sensitivity must be measured and set.	This step is omitted if the patient has no intrinsic rhythm. In determining a sensitivity threshold, the mA should be turned to the lowest level to avoid the possibility of a pacemaker stimulus falling on the T wave (R-on-T phenomenon) and inducing a potentially lethal dysrhythmia.	
A. Gradually turn the sensitivity dial counterclockwise (or to a higher numeric setting), and observe the sense indicator light for flashing. The sense indicator light stops flashing when the device is unable to sense the patient's intrinsic rhythm.			
B. Slowly turn the sensitivity dial clockwise (or to a lower numeric setting) until the sense indicator light flashes with each complex and the pace indicator light stops. This value is the sensing threshold.		If the sensitivity is set to the most sensitive, the pacemaker may be inappropriately inhibited because it may detect and interpret extramyocardial activity (e.g., muscle movement, artifact) as actual myocardial activity.	
C. Set the sensitivity dial to the number that was half the sensing threshold to provide a 2:1 safety margin.[1,6,7]			

*Level M: Manufacturer's recommendations only.

Procedure continues on following page

Procedure for Temporary Transvenous and Epicardial Pacing—*Continued*

Steps	Rationale	Special Considerations
5. Determine the stimulation threshold (for each chamber as necessary).[1,6,7] Follow institution standards.	The output dial regulates the amount of electrical current (mA) that is delivered to the myocardium to initiate depolarization. The output (mA) is set at least two times above the stimulation threshold to allow for increases in the stimulation threshold without loss of capture.[1,6,7] The output (mA) is recommended to be ≤15 mA to prevent fibrosis at the lead/myocardium interface.[3]	This step should be performed by a physician or advanced practice nurse in a patient who is pacemaker dependent for bradyarrhythmias. Individual institutional standards govern when threshold determination should be done and whether a nurse may test the stimulation threshold; thresholds may not be determined if sensitivity is poor or if the patient's inherent heart rate is >90 beats/min. Threshold may increase or decrease within hours of electrode placement as a result of fibrosis at the tip of the catheter, medication administration (e.g., some antidysrhythmics), alteration of position, or underlying pathology.[1,4,6-8] In the case of dual-chamber pacing, the threshold for each chamber is assessed. Pacing rates vary depending on the indication for pacing.
A. Set the pacing rate to approximately 10 beats/min above the patient's intrinsic rate.		
B. Gradually decrease the output from 20 mA until capture is lost.		
C. Gradually increase the mA until 1:1 capture is established. This is the stimulation threshold. The pace light will be flashing.		
D. Set the mA at least two times higher than the stimulation threshold.[1,6,7,12]	The output (mA) is recommended to be ≤15 mA to prevent fibrosis at the lead/myocardium interface.[2]	This output setting is sometimes referred to as the *maintenance threshold*.
6. Set the prescribed pacemaker rate.	Ensures adequate cardiac output.	
7. Assess the cardiac rate and rhythm for appropriate pacemaker function:	The ECG tracing should reflect an appropriate response to the pacemaker settings if functioning properly.	
A. Capture: Is there a QRS complex for every ventricular pacing stimulus? Is there also a P wave for every atrial pacing stimulus? (Fig. 46.10).	Sometimes atrial activity may not be visible because of low-voltage amplitude. If the patient is paced solely via atrial pacing, ventricular tracking and response should follow the atrial rate setting.	

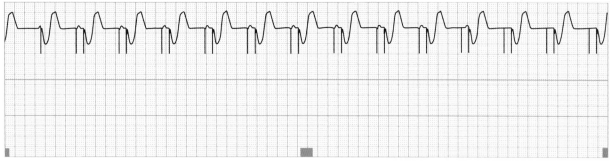

Figure 46.10 Pacemaker electrocardiogram (ECG) strip of atrioventricular pacing. Note the atrial pacing spike before each P wave and the ventricular pacing spike before each QRS complex.

Procedure for Temporary Transvenous and Epicardial Pacing—*Continued*

Steps	Rationale	Special Considerations
B. Rate: is the rate at or above the pacemaker rate if in the demand mode? C. Sensing: does the sense light indicate that every QRS complex is sensed?		
8. After the settings are adjusted for optimal patient response, place the protective plastic cover over the pacemaker controls, or place the controls in the locked position.	Pacemaker settings may be inadvertently altered by patient movement or handling if the controls are not covered or locked.	The patient may need to be reminded not to touch the pulse generator.
9. Assess the patient's response to pacing, including blood pressure, level of consciousness, heart rhythm, and other hemodynamic parameters.	Pacemaker settings are determined by patient response.	
10. Apply a sterile occlusive dressing over the insertion site.	Prevents infection.	The epicardial electrodes and the insertion sites may be covered with a 4 × 4–inch dressing and taped to the chest. The wires may be placed over the dressing and covered with gauze.
11. Secure the necessary equipment to provide some stability for the pacemaker, such as hanging the pulse generator on an intravenous pole, strapping the pulse generator to the patient's torso, or hanging the pulse generator around the patient's neck.	The pulse generator should be protected from falling or becoming inadvertently detached by patient movement.	Exposed wires should be secured in an insulated material (e.g., finger cots, glove, plastic needle cap, ear plug).[9,13] Care must be taken to avoid bending or kinking the wires because this can lead to fractured wires.
12. Remove gloves, and discard used supplies in appropriate receptacles.	Reduces the transmission of microorganisms; standard precautions.	
13. 🅷🅷		
14. Obtain a chest radiograph as prescribed.	In the absence of fluoroscopy, a radiograph is essential to detect potential complications associated with insertion and to visualize lead position.	Not necessary for epicardial pacing.
15. Selectively restrict patient mobility depending on the insertion site.	Prevents electrode dislodgment.	Follow institutional policy regarding ambulation for the patient with a temporary pacemaker.

Expected Outcomes

- Paced rhythm on ECG is consistent with parameters set on the pacemaker, as evidenced by appropriate heart rate, sensing, and capture
- Patient exhibits hemodynamic stability, as evidenced by a systolic blood pressure >90 mm Hg, a mean arterial blood pressure >60 mm Hg, baseline mental status, and no syncope or ischemia
- All pacemaker wires are securely connected to the pulse generator

Unexpected Outcomes

- Failure of the pacemaker to sense, causing competition between the pacemaker-initiated impulses and the patient's intrinsic cardiac rhythm
- Failure of the pacemaker to capture the myocardium
- Pacemaker oversensing that causes the pacemaker to be inappropriately inhibited
- Stimulation of the diaphragm that causes hiccupping, which may be related to pacing the phrenic nerve, perforation, wire dislodgment, or an excessively high pacemaker mA setting
- Phlebitis, thrombosis, embolism, or bacteremia
- Ventricular dysrhythmias
- Pneumothorax or hemothorax
- Myocardial perforation, pericardial effusion, and cardiac tamponade
- Air embolism
- Lead dislodgment
- Pacemaker syndrome as a result of loss of AV synchrony
- Continual hiccups (may indicate wire perforation)
- Pain

Patient Monitoring and Care

Steps	Rationale	Reportable Conditions
		These conditions should be reported to the provider if they persist despite nursing interventions.
1. Monitor vital signs and hemodynamic response to pacing following institution standards and as often as the patient condition warrants.	The goal of cardiac pacing is to improve cardiac output by increasing heart rate or by overriding life-threatening dysrhythmias.	• Abnormal vital signs associated with signs and symptoms of hemodynamic deterioration
2. Evaluate the ECG for the presence of the paced rhythm or resolution of the initiating dysrhythmia.	Proper pacemaker functioning is assessed by observing the ECG for pacemaker activity consistent with the parameters set.	• Inability to obtain a paced rhythm (loss of capture or failure to capture) (Fig. 46.11) • Oversensing • Undersensing (Fig. 46.12)

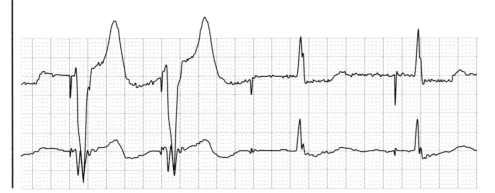

Figure 46.11 Failure to capture on ECG.

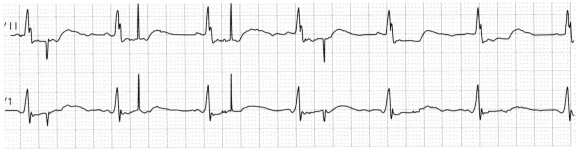

Figure 46.12 Pacemaker undersensing on ECG.

Patient Monitoring and Care —*Continued*

Steps	Rationale	Reportable Conditions
3. Follow institutional standards for assessing pain. Administer analgesia as prescribed.	Identifies the need for pain interventions.	• Continued pain despite pain interventions • Continual hiccups
4. Check and document the sensitivity and stimulation threshold according to institutional standards (e.g., usually at least every 24 hours).[8,9] The threshold may be checked by physicians and/or advanced practice nurses in patients at high risk (e.g., if pacemaker dependent).	Ensures proper pacemaker functioning and prevents high levels of energy delivery to the myocardium. The threshold may be checked more frequently if the patient's condition changes or pacemaker function is questioned.	• Problems or significant changes with sensitivity or threshold
5. Replace gauze dressings every 2 days and transparent dressings at least every 7 days[2,6] Cleanse the site with an antiseptic solution (e.g., 2% chlorhexidine-based preparation). Follow institutional standards. **(Level D*)**	Although guidelines specific to epicardial wires and transvenous pacemaker sites do not exist, the U.S. Centers for Disease Control and Prevention (CDC) recommend replacing dressings on intravascular catheters when the dressings become damp, loosened, or soiled or when inspection of the site is necessary.[2,6]	• Increased temperature • Increased white blood cell count • Drainage at the insertion site • Warmth or pain at the insertion site
6. Monitor for other complications.	Early recognition leads to prompt treatment.	• Embolus • Thrombosis • Perforation of the myocardium • Pneumothorax • Hemothorax • Phlebitis
7. Monitor electrolyte levels as prescribed.	Electrolyte imbalances may precipitate dysrhythmias or change stimulation thresholds.	• Abnormal electrolyte values
8. Ensure that all connections are secure and the low-battery indicator is not present.	Maintenance of tight connections is necessary to ensure proper pacemaker functioning. Battery life varies with the amount of pacing energy needed. Follow institutional guidelines for assessing the low-battery indicator.	• Inability to maintain tight connections with available equipment, jeopardizing pacing therapy
9. If the pulse generator is no longer needed for a patient with epicardial pacing wires, isolate and contain the tips to avoid microshocks (e.g., finger cot, needle cap, needle barrel, glove, ear plug).[9,13]	Microshocks can lead to lethal dysrhythmias. Epicardial wires are often left in place after pacing is no longer needed (generator is disconnected).	• Microshocks

*Level D: Peer-reviewed professional and organizational standards with the support of clinical study recommendations.

UNIT II

Documentation

Documentation should include the following:
- Patient and family education
- Signed informed consent form
- Universal protocol requirements
- Date and time of initiation of pacing
- Description of events that warranted intervention
- Vital signs and hemodynamic parameters before, during, and after the procedure
- ECG monitoring strip recording before and after pacemaker insertion
- Type of pacemaker wire inserted and location
- Pacemaker settings: mode, rate, output, sensitivity, threshold measurements, and whether the pacemaker is on or off
- Presence of underlying rhythm
- Patient response to the procedure
- Complications and interventions
- Medications administered and patient response to the medications
- Pain assessment, interventions, and patient response
- Date and time of battery-status assessments
- Date and time pacing was discontinued
- Adjustment to monitoring system settings to ensure detection of paced rhythms

References and Additional Readings

For a complete list of references and additional readings for this procedure, scan this QR code with your smartphone, or visit https://www.elsevier.com/__data/assets/pdf_file/0007/1319821/Chapter0046.pdf

PROCEDURE

47 Intraaortic Balloon Pump Management

Brandi L. Holcomb

PURPOSE Intraaortic balloon pump (IABP) therapy is designed to increase coronary artery perfusion and myocardial oxygen supply and to decrease myocardial afterload and myocardial oxygen demand.

PREREQUISITE NURSING KNOWLEDGE

- Knowledge of the anatomy and physiology of the cardiovascular system
- Understanding of the principles of hemodynamic monitoring, electrophysiology, dysrhythmias, and coagulation
- Clinical and technical competence related to the use of IABP
- Advanced cardiac life support knowledge and skills
- Indications for IABP therapy are as follows:
  - Cardiogenic shock[2,6,29]
  - Refractory unstable angina
  - Acute myocardial infarction (MI) complicated by left-ventricular failure[21,29]
  - Ischemia-induced recurrent ventricular dysrhythmias[19]
  - Support before, during, and after coronary artery bypass graft surgery[9,30,31]
  - Support before, during, and after coronary artery angioplasty or additional interventional cardiology procedures for patients at high risk[13,30]
  - Mechanical complications of acute MI, including aortic stenosis, mitral stenosis, mitral valvuloplasty, mitral insufficiency, ventricular septal defect, and left-ventricular aneurysm[29]
  - Intractable ventricular dysrhythmias
  - Bridge to cardiac transplantation, ventricular-assist devices, or total artificial hearts
  - Cardiac injury, including contusion and coronary artery tears
  - Septic shock
  - Patient at high risk undergoing noncardiac surgery
- Contraindications to IABP therapy are as follows:
  - Moderate to severe aortic insufficiency
  - Thoracic and abdominal aortic aneurysms
- The relative value of IABP therapy in the presence of severe aortoiliac disease, major coagulopathies, and terminal disease should be evaluated individually.
- IABP therapy is an acute short-term therapy for patients with reversible left-ventricular failure or an adjunct to other therapies for irreversible heart failure. Cardiac

assistance with the IABP is performed to improve myocardial oxygen supply and reduce myocardial workload. IABP therapy is based on the principles of counterpulsation (Fig. 47.1).
- The events of the cardiac cycle provide the stimulus for balloon function, and the movement of helium gas between the balloon and the control console gas source produces inflation and deflation of the balloon.
- Recognition of the R wave or the QRS complex on the electrocardiogram (ECG) is the most commonly used trigger source.[4,12]
- Inflation occurs during ventricular diastole and causes an increase in aortic pressure. This increased pressure displaces blood proximally to the coronary arteries and distally to the peripheral circulation. The result is an increase in myocardial oxygen supply and subsequent improvement in cardiac output.
- Deflation occurs just before ventricular systole or ejection, which decreases the pressure within the aortic root, reducing afterload and myocardial workload.
- Insertion and placement verification
  - The IAB catheter is commonly placed in the femoral artery via percutaneous puncture or arteriotomy.
  - The IAB catheter can also be placed in the left-axillary artery.[18]
  - The IAB catheter lies approximately 2 cm inferior to the left subclavian artery and superior to the renal arteries. This position allows for maximum balloon effect without occlusion of other arterial supplies (Fig. 47.2).
  - The IAB should not fully occlude the aorta during inflation. It should be 85% to 90% occlusive.
  - Fluoroscopy is recommended to aid in IAB catheter positioning, especially for patients with a tortuous aorta.
  - Correct catheter position is verified via radiography if fluoroscopy is not used during catheter insertion. The visibility of the IAB catheter tip may be enhanced when the IABP is temporarily placed on stand-by (follow the manufacturer's guidelines).
  - The central lumen of many IAB catheters provides a means for monitoring aortic pressure.

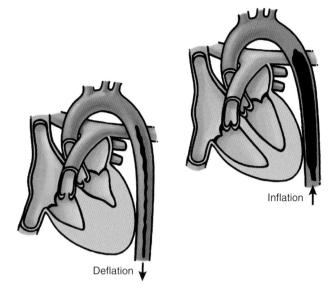

Figure 47.1   Counterpulsation. *(Courtesy Datascope Corporation, Montvale, NJ.)*

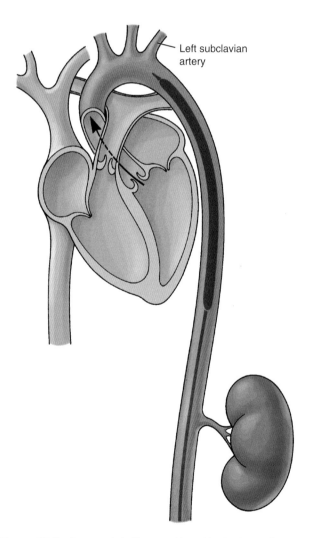

Left subclavian artery

Figure 47.2   Intraaortic balloon positioned in the descending thoracic aorta, just below the left subclavian artery but above the renal artery. *(From Quaal SJ: Comprehensive intraaortic balloon counterpulsation, ed 2, St. Louis, 2000, Mosby.)*

❖ Some IAB catheters use fiber-optic technology. These catheters have a fiber-optic sensor located at the tip of the IAB catheter. The sensor transmits the pressure signal to the IAB console, where it is displayed as an aortic pressure waveform.[23,30]

- Timing methods of IABP therapy vary slightly from manufacturer to manufacturer. With the traditional or conventional method, the IAB deflates at the QRS complex, before isovolumetric contraction. The IAB also deflates at the QRS complex with the real-time method. An important principle of real timing is the duration of the balloon deflation during cardiac systole. During real timing, the IAB is timed to deflate at the onset of each QRS complex and to remain deflated throughout systole. A constant diastolic interval is not necessary for real timing.[4,23,24]

- The development of fiber-optic catheters and changes in the design of the IABP console has produced timing algorithms that automatically adjust timing. The algorithms identify markers, including the initial trigger event, the dicrotic notch, and end-diastolic pressure. The timing algorithms are updated on a continual basis, allowing for optimal inflation and deflation. Timing adapts to changes in both heart rate and ECG rhythm on a beat-to-beat basis.[4,23,24]

- The mechanics of the IABP control console vary from manufacturer to manufacturer.

- Specific information concerning controls, alarms, troubleshooting, and safety features is available from each manufacturer and should be read thoroughly by the nurse before use of the equipment.

EQUIPMENT

- IABP, helium gas supply
- ECG and arterial pressure monitoring supplies
- IAB catheter (size range, 7 to 10F for adults; balloon catheters vary in balloon volumes, 25 to 50 mL)
- IAB catheter insertion kit
- Antiseptic solution (e.g., 2% chlorhexidine-based preparation)
- Caps, goggles or face shields, masks, sterile gowns, gloves, and drapes
- Sterile dressing supplies
- O-silk suture on a cutting needle or a sutureless securement device
- No. 11 scalpel, used for skin entry
- 1% lidocaine without epinephrine, one 30-mL vial
- Stopcocks, one two-way and one three-way
- One Luer-Lok plug
- 500 mL of normal saline flush solution (add heparin if prescribed or according to institutional standards)
- Single-pressure transducer system (see Procedure 60, Single-Pressure and Multiple-Pressure Transducer Systems)

Additional equipment, to have available as needed, includes the following:

- Analgesics and sedatives as prescribed
- Lead apron/collar and radiation dosimeter badge (needed if procedure is performed with fluoroscopy)
- Intravenous (IV) solutions as prescribed
- Emergency medications and resuscitation equipment
- Vasopressors as prescribed
- Antibiotics as prescribed
- Heparin infusion or dextran if prescribed

PATIENT AND FAMILY EDUCATION

- Assess patient and family understanding of IABP therapy and the reason for its use. *Rationale:* Clarification or reinforcement of information is an expressed family need.
- Explain the standard care to the patient and family, including the insertion procedure, IABP sounds, frequency of assessment, alarms, dressings, need for immobility of the affected extremity, expected length of therapy, and parameters for discontinuation of therapy. *Rationale:* This explanation encourages the patient and family to ask questions and prepares the patient and family for what to expect.
- After catheter removal, instruct the patient to report any warm or wet feeling on the leg and any dizziness or lightheadedness. *Rationale:* These feelings may be indicative of bleeding at the insertion site.

PATIENT ASSESSMENT AND PREPARATION

Patient Assessment

- Assess the patient's medical history, specifically related to competency of the aortic valve, aortic disease, or peripheral vascular disease. *Rationale:* This assessment provides baseline data regarding cardiac functioning and identifies contraindications to IABP therapy.
- Assess the patient's cardiovascular, hemodynamic, peripheral vascular, and neurovascular status. *Rationale:* This assessment provides baseline data.
- Assess the extremity for the intended IAB catheter placement for the quality and strength of the femoral, popliteal, dorsalis pedal, and posterior tibial pulses.[7,27]
- Assess the ankle/arm index as follows. *Rationale:* The IAB catheter is inserted into the vasculature of the extremity that exhibits the best perfusion. Also, this assessment provides baseline data related to peripheral blood flow, which may be compromised by the IAB.
  - ❖ Record the brachial systolic pressure with a Doppler scan signal.
  - ❖ Locate the posterior tibial or dorsalis pedal pulse with a Doppler scan signal.
  - ❖ Apply the blood pressure cuff around the ankle, above the malleolus.
  - ❖ Inflate the cuff to 20 mm Hg above the brachial systolic pressure.
  - ❖ Note the reappearance of the Doppler scan signal as the cuff deflates.
  - ❖ Divide the ankle systolic pressure by the brachial systolic pressure to determine the ankle/arm index (normal range, 0.8 to 1.2).

- Assess the patient's current laboratory profile, including complete blood count, platelet count, prothrombin time, international normalized ratio, partial thromboplastin time, and bleeding time. *Rationale:* Provides baseline data. Baseline coagulation studies are helpful in determining the risk for bleeding. Platelet function may be affected by the mechanical trauma from balloon inflation and deflation.[3]
- Assess for signs and symptoms of heart failure that necessitate IABP therapy, including the following. *Rationale:* Physical signs and symptoms result from the heart's inability to adequately contract and from inadequate coronary or systemic perfusion.
  - ❖ Unstable angina
  - ❖ Altered mental status
  - ❖ Heart rate greater than 110 beats/min
  - ❖ Dysrhythmias
  - ❖ Systolic blood pressure less than 90 mm Hg
  - ❖ Mean arterial pressure (MAP) less than 70 mm Hg with vasopressor support
  - ❖ Cardiac index less than 2.4
  - ❖ Pulmonary artery occlusion pressure (pulmonary capillary wedge pressure) greater than 18 mm Hg
  - ❖ Decreased mixed venous oxygen saturation (Svo_2)
  - ❖ Inadequate peripheral perfusion
  - ❖ Urine output less than 0.5 mL/kg/hour

Patient Preparation

- Verify the correct patient with two identifiers. *Rationale:* Before performing a procedure, the nurse should ensure the correct identification of the patient for the intended intervention.
- Ensure that the patient and family understand the preprocedural teaching. Answer questions as they arise, and reinforce information as needed. *Rationale:* Understanding of previously taught information can be evaluated and reinforced.
- Validate that the informed consent form has been signed. *Rationale:* Informed consent protects the rights of the patient and makes a competent decision possible for the patient; however, in emergency circumstances, time may not allow the form to be signed.
- Perform a preprocedure verification and final time out. *Rationale:* Ensures patient safety.
- Validate the patency of central and peripheral intravenous access. *Rationale:* Central access is needed for vasopressor administration; peripheral access is needed for fluid administration.
- Assist the patient to the supine position. *Rationale:* Positions the patient for IAB insertion.

Procedure	for Assisting With Intraaortic Balloon Catheter Insertion	
Steps	**Rationale**	**Special Considerations**
1. 🅷🅷		
2. 🅿🅴		
3. Turn on the IABP console and the helium gas.	Provides power source and activates the gas that drives the IABP.	Follow the manufacturer's recommendations.
4. Sedate the patient as prescribed and as needed; the affected extremity may need to be restrained.	Movement of the lower extremity may inhibit insertion of the catheter or contribute to catheter kinking once the IAB is in place.	A knee immobilizer or a sheet placed over the affected leg and tucked in may minimize movement of the affected leg.
5. Establish ECG input to the IABP console, and obtain an ECG configuration with optimal R-wave amplitude and absence of artifact. Indirect ECG input can be obtained via a "slave" of the bedside ECG to the IABP console.	The R wave is the preferred trigger signal from which the IABP can reference systole and diastole and therefore establish inflation and deflation points.	Usually, one set of ECG electrodes connects to the bedside monitoring system, and the second set of ECG electrodes connects to the IABP console. With use of a slave signal, refer to the bedside monitor manufacturer's instructions for optimizing the ECG and pacemaker recognition.
6. Assist with placement of hemodynamic monitoring catheters if they are not already present (see Procedures 58, Pulmonary Artery Catheter Insertion [Perform], and 59, Pulmonary Artery Catheter Insertion [Assist] and Pressure Monitoring).	Hemodynamic monitoring aids in the assessment and management of the patient who needs IABP therapy.	A radial arterial catheter is commonly inserted (see Procedure 53, Arterial Catheter Insertion [Assist], Care, and Removal)
7. Complete the IABP console preparation. Refer to the instruction manual. (**Level M***)	Ensures adequate functioning of the IABP device.	Models of the pump console vary. Review of the manufacturer's instructions is recommended.
8. All personnel performing and assisting with the procedure should apply personal protective equipment (e.g., masks, head covers, goggles or face shields, sterile gowns, and gloves).	Minimizes the risk of infection and maintains standard and sterile precautions.	
9. Wear a lead apron/collar and radiation dosimeter badge if inserted under fluoroscopy.	A lead apron/collar minimizes radiation exposure. A radiation dosimeter badge tracks radiation exposure.	
10. Assist if needed with prepping and draping the intended insertion site with sterile drapes.	Provides a sterile field and reduces transmission of microorganisms.	
11. Assist as needed with removing the IAB catheter from the sterile packing, and place the catheter and insertion tray on the sterile field.	Makes supplies available and maintains sterility.	Catheters vary in balloon volumes. An adequate volume is necessary to achieve optimal hemodynamic effects from IABP therapy. Patient height may be used as a guideline for selection of balloon volume. Clinical judgment and patient factors, such as patient torso length, are considered.
12. Administer a heparin bolus before arterial puncture if clinically indicated and prescribed.	Anticoagulation therapy may decrease the incidence of thromboembolism related to the indwelling IAB catheter.	Systemic anticoagulation therapy may not be used in all patients.[3]
13. Attach the supplied one-way valve to the Luer-tip of the distal end of the balloon helium lumen.	Creates a device for removing air from the balloon catheter.	

*Level M: Manufacturer's recommendations only.

Procedure	for Assisting With Intraaortic Balloon Catheter Insertion—*Continued*	
Steps	Rationale	Special Considerations
14. Pull back slowly on the syringe until all air is aspirated.	Removes air from the balloon, creating a vacuum.	Maintains the wrap of the balloon for insertion.
15. Disconnect the syringe only, leaving the one-way valve in place.	Prevents air entry back into the balloon.	
16. Follow the manufacturer's recommendations for lubricating the catheter before insertion. **(Level M*)**	May decrease the drag on the catheter during insertion.	Not all IAB catheters need lubrication. Review the manufacturer's instructions.
17. Flush the inner lumen of the IAB catheter before insertion.	Removes air from the central lumen.	If the catheter is not flushed before insertion, allow the backflow of arterial blood before connection to the flush system.[4,25] Follow institutional policy or physician's or advanced practice nurse's prescription regarding the use of heparinized normal saline solution.
18. Assist as needed with the introducer sheath or dilator assembly and insertion.	Prepares for balloon catheter entry.	Some IABs are inserted without a sheath.[8] If the IAB is inserted via the sheathless method, only the vessel dilator is used.[8]
19. Assist with balloon catheter insertion.	Catheter placement is a necessary part of IAB setup.	Some fiber-optic IAB catheters must be calibrated before insertion. Follow the manufacturer's guidelines.[30]
20. Assist with removal of the one-way valve according to the manufacturer's recommendations.	Releases the vacuum and readies the balloon for counterpulsation.	
21. If the inner lumen of a double-lumen catheter is used to monitor arterial pressure, attach a three-way stopcock with a single-pressure transducer system (see Procedure 60, Single-Pressure and Multiple-Pressure Transducer Systems) connected to the monitor, and set the alarms.	Monitors the arterial pressure.	Follow institutional policy or physician's or advanced practice nurse's prescription regarding the use of heparinized normal saline solution. The inner lumen, if used, must be attached to an alarm system because undetected disconnection could result in life-threatening hemorrhage. The proximal tip of the inner lumen used for arterial pressure monitoring is at the level of the left subclavian artery, not at the aortic arch; therefore this location is not the same as a central line placed at the aortic root.[24,25]
22. Avoid fast flush and blood sampling from the central aortic lumen.	Air may enter the system during fast flush and also during blood sampling, resulting in air emboli.	Some manufacturers and institutions recommend hourly fast flush of central lumen lines. If fast flush is required and prescribed, ensure that the IABP is on stand-by (not pumping) during the flush. However, the risk of air embolus entry or dislodging a thrombus at the lumen tip is a major concern. Refer to institutional policy regarding fast flush of central lumen catheters.

*Level M: Manufacturer's recommendations only.

Procedure continues on following page

UNIT II

Procedure for Assisting With Intraaortic Balloon Catheter Insertion—*Continued*		
Steps	Rationale	Special Considerations
23. Attach the helium tubing to the balloon helium lumen, and connect the helium tubing to the IABP console.	Attachment is necessary to initiate therapy.	The helium tubing is packaged with the IAB.
24. Follow the steps for timing, troubleshooting, and patient monitoring.[10,20]	Provides for appropriate operation of counterpulsation.	Many IABP consoles have features for automatic timing. Refer to the specific manufacturer's instructions.
25. Conventional IAB: A. Level the air-fluid interface of the stopcock. B. Zero the hemodynamic monitoring system.	Ensures accurate arterial pressure measurement. Negates the effects of atmospheric pressure.	
26. Fiber-optic IAB: A. Calibrate the system. B. Follow the manufacturer's instructions for calibration.[20,22]	Prepares the equipment. Prepares the equipment.	Refer to the specific manufacturer's instructions for fiber-optic IAB catheters. Some fiber-optic IAB catheters perform automatic in vivo calibration.
27. Ensure that a portable chest radiograph is obtained. Note: Temporarily place the IABP on stand-by while obtaining the chest radiograph.	The correct IAB catheter position must be confirmed to prevent complications associated with interference of the arterial blood supply. Placing the IABP on stand-by enhances visibility of the balloon on the radiograph. Some IAB catheters have radiopaque markers at the tip and base of the IAB membrane to identify the position of the catheter.	If fluoroscopy is used for insertion of the catheter, a radiograph immediately after placement is not necessary. Some patients may have hemodynamic instability when the IABP is on stand-by for more than a few seconds; assess each patient's hemodynamic response to IABP therapy.
28. Ensure that the IAB is secured to the patient's skin.	Maintains optimal position and reduces the risk of IAB catheter migration.	The IAB catheter may be sutured, or a sutureless securement device may be used to secure the catheter.
29. Assist as needed with applying a sterile dressing to the catheter insertion site.	Minimizes the risk of infection.	The IAB catheter may have a sleeve to allow for repositioning of the catheter under aseptic conditions.
30. Ensure that sharps are discarded in a sharps container; remove **PE** and sterile equipment, and discard used supplies in appropriate receptacles.	Reduces the risk of injury and the transmission of microorganisms; standard precautions.	
31. **HH**		

Procedure for Timing of the Intraaortic Balloon Pump

Steps	Rationale	Special Considerations
1. Select an ECG lead that optimizes the R wave. **(Level M*)**	The R wave of the ECG is the preferred trigger source for identifying the cardiac cycle.	Refer to the manufacturer's instructions for trigger options.
2. Assess the timing of the IABP with the arterial waveform.	The arterial waveform assists in identifying accurate IAB inflation and deflation.[20-22]	Refer to the specific manufacturer's instructions for automatic timing.
3. Set the IABP to auto mode.	The IABP console automatically adjusts the timing of inflation and deflation.	Some IABP consoles have this feature. Fiber-optic catheters have a sensor at the tip of the IAB catheter that transmits the pressure signal back to the IABP console, producing an aortic pressure waveform. Timing algorithms adjust inflation and deflation automatically.
4. Timing can be checked by setting the IABP frequency to the every-other-beat setting (1:2 or 50%; Fig. 47.3).	Comparison can be made between the assisted and unassisted arterial waveforms.	

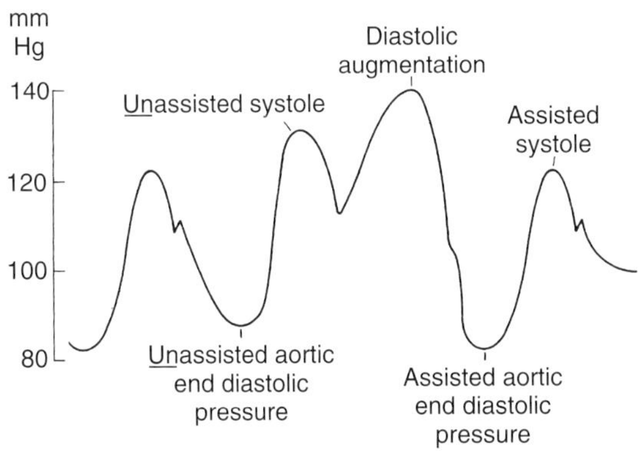

Figure 47.3 Intraaortic balloon pump frequency of 1:2. *(Courtesy Datascope Corporation, Montvale, NJ.)*

Steps	Rationale	Special Considerations
5. Inflation:	The dicrotic notch represents closure of the aortic valve.[23]	
A. Identify the dicrotic notch of the assisted systolic waveform (see Fig. 47.3).		
B. Adjust inflation later to expose the dicrotic notch.	Identifies the landmark for accurate inflation.	
C. Slowly adjust inflation earlier until the dicrotic notch disappears and a sharp V wave forms (see Fig. 47.3).	Balloon augmentation should occur after the aortic valve closes.[8,10,11]	A sharp V wave may not be seen in patients with low systemic vascular resistance.
D. Compare the augmented pressure with the patient's unassisted systolic pressure.	Balloon augmentation ideally is equal to or greater than the patient''s unassisted systolic blood pressure.[4]	If balloon augmentation is less than the patient's systolic pressure, consider the possibility that the patient is hypovolemic or tachycardic, the balloon is positioned too low, or the balloon volume is set too low.[4,25] Low volume may also be the result of an inadequate fill volume or an IAB catheter that is too small for the patient.

*Level M: Manufacturer's recommendations only.

Procedure continues on following page

Procedure for Timing of the Intraaortic Balloon Pump—*Continued*

Steps	Rationale	Special Considerations
E. Adjust inflation if needed.	Necessary to achieve optimal diastolic augmentation.	Timing of inflation varies slightly depending on the location of the arterial catheter and resulting physiological delays.[4,22] Radial: Inflate 40–50 ms before the dicrotic notch. Femoral: Inflate 120 ms before the dicrotic notch (Fig. 47.4). The radial artery is recommended for use for pressure monitoring for IABP timing.[4,22]

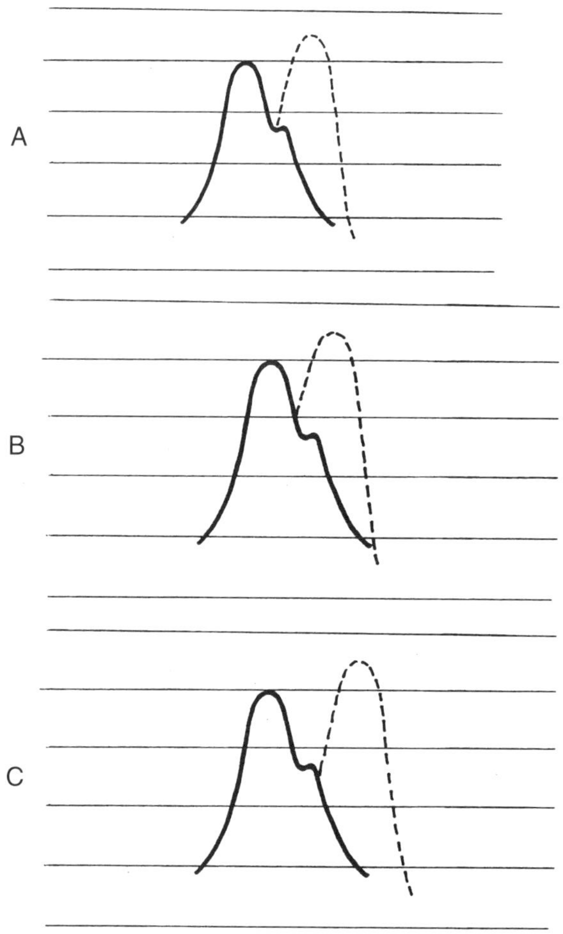

Figure 47.4   Intraaortic balloon pump inflation. **A,** Radial. **B,** Femoral. **C,** Central aortic.

6. Deflation:

Steps	Rationale	Special Considerations
A. Identify the assisted and unassisted aortic end-diastolic pressures and the assisted and unassisted systolic pressures (see Fig. 47.3).[4,21,23]	These landmarks are important in determination of accurate IAB deflation.	IABP frequency is set at 1:2 (50%).
B. Set the balloon to deflate so the assisted aortic end-diastolic pressure is as low as possible (lower than the patient's unassisted diastolic pressure) while still maintaining optimal diastolic augmentation and not impeding the next systole (the assisted systole).	The assisted systolic pressure is less than the unassisted systolic pressure as a result of a decrease in afterload, thus reducing the myocardial workload.[11,13]	Reduction of afterload decreases the energy required by the heart during systole. Afterload reduction without diminishment of diastolic augmentation is important to achieve.[4]

Procedure for Timing of the Intraaortic Balloon Pump—*Continued*		
Steps	Rationale	Special Considerations
7. Set the IABP frequency to 1:1 (100%; Fig. 47.5).	Ensures that each heartbeat is assisted.	

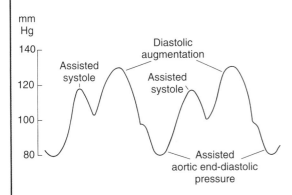

1:1 IABP Frequency

Figure 47.5 Correct intraaortic balloon pump timing (1:1). *(Courtesy Datascope Corporation, Montvale, NJ.)*

Steps	Rationale	Special Considerations
8. Assess timing every hour, whenever the heart rate changes by more than 10 beats/min, and when the rhythm changes.	Inappropriate timing prevents effective IABP therapy.	Many IABP models use algorithms to automatically adjust timing for changes in heart rate and rhythm. Refer to the specific manufacturer guidelines for a description of automatic timing modes and their specific features.
9. Assess and intervene to correct inappropriate timing. A. Problem: early inflation (Fig. 47.6). Intervention: adjust inflation later.	Ensures accurate timing and optimal functioning of the IABP. Inflation occurs before closure of the aortic valve, leading to premature aortic valve closure, increased left-ventricular volume, and decreased stroke volume.[21]	Early inflation is the worst timing error, reducing left-ventricular performance and IABP efficiency.[4,22]

Timing Errors
Early Inflation

Inflation of the IAB prior to aortic valve closure

Waveform Characteristics:
• Inflation of IAB prior to dicrotic notch
• Diastolic augmentation encroaches onto systole (may be unable to distinguish)

Physiologic Effects:
• Potential premature closure of aortic valve
• Potential increased in LVEDV and LVEDP or PCWP
• Increased left ventricular wall stress or afterload
• Aortic regurgitation
• Increased MVo₂ demand

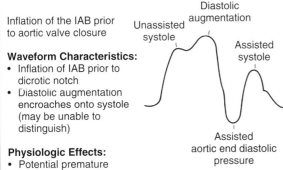

Figure 47.6 Early inflation. *(Courtesy Datascope Corporation, Montvale, NJ.)*

Procedure continues on following page

UNIT II

Procedure	for Timing of the Intraaortic Balloon Pump—*Continued*	
Steps	Rationale	Special Considerations
B. Problem: late inflation (Fig. 47.7). Intervention: adjust inflation earlier.	A delay in inflation leads to a decrease in coronary artery perfusion.	

Timing Errors
Late Inflation

Inflation of the IAB markedly after closure of the aortic valve

Waveform Characteristics:
- Inflation of the IAB after the dicrotic notch
- Absence of sharp V
- Suboptimal diastolic augmentation

Physiologic Effects:
- Suboptimal coronary artery perfusion

Unassisted systole • Diastolic augmentation • Assisted systole • Dicrotic notch • Assisted aortic end-diastolic pressure

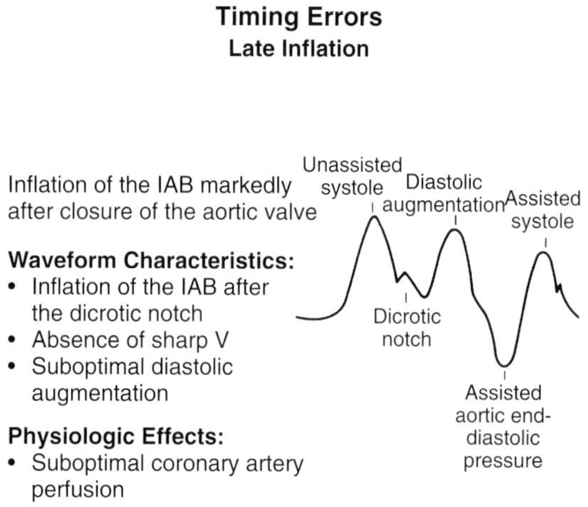

Figure 47.7 Late inflation. *(Courtesy Datascope Corporation, Montvale, NJ.)*

C. Problem: early deflation (Fig. 47.8). Intervention: adjust deflation later.	Deflation occurs before the aortic valve opens, leading to decreased balloon augmentation and less or no afterload reduction; coronary artery perfusion may also be decreased.	Note the sharp diastolic wave after augmentation and the increase in the assisted systolic pressure.

Timing Errors
Early Deflation

Premature deflation of the IAB during the diastolic phase

Waveform Characteristics:
- Deflation of IAB is seen as a sharp drop following diastolic augmentation
- Suboptimal diastolic augmentation
- Assisted aortic end diastolic pressure may be equal to or less than the unassisted aortic end diastolic pressure
- Assisted systolic pressure may rise

Physiologic Effects:
- Suboptimal coronary perfusion
- Potential for retrograde coronary and carotid blood flow
- Angina may occur as a result of retrograde coronary blood flow
- Suboptimal afterload reduction
- Increased MVO_2 demand

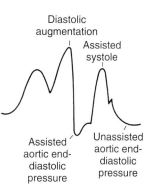

Diastolic augmentation • Assisted systole • Assisted aortic end-diastolic pressure • Unassisted aortic end-diastolic pressure

Figure 47.8 Early deflation. *(Courtesy Datascope Corporation, Montvale, NJ.)*

Procedure for Timing of the Intraaortic Balloon Pump—*Continued*

Steps	Rationale	Special Considerations
D. Problem: late deflation (Fig. 47.9). Intervention: adjust deflation earlier.	Deflation occurs after the aortic valve has opened, leading to an increase in the aortic end-diastolic pressure and an increase in afterload.	Note the delayed diastolic wave after augmentation and the diminished assisted systole. Late deflation is identified by a diminished assisted systolic pressure, an increase in heart rate, an increase in filling pressures, a decrease in cardiac output and cardiac index, and an increased afterload. Maintaining a reliable trigger minimizes the risk of late deflation.[4,22-25]

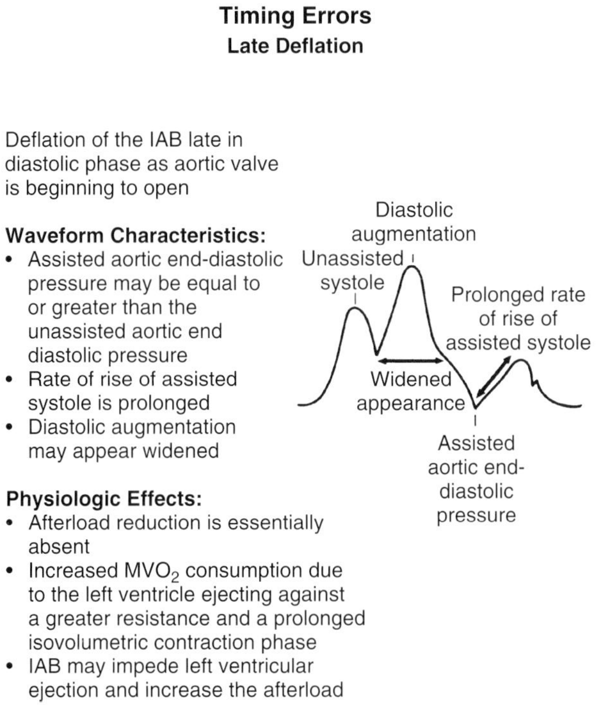
Timing Errors
Late Deflation
Deflation of the IAB late in diastolic phase as aortic valve is beginning to open
Waveform Characteristics:
• Assisted aortic end-diastolic pressure may be equal to or greater than the unassisted aortic end diastolic pressure
• Rate of rise of assisted systole is prolonged
• Diastolic augmentation may appear widened
Physiologic Effects:
• Afterload reduction is essentially absent
• Increased MVO_2 consumption due to the left ventricle ejecting against a greater resistance and a prolonged isovolumetric contraction phase
• IAB may impede left ventricular ejection and increase the afterload
Diastolic augmentation
Unassisted systole
Prolonged rate of rise of assisted systole
Widened appearance
Assisted aortic end-diastolic pressure

Figure 47.9 Late deflation. *(Courtesy Datascope Corporation, Montvale, NJ.)*

Procedure for Balloon-Pressure Waveform

Steps	Rationale	Special Considerations
1. Determine whether the IABP console has a balloon-pressure waveform.	Helium is shuttled in and out of the IAB catheter, and the balloon-pressure waveform represents this movement.	Refer to the specific manufacturer's instructions regarding the balloon-pressure waveform.
2. Assess the balloon-pressure waveform.	Reflects pressure that is in the IAB.	
3. Determine whether the balloon pressure waveform is normal (Fig. 47.10). A normal balloon pressure waveform:	A normal balloon-pressure waveform reflects that the IAB is inflating and deflating properly.[4,22]	

Procedure continues on following page

UNIT II

Procedure	for **Balloon-Pressure Waveform**—*Continued*	
Steps	Rationale	Special Considerations

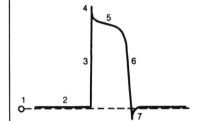

Figure 47.10   Normal balloon gas waveform. *1,* zero baseline; *2,* fill pressure; *3,* rapid inflation; *4,* peak inflation artifact; *5,* plateau pressure or inflation plateau pressure; *6,* rapid deflation; *7,* peak deflation pressure and return to fill pressure. *(Courtesy Arrow International.)*

Steps	Rationale	Special Considerations
A. Has a fill pressure (baseline pressure) slightly above zero.	Reflects pressure in the tubing between the IAB and the IABP driving mechanism.	
B. Has a sharp upstroke.	Occurs as helium inflates the IAB catheter.	
C. Has peak inflation artifact.	This overshoot pressure artifact is caused by helium gas pressure in the pneumatic line.[4]	
D. Has a pressure plateau.	This plateau is created as the IAB remains inflated during diastole.	The plateau indicates the length of time of inflation and whether full inflation (volume) has been delivered to the IAB. If no plateau pressure is found, the IAB may not be fully inflated.
E. Has a rapid deflation.	Helium is quickly shuttled from the IAB.	
F. Has a negative deflection below baseline and then returns to baseline.	Helium returns to the IABP console and then stabilizes within the system.	
4. Compare the balloon-pressure waveform with the arterial pressure waveform (Fig. 47.11).	Demonstrates the relationship between the balloon-pressure waveform and the arterial waveform. Reflects the effect of the balloon on the augmented arterial pressure.	Note the similarity in the width of the balloon-pressure waveform and the augmented arterial waveform.[4,22]

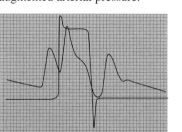

A

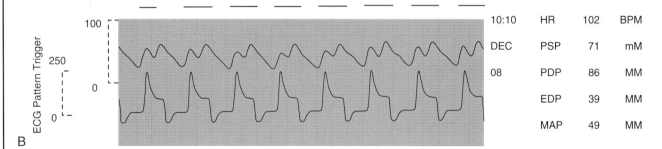

B

Figure 47.11   A, Balloon-pressure waveform superimposed on an arterial pressure waveform. **B,** Actual recording of an arterial pressure waveform *(top)* and balloon gas waveform *(bottom)* from a patient with a balloon pump. *(Courtesy Arrow International.)*

Procedure for Balloon-Pressure Waveform—*Continued*		
Steps	Rationale	Special Considerations
5. Determine whether the balloon pressure waveform meets the previous description.	Abnormal balloon-pressure waveforms may indicate restriction to helium shuttle.	Refer to the specific manufacturer's instructions regarding troubleshooting abnormal balloon-pressure waveforms.

Procedure for Troubleshooting		
Steps	Rationale	Special Considerations
1. Atrial fibrillation: A. Assess and treat the underlying cause.	The underlying cause of the dysrhythmia should be treated.	
B. Set the IABP to inflate and deflate most of the patient's beats.		Inflation of the IAB should correspond to the diastolic interval of each cardiac cycle. The IAB automatically deflates on the R wave.
C. Refer to the manufacturer's instructions for the appropriate IABP console settings for atrial fibrillation (e.g., the atrial fibrillation trigger mode).	Select a mode on the IABP console for optimal R wave tracking.	The real-time method of timing may track dysrhythmias better than traditional or conventional IABP timing.[4,22]
2. Tachycardia: A. Assess and treat the underlying cause.	The underlying cause of the tachycardia should be treated.	Because diastole is shortened during tachycardia, the IAB inflation time also is shortened. The IABP may need to be changed to a 1:2 frequency. Pumping every other beat may improve the patient's hemodynamic status. Some IABPs with automatic timing can track rates as high as 220 beats/min.
B. Set the timing and the frequency of the IABP to optimize hemodynamic response.	IAB timing and frequency should be set to optimize coronary perfusion and afterload reduction.	
3. Asystole: A. Switch the trigger to arterial pressure.	This trigger can be used if an arterial pressure is generated from chest compressions.	Follow advanced cardiac life support (ACLS) standards for emergency care.
B. If the IABP console is not in the auto-operation mode: i. Set inflation to provide diastolic augmentation. ii. Set deflation to occur before the upstroke of the next systole.	Sets the IABP timing.	Refer to the manufacturer's manual. Preliminary research suggests that when used during cardiopulmonary resuscitation, IAB counterpulsation increases cerebral and coronary perfusion.[4]
C. If chest compressions do not provide an adequate trigger:		Refer to the manufacturer's guidelines for recommendations for minimal balloon volume.
i. Turn or push the control to internal trigger.	The internal trigger keeps the IAB catheter moving so clot formation is minimized.[4]	
ii. Set the rate at 60–80 beats/min.	Maintains consistent movement of the IAB catheter.	
iii. Set the IABP frequency to 1:2.	A 1:2 frequency is adequate to prevent thrombus formation on the IAB catheter.	
iv. Turn the balloon augmentation down to 50%.	Slight inflation and deflation of the IAB catheter prevents clot formation.	

Procedure continues on following page

UNIT II

Procedure	for Troubleshooting—*Continued*	
Steps	Rationale	Special Considerations
D. If the IABP console is in the auto-timing mode, the console automatically attempts to self-time if an arterial pressure is generated, or switches to an internal trigger.	Sets the IABP timing and maintains consistent movement of the IAB catheter.	
4. Ventricular tachycardia or ventricular fibrillation:		
A. Assess and treat the underlying cause.	The underlying cause of the tachycardia should be treated.	
B. Cardiovert or defibrillate as necessary (see Procedures 32, Cardioversion, and 33, Defibrillation [External]).	Attempts to convert the dysrhythmia.	Follow ACLS standards for emergency care. Ensure that personnel are cleared from the patient and equipment before cardioversion or defibrillation. The IABP console is electrically isolated.
5. Loss of vacuum or IABP failure:		
A. Check and tighten the connections on the pneumatic tubing.	A loose connection may contribute to a loss of vacuum.	
B. Check the compressor power source.	Ensures that power is available to drive the helium.	
C. Hand inflate and deflate the balloon every 5 minutes if necessary. (**Level M***)	Prevents clot formation along the dormant balloon.	Refer to the specific manufacturer's guidelines for manually inflating and deflating the IAB. Ensure that the correct syringe is kept with the IABP console for this emergency; check the manufacturer's guidelines for frequency of hand inflation.
D. Change the IAB console. (**Level M***)	Establishes a power source and effective IABP therapy.	
6. Suspected balloon perforation:		
A. Observe for loss of augmentation.	Helium may be gradually leaking from the balloon catheter.	Set the alarm limits so the alarms sound with a decrease of 10 mm Hg in diastolic augmentation.
B. Check for blood in the balloon lumen tubing.	Blood or any discoloration in the helium tubing indicates that the balloon has perforated and that arterial blood is present.	It is possible for a balloon leak to be self-sealing as a result of the surface tension between the inside and the outside of the IAB membrane. This may be evidenced by the presence of dried blood in the balloon lumen tubing. The dried blood may appear as a brownish, coffee-ground–like substance.
C. Assess for changes or lack of a normal balloon-pressure waveform.	The balloon-pressure waveform may be absent if the balloon is unable to retain helium, or the pressure plateau may gradually decrease if the IAB is leaking helium.	

*Level M: Manufacturer's recommendations only.

Procedure for Troubleshooting—*Continued*		
Steps	Rationale	Special Considerations
7. Balloon perforation: A. Place the IABP on stand-by.	Prevents further IAB pumping and continued helium exchange.	Some IABP consoles automatically shut off if a leak is detected. The IAB catheter should be removed within 15–30 minutes.[4]
B. Clamp the IAB catheter.	Prevents arterial blood backup.	
C. Disconnect the IAB catheter from the IABP console.	Prevents blood from backing up into the IABP console.	
D. Notify the provider.	The IAB catheter must be removed or replaced immediately.	If the IAB leak has sealed itself off, this may result in entrapment of the IAB in the vasculature. Surgical removal may be necessary.
E. Prepare for IAB catheter removal or replacement.	The IAB catheter should not lie dormant for longer than 30 minutes.	Do not manually inflate and deflate the IAB if balloon perforation is suspected. Perforation of a balloon membrane may indicate that the patient's vascular condition may induce abrasion or perforation in subsequent balloon membranes.
F. Discontinue anticoagulation therapy as prescribed.	Clotting occurs more readily if anticoagulation therapy is stopped (necessary if removing the catheter).	

Procedure for Weaning and Intraaortic Balloon Catheter Removal		
Steps	Rationale	Special Considerations
1. **HH**		
2. **PE**		
3. Assess clinical readiness for weaning.	Optimal clinical and hemodynamic parameters validate readiness for weaning.	Patient hemodynamic status should be optimal before weaning from IABP therapy. Signs of clinical readiness include the following: no angina, heart rate <110 beats/min, absence of unstable dysrhythmias, MAP >70 mm Hg with minimal or no vasopressor support, pulmonary artery occlusion pressure <18 mm Hg, cardiac index >2.4, mixed venous oxygen saturation between 60% and 80%, capillary refill <2 seconds, and urine output >0.5 mL/kg/hour.
4. Change the assist ratio to 1:2 (50%), and monitor the patient's response for 1–6 hours, as prescribed, or per the institution's protocol.	The length of time required to wean from IABP therapy depends on the hemodynamic response of the patient and the length of time the patient has received IABP therapy.[7]	Follow physician's or advanced practice nurse's prescription or institutional policy on IABP weaning.
5. If hemodynamic parameters remain stable, further change the ratio (depending on the patient and the balloon-console assist frequencies, or as prescribed).	IABP consoles vary in assist ratios.	Follow physician's or advanced practice nurse's prescription or institutional policy on IABP weaning.

Procedure continues on following page

UNIT II

Procedure	for Weaning and Intraaortic Balloon Catheter Removal—*Continued*		
Steps	**Rationale**	**Special Considerations**
6. Discontinue heparin or dextran 4–6 hours before IAB catheter removal, or reverse heparin with protamine (as prescribed) just before catheter removal.	Decreases the likelihood of bleeding after balloon removal.	
7. Turn the IABP to stand-by or off, and disconnect the IAB from the console.	Ensures deflation of the IAB catheter.	The patient's arterial pressure collapses the balloon membrane in preparation for withdrawal.
8. Assist with removing sutures or the sutureless securement device.	Prepares for IAB removal.	
9. Assist the physician or advanced practice nurse with removal of the percutaneous catheter.	Facilitates removal.	The IAB catheter is not withdrawn into the sheath but removed as an entire unit to avoid shearing the balloon.
10. Ensure that pressure is held on the insertion site for 30–45 minutes after the IAB catheter is withdrawn.	Ensures that hemostasis is obtained and decreases the incidence of bleeding and hematoma formation.	A femoral compression system can be used to achieve hemostasis (see Procedure 69, Femoral Arterial and Venous Sheath Removal). Pressure may be needed for a longer period if the patient has been receiving anticoagulant therapy or if coagulation study results are abnormal.
11. Assess the insertion site for signs of bleeding or hematoma formation before application of a sterile pressure dressing.	Assists in the detection of bleeding.	
12. Apply a pressure dressing to the insertion site for 2–4 hours or as prescribed.	Minimizes bleeding from the insertion site.	
13. Obtain vital signs and hemodynamic parameters every 15 minutes × 4, every 30 minutes × 2, then every hour as the patient's condition warrants, or as prescribed.	Determines patient stability or instability.	
14. Assess the quality of perfusion to the decannulated extremity immediately after removal and every 1 hour × 2, then every 2 hours, or as prescribed.	Removal of the IAB catheter may dislodge thrombi on the catheter and lead to arterial occlusion.	
15. Maintain immobility of the decannulated extremity, and maintain bed rest with the head of the bed elevated no greater than 30 degrees for 8 hours, as prescribed or according to institutional protocol.	Promotes healing and decreases stress at the insertion site.	
16. Remove **PE**, and discard used supplies in an appropriate receptacle.	Reduces the transmission of microorganisms and body secretions; standard precautions.	
17. **HH**		

Expected Outcomes

- Increased myocardial oxygen supply
- Decreased myocardial oxygen demand
- Increased cardiac output
- Increased tissue perfusion, including cerebral, renal, and peripheral circulation

Unexpected Outcomes

- Impaired perfusion to the extremity with the IAB catheter in place
- Balloon perforation
- Inappropriate IAB placement
- Pain
- Bleeding or coagulation disorders
- Aortic dissection
- Infection

Patient Monitoring and Care

Steps	Rationale	Reportable Conditions
		These conditions should be reported to the provider if they persist despite nursing interventions.
1. Perform systematic cardiovascular, peripheral vascular, and hemodynamic assessments every 15–60 minutes as patient status requires or as prescribed.		
A. Level of consciousness	Assesses for adequate cerebral perfusion; thrombi may develop and dislodge during IABP therapy; the IAB may migrate, decreasing blood flow to the carotid arteries.[4]	• Change in level of consciousness
B. Vital signs and pulmonary artery pressures	Demonstrates effectiveness of IABP therapy.	• Unstable vital signs • Significant changes in hemodynamic pressures • Lack of response to IABP therapy
C. Arterial and balloon pressures	Ensures effectiveness of IABP timing and therapy.	• Difficulty achieving effective IABP therapy
D. Cardiac output, cardiac index, and systemic vascular resistance values	Demonstrates effectiveness of IABP therapy.	• Abnormal cardiac output, cardiac index, and systemic vascular resistance values
E. Circulation to extremities	Determines peripheral perfusion. If reportable conditions are found, they may indicate catheter or embolus obstruction of perfusion to the extremity. Specifically, decreased perfusion to the left arm may indicate misplacement of the IAB catheter.[15,25,27]	• Capillary refill >2 seconds • Diminished or absent pulses (e.g., antecubital, radial, femoral, popliteal, tibial, pedal) • Color pale, mottled, or cyanotic • Diminished or absent sensation • Pain • Diminished or absent movement • Cool or cold to the touch
F. Urine output	Determines perfusion to the kidneys.	• Urine output <0.5 mL/kg/hour
2. Assess heart and lung sounds every 4 hours and as needed.	Abnormal heart and lung sounds may indicate the need for additional treatment. *Special note:* When the patient's condition permits, place the IABP on stand-by to accurately auscultate heart and lung sounds because IABP therapy creates extraneous sounds and impairs heart and lung sound assessment.	• Abnormal heart and lung sounds
3. Maintain the head of the bed at less than 30 degrees.	Prevents kinking of the IAB catheter and migration of the catheter.	

Procedure continues on following page

UNIT II

Patient Monitoring and Care —*Continued*

Steps	Rationale	Reportable Conditions
4. Monitor for signs of balloon perforation by assessing the balloon tubing on a regular basis for evidence of discoloration or blood in the tubing.	In the event of balloon perforation, a very small amount of helium could be released into the aorta, potentially causing an embolic event. Because of pressure gradients in the aorta, blood is more likely to enter the balloon membrane and be dehydrated by the helium.	• Blood or brown flecks in the tubing • Loss of IABP augmentation • Control-console alarm activation (e.g., gas loss)
5. Maintain accurate IABP timing.	If timing is not accurate, cardiac output may decrease rather than increase.	• Signs and symptoms of hemodynamic instability
6. Log-roll the patient every 2 hours. Prop up pillows to support the patient and to maintain alignment. Consider use of pressure-relief devices. **(Level E*)**	Promotes comfort and skin integrity and prevents kinking of the IAB catheter. *Special note:* Log-rolling may not be tolerated in patients with severe hemodynamic compromise; low-pressure beds are necessary for these patients. Low-pressure beds can decrease the occurrence of pressure ulcers in patients who need IABP therapy.[4,25]	
7. Immobilize the cannulated extremity with a draw sheet tucked under the mattress or with a soft ankle restraint or a knee immobilizer as prescribed.	Prevents dislodgment and migration of the IAB catheter. *Special note:* Assess skin integrity and perfusion distal to the restraint every hour.	• Alteration in skin integrity • Alteration in peripheral perfusion
8. Initiate passive and active range-of-motion exercises every 2 hours to extremities that can be mobilized.	Prevents venous stasis and muscle atrophy.	
9. Assess the area around the IAB catheter insertion site every 2 hours and as needed for evidence of hematoma or bleeding.[25]	IAB catheter inflation and deflation traumatizes red blood cells and platelets.	• Bleeding at insertion site • Hematoma at insertion site
10. Maintain anticoagulation therapy as prescribed; monitor coagulation studies.	Prophylactic anticoagulation therapy may be used to prevent thrombi and emboli development. Anticoagulation therapy may alter hemoglobin, hematocrit, and coagulation values.[3]	• Abnormal coagulation study results • Abnormal hemoglobin and hematocrit study results
11. Monitor the patient for systemic evidence of bleeding or coagulation disorders.	Hematological and coagulation profiles may be altered as a result of blood loss during balloon insertion, anticoagulation, and platelet dysfunction as a result of mechanical trauma by balloon inflation and deflation.[3]	• Bleeding from IAB insertion site • Bleeding from incisions or mucous membranes • Petechiae or ecchymosis • Guaiac-positive nasogastric aspirate or stool • Hematuria • Decreased hemoglobin or hematocrit • Decreased filling pressures • Increased heart rate • Retroperitoneal hematoma • Pain in the lower abdomen, flank, thigh, or lower extremity

*Level E: Multiple case reports, theory-based evidence from expert opinions, or peer-reviewed professional organizational standards without clinical studies to support recommendations.

Patient Monitoring and Care —*Continued*

Steps	Rationale	Reportable Conditions
12. Follow institutional standards for assessing pain. Administer analgesia as prescribed.	Promotes comfort.	• Continued pain despite pain interventions
13. Replace gauze dressings at the IAB catheter site every 2 days and transparent dressings at least every 7 days. Cleanse the site with an antiseptic solution (e.g., 2% chlorhexidine solution). **(Level D*)**	Decreases the incidence of infection and allows an opportunity for site assessment. Although guidelines do not exist specifically for IAB site dressings, the U.S. Centers for Disease Control and Prevention (CDC) recommend replacing invasive line dressings when the dressing becomes damp, loosened, or soiled or when inspection of the site is necessary.[20]	• Signs or symptoms of infection
14. Assess for balloon migration.	The IAB should be positioned 2 cm below the left subclavian artery and just above the renal arteries. If the IAB migrates proximally, it may occlude the subclavian or carotid arteries. If the IAB migrates too low, it could occlude the renal or mesenteric arteries.	• Signs of possible subclavian artery occlusion: unequal or absent radial pulse and dampening or loss of the arterial pressure waveform in the ipsilateral radial artery (radial artery on the same side as the IAB catheter) • Signs of possible carotid artery occlusion include change in level of consciousness and orientation or unilateral neurological deficit • Signs of renal artery occlusion: oliguria or anuria, back or flank pain, nausea, and anorexia • Signs of mesenteric artery occlusion: abdominal pain, diarrhea, nausea, and decreased bowel sounds
15. Identify parameters that demonstrate clinical readiness to wean from IABP therapy.	Close observation of the patient's tolerance to weaning procedures is necessary to ensure that the body's oxygen demands can be met. The presence of these reportable conditions indicates that consideration should be given to weaning the patient from the IABP.	• No angina • Heart rate <110 beats/min • Absence of unstable dysrhythmias • MAP >70 mm Hg with little or no vasopressor support • Pulmonary artery occlusion pressure <18 mm Hg • Cardiac index >2.4 • SvO_2 between 60% and 80% • Capillary refill <2 seconds • Urine output >0.5 mL/kg/hour

*Level D: Peer-reviewed professional and organizational standards with the support of clinical study recommendations.

Procedure continues on following page

Documentation

Documentation should include the following:

- Patient and family education
- Informed consent
- Universal protocol requirements
- Insertion of the IAB catheter (including size of catheter used and balloon volume)
- Peripheral pulses and neurovascular assessment of the affected extremity
- Any difficulties with insertion
- IABP frequency
- Patient response to the procedure and to IABP therapy
- Assessment of pain, interventions, and response to interventions
- Confirmation of placement (e.g., chest radiograph)
- Insertion site assessment
- Hemodynamic status
- IABP pressures (unassisted end-diastolic pressure, unassisted systolic pressure, balloon-augmented pressure, assisted systolic pressure, assisted end-diastolic pressure, and MAP)
- Occurrence of unexpected outcomes
- Additional nursing interventions taken

References and Additional Readings

For a complete list of references and additional readings for this procedure, scan this QR code with your smartphone, or visit https://www.elsevier.com/__data/assets/pdf_file/0008/1319822/Chapter0047.pdf

PROCEDURE
48

Ventricular Assist Devices

Laura A. Wilson

PURPOSE Ventricular assist devices, depending on the device, can be used for cardiogenic shock and postcardiotomy support to allow for myocardial recovery, for bridge to cardiac transplantation, or for destination therapy (permanent implantation in patients who are not transplant candidates). Temporary devices are used as a bridge from one device to another, as a bridge to a decision for cardiac transplant, or as a bridge to recovery. Patients should be in New York Heart Association class IIIB or IV heart failure, have a left ventricular ejection fraction of 25% or less, an oxygen treadmill test of 14 or less, or be inotrope-dependent for 14 days or intraaortic balloon pump–dependent for 7 days.[1-6,12,18,23,25-27]

PREREQUISITE NURSING KNOWLEDGE

- Normal anatomy and physiology of the cardiovascular, peripheral vascular, and pulmonary systems.
- Management of heart failure.
- Principles of hemodynamic monitoring, cardiopulmonary bypass, electrophysiology and dysrhythmias, and coagulation.
- Clinical and technical competence related to use of ventricular assist devices (VADs).
- Advanced cardiac life support knowledge and skills.
- Complications of VAD therapy, including, but not limited to, bleeding, cardiac tamponade, right ventricular failure, myocardial infarction, cardiac arrhythmias, hepatic dysfunction, pulmonary dysfunction, renal dysfunction, infection, neurological dysfunction, thrombosis, and VAD malfunction.[2,3,10,13]
- The effect of preload, afterload, right ventricular failure, cardiac tamponade, and cardiac dysrhythmias on the function of the device.
- Interaction between the patient and the device.
- Specific information concerning controls, alarms, troubleshooting, and safety features is available from each manufacturer and should be read thoroughly by the nurse before use of the equipment. Please refer to the operator's instructions for use (IFU), which are available for each system, for more details.
- Anticoagulation goals specific to the VAD that is being used are necessary. Competence in testing coagulability and titrating medication to maintain optimal anticoagulation according to institutional protocols.
- Indications for VAD therapy include the following[22]:
  - Inability to wean from cardiopulmonary bypass
  - Bridge to cardiac transplant

- Destination therapy: New York Heart Association class IIIB or IV status in a patient whose condition does not respond to optimal medical therapy and who is not a transplant candidate[4,9]
  - Bridge to myocardial recovery after cardiogenic shock
- Relative contraindications of VAD therapy include the following[6,23]:
  - Body surface area (BSA) less than 1.2 m² (HeartMate II left ventricular assist device LVAD; Abbott Corporation, Abbott Park, IL)[6,23]
  - Patients with irreversible end-stage organ damage[6,23]
  - Unrepairable ventricular septal defect or free wall rupture with those receiving an LVAD alone[6,23]
  - Comorbidity that limits life expectancy to less than 3 years (e.g., cancer, liver disease)[6,23]
  - Active infection (valvular endocarditis, implantable cardioverter defibrillator [ICD] infection with bacteremia)[6,23]
  - Diabetes-related proliferative retinopathy, very poor glycemic control, or severe nephropathy, vasculopathy, or peripheral neuropathy[6,23]
  - Active pregnancy[6,23]
  - Active psychiatric illness that requires long-term institutionalization or a patient's inability to care for or maintain the device[6,23]
  - Neuromuscular disease that severely compromises a patient's ability to use and care for the external system components or to ambulate or exercise[6,23]
  - Psychosocial and cognitive conditions may limit the use of a VAD except in bridge to recovery because the patient must have the cognitive skills to manage the VAD[6,23]
  - Significant caregiver burden or lack of any caregiver[6,23]
  - Active substance abusers[6,11,23]
  - Medical noncompliance[6,11,23]

Temporary Devices

- Impella (Abiomed, Danvers, MA)[16,12,23]:
  - The Impella system is a minimally invasive temporary percutaneous VAD (p-VAD), which is a nonpulsatile microaxial flow device that delivers cardiovascular support with different access and different capabilities.[16,12,23]

❖ These catheter-based pumps are implanted percutaneously or by arterial cutdown (usually the femoral or axillary artery).

  ○ Impella 2.5 (2.5 L/min), Impella CP with SmartAssist (4.3 L/min), and Impella 5.0 (5 L/min) catheters provide short-term support of blood flow for 4 to 14 days.[16,12,23]

❖ Impella 5.5 with SmartAssist, and Impella LD Catheters are surgically implanted catheters. LD is a direct access into the aorta surgically via sternotomy with a 5 L/min flow rate for up to 14 days.[16,12,23]

❖ Once in position, the Impella sits across the aortic valve with the inlet area in the left ventricle and the outlet area in the ascending aorta.[16,12,23]

❖ Transthoracic echocardiography (TTE) is used to confirm proper placement.

❖ The console continuously monitors pump placement and alerts the physician, advanced practice nurses, and other healthcare professionals to issues with catheter displacement and other alarm states.

❖ In addition to the aforementioned configurations, there is an Impella RP catheter, which is inserted via the femoral vein across the pulmonary valve to the left pulmonary artery for right ventricle support with a 4 L/min flow rate for up to 14 days.[16,12,23]

• CentriMag. The CentriMag Ventricular Assist Device: temporary external VAD that can support the right, left, or both ventricles. Extracorporeal life support (ECLS/ECMO) indicated for temporary use (Abbott Corporation).[1,23]

• CentriMag use is not considered ECMO unless an artificial lung is placed with the pump; without the lung it is simply an external temporary VAD and using the word ECMO here is not necessary (Abbott Corporation)[1,23]

❖ The CentriMag VAD is a continuous centrifugal flow device that delivers up to 9.9 L/min of blood flow.[23]

❖ The pump is placed via catheters by a thoracotomy approach (the catheters are placed internally, but the pump is external to the body).[23]

❖ The CentriMag operates via an electromagnetic rotor that operates at a range of 0 to 5500 rpm.[23]

❖ The pump is driven by a primary console. Intraoperative cannulation can be accomplished via left atrial or left ventricular cannulation (inflow) to the aorta (outflow), accomplishing left ventricular support for short-term use.[23]

❖ Intraoperative cannulation can also be accomplished via right atria (inflow) to the pulmonary artery (outflow), accomplishing right ventricular support for short-term use.[23]

❖ Using two devices, biventricular support can be accomplished.[23]

• The Tandem Heart (TandemLife Corp., Pittsburgh, PA) (temporary)[19,20,24]:

❖ The Tandem Heart is a continuous centrifugal flow device that delivers up to 5 L/min of blood flow at 7500 rpm.[19,24] This device can be configured for right, left, or both ventricles or an extracorporeal life support (ECLS/ECMO) system indicated for short-term use up to 6 hours.[24]

❖ The pump is implanted via a percutaneous approach. Depending on configuration for right ventricle, left ventricle, or biventricular, the access would be arterial or venous.

❖ Biventricular support is accomplished transseptally via femoral vein access.[19,20,24]

❖ The Tandem Heart operates via an electromagnetic rotor that operates at a range of 3000 to 7500 rpm.[19,20,24]

❖ The pump is driven by a microprocessor controller.[19,20,24]

❖ The Tandem Heart has a dual-chamber pump. The upper housing allows for the movement of blood. The lower housing communicates with the controller and contains a continuous flow of saline to decrease the risk of thrombus formation and provide lubrication.[19,20,24]

❖ Using the ProtekDuo RA-PA catheter, percutaneous right ventricular support can be achieved.

Durable Devices

• The HeartMate II and III Left Ventricular Assist Device (LVAD) are long term (Thoratec/Abbott Corporation, Pleasanton, CA):[1,23,22,25]

❖ The HeartMate II LVAD is a continuous axial flow pump, and the HeartMate III is a pulsatile-flow system without mechanical bearings. They are approved as a bridge to transplant and destination therapy in patients with advanced heart failure.[1,23,22,25]

❖ The Heartmate II LVAD is implanted just below the diaphragm in the abdomen, whereas the Heartmate III is implanted above the diaphragm.[1,22,23,25]

❖ Blood flows from the left ventricle through the pump and back to the patient's circulation via the outflow graft.[1,23,22,25]

❖ Continuous flow is generated by a small rotor inside the pump.

❖ The speed of the pump is set by the LVAD team and does not change in response to preload.[1,22,23,25]

❖ In the HeartMate II, the controller sends power and operating signals to the pump and collects information, whereas in the HeartMate III the internal pump controls the information and sends information to the controller.

❖ The percutaneous driveline is passed underneath the skin and exits the right or left upper quadrant of the abdomen. The driveline connects the LVAD to a controller and a power source (batteries or power module).[1,23,22,25]

❖ The HeartMate III has a modular driveline to facilitate replacement of the external portion if it becomes damaged.

• HeartWare LVAD (HeartWare Corporation, Framingham, MA):[11]

❖ The HeartWare devices are not used for new implantation, so this device may be present in patients who had the device placed before admission. The HeartWare Left Ventricular Assist System consists of a continuous-flow centrifugal force blood pump with an integrated, partially centered inflow cannula; a 10-mm diameter gel-impregnated polyester outflow graft; and a percutaneous driveline.[4,22,25]

❖ The pump has one moving part, an impeller, that spins blood to generate up to 10 L/min of flow.[4,22,25]

- A short-integrated inflow cannula is inserted into the left ventricle, and the outflow graft connects the pump to the aorta.[4,22,25]
- The device is implanted in the thoracic cavity above the diaphragm.[4,22,25]
- The controller is a microprocessor unit that controls and manages the HeartWare System operation. The controller sends power and operating signals to the blood pump and collects information from the pump.[4,22,25]

EQUIPMENT

Impella Percutaneous Ventricular Assist Device

- Impella device
- Automated Impella controller (console)
- Impella purge cassette
- Purge fluid (dextrose/heparin solution prepared by pharmacy)
- Normal saline (NS) 500 mL infusion bag
- Straight IV tubing (nonpump tubing)
- Pressure bag
- Knee immobilizer (if Impella is placed femorally)
- Sterile gauze
- Straight IV tubing in the cage of the Impella controller
- Connector cable
- Impella "instructions for use" with alarm explanation

CentriMag Ventricular Assist Device

- CentriMag device
- Automated CentriMag controller
- Backup CentriMag controller
- Two chest tube clamps
- CentriMag "instructions for use" with alarm explanation

TandemHeart Ventricular Assist Device

- TandemHeart device
- TandemHeart controller
- Backup TandemHeart controller
- 1000-mL bag of NS solution
- TandemHeart infusion tubing
- Two chest tube clamps
- Kelly clamp
- TandemHeart "instructions for use" with alarm explanation

LVAD: Heartmate II and III and HeartWare

- VAD device and system controller
- Driveline
- Backup system controller and batteries (6 to 8 batteries, battery charger); wall power (wall power module or AC power adapter); backup controller
- Device-specific equipment (Doppler)

Additional equipment to have available for LVAD driveline dressing changes includes the following:
- Emergency equipment and medications
- Sterile dressing supplies for acute dressing change
- Preslit 4 × 4 sterile gauze pads (alternatively, round preslit island dressing)
- Sterile 2 × 2 sterile gauze
- ChrorPrep applicator, 3 mL in size

- Tape, 1-inch and 2-inch
- Sterile gloves
- Head covers (until driveline ingrowth occurs)
- Masks (until driveline ingrowth occurs)
- Sterile gowns (until driveline ingrowth occurs)
- Sterile drapes
- Driveline fixation device
- Sterile dressing supplies for chronic dressing change:
  - LVAD prepackaged driveline management system consisting of:
    - Sterile 4 × 4 gauze and/or sterile 4 × 4 split gauze
    - Antiseptic cleaning solution
    - Sterile gloves
    - Masks
    - Driveline fixation device
    - Biopatch (based on institutional protocol)
    - Clear Tegaderm dressing shield

PATIENT AND FAMILY EDUCATION

- Assess patient and family understanding of VAD therapy and the reason for its use. *Rationale:* Clarification or reinforcement of information is an expressed patient and family need during times of stress and anxiety.
- Explain the environment and plan of care to the patient and family, including the frequency of assessment, sounds and function of equipment, placement of the device, explanation of alarms, dressings and therapy, anticoagulation needs, decreased or assisted mobility, and parameters for discontinuation of therapy. *Rationale:* This communication provides information and encourages the patient and family to ask questions or voice concerns or fears related to the therapy.
- Before surgery, a meeting with another patient receiving VAD therapy may be helpful for the patient and family, if both patients agree. *Rationale:* Meeting with another patient with a VAD provides social support.
- If appropriate, begin discharge teaching to include operation of the LVAD, dressing changes, battery changes, placement of self on and off of the battery and the power module, changing of the controller, and appropriate bathing techniques with use of shower equipment (when approved by the VAD team). It is recommended that patients and their families be provided with comprehensive education regarding the care and maintenance of their VAD with the expectation they will be able to perform a return demonstration of these key components. *Rationale:* This teaching provides information and ensures that the patient will be safe at home. It also allows the patient and family to ask questions as needed.

PATIENT ASSESSMENT AND PREPARATION

Patient Assessment

- Assess the patient's medical history, history of heart failure, competency of the aortic/pulmonic valves, competency of the mitral/tricuspid valves, pulmonary hypertension, right ventricular function, left ventricular function, and peripheral vascular disease. ***Rationale:*** This assessment provides baseline data regarding cardiac functioning and facilitates decision making regarding insertion of the appropriate device and postoperative management.

- Perform a cardiovascular, hemodynamic, peripheral vascular, neurovascular, and psychosocial assessment and assessment of body mass index (height, weight, BSA). ***Rationale:*** These assessments provide baseline data and help with determination of the type of device to use.
- Assess the patient's current laboratory profile, including complete blood count, platelet count, prothrombin time, partial thromboplastin time (PTT), international normalized ratio (INR), blood chemistry, liver profile, protein, and albumin levels. ***Rationale:*** This assessment provides baseline data and may indicate end-organ dysfunction related to low-flow state. It also may be used to predict the patient's risk of bleeding.

Patient Preparation

- Verify the correct patient with two identifiers. ***Rationale:*** Before performing the procedure, the nurse should ensure the correct identification of the patient for the intended intervention.

- Ensure that the patient and family understand the preoperative teaching. Answer questions as they arise, and reinforce information as needed. ***Rationale:*** This communication evaluates and reinforces understanding of previously taught information.
- Ensure that an informed consent form has been signed (if it is known before surgery that the VAD will be placed). ***Rationale:*** Informed consent protects the rights of the patient and makes a competent decision possible for the patient and family.
- For the LVAD HeartMate and HeartWare, the driveline exit site may need to be marked and verified with the implanting surgeon. Patient position, surgical history (gastric surgery), and daily habits are assessed to determine the best placement of the driveline exit site. ***Rationale:*** If the patient wears suspenders or high-waisted pants, previous surgical sites can rub and irritate the driveline site, decreasing the patient's quality of life and increasing the risk of infection.
- Perform a preprocedural verification and time out. ***Rationale:*** This ensures patient safety.
- Provide emotional support to the patient and family. ***Rationale:*** The patient and family are under an extreme amount of stress.

Procedure **for Ventricular Assist Devices (Temporary/Short Term)**

Steps	Rationale	Special Considerations
Impella Percutaneous Ventricular Assist Device (Abiomed)		
1. Verify the presence of the backup motor and console.	In the event of device failure, support can rapidly be reestablished.	
2. **HH**		
3. **PE**		
4. Once the patient is stable after admission to the critical care unit, transition from initial setup to standard configuration on the Impella controller:	Prepares the system.	
A. Attach NS with straight tubing to the red side arm of the Impella 2.5 and Impella CP catheter.		
B. Pressurize the NS with the pressure bag to 300 mm Hg (do not use pressure tubing).		
C. Press "PURGE SYSTEM" on the Impella CP controller, and then select "Transfer to Standard Configuration."		
D. Create a slow drip from the pressurized NS to flood the Luer-Lok connector of the red pressure side arm and make a wet-to-wet connection.		
E. Fully open the roller clamp once connected.		
F. Select OK to confirm transfer.		

Procedure for Ventricular Assist Devices (Temporary/Short Term)—*Continued*

Steps	Rationale	Special Considerations
5. Change the purge fluid as prescribed or based on institutional standards (e.g., heparin 25,000 units/D5W 500 mL).	Heparin and dextrose are specific to the function of the Impella device and longevity of the catheter.	The rate will be preset by the Automatic Impella Controller (AIC) flow rate. Change the pressurized NS bag every 24 hours; change the purge cassette and tubing every 96 hours; follow institutional protocols.
6. Check the ACT as prescribed (e.g., 2 hours after the purge solution is initiated).	Determines whether the desired level of anticoagulation is achieved.	Additional heparin may be needed in the purge fluid to achieve the desired ACT range. The range will be determined by the provider.
7. Ensure that the Impella device is in the proper position.		
A. Ensure that a transthoracic echocardiogram is obtained as prescribed.	Determines whether the device is across the aortic valve.	
B. Ensure that the Tuohy-Borst valve is locked.	Maintains the position of the device across the aortic valve.	May need to remove the initial dressing to assess whether the valve is locked. Follow institutional protocols. Document the centimeter marker on the Impella CP catheter closest to the sheath.
C. Apply the knee immobilizer (for femoral insertion).	Prevents catheter migration.	
D. Assess Impella position using the "Placement Signal" as displayed by the Automatic Impella.	Ensures that the catheter has not migrated.	
8. Confirm that the mode of operation is P-level mode.	Ensures that equipment is set as prescribed.	Verify the prescribed P-level.
9. If the P-level must be changed, push the menu button and choose P-level mode.		
10. Ensure that the white introducer side arm is capped off and marked "DO NOT USE."	Accessing the introducer could compromise the position of the Impella.	
11. Troubleshooting:		
A. Resuscitation:		
i. For CPR, decrease the performance level to P2.		
ii. Defibrillate as needed.		There is no need to stop or disconnect the device.
iii. Consider compressions	Compressions may dislodge cannulation, causing loss of support and/or bleeding.	Provide compressions only if prescribed by the provider. Follow institutional protocols.
iv. ROSC		
a. Verify the position of the device with an echocardiogram	Determines whether the position of the device is correct.	
b. Resume P-level as prescribed.	Continues treatment as prescribed.	
B. Respond to device alarms:	Corrects the alarm condition.	Refer to the IFU for specific interventions needed for each alarm.
i. Rapidly assess the alarm condition.		
ii. Respond to each alarm.		
iii. Notify the physician or advanced practice nurse if assistance is needed.		

Procedure continues on following page

Procedure for Ventricular Assist Devices (Temporary/Short Term)—*Continued*

Steps	Rationale	Special Considerations
12. Weaning and removal:		Discontinue anticoagulation as prescribed.
A. Follow the weaning process as prescribed. Follow institutional protocols.		
B. Decrease the performance level by 2 P-levels every 3 hours, or as prescribed, until at P2.		
C. Maintain the Impella at P2 for the prescribed amount of time.		This is typically at least 2 hours.
D. Assess the patient's response to P2.		Some institutional protocols require the laboratory tests and echocardiogram to be performed to assess the patient's toleration to P2.
E. Assist as needed with device removal.	The patient must demonstrate ventricular recovery before removal.	
F. Assist as needed as pressure is maintained at the insertion site.		Manual pressure may be maintained at the insertion site for a minimum of 20 minutes or until hemostasis is achieved. Follow institutional protocols.
G. Compression devices may be utilized after manual compression.		
H. Monitor for hematoma formation or overt bleeding at the site.		
I. Assess for retroperitoneal bleeding (HCT dropping, abdominal/flank pain) or hemodynamic compromise.		
13. Remove **HH**, and discard used supplies.	Reduces the transmission of microorganisms; standard precautions.	
14. **PE**		

CentriMag Ventricular Assist Device (Left, Right, or Biventricular Device) (Thoratec/Abbott Corporation)

Steps	Rationale	Special Considerations
1. Verify the presence of the backup motor, console, and chest tube clamps.	In the event of device failure, support can rapidly be established.	
2. **HH**		
3. **PE**		
4. Assess pump function.	Ensures that the device is functioning appropriately.	Low-flow alarms should be a part of initial checks.
5. Assess the pump insertion site.	Determines whether bleeding or hematoma is present.	
6. Assess for VAD chatter.	VAD chatter indicates that the device is running too fast for the amount of blood being delivered to it (or that the patient's fluid status is low).	Assess for volume, VAD rate, right ventricular function, arrhythmia, and position of the cannula.
7. Adjust the flow probe 1 cm every 8 hours, ensuring that the arrows on the probe point in the direction of blood flow.	The flow probe can contribute to thrombus formation if left in place too long.	Check institutional protocols.

Procedure	for Ventricular Assist Devices (Temporary/Short Term)—*Continued*	
Steps	**Rationale**	**Special Considerations**
8. Anticoagulation:		
A. Administer anticoagulation as prescribed (e.g., heparin 25,000 units/500 mL D5W).	Maintains the patency of the device and decreases thrombus formation.	There are special circumstances, but typically this device with an external pump and cannula tubing requires systemic anticoagulation
B. Check the ACT as prescribed (e.g., hourly).	Determines whether the desired level of anticoagulation is achieved.	Some institutional protocols may include PTT or Xa
C. Additional anticoagulation may be needed as prescribed.	The ACT range will be determined by the physician or advanced practice nurse.	
9. Troubleshooting:		
A. CPR: Compressions may be contraindicated.	Compressions may dislodge the cannula(ae).	Only provide compressions if prescribed by the provider. Follow institutional protocols.
B. Defibrillate as necessary.		There is no need to stop or disconnect the device.
C. Respond to device alarms:		
i. Rapidly assess the alarm condition.	If the device is stopped for longer than 5 minutes, it may not be safe to restart.	Refer to the IFU for specific interventions needed for each alarm.
ii. Respond to each alarm.		
iii. Notify the provider if assistance is needed.		
iv. If an equipment change is necessary, clamp the return tubing before switching to the backup equipment.	Prevents backflow of the device.	Switching to a backup console should only be done by trained personnel.
v. Always unclamp the tubing after restarting the device.		
10. Weaning and removal:		Discontinue anticoagulation as prescribed.
A. Follow the physician or advanced practice nurse prescription for weaning.		
B. Decrease the device rate as prescribed.		
C. Assess the patient's response to the decrease in the device rate.	The patient needs to demonstrate ventricular recovery before removal.	
D. The device will be removed in the operating room.		
E. Assess for bleeding, hematoma, and hemodynamic status after return from the operating room.	Determines patient stability.	
11. Remove **PE**, and discard used supplies.	Reduces the transmission of microorganisms; standard precautions.	
12. **HH**		

TandemHeart Ventricular Assist System (Left, Right, or Biventricular Device) (TandemLife Corporation)

1. Verify the presence of the backup console and tubing clamps.	In the event of device failure, support can be rapidly reestablished.	
2. **HH**		
3. **PE**		

Procedure continues on following page

Procedure	for Ventricular Assist Devices (Temporary/Short Term)—*Continued*	
Steps	**Rationale**	**Special Considerations**
4. Assess pump function.	Ensures that the device is functioning appropriately.	
5. Assess the pump insertion site.	Determines whether bleeding or hematoma is present.	
6. Assess the VAD for chatter.	VAD chatter indicates that the device is running too fast for the amount of blood being delivered to it.	Assess for volume, VAD rate, right ventricular function, arrhythmia, and malposition of the cannula.
7. Assess the insertion depth.	Determines the position of the cannula(ae).	
8. Immobilize the affected limb.	Prevents catheter migration.	
9. Anticoagulation:		
A. Administer anticoagulation as prescribed (e.g., heparin 25,000 units/500 mL D5W).	Maintains the patency of the device and decreases thrombus formation.	A heparin infusion is prescribed along with the TandemHeart infusate.
B. Check the activated clotting time as prescribed (e.g., hourly).	Determines whether the desired level of anticoagulation is achieved.	Some institutional protocols require monitoring PTT or Xa.
C. Additional anticoagulation may be needed as prescribed.	The ACT range will be determined by the physician or advanced practice nurse.	
D. Heparin may also be used as an infusate through the device.	Maintains the patency of the device and decreases thrombus formation.	Do not use heparin in D5W through the device.
10. Troubleshooting:		
A. CPR: Compressions may be contraindicated.	Compressions may dislodge the cannula(ae).	Only provide compressions if prescribed by the provider. Follow institutional protocols.
B. Defibrillate as necessary.		There is no need to stop or disconnect the device.
C. Respond to device alarms:		
i. Rapidly assess the alarm condition.	If the device is stopped for longer than 5 minutes, it may not be safe to restart.	Refer to the IFU for specific interventions needed for each alarm.
ii. Respond to each alarm.		
iii. Notify the provider if assistance is needed.		
iv. If an equipment change is necessary, clamp the return tubing before switching to the backup equipment.	Prevents backflow of blood into the device.	Switching to a backup device should only be done by trained personnel.
v. Always unclamp the tubing after restarting the device.		
11. Weaning and removal:		Discontinue anticoagulation as prescribed.
A. Follow the weaning process as prescribed. Follow institutional protocols.		
B. Decrease the device rate as prescribed.		
C. Assess the patient's response to the decrease in device rate.	The patient must demonstrate ventricular recovery before removal.	
D. Assist as needed with device removal.		
E. Assist as needed as pressure is maintained at the insertion site.		Manual pressure may be maintained at the insertion site for a minimum of 20 minutes or until hemostasis is achieved. Follow institutional protocols.

Procedure for Ventricular Assist Devices (Temporary/Short Term)—*Continued*

Steps	Rationale	Special Considerations
F. Compression devices may be utilized after manual compression.		
G. Monitor for hematoma formation or overt bleeding at the site.		
H. Assess for retroperitoneal bleeding (HCT decreasing, abdominal/flank pain) or hemodynamic compromise.		
12. Remove **PE**, and discard used supplies.	Reduces the transmission of microorganisms; standard precautions.	
13. **HH**		

Procedure for Ventricular Assist Devices (Durable/Long Term)

Steps	Rationale	Special Considerations
HeartMate II and HeartMate III LVAD (Abbott/Thoratec Corporation)		
1. **HH**		
2. **PE**		
3. Changing from the power module to batteries:		
A. Check the battery life by pushing down the alarm silence button.	Ensures that the battery is charged.	Batteries are fully charged when four green lights appear. Batteries are changed when one green light is lit.
B. Place a battery into each battery clip by lining up the arrow on the large battery and battery clip and inserting until the battery clicks securely into the holder.	Allows patient ambulation.	Assist the patient with equipment during ambulation, or provide a holster to hold the batteries and controller.
C. Disconnect the white controller cable from the power module cable by loosening the white nut and then pulling them apart.	An alarm sounds once per second, and a yellow crescent flashes, indicating disconnection from the power module.	NEVER disconnect both power sources at the same time.
D. Connect the white controller cable to the battery clip, and tighten the white nut.	The alarm is resolved.	Line up arrows to each other on the cable and battery clip for connection to prevent damage to prongs.
E. Disconnect the black controller cable from the power module cable by loosening the black nut and then pulling them apart.	An alarm sounds once per second, and the yellow crescent flashes, indicating disconnection from the power module.	
F. Connect the black controller cable to the battery clip, and tighten the black nut.	The alarm resolves after the cable is connected properly.	Line up arrows to each other on the cable and battery clip for connection to prevent damage to prongs.
4. Changing from batteries to the power module:		
A. Disconnect the white controller cable from the battery clip by loosening the white nut and then pulling them apart.	An alarm sounds once per second, and the yellow crescent flashes, indicating disconnection from the battery.	Do not disconnect both cables at the same time because power failure may occur, resulting in the need to use the emergency backup battery.

Procedure continues on following page

Procedure for Ventricular Assist Devices (Durable/Long Term)—*Continued*

Steps	Rationale	Special Considerations
B. Connect the white controller cable to the white power module cable connection, and tighten the white nut.	The alarm is resolved.	Line up arrows to each other on the cable and battery clip for connection to prevent damage to prongs.
C. Disconnect the black controller cable from the battery clip by loosening the black nut and then pulling them apart.	An alarm sounds once per second, and the yellow crescent flashes, indicating disconnection from the power module.	
D. Connect the black controller cable to the black power module cable connection, and tighten the black nut.	Returns the power connection to the power module cable to allow power to be obtained from an AC source. The alarm is resolved.	Line up arrows to each other on the cable and battery clip for connection to prevent damage to prongs.
E. Remove the batteries from the clips, and place the batteries back into the universal battery charger.	Allows the batteries to recharge.	Batteries will be fully charged when lit green on the universal battery charger.
5. Troubleshooting (general):		
A. Power module alarm: AC fail:	The external power to the power module is off. The internal battery of the power module powers the pump for 30 minutes.	The power module emits a steady tone.
i. Change the power source.		
ii. Switch from the power module to the batteries.		
iii. Ensure that the power module is plugged into an outlet with emergency power backup.		
B. Power module alarm: Low battery:	The power module internal battery is almost depleted.	This alarm is a steady tone.
i. Change the power source.		
ii. Switch from the power module to batteries.		Ensure that the power module is plugged into an outlet with emergency power backup
C. Power module alarm: Alarm reset:	Used to silence the power module fail alarm.	If the patient is connected to the power module, all alarms sound at the power module and controller; both must be silenced.
i. Press the alarm reset switch.		
ii. The AC fail alarm is silenced and does not come back on.		
6. Troubleshooting (HeartMate II and HeartMate III controller alarms):		Always check the patient, then check connections from the patient to the controller, and then check connections from the controller to the patient. If the patient is on \the monitor, the alarm is visible on the monitor.
A. Alarm: Red heart:	The VAD may not be functioning adequately.	Emits a steady tone. Notify the provider and LVAD team.

Procedure for Ventricular Assist Devices (Durable/Long Term)—*Continued*

Steps	Rationale	Special Considerations
i. Check whether the LVAD is still pumping by listening for a VAD hum with a stethoscope, and look for the green power light on the controller. Assess the patient.	If the VAD is not functioning adequately, emergency interventions may be needed.	"RED HEART: GREEN POWER LIGHT ON" can occur if the LVAD flow is <2.5 L/min. If the pump is running, administer IV fluids, and treat arrhythmias and hypertension as prescribed. If the pump is not running, change the controller per the IFU procedure. If the pump is not running and the patient is in cardiovascular arrest, begin basic life support (BLS) and advanced cardiac life support (ACLS). (Do not start compressions without a specific order.)
ii. Check that the controller is connected securely to the driveline.		
iii. Change the power source: change batteries or, if on the power module, switch to a battery source.		
B. Alarm: Red battery:	Fewer than 5 minutes of battery power remain.	Emits a steady tone.
	After the batteries are depleted, the emergency battery will give an additional 15 minutes of power.	Batteries should not be permitted to get this low.
i. Immediately replace the batteries. *Or*		
ii. Change to an alternate power source.		
C. Alarm: Yellow diamond:	Fewer than 15 minutes of battery power remain.	Emits 1 beep per second.
i. Change batteries. *Or*		
ii. Change to power module.		
D. Alarm: Yellow wrench:	Assess for interruption of the driveline (driveline fault), emergency battery not installed or expired, or controller not synchronized with monitor time.	Refer to the IFU for specific interventions.
i. Read the LCD screen, and follow instructions.		
ii. Consult your hospital contact or Abbott representative.		
7. Self-test:		
A. Place the patient on the power module, and then hold down the battery button until all the lights on the controller light and a loud alarm sounds.	A self-test is done each day to check the function of the pump, controller, and the emergency backup battery.	
B. All lights should go off except for the power light, and all alarms should silence if the controller passes the test.		

Procedure continues on following page

Procedure for Ventricular Assist Devices (Durable/Long Term)—*Continued*		
Steps	Rationale	Special Considerations
8. Changing the controller:		Refer to the IFU for specific interventions.
A. Lay out the new controller next to the old controller. Connect a battery or the power module to the new controller.	Eases the changing of the controllers. Allows power to the new controller	The patient should be in a sitting or lying position.
B. Open the latch on the back of the controller. Push the red button down, and pull the driveline out of the controller at the same time.	Allows for the controller change.	The device will stop when you disconnect the patient from the controller. Monitor the patient closely.
C. Connect the batteries to the new controller. Connect the driveline to the new controller by lining up the "black triangles or black lines" and pushing to engage. Close the controller lock to ensure that the driveline stays engaged.	Allows the power to be restored.	The controller will have the backup battery powering the controller but must have both batteries replaced to continue safely. The controller starts the pump at the preset rate.
D. Connect the second battery to the new controller.	Restores power.	
E. The original controller must be placed in standby mode by pushing and holding the battery button for a count of five after both power cables have been disconnected.	Silences the alarms on the disconnected controller.	The controller will stop alarming.
9. Remove **PE**, and discard used supplies.	Reduces transmission of microorganisms; standard precautions.	
10. **HH**		
HeartWare LVAD (HeartWare)		
1. **PE**		
2. **HH**		
3. Changing from the AC power to batteries:		
A. Ensure that the battery to which you are connecting is fully charged by pressing the battery button. One battery will remain connected to the controller while on the AC power cable as a backup.	Ensures that the new battery will power the LVAD during disconnect from the AC source.	Batteries are fully charged when four green lights appear. Make certain that the backup battery is available and is fully charged. Verify that the battery currently connected is fully charged before changing the power source.
B. Remove the AC power cable from the controller by turning the connector toward the arrow and pulling straight out.		
C. Connect the new battery to the controller by grasping the connector of the battery, lining up the arrows, and pushing straight in.	The patient is now on total battery power.	There will be an audible click when the battery is engaged.
4. Changing from batteries to AC power:		
A. Connect the power cable to the AC outlet (be sure that it is grounded).	Ensures safety.	
B. Remove one of the batteries from the controller by turning the connector toward the arrow and pulling straight out.		
C. Connect the AC power cable to the controller by grasping at the connector of the battery, lining up the arrows, and pushing straight in.	Connects the VAD to AC power.	There will be an audible click when the battery is engaged. One battery will remain connected to the controller as a backup.

Procedure for Ventricular Assist Devices (Durable/Long Term)—*Continued*

Steps	Rationale	Special Considerations
5. Troubleshooting HeartWare Alarms:		
A. VAD stopped		Assess the patient, and implement emergency care if needed.
B. Look at the LED screen. The LED screen displays "connect driveline," and the red alarm indicator will be flashing red.	If the driveline disconnects, the device will stop.	
C. Check connections.		
D. Reconnect the driveline to the controller.	Continues VAD function.	
E. If the LED screen displays, "change controller" or "controller failure.		
F. Immediately change the controller.	Replaces equipment.	Notify the VAD coordinator.
6. Battery alarms:		
A. If the alarm is "Critical Battery 1 or 2," change the battery that is depleted.	Ensures that the battery is fully charged.	
B. If there is a continuous high-pitched alarm with no LED message, replace the power immediately.	All power has been lost, necessitating a new power source.	This will result in the VAD stopping. Assess the patient, and implement emergency care if needed.
7. Changing the controller:		Refer to the IFU.
A. Place the new controller next to the old controller.	Eases the transition when connecting the new controller.	The patient should lie or sit down because the patient will lose support momentarily as the controller is changed.
B. Connect the backup power source to the new controller. A backup power source is the AC power cable and battery or two batteries.	Provides power to the new controller.	The power-disconnect alarm and the VAD-stopped alarm will sound until the controller is connected to the driveline.
C. Pull back the white driveline cover on the old controller's silver connector.	Exposes the driveline connector to the controller.	
D. Grasp the driveline connector, and pull straight out to disconnect the patient from the controller.		The device will stop when the driveline is disconnected from the controller. Monitor the patient closely.
E. Align the black dot on the driveline connector with the black dot on the new controller driveline port, and push in until a click is heard.	The device will restart.	
F. Replace the white driveline cover over the silver connector.		
G. Place the red adapter into the old controller, and remove all power.		The controller should stop alarming.
H. If no red alarm adapter is available, press both the alarm silence and the scroll buttons together for 5 seconds.		
8. Remove 🅿🅴, and discard used supplies.	Reduces the transmission of microorganisms; standard precautions.	
9. 🅷🅷		

UNIT II

Procedure   for Acute Driveline Dressing[4]

Steps	Rationale	Special Considerations
1. Gather supplies and protective equipment for dressing change.	Prepares for the procedure.	Position the patient, and raise the head of the bed as needed to provide access to the driveline for the procedure.
2. **HH**		
3. **PE**		
4. Create a sterile field with the sterile drape.		
5. Drop the sterile dressing supplies onto the sterile drape.		
6. Place a mask on the patient unless the patient is intubated.	Decreases contamination of the wound.	Everyone in the room should apply a mask. This is required until tissue ingrowth occurs.
7. Apply a cap.	Prepares for the procedure.	This is required until tissue ingrowth occurs.
8. Remove gloves, wash hands, and apply clean gloves	Prepares for the procedure.	
9. Carefully remove the old dressing.		
10. Assess the driveline site for drainage and redness.	Determines early signs of infection.	
11. Remove clean gloves, and wash hands.		
12. Apply sterile gloves.	Prepares for the sterile procedure.	
13. Gently cleanse around the exit site from the center out with antiseptic solution (e.g., 2% chlorhexidine-based preparation or 70% isopropyl alcohol swab sticks) as per institutional policy.	Deceases the risk of infection.	
14. Allow the antiseptic solution to dry.	Increases the effectiveness of the antiseptic.	
15. Never use Betadine ointment, skin prep, Uni-Solve, or acetone around the driveline.	These products can cause damage to the driveline.	
16. Place a folded 2 × 2 gauze pad under the driveline or per institutional protocols.	Relieves pressure at the edge of the exit site under the driveline, preventing erosion.	
17. Apply a preslit 4 × 4 gauze pad (for excessive drainage) or preslit island dressing (for normal drainage) or per institutional protocols.	Decreases strikethrough.	
18. Use breathable tape to secure the 4 × 4 or to close the preslit island dressing, or per institutional protocols.	Decreases strikethrough.	
19. Secure the driveline with a driveline fixation device or an abdominal binder, or per institutional protocols.	An immobilized driveline allows for faster tissue ingrowth and decreases the risk of infection.	
20. Remove **PE**, and discard used supplies.	Reduces the transmission of microorganisms; standard precautions.	
21. **HH**		

Procedure	for Chronic Driveline Dressing[4]		
Steps	**Rationale**		**Special Considerations**
1. Gather supplies and protective equipment for a dressing change.			Use the acute dressing if any drainage or redness appears.
2. 🅷🅷			
3. 🅿🅴			
4. Open the dressing kit.			
5. Place a mask on the patient unless the patient is intubated.	Decreases contamination of the wound.		Everyone in the room should apply a mask.
6. Remove gloves, wash hands, and apply clean gloves.			
7. Remove the old dressing.			
8. Assess the driveline site for drainage and redness.	Determines whether signs of infection are present.		
9. Remove clean gloves, wash hands, and apply sterile gloves.	Prepares for the procedure.		
10. Gently cleanse around the exit site from the center out with antiseptic solution (e.g., 2% chlorhexidine-based preparation or 70% isopropyl alcohol swab sticks) as per institutional policy. Allow the antiseptic solution to dry.	Never use Betadine ointment, skin prep, Uni-Solve, or acetone around the driveline. These products can cause damage to the driveline.		
11. Place a Biopatch around the driveline. Follow institutional standards.	May decrease the risk of infection.		Placing the Biopatch on damp skin can cause irritation. The site must be dry.
12. Place a clear dressing (e.g., Tegaderm) over the driveline exit site.			
13. Secure the driveline with a driveline fixation device or abdominal binder.			
14. Remove 🅿🅴, and discard used supplies.	Reduces the transmission of microorganisms; standard precautions.		
15. 🅷🅷			

Expected Outcomes

- Increased myocardial oxygen supply and decreased myocardial oxygen demand
- Increased cardiac output and index
- Increased tissue perfusion
- Safe bridge to heart transplant
- Improved activity tolerance and quality of life

Unexpected Outcomes

- Device failure
- VAD infection
- Neurological dysfunction
- Bleeding and coagulation disorders
- Multisystem organ failure
- Thrombotic event
- Pain
- Depression, decreased activity tolerance, or decreased quality of life

Procedure continues on following page

UNIT II

Patient Monitoring and Care

Steps	Rationale	Reportable Conditions
		These conditions should be reported to the provider if they persist despite nursing interventions.
1. Perform systematic cardiovascular, respiratory, peripheral vascular, and hemodynamic assessments as patient status necessitates. Follow institutional protocols.		
A. Level of consciousness.	Assesses for the adequacy of cerebral perfusion; thrombi may develop and dislodge during VAD therapy.	• Decreased level of consciousness • Agitation • Confusion
B. Vital signs and pulmonary artery pressures.	Demonstrates the effectiveness of VAD therapy and evaluates ventricular function. Nonpulsatile pumps will produce only a single BP value (not systolic and diastolic).	• Unstable vital signs • Hemodynamic instability
C. VAD flow and mixed venous oxygen saturation.	Demonstrates the effectiveness of VAD therapy.	• Abnormal values
D. Circulation to the extremities.	Demonstrates adequate peripheral perfusion. If reportable conditions are found, they may indicate thrombotic or embolic obstruction of perfusion to an extremity. Nonpalpable pulses may be a normal finding in the continuous-flow devices. Doppler should be used in these cases to verify continuous flow. May only have "wind tunnel" pulses if continuous flow pump (e.g., Impella).	• Extremities: Cool or cold to the touch • Capillary refill >2 seconds • Diminished or absent pulses (radial, popliteal, tibial, pedal) • Color pale, mottled, or cyanotic • Diminished or absent sensation • Pain • Diminished or absent movement
E. Urine output.	Demonstrates adequate perfusion to the kidneys.	• Urine output <0.5 mL/kg/hour.
2. Assess VAD, heart, and lung sounds every 4 hours and as needed. Follow institutional protocols.	Abnormal VAD, heart, and lung sounds may indicate the need for additional treatment.	• Abnormal VAD sounds, such as grinding or sputtering • Diastolic murmur • Crackles or rhonchi
3. Monitor for signs and symptoms of inadequate preload.	Adequate VAD function depends on an appropriate volume status.	• Inadequate VAD output • Abnormal hemodynamic data
4. Logroll the patient every 2 hours until hemodynamic stability is obtained, and then advance activity as prescribed and tolerated. Prop pillows or a positioning wedge to support the patient and maintain alignment. Consider specialty beds as needed.	Promotes comfort and skin integrity and prevents kinking of the VAD drivelines.	• Disruption of skin integrity
5. Initiate passive and active range-of-motion exercises every 2 hours.	Prevents venous stasis and muscle atrophy.	• Mobility concerns • Developing contractures

Patient Monitoring and Care —*Continued*

Steps	Rationale	Reportable Conditions
6. Assess the area around the VAD cannulates/drivelines exit site(s) for evidence of bleeding. Ensure that each driveline is positioned properly and secured. Use of a VAD driveline securement device or stabilizer belt may help. Follow institutional protocols.	Anticoagulation therapy increases the risk of bleeding.	• Bleeding from the driveline exit site • Any signs of cracking or wear in the driveline
7. Assess prothrombin time, PTT, INR, CBC, platelets, haptoglobin, and plasma-free hemoglobin as prescribed.	Monitors for coagulation problems and hemolysis. All VADs require prophylactic anticoagulation therapy to prevent thrombi and emboli development.	• Bleeding from cannulation sites, mucus membranes, or wounds • Abnormal laboratory values and coagulation levels outside of goal range • Signs and symptoms of emboli
8. Change the VAD site dressing per institutional protocols. Do not use prophylactic topical agents because they may increase maceration and increase the risk of resistant microorganisms.[6,11,19,20]	Decreases the incidence of infection and allows an opportunity for site assessment. Special note: Most manufacturers do not recommend the use of povidone-iodine because of degradation of the drivelines. In addition, no acetone should be in the patient's room. Patients with an open sternotomy may need a physician or an advanced practice nurse at the bedside during dressing changes.	• Signs and symptoms of infection • Alterations in wound healing
1. Follow institutional protocols for assessing pain. Administer analgesia as prescribed.	Identifies the need for pain interventions.	• Continued pain despite pain interventions

Documentation

Documentation should include the following:
- Patient and family education
- Universal protocol requirements
- Informed consent
- VAD parameters (e.g., flow, pump speed)
- VAD power source
- Patient response to the VAD
- Confirmation of placement
- Hemodynamic status
- Pain assessment, interventions, and effectiveness
- Activity level
- Unexpected outcomes
- Additional interventions
- Assessment of driveline site
- Backup equipment (e.g., system controller)
- Dressing changes
- Skin integrity
- Device-specific documentation:
  - HeartMate II: pump speed, flow, motor power, and pulse index
  - HeartWare: pump speed, flow, and motor power

References and Additional Readings
For a complete list of references and additional readings for this procedure, scan this QR code with your smartphone, or visit https://www.elsevier.com/__data/assets/pdf_file/0009/ 1319823/Chapter0048.pdf

PROCEDURE

49

Electrocardiographic Leads and Cardiac Monitoring

Barbara "Bobbi" Leeper

PURPOSE Continuous physiological monitoring is performed routinely for patients with acute and critical illnesses. A key component of physiological monitoring is electrocardiographic or ECG monitoring. The electrocardiogram provides a graphic picture of cardiac electrical activity and can be used continuously to assess dynamic changes. The electrocardiogram is used for diagnostic purposes and to guide treatment.

PREREQUISITE NURSING KNOWLEDGE

- Anatomy and physiology of the cardiovascular system, principles of cardiac conduction, principles of electrophysiology, electrocardiographic lead placement, basic dysrhythmia interpretation, and electrical safety.
- Knowledge of cardiac pathophysiology.
- Electrocardiographic monitoring is indicated for patients in critical care units and for those in select acute-care settings, including progressive care, medical surgical units, postanesthesia care units, operating rooms, procedural areas, and emergency departments. Electrocardiographic monitoring may also be used during patient transport in the acute-care setting.
- Electrocardiographic monitoring is designed to provide clinicians with a graphic display of the electrical activity of the heart and is generated by depolarization and repolarization of cardiac tissue. Cardiac depolarization and repolarization is the result of electrolytes shifting in and out of the myocardial cells, which is captured on the body surface in the form of an ECG. Both normal and abnormal cardiac activity can be assessed with the ECG.
- Hardwire ECG monitors display the ECG using skin electrodes that are placed on the patient's torso and lead wires that are attached to the skin electrodes. This type of monitoring system means patients cannot move further than the length of the lead wires; consequently patients are tethered to the monitoring system, which may be bedside or portable (Fig. 49.1). ECG abnormalities generate an audible alarm and are transmitted and stored in a central monitoring system, which may or may not be assessed by a dedicated monitor observer. Alarms can and should be adjusted for each patient from either the bedside monitor or central monitoring station to minimize false alarms.[3]
- Telemetry ECG monitoring systems also use skin electrodes and leads wires, but they are designed to transmit the ECG waveforms, via telemetry, to a central monitoring system for analysis (Figs. 45.2 and 45.3). This wireless system allows patients to ambulate freely. Some telemetry

systems can monitor patients' ECGs during transport to other hospital units such as radiology, the cardiac catheterization laboratory, and other diagnostic areas of the hospital.
- With both hardwire and telemetry monitoring systems, it is important to appreciate that ECG waveforms can be altered from body-position changes and artifact, which can cause false alarms.
- Electrocardiographic leads are placed at specific locations on the torso to "view" different aspects of the heart. The number of ECG leads available varies by manufacturer and age of the ECG system; there are 3-, 5-, 6- or even 12-lead systems. Some ECG monitoring systems "derive" more views of the heart using a reduced number of lead wires, and then mathematically generate additional views of the heart. One example is the EASI lead configuration, which uses five lead wires to generate a "derived" 12-lead ECG (Phillips Healthcare, Andover, MA). EASI-derived 12-lead ECGs and their measurements are approximations to standard 12-lead ECGs and should not be used for diagnostic interpretations; instead, a standard 12-lead ECG that applies electrodes on the chest, wrist, and ankles should be obtained.
- Accurate ECG interpretation is based on precise placement of skin electrodes on the torso; hence, correct and consistent placement of skin electrodes during ECG monitoring is critical. Incorrect placement of skin electrodes can distort the appearance of the ECG waveform enough that misdiagnosis and therefore inappropriate treatment can occur. Figure 49.4 illustrates the location of skin electrodes for three- and five-lead ECG systems, which are shown because these two lead systems are commonly used in the hospital setting.
- Correct attachment of the lead wires to the skin electrodes is of critical importance as well. Lead wires are labeled by the manufacturer to assist with placement. Labels typically used are RA (right arm), RL (right leg), LA (left arm), LL (left leg), and V or C (V or precordial vector and C or chest lead) in systems that provide this lead(s). Lead wires may also be color-coded, but these can vary by manufacturer. Figures 49.5 and 49.6 show lead wires for three- and five-lead systems.

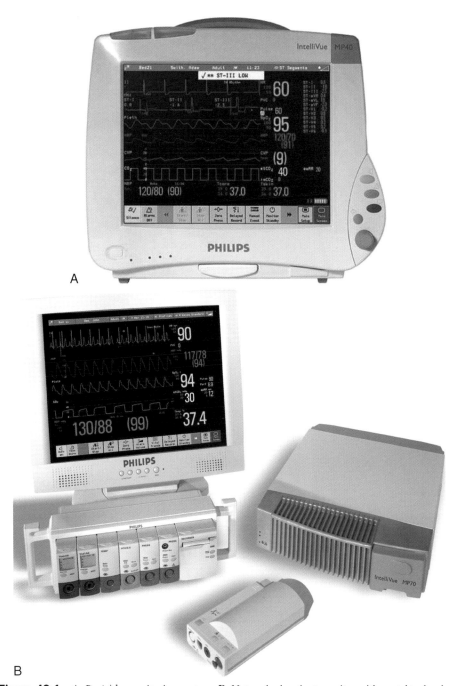

Figure 49.1 **A,** Bedside monitoring system. **B,** Networked patient monitor with portal technology for critical and intermediate care. *(Courtesy Philips Medical Systems, Andover, MA.)*

- Electrocardiographic waveforms are described as either positive (i.e., upward direction) or negative (i.e., downward direction). The factors that determine the direction of the ECG waveforms are (1) lead location, (2) lead polarity (positive or negative), and (3) the direction of the cardiac impulse generated by the heart. Normal cardiac conduction proceeds from the atria (superior part of the heart) to the ventricles (inferior part of the heart). When cardiac conduction flows toward a positive electrode, an upright QRS complex, or positive, waveform is produced (Fig. 49.7A).
- The number of ECG leads displayed visually on the bedside or central monitor varies by clinician preference, manufacturer, or lead system type (i.e., hardwire versus telemetry). It is important to note that the ECG monitoring

system may analyze more leads than are visible on the monitoring screen, thus providing clinicians with more ECG information. Variations among cardiac monitors should be communicated in the unit's educational program and included in each unit's policies and procedures. Optimal ECG lead selection for analysis and display is based on the goals of monitoring for each patient's clinical situation (e.g., heart rate, rhythm changes, ischemia).[2,3,6,7]

EQUIPMENT

- ECG monitor (i.e., hardwire or telemetry), which may also include transport ECG monitor
- ECG lead wires, which may or may not be disposable

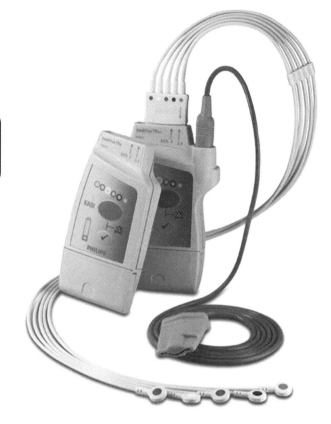

Figure 49.2   Telemetry monitoring system. *(Courtesy Philips Medical Systems, Andover, MA.)*

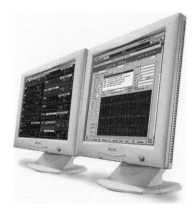

Figure 49.3   Central station. *(Courtesy Philips Medical Systems, Andover, MA.)*

- Skin electrodes, pregelled and disposable
- Nonsterile gloves
- Skin-preparation supplies, which vary based on the hospital protocol, to include
  ❖ Dry gauze pads
  ❖ Terrycloth with soap and water

Additional equipment, to have available as needed, includes the following:

- Pouch or pocket gown to hold telemetry device
- Clippers or scissors, used with caution in patients on anticoagulants, to clip hair from the chest as needed to ensure adequate adhesion of skin electrodes
- Indelible marker to mark precordial sites where skin electrodes are placed, to ensure electrodes are replaced in the correct location and thus maintain consistent lead locations

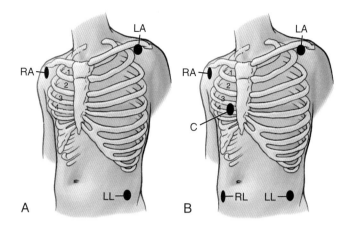

Figure 49.4   Three-lead (**A**) and five-lead (**B**) wire system locations on the torso.

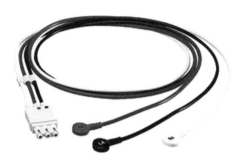

Figure 49.5   Three-lead wire system. *(Courtesy Philips Medical Systems, Andover, MA.)*

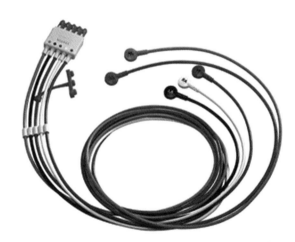

Figure 49.6   Five-lead wire system. *(Courtesy Philips Medical Systems, Andover, MA.)*

- ECG calipers for measuring waveforms, which may be available electronically via the central monitor
- Telemetry batteries

PATIENT AND FAMILY EDUCATION

- Assess the readiness of the patient and family to learn. *Rationale:* Anxiety and concerns of the patient and family may inhibit the ability to learn.
- Provide explanation to the patient and family regarding ECG equipment, the purpose of ECG monitoring, and the possibility of alarms. *Rationale:* These explanations assist

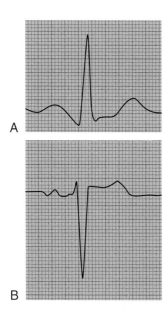

Figure 49.7   Positive (**A**) and negative (**B**) waveforms.

in making the patient and family feel more comfortable with monitoring and may reduce anxiety.

- Reassure the patient and family that ECG monitoring is continuous and that the patient's heart rate and rhythm will be monitored and treated as indicated. ***Rationale:*** This reassures the patient and family that immediate care is available.
- Teach the patient and family about the ability to move and or ambulate based on activity prescriptions and the monitoring type (i.e., hardwire versus telemetry). ***Rationale:*** This emphasis encourages mobility on the part of the patient and allays fear about disruption of the monitoring system.
- Explain the importance of reporting any symptoms, such as pain, dizziness, palpitations, or chest discomfort.

Rationale: Reporting of symptoms ensures appropriate and timely assessment and intervention if indicated.

PATIENT ASSESSMENT AND PREPARATION

Patient Assessment

- Assess whether the patient has a history of, or is at risk for, cardiac dysrhythmias or cardiac problems. ***Rationale:*** The history provides baseline data and may guide selection of monitoring leads.
- Assess landmarks on the torso for identification of correct placement of skin electrodes. ***Rationale:*** This assessment ensures that accurate ECG data will be obtained for interpretation.

Patient Preparation

- Verify the correct patient with two identifiers. ***Rationale:*** Before performing a procedure, the nurse should ensure the correct identification of the patient for the intended procedure.
- Ensure that the patient and family understand the preprocedural teaching. Answer questions as they arise, and reinforce information as needed. ***Rationale:*** This communication evaluates and reinforces the understanding of previously taught information.
- Assist the patient to the supine position. If the patient unable to lie supine, the semi-Fowler's position is acceptable. ***Rationale:*** This position enables easy access to the chest for electrode placement.
- Assist the patient in removing clothing that covers the chest and limbs. but provide for the patient's privacy. ***Rationale:*** Clothing removal provides a clear view of the chest and allows for identification of landmarks and proper placement of leads as the patient's privacy is maintained.

Procedure	for Cardiac Monitoring: Hardwire and Telemetry	
Steps	Rationale	Special Considerations
1. 🄷🄷		
2. Verify that the central monitor system is on, if applicable.	When activated, the central monitoring system will turn on ECG software that will sound an alarm when ECG parameters are exceeded.	When an alarm is generated, the nurse must assess the patient to confirm findings, verify patterns, and carefully evaluate computer software interpretations for accuracy.
3. For telemetry monitoring, insert a battery (or batteries) into the telemetry device.	Batteries can fail if left sitting for long periods in the unit.	Refer to the manufacturer's recommendations regarding battery storage and replacement.
4. Check the cable and lead wires for fraying, broken wires, or discoloration.	Detects conditions that may interfere with the ECG signal.	Safety must be maintained; if equipment is damaged, obtain alternative equipment, and notify the biomedical engineer for repair. Disposable lead wire systems are available.
5. Plug the patient cable into the monitor. Identify the number of lead wires available for the system being used.	Assists with determining placement of skin electrodes and the number of lead wires available for monitoring.	Optimal lead selection should be based on the type of lead system available and the goals of monitoring for each patient's clinical situation (i.e., heart rate, arrhythmia, ischemia, QT-interval monitoring).[2,3,6,7]

Procedure continues on following page

Procedure for Cardiac Monitoring: Hardwire and Telemetry—*Continued*

Steps	Rationale	Special Considerations
A. Three-lead systems use the following lead wires; RA, LA, and LL (see Figs. 49.4A and 49.5).	Assists with determining placement of skin electrodes and lead wires available.	The three-lead system is the simplest ECG monitoring lead system. With this lead configuration, leads I, II, or III can be displayed. This system is often used for portable monitor defibrillators.
B. Five-lead systems use the following lead wires; RA, LA, RL, LL, and a chest lead labeled "C" or "V" (see Figs. 49.4B and 49.6).	Assists with determining placement of skin electrodes and lead wires available.	This lead system provides the following leads; the six limb leads I, II, III, aVR (augmented unipolar [vector] right arm), aVL (augmented unipolar [vector] left arm), aVF (augmented unipolar [vector] foot [i.e., left leg]), and one precordial or chest lead labeled V unipolar [vector] or C (chest). Select the V or chest lead based on goals of ECG monitoring.[2,7]
6. If lead wires are designed with a "snap" connection, connect the lead wires to each electrode before placing the skin electrode on the patient's torso.	Prepares monitoring.	Pushing the snap type lead wires onto the skin electrodes already placed on the torso can be uncomfortable for the patient.
7. 🔲		
8. 🔲		
9. Identify skin electrode locations (see Fig. 49.4), and then cleanse and slightly abrade the skin where the electrodes will be applied. A. Wash the skin with soap and water. B. Clipping of chest hair may be necessary to ensure that adequate skin contact with the skin electrodes is made. C. Abrade the skin with a gauze pad. D. Ensure that the skin is dry before skin electrodes are applied. **(Level C*)**	Removes dead skin cells, promoting impulse transmission. Moist skin is not conducive to electrode adherence. Failure to properly prepare the skin may cause artifacts and interfere with interpretation.	Clipping hair should be done with caution in patients at risk for bleeding. Quality improvement projects have shown that changing skin electrodes daily can reduce artifacts, but considerations for skin breakdown should be made. Some electrodes have a built-in skin abrader on the backing of the electrode. Avoid the use of isopropyl alcohol to prepare the skin as this may cause irritation.
10. If possible, mark any precordial location with an indelible marker.	Ensures that skin electrodes are replaced to the correct location to maintain consistent lead locations.	
11. Remove the backing from the pregelled electrodes, and assess the center of the pads for moistness.	The gel should be moist to allow for maximal impulse transmission.	Skin electrodes should be stored in a dry area and not exposed to direct sunlight because this can dry out the conductive gel. Ensure that electrodes are within the manufacturer's expiration dates.
12. Apply electrodes to the correct location on the torso. Ensure that the skin electrodes are completely adhering to the skin.	Electrodes must be applied firmly to the skin to prevent external influences from affecting the ECG.	Electrode failure due to loss of contact with the skin or dried-out gel can result in excessive false alarms.

*Level C: Qualitative studies, descriptive or correlation studies, integrative reviews, systematic reviews, or randomized controlled trials with inconsistent results.

Steps	Rationale	Special Considerations

13. Place electrodes as follows:
  A. Three-lead system (see Figs. 49.4A and 49.5):
    • Apply the RA electrode just below the clavicle close to the junction of the right arm and torso.
    • Apply the LA electrode just below the clavicle close to the junction of the left arm and torso.
    • Apply the LL electrode below the level of the umbilicus, on the left abdominal region. **(Level C*)**
	Proper positioning is essential to ensure that accurate waveforms are generated for analysis.[2,4,7]	Lead selection for display and analysis by the central monitoring station is based on the aims of cardiac monitoring and chest wall constraints (e.g., wounds, dressings).[2,4,7]

B. Five-lead system (Figs. 49.4B and 49.6):
    • Apply the RA electrode just below the clavicle close to the junction of the right arm and torso.
    • Apply the LA electrode just below the clavicle close to the junction of the left arm and torso.
    • Apply the RL electrode below the level of the umbilicus, on the right abdominal region.
    • Apply the LL electrode below the level of the umbilicus, on the left abdominal region.
    • Apply the chest (precordial) lead electrode to the selected site based on the goals of monitoring:
      • Lead V_1 is the single best chest, or precordial lead for arrhythmia monitoring.[5] This lead is located in the fourth intercostal space on the right sternal border.
      • Lead V_6 can be substituted when V_1 cannot be applied (e.g., dressings, wounds). Lead V_6 is located at the midaxillary line in the fifth intercostal space.
      • Lead V_3 is the single best precordial lead for detection of transient myocardial ischemia[7]
    • On the central monitoring station, ensure that the chest lead placed on the patient is correctly identified on the monitor. **(Level D*)**
	Arm electrodes that are not placed on the outer chest and under the clavicle or leg electrodes that are placed above the umbilicus can alter the ECG waveforms and result in inaccurate recordings.[2,3] In five-lead systems, only one precordial lead can be selected. The central monitoring station should be programmed to indicate the chest (precordial) lead selected.	Many hospitals set the default precordial lead to V_1. If another chest lead is selected, the central monitoring station should be edited to reflect the correct chest lead being monitored because the V lead selected will be printed on any rhythm strips printed or stored.

*Level C: Qualitative studies, descriptive or correlation studies, integrative reviews, systematic reviews, or randomized controlled trials with inconsistent results.
*Level D: Peer-reviewed professional and organizational standards with the support of clinical study recommendations.

Procedure continues on following page

Procedure for Cardiac Monitoring: Hardwire and Telemetry—*Continued*

Steps	Rationale	Special Considerations
14. Reduce tension on the lead wires and cables.	Decreased tension on the lead wires will minimize the leads becoming disconnected. This will also minimize pulling on the electrodes, which can be uncomfortable for the patient.	Software analysis will cease when the lead wires are not connected or the skin electrodes are not in contact with the torso.
15. For telemetry monitoring, secure the recorder in a pouch or pocket in the patient's gown.	The recorder must be secure so it is not dropped or damaged and to minimize pulling on the electrodes.	
16. Examine the ECG tracing on the monitor for quality waveforms.	The QRS complex should be approximately twice the height of the other waveforms (e.g., P wave, T wave) to ensure proper detection of heart rate by the ECG software. If the T wave is nearly equal to the R wave, each complex may be double counted, resulting in false heart rate alarms.	Most calibration is set to default settings by each facility's biomedical department. Typically, calibration of the ECG should be set to 10 mm/mV; at this calibration, 1 mV is expected to produce a rectangle of 10-mm height and 5-mm width. Calibration for ECG time (speed of paper recording) is typically set to 25 mm/sec. Some cardiac monitors have size adjustments that can be used to increase or decrease the size (gain) of complexes along with speed adjustments to slow or speed up the rate of the paper recording of the ECG. Alteration of these settings can affect waveform analysis; it should be done with careful consideration and noted in the medical record.
17. Obtain a baseline ECG strip, and interpret for rhythm, heart rate, presence of P waves, length of PR interval, width of QRS complexes, ST-segment deviation, presence of T waves, and length of QT and QTc intervals.	Review the normal conduction sequence, and identify abnormalities that may necessitate further evaluation or treatment.	
18. Set alarm parameters. Upper and lower alarm limits are set on the basis of the patient's current clinical status and heart rate.	For hardwire monitoring systems, alarms can be adjusted at the bedside or at the central monitoring station. For telemetry monitoring systems, alarm parameters are typically adjusted at the central monitoring station.	Monitoring systems allow for setting and adjusting alarms at the bedside or the central console. The types of alarms may include heart rate (i.e., high or low), abnormal rhythms or waveforms, pacemaker recognition, and others, depending on the manufacturer. *Caution:* alarms should not be disabled except in specific circumstances (e.g., anticipated end of life). To reduce alarm burden (false alarms), alarms should be adjusted according to the known clinical status of the patient to minimize false alarms.[3,7]
19. Set ST-segment parameters if indicated (see Procedure 50, ST-Segment Monitoring [Continuous]).	Transient myocardial ischemia can be assessed with ST-segment software in select patients when indicated.	ST-segment monitoring should not be used in patients with left bundle branch block or patients with ventricular pacing because a high number of false alarms are likely to occur.[7]
20. Remove **PE**, and discard used supplies in appropriate receptacles.	Reduces the transmission of microorganisms; standard precautions.	
21. **HH**		

Expected Outcomes

- Properly applied skin electrodes and lead wires
- A clear ECG tracing displayed (Fig. 49.8)
- Alarms are adjusted to the patient's current clinical status
- Prompt identification of heart rate changes, dysrhythmias, ischemia, and lengthening of the QT-interval based on the goals of monitoring
- False alarms that require human overreading

Unexpected Outcomes

- Altered skin integrity
- Alternating current interference, also called *60-cycle interference* (Fig. 49.9)
- Wandering baseline (Fig. 49.10)
- Artifact (Fig. 49.11)

UNIT II

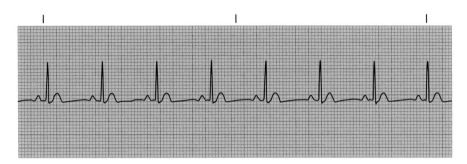

Figure 49.8 Monitor strip of clear ECG pattern.

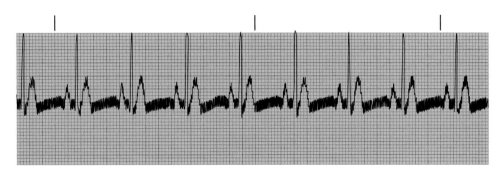

Figure 49.9 Monitor strip with 60-cycle interference.

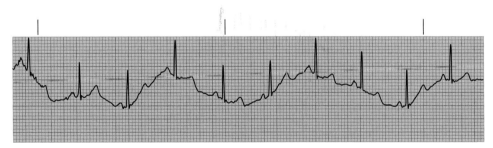

Figure 49.10 Monitor strip with wandering baseline.

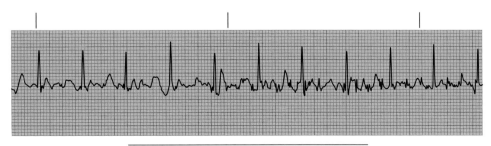

Figure 49.11 Monitor strip with motion artifact.

UNIT II

Patient Monitoring and Care

Steps	Rationale	Reportable Conditions
		These conditions should be reported to the provider if they persist despite nursing interventions.
1. Evaluate the ECG routinely for the presence of P waves, QRS complexes, clear interpretable baseline, and absence of artifact or distortion. Obtain and analyze visually a rhythm strip on admission, every shift (as per institutional protocol), and following any changes from the patient's baseline.	Continuous evaluation of ECG waveforms and following any changes can promptly identify alterations in the patient's condition so treatment can be initiated if indicated.[1,2,7]	• Abnormal ECG waveforms, heart rate changes from the patient's baseline level, and rhythm changes
2. Evaluate the ECG pattern continually for dysrhythmias, assess the patient's clinical tolerance following any changes, and provide prompt nursing interventions.	Changes in the ECG pattern may indicate significant problems for the patient and may necessitate immediate intervention or additional diagnostic tests, such as a 12-lead ECG, or laboratory tests.	• Abnormal cardiac rate and rhythm • Hemodynamic instability
3. Evaluate skin integrity around the electrodes on a daily basis, and change the electrodes according to institutional protocols.	Skin integrity must be maintained in patients while ensuring that ECG quality is high. Replace electrodes quickly so that continuous monitoring is ensured. Skin electrodes may require slight relocation if skin integrity is compromised. Place the skin electrode as close to the correct site as possible, and note this in the medical record.	• Alteration in skin integrity
4. Verify accurate electrode placement and that lead wires are correctly attached every shift or when leads are removed (e.g., following transport to another department, shower).	Accurate interpretation of waveforms and dysrhythmias depends on proper placement of the electrodes and knowledge of leads being viewed.	

Documentation

Documentation should include the following:
- Patient and family education
- An initial or baseline ECG strip
- Routine ECG strips every shift and per institutional protocol
- An ECG strip should be printed and placed in the medical record following changes in heart rate or rhythm, when the patient experiences symptoms, when there is a change in lead placement, when there are changes in electrolytes, or following administration of medications that can affect the QT interval.[6]
- Unexpected outcomes

References and Additional Readings

For a complete list of references and additional readings for this procedure, scan this QR code with your smartphone, or visit https://www.elsevier.com/__data/assets/pdf_file/0010/1319824/Chapter0049.pdf

PROCEDURE

50 ST-Segment Monitoring (Continuous)

Shelley K. Welch

PURPOSE Bedside ST-segment monitoring provides ongoing analysis for detection of transient myocardial ischemia. This technology should be applied to patients who are being evaluated or are diagnosed with acute coronary syndrome (ACS), including acute myocardial infarction (MI) and unstable angina. For these patients, continuous ST-segment monitoring is crucial to detect recurrent or transient ischemia and to determine the success of thrombolytic therapy and percutaneous coronary intervention.

PREREQUISITE NURSING KNOWLEDGE

- Anatomy and physiology of the cardiovascular system, coronary arteries and associated location of the heart perfused by the coronary arteries, principles of cardiac conduction, electrocardiogram (ECG) lead placement, basic dysrhythmia interpretation, ECG leads and location of each lead or lead views, and electrical safety.
- ACS and associated terms: ST-elevation myocardial infarction (STEMI); non-STEMI, and unstable angina.
- Advanced cardiac life support (ACLS) knowledge and skills.
- The ST segment of the ECG complex represents ventricular repolarization (the "resting" period for the ventricles). Changes in the ST segment can be one of the earliest indications of myocardial ischemia.[1] This is helpful in patients who may not recognize or experience chest pain.
- According to the American Heart Association, ST elevation or depression of 1 to 2 mm captured on a rhythm strip that lasts for at least 1 minute with or without symptoms merits further clinical assessment.[4]
- Patients who have transient ischemia detected with continuous ST segment monitoring are more likely to have unfavorable outcomes, including MI and death, compared with patients without such events.[2-4]
- Given the dynamic, unpredictable, and silent nature of myocardial ischemia, continuous ECG monitoring of patients for ischemia is essential. Clinicians should monitor the trend of the ST segments and the part of the ECG that changes during acute ischemia and evaluate any ST-segment changes (elevation or depression) for possible myocardial ischemia.[5]
- Nonischemic ST-segment changes can occur and should be considered when evaluating ST-segment trend changes. These may include movement of the skin electrodes, dysrhythmias, intermittent bundle-branch block pattern, body position changes, and ventricular paced rhythms.
- One type of myocardial ischemia seen in patients with ACS is supply-related ischemia, which results from complete coronary artery occlusion. Coronary occlusion is

brought on by disruption of an atherosclerotic plaque followed by cycles of plaque rupture, coronary vasospasm, platelet stimulation, and thrombus formation with resultant loss of blood flow. Because this type of ischemia threatens the entire thickness or transmural, part of the myocardium, immediate treatment to reestablish blood flow to the heart is essential. The typical ECG manifestation of total supply-related ischemia is ST-segment elevation, which is visible in the ECG leads that lie directly over the ischemic myocardial zone.

- Occlusion of the right coronary artery typically produces ST-segment elevation in leads II, III, and aVF (Fig. 50.1). Occlusion of the left anterior descending coronary artery typically produces ST-segment elevation in leads V_2, V_3, and V_4 (Fig. 50.2). Diagnosis of total coronary occlusion of the left circumflex coronary artery (LCX) is more complex because placement of the standard ECG electrodes is on the anterior chest, opposite the wall that this coronary artery supplies. Occlusion of the LCX may produce ST-segment depression in leads V_1, V_2, or V_3, which reflects the reciprocal, or mirror-image, ST-segment elevation occurring in the posterior wall of the left ventricle. In some patients, ST-segment changes may also be seen in leads I and aVL.
- A second type of ischemia for which patients with ACS or stable angina are at risk is demand-related ischemia. This type of ischemia occurs when the demand for oxygen (i.e., exercise, tachycardia, or stress) exceeds the flow capabilities of a coronary artery. Patients with this type of ischemia are likely to have a stable atherosclerotic plaque. The ST-segment pattern of demand-related ischemia is ST-segment depression, often appearing in several ECG leads (Fig. 50.3).
- Ideally, diagnosis of myocardial ischemia should be done with continuous monitoring of all 12 ECG leads because the mechanism of ischemia may vary (i.e., supply- [occlusion] versus demand-related ischemia). This may result in distinctly different ST-segment patterns (e.g., elevation or depression) in specific ECG leads. Knowledge of the patients "ST-segment fingerprint" is essential in selecting lead placement that is specific to the patient's condition

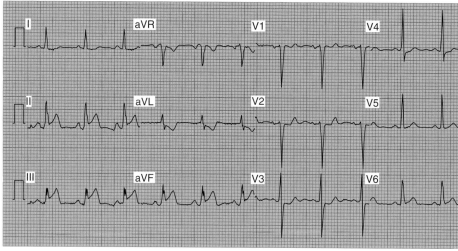

Figure 50.1 The typical ST-segment pattern of supply-related ischemia in the inferior wall. The right coronary artery is likely occluded, resulting in ST-segment elevation in leads II, III, and aVF.

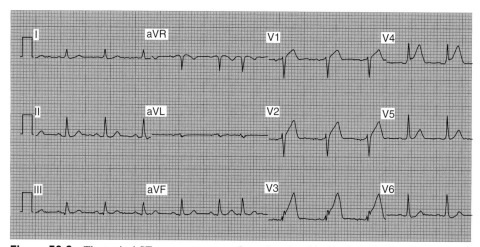

Figure 50.2 The typical ST-segment pattern of supply-related ischemia in the anterior wall. The left anterior descending artery is likely occluded, resulting in ST-segment elevation in leads V_2 to V_4.

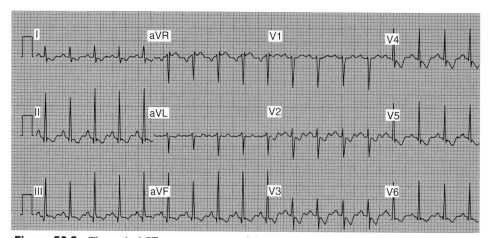

Figure 50.3 The typical ST-segment pattern of demand-related ischemia. Note the ST-segment depression appearing in nearly every ECG lead, with the exception of V_1 and aVR. Note also that this patient is experiencing tachycardia, a common cause of demand-related ischemia.

and cardiac history. Although there is no strong evidence to support the practice, it is generally accepted that if only two ECG leads are available, the best two for ischemia detection are leads III and V_3. Patient-specific monitoring also may be done if a prior 12-lead ECG was obtained during acute ischemia (i.e., STEMI, percutaneous coronary intervention [PCI], or treadmill test). In this scenario, the ECG lead(s) showing maximal ST-segment deviation should be selected for continuous monitoring to detect recurrent ischemia.

- According to current guidelines,[4] multilead ST-segment monitoring is indicated in most patients with the following diagnoses:
  - Early phase of acute coronary syndrome (ACS) less than 24 hours if the patient is high risk for Non-STEMI ACS (NSTE-ACS) or STEMI: patients should be monitored for 24 to 48 hours or until "ruled out" or negative biomarkers.
  - Post-acute MI without revascularization or with residual lesions, continuous ST segment monitoring should occur immediately and continue for greater than 24 to 48 hours when there is no evidence of ongoing modifiable ischemia and the patient is hemodynamically stable.
  - After nonurgent PCI procedures with suboptimal results, or complications, for greater than 24 hours or resolution of the complication.
  - During and after cardiac surgery.
  - Variant angina resulting from coronary vasospasm.
- ST-segment monitoring may be considered for the following cases:[4]
  - Postacute MI with revascularization of all ischemic lesions, continuing for greater than 12 to 24 hours after revascularization, confirmation of biomarker levels.
  - During therapeutic hypothermia post–cardiac arrest.
  - Acute stroke with increased risk for cardiac events for greater than 24 to 28 hours.
  - Stress cardiomyopathy from apical ballooning until symptoms subside.
- There is no evidence of benefit for continuous ST segment monitoring for the following:[4]
  - Fully awake patients who can recognize and verbalize symptoms of angina.
  - After nonemergent, noncomplicated PCI.
  - After femoral sheath removal of routine coronary angiography.
  - Low-risk noncardiac chest pain with risk score using an established scoring tool.
- A variety of bedside and telemetry cardiac monitors are currently available for use in clinical practice. Not all monitoring systems are equipped with ST-segment monitoring software. Clinicians must determine whether their cardiac monitoring system has ST-segment monitoring capabilities.[4]

EQUIPMENT

- ECG monitor with ST-segment monitoring capacity
- ECG lead wires (may or may not be disposable)

- Skin electrodes, pre-gelled and disposable
- Nonsterile gloves
- Skin-preparation supplies, which vary based on the hospital protocol; these may include a washcloth, soap and water, or gauze pads

Additional equipment, to have available as needed, includes the following:

- Clippers or scissors, used with caution in patients on anticoagulants, to clip hair from the chest as needed to ensure adequate adhesion of skin electrodes
- Black indelible marker to mark precordial skin electrode site placement to maintain consistent electrode locations
- ECG calipers for measuring waveforms (may be available electronically via the central monitor)

PATIENT AND FAMILY EDUCATION

- Explain the purpose of ST-segment monitoring. *Rationale:* This explanation decreases patient and family anxiety.
- Encourage the patient to report any symptoms of chest pain or anginal equivalent (e.g., arm pain, jaw pain, shortness of breath, or nausea). *Rationale:* This education heightens the patient's awareness of cardiac sensations and encourages communication of anginal symptoms.

PATIENT ASSESSMENT AND PREPARATION

Patient Assessment

- Assess if the patient is at high risk for ischemia. *Rationale:* Patients at risk for myocardial ischemia must be identified.
- Assess the patient's cardiac rhythm. *Rationale:* This assessment provides baseline data and ensures that the patient has a cardiac rhythm suitable for ST-segment monitoring.
- Identify the patient's baseline ST-segment levels before initiating ST-segment monitoring. *Rationale:* The patient's baseline ST-segment level is identified for comparison with subsequent changes.

Patient Preparation

- Verify the correct patient with two identifiers. *Rationale:* Before performing a procedure, the nurse should ensure the correct identification of the patient for the intended intervention.
- Ensure that the patient and family understand the preprocedural teaching. Answer questions as they arise, and reinforce information as needed. *Rationale:* This communication evaluates and reinforces understanding of previously taught information.
- Place the patient in a resting supine position in bed, and expose the patient's torso while maintaining modesty. *Rationale:* This preparation provides access to the patient's chest for electrode placement and ensures that an artifact-free ECG is obtained.

UNIT II

Procedure for Continuous ST-Segment Monitoring

Steps	Rationale	Special Considerations
1. **HH** 2. **PE** 3. Identify accurate electrode placement (Fig. 50.4).	Ensures accurate ECG data.	Electrodes (V_3 to V_5) should be placed immediately below a pendulous breast so the breast lies on top of the electrode, preventing motion artifact.

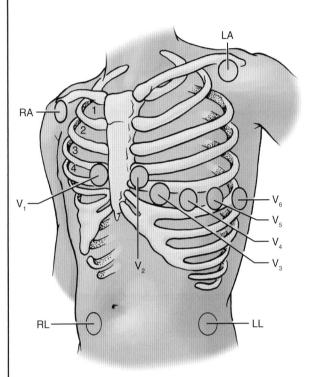

Figure 50.4 Correct lead placement for 12-lead ST-segment monitoring. Limb electrodes must be located as close as possible to the junction of the limb and the torso. To ensure an inferior view of the myocardium, the left leg *(LL)* electrode must be placed well below the level of the umbilicus. For V_1, the electrode is located at the fourth intercostal space to the right of the sternum. V_2 is in the same fourth intercostal space just to the left of the sternum, and V_4 is in the fifth intercostal space on the midclavicular line. Placement of lead V_3 is halfway on a straight line between leads V_2 and V_4. Leads V_5 and V_6 are positioned on a straight line from V_4, with V_5 in the anterior axillary line and V_6 in the midaxillary line. *RA*, Right arm; *LA*, left arm; *RL*, right leg.

Steps	Rationale	Special Considerations
4. Cleanse and slightly abrade the skin where the electrodes will be applied.[1] A. Wash the skin with soap and water. B. Abrade the skin with a gauze pad. C. Ensure that the skin is dry before skin electrodes are applied. D. Clipping chest hair may be necessary to ensure that adequate skin contact with the skin electrodes is made. (**Level C***)	Removes dead skin cells, promoting impulse transmission. Moist skin is not conducive to electrode adherence. Failure to properly prepare the skin may cause artifacts and interfere with interpretation.[1]	Clipping hair should be done with caution in patients at risk for bleeding. Quality improvement projects have shown that changing skin electrodes daily can reduce artifacts.
5. If possible, mark any precordial locations with a black indelible marker.[1]	Ensures that skin electrodes are replaced to the correct location to maintain consistent lead locations.	Continuous ST-segment monitoring trends depend on stable electrode placement. Sudden changes in ST-segment trends often indicate electrode movement.
6. Remove the backing from the pregelled electrodes, and assess the center of the pads for moistness.	Gel should be moist to allow for maximal impulse transmission.	Skin electrodes should be stored in a dry area and not exposed to direct sunlight because this can dry out the conductive gel.
7. Connect the ECG leads to the electrodes before placing the electrodes on the patient.	Prepares the monitoring system and prevents unnecessary pressure on the patient's chest when connecting the lead wires to the electrodes.	

Procedure	for Continuous ST-Segment Monitoring—*Continued*	
Steps	**Rationale**	**Special Considerations**
8. Select the monitoring leads.	Although any ECG lead can be used for ST-segment monitoring, monitoring of all 12 ECG leads or the selection of a lead or leads based on the myocardial zone at risk is desirable (e.g., inferior or anterior).	If continuous 12-lead ECG monitoring is unavailable, lead-specific ischemia monitoring is encouraged. Lead III is sensitive to inferior ischemia, and V_3 is sensitive to anterior or posterior ischemia.
9. If required by the bedside monitor manufacturer, identify the ECG complex landmarks, and select the J point + 60-ms landmark. (**Level M***)	Prepares the monitoring system and ensures accurate monitoring.	Refer to the manufacturer's recommendations.
10. Set the ST-segment alarm.	Maximizes the sensitivity and specificity of ST-segment monitoring and may reduce unnecessary false alarms.	For bedside cardiac monitoring, the alarm threshold should be set 1–2 mm above and below the patient's baseline ST-segment level (Fig. 50.5). Recently, a wider threshold of 2 mm for triggering an alarm has been used to reduce false positives and alarm fatigue. Establishing a patient-specific ST-segment level, rather than an isoelectric ST-segment level, is important because the patient's baseline ST-segment level is rarely isoelectric.

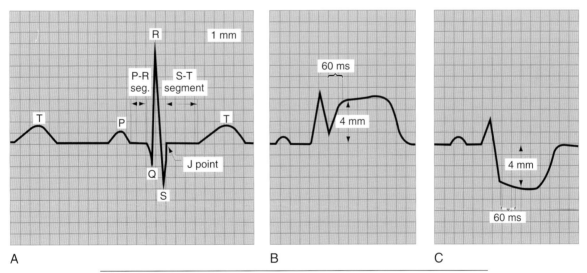

Figure 50.5 **A,** Normal electrocardiograph complex. Measurement points used in ST-segment analysis are indicated. The PR segment is used to identify the iso-electric line. The ST segment begins at the J point, which is the end of the QRS complex. The ST-segment measurement point can be measured at 60 or 80 ms past the J point. **B,** ST-segment elevation. The ST segment shown measures +4 mm. **C,** ST-segment depression. The ST segment shown measures −4 mm. *(Modified from Tisdale LA, Drew BJ: ST segment monitoring for myocardial ischemia, AACN Clin Issues Crit Care Nurs 4:36, 1993.)*

*Level C: Qualitative studies, descriptive or correlational studies, integrative reviews, systematic reviews, or randomized controlled trials with inconsistent results.
*Level M: Manufacturer's recommendations only.

Procedure continues on following page

UNIT II

Procedure for Continuous ST-Segment Monitoring—*Continued*

Steps	Rationale	Special Considerations
11. Print the baseline ECG tracing to evaluate the quality of the signal, and secure it for future reference.	Ensures a quality baseline ECG for comparing subsequent changes because ST-segment monitoring is based on continuous trending.	Verify that lead wires are not reversed, especially the limb leads.
12. If possible, obtain an ECG with the patient in the right and left side-lying positions, and secure them for future reference.[1]	Comparison of side-lying ECGs with ECGs from subsequent alarms may prevent interpreting as ischemia false-positive ST-segment deviations caused by changes in body position.	Because a change in body position (lying on the left or right side) can alter the ST segment, mimicking ischemia, when an ST alarm sounds and the patient is found in a side lying position, the patient should be returned to the supine position.[1]
13. Remove **PE**, and discard used supplies in appropriate receptacles.	Reduces the transmission of microorganisms; standard precautions.	
14. **HH**		

Expected Outcomes

- Accurate ECG monitoring that allows clinicians to detect and interpret ST-segment changes
- Timely detection of myocardial ischemia
- An increase in the number of bedside alarms when the ST-segment software is initiated, which may be caused by actual ischemia, body-position changes, transient dysrhythmias, heart rate changes, artifacts, or lead misplacement

Unexpected Outcomes

- Altered skin integrity
- Alternating current (AC) interference, also called *60-cycle interference*
- Wandering baseline
- Artifacts
- Inappropriate diagnosis of ischemia in nonischemic conditions (i.e., bundle-branch block, early repolarization)
- Inappropriate intervention based on a false ST-segment alarm

Patient Monitoring and Care

Steps	Rationale	Reportable Conditions
		These conditions should be reported to the provider if they persist despite nursing interventions.
1. Check electrode placement every shift. There are inadequate data on disposable electrodes and how often they should be changed to prevent false alarms due to electrode failure.	Enhances the quality of ST-segment monitoring.	
2. Evaluate ST-segment trends routinely while obtaining vital signs.	Ensures that no significant deviations in the ST-segment trend occur. Requiring the ST change to last at least 1 minute and to be present in two contiguous leads may drastically reduce the number of false ST-segment monitor alarms. Contiguous leads in the limb leads should be defined using the following sequence: aVL, I, minus aVR, II, aVF, III. ST changes in two of these side-by-side leads would meet the criteria for ischemia.	• ST-segment trend changes more than 1 mm • ST amplitude change lasting at least 1 minute

Steps	Rationale	Reportable Conditions
3. Interpret all ST-segment alarms, and determine the cause. If actual ischemia is noted, assess the patient for signs and symptoms that suggest acute ischemia, anginal equivalents, hemodynamic changes, or dysrhythmias, and then obtain a 12-lead ECG.	Ensures accurate interpretation. A 12-lead resting ECG assists with determining ischemia location and type (i.e., supply versus demand). Determines the patient's response to ischemia.	• ST-segment changes • Onset of symptoms or anginal equivalent
4. Assess the patient for signs and symptoms that suggest acute ischemia, even if no new ST-segment changes are identified, and obtain a 12-lead ECG as needed.	Determines the presence of ischemia. Because ischemia can be clinically silent, a 12-lead ECG assists with determining ischemia location and type (i.e., supply versus demand).	• ST-segment changes • Onset of symptoms or anginal equivalent
5. Follow institutional standards for assessing pain. Administer analgesia and nitrates as prescribed.	Identifies need for pain interventions.	• Continued pain despite pain interventions

Documentation

Documentation should include the following:
- Patient and family education
- Initiation of ST-segment bedside monitoring
- Initial ECG strip with baseline ST segment
- Any ST-segment changes or any symptoms that suggest acute ischemia
- Presence and intensity of chest pain or anginal equivalent, interventions, and effectiveness
- Additional interventions taken
- Unexpected outcomes

References and Additional Readings

For a complete list of references and additional readings for this procedure, scan this QR code with your smartphone, or visit https://www.elsevier.com/__data/assets/pdf_file/0011/1319825/Chapter0050.pdf

51

Twelve-Lead Electrocardiogram With Right and Left Posterior Leads

Angela Muzzy

PURPOSE A 12-lead electrocardiogram (ECG) provides information about the conduction system of the heart from 12 different views. One can also use extra ECG leads in conjunction with the standard 12-lead ECG for a larger view of the heart's electrical conduction system. The use of a 12-lead ECG is to first assess for cardiac etiologies for broad symptoms including chest pain, shortness of breath, palpitations, dyspnea on exertion, dizziness, fatigue, and syncope to further aid in the diagnosis of acute coronary syndromes, arrhythmias, electrolyte abnormalities, adverse medication responses, or conduction abnormalities.

PREREQUISITE NURSING KNOWLEDGE

- Anatomy and physiology of the cardiovascular system, principles of electrophysiology, and basic rhythm identification.
- A 12-lead ECG provides different views of the conduction system of the heart. These views are seen by 12 standard leads and additional leads from the right and left precordial leads. These include six limb leads (I, II, III, augmented vector right [aVR], augmented vector foot [aVF], and augmented vector left [aVL]), six precordial leads (V_1 to V_6), right ventricular (RV) leads V_{1R} to V_{6R}, and left posterior leads V_7 to V_9.
- The limb leads view the heart from the frontal or vertical plane (Fig. 51.1), and the chest leads view the heart from the horizontal plane (Fig. 51.2). Right precordial leads are useful in diagnosing an RV myocardial infarction (MI). The left posterior leads are used to aid in the detection of posterior wall MI.
- Indications for recording a right-precordial ECG include suspected inferior-wall MI (ST-segment elevation in leads II, III, and aVF). This offers a prediction of the site of coronary artery occlusion (RV infarction occurs with proximal right coronary artery [RCA] occlusion).[2]
- Posterior wall infarctions may account for up to 21% of all myocardial infarctions. Therefore it is important to remember that standard 12-lead ECGs do not include posterior leads.[10] Indications for recording a left-posterior ECG include suspected MI with isolated ST-segment depression in the precordial leads V_1 to V_3 and patients with a nondiagnostic ECG. Left-posterior ECG can also help differentiate true posterior MI from other conditions that can cause tall R waves in lead V_1, such as RV hypertrophy, right bundle-branch block, Wolff-Parkinson-White syndrome, and ventricular septal hypertrophy.[5]

- In patients with RV infarction who exhibit shock, volume expansion is used to provide adequate RV and left ventricular (LV) filling pressures to restore arterial pressure and peripheral blood flow. Positive inotropic agents also may be indicated to augment the residual contractile force of the damaged RV if unresponsive to fluids. Use of vasodilators (e.g., nitroglycerin) should generally be avoided because they cause venous dilation and reduced preload. Use of diuretics (e.g., furosemide) should also be avoided because they reduce preload and LV filling pressures.[2]
- Progressive and critical care nurses should be able to evaluate the standard 12-lead ECG for the location of myocardial ischemia or infarction and assess the possibility of RV and posterior involvement (Fig. 51.3)
- The morphology of the basic ECG waveform includes P, Q, R, S, and T waves, which represent the conduction system in the heart.
- Accuracy in identification of anatomic landmarks for location of electrode sites and knowledge of the importance of accurate electrode placement are needed. Accurate ECG interpretation is possible only when the recording electrodes are placed in the proper positions. Slight alterations of the electrode positions may significantly distort the appearance of the ECG waveforms and can lead to misdiagnosis of an acute coronary syndrome.[7]
- Nurses should be aware of changes in body position that can alter ECG recordings. Serial ECGs should be recorded with the patient in the supine position to ensure that all recordings are done in a consistent manner. Side-lying positions and elevation of the torso may change the position of the heart within the chest and can change the waveforms on the ECG recording.[3] If a position other than supine is clinically necessary, notation of the altered position should be made on the tracing.
- Nurses should be able to operate the 12-lead ECG machine. Calibration of 1 mV equals 10 mm and paper speed of

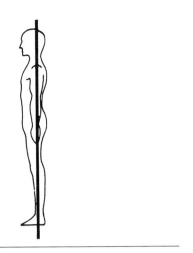

Figure 51.1 Vertical plane leads: I, II, III, aVR, aVL, aVF

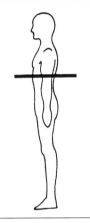

Figure 51.2 Horizontal plane leads: V_1 to V_6.

25 mm/sec are standards used in clinical practice. Any variation used for particular clinical purposes should be noted on the tracing. Specific information regarding configuring the ECG machine, troubleshooting, and safety features is available from the manufacturer and should be read before use of the equipment. Nurses should be able to interpret recorded ECGs for the presence or absence of myocardial ischemia/infarction and arrhythmias so patients can be treated appropriately.

EQUIPMENT

- ECG electrodes
- 12-lead ECG machine with patient cable and lead wires
- Gauze pads or terrycloth washcloth
- Cleansing pads or non-emollient soap and water
- Skin preparation solution (e.g., skin barrier wipe)
- Clippers or scissors to clip hair from the patient's chest if needed

PATIENT AND FAMILY EDUCATION

- Describe the procedure and reasons for obtaining the 12-lead ECG. Reassure the patient that the procedure is painless.

Rationale: This communication clarifies information, reduces anxiety, and gains cooperation from the patient.
- Explain the patient's role in assisting with the ECG recording, and emphasize actions that improve the quality of the ECG tracing, such as avoiding conversation, avoiding body movement, and breathing normally. *Rationale:* This explanation ensures the patient's cooperation to improve the quality of the tracing and avoids unnecessary repeating of the ECG because of muscle artifact.

PATIENT ASSESSMENT AND PREPARATION

Patient Assessment

- Assess and immediately address the presence of symptoms, such as chest pain, pressure, tightness, palpitations, heaviness, fullness, squeezing sensation, radiating pain, shortness of breath, nausea, or extreme fatigue.
- Attempt to locate previously recorded ECGs. *Rationale:* Each patient has an individual baseline ECG. Previous ECG recordings can help clinicians determine whether a change is acute or chronic.
- Assess the patient's history of cardiac conditions and medications. Knowledge about the patient's cardiac history and medications can help in interpretation of ECG recordings. For example, digitalis therapy causes chronic ST-segment depression that does not indicate acute myocardial ischemia. A normal-looking isoelectric ST segment in a patient on digitalis therapy may indicate acute myocardial ischemia.
- Upon completion, interpret the patient's standard 12-lead ECG for any signs of myocardial ischemia, infarction, or dysrhythmias. Nurses should be able to evaluate the standard 12-lead ECG for the location of myocardial ischemia or infarction and assess the possibility of RV and posterior wall involvement (see Fig. 51.3).

Patient Preparation

- Verify the correct patient with two identifiers. *Rationale:* Before performing any procedure, the nurse should ensure the correct identification of the patient for the intended intervention.
- Ensure that the patient and family understand the preprocedural teaching. Answer questions as they arise, and reinforce information as needed. *Rationale:* This communication evaluates and reinforces the understanding of previously taught information.
- Assist the patient to the supine position, and expose the patient's torso while maintaining the patient's modesty as well as privacy. *Rationale*: This position enables recording of the ECG and allows comparison of serial ECGs and comparison with standard waveforms. Changes in body position, such as elevation and rotation, can change recorded amplitudes and axes.

UNIT II

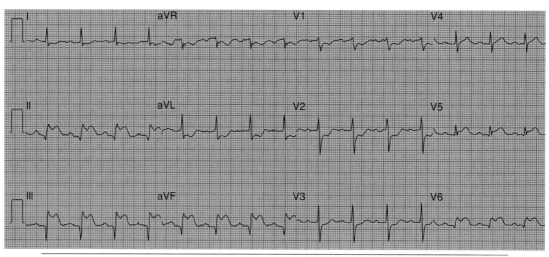

Figure 51.3   Initial ECG in a patient admitted to the emergency department with an acute inferior MI (elevated ST segments and Q waves in leads II, III, and aVF) with apical involvement (elevated ST segment in leads V_4, V_5, and V_6). ST-segment depression in leads V_1, V_2, and V_3 suggests posterior involvement. Left posterior and right precordial leads should be recorded to assess posterior and RV involvement.

Procedure   for 12-Lead Electrocardiogram

Steps	Rationale	Special Considerations
1. **HH**		
2. Check cables and lead wires for fraying or broken wires.	Detects faulty equipment.	If the equipment is damaged, obtain alternative equipment and notify a biomedical engineer for repair.
3. Check the lead wires for accurate labels.	Obtains accurate ECG recordings and proper placement of leads.	
4. Plug the ECG machine into a grounded alternating current (AC) wall outlet, or ensure functioning if battery operated.	Maintains electrical safety.	Follow manufacturer's recommendations and institutional protocol on electrical safety per the biomedical department.
5. Turn on the ECG machine, and program the ECG machine: paper speed, 25 mm/sec; calibration, 10 mm/mV; filter settings, 0.05–100 Hz. (**Level E***)	Equipment may require self-test and warm-up time. The American Heart Association (AHA) along with other leading cardiology organizations have specific guidelines on calibration standards for ECG equipment.[8] Multichannel machines may require input of information (e.g., data about the patient) to store the ECG appropriately.	Manufacturers provide a calibration check in the machine to identify the sensitivity setting. Most machines have automatic settings.
6. **PE**		
7. Place the patient in the supine position. (**Level B***)	Provides adequate support for limbs so muscle activity is minimal. Changes in body position can cause ST-segment deviation and QRS waveform alteration.[3]	ECGs should be recorded in the same body position each time to ensure ECG changes are not caused by a change in body position. If another position is clinically necessary, note the altered position on the ECG recording.
8. Expose only the necessary body parts of the patient (legs, arms, and chest) for electrode placement.	Provides privacy and warmth, which reduces shivering.	Ensuring privacy may reduce anxiety. Shivering may interfere with the quality of recording.

*Level B: Well-designed, controlled studies with results that consistently support a specific action, intervention, or treatment.
*Level E: Multiple case reports, theory-based evidence from expert opinions, or peer-reviewed professional organizational standards without clinical studies to support recommendations.

Procedure for 12-Lead Electrocardiogram—*Continued*

Steps	Rationale	Special Considerations

9. Identify skin electrode locations.
 	
A. Limb leads (Fig. 51.4)
• Right arm (RA): inside right forearm
• Left arm (LA): inside left forearm
• Right leg (RL): anywhere on the body; by convention, usually on the right ankle or inner aspect of the calf
• Left leg (LL): left ankle or inner aspect of the calf
B. Precordial leads (Fig. 51.5)
• Identify the sternal notch. Slide fingers down the center of the sternum to the obvious bony prominence, the angle of Louis, which identifies the second rib and provides a landmark for noting the second intercostal space (ICS).
  • V_1: fourth ICS at right sternal border
  • V_2: fourth ICS at left sternal border
  • V_4: fifth ICS at midclavicular line
  • V_3: halfway between V_2 and V_4
  • V_5: horizontal level to V_4 at the anterior axillary line
  • V_6: horizontal level to V_4 at the midaxillary line
	Ensures the accuracy of the lead placements.
	
	Accurate electrode placement is essential for obtaining valid and reliable data for ECG recordings. The RL electrode is a ground electrode that does not contribute to the ECG tracings.
	
	The angle of Louis assists with identifying the second rib for correct placement of precordial leads in the appropriate ICS. Slight alterations in the position of any of the precordial leads may alter the ECG significantly and can affect diagnosis and treatment.[7]
		Limb leads should be placed in fleshy areas; bony prominences should be avoided. The limb leads need to be placed equidistant from the heart and should be positioned in approximately the same place on each limb.
		
		Variations in precordial lead placement of as little as 2 cm can result in important diagnostic errors, particularly in anteroseptal infarction and ventricular hypertrophy.[5]
		If precordial leads cannot be accurately placed because of chest wounds, placement of defibrillator pads, or other reasons, the alternative site should be clearly documented on the ECG.
		In women, place electrodes V_4, V_5 and V_6 under the breast tissue. Explain to the patient the importance of an accurate tracing and the reduction of interference when placed closest to the heart.

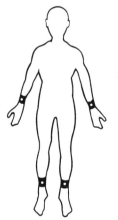

Figure 51.4 Limb lead placement in a 12-lead ECG.

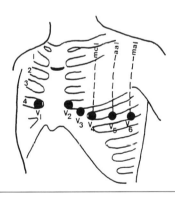

Figure 51.5 Precordial or chest lead placement.

Steps	Rationale	Special Considerations
10. Cleanse and slightly abrade the skin where the electrodes will be applied. A. Wash the skin with soap and water, if needed. B. Abrade the skin with a gauze pad. C. Ensure that the skin is dry before skin electrodes are applied. D. Clipping of chest hair may be necessary to ensure adequate skin contact with the skin electrodes. (**Level C***)	Preparing the skin by removing dead skin cells, lotions, moisture, and hair will promote impulse transmission.	Failure to properly prepare the skin may cause artifacts and interfere with interpretation.

*Level C: Qualitative studies, descriptive or correlational studies, integrative reviews, systematic reviews, or randomized controlled trials with inconsistent results.

Procedure continues on following page

Procedure for 12-Lead Electrocardiogram—*Continued*

Steps	Rationale	Special Considerations
11. Identify the electrode sites, and mark them with an indelible marker.	Minimizes ECG changes caused by changes in electrode placement.[7]	After accurate identification of the locations, an indelible marker should be used to mark the electrode sites if serial ECGs are anticipated; For example, when chest pain is being actively treated.
12. For pre-gelled electrodes, remove the backing and test for moistness. For adhesive electrodes, remove the backing and check each adhesive pad, as each should be sticky or moist.	Allows for appropriate conduction of impulses.	Gel must be moist. If pre-gelled electrodes are not moist or adhesive electrodes are not sticky, replace the electrodes.
13. Apply the electrodes securely, and place the electrodes on the marked locations.	Electrodes must be secure to prevent external influences from affecting the ECG. Secure the electrodes to obtain quality ECG recordings.	If limb plate electrodes are used, do not overtighten to minimize discomfort.
14. Fasten the designated lead wires to the limb electrodes, avoiding bending or strain on the wires, and use the correct lead-to-electrode connection.	Provides for correct lead-to-limb connection.	
15. Identify the multiple-channel machine recording setting (Fig. 51.6).	Multiple-channel machines run several leads simultaneously and can be set to run leads in different configurations.	

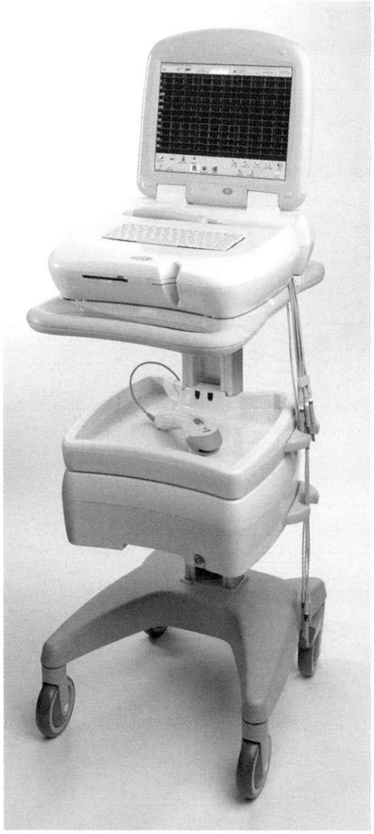

Figure 51.6   Multiple-channel ECG machine. *(Courtesy Philips Medical Systems, Andover, MA.)*

Procedure | **for 12-Lead Electrocardiogram—*Continued***

Steps	Rationale	Special Considerations
16. Obtain a 12-lead ECG recording. Most systems record each lead for 3–6 seconds and automatically mark the correct lead.	Three to six seconds are all that is needed for a permanent record; a longer strip may be obtained if a rhythm strip is needed.	A multiple-channel machine runs the limb and chest leads simultaneously. Many machines will indicate when an acceptable tracing is complete.
17. Examine the quality of the 12-lead ECG tracing.	While the patient is still connected to the machine, the nurse should examine the ECG to see whether any leads need to be repeated.	Reviews the normal conduction sequence and identifies abnormalities that may necessitate further evaluation or treatment.
18. Disconnect the equipment; cleanse the gel off the patient (if necessary), remove **PE**, discard used supplies, and prepare the equipment for future use.	Increases patient comfort. Reduces the transmission of microorganisms; standard precautions.	Some pre-gelled electrodes can be left in place for repeat ECGs. Follow the manufacturer's directions and institutional protocols for electrode use and removal in these cases.

19. **HH**
Right Precordial Leads (Fig. 51.7)

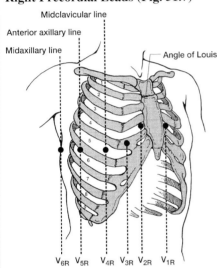

Midclavicular line
Anterior axillary line
Midaxillary line
Angle of Louis

V_{6R} V_{5R} V_{4R} V_{3R} V_{2R} V_{1R}

V_{1R}: 4th intercostal space (ICS) at left sternal border

(same as V_2)

V_{2R}: 4th ICS at right sternal border (same as V_1)

V_{3R}: halfway between V_{2R} and V_{4R}

V_{4R}: right midclavicular line in the 5th ICS

V_{5R}: right anterior axillary line at the same horizontal

level as V_{4R}

V_{6R}: right midaxillary line at the same horizontal

level as V_{4R}

Figure 51.7 Electrode locations for recording a right precordial ECG. *(From Drew BJ, Ide B: Right ventricular infarction, Prog Cardiovasc Nurs 10:46, 1995.)*

- V_{1R}: fourth intercostal space (ICS) at the left sternal border (same as V_2)
- V_{2R}: fourth ICS at the right sternal border (same as V_1)
- V_{3R}: halfway between V_{2R} and V_{4R}
- V_{4R}: right midclavicular line in the fifth ICS
- V_{5R}: right anterior axillary line at the same horizontal level as V_{4R}
- V_{6R}: right midaxillary line at the same horizontal level as V_{4R}

All patients with a suspected/actual acute inferior wall MI should have right precordial leads recorded in addition to precordial leads V_1 to V_6.

Slight alterations in the position of one precordial electrode may distort significantly the appearance of the cardiac waveforms and can have a significant impact on the diagnosis.[1]

These right precordial leads are placed across the right precordium with the same landmarks that are used for the precordial leads V_1 to V_6.[8]

V_{1R} is at the same location as V_2, and V_{2R} is at the same location as V_1 in the standard 12-lead ECG (Fig. 51.8). The redundancy of V_1 (or V_{2R}) and V_2 (or V_{1R}) can be used to ensure that the ECGs are recorded accurately. Identify the sternal notch, and move downward to locate the angle of Louis; the second ICS is located right below the angle of Louis.

Procedure continues on following page

Procedure	**for 12-Lead Electrocardiogram—*Continued***	
Steps	Rationale	Special Considerations

Left Posterior Leads (Fig. 51.9)

- V_7: posterior axillary line at the same level as V_4 to V_6
- V_8: halfway between V_7 and V_9
- V_9: left paraspinal line at the same level as V_4 to V_6

Left posterior leads are placed to view the posterior wall of the left ventricle. Left posterior leads should be recorded in patients admitted with a suspected posterior MI or known to have left circumflex artery disease.[10]

Help the patient turn to the right side to expose the left side of the back. Ensure that the patient is safely turned. Leads V_4 to V_6 are located at the midclavicular line in the fifth ICS; leads V_7 to V_9 are at the same horizontal level as V_4 to V_6.

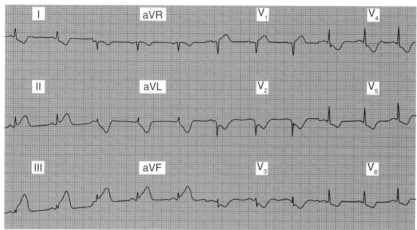
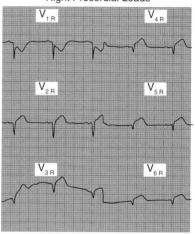

Conventional 12-Lead ECG

Right Precordial Leads

Figure 51.8   ST-segment elevation in leads II, III, and aVF indicates acute inferior wall MI. These characteristics on the standard 12-lead electrocardiogram (ECG) *(left panel)* suggest RV infarction: diagnosis of an inferior MI; ST-segment elevation in lead III exceeding that of lead II; ST-segment elevation confined to V_1 without elevation in the remaining precordial leads; and ST depression in lead aVL. Definitive diagnosis of RV infarction is made by observing ST-segment elevation greater than or equal to 1 mm in one or more of the right precordial leads. In the *right panel*, ST-segment elevation is seen in V_{2R} (V_1) to V_{6R}. *(From Drew BJ, Ide B: Right ventricular infarction, Prog Cardiovasc Nurs 10:46, 1995.)*

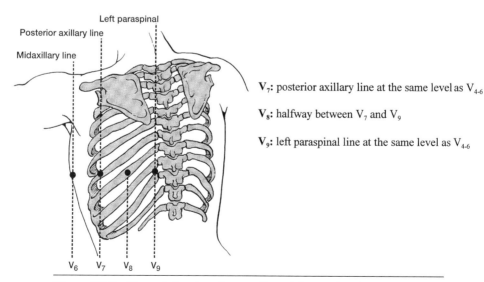

V_7: posterior axillary line at the same level as V_{4-6}

V_8: halfway between V_7 and V_9

V_9: left paraspinal line at the same level as V_{4-6}

Figure 51.9   Electrode locations for recording a left posterior electrocardiogram.

Procedure	for 12-Lead Electrocardiogram—*Continued*	
Steps	Rationale	Special Considerations

Follow **Steps 10–19** above
   A. For recording RV leads with a 12-lead ECG machine, connect as follows:
• V_1 wire to electrode V_{1R}
• V_2 wire to electrode V_{2R}
• V_3 wire to electrode V_{3R}
• V_4 wire to electrode V_{4R}
• V_5 wire to electrode V_{5R}
• V_6 wire to electrode V_{6R}
   B. For recording of left posterior leads with a 12-lead ECG machine, connect as follows:
• V_4 wire to electrode V_7
• V_5 wire to electrode V_8
• V_6 wire to electrode V_9
	When the unipolar precordial lead wires V_1 to V_6 are connected to the RV or left posterior electrodes, the ECG machine records signals from where the electrodes are placed.	It is important to change the labels on the ECG printouts from V_1 to V_{1R}, V_2 to V_{2R}, V_3 to V_{3R}, V_4 to V_{4R}, V_5 to V_{5R}, and V_6 to V_{6R}.
		
		Make a notation of "left posterior leads," and relabel appropriately on the printouts: change V_4 to V_7, V_5 to V_8, and V_6 to V_9.

Assess the quality of the tracing.	Ensures that a clear tracing is obtained and no lead is off.	
Disconnect the equipment; cleanse the gel off the patient (if necessary), remove **PE**, discard used supplies, and prepare the equipment for future use. 20. **HH**	Reduces the transmission of microorganisms; standard precautions.	Some pre-gelled electrodes can be left in place for repeat ECGs. Follow the manufacturer's directions and hospital policy for electrode use and removal in these cases.

Expected Outcomes

- A clear and accurate 12-lead ECG recording that allows clinicians to diagnose dysrhythmias, ischemia, injury, and infarction (Fig. 51.10).
- Prompt identification of abnormalities that lead to applicable and timely patient intervention(s).

Unexpected Outcomes

- Altered skin integrity
- Inaccurate lead placement or connection (Fig. 51.11)
- AC interference, also called *60-cycle interference* (Fig. 51.12)
- Wandering baseline (Fig. 51.13)
- Artifact or waveform interference (Fig. 51.14)

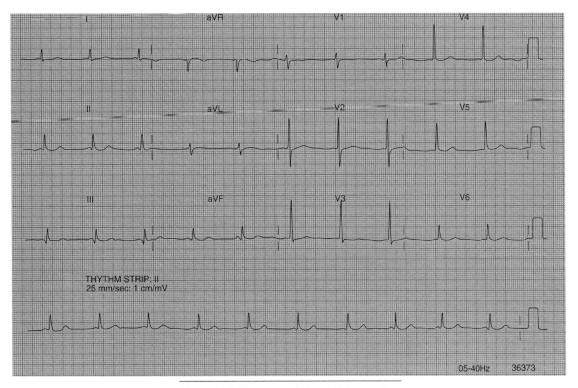

Figure 51.10   Clear 12-lead ECG recording.

Expected Outcomes   **Unexpected Outcomes**

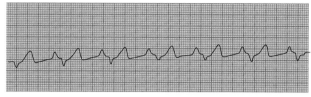

A

B

Figure 51.11   Limb lead reversal on 12-lead electrocardiogram (ECG) in lead I. **A,** Correct placement. **B,** Incorrect placement.

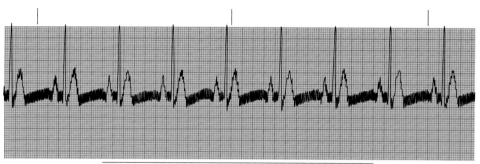

Figure 51.12   Monitor strip with 60-cycle interference.

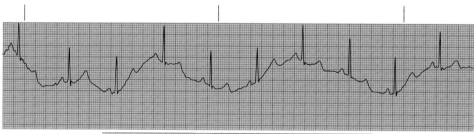

Figure 51.13   Monitor strip with a wandering baseline.

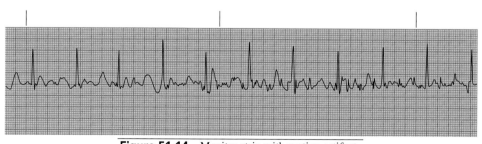

Figure 51.14   Monitor strip with motion artifact.

UNIT II

Patient Monitoring and Care

Steps	Rationale	Reportable Conditions
1. Obtain a 12-lead ECG as ordered. (e.g., for angina or dysrhythmias).	Provides determination of myocardial ischemia, injury, and infarction. Aids in diagnosis of dysrhythmias.	*These conditions should be reported to the provider if they are new or persist despite nursing interventions.*
2. Compare the 12-lead ECG with the previous 12-lead ECGs.	Determines normal and abnormal findings.	• Angina, dysrhythmias, or abnormal 12-lead ECG. • Any abnormal changes in the 12-lead ECG
3. Record whether the patient has chest pain on the ECG tracing. Use a 0–10 score to quantify pain severity (e.g., 8/10 chest pain).	Matching the ECG results to patient symptoms assists in gathering important data and evaluating interventions.[4]	

Specific Patient Monitoring and Care for Right Ventricular or Posterior Myocardial Infarction

1. Evaluate the ECG recordings for acute RV or posterior myocardial ischemia or infarction.	Promptly initiates appropriate interventions, such as reperfusion treatment or vasodilators. A criterion of 0.5 mm ST elevation in V_{7-9} may suggest acute myocardial ischemia in the posterior wall of the left ventricle.[6]	• Abnormal ST-segment deviation (elevation or depression) may indicate acute myocardial ischemia, injury, or infarction
2. Evaluate the patient's ECG for signs of AV node conduction disturbances in patients with RV infarction (e.g., second-degree or third-degree AV block).	The RCA supplies blood to the AV node in 90% of patients. Occlusion of the RCA proximal to the RV branch decreases the blood supply to the AV nodal artery.	• Patients with an acute MI with RV involvement, as evidenced by a QRS pattern or ST-segment elevation greater than or equal to 1 mm in the right precordial leads.[9]
3. Assess the patient's hemodynamic status.	Hypotension and reduced cardiac output in patients with RV infarction could be attributed to inadequate LV filling.[2]	• Cardiovascular and hemodynamic changes associated with RV ischemia, injury, or infarction (e.g., elevated mean arterial pressure and central venous pressure, reduced cardiac output, hypotension, and prominent venous engorgement).

Documentation

Documentation should include the following:
• Patient and family education
• The fact that a 12-lead ECG was obtained
• Any altered lead placement and indication
• Symptoms that the patient experienced (e.g., chest pain, syncope, dizziness, or palpitations)
• Pain assessment, interventions, and patient response to interventions
• Follow-up to the 12-lead ECG as indicated
• Unexpected outcomes
• Additional interventions

References and Additional Readings

For a complete list of references and additional readings for this procedure, scan this QR code with your smartphone, or visit https://www.elsevier.com/__data/assets/pdf_file/0003/1319826/Chapter0051.pdf.

PROCEDURE

52 Arterial Catheter Insertion AP (Perform)

Hillary Crumlett, Katie Neil, and Veronica Ann Lock

PURPOSE Arterial catheters are used for continuous monitoring of blood pressure, assessment of cardiovascular effects of vasoactive drugs, and frequent arterial blood gas and laboratory sampling. In addition, arterial catheters provide access to blood samples supporting the diagnostics related to oxygen, carbon dioxide, and bicarbonate levels (oxygenation, ventilation, and acid-base status).

PREREQUISITE NURSING KNOWLEDGE

- Knowledge of anatomy and physiology of the vasculature and adjacent structures.
- Knowledge of the principles of sterile technique.
- Understanding of the principles of hemodynamic monitoring.
- Clinical competence in suturing.
- Conditions warranting the use of arterial pressure monitoring include patients with the following:
  - ❖ Frequent blood sampling:
    - · Respiratory conditions requiring arterial blood gas monitoring (oxygenation, ventilation, acid-base status)
    - · Bleeding, actual or potential
    - · Electrolyte or glycemic abnormalities, actual or potential
    - · Metabolic abnormalities (acid-base, tissue perfusion), actual or potential
    - · Monitoring serum levels related to therapeutic interventions (e.g., renal replacement therapy, chemotherapy, biotherapy, apheresis therapy)
  - ❖ Continuous blood pressure monitoring:
    - · Hypotension or hypertension
    - · Shock: cardiogenic, septic, hypovolemic, neurogenic
    - · Mechanical circulatory support
    - · Vasoactive medication administration
- Noninvasive indirect blood pressure measurements determined with auscultation of Korotkoff sounds distal to an occluding cuff consistently average 10 to 20 mm Hg lower than simultaneous direct measurement.[15]
- Arterial waveform inspection can help with rapid diagnosis of the presence of valvular disorders and can determine

the effects of dysrhythmias on perfusion, the effects of the respiratory cycle on blood pressure, and the effects of intra-aortic balloon pump therapy or ventricular-assist device therapy on blood pressure.

- The most common complications associated with arterial puncture include pain, vasospasm (artery spasm), hematoma formation, thrombosis, embolism, infection, hemorrhage, vascular insufficiency, ischemia, direct nerve trauma, and fistula formation.[4] It has been found that major complications occurred in less than 1% of patients with arterial catheters, regardless of site selection.[23] Arterial catheter sites are a source of bloodstream infections, with the femoral site being more heavily associated with colonization compared with other sites. The infective potential of the arterial catheter is equivalent to the short-term central venous device regarding colonization and bloodstream infections and should be assessed together for signs and symptoms of infection.[12]
- Causes of failure to cannulate the artery include a tangential approach to the artery, tortuosity of the artery, arterial spasm, and impingement of the needle tip on the posterior wall.[24]
- Site selection should include the following considerations:
  - ❖ The preferred artery for arterial catheter insertion is the radial artery.[9,16] Although this artery is smaller than the ulnar artery, it is more superficial and can be more easily stabilized during the procedure.[12] Conduct the modified Allen's test before performing an arterial puncture on the radial artery (see Fig. 73.3). Normal palmar blushing is complete before 7 seconds, indicating a positive result; 8 to 14 seconds is considered equivocal; and 15 or more seconds indicates a negative test result. Doppler flow studies or plethysmography can also be performed to ensure the presence of collateral flow. Research shows these studies to be more reliable than the modified Allen's test.[1,24] Thrombosis of the arterial cannula is a possible complication. Ensuring collateral flow distal to the puncture site is important for prevention of ischemia. Puncture of both the radial and ulnar

---

AP   This procedure should be performed only by clinicians who have demonstrated competence and are credentialed to perform it. In addition, the procedure must be within the scope of practice defined by their professional licensure, and in accordance with professional practice acts. Physicians, advanced practice nurses, and physician assistants may be credentialed to perform this procedure.

arteries on the same hand is never recommended to prevent compromising blood supply to the hand.[5,9,18]

❖ The brachial artery is a potential insertion site. Before using this site, consider the brachial artery as the main artery supplying the arm; it branches into the radial and ulnar arteries, and it has no collateral circulation.[22] Hemostasis after arterial cannulation is enhanced by its proximity to the bone if the entry point is approximately 1.5 inches above the antecubital fossa.

❖ Use the femoral artery in the case of cardiopulmonary arrest or altered perfusion to the upper extremities. The femoral artery is a large superficial artery located in the groin. It is easily palpated and punctured; however, risk is associated with accessing the arterial vessel due to the proximity of the femoral artery to the femoral vein (see Fig. 73.2). Complications related to femoral artery puncture include hemorrhage and hematoma formation (because bleeding can be difficult to control), inadvertent puncture of the femoral vein (because of its close proximity to the artery), infection (because aseptic techniques are difficult to maintain in the groin area), and limb ischemia (if the femoral artery is damaged).

❖ The dorsalis pedis and posterior tibial arteries are typically avoided when selecting an arterial catheter site; however, they may be considered because they are supported by collateral circulation, which can prevent ischemic injury.[13] The dorsalis pedis is typically avoided because of the risk of dislodgement and inability to secure the catheter well. The posterior tibial artery has been associated with ischemic injuries that have resulted in amputation.[22]

• In adults, use of the radial, brachial, or dorsalis pedis sites is preferred over the femoral or axillary sites of insertion to reduce the risk of infection.[16,20]

• Ultrasound guidance is recommended to place arterial catheters if the technology is available.[11,16]

EQUIPMENT

• 2-inch, 20-gauge, nontapered Teflon cannula-over-needle or prepackaged kit that includes a 6-inch, 18-gauge Teflon catheter with appropriate introducer and guidewire (or the specific catheter for the intended insertion site)

• Pressure module and cable for interface with the monitor

• Pressure transducer system, including flush solution recommended according to institutional standards, a pressure bag or device, pressure tubing with transducer, and flush device (see Procedure 60, Single-Pressure and Multiple-Pressure Transducer Systems)

• Wasteless blood sampling system, if available. If available, then stopcocks are needed and must have dead-end Luer-lock caps for accuracy of monitoring.[17]

• Dual-channel recorder

• Nonsterile gloves, head covering, goggles, and mask

• Sterile gloves

• Sterile gown

• Large sterile fenestrated drape

• Skin antiseptic solution (e.g., 2% chlorhexidine-based preparation)

• Sterile 4 × 4 gauze pads

• Transparent occlusive dressing

• 1% lidocaine without epinephrine, 1 to 2 mL

• Sterile sodium chloride 0.9%

• 3-mL syringe with 25-gauge needle

• Waterproof pad

• Point-of-care ultrasound machine with vascular probe

• Sterile ultrasound probe cover

• Sterile ultrasound gel

Additional equipment to have available as needed includes the following:

• Bath towel

• Small wrist board

• Suture or sutureless securement device

• Chlorhexidine-impregnated sponge

• Additional transparent adhesive dressing with tape (if dressing has no tape, consider the use of ½-inch Steri-Strips)

• Transducer holder, intravenous pole, and laser or carpenter level for pole-mounted arterial catheter transducers

PATIENT AND FAMILY EDUCATION

• Explain the procedure and the purpose of the arterial catheter. **Rationale:** This explanation decreases patient and family anxiety.

• Explain to the patient that the procedure may be uncomfortable but a local anesthetic will be used first to alleviate most of the discomfort. **Rationale:** Patient cooperation is elicited, and insertion is facilitated.

• Explain the patient's role in assisting with catheter insertion. **Rationale:** This explanation elicits patient cooperation and facilitates insertion.

PATIENT ASSESSMENT AND PREPARATION

Patient Assessment

• Obtain the patient's medical history, including history of diabetes, hypertension, peripheral vascular disease, vascular grafts, arterial vasospasm, thrombosis, or embolism. Obtain the patient's history of coronary artery bypass graft surgery in which radial arteries were removed for use as conduits or for the presence of arteriovenous fistulas or shunts. **Rationale:** Extremities with any of these problems should be avoided as sites for cannulation because of the potential for complications. Patients with diabetes mellitus or hypertension are at higher risk for arterial or venous insufficiency. Previously removed radial arteries are a contraindication for ulnar artery cannulation.

• Assess the patient's medical history of coagulopathies, use of anticoagulant therapy, vascular abnormalities, or peripheral neuropathies. **Rationale:** This assessment assists in determining the safety of the procedure and aids in site selection.

• Assess the patient's allergy history (e.g., allergy to lidocaine, topical anesthetic cream, antiseptic solutions, or tape). **Rationale:** This assessment decreases the risk for allergic reactions.

• Assess the patient's current anticoagulation therapy, known blood dyscrasias, and pertinent laboratory values

492 **Unit II** Cardiovascular System

UNIT II

(e.g., platelet levels, partial thromboplastin time, prothrombin time, and international normalized ratio) before the procedure. ***Rationale:*** Anticoagulation therapy, blood dyscrasias, or alterations in coagulation studies could increase the risk for hematoma formation or hemorrhage.

- Assess the intended insertion site for the presence of a strong pulse. ***Rationale:*** Identification and localization of the pulse increases the chance of successful arterial cannulation.
- Before the artery is cannulated, evaluate for the presence of collateral flow to the area distal to the arterial catheter. For radial arterial lines, the modified Allen's test should be performed. ***Rationale:*** This assessment determines the presence of collateral flow to the hand to reduce vascular complications including ischemia.
- If available, assess the intended artery with a Doppler ultrasound scan. ***Rationale:*** This assessment aids in determination of the patency of the artery and blood flow.[1,2] Identification and localization of the artery to be cannulated increases the chance of a successful cannulation and reduces the complication rate and need for multiple attempts at placement.[11,19]

Patient Preparation

- Verify the correct patient with two identifiers. ***Rationale:*** Before performing a procedure, the nurse should ensure the correct identification of the patient for the intended intervention.
- Perform a preprocedure verification and time out, if nonemergent. Consider the use of an arterial line placement checklist to ensure that all equipment and supplies are available preprocedure.[3] ***Rationale:*** Ensures patient safety.
- Ensure that the patient and family understand the preprocedural teaching. Answer questions as they arise, and reinforce information as needed. ***Rationale:*** Understanding of previously taught information is evaluated and reinforced.
- Obtain informed consent. ***Rationale:*** Informed consent protects the rights of the patient and makes a competent decision possible for the patient; however, in emergency circumstances, time may not allow the form to be signed.
- Place the patient supine with the head of the bed at a comfortable position. The limb into which the arterial catheter will be inserted should be resting comfortably on the bed. ***Rationale:*** This placement provides patient comfort and facilitates insertion.
- If the radial artery is selected, position the hand to allow for palpation of the artery (a pillow or towel may be used to support the wrist). ***Rationale:*** This placement positions the arm and brings the artery closer to the surface.
- If the brachial artery is selected, elevate and hyperextend the patient's arm, and palpate the artery (a pillow or towel may be used to support the arm). ***Rationale:*** This action increases accessibility of the artery.
- If the femoral artery is selected, position the patient supine with the head of the bed at a comfortable angle. The patient's leg should be straight with the femoral area easily accessible. Palpate the artery (a small towel may be needed to support the hip in some cases). ***Rationale:*** This position is the best for localizing the femoral artery pulse.

Procedure for Performing Arterial Catheter Insertion

Steps	Rationale	Special Considerations
1. Obtain ultrasound equipment.	Prepares equipment.	Assistance may be needed from radiology.
2. Ensure that a pressure transducer system is prepared (see Procedure 60, Single-Pressure and Multiple-Pressure Transducer Systems).	Prepares equipment.	
3. **HH**		
4. **PE**		
5. Place a waterproof pad under the selected site.	Avoids soiling of bed linens.	
6. Determine the anatomy of the artery. (**Level E***)	Helps ensure proper placement of the arterial catheter and guides the area to be prepped.[16]	
7. If the radial artery is to be used, perform the modified Allen's test before arterial catheter insertion (see Fig. 73.3). (**Level C***)	Although evidence is found in support of and against the use of the modified Allen's test, the test can be performed before a radial artery puncture in an attempt to assess the patency of the ulnar artery and to assess for an intact superficial palmar arch.[4,5,7,10,18,19]	The modified Allen's test does not always ensure adequate flow through the ulnar artery. A Doppler ultrasound flow indicator can also be used to further verify blood flow.[1,7]

*Level E: Multiple case reports, theory-based evidence from expert opinions, or peer-reviewed professional organizational standards without clinical studies to support recommendations.

*Level C: Qualitative studies, descriptive or correlational studies, integrative reviews, systematic reviews, or randomized controlled trials with inconsistent results.

Procedure	for Performing Arterial Catheter Insertion—*Continued*	
Steps	**Rationale**	**Special Considerations**
A. With the patient's hand held overhead, instruct the patient to open and close the hand several times.	Forces the blood from the hand.	
B. With the patient's fist clenched, apply direct pressure on both the radial and the ulnar arteries.	Obstructs blood flow to the hand.	If the patient is unconscious or unable to perform the procedure, clench the fist passively for the patient.
C. Instruct the patient to lower and open the hand.	Allows observation for pallor.	Performed passively if the patient is unconscious or unable to assist.
D. While maintaining pressure on the radial artery, release the pressure over the ulnar artery, and observe the hand for the return of color.	Return of color within 7 seconds indicates patency of the ulnar artery and an intact superficial palmar arch; this is interpreted as a normal Allen's test result. If color returns between 8 and 14 seconds, the test is considered equivocal, and the healthcare provider must consider the risk and benefits of continuing with performing this procedure. If 15 or more seconds are needed for color to return, test results are considered abnormal, and another site should be considered.	If the test results are abnormal, perform the modified Allen's test on the opposite hand. If results for both hands are abnormal, consider use of a site other than the radial arteries.
8. **HH**		
9. **PE**	Reduces the transmission of microorganisms.	

10. Prepare the site with the antiseptic solution (e.g., 2% chlorhexidine-based preparation).
  A. Cleanse the site with a back-and-forth motion while applying friction for 30 seconds.
  B. Allow the antiseptic solution to dry.
	Limits the introduction of potentially infectious skin flora into the vessel during the puncture.	There should be special consideration to avoid the femoral artery due to lack of associated collateral circulation for the lower extremity.[21] This poses a significant risk to the patient if the femoral artery becomes occluded or obstructed.[21]

11. Remove gloves, and perform **HH**		
12. Open the arterial cannula insertion kit.	Prepares for the procedure.	
13. Apply sterile gloves.	Arterial catheter insertion is a sterile procedure.	Personal protective equipment (e.g., head cover, mask, goggles) is needed as well as sterile equipment. If the arterial catheter will be placed in a femoral artery, a sterile gown should be worn.[20]
14. Drape the area around the site with sterile drapes.	Provides a sterile field and minimizes the transmission of organisms.	A large sterile fenestrated drape should be used during peripheral arterial catheter insertion.[16,20] Maximal sterile barrier precautions should be used for femoral artery catheter insertion; however, this site should be avoided if possible.[16,20]

Procedure continues on following page

Procedure for Performing Arterial Catheter Insertion—*Continued*

Steps	Rationale	Special Considerations
15. Locally anesthetize the puncture site.[5,10,13,14,18] **(Level C*)**	Provides local anesthesia for the arterial puncture.	Most patients experience pain during arterial puncture.[8,10]
A. Use a 1-mL syringe with a 25-gauge needle to draw up 0.5 mL of 1% lidocaine without epinephrine.	Minimizes vessel trauma. Absence of epinephrine decreases the risk for peripheral vasoconstriction.	Medications such as lidocaine ointment, amethocaine gel, and EMLA cream may reduce pain.[12,15,18,25] If these medications are used, follow the manufacturer's recommendations.
B. Aspirate before injecting the local anesthetic.	Determines whether or not a blood vessel has been inadvertently entered.	
C. Inject intradermally and then with full infiltration around the intended arterial insertion site. Use approximately 0.2–0.3 mL for an adult.	Decreases the incidence of localized pain during injection of all skin layers. Patients report reduced pain when a local intradermal anesthetic agent is used before arterial puncture.	
16. Perform the percutaneous puncture of the selected artery.		Use of ultrasound technology may be used to assist with catheter insertion.
A. Palpate and stabilize the artery with the index and middle fingers of the nondominant hand.	Increases the likelihood of correctly locating the artery and decreases the chance of the vessel rolling.	
B. With the needle bevel up and the syringe at a 30-degree to 60-degree angle to the radial or brachial artery, puncture the skin slowly. Adjust the angle to a 60-degree to 90-degree angle to the femoral artery.	A slow, gradual thrust promotes entry into the artery without inadvertently passing through the posterior wall.	
17. Advance the needle and the cannula until a blood return is noted in the hub, and then slowly advance the catheter about ¼ to ½ inch farther to ensure that the cannula is in the artery.	Advancing the cannula farther ensures that the entire cannula is in the artery and not just the tip of the stylet.	
18. If, on initial insertion, blood return is not noted, a 3-mL syringe may be placed at the end of the cannula. While advancing the catheter, gentle withdrawing of the syringe plunger may be performed in an effort to determine proper placement in the artery.	Some arteries may vasospasm as a result of sudden insertion of the catheter. Taking the time to place a syringe on the catheter and withdrawing slightly during insertion may allow the artery to relax and help determine whether proper placement within the artery has been achieved.	
19. Level the catheter to the skin; then continue to advance the cannula to its hub with a steady rotary action.	The rotary action helps advance the catheter through the skin.	If an over-the-wire catheter is used, advance the wire completely to the hub, and then advance the catheter over the wire.
20. Once positioning is confirmed, remove the stylet, connect the catheter to the pressure transducer system, and flush the system.	Maintains catheter patency and prepares the system for arterial blood pressure monitoring.	Arterial blood is pulsatile.

*Level C: Qualitative studies, descriptive or correlational studies, integrative reviews, systematic reviews, or randomized controlled trials with inconsistent results.

Procedure for Performing Arterial Catheter Insertion—*Continued*

Steps	Rationale	Special Considerations
21. Observe the arterial waveform.	Confirms arterial catheter placement.	
22. Secure the arterial catheter in place.	Maintains arterial catheter positioning; reduces the chance of accidental dislodgment.	The catheter may be sutured in place, or a sutureless securement device may be used to secure the catheter. Follow institutional standards.
23. Apply an occlusive sterile dressing to the insertion site.	Reduces the risk for infection.	For patients older than 18 years of age, the use of FDA-approved chlorhexidine-impregnated dressings is currently recommended by the U.S. Centers for Disease Control and Prevention (CDC).[6] Refer to institutional standards on use of this type of dressing.
24. Level the air-fluid interface (zeroing stopcock) to the phlebostatic axis, zero the monitoring system, verify the arterial waveform through a square wave test, and activate the alarm system (see Procedure 53, Arterial Catheter Insertion [Assist], Care, and Removal).	Prepares the monitoring system.	
25. Remove **PE** and discard used supplies in appropriate receptacles; dispose of needles and other sharp objects in appropriate containers.	Reduces the transmission of microorganisms; standard precautions. Safely removes sharp objects.	
26. **HH**		

Expected Outcomes

- Successful cannulation of the artery
- Ability to obtain blood samples from the arterial catheter
- Peripheral vascular and neurovascular systems intact
- Alterations in blood pressure stability identified and treated accordingly

Unexpected Outcomes

- Pain
- Complications of puncture or vasospasm
- Complications after the procedure, such as change in color, temperature, sensation, or movement of the cannulated extremity; hematoma, hemorrhage, infection, or thrombus at the insertion site
- Inability to cannulate the artery

Patient Monitoring and Care

Steps	Rationale	Reportable Conditions
		These conditions should be reported to the provider if they persist despite nursing interventions.
1. Observe the insertion site for signs of hemostasis after the procedure.	Postinsertion bleeding can occur in any patient but is more likely to occur in patients with coagulopathies or patients undergoing anticoagulation therapy.	• Bleeding • Hematoma • Changes in vital signs
2. Assess the arterial catheter insertion site and involved extremity for signs of postinsertion complications.[18]	Arterial catheter insertion can result in peripheral vascular and neurovascular compromise of the extremity distal to the puncture site.	• Changes in pulse, color, size, temperature, sensation, or movement in the extremity used for the arterial catheter insertion

Procedure continues on following page

Patient Monitoring and Care —*Continued*

Steps	Rationale	Reportable Conditions
3. Ensure that the catheter is clearly labeled as "arterial."	Alerts physicians, advanced practice nurses, and other healthcare professionals that the catheter is arterial, not venous.	
4. Assess the arterial catheter insertion site for signs or symptoms of infection.	Determines the necessity for catheter removal and further treatment.	• Erythema, warmth, hardness, tenderness, or pain at the arterial line insertion site • Presence of purulent drainage from the arterial line insertion site
5. Follow institutional standards for assessing pain. Administer analgesia as prescribed.	Identifies the need for pain interventions.	• Continued pain despite pain interventions

Documentation

Documentation should include the following:
- Patient and family education
- Performance of the modified Allen's test before insertion and its results (when using the radial artery)
- Preprocedure verifications and time out
- Signed consent form
- Arterial site accessed
- Insertion of the arterial catheter (date, time, and initials marked on the dressing itself)
- Size of cannula-over-needle catheter used
- Any difficulties in the insertion; number of attempts
- Patient tolerance of the procedure
- Pain assessment, interventions, and effectiveness
- Appearance of the site
- Appearance of the limb, color, pulse, sensation, movement, capillary refill time, and temperature of the extremity after insertion is complete
- Occurrence of unexpected outcomes
- Nursing interventions performed before, during, and after the procedure.

References and Additional Readings

For a complete list of references and additional readings for this procedure, scan this QR code with your smartphone, or visit https://www.elsevier.com/__data/assets/pdf_file/0004/1319827/Chapter0052.pdf

53

Arterial Catheter Insertion (Assist), Care, and Removal

Hillary Crumlett and Deborah Thorgesen

PURPOSE Arterial catheters are used for continuous monitoring of blood pressure, assessment of cardiovascular effects of vasoactive drugs, and frequent arterial blood gas and laboratory sampling. Additionally, arterial catheters provide access to blood samples that support the diagnostics related to oxygen, carbon dioxide, and bicarbonate levels (oxygenation, ventilation, and acid-base status).

PREREQUISITE NURSING KNOWLEDGE

- Knowledge of the anatomy and physiology of the vasculature and adjacent structures.
- Knowledge of the principles of hemodynamic monitoring.
- Understanding of the principles of aseptic technique.
- Conditions that warrant the use of arterial pressure monitoring include patients with the following:
  - Frequent blood sampling:
    - Respiratory conditions requiring arterial blood gas monitoring (oxygenation, ventilation, acid-base status)
    - Bleeding, actual or potential
    - Electrolyte or glycemic abnormalities, actual or potential
    - Metabolic abnormalities (acid-base, tissue perfusion), actual or potential
    - Monitoring serum levels related to therapeutic interventions (e.g., renal replacement therapy, chemotherapy, biotherapy, apheresis therapy)
  - Continuous blood pressure monitoring:
    - Hypotension or hypertension
    - Shock: cardiogenic, septic, hypovolemic, neurogenic
    - Mechanical circulatory support
    - Vasoactive medication administration
- Arterial pressure represents the forcible ejection of blood from the left ventricle into the aorta and the arterial system. During ventricular systole, blood is ejected into the aorta, generating a pressure wave. Because of the heart's intermittent pumping action, this arterial pressure wave is generated in a pulsatile manner (Fig. 53.1). The ascending limb of the aortic pressure wave (anacrotic limb) represents an increase in pressure because of left-ventricular ejection. This ejection is the peak systolic pressure, which should be less than 120 mm Hg in adults.[23] After reaching this peak, the ventricular pressure declines to a level below aortic pressure, and the aortic valve closes, marking the end of ventricular systole. Closure of the aortic valve produces a small rebound wave that creates a notch known as the *dicrotic notch.* The descending limb of the curve (diastolic downslope) represents diastole and is characterized

by a long declining pressure wave during which the aortic wall recoils and propels blood into the arterial network. The diastolic pressure is measured as the lowest point of the diastolic downslope, which should be less than 80 mm Hg in adults.[23]

- The difference between the systolic and diastolic pressures is the pulse pressure, with a normal value of about 40 mm Hg.
- Arterial pressure is determined by the relationship between blood flow through the vessels (cardiac output) and the resistance of the vessel walls (systemic vascular resistance). The arterial pressure therefore is affected by any factors that change either cardiac output or systemic vascular resistance.
- The average arterial pressure during a cardiac cycle is called the *mean arterial pressure* (MAP). MAP is not the average of the systolic plus the diastolic pressures because, during the cardiac cycle, the pressure remains closer to diastole than to systole for a longer period (at normal heart rates). The MAP is calculated automatically by most patient monitoring systems; however, it can be calculated with the following formula:

$$MAP = \frac{(\text{systolic pressure}) + (\text{diastolic pressure} \times 2)}{3}$$

- MAP represents the driving force (perfusion pressure) for blood flow through the cardiovascular system. MAP is at its highest point in the aorta. As blood travels through the arterial system away from the aorta, systolic pressure increases and diastolic pressure decreases, with an overall decline in MAP (Fig. 53.2).
- The location of arterial catheter placement depends on the condition of the arterial vessels and the presence of other catheters (e.g., the presence of a dialysis shunt is a contraindication for placement of an arterial catheter in the same extremity). Once inserted, the arterial catheter causes little or no discomfort to the patient and allows continuous blood pressure assessment and intermittent blood sampling. If intra-aortic balloon pump therapy is necessary, arterial pressure may be directly monitored from the tip of the balloon catheter in the aorta.

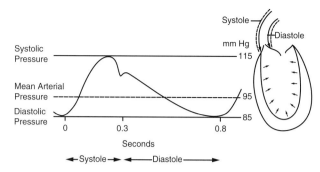

Figure 53.1   The generation of a pulsatile waveform. This is an aortic pressure curve. During systole, the ejected volume distends the aorta, and aortic pressure increases. The peak pressure is known as the *aortic systolic pressure*. After the peak ejection, the ventricular pressure decreases; when it drops below the aortic pressure, the aortic valve closes, which is marked by the dicrotic notch, the end of the systole. During diastole, the pressure continues to decrease and the aortic wall recoils, pushing blood toward the periphery. The trough of the pressure wave is the diastolic pressure. The difference between the systolic and diastolic pressure is the pulse pressure. *(From Smith JJ, Kampine JP: Circulating physiology, Baltimore, 1980, Williams & Wilkins, 55.)*

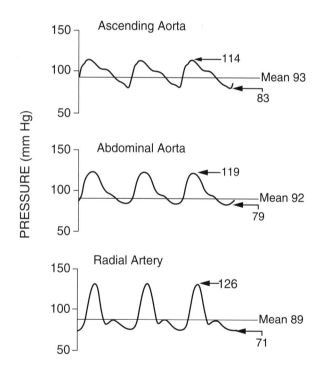

Figure 53.2   Arterial pressure from different sites in the arterial tree. The arterial pressure waveform varies in configuration, depending on the location of the catheter. With transmission of the pressure wave into the distal aorta and large arteries, the systolic pressure increases and the diastolic pressure decreases; with a resulting heightening of the pulse, pressure declines steadily. *(From Smith JJ, Kampine JP: Circulating physiology. Baltimore, 1980, Williams & Wilkins, 57.)*

- The radial artery is the most common site for arterial pressure monitoring. Arterial pulse waveforms recorded from a peripheral site (compared with a central site) changes the waveform morphology. The anacrotic limb becomes more peaked and narrowed, with increased amplitude; therefore the systolic pressure in peripheral sites is higher than the systolic pressure recorded from a more central site (see Fig. 53.2). Also the diastolic pressure decreases, the diastolic downslope may show a secondary wave, and the dicrotic notch becomes less prominent from distal sites.

- Vasodilators and vasoconstrictors may change the appearance of the waveforms from distal sites. Vasodilators may cause the waveform to take on a more central appearance. Vasoconstrictors may cause the systolic pressure to become more exaggerated because of enhanced resistance in the peripheral arteries.

- Several potential complications are associated with arterial pressure monitoring. Infection at the insertion site can develop and cause sepsis. Clot formation in the catheter can lead to arterial embolization. The catheter can cause a pseudoaneurysm or vessel perforation with extravasation of blood and flush solution into the surrounding tissue. Finally, the distal extremity can develop circulatory or neurovascular impairment.

- Ultrasound guidance is recommended to place arterial catheters if the technology is available.[8,4]

EQUIPMENT

- Consider the use of an arterial line placement checklist to ensure that all equipment and supplies are available preprocedure.[5]
- 2-inch, 20-gauge, nontapered Teflon cannula-over-needle or prepackaged kit that includes a 6-inch, 18-gauge Teflon catheter with appropriate introducer and guidewire (or the specific catheter for the intended insertion site)
- Pressure module and cable for interface with the monitor
- Pressure transducer system, including flush solution recommended according to institutional standards, a pressure bag or device, pressure tubing with transducer, and flush device (see Procedure 60, Single-Pressure and Multiple-Pressure Transducer Systems)
- Wasteless blood sampling system if available. When used, stopcocks are needed and must have dead-end Luer-lock caps for accuracy of monitoring.[23]
- Dual-channel recorder
- Nonsterile gloves, head covering, goggles, and mask
- Sterile gloves and large sterile fenestrated drape
- Skin antiseptic solution (e.g., 2% chlorhexidine-based preparation)
- Sterile 4 × 4 gauze pads
- Transparent occlusive dressing
- 1% lidocaine without epinephrine, 1 to 2 mL
- Sterile sodium chloride 0.9% for the pressure bag
- 3-mL syringe with 25-gauge needle
- Sheet protector
- Bedside ultrasound machine with vascular probe
- Sterile ultrasound probe cover
- Sterile ultrasound gel
  Additional equipment to have available as needed includes the following:
- Sterile gown and full drape
- Bath towel
- Small wrist board
- Sutureless securement device
- Suture material

- Chlorhexidine-impregnated sponge
- Additional transparent adhesive dressing with tape (if dressing has no tape, consider the use of ½-inch Steri-Strips)
- Transducer holder, intravenous (IV) pole, and laser lever for pole-mounted arterial catheter transducers

PATIENT AND FAMILY EDUCATION

- Explain the procedure and the purpose of the arterial catheter. *Rationale:* This explanation decreases patient and family anxiety.
- Explain the standard of care to the patient and family, including insertion procedure, alarms, dressings, and length of time the catheter is expected to be in place. *Rationale:* This explanation encourages the patient and family to ask questions and voice concerns about the procedure and decreases patient and family anxiety.
- Explain the patient's expected participation during the procedure. *Rationale:* Patient cooperation during insertion is encouraged.
- Explain the importance of keeping the affected extremity immobile. *Rationale:* This explanation encourages patient cooperation to prevent catheter dislodgment and maintains catheter patency and function.
- Instruct the patient to report any warmth, redness, pain, or wet feeling at the insertion site at any time. *Rationale:* These symptoms may indicate infection, bleeding, or disconnection of the tubing or catheter.

PATIENT ASSESSMENT AND PREPARATION

Patient Assessment

- Obtain the patient's medical history, including a history of diabetes, hypertension, peripheral vascular disease, vascular grafts, arterial vasospasm, thrombosis, or embolism. Obtain the patient's history of coronary artery bypass graft surgery and the use of radial arteries as conduits or presence of arteriovenous fistulas or shunts. *Rationale:* Avoid cannulation to extremities with a history of previously mentioned procedures related to potential complications. Patients with diabetes mellitus or hypertension are at higher risk for arterial or venous insufficiency. Previously removed radial arteries are a contraindication for ulnar artery cannulation.
- Review the patient's current anticoagulation therapy, history of blood dyscrasias, and pertinent laboratory values (prothrombin time [PT], international normalized ratio [INR], partial thromboplastin time [PTT], and platelets) before the procedure. *Rationale:* Anticoagulation therapy, blood dyscrasias, or alterations in coagulation studies could increase the risk of hematoma formation or hemorrhage.

- Review the patient's allergy history (e.g., allergy to heparin, lidocaine, antiseptic solutions, or adhesive tape). *Rationale:* This assessment decreases the risk for allergic reactions. Patients with heparin-induced thrombocytopenia should not receive heparin in the flush solution.
- Assess the neurovascular and peripheral vascular status of the extremity to be used for the arterial cannulation, including color, temperature, presence and fullness of pulses, capillary refill, presence of bruit (in larger arteries such as the femoral artery), and motor and sensory function (compared with the opposite extremity). Note: A modified Allen's test should be performed before cannulation of the radial artery. *Rationale:* This assessment may help identify any neurovascular or circulatory impairment before cannulation to avoid potential complications, including ischemia.[2,24,21]

Patient Preparation

- Verify the correct patient with two identifiers. *Rationale:* Before performing a procedure, the nurse should ensure the correct identification of the patient for the intended intervention.
- Ensure that the patient and family understand the preprocedural teaching. Answer questions as they arise, and reinforce information as needed. *Rationale:* Understanding of previously taught information is evaluated and reinforced.
- Ensure that informed consent is obtained. *Rationale:* Informed consent protects the rights of the patient and allows a competent decision to be made by the patient; however, in emergency circumstances, time may not allow the form to be signed.
- Nonemergent procedures require a preprocedure verification and time out. *Rationale:* Ensures patient safety.
- Place the patient supine with the head of the bed in a comfortable position. The limb selected for arterial line insertion should be resting comfortably on the bed. *Rationale:* This placement provides patient comfort and facilitates insertion.
- If the radial artery is selected, position the hand to allow for palpation of the artery (support the wrist with a small pillow or towel if necessary). *Rationale:* This placement positions the arm and brings the artery closer to the surface.
- If the brachial artery is selected, elevate and hyperextend the patient's arm, and palpate the artery (support the arm with a small pillow or towel if necessary). *Rationale:* This increases the accessibility of the artery.
- If the femoral artery is selected, position the patient supine with the head of the bed in a comfortable position. The patient's leg should be straight with the femoral area easily accessible and for palpation the artery (support the hip with a small pillow or towel if necessary). *Rationale:* This position is the best for localizing the femoral artery pulse.

Procedure for Assisting With Insertion of an Arterial Catheter

Steps	Rationale	Special Considerations
1. **HH**		
2. Prepare the flush solution (see Procedure 60, Single-Pressure and Multiple-Pressure Transducer Systems). A. Use an IV solution of normal saline. B. Follow institutional standards for adding heparin to the IV solution, if heparin is not contraindicated. **(Level B*)**	Heparinized flush solutions are commonly used to minimize thrombi and fibrin deposits on catheters that might lead to thrombosis or bacterial colonization of the catheter.	Although heparin may prevent thombosis,[9,15,18] it has been associated with thrombocytopenia and other hematological complications.[6] Other factors that promote patency of the arterial line besides heparinized saline solution include male gender, longer arterial catheters, larger vessels cannulated, patients receiving other anticoagulants or thrombolytics, and short-term use of the catheter.[1]
3. Consider the use of a blood-conservation arterial line system. **(Level B*)**	Reduces the risk of nosocomial anemia.[11,13,17,19,20]	
4. Prime or flush the entire single-pressure transducer system, including the wasteless blood-draw system if using (see Procedure 60, Single-Pressure and Multiple-Pressure Transducer Systems).	Removes air bubbles. Air bubbles introduced into the patient's circulation can cause air embolism. Air bubbles within the tubing damp the waveform.	Air is more easily removed from the hemodynamic tubing when the system is not under pressure.
5. Apply and inflate the pressure bag or device to 300 mm Hg.	Each flush device delivers 1–3 mL/hour to maintain patency of the hemodynamic system.	
6. Connect the pressure cable to the bedside monitor.	Connects the pressure transducer system to the bedside monitoring system.	
7. Set the scale on the bedside monitor for the anticipated pressure waveform.	Prepares the bedside monitor.	
8. Level the air-fluid interface (zeroing stopcock) to the phlebostatic axis (see Figs. 60.7 and 60.9).	Leveling ensures that the air-fluid interface of the monitoring system is level with a reference point on the body. The phlebostatic axis reflects central arterial pressure.[14]	Use a pole mount or patient mount according to institutional protocol (see Procedure 60, Single-Pressure and Multiple-Pressure Transducer Systems). The tip of the arterial catheter is not used as the reference point because it measures transmural pressure of a specific area in the arterial tree, which may be increased by hydrostatic pressure.[14]
9. Zero the system by turning the stopcock off to the patient, opening it to air, and zeroing the monitoring system (see Procedure 60, Single-Pressure and Multiple-Pressure Transducer Systems).	Prepares the monitoring system.	
10. **HH**		
11. **PE**		
12. Assist as needed with skin preparation.	Helps the provider inserting the catheter.	
13. Assist as needed with immobilizing the extremity during catheter insertion.	Facilitates insertion.	Personal protective equipment (e.g., head cover, mask, goggles) is needed as well as sterile equipment. Maximal sterile barrier precautions should be used for femoral artery catheter insertion.[8,15]

*Level B: Well-designed, controlled studies with results that consistently support a specific action, intervention, or treatment.

Procedure for Assisting With Insertion of an Arterial Catheter—*Continued*

Steps	Rationale	Special Considerations
14. Connect the pressure cable from the arterial transducer to the bedside monitor.	Connects the arterial catheter to the bedside monitoring system.	
15. Reassess accurate leveling, and secure the transducer (see Procedure 60, Single-Pressure and Multiple-Pressure Transducer Systems).	Ensures that the air-filled interface (zeroing stopcock) is maintained at the level of the phlebostatic axis. If the air-fluid interface is above the phlebostatic axis, arterial pressures are falsely low. If the air-fluid interface is below the phlebostatic axis, arterial pressures are falsely high.	Leveling ensures accuracy. The point of the phlebostatic axis should be marked with an indelible marker, especially when the transducer is secured in a pole-mount system.
16. Zero the system again (see Procedure 60, Single-Pressure and Multiple-Pressure Transducer Systems).	Ensures accuracy of the system with the established reference point.	
17. Turn the stopcock off to the top port of the stopcock. Place a sterile cap or a needleless cap on the top port of the stopcock.	Prepares the system for monitoring and ensures a closed system.	
18. Observe the waveform, and perform a dynamic response test (square wave test; Fig. 53.3).	Determines whether the system is damped. This will ensure that the pressure waveform components are clearly defined. This aids in accurate measurement.	The square wave test can be performed by activating and quickly releasing the fast flush. A sharp upstroke should terminate in a flat line at the maximal indicator on the monitor. This should be followed by an immediate rapid downstroke extending below the baseline with 1–2 oscillations within 0.12 second and a quick return to baseline (see Fig. 53.3).
19. Ensure that the provider inserting the catheter has secured the arterial catheter in place.	Maintains arterial catheter position; reduces the chance of accidental dislodgement.	A sutureless securement device can be used.
20. Ensure that the provider inserting the catheter has applied an occlusive, sterile dressing to the insertion site.	Reduces the risk of infection.	
21. Apply an arm board, if necessary.	Ensures the correct position of the extremity for an optimal waveform.	
22. Set the alarm parameters according to the patient's current blood pressure and institutional policy.	Activates the bedside and central alarm system.	
23. Remove **PE**, and discard used supplies in appropriate receptacles; ensure that all needles and other sharp objects are disposed of in appropriate containers.	Reduces the transmission of microorganisms; standard precautions. Safely removes sharp objects.	
24. **HH**		

Procedure continues on following page

UNIT II

Procedure   for Assisting With Insertion of an Arterial Catheter—*Continued*

Steps	Rationale	Special Considerations

When the fast flush of the continuous flush system is activated and quickly released, a sharp upstroke terminates in a flat line at the maximal indicator on the monitor and hard copy. This is then followed by an immediate rapid downstroke extending below baseline with just 1 or 2 oscillations within 0.12 second (minimal ringing) and a quick return to baseline. The patient's pressure waveform is also clearly defined with all components of the waveform, such as the dicrotic notch on an arterial waveform, clearly visible.

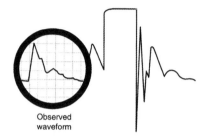

Square wave test configuration

Observed waveform

Intervention

A   There is no adjustment in the monitoring system required.

The upstroke of the square wave appears somewhat slurred, the waveform does not extend below the baseline after the fast flush and there is no ringing after the flush. The patient's waveform displays a falsely decreased systolic pressure and false high diastolic pressure as well as poorly defined components of the pressure tracing such as a diminished or absent dicrotic notch on arterial waveforms.

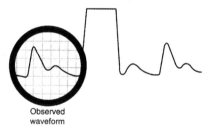

Square wave test configuration

Observed waveform

Intervention

To correct for the problem:
1. Check for the presence of blood clots, blood left in the catheter following blood sampling, or air bubbles at any point from the catheter tip to the transducer diaphragm and eliminate these as necessary.
2. Use low compliance (rigid), short (less than 3 to 4 feet) monitoring tubing.
3. Connect all line components securely.
B   4. Check for kinks in the line.

The waveform is characterized by numerous amplified oscillations above and below the baseline following the fast flush. The monitored pressure wave displays false high systolic pressures (overshoot), possibly false low diastolic pressures, and "ringing" artifacts on the waveform.

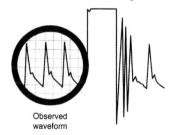

Square wave test configuration

Observed waveform

Intervention

To correct the problem, remove all air bubbles (particularly pinpoint air bubbles) in the fluid
C   system, use large-bore, shorter tubing, or use a damping device.

Figure 53.3   Dynamic response test (square wave test) using the fast flush system. **A,** Optimally damped system. **B,** Overdamped system. **C,** Underdamped system. *(From Darovic GO, Zbilut JP: Fluid-filled monitoring systems. In Hemodynamic monitoring, ed 3, Philadelphia, 2002, Saunders, 122.)*

UNIT II

Procedure for Assisting With Insertion of an Arterial Catheter—*Continued*		
Steps	Rationale	Special Considerations
25. Obtain a blood pressure.	Obtains baseline data.	Do not compare manual (noninvasive) with arterial (invasive) blood pressures. No direct relationship exists between noninvasive and invasive blood pressures because noninvasive techniques measure blood flow, and invasive techniques measure pressure.[14]
26. Run a waveform strip, and record the patient's baseline arterial pressures.	Obtains baseline data.	

Procedure for Troubleshooting an Overdamped Waveform		
Steps	Rationale	Special Considerations
1. HH		
2. PE		
3. Identify the overdamped waveform (Fig. 53.4).	Identifies the problem.	An overdamped waveform results in a falsely low systolic pressure and a falsely high diastolic pressure.

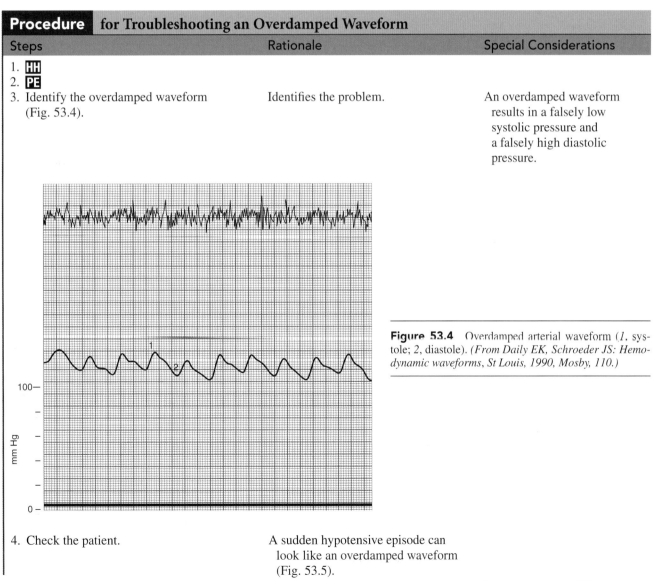

Figure 53.4 Overdamped arterial waveform (*1*, systole; *2*, diastole). (*From Daily EK, Schroeder JS: Hemodynamic waveforms, St Louis, 1990, Mosby, 110.*)

4. Check the patient.	A sudden hypotensive episode can look like an overdamped waveform (Fig. 53.5).	

Procedure continues on following page

UNIT II

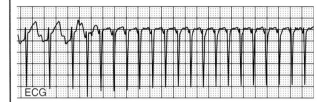

ECG

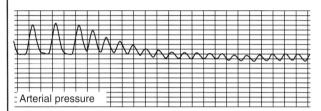

Arterial pressure

Figure 53.5 Patient developed supraventricular tachycardia (SVT) with a decrease in arterial pressure. Note how the arterial waveform appears overdamped but is in fact reflecting a severe hypotensive episode associated with the tachycardia.

5. If the waveform is overdamped, follow these steps:

A. Check the arterial line insertion site for catheter positioning.

Wrist movement in the radial site or leg flexion in the femoral site can cause catheter kinking or dislodgment, resulting in an overdamped waveform.

B. Check the system for air bubbles and eliminate them if they are found.

Air bubbles can be a cause of an overdamped system; air bubbles can also cause emboli.

C. Check the tubing system for leaks or disconnections, and correct the problem if it is found.

Ensures all connections are tight.

D. Check the flush bag to ensure fluid is present in the bag and that pressure is maintained at 300 mm Hg.

An empty flush bag or a pressure of less than 300 mm Hg may result in an overdamped system.

E. A catheter with an overdamped waveform should always be aspirated before flushing.

Use of the fast-flush device or flushing with a syringe first may force a clot at the catheter tip into the arterial circulation.

Attempt to aspirate and flush the catheter as follows:

Assists with the withdrawal of air in the tubing or clots that may be at the catheter tip.

- Using the stopcock closest to the patient, remove the nonvented cap from the blood sampling port or cleanse the needleless port and attach a 5- or 10-mL syringe to the top port of the stopcock (see Fig. 61.1).

A 5-mL syringe generates less pressure and may prevent arterial spasm in smaller arteries (e.g., radial artery).

A 10-mL syringe may be needed for larger arteries (e.g., the femoral artery). A needleless system can also be used.

- Turn the stopcock off to the flush solution (see Fig. 61.4B).

Opens the system from the patient to the syringe. Assesses catheter patency. Normally, blood should be aspirated into the syringe without difficulty.

- Gently attempt to aspirate; if resistance is felt, reposition the extremity and reattempt aspiration.
- If resistance is still felt, stop and notify the physician or advanced practice nurse.

Procedure | **for Troubleshooting an Overdamped Waveform—*Continued***

Steps	Rationale	Special Considerations
• If blood is aspirated, remove 3 mL, turn the stopcock off to the patient, and discard the 3-mL sample.	Removes any clotted material within the catheter.	All blood wastes should be disposed using standard precautions.
• Fast-flush the remaining blood from the stopcock onto a sterile gauze pad or into another syringe and remove the syringe.	Removes blood residue from the stopcock, where it could be a reservoir for bacterial growth, and prevents clotting in the blood sampling port.	
• Turn the stopcock off to the blood sampling port (see Fig. 61.1) and place a new sterile nonvented cap (not needed if using a needleless port).	Maintains sterility and a closed system.	
• Use the fast-flush device to clear the line of blood.	Prevents the arterial line from clotting.	
6. Remove **PE** and discard used supplies in the appropriate receptacles.	Reduces the transmission of microorganisms; standard precautions.	
7. **HH**		

Procedure | **for Troubleshooting an Underdamped Waveform**

Steps	Rationale	Special Considerations
1. **HH**		
2. **PE**		
3. Identify the underdamped waveform.	Identifies the problem.	An underdamped waveform results in a falsely high systolic pressure and a falsely low diastolic pressure.
4. Check the system for air bubbles and eliminate them if they are found.	Air bubbles can contribute to underdamping; air bubbles can also cause emboli.	
5. Check the length of the tubing of the pressure transducer system.	Ensures that the tubing length is minimized.	
6. Observe the waveform and perform a dynamic response test (square wave test; see Fig. 53.3).	Determines whether the system is damped. This will ensure that the pressure waveform components are clearly defined and accurate measurements are obtained. This aides in accurate measurement.	
7. Remove **PE** and discard used supplies in appropriate receptacles.	Reduces the transmission of microorganisms; Standard Precautions.	
8. **HH**		

UNIT II

Procedure for Arterial Catheter Dressing Change

Steps	Rationale	Special Considerations
1. **HH**		
2. **PE**		
3. Carefully remove and discard the arterial line dressing.	Removes the previous dressing without disrupting the integrity of the catheter.	If present, remove the securement device.
4. Inspect the catheter, insertion site, and surrounding skin.	Assesses for signs of infection, catheter dislodgement, or leakage.	
5. Remove nonsterile gloves, discard dressings, and perform hand hygiene.	Reduces the transmission of microorganisms	
6. Don sterile gloves	Maintains aseptic and sterile technique.	
7. Cleanse the skin and catheter with 2% chlorhexidine-based preparation.[15]	Reduces the rate of recolonization of skin flora. Decreases the risk for bacterial growth at the insertion site.	Allow time for the solution to air dry.
8. Apply a new stabilization device.	Secures the catheter.	
9. Apply a chlorhexidine-impregnated sponge to the site.[12,15,4] **(Level D*)**	Reduces the transmission of microorganisms.	Follow institutional standards. A chlorhexidine-impregnated sponge dressing is recommended if an institution's central line–associated bloodstream infection rate is not decreasing despite adherence to basic prevention measures, including education and training, appropriate use of chlorhexidine for skin antisepsis, and maximum sterile barrier.[8,12,15] Use with caution in patients predisposed to local skin necrosis, such as burn patients or patients with Stevens-Johnson syndrome.[22]
10. Apply a sterile air-occlusive dressing. Dressings may be a sterile gauze or a sterile, transparent, semipermeable dressing.[15]	Provides a sterile environment.	Write the date and time of the dressing change on a label, and tape it to the dressing.
11. Remove gloves and discard used supplies in appropriate receptacles.	Reduces the transmission of microorganisms; standard precautions.	
12. **HH**		

*Level D: Peer-reviewed professional and organizational standards with the support of clinical study recommendations.

Procedure	for Removal of the Arterial Catheter		
Steps	**Rationale**		**Special Considerations**
1. Review the patient's coagulation profile (PT, INR, PTT, platelets) and anticoagulation medication profile before removal of the arterial catheter.	Elevated PT, INR, PTT, and decreased platelets affect time to hemostasis.		If laboratory values are abnormal, pressure must be applied for a longer period to achieve hemostasis.
2. ▣ HH			
3. ▣ PE			
4. Turn off the arterial monitoring alarms.	The alarm system is no longer needed.		
5. Remove the dressing.	Prepares for catheter removal.		
6. Remove the stabilizing device.	Prepares for catheter removal.		
7. Turn the stopcock off to the flush solution (see Fig. 62.4B).	Turns the monitoring system off to the flush solution.		
8. Apply pressure 1–2 finger widths above the insertion site.	The arterial puncture site is above the skin puncture site because the catheter enters the skin at an angle.		
9. Remove the arterial catheter, and place a sterile 4 × 4 gauze pad over the catheter site.	Prevents splashing of blood.		
10. Continue to hold proximal pressure, and immediately apply firm pressure over the insertion site as the catheter is removed.	Prevents bleeding.		
11. Continue to apply pressure for a minimum of 5 minutes for the radial artery.	Achieves hemostasis.		Follow institutional standards. Longer periods of direct pressure may be needed to achieve hemostasis (e.g., patients receiving systemic heparin or thrombolytics, patients with catheters in larger arteries such as the femoral artery, or patients with abnormal coagulation values).
12. Apply a pressure dressing to the insertion site.	A pressure dressing helps prevent rebleeding.		The dressing should not encircle the extremity (prevents ischemia of the extremity).
13. Remove ▣ PE, and discard used supplies in appropriate receptacles.	Reduces the transmission of microorganisms; standard precautions.		
14. ▣ HH			

Expected Outcomes

- Successful cannulation of the artery
- Peripheral vascular and neurovascular systems intact
- Alterations in blood pressure identified and treated
- Ability to continuously monitor blood pressure
- Maintenance of baseline hemoglobin and hematocrit levels
- Adequate circulation to the involved extremity
- Adequate sensory and motor function to the involved extremity
- Maintenance of the catheter site without infection
- Removal of the catheter when no longer needed

Unexpected Outcomes

- Pain
- Insertion complications
- Inability to cannulate the artery
- Change in color, temperature, sensation; movement of the extremity used for insertion
- Hematoma, hemorrhage, infection, or thrombosis at the insertion site
- Decreased hemoglobin and hematocrit values
- Catheter disconnection with significant blood loss
- Presence of a new bruit
- Impaired sensory or motor function of the extremity
- Elevated temperature or elevated white blood cell count
- Redness, warmth, edema, or drainage at or from the insertion site

Procedure continues on following page

Patient Monitoring and Care

Steps	Rationale	Reportable Conditions
		These conditions should be reported to the provider if they persist despite nursing interventions.
1. Assess the neurovascular and peripheral vascular status of the cannulated extremity immediately after catheter insertion and every 4 hours, or more often if warranted, according to institutional standards.	Validates adequate peripheral vascular and neurovascular integrity. Changes in sensation, motor function, pulses, color, temperature, or capillary refill may indicate ischemia, thrombosis, arterial spasm, or neurovascular compromise.	• Diminished or absent pulses • Pale, mottled, or cyanotic appearance of the distal extremity • Extremity that is cool or cold to the touch • Capillary refill time greater than 2 seconds • Diminished or absent sensation or pain at the site or distal extremity • Diminished or absent motor function
2. Check the arterial line flush system every 4 hours to ensure the following: • Pressure bag or device is inflated to 300 mm Hg. • Fluid is present in the flush solution.	Ensures that approximately 1–3 mL/hour of flush solution is delivered through the catheter, thus maintaining patency and preventing backflow of blood into the catheter and tubing. The risk of catheter occlusion related to fibrin sheath or clot formation increases if the flush solution is not continuously infusing.	
3. Perform a dynamic response test (square wave test) at the start of each shift, with a change of the waveform, or after the system is opened to air (see Fig. 53.3).	An optimally damped system provides an accurate waveform.	• Overdamped or underdamped waveforms that cannot be corrected with troubleshooting procedures
4. Monitor for overdamped or underdamped waveforms. An overdamped waveform is characterized by a flattened waveform, a diminished or absent dicrotic notch, or a square wave that does not fall to baseline or below baseline (see Fig. 53.4). An underdamped waveform is characterized by catheter fling or artifacts on the waveform (see Fig. 53.3C).	An optimally damped system provides an adequate waveform that facilitates accuracy of blood pressure monitoring. An overdamped waveform can result in inaccurate blood pressure measurement. The patient's blood pressure measurement may be inaccurately low. An overdamped system can be caused by air bubbles in the system; use of compliant tubing versus stiff, loose tubing connections in the system; too many stopcocks in the system; a cracked tubing or stopcock; arterial catheter occlusion or a kink; the catheter tip being against the arterial wall; blood in the transducer; and insufficient pressure of the flush solution. An underdamped waveform can also result in an inaccurate blood pressure measurement. The patient's blood pressure measure may be inaccurately high. Common causes of an underdamped waveform include excessive tubing length, movement of the catheter in the artery, patient movement, and air bubbles in the system.	• Overdamped or underdamped waveforms that cannot be corrected with troubleshooting procedures

Patient Monitoring and Care —*Continued*

Steps	Rationale	Reportable Conditions
5. Zero the transducer during the initial setup, after insertion, if disconnection occurs between the transducer and the monitoring cable, if disconnection occurs between the monitoring cable and the monitor, and when the values obtained do not fit the clinical picture. Follow the manufacturer's recommendations for disposable systems.	Ensures accuracy of the hemodynamic monitoring system.	
6. Recheck the level of the air-fluid interface (zeroing stopcock) to the phlebostatic axis whenever patient position changes (see Procedure 60, Single-Pressure and Multiple-Pressure Transducer Systems).	Ensures an accurate reference point for the left atrium and accuracy of blood pressure measurements.	
7. Place sterile injectable or noninjectable caps on all stopcocks. Replace with new sterile caps whenever the caps are removed.	Stopcocks can be a source of contamination. Stopcocks that are part of the initial setup are packaged with vented caps. Vented caps must be replaced with sterile injectable or noninjectable caps to maintain a closed system and reduce the risk of contamination and infection.	
8. Continuously monitor the arterial catheter values and waveform.	Provides for continuous waveform analysis and assessment of patient status.	
9. Observe the insertion site for signs and symptoms of infection.	Infected catheters must be removed as soon as possible to prevent bacteremia. The CDC does not recommend routinely replacing peripheral arterial catheters to prevent catheter-related infections.[15]	• Redness at the insertion site • Purulent drainage • Tenderness or pain at the insertion site • Elevated temperature • Elevated white blood cell count
10. Change the pressure transducer system (flush solution, pressure tubing, transducers, and stopcocks) every 96 hours. **(Level B*)** The flush solution may need to be changed more frequently.	The CDC,[15] the Infusion Nurses Society,[8] and research findings[10,16] recommend that the hemodynamic flush system can be used safely for 96 hours. This recommendation is based on research conducted with disposable pressure monitoring systems used for peripheral and central lines.	
11. Label the tubing: A. Arterial B. Date and time prepared	Identifies that the catheter is arterial and when the system must be changed.	
12. Maintain the pressure bag or device at 300 mm Hg.	Maintains catheter patency.	
13. Print a strip of the arterial pressure waveform, and obtain measurement of the arterial pressures. Note if there are respiratory variations.	Ensures an accurate blood pressure measurement.	

*Level B: Well-designed, controlled studies with results that consistently support a specific action, intervention, or treatment.

Procedure continues on following page

UNIT II

Patient Monitoring and Care —*Continued*

Steps	Rationale	Reportable Conditions
14. Obtain an arterial pressure waveform strip to place on the patient's chart at the start of each shift and whenever a change is found in the waveform.	The printed waveform allows assessment of the adequacy of the waveform, damping, or respiratory variation.	
15. Monitor hemoglobin or hematocrit values daily or as prescribed.	Allows assessment of nosocomial anemia.	• Abnormal hemoglobin values • Abnormal hematocrit values
16. Replace gauze dressings every 2 days and transparent dressings at least every 5–7 days and more frequently as needed.[7,8,15,22] **(Level D*)**	Decreases the risk for infection at the catheter site. The CDC[15] and the Infusion Nurses Society[7,8] recommends replacing the dressing when it becomes damp, loosened, or soiled or when inspection of the site is necessary.	
17. Assess the need for the arterial catheter daily. **(Level D*)**	The CDC[15] does not recommend routine replacement of arterial catheters. Catheters should be removed when no longer needed and should be replaced when there is a clinical indication.	• Signs and symptoms of infection at the arterial catheter insertion site
18. Follow institutional standards for assessing pain. Administer analgesia as prescribed.	Identifies the need for pain interventions.	• Pain at the catheter insertion site.

*Level D: Peer-reviewed professional and organizational standards with the support of clinical study recommendations.

Documentation

Documentation should include the following:
- Patient and family education
- Completion of informed consent
- Preprocedure verifications and time out
- Performance of the modified Allen's test before insertion and its results (when using the radial artery)
- Insertion of the arterial catheter
- Size of the arterial catheter inserted
- Number of insertion attempts
- Date and time of arterial catheter site care and dressing change
- Pain assessment, interventions, and effectiveness
- Site assessment
- Arterial site dressing change
- Intake of flush solution volume
- Printed strip of the arterial pressure waveform
- Appearance of the limb, color, pulse, sensation, movement, capillary refill time, and temperature of the extremity after insertion is complete
- Arterial pressures
- Waveforms
- Occurrence of unexpected outcomes and interventions

References and Additional Readings

For a complete list of references and additional readings for this procedure, scan this QR code with your smartphone, or visit https://www.elsevier.com/__data/assets/pdf_file/0005/1319828/Chapter0053.pdf

PROCEDURE

54 Blood Sampling From an Arterial Catheter

Hillary Crumlett, Katie Neil, and Veronica Ann Lock

PURPOSE: Blood sampling from an arterial catheter is performed to obtain blood specimens for arterial blood gas (ABG) analysis or other laboratory testing.

PREREQUISITE NURSING KNOWLEDGE

- Knowledge of aseptic and sterile technique.
- Knowledge of vascular anatomy and physiology.
- Understanding of gas exchange and acid-base balance.
- Technique for specimen collection and labeling.
- Principles of hemodynamic monitoring.
- Knowledge about the care of patients with an arterial catheter (see Procedure 53, Arterial Catheter Insertion [Assist], Care, and Removal) and stopcock manipulation (see Procedure 60, Single-Pressure and Multiple-Pressure Transducer Systems).
- Understanding of the closed arterial line blood sampling system.
- Closed blood-sampling systems provide the opportunity to reinfuse blood to the patient after the laboratory sample is obtained to help reduce the risk of nosocomial anemia.[3,9-11,15,20,21,25]

EQUIPMENT

- Nonsterile gloves
- Sterile 4 × 4–inch gauze pads
- ABG kit and blood specimen tubes
- Labels with the patient's name and appropriate identifying data
- Laboratory form/electronic laboratory ordering process and specimen labels
- Goggles or fluid-shield face mask
- Needleless blood-sampling access device (blood-transfer device)
- Extra blood-specimen tube (for discard)
- Sterile injectable or noninjectable caps
- Antiseptic solution (i.e., 2% chlorhexidine–based preparation)
- Specimen transport bag(s)
  Additional equipment to have available as needed includes the following:
- Bag of ice

- 5- and 10-mL syringes
- Needleless cannula (for closed arterial blood-sampling system)

PATIENT AND FAMILY EDUCATION

- Explain the procedure to the patient and family. ***Rationale:*** Teaching provides information and may reduce anxiety and fear.
- Explain the importance of keeping the affected extremity immobile. ***Rationale:*** This explanation encourages patient cooperation during blood withdrawal.
- Explain the patient's expected participation during the procedure. ***Rationale:*** Patient cooperation during insertion is encouraged.

PATIENT ASSESSMENT AND PREPARATION

Patient Assessment

- Assess the patency of the arterial catheter. ***Rationale:*** This ensures a functional arterial catheter.
- Assess the patient's previous laboratory results. ***Rationale:*** This assessment provides data for comparison.

Patient Preparation

- Verify the correct patient with two identifiers. ***Rationale:*** Before performing a procedure, the nurse should ensure the correct identification of the patient for the intended intervention.
- Ensure that the patient and family understand the preprocedural teaching. Answer questions as they arise, and reinforce information as needed. ***Rationale:*** Understanding of previously taught information is evaluated and reinforced.
- Expose the stopcock to be used for blood sampling, and position the patient's extremity so the site can easily be accessed. ***Rationale:*** This prepares the site for blood withdrawal.

511

Procedure   for Blood Sampling From an Arterial Catheter

Steps	Rationale	Special Considerations
1. **HH**		
2. **PE**		
3. When obtaining an ABG sample, open the ABG kit, and use the plunger to rid the excess heparin and air from the syringe.	Prepares the ABG syringe.	Heparin is usually in powdered form. If prepackaged ABG kits are not available, draw 0.5 mL of a 1:1000 dilution of heparin in a 3-mL syringe. Pull back on the plunger to coat the inside of the syringe and the needle. Rid the excess heparin and air from the syringe.[2,6]
4. Temporarily suspend the arterial alarms.	Prevents the alarm from sounding as the pressure waveform is lost during the blood draw.	

Blood Sampling With a Needleless Blood-Sampling Access Device (Blood-Transfer Device) or a Syringe

1. Arterial stopcock:		
A. Remove the sterile cap from the port of the three-way stopcock closest to the patient, and attach the needleless blood-sampling access device (blood-transfer device) (Fig. 54.1A) or syringe (see Fig. 54.1B) to the stopcock. *Or*	Prepares for blood sampling.	

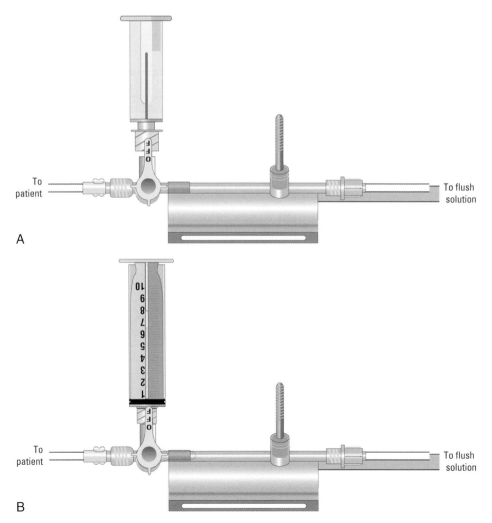

Figure 54.1 **A,** Needleless blood-sampling access device (blood-transfer device) attached to the port of the three-way stopcock. The stopcock is turned "off" to the port of the stopcock. **B,** A syringe attached to the port of the three-way stopcock. The stopcock is turned "off" to the port of the stopcock). *(Courtesy Paul W. Schiffmacher, Thomas Jefferson University Hospital, Philadelphia, PA.)*

UNIT II

Procedure for Blood Sampling From an Arterial Catheter—*Continued*

Steps	Rationale	Special Considerations
B. Cleanse the injectable cap at the top of the stopcock closest to the patient with an antiseptic solution[1,11,13,14,22,23] **(Level B*),** and attach the needleless blood-sampling access device (blood-transfer device) (Fig. 54.2).		
2. Turn the stopcock off to the flush solution (Fig. 54.3).	The needleless blood-sampling access device (blood-transfer device) or syringe is then in direct contact with the blood in the arterial catheter.	
3. When using a needleless blood sampling access device (blood-transfer device), engage the blood specimen tube to obtain the discard volume, or, if using a syringe, slowly and gently aspirate the discard volume.	Clears the catheter of flush solution.	

*Level B: Well-designed, controlled studies with results that consistently support a specific action, intervention, or treatment.

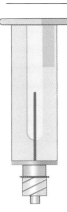

Figure 54.2 Needleless blood-sampling access device (blood-transfer device). *(Courtesy Paul W. Schiffmacher, Thomas Jefferson University Hospital, Philadelphia, PA.)*

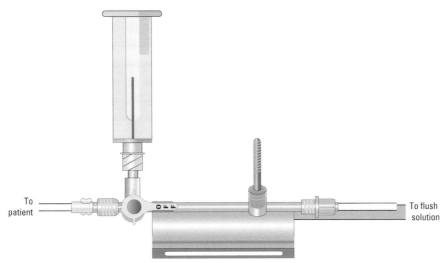

Figure 54.3 Needleless blood-sampling access device (blood-transfer device) attached to the port of the three-way stopcock. The stopcock is turned "off" to the flush solution. *(Courtesy Paul W. Schiffmacher, Thomas Jefferson University Hospital, Philadelphia, PA.)*

Procedure continues on following page

Procedure   for Blood Sampling From an Arterial Catheter—*Continued*

Steps	Rationale	Special Considerations
A. When obtaining blood for an ABG sample, discard a blood sample that is two times the dead space volume. **(Level B*)**	The discard volume includes the dead space and the blood diluted by the flush solution (e.g., dead space of 0.8 mL = 1.6 mL discard).[16,17]	The dead space is the space between the tip of the arterial catheter to the top port of the stopcock.
B. When obtaining blood for coagulation studies (particularly those affected by heparin such as activated partial thromboplastin time and antifactor Xa) from a heparinized arterial line, use a discard volume of six times the dead-space volume. **(Level B*)**	Additional discard is needed to prevent contamination of the specimen with heparin to ensure accurate laboratory results (e.g., dead space of 0.8 mL = 4.8 mL discard).[4,5,8,12,18]	This recommendation does not apply to patients undergoing systemic heparin therapy. More research is needed with this patient population.
4. Turn the stopcock off to the syringe.	Stops blood flow and closes the top port of the stopcock.	Not necessary if using a needleless blood-sampling device.
5. Remove the syringe or the blood-specimen tube, and discard it in the appropriate receptacle.	Removes and safely disposes of the discard.	If unable to dispose of the discard specimen immediately, place it away from the field so it is not mistaken for the actual blood specimen(s) for laboratory analysis.
6. Obtain the blood sample:	Obtains the appropriate blood specimens.	If obtaining multiple laboratory specimens in addition to an ABG and coagulation studies, obtain the laboratory studies according to laboratory specimen order of draw recommendations to minimize the heparin effect and other laboratory tube additive contamination.[7,24,26] Specimen volume should be the amount required for the blood test(s).[7,24,26]
A. If using the needleless system, the stopcock should remain off to the flush solution as each blood specimen tube is engaged.	The needleless blood-sampling access device (blood-transfer device) is a nonvented system, so no backflow of arterial blood from the patient occurs.	
B. If using syringes to obtain blood specimens, turn the stopcock off to the patient before changing each syringe (Fig. 54.4A).	Prevents backflow of arterial blood through the open blood sampling port.	Transfer the specimen to the appropriate laboratory tubes or specimen collection containers in the recommended order when more than one laboratory tube is being filled.[7,24,26]
After each new syringe is attached to the blood-sampling port, turn the stopcock off to the flush solution (see Fig. 54.4B).	Opens the arterial line from the patient to the syringe.	
C. When obtaining an ABG sample, turn the stopcock off to the patient, and attach the ABG syringe directly to the top port of the stopcock, or place the ABG syringe inside of the needleless access device.	Prepares for connection of the ABG syringe.	
D. Turn the stopcock off to the flush solution.	Opens the arterial line to the ABG syringe.	
E. Gently aspirate the ABG sample.	Obtains the ABG sample while minimizing vessel trauma.	

*Level B: Well-designed, controlled studies with results that consistently support a specific action, intervention, or treatment.

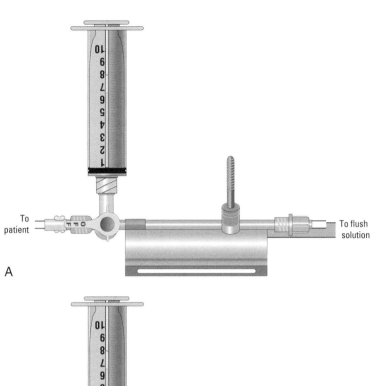

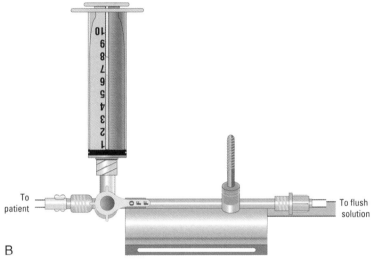

Figure 54.4 A, Syringe attached to the port of the three-way stopcock. The stopcock is turned "off" to the patient. **B,** Syringe attached to the top of the three-way stopcock. The stopcock is turned "off" to the flush solution. *(Courtesy Paul W. Schiffmacher, Thomas Jefferson University Hospital, Philadelphia, PA.)*

Procedure	for Blood Sampling From an Arterial Catheter—*Continued*	
Steps	Rationale	Special Considerations
F. Turn the stopcock off to the patient before removing the ABG syringe.	Prevents the backflow of arterial blood.	
G. Expel any air bubbles from the ABG syringe, and cap the syringe.	Ensures accuracy of the ABG results.	
7. After the last specimen is obtained, turn the stopcock off to the patient.	Detaches the specimen and ensures no backflow of arterial blood from the patient.	
8. Using the fast-flush device, flush the remaining blood from the top port of the stopcock onto a sterile gauze pad, into a discard syringe, or into a blood-specimen tube.	Clears blood from the system.	Follow institutional standards.
9. Turn the stopcock off to the top port of the stopcock.	Opens the system for continuous arterial pressure monitoring.	Remove the needleless blood-sampling access device (blood-transfer device) if used.

Procedure continues on following page

Procedure   for Blood Sampling From an Arterial Catheter—*Continued*

Steps	Rationale	Special Considerations
10. Place a new, sterile, injectable or noninjectable cap to the top port of the stopcock.	Maintains a closed sterile system.	
11. Using the fast-flush device, flush the remaining blood in the arterial catheter back into the patient.	Promotes patency of the arterial catheter.	
Blood Sampling With a Closed Arterial Blood-Sampling System		
1. Slowly and gently pull back on the blood-withdrawal reservoir plunger until it fills to full capacity (Fig. 54.5).	Withdraws and stores blood from the patient until it is ready to be reinfused after blood sampling is complete.	Temporarily silence the arterial alarm.
2. Close the stopcock by turning it perpendicular to the tubing (Fig. 54.6).	Closes the system.	
3. Attach a needleless cannula (Fig. 54.7) to the needleless blood-sampling access device (blood-transfer device) (Fig. 54.8A) or a syringe (see Fig. 54.8B).	Prepares for blood sampling.	
4. Cleanse the blood-sampling port with an antiseptic solution.[1,13,14,19,22,23] **(Level B*)**	Prepares for blood sampling and reduces the risk for infection.	Follow institutional standards.
5. While holding the base of the blood sampling port, engage (push) the needleless cannula (with the attached needleless blood-sampling access dVevice or syringe) into the blood-sampling port (Fig. 54.9).	Prepares for blood sampling.	

*Level B: Well-designed, controlled studies with results that consistently support a specific action, intervention, or treatment.

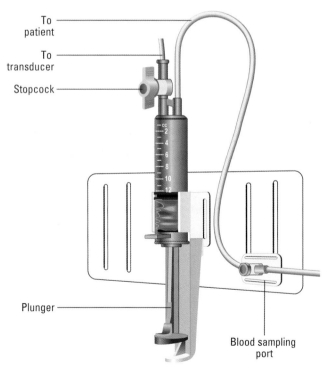

Figure 54.5   Closed blood-sampling system. *(Courtesy Paul W. Schiffmacher, Thomas Jefferson University Hospital, Philadelphia, PA.)*

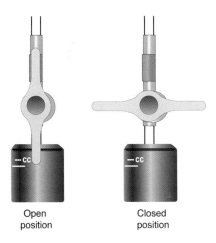

Figure 54.6 The stopcock of a closed blood-sampling system in the open and closed positions. *(Courtesy Paul W. Schiffmacher, Thomas Jefferson University Hospital, Philadelphia, PA.)*

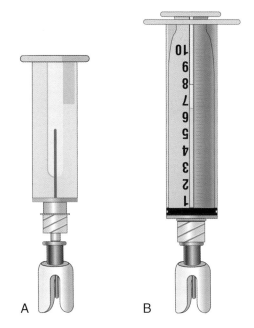

Figure 54.8 **A,** Needleless cannula attached to a needleless blood-sampling access device. **B,** Needleless cannula attached to a syringe. *(Courtesy Paul W. Schiffmacher, Thomas Jefferson University Hospital, Philadelphia, PA.)*

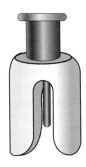

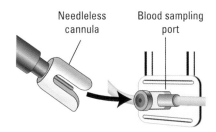

Figure 54.9 Attachment of the needleless cannula into the blood-sampling port of a closed blood-sampling system. *(Courtesy Paul W. Schiffmacher, Thomas Jefferson University Hospital, Philadelphia, PA.)*

Figure 54.7 Needleless cannula for a closed blood-sampling system. *(Courtesy Paul W. Schiffmacher, Thomas Jefferson University Hospital, Philadelphia, PA.)*

Procedure	**for Blood Sampling From an Arterial Catheter—*Continued***	
Steps	Rationale	Special Considerations
6. Engage each blood tube into the needleless blood-sampling access device (blood-transfer device), or obtain an ABG sample.	Obtains the sample.	If obtaining both blood samples and an ABG sample, remove the entire unit (needleless cannula with the needleless blood-sampling access device) before engaging the needleless cannula with the ABG syringe.
7. After the blood samples are obtained, hold the base of the blood-sampling port, and remove the needleless cannula (with attached needleless blood-sampling access device or ABG syringe) from the sampling port by pulling it straight out (Fig. 54.10).	Removes the needleless cannula.	

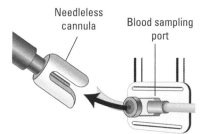

Figure 54.10   Removal of the needleless cannula from the blood-sampling port of the closed blood-sampling system. *(Courtesy Paul W. Schiffmacher, Thomas Jefferson University Hospital, Philadelphia, PA.)*

Procedure   for Blood Sampling From an Arterial Catheter—*Continued*

Steps	Rationale	Special Considerations
8. Open the stopcock by turning it to the open position (parallel to the tubing) (see Fig. 54.6).	Opens the system to prepare for reinfusion of the stored withdrawn blood sample.	
9. Slowly and smoothly reinfuse the discard volume.[3,9,15,20,21] **(Level B*)**	Returns blood to the patient to help reduce the risk of nosocomial anemia.[2,3,12]	
10. Swab the blood sampling port with antiseptic solution.	Removes excess blood and fluid from the sampling port to prevent bacterial growth.	
11. Flush the system with the fast-flush device until the tubing is cleared of blood.	Promotes patency of the arterial catheter.	
After Blood Specimens Are Obtained		
1. Remove **PE**, and discard used supplies in appropriate receptacles.	Reduces transmission of microorganisms; Standard Precautions.	
2. **HH**		
3. Turn the alarms on, and ensure that the waveform returns.	Provides accurate waveform and safe blood pressure monitoring.	
4. Label the specimens, and place them in a transport bag. Complete the laboratory form or laboratory electronic collection per institutional protocol.	Properly identifies the patient and laboratory tests to be performed.	Confirm identifying information. For ABG samples, note the time the specimen was drawn and the percentage of oxygen therapy, patient temperature. and any other data required by institutional protocol.
5. Send the specimens for analysis.	Allows the laboratory to conduct the analysis.	Follow institutional standards regarding the use of ice for ABG samples.

*Level B: Well-designed, controlled studies with results that consistently support a specific action, intervention, or treatment.

Expected Outcomes

- Adequate blood sample with minimal blood loss
- No hemolysis of specimens
- No arterial spasm
- Arterial line patency maintained

Unexpected Outcomes

- Inadequate blood sample
- Hemolysis of specimens
- Arterial spasm
- Dilution of specimens that causes inaccurate laboratory results
- Anemia
- Clotting of the arterial catheter

UNIT II

Patient Monitoring and Care

Steps	Rationale	Reportable Conditions
		These conditions should be reported to the provider if they persist despite nursing interventions.
1. Use the minimal volume of blood discard.	Helps prevent nosocomial anemia.	• Decrease in hemoglobin or hematocrit levels
2. Monitor hemoglobin or hematocrit daily or as prescribed.	Allows early detection of nosocomial anemia.	• Decrease in hemoglobin or hematocrit levels
3. Attempt to group blood draws together whenever possible.	Diminishes the number of times the system is entered to help minimize the risk for infection. Decreases blood discard volume to prevent nosocomial anemia.	• Signs of catheter-related infection • Decrease in hemoglobin or hematocrit levels
4. Before and after the blood withdrawal, assess and evaluate the arterial waveform.	Ensures accurate arterial pressure monitoring.	
5. Turn on arterial blood pressure alarms after blood withdrawal, and review parameters.	Ensures safe arterial pressure monitoring.	
6. Obtain laboratory specimen results.	Monitors test results.	• Abnormal specimen results

Documentation

Documentation should include the following:
• Patient and family education
• Date, time, and type of specimen drawn
• Unexpected outcomes
• Additional nursing interventions
• Results of laboratory tests, when available

References and Additional Readings

For a complete list of references and additional readings for this procedure, scan this QR code with your smartphone, or visit https://www.elsevier.com/__data/assets/pdf_file/0006/1319829/Chapter0054.pdf.

55 Arterial Pressure–Based Cardiac Output Monitoring

Susan Scott

PURPOSE Arterial pressure–based cardiac output monitoring is a minimally invasive technology that can be used to obtain hemodynamic data on a continuous basis.

PREREQUISITE NURSING KNOWLEDGE

- Anatomy and physiology of the cardiovascular system.
- Anatomy and physiology of the vasculature and adjacent structures.
- Pathophysiological changes that occur in heart disease and affect flow dynamics.
- Aseptic technique.
- Hemodynamic effects of vasoactive medications and fluid resuscitation.
- Principles involved in hemodynamic monitoring.
- Invasive cardiac output (CO) monitoring.
- Arterial waveform interpretation.
- Definitions and norms for CO, cardiac index, systemic vascular resistance, stroke volume, stroke index, stroke volume variation, preload, afterload, and contractility.
- Arterial pressure represents the forcible ejection of blood from the left ventricle into the aorta and out into the arterial system. During ventricular systole, blood is ejected into the aorta, generating a pressure wave. Because of the intermittent pumping action of the heart, this arterial pressure wave is generated in a pulsatile manner (see Fig. 53.1). The ascending limb of the aortic pressure wave (anacrotic limb) represents an increase in pressure because of left-ventricular ejection. The peak of ejection is the peak systolic pressure, which is normally 100 to 140 mm Hg in adults. After reaching this peak, the ventricular pressure decreases to a level below aortic pressure and the aortic valve closes, marking the end of ventricular systole. The closure of the aortic valve produces a small rebound wave that creates a notch known as the *dicrotic notch.* The descending limb of the curve (diastolic downslope) represents diastole and is characterized by a long declining pressure wave, during which the aortic wall recoils and propels blood into the arterial network. The diastolic pressure is measured at the lowest point of the diastolic down slope and is normally 60 to 80 mm Hg.
- The difference between the systolic and diastolic pressures is called the *pulse pressure,* with a normal value of 40 mm Hg.

- Arterial pressure is determined by the relationship between blood flow through the vessels (stroke volume), the compliance of the aorta and larger vessels, and the resistance of the more peripheral vessel walls (systemic vascular resistance). The arterial pressure is therefore affected by factors that change either CO, compliance, or systemic vascular resistance.
- The average arterial pressure during a cardiac cycle is called the *mean arterial pressure* (MAP). It is not the average of the systolic plus the diastolic pressures because at normal heart rates, systole accounts for one-third of the cardiac cycle, and diastole accounts for two-thirds of the cardiac cycle. The MAP is calculated automatically by most patient monitoring systems; however, it can be calculated manually using the following formula:

$$\frac{systolic\ BP + (2 \times diastolic\ BP)}{3}$$

- MAP represents the driving force (perfusion pressure) for blood flow through the cardiovascular system. MAP is at its highest point in the aorta. As blood travels through the circulatory system, systolic pressure increases and diastolic pressure decreases, with an overall decline in the MAP (see Fig. 53.2).
- Arterial pressure–based cardiac output (APCO) is obtained from the analysis of the pressure waveform of an arterial catheter.[1,2]
- Stroke volume and heart rate are key determinants of CO.
- Although systemic vascular resistance affects CO, the location of this effect is global and not limited by location of the measurement, because CO is measured as flow per minute throughout the body. Manufacturers of arterial pressure–based CO systems have factored in variance for both radial artery catheters and femoral artery catheters.[2,5]
- Ultrasound guidance is recommended to place arterial catheters if the technology is available.[6-8]

EQUIPMENT

- Invasive arterial catheter and insertion kit
- Specialized sterile transducer and sensor kit (manufacturer specific)

- Intravenous (IV) pole and transducer holder (manufacturer specific)
- Pressure-transducer system, including flush solution recommended according to institutional standards, a pressure bag or device, pressure tubing with transducer, and flush device
- Pressure module and cable for interface with the monitor
- Normal saline-flush solution
- Monitoring system (central and bedside monitor)
- Special monitor to interface with the bedside monitor for trending and display of hemodynamic values (manufacturer specific)
- Dual-channel recorder
- Indelible marker
- Nonvented (noninjectable) caps
- Leveling device (low-intensity laser or carpenter level)
- Sterile and nonsterile gloves
  Additional equipment to have available as needed includes the following:
- Heparin, if prescribed
- 3-mL syringe
- Dressing supplies
- Tape
- Sterile ultrasound probe cover
- Sterile ultrasound gel

PATIENT AND FAMILY EDUCATION

- Explain the rationale for arterial line insertion, including how the arterial pressure is displayed on the bedside monitor. *Rationale:* This explanation may decrease patient and family anxiety and increase understanding.
- Explain the standard of care to the patient and family, including the insertion procedure, alarms, dressings, and length of time the catheter is expected to be in place. *Rationale:* This explanation encourages the patient and family to ask questions and voice concerns about the procedure and may decrease patient and family anxiety.
- Explain the patient's expected participation during the procedure. *Rationale:* Patients will know how they can help with the procedure.
- Explain the importance of keeping the affected extremity immobile. *Rationale:* This explanation encourages patient cooperation to prevent catheter dislodgment and ensures a more accurate waveform.
- Instruct the patient to report any warmth, redness, pain, numbness, or wet feeling at the insertion site at any time, including after catheter removal. *Rationale:* These symptoms may indicate infection, bleeding, or disconnection of the tubing or catheter.

PATIENT ASSESSMENT AND PREPARATION

Patient Assessment

- Obtain the patient's medical history, including a history of peripheral vascular disease, diabetes, and hypertension. *Rationale:* These conditions increase the patient's risk for arterial or venous insufficiency.
- Obtain the patient's medical history for peripheral vascular disease, vascular grafts, arteriovenous fistulas or shunts, arterial vasospasm, thrombosis, or embolism. In addition, obtain the patient's history of coronary artery bypass graft surgery in which radial arteries were removed for use as conduits. *Rationale:* Extremities with any of these problems should be avoided as sites for cannulation because of the potential for complications.
- Assess the neurovascular and peripheral vascular status of the extremity to be used for the arterial cannulation, including color, temperature, presence and fullness of pulses, capillary refill, presence of bruit, and motor and sensory function (compared with the opposite extremity). Note: A modified Allen's test may be performed before cannulation of the radial artery. *Rationale:* This assessment may identify neurovascular or circulatory impairment so potential complications related to radial artery cannulation may be avoided.
- Assess the patient's vital signs and compliance factors (e.g., age, gender, height, weight). *Rationale:* This assessment provides baseline data. The compliance factors allow for the individual variables that ultimately dictate pulse pressure and its relevance (proportionality) to stroke volume.

Patient Preparation

- Verify the correct patient with two identifiers. *Rationale:* Before performing a procedure, the nurse should ensure the correct identification of the patient for the intended intervention.
- Ensure that the patient and family understand preprocedural teaching. Answer questions as they arise, and reinforce information as needed. *Rationale:* Understanding of previously taught information is evaluated and reinforced.
- Ensure that informed consent has been obtained. *Rationale:* Informed consent protects the rights of the patient and makes a competent decision possible for the patient.
- Perform a preprocedure verification and time-out, if nonemergent. *Rationale:* This ensures patient safety.
- Validate the patency of IV access. *Rationale:* Access may be needed for administration of emergency medications or fluids.
- Place the patient's extremity in the appropriate position with adequate lighting of the insertion site. *Rationale:* This placement prepares the site for cannulation and facilitates accurate insertion.

Procedure | for Arterial Pressure–Based Cardiac Output Monitoring

Steps	Rationale	Special Considerations
Initiating the Procedure		
1. HH		
2. PE		
3. If the radial artery is to be used, perform the modified Allen's test before the puncture. **(Level C*)**	The modified Allen's test has been recommended before a radial artery puncture to assess the patency of the ulnar artery and an intact superficial palmar arch.	The modified Allen's test does not always ensure adequate flow through the ulnar artery.[4,15] A Doppler ultrasound flow indicator or pulse oximeter waveform can also be used to further verify blood flow.[3,6,7,10,13]
4. Prepare the flush solution (see Procedure 60, Single-Pressure and Multiple-Pressure Transducer Systems). A. Use an IV solution of normal saline or solution based on institutional standards		Some institutional standards may include using heparin.
5. Gather the equipment needed for obtaining an arterial pressure–based CO.	Prepares supplies.	Refer to the manufacturer's recommendations for additional required equipment for setup and maintenance. Some technologies require additional calibration procedures and equipment.[14]
6. Obtain the patient's baseline compliance factors (e.g., age, gender, height, weight). **(Level M*)**	This information may be needed to allow for the individual variables that ultimately dictate pulse pressure and its relevance (proportionality) to stroke volume.	Follow manufacturer's guidelines. Some manufacturers require calibration. Manufacturers that do not require calibration use age, gender, height, and weight to determine vascular compliance. An accurate height and weight reflecting perfused tissue is important in the determination of body surface area (BSA) and cardiac index. Fluid weight gain often is discounted because it is not perfused tissue. Medications are generally based on perfused weight in the case of morbidly obese patients. Because adipose tissue is highly vascular, actual weight and height are necessary to determine BSA. BSA is needed for calculating indexed values.
7. Remove PE, and discard used supplies.	Reduces transmission of micro-organisms; standard precautions.	
8. HH		
Setting Up the Arterial Pressure–Based Cardiac Output (APCO) System		
1. HH		
2. PE		
3. Open the APCO sensor kit.	Prepares equipment.	Follow manufacturer's recommendations.
4. Secure all connections.	Tight connections ensure the integrity of the system.	Vented caps are standard with transducer sets and allow for initial priming of the system.
5. Insert the APCO sensor into the transducer holder that is secured on the IV pole next to the patient.	Stabilizes the sensor.	

*Level C: Qualitative studies, descriptive or correlational studies, integrative reviews, systematic reviews, or randomized controlled trials with inconsistent results.
*Level M: Manufacturer's recommendations only.

Procedure for Arterial Pressure–Based Cardiac Output Monitoring—*Continued*

Steps	Rationale	Special Considerations
6. Level the vent port near the sensor to the phlebostatic axis.	The reference point is the phlebostatic axis because it accurately reflects central arterial pressure.[11]	
7. Prime or flush the entire APCO system:	Removes air bubbles.	Prime the system using gravity to minimize small bubbles. In-line reservoir systems are available to avoid wasting blood during blood draws.
A. Activate the flush device to deliver the flush solution through the sensor and out through the vent port.	Removes air from the system.	
B. Close the vent port by turning the stopcock to the neutral position.		
C. Place a sterile nonvented (noninjectable) cap on the top of the stopcock.	Maintains a closed sterile system.	
D. Purge air from the remaining part of the tubing.	Prepares the monitoring system.	
8. Inflate the pressure bag or device to 300 mm Hg.	Inflating the pressure bag to 300 mm Hg allows approximately 1–3 mL/hour of flush solution to be delivered through the catheter, thus maintaining catheter patency and minimizing clot formation.	
9. Assist as needed with insertion of the arterial catheter (see Procedures 52, Arterial Catheter Insertion [Perform], and 53, Arterial Catheter Insertion [Assist], Care, and Removal).	Provides needed assistance.	
10. Connect the bedside monitor cable to the APCO sensor.	Information can then be transferred from the sensor to the monitor.	Follow manufacturer's guidelines. Some cables are color coded.
11. Enter the patient's gender, age, height, and weight. **(Level M*)**	This information is needed to allow for the individual variables that ultimately dictate pulse pressure and its relevance (proportionality) to stroke volume. The result is stroke volume variability.	Follow manufacturer's guidelines. Some manufacturers require calibration.
12. Set up the monitor.	Prepares equipment.	Follow the manufacturer's guidelines as the setup may vary.
13. Observe the CO display.	Provides assessment data.	The CO value is updated regularly based on the manufacturer.
14. Set the alarm parameters according to the patient's current blood pressure and institutional protocols.	Activates the bedside and central alarm system.	Follow manufacturer's guidelines.
15. Remove **PE**, and discard used supplies in appropriate receptacles.	Reduces transmission of microorganisms; standard precautions.	Ensure that sharps are safely disposed.
16. **HH**		

*Level M: Manufacturer's recommendations only.

Procedure continues on following page

UNIT II

Expected Outcomes

- Accurate measurement of CO
- Maintenance of catheter patency
- Minimal discomfort from the arterial catheter
- Maintenance of baseline hemoglobin and hematocrit levels
- Adequate circulation to the involved extremity
- Adequate sensory and motor function of the extremity
- Maintenance of the catheter site without infection

Unexpected Outcomes

- Poor-quality arterial pressure wave leading to the inability to obtain an accurate CO
- Infection
- Impaired peripheral tissue perfusion (e.g., edema, coolness, pain, paleness, or slow capillary refill of the fingers of the cannulated extremity)
- Perforated or lacerated artery
- Hematoma at the insertion site
- Pain or discomfort from the arterial catheter insertion site
- Decreased hemoglobin and hematocrit values
- Catheter disconnection with significant blood loss

Patient Monitoring and Care

Steps	Rationale	Reportable Conditions
		These conditions should be reported to the provider if they persist despite nursing interventions.
1. Assess the neurovascular and peripheral vascular status of the cannulated extremity immediately after catheter insertion and every 4 hours, or more often if needed. Follow institutional standards.	Determines peripheral vascular and neurovascular integrity. Changes in sensation, motor function, pulses, color, temperature, or capillary refill may indicate ischemia, arterial spasm, or neurovascular compromise.	• Diminished or absent pulses • Pale, mottled, or cyanotic appearance of the extremity • Extremity that is cool or cold to the touch • Capillary refill time of more than 2 seconds (or longer than the patient's baseline) • Diminished or absent sensation • Diminished or absent motor function
2. Assess the arterial catheter insertion site for signs and symptoms of infection.	Identifies the possibility of site infection.	• Redness at the site • Purulent drainage • Tenderness or pain at the insertion site • Elevated temperature • Elevated white blood cell count
3. Continuously monitor heart rate, blood pressure, and cardiac indices.	Provides an assessment of patient status.	• Abnormal vital signs • Abnormal CO • Abnormal cardiac index
4. Follow institutional standards for assessing pain. Administer analgesia as prescribed.	Identifies the need for pain interventions.	• Continued pain despite pain interventions
5. Assess the patient's response to prescribed interventions.	The hemodynamic management of the patient requires close monitoring and interventions based on the parameters obtained from the APCO data.	• Abnormal CO • Abnormal cardiac index • Abnormal vital signs
6. Replace gauze dressings every 2 days and transparent dressings at least every 5–7 days and more frequently as needed[6,7,9] May use a chlorhexidine sponge per institutional policy. **(Level D*)**	Decreases the risk for infection at the catheter site. The CDC and the Infusion Nurses Society recommend replacing the dressing when the dressing becomes damp, loosened, or soiled or when inspection of the site is necessary.[6,7]	

*Level D: Peer-reviewed professional and organizational standards with the support of clinical study recommendations.

Documentation

Documentation should include the following:
- Patient and family education
- Informed consent
- Preprocedure verification and time-out
- Patient tolerance of the procedure
- Peripheral vascular and neurovascular assessment before and after the procedure
- Assessment of the insertion site
- Patient response to the insertion procedure
- Pain assessment, interventions, and effectiveness
- Type of flush used
- Amount of flush solution on the intake and output record
- Vital signs, CO, cardiac index, and other hemodynamic parameters
- Positive flow by modified Allen's test if the radial artery is used
- Site assessment
- Unexpected outcomes
- Additional nursing interventions

References and Additional Readings

For a complete list of references and additional readings for this procedure, scan this QR code with your smartphone, or visit https://www.elsevier.com/__data/assets/pdf_file/0007/1319830/Chapter0055.pdf.

56 Central Venous/Right Atrial Pressure Monitoring

Carrie Boom

PURPOSE Right atrial pressure (RAP), when measured accurately, reflects the right ventricular end-diastolic pressure. Central venous pressure (CVP) monitoring, which may be measured in the distal superior or inferior vena cava, is identical to right-atrial pressure in the absence of vena caval obstruction. If CVP monitoring of the inferior vena cava (femoral catheterization) is utilized, the absence of elevated abdominal pressure is clinically necessary for accuracy.[1,8] By reflecting right ventricular end-diastolic pressure, CVP/RAP monitoring allows for evaluation of right-sided heart hemodynamics, right ventricular preload, and patient response to therapy.[4] In addition to being responsive to changes in pulmonary vascular resistance, CVP/RAP influences and is influenced by venous return and cardiac function. Although the CVP/RAP is used as a measure of changes in the right ventricle, the relationship is not linear because the right ventricle is able to expand and alter its compliance. Hence, changes in volume can occur with little change in pressure.[2] Evaluating the pressure number in the context of the patient's clinical condition is imperative.

PREREQUISITE NURSING KNOWLEDGE

- Knowledge of the normal anatomy and physiology of the cardiovascular system.
- Knowledge of the principles of aseptic technique and infection control.
- Principles of hemodynamic monitoring.
- The CVP/RAP represents right-sided preload by reflecting right-ventricular pressure at the end of diastole.
- The CVP/RAP normally ranges from 2 to 8 mm Hg in the adult.
- A CVP/RAP is obtained through a central venous catheter inserted in a central vein with the tip of the catheter placed in the distal superior vena cava (SVC) or in the distal inferior vena cava (IVC) close to the right atrium.
- Use of femoral venous pressure (inferior vena caval or iliac venous pressure) has been found to correlate with CVP/RAP if the abdominal pressure (i.e., bladder pressure) is less than 15 mm Hg.[1]
- Knowledge is needed of the setup, leveling, and zeroing of the hemodynamic monitoring system (see Procedure 60, Single-Pressure and Multiple-Pressure Transducer Systems).
- Interpretation of CVP/RAP waveforms including identification of *a*, *c*, and *v* ascending waves is important. The *a* wave reflects right atrial contraction and is followed by an *x* descent. The *c* wave reflects closure of the tricuspid valve. The *v* wave reflects passive filling of the atria during right-ventricular systole and is followed by a *y* descent (Fig. 56.1). Accurate CVP/RAP measurement is the mean of the *a* wave (when present) or the base of the *c* wave (when an *a* wave is not present) (Table 56.1).
- Some pathology can alter the waves and must be considered when interpreting the CVP/RAP waveform (see Table 56.1).

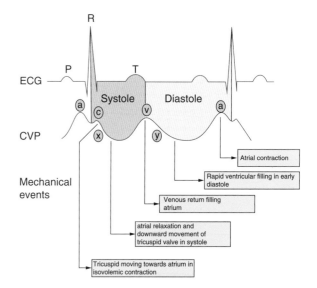

Figure 56.1 The relationship of the central venous pressure (CVP) tracing to the electrocardiogram (ECG) in normal sinus rhythm. The normal CVP waveform consists of three upward deflections (*A*, *C*, and *V* waves) and two downward deflections (*X* and *Y* descents). The *A* wave is produced by right atrial contraction and occurs just after the P wave on the ECG. The C wave occurs because of the isovolumic ventricular contraction forcing the tricuspid valve to bulge upward into the right atrium. The pressure within the right atrium then decreases as the tricuspid valve is pulled away from the atrium during right ventricular ejection, forming the X descent. The right atrium continues to fill during late ventricular systole, forming the V wave. The Y descent occurs when the tricuspid valve opens and blood from the right atrium empties rapidly into the right ventricle during early diastole. *(From Raut MS, Maheshwari A: "x" descent of CVP: An indirect measure of RV dysfunction?. J Anaesthesiol Clin Pharmacol 30[3]:430–431, 2014.)*

TABLE 56.1 | **Pathologies That Can Alter CVP/RAP Measurement Strategies**

The *red dashed mark* indicates where the mean of the *a* wave would be obtained at end expiration. In all but the second example, the mean of the *a* wave is obtained by placing this monitoring line with approximately two-thirds of the area of the triangular wave above the monitoring line and one-third of the area of the triangular wave below the monitoring line (with the cannon wave excluded from example 5). In the second example, the measurement is taken at the base of the c wave.

Pathology/ condition	Findings and Measurement Strategy	Example
Sinus Rhythm	Measure the mean of the *a* wave at end expiration To estimate the mean of the *a* wave estimate 2/3 of wave above cursor, 1/3 of wave below cursor	
Atrial fibrillation Atrial Flutter	Absence or abnormal timing of *a* wave(s) Measure the CVP/RAP at the base of the *c* wave at end expiration	
Tricuspid stenosis	Enlargement of the *a* wave due to atrial contraction against a stenotic tricuspid valve No measurement change	
Tricuspid regurgitation	Increased *v* wave due to regurgitant pressure back into the atria during systole due to valvular incompetence. The enlarged *v* wave should be excluded in the measurement of the mean of the *a* wave.	
Complete heart block Premature ventricular/ junctional contraction Junctional rhythm	Can result in a simultaneous merge of the *a* and *v* waves (referred to as a "cannon" *a* wave) If possible, care should be taken to exclude the abnormal *a* waves in the measurement of the mean of the *a* wave.	Common
Pericardial tamponade	Decreased *y* descent following the *v* wave due to poor ventricular filling during early diastole.	
Cardiomegaly	In the setting of correctly positioned PA catheter, the CVP monitoring port may be advanced past the tricuspid valve and will read a right ventricular waveform (with a *v* wave which emulates the PA systolic pressure) Exclude the *v* wave and read the waveform just prior to the ventricular upstroke.	Equiv to PA syst

CVP, Central venous pressure; *LVEDP,* left ventricular end diastolic pressure; *RAP,* right atrial pressure
Modified from *Atlas of cardiovascular monitoring,* New York, 1998, Churchill Livingstone.

EQUIPMENT

- Pressure transducer system, including flush solution recommended according to institutional standards, a pressure bag or device, pressure tubing with a transducer, and a flush device (see Procedure 60, Single-Pressure and Multiple-Pressure Transducer Systems)
- Pressure module and cable for interface with the monitor
- Dual-channel recorder
- Leveling device (low-intensity laser or carpenter level)
- Nonsterile gloves
- Sterile injectable or noninjectable caps
- Indelible skin marker (to mark the phlebostatic axis)

PATIENT AND FAMILY EDUCATION

- Discuss the purpose of the central venous catheter and monitoring with both the patient and family. ***Rationale:*** This discussion reduces anxiety and includes the patient and family in the plan of care.
- Explain the patient's expected participation during the procedure. ***Rationale:*** This explanation encourages patient assistance.

PATIENT ASSESSMENT AND PREPARATION

Patient Assessment

- Determine hemodynamic, cardiovascular, and peripheral vascular status. ***Rationale:*** This assessment provides baseline data.
- Determine the patient's baseline pulmonary status. If the patient is mechanically ventilated, note the type of support, ventilator mode, presence or absence of positive end-expiratory pressure (PEEP) or continuous positive airway pressure (CPAP), and patient effort (i.e., initiating breaths,

overbreathing the ventilator). ***Rationale:*** The presence of mechanical ventilation alters hemodynamic waveforms and pressures.

- Assess for signs and symptoms of fluid volume deficit. Signs and symptoms may include thirst, oliguria, tachycardia, and dry mucous membranes. ***Rationale:*** Assessment data may correlate with a decreased CVP/RAP value.
- Assess for signs and symptoms of fluid volume excess. Signs and symptoms may include dyspnea, abnormal breath sounds (i.e., crackles), S_3 heart sounds, peripheral edema, tachycardia, and jugular vein distention. ***Rationale:*** Assessment data may correlate with an increased CVP/RAP value.

Patient Preparation

- Verify the correct patient with two identifiers. ***Rationale:*** Before performing a procedure, the nurse should ensure the correct identification of the patient for the intended intervention.
- Ensure that the patient and family understand the preprocedural teaching. Answer questions as they arise, and reinforce information as needed. ***Rationale:*** Understanding of previously taught information is evaluated and reinforced.

Procedure for Central Venous/Right Atrial Pressure Monitoring		
Steps	Rationale	Special Considerations
1. HH 2. PE 3. Position the patient in the supine position with the head of the bed at any angle between 0 and 60 degrees.[1] **(Level B*)**	Standardized positioning may improve the accuracy of identifying the phlebostatic axis and the consistency of serial trending of CVP/RAP.	For those unable to tolerate supine positioning with the head of the bed elevated 0 to 45 degrees, CVP/RAP may be obtained with the head of the bed elevated up to 60 degrees with the patient in an up to 90-degree lateral position, or prone after allowing stabilization of 5–15 minutes (or longer for prone positioning).[1,8] With each of these maneuvers, the level of the right atrium will be altered from the previously identified phlebostatic axis.[3]
4. Level the air-fluid interface of the monitoring system to the phlebostatic axis (see Procedure 60, Single-Pressure and Multiple-Pressure Transducer Systems)	The phlebostatic axis is used as the reference point for the air-fluid interface. It is located at the fourth intercostal space (ICS) midway between the anterior and posterior thorax (not the mid-axillary line) and represents the approximate level of the atria.	Mark the location of the phlebostatic axis if not already identified. It is recommended to use a leveling device such as a low-intensity laser or carpenter level. Great variability exists with or without these assistive devices.[9] Great care must be taken to ensure proper identification of the phlebostatic axis and leveling location.
5. Zero the transducer (see Procedure 60, Single-Pressure and Multiple-Pressure Transducer Systems).	Allows the monitor to use atmospheric pressure as a reference for zero.	
6. Ensure that the CVP/RAP line is a closed system before measuring and documenting (i.e., without open stopcocks or infusing solutions).	Open stopcocks or infusing solutions will adversely affect accuracy of the CVP/RAP measurement.	

Procedure for Central Venous/Right Atrial Pressure Monitoring—*Continued*

Steps	Rationale	Special Considerations
7. Identify the scale of the CVP/RAP tracing (Figs. 56.2 and 56.3).	Aids in determining the pressure measurement.	The CVP/RAP scale commonly is set at 10–30 mm Hg depending on the patient's CVP/RAP (recommend setting the scale just slightly above the highest wave on the CVP/RAP tracing to enable well-visualized waves). The CVP/RAP may be best appreciated in an "Optimum Scale" setting on the monitor, if available.
8. Observe the waveform, and perform a dynamic response test (square wave test) (see Fig. 56.4).	Determines whether the system is damped. This will ensure that the pressure waveform components are clearly defined. This aids in accurate measurement.	The square wave test can be performed by activating and quickly releasing the fast flush. A sharp upstroke should terminate in a flat line at the maximal indicator on the monitor. This should be followed by an immediate rapid downstroke extending below baseline with 1–2 oscillations within 0.12 second and a quick return to baseline (Fig. 56.4).

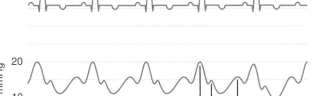

Figure 56.2 Example of measuring a CVP/RAP from a paper printout at end-expiration in a spontaneously breathing patient. While observing the patient, identify inspiration. The point just before inspiration is end-expiration. The *arrow* indicates the point of end-expiration. Reading is taken as a mean value of the *a* wave. The RAP value for this patient is 16 mm Hg.

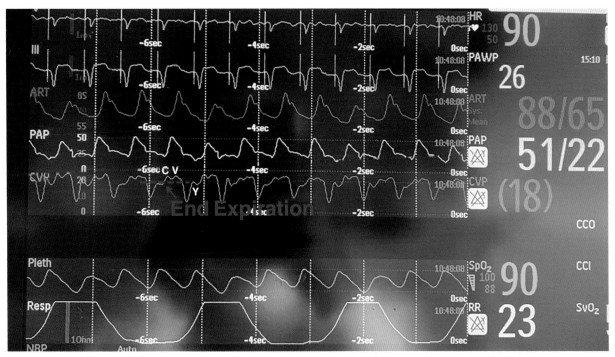

Figure 56.3 From personal photo. The above screen shot shows a patient in atrial fibrillation, with ventricular pacing. End-expiration is challenging in the CVP/RAP waveform but can be seen more easily in the PA pressure waveform, and the respiratory waveform also provides clues to end-expiration. Note that there is no *a* wave, only *c* and *v* waves with a steep y descent. Measurement at the base of the c wave at end-expiration shows a CVP/RAP of 18.

Procedure continues on following page

Procedure | for Central Venous/Right Atrial Pressure Monitoring—*Continued*

Steps	Rationale	Special Considerations

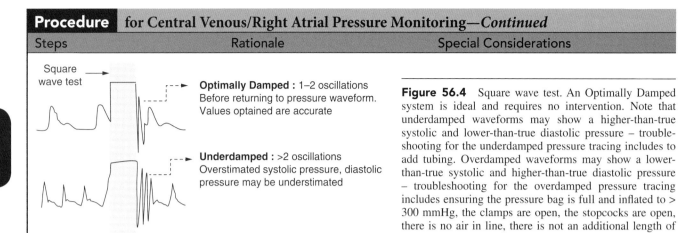

Optimally Damped : 1–2 oscillations
Before returning to pressure waveform.
Values optained are accurate

Underdamped : >2 oscillations
Overstimated systolic pressure, diastolic
pressure may be understimated

Overdamped : <1.5 oscillations
Understimation of systolic pressure,
diastolic may not be affected

Figure 56.4   Square wave test. An Optimally Damped system is ideal and requires no intervention. Note that underdamped waveforms may show a higher-than-true systolic and lower-than-true diastolic pressure – troubleshooting for the underdamped pressure tracing includes to add tubing. Overdamped waveforms may show a lower-than-true systolic and higher-than-true diastolic pressure – troubleshooting for the overdamped pressure tracing includes ensuring the pressure bag is full and inflated to > 300 mmHg, the clamps are open, the stopcocks are open, there is no air in line, there is not an additional length of tubing added. *(From Comisso I, Lucchini A: Cardiovascular assessment. In Nursing in critical care setting, Cham, 2018, Springer.)*

Steps	Rationale	Special Considerations
9. Run a dual-channel strip of, or "freeze" the monitor including the electrocardiogram (ECG) and CVP/RAP waveform (see Figs. 56.2 and 56.3).	Right atrial pressures should be determined in coordination with the real-time ECG tracing from the graphic recording or the monitor stop-cursor option so end-expiration can be properly identified.	Many monitors are capable of "freeze framing" waveforms to include ECG and CVP/RAP waveforms in real time, and most allow both vertical and horizontal cursors that can be used to identify the *a, c,* and *v* waves and to determine the best location for end-expiration measurements. Caution: the use of portable telemetry monitoring may create a "lag" of several seconds between the ECG and pressure waveform tracings. Refer to institutional policies regarding the appropriate use of telemetry to ensure accuracy.
10. Measure all hemodynamic pressures at end-expiration. **(Level B*)**	Atmospheric and alveolar pressures are approximately equal at end-expiration. Intrathoracic pressure is closest to zero at end-expiration. Measurement of hemodynamic pressures is most accurate at end-expiration because pulmonary pressures have minimal effect on intracardiac pressures.	Extubated patients and patients on ventilators who spontaneously breathe have diaphragmatic drive of their respirations, which creates a negative pressure on inspiration. Intubated patients who are on significant positive support or who are not spontaneously breathing have breath delivered, which creates a positive pressure during inspiration[5] (Table 56.2).
11. Determine end-expiration by observing the rise and fall of the chest during breathing. This may be combined with printed graphics of hemodynamic, respiratory, capnography, or continuous airway pressure waveforms.	Aids in determination of the end-expiratory phase of ventilation.	

TABLE 56.2	General Respiratory Variation Patterns in Central Line Tracings

This table reviews the general respiration variability that occurs in different modes of ventilation from extubated to full ventilator support without respiratory effort. The *red circles* indicate end-expiration, the general area where a measurement from the CVP/RAP can be accurately found.

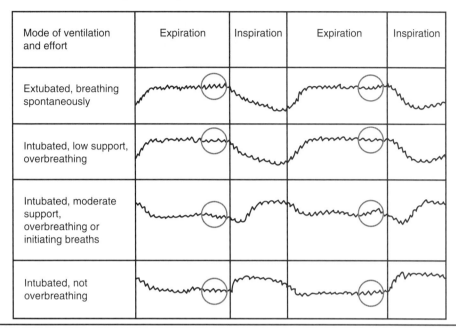

Mode of ventilation and effort	Expiration	Inspiration	Expiration	Inspiration
Extubated, breathing spontaneously				
Intubated, low support, overbreathing				
Intubated, moderate support, overbreathing or initiating breaths				
Intubated, not overbreathing				

CVP, Central venous pressure; *RAP,* right atrial pressure.
Modified from *Atlas of cardiovascular monitoring,* New York, 1998, Churchill Livingstone.

Procedure	for Central Venous/Right Atrial Pressure Monitoring—*Continued*

Steps	Rationale	Special Considerations
12. Identify the *a* (if present), *c*, and *v* waves in the area of the waveform identified as end-expiration.	Electrical activity (ECG) precedes mechanical activity. The first wave on the CVP/RAP waveform that follows the *p* wave on the ECG usually represents the *a* wave. The next wave generally represents the *c* wave, and the next wave in series represents the *v* wave (see Fig. 56.1).	See Table 56.1 for CVP/RAP measurement strategies in several common conditions/pathologies.
13. Obtain the CVP/RAP measurement by finding the mean of the *a* wave (or in the setting of an absent or abnormal *a* wave, obtain the measurement at the base of the *c* wave) at end-expiration.	The *a* wave represents the open tricuspid valve in diastole, therefore left ventricular end-diastolic pressure (see Fig. 56.1).	Monitors average the CVP/RAP waveform throughout the cycle of breathing; this can result in incorrect monitor (and documented) readings. Inaccurate readings may result in adverse medical therapy.
14. Document the CVP/RAP measurement that you obtained per your hospital documentation guidelines.	Trending CVP/RAP can affect medical decisions.	Documenting special circumstances (cannon *a* waves in the setting of junctional rhythm, large *v* waves in the setting of tricuspid regurgitation) assists other providers to know if changes are found in future CVP/RAP measurements.
15. Remove **PE**, and discard used supplies in appropriate receptacles.	Reduces the transmission of microorganisms; standard precautions.	
16. **HH**		

Procedure continues on following page

UNIT II

Expected Outcomes

- Accurate CVP/RAP measurements
- Adequate and appropriate waveforms
- CVP/RAP readings that correlate with physical findings
- Evaluation of information obtained to guide therapeutic interventions

Unexpected Outcomes

- Inaccurate readings
- CVP/RAP readings that do not correlate with physical findings
- Infection
- Sepsis
- Air embolism
- Occluded catheter

Patient Monitoring and Care

Steps	Rationale	Reportable Conditions
		These conditions should be reported to the provider if they persist despite nursing interventions.
1. Recheck leveling whenever the patient position changes.	Ensures an accurate reference point at the phlebostatic axis. A transducer below the phlebostatic axis will read a falsely elevated CVP/RAP, while a transducer placed above the level of the phlebostatic axis will read a falsely low CVP/RAP.	
2. Zero the transducer during initial setup or before insertion, if disconnection occurs between the transducer and the monitoring cable, if disconnection occurs between the monitoring cable and the monitor, at least once per shift, and when the values obtained do not fit the clinical picture. Follow the manufacturer's recommendations regarding routine zeroing of the system.	Ensures accuracy of the hemodynamic monitoring system; minimizes the risk for contamination of the system.	
3. Monitor the pressure transducer system (pressure tubing, transducer, stopcocks) for air, and eliminate air from the system.	Avoid air entry into the system. Air emboli are potentially fatal.	• Suspected air entry into the patient's central line
4. Assess central venous catheter patency every 8 hours, and administer thrombolytics as prescribed if the catheter is occluded.[7]	Ensures catheter patency. Evidence suggests correlation with thrombosed central venous catheter (CVC) and line infection.[11]	• Occluded catheter
5. Continuously monitor the CVP/RAP waveform, and obtain the hemodynamic value hourly (or per institutional standards) and as necessary with changes in the patient's condition.	Provides for continuous waveform analysis and assessment of patient status.	• Abnormal or unexpected appearance of CVP/RAP waveforms • Change in waveform • Unexpected or significant change in CVP/RAP measurement
6. Change the hemodynamic monitoring system (flush solution, pressure tubing, transducer, and stopcocks) every 96 hours. The flush solution may need to be changed more frequently if the volume of solution is decreased.	The U.S. Centers for Disease Control and Prevention (CDC) and the Infusion Nurses Society recommend that the hemodynamic flush system can be used safely for 96 hours.[6,10]	

Patient Monitoring and Care —*Continued*

Steps	Rationale	Reportable Conditions
7. Perform a dynamic response test (square wave test) at the start of each shift, with a change of the waveform, or when the system is opened to air (see Fig. 56.2).	An optimally damped system provides an accurate waveform.	• Overdamped or underdamped waveforms that cannot be corrected with troubleshooting procedures
8. Maintain the pressure bag or device at 300 mm Hg.	At 300 mm Hg, each flush device delivers approximately 1–3 mL/hour to maintain patency of the system.	
9. Follow the procedure above to obtain an accurate CVP/RAP measurement on the monitor at the start of each shift and whenever there is a change in the waveform or the patient's condition. Follow institutional policy regarding printing and documenting the CVP/RAP.	Saving the measurement location on the monitor or documenting the location of measurement on the recording may enhance accuracy and reproducibility. Reviewing waveforms and measurement decisions may advance clinician knowledge.	• Significant change in waveform (e.g., from RA to RV tracing). • Significant change in CVP/RAP result (may represent significant clinical change)

Documentation

Documentation should include the following:
- Patient and family education
- CVP/RAP pressures and waveform
- Site assessment
- Occurrence of unexpected outcomes and interventions

References and Additional Readings

For a complete list of references and additional readings for this procedure, scan this QR code with your smartphone, or visit https://www.elsevier.com/__data/assets/pdf_file/0008/1319831/Chapter0056.pdf.

57 Blood Sampling From a Central Venous Catheter

Kayla Little

PURPOSE To obtain blood from the central venous catheter (CVC) for laboratory analysis.

PREREQUISITE NURSING KNOWLEDGE

- Anatomy and physiology of the cardiovascular system.
- Principles and performance of sterile and aseptic technique and infection control.
- Technique for specimen collection and labeling.
- Signs and symptoms of central-line–associated bloodstream infection (CLABSI) and sepsis.
- CLABSIs are associated with increased hospital length of stay, a 10% to 30% mortality rate, and additional healthcare costs between $300 million and $2.3 billion per year.[1,5,10,12,14]
- Strategies to prevent CLABSI.
- Skill and knowledge of caring for patients with CVCs (see Procedure 75, Central Venous Catheter Insertion [Assist], Nursing Care and Removal).
- Awareness of the effect of heparin, intravenous medication infusions, and hemolysis on various blood tests and the need for appropriate discard volumes.[7]
- Alternate routes of blood specimen collection such as venipuncture or arterial catheters should be considered to minimize the risk of CLABSI.[7,12]
- Ideally a needleless system should be used for capping and accessing CVC ports. Needleless systems reduce needle-stick injuries and risk of blood-borne infection transmission to healthcare professionals and may also reduce CLABSIs.[4,7]

EQUIPMENT

- Nonsterile gloves
- Goggles or fluid shield face mask
- 70% isopropyl alcohol or alcohol-based chlorhexidine suitable for use with medical devices
- Needleless blood-sampling access device (blood-transfer device)
- Blood specimen tube(s) for specimen collection
- Blood-specimen tubes for discard
- Sterile 10-mL 0.9% sodium chloride solution for injection
- Laboratory form
- Patient identification specimen labels
- Needleless connector (injectable caps)
- Specimen transport bag(s)
- Sterile end cap or antiseptic-containing end cap

Additional equipment, to have available as needed, includes the following:
- 3-mL, 5-mL, or 10-mL syringe; type of syringe depends on discard volume
- 10-mL sterile 0.9% sodium chloride solution for injection

PATIENT AND FAMILY EDUCATION

- Explain the purpose for blood sampling to the patient and family. *Rationale:* Provision of information helps the patient and family make informed decisions, reduces anxiety, and facilitates cooperation.
- Explain the patient's expected participation during the procedure. *Rationale:* Discussion of the patient's participation supports patient autonomy and sense of control and increases patient cooperation.[2,7]

PATIENT ASSESSMENT AND PREPARATION

Patient Assessment

- Assess the patency of the CVC. *Rationale:* Ensures function of the CVC catheter.
- Evaluate previous laboratory results. *Rationale:* These results provide baseline data for comparison.
- Determine whether intravenous solutions or medications are infusing through the CVC. *Rationale:* Intravenous solutions and medications must be temporarily discontinued before blood sampling to reduce interference with the laboratory analysis.[7,15] Critical infusions (e.g., vasoactive medications) may not be able to be stopped; additional blood access sites must be considered.

Patient Preparation

- Verify the correct patient with two identifiers. *Rationale:* Before performing a procedure, the nurse should ensure the correct identification of the patient for the intended intervention.
- Confirm that the patient and family understand the preprocedural teaching by having them verbalize understanding. Clarify key points by reinforcing important information, and answer all questions. *Rationale:* Preprocedure communication provides a framework of

patient expectations, enhances cooperation, and reduces anxiety.[2,7]

- Position the patient in a seated or recumbent position with the intended blood sampling port exposed.[7] ***Rationale:***

Optimal positioning improves the ease of obtaining the blood sample and reduces potential contamination of the port.

Procedure	**for Blood Sampling From Central Venous Catheters**	
Steps	**Rationale**	**Special Considerations**
1. 🅷🅷		
2. 🅿🅴		

Blood Sampling From the CVC With a Transducer

Steps	Rationale	Special Considerations
1. Remove the antiseptic-containing end cap or dead-end cap, and cleanse the blood sampling port of the stopcock with 70% isopropyl alcohol or alcohol-based chlorhexidine suitable for use with medical devices. Allow to dry.[4,5,7-9,13,15] **(Level B*)**	Reduces the risk for infection.	Follow institutional protocols. Dry time is 5 seconds for 70% isopropyl alcohol and 20 seconds for alcohol-based chlorhexidine.[7]
2. Attach the needleless blood sampling device (blood transfer device) to the blood sampling port of the stopcock (Fig. 57.1).	Prepares for blood sampling.	
3. If applicable, temporarily suspend the right-atrial pressure/central venous pressure (RAP/CVP) monitoring alarm.	Prevents the alarm from sounding because the RAP/CVP waveform is lost during the blood sampling.	

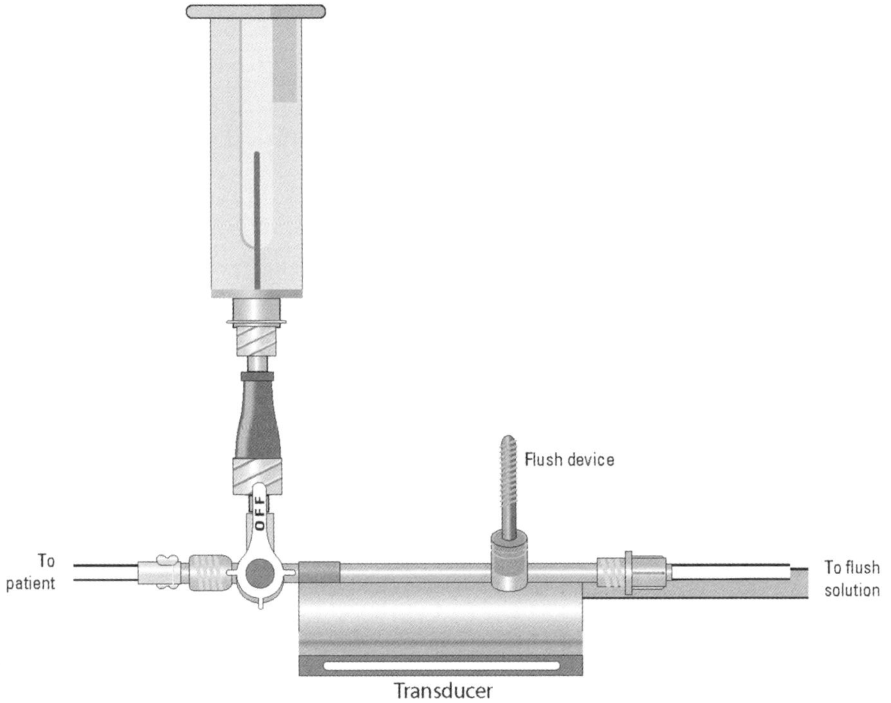

Figure 57.1 Needleless blood-sampling device (blood-transfer device) attached to the blood sampling port of the stopcock of the hemodynamic monitoring system. The stopcock is open to the transducer system. (*Drawing by Paul W. Schiffmacher, Thomas Jefferson University, Philadelphia, PA.*)

Steps	Rationale	Special Considerations
4. Turn the stopcock off to the monitoring system, and flush the solution (Fig. 57.2).	The needleless blood sampling device is now in contact with the central venous blood.	

*Level B: Well-designed, controlled studies with results that consistently support a specific action, intervention, or treatment.

Procedure continues on following page

Procedure | **for Blood Sampling From Central Venous Catheters—*Continued***

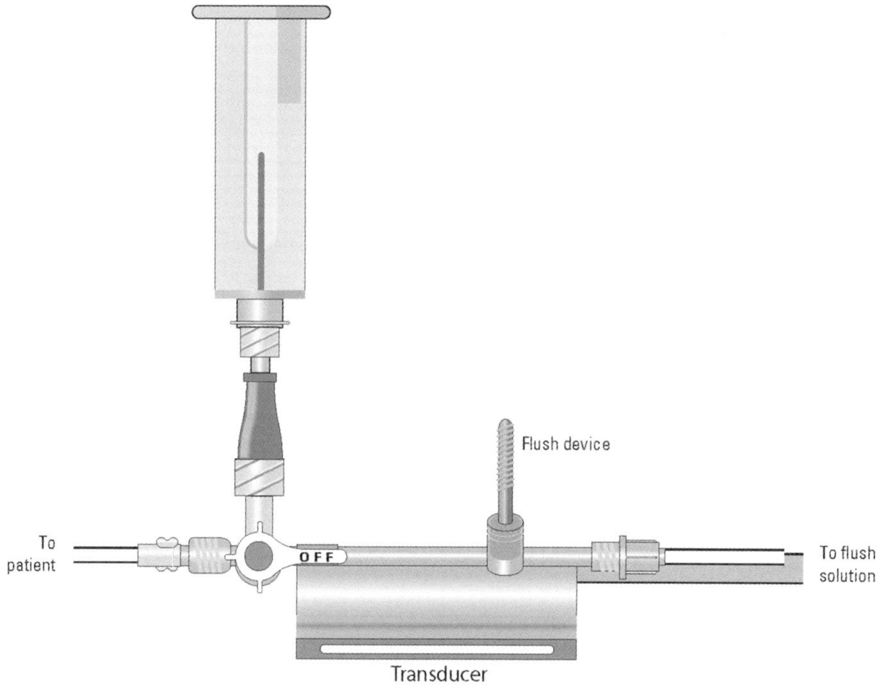

Steps	Rationale	Special Considerations

Figure 57.2   Needleless blood-sampling device (blood-transfer device) attached to the blood sampling port of the stopcock of the hemodynamic monitoring system. The stopcock is turned "off" to the monitoring system and flush solution. *(Drawing by Paul W. Schiffmacher, Thomas Jefferson University, Philadelphia, PA.)*

Steps	Rationale	Special Considerations
5. Insert a blood-specimen tube into the blood-sampling device (blood-transfer device) to obtain the discard volume.[4,7] **(Level B*)**	Clears the catheter of flush solution. The discard volume includes the dead space (from the tip of the lumen to the top port of the needleless capped stopcock) and the blood diluted by the flush solution (ranging from 2–25 mL).[7,15]	Dead-space information for the CVC is usually listed in the information that comes with the CVC.
6. Remove the discard blood-specimen tube, and discard it in the appropriate receptacle.	Removes discard safely.	
7. Insert the blood-specimen tube into the blood-sampling device to obtain the specimen.	Obtains the blood specimen.	Collection tubes contain different additives as indicated by the colored top of the tube. Verify that the correct tube is used for the ordered blood sample.[7]
8. Remove the blood-specimen tube, and label the specimen at the time of collection in the presence of the patient.[7]	Properly identifies the patient and laboratory tests to be performed.	Confirm identifying information.
9. Insert a discard blood-specimen tube to clear the blood sampling port of the stopcock.		The blood in the needleless cap can be cleared by fast-flushing the blood into a blood-specimen tube or syringe (Fig. 57.3).
10. Activate the fast-flush to clear the sampling port of the stopcock.		
11. Remove the discard blood-specimen tube, and discard it in the appropriate receptacle.	Removes discard safely.	

*Level B: Well-designed, controlled studies with results that consistently support a specific action, intervention, or treatment.

UNIT II

Procedure for Blood Sampling From Central Venous Catheters—*Continued*		
Steps	**Rationale**	**Special Considerations**

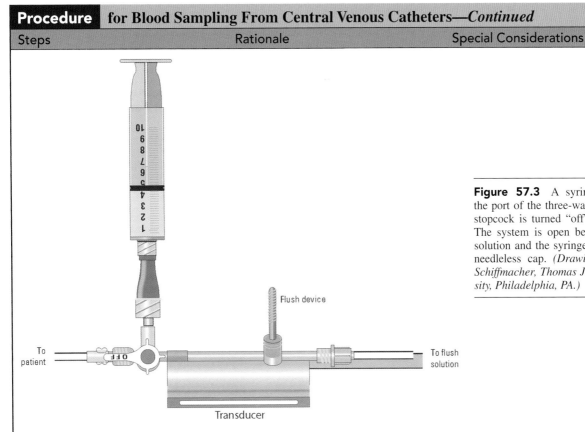

Flush device

To patient

To flush solution

OFF

Transducer

Figure 57.3 A syringe attached to the port of the three-way stopcock. The stopcock is turned "off" to the patient. The system is open between the flush solution and the syringe attached to the needleless cap. *(Drawing by Paul W. Schiffmacher, Thomas Jefferson University, Philadelphia, PA.)*

12. Turn the stopcock off to the blood sampling port, detach the blood-sampling device from the stopcock, and discard it in the appropriate receptacle. **(Level B*)**	Opens the system for continuous RAP/CVP pressure monitoring.[11] Removes and safely discards equipment.	
13. Apply a sterile dead-end cap or antiseptic-containing end cap to the blood sampling port.[4,15]	Reduces the risk for infection.	
14. Fast-flush the remaining blood in the CVC back into the patient.	Promotes patency of the CVC.	
15. Observe the monitor for return of the RAP/CVP waveform.[11]	Ensures continuous monitoring of the waveform.	
16. Remove **PE**, and discard used supplies in appropriate receptacles.	Reduces the transmission of microorganisms; standard precautions.	
17. **HH**		
18. Turn the alarms back on.	Activates the alarm system.	
19. Place the laboratory specimen in a transport bag. Complete the laboratory form.	Properly identifies the patient and laboratory tests to be performed.	Confirm identifying information.
20. Send the specimen for analysis.	Ensures analysis.	

Blood Sampling From a Single CVC Port Without a Transducer

1. **HH**
2. **PE**

*Level B: Well-designed, controlled studies with results that consistently support a specific action, intervention, or treatment.

Procedure continues on following page

Procedure for Blood Sampling From Central Venous Catheters—*Continued*

Steps	Rationale	Special Considerations
3. Temporarily discontinue intravenous solutions and medications before blood sampling.	Minimizes the risk of diluting the blood specimen, which may affect the accuracy of the laboratory results.[3]	If the blood sample is obtained from a multiple-lumen catheter (e.g., triple lumen), ensure that temporarily discontinuing intravenous medications does not affect hemodynamic stability, and discontinue intravenous medication infusions from all of the CVC ports. The length of time for discontinuing intravenous medications before blood sampling is unknown and dependent on the internal volume of the CVC.[7] Obtain the blood sample from the distal lumen.
4. Remove and cap the intravenous solution infusing through the intended blood-sampling port.	Prepares equipment and maintains asepsis of the intravenous system.	If possible, obtain the blood sample from a dedicated lumen that is not used for administration of the drug being monitored.[7]
5. Clean the needleless connector (injectable cap) at the end of the CVC sampling port with 70% isopropyl alcohol or alcohol-based chlorhexidine suitable for use with medical devices. Allow it to dry.[4,5,7-9,13,15] **(Level B*)**	Reduces the risk for infection.	Follow institutional protocols. Dry time is 5 seconds for 70% isopropyl alcohol and 20 seconds for alcohol-based chlorhexidine.[7]
6. Attach a 10-mL syringe filled with sterile 0.9% sodium chloride solution to the needleless connector (injectable cap) of the CVC port.	Prepares the flush solution.	
7. Gently flush the 0.9% sodium chloride solution into the needleless connector (injectable cap).	Removes fibrin deposits, drug precipitate, and other debris from the lumen.	Consider the size of the CVC and the type of infusion therapy when determining the flush volume. Use a minimum volume equal to twice the internal volume of the CVC.[6,7]
8. Remove the 0.9% sodium chloride solution syringe, and discard it in the appropriate receptacle.	Removes and safely discards equipment.	
9. Clean the needleless connector (injectable cap) at the end of the CVC sampling port with 70% isopropyl alcohol or alcohol-based chlorhexidine suitable for use with medical devices. Allow it to dry.[4,5,7-9,13,15]	Reduces the risk for infection.	Dry time is 5 seconds for 70% isopropyl alcohol and 20 seconds for alcohol-based chlorhexidine.[7]
10. Attach the needleless blood-sampling device (blood-transfer device) to the needleless connector (injectable cap) of the CVC port (Fig. 57.4).	Prepares for blood sampling.	

*Level B: Well-designed, controlled studies with results that consistently support a specific action, intervention, or treatment.

Procedure	**for Blood Sampling From Central Venous Catheters—*Continued***	
Steps	**Rationale**	**Special Considerations**

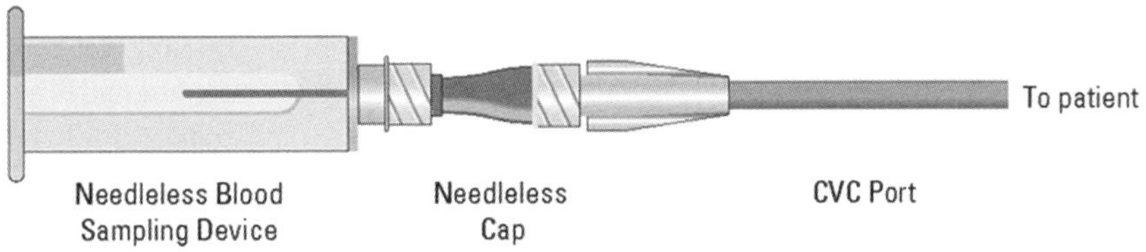

To patient

Needleless Blood Sampling Device

Needleless Cap

CVC Port

Figure 57.4 The needleless blood-sampling device (blood-transfer device) attached to the needleless (injectable) cap of the central venous catheter (CVC) port. *(Drawing by Paul W. Schiffmacher, Thomas Jefferson University, Philadelphia, PA.)*

Steps	Rationale	Special Considerations
11. Insert a blood-specimen tube into the blood-sampling device to obtain the discard volume.	Clears the catheter of flush solution. The discard volume includes the dead space (from the tip of the lumen to the top port of the needleless capped stopcock) and the blood diluted by the flush solution (ranging from 2–25 mL).[3]	Dead-space information for a CVC is usually listed in the information that comes with the CVC.
12. Remove the discard blood-specimen tube, and discard it in the appropriate receptacle.	Removes discard safely.	
13. Insert the blood-specimen tube into the blood-sampling device to obtain the specimen.	Obtains the blood specimen.	Obtain additional specimens as prescribed. Specimen size should be the amount required for the blood test(s). Collection tubes contain different additives as indicated by the colored top of the tube. Verify that the correct tube is used for the ordered blood sample.[7]
14. After obtaining the specimen, detach the blood-sampling device from the CVC, and discard it in the appropriate receptacle.	Removes and safely discards equipment.	
15. Clean the needleless connector (injectable cap) of the CVC port with 70% isopropyl alcohol or alcohol-based chlorhexidine suitable for use with medical devices. Allow it to dry.[4,5,7-9,13,15] **(Level B*)**	Reduces the risk for infection.	Follow institutional protocols. Dry time is 5 seconds for 70% isopropyl alcohol and 20 seconds for alcohol-based chlorhexidine.[7]
16. Attach a 10-mL syringe filled with sterile 0.9% sodium chloride solution to the needleless connector (injectable cap) of the CVC port.	Prepares flush solution.	
17. Gently flush the 0.9% sodium chloride solution into the needleless connector (injectable cap).	Clears blood from the needleless connector (injectable cap) and the CVC port.	
18. Remove the 0.9% sodium chloride solution syringe, and discard it in the appropriate receptacle.	Removes and safely discards equipment.	

*Level B: Well-designed, controlled studies with results that consistently support a specific action, intervention, or treatment.

Procedure continues on following page

UNIT II

Procedure   for Blood Sampling From Central Venous Catheters—*Continued*

Steps	Rationale	Special Considerations
19. Clean the needleless connector (injectable cap) of the CVC port with 70% isopropyl alcohol or alcohol-based chlorhexidine suitable for use with medical devices. Allow it to dry.[2,5,7-9,13,15] **(Level B*)**	Reduces the risk for infection.	Follow institutional protocols. Dry time is 5 seconds for 70% isopropyl alcohol and 20 seconds for alcohol-based chlorhexidine.[7]
20. Reattach and resume the intravenous solution or medication infusion.	Continues treatment.	
21. Remove **PE**, and discard used supplies in appropriate receptacles.	Reduces the transmission of microorganisms; standard precautions.	
22. **HH**		
23. Label the specimen at the time of collection and in the presence of the patient, and place it in a transport bag. Complete the laboratory form.[7]	Properly identifies the patient and laboratory tests to be performed.	Confirm identifying information.
24. Send the specimen for analysis.	Allows the laboratory to conduct the analysis.	

*Level B: Well-designed, controlled studies with results that consistently support a specific action, intervention, or treatment.

Expected Outcomes

- CVC remains patent with good waveform if a monitoring system is used
- CVC insertion site remains free from infection
- Adequate blood sample with minimal blood loss
- No hemolysis of the specimen

Unexpected Outcomes

- Clotting of the CVC
- CLABSI
- Inability to obtain a blood sample
- Hemolysis of specimens
- Dilution of specimens that causes inaccurate laboratory results

Patient Monitoring and Care

Steps	Rationale	Reportable Conditions
		These conditions should be reported to the provider if they persist despite nursing interventions.
1. Use the minimal volume of blood discard.[3,7]	Helps prevent hospital-acquired anemia.	- Decreased hemoglobin level and hematocrit level
2. Monitor hemoglobin and hematocrit values if frequent blood sampling is needed.	Allows early detection of hospital-acquired anemia.	- Decreased hemoglobin level and hematocrit level
3. Attempt to obtain all blood samples at one time when possible.[7]	Diminishes the number of times the system is entered to help minimize the risk of infection.	- Signs of catheter-related sepsis
4. Before and after the blood withdrawal, assess and evaluate the RAP/CVP waveform if monitored.	Ensures accurate RAP/CVP monitoring.	- Abnormal RAP/CVP waveforms
5. Obtain laboratory specimen results.	Assesses patient condition.	- Abnormal specimen results

Documentation

Documentation should include the following:
- Patient and family education
- Time and type of specimen drawn
- Results of laboratory tests when available
- Unexpected outcomes
- Inability to obtain sample

References and Additional Readings

For a complete list of references and additional readings for this procedure, scan this QR code with your smartphone, or visit https://www.elsevier.com/__data/assets/pdf_file/0009/1319832/Chapter0057.pdf

58 Pulmonary Artery Catheter Insertion (Perform)

Nikki J. Taylor

PURPOSE Pulmonary artery (PA) catheters are used to determine hemodynamic status in critically ill patients.[3] PA catheters provide information about right-sided and left-sided intracardiac pressures and cardiac output. Additional functions available are fiberoptic monitoring of mixed venous oxygen saturation (Sv_{O2}), intracardiac pacing,[10] and assessment of right-ventricular volumes and ejection fraction. Hemodynamic information obtained with a PA catheter is used to aid diagnosis and guide therapeutic intervention, including administration of fluids and diuretics and titration of vasoactive and inotropic medications.[10]

PREREQUISITE NURSING KNOWLEDGE

- Knowledge of the normal anatomy and physiology of the cardiovascular and pulmonary systems.
- Knowledge of the normal anatomy and physiology of the vasculature and adjacent structures of the neck.
- Knowledge of the principles of sterile technique.
- Clinical and technical competence in central line insertion and suturing.
- Competence in chest radiograph interpretation.
- Basic dysrhythmia recognition and treatment of life-threatening dysrhythmias.
- Advanced cardiac life support (ACLS) knowledge and skills.
- Understanding of PA pressure monitoring (see Procedure 59).
- Hemodynamic information obtained with a PA catheter is routinely used to guide therapeutic interventions, including administration of fluids and diuretics as well as titration of vasoactive and inotropic medications.[1,2,6,14]
- Interpretation of right-atrial pressure/central venous pressure (RAP/CVP) and pulmonary arterial occlusion pressure (PAOP) waveforms including identification of *a, c,* and *v* waves is needed. The *a* wave reflects atrial contraction. The *c* wave reflects closure of the atrioventricular valves. The *v* wave reflects passive filling of the atria during ventricular systole.
- Directly measured or calculated hemodynamic data obtained from the PA catheter include cardiac output (CO), cardiac index (CI), systemic vascular resistance (SVR), pulmonary vascular resistance (PVR), stroke volume/stroke index), Sv_{O2}, right-heart pressures (pulmonary artery pressure [PAP] and RAP), and PAOP, a reflection of left-ventricular

end-diastolic pressure and volume. Also, information regarding right-ventricular ejection fraction and end-diastolic volume can be determined with specific PA catheters.
- CO, CI, and Sv_{O2} can be measured intermittently or continuously.
- There are several types of PA catheters with different functions (e.g., pacing, Sv_{O2} monitoring, continuous CO, or right-ventricular volume monitoring). Catheter selection is based on patient need.
- The PA catheter contains a proximal lumen port, a distal lumen port, a thermistor connector, and a balloon inflation lumen port (see Fig. 59.1). Some catheters also have additional infusion ports that can be used for infusion of medications and intravenous fluids.
- The distal lumen port is connected to a transducer system to monitor systolic, diastolic, and mean PA pressures, and it can be accessed to obtain mixed venous blood samples for analysis or calibration of Sv_{O2} for continuous monitoring. The proximal lumen (or injectate lumen) port is connected to a transducer system to monitor the right-atrial pressure and is accessed to inject solution when measuring thermodilution cardiac outputs. The balloon inflation lumen port is accessed to inflate the balloon with air to advance (float) the catheter tip to occlude forward flow through the PA and measure PAOP or pulmonary artery wedge pressure.
- The standard 7.5F PA catheter is 110 cm long and has black markings at 10-cm increments and wide black markings at 50-cm increments to facilitate insertion and positioning (see Fig. 59.1). The catheter should reach the PA after advancing 40 to 55 cm from the internal jugular vein, 35 to 50 cm from the subclavian vein, 60 cm from the femoral vein, 70 cm from the right antecubital fossa, and 80 cm from the left antecubital fossa.
- Central venous access for PA catheter insertion may be obtained at a variety of sites (see Procedure 74, Central Venous Catheter Insertion [Assist]).
- The right subclavian vein is a more direct route than the left subclavian vein for placement of a PA catheter because the catheter does not cross the midline of the thorax.[1,2,6,14]

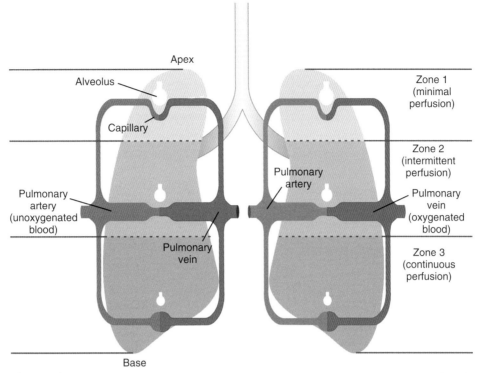

Figure 58.1   West's lung zones. Schema of the heart and lungs demonstrating the relationship between the cardiac chambers and the blood vessels and the physiological zones of the lungs. *Zone 1* (PA > Pa > Pv): Absence of blood flow. *Zone 2* (Pa > PA > Pv): Intermittent blood flow. *Zone 3* (Pa > Pv > PA): Continuous blood flow, resulting in an open channel between the pulmonary artery catheter and the left atrium. *PA,* Pulmonary artery; *Pa,* pressure arterial; *Pv,* pressure venous. *(From Copstead LC, Banasik JL: Pathophysiology, ed 5, Philadelphia, 2014, Saunders.)*

- Use of an internal jugular vein minimizes the risk for a pneumothorax. The preferred site for catheter insertion is the right internal jugular vein. The right internal jugular vein is a "straight shot" to the right atrium.
- Knowledge of West's lung zones helps identify optimal physiological zones to obtain data from the PA catheter (Fig. 58.1). The PA catheter tip should be positioned in lung zone 3, below the level of the left atrium in the dependent portion of the lung.[7] In lung zone 3, both pulmonary arterial and venous pressures exceed alveolar pressure, resulting in the PAOP reflecting left-atrial pressures rather than alveolar pressures.[7]
- Common indications for insertion of a PA catheter include the following:[1,2,6-9,14,16,18,19]
  - ❖ Acute coronary syndrome or myocardial infarction (MI) complicated by hemodynamic instability, heart failure, cardiogenic shock, mitral regurgitation, ventral septal rupture, subacute cardiac rupture with tamponade, postinfarction ischemia, papillary muscle rupture, or severe heart failure (e.g., cardiomyopathy, constrictive pericarditis)
  - ❖ Preoperative and postoperative management in high-risk patients with cardiac, pulmonary, or renal dysfunction
  - ❖ Hypotension unresponsive to fluid replacement or with heart failure
  - ❖ Cardiac tamponade, significant dysrhythmias, right-ventricular infarct, acute pulmonary embolism, and tricuspid insufficiency

- ❖ Anesthesia in cardiac surgery with any of the following:
  - ○ Evidence of previous MI
  - ○ Resection of ventricular aneurysm
  - ○ Coronary artery bypass graft (reoperation)
  - ○ Coronary artery bypass graft (left main or complex coronary disease)
  - ○ Complex cardiac surgery (multivalvular surgery)
  - ○ High-risk surgery (e.g., pulmonary hypertension)
- ❖ General surgery:
  - ○ Vascular procedures (abdominal aneurysm repair, aortobifemoral bypass)
  - ○ Patients at high risk[1,2,14]
  - ○ Hypotensive anesthesia
- ❖ Cardiac disorders:
  - ○ Unstable angina that necessitates vasodilator therapy
  - ○ Heart failure unresponsive to conventional therapy (cardiomyopathy)[2]
  - ○ Management of heart failure
  - ○ Cardiogenic shock
  - ○ Potentially reversible systolic heart failure, such as fulminant myocarditis and peripartum cardiomyopathy
  - ○ Pulmonary hypertension during acute medication therapy
  - ○ Distinguishing cardiogenic from noncardiogenic pulmonary edema
  - ○ Constrictive pericarditis or cardiac tamponade
  - ○ Evaluation of pulmonary hypertension for a precardiac transplant workup
- ❖ Patients who need mechanical circulatory support

- ❖ Pulmonary disorders:
  - ○ Acute respiratory failure with chronic obstructive pulmonary diseases
  - ○ Cor pulmonale with pneumonia
  - ○ Optimization of positive end-expiratory pressure and volume therapy in patients with acute respiratory distress syndrome
- ❖ Critically ill pregnant patients (e.g., severe preeclampsia with unresponsive hypertension, pulmonary edema, persistent oliguria)
- ❖ Severe shock states
- ❖ Major trauma or burn
- ❖ Systemic inflammatory response syndrome
- ❖ Patients undergoing liver transplantation workup
- Relative contraindications to PA catheter insertion include the following:
  - ❖ Preexisting left bundle-branch block
  - ❖ Presence of fever (>101°F [38°C])
  - ❖ Right-sided endocarditis
  - ❖ Right heart mass (thrombus or tumor)
  - ❖ Mechanical tricuspid valve
  - ❖ Severe coagulopathy
  - ❖ Presence of an endocardial pacemaker
  - ❖ History of heparin-induced thrombocytopenia if only heparin-coated PA catheters are available

EQUIPMENT

- Percutaneous sheath introducer kit and sterile catheter sleeve
- PA catheter (non–heparin-coated catheters and latex-free PA catheters are available)
- Bedside hemodynamic monitoring system with pressure and cardiac output monitoring capability
- Pressure modules and cables for interface with the monitor
- Cardiac output cable with a thermistor/injectate sensor
- Pressure transducer system, including flush solution recommended according to institutional standards, a pressure bag or device, pressure tubing with transducers, and a flush device (see Procedure 60, Single-Pressure and Multiple-Pressure Transducer Systems)
- Dual-channel recorder
- Sterile normal saline intravenous fluid for flushing the introducer and catheter-infusion ports
- Antiseptic solution (e.g., 2% chlorhexidine-based preparation)
- Head covering, protective eyewear, fluid-shield masks, sterile gowns, sterile gloves, nonsterile gloves, and full sterile drapes
- 1% lidocaine without epinephrine
- Sterile basin or cup
- Sterile water or normal saline solution for checking balloon integrity
- Sterile dressing supplies
- Stopcocks (may be included with pressure tubing systems)
- Sterile caps (injectable or noninjectable)
- Leveling device (low-intensity laser or carpenter level)

Additional equipment, to have available as needed, includes the following:

- Fluoroscope
- Lead apron and thyroid guard
- Emergency equipment
- Temporary pacing equipment
- Indelible marker
- Transducer holder and intravenous pole
- Heparin (for flush solution if prescribed)
- 3-mL syringe
- Chlorhexidine-impregnated sponge/dressing

PATIENT AND FAMILY EDUCATION

- Explain the procedure and the reason for the PA catheter insertion. **Rationale:** Explanation may decrease patient and family anxiety.
- Explain the need for sterile technique, and explain that the patient's face may be covered. **Rationale:** This explanation decreases patient anxiety and elicits cooperation.
- Inform the patient of expected benefits and potential risks. **Rationale:** The patient is given information to make an informed decision.
- Explain the patient's expected participation during the procedure. **Rationale:** This encourages patient assistance.

PATIENT ASSESSMENT AND PREPARATION

Patient Assessment

- Determine the patient's medical history of cervical disk disease or difficulty with vascular access. **Rationale:** Baseline data are provided.
- Determine the patient's medical history of pneumothorax or emphysema. **Rationale:** Patients with emphysematous lungs may be at higher risk for puncture and pneumothorax depending on the approach.
- Determine the patient's medical history of anomalous veins. **Rationale:** Patients may have a history of dextrocardia or transposition of the great vessels, which leads to greater difficulty in catheter placement.
- Assess the intended insertion site. **Rationale:** Scar tissue may impede placement of the catheter.
- Assess the patient's cardiac and pulmonary status. **Rationale:** Some patients may not tolerate the supine position or Trendelenburg position for extended periods.
- Assess vital signs and pulse oximetry. **Rationale:** This provides baseline data.
- Assess for electrolyte imbalances (potassium, magnesium, and calcium). **Rationale:** Electrolyte imbalances may increase cardiac irritability.
- Assess the electrocardiogram (ECG) for left bundle-branch block. **Rationale:** Right bundle-branch block has been associated with PA catheter insertion. Caution should be used because complete heart block may ensue.[1,17]
- Assess for heparin and latex sensitivity or allergy. **Rationale:** PA catheters are heparin bonded and contain latex. If the patient has a heparin allergy or a history of heparin-induced thrombocytopenia, consider the use of a non–heparin-coated catheter. If the patient has a latex allergy, use a latex-free PA catheter.
- Assess for a coagulopathic state, and determine whether the patient has recently received anticoagulant or

thrombolytic therapy. **Rationale:** These patients are more likely to have complications related to bleeding and may need interventions before insertion of the PA catheter.

Patient Preparation

- Verify the correct patient with two identifiers. **Rationale:** Before performing a procedure, the inserting provider should ensure the correct identification of the patient for the intended intervention.
- Ensure that the patient understands the preprocedural teaching. Answer questions as they arise, and reinforce information as needed. **Rationale:** Understanding of previously taught information is evaluated and reinforced.

- Obtain informed consent. **Rationale:** Informed consent protects the rights of a patient and makes a competent decision possible for the patient.
- Perform a pre-procedure verification and time out. **Rationale:** This ensures patient safety.
- Prescribe sedation or analgesics as needed. **Rationale:** Sedation and analgesics minimize anxiety and discomfort. Movement of the patient may inhibit insertion of the PA catheter.
- If the patient is obese or muscular and the preferred site is the internal jugular vein or subclavian vein, place a towel posteriorly between the shoulder blades. **Rationale:** This action helps extend the neck and provide better access to the subclavian and internal jugular veins.

Procedure for Performing Pulmonary Artery Catheter Insertion

Steps	Rationale	Special Considerations
1. HH		
2. PE		
3. Place the patient in the supine position, and prepare the area with the antiseptic solution (e.g., 2% chlorhexidine–based preparation).[5,13]	The site access is prepared for PA catheter insertion.	Ensure that the patient is in the Trendelenburg position (see Procedure 74, Central Venous Catheter Insertion [Assist]).
4. Perform hand hygiene, and apply a sterile gown and gloves.	Minimizes the risk of infection and maintains standard and sterile precautions.	All healthcare personnel involved in the procedure must apply head coverings, fluid-shield masks, sterile gowns, and gloves.
5. Place sterile drapes over the prepared area.	Prepares the sterile field.	Fully drape the patient with exposure of only the insertion site.
6. With assistance, open the sterile kits.	Prepares the equipment.	
7. Obtain central venous access with an introducer (see Procedure 74, Central Venous Catheter Insertion [Assist]).	The PA catheter is inserted into a central vein.	
8. Hand off the ports of the PA catheter to the critical care nurse assisting with connection to the hemodynamic monitoring system (see Procedure 59, Pulmonary Artery Catheter Insertion [Assist] and Pressure Monitoring).	Connects the ports to the flush system; connects the transducer systems to the bedside monitor.	
9. Flush all open lumens with normal saline solution, and attach sterile injectable or noninjectable caps to retain the flush.	Removes air from the PA catheter.	
10. Insert the recommended amount of air (1.5 mL) into the balloon port, and immerse the inflated balloon in the sterile bowl with water or normal saline solution.	Checks for integrity of the balloon.	If an air leak is present, air bubbles are noted.
11. Remove the balloon syringe, and let the balloon passively deflate; empty the syringe, and reattach the syringe to the balloon port.	Prepares for insertion.	
12. Insert the PA catheter through the sterile catheter sleeve. (**Level B***)	Maintains sterility of the PA catheter to allow repositioning of the catheter.[4]	

*Level B: Well-designed, controlled studies with results that consistently support a specific action, intervention, or treatment.

Procedure continues on following page

Procedure	for Performing Pulmonary Artery Catheter Insertion—*Continued*		
Steps	**Rationale**	**Special Considerations**	
13. If a PA catheter with the ability to monitor Svo$_2$ is being inserted, the fiberoptics are calibrated before removal from the package (see Procedure 63, Continous Venous Oxygen Saturation Monitoring). **(Level M*)**	Calibrates the system.	Calibrate the catheter according to the manufacturer's guidelines.	
14. Ensure that the critical care nurse has leveled and zeroed the hemodynamic monitoring system (see Procedure 60, Central Venous Catheter Insertion [Assist]).	Prepares the monitoring system so right-heart pressures and PA pressures can be visualized and measured during catheter insertion.		
15. Wiggle the PA catheter, and observe the monitor. Wiggling (sometimes called *whipping*) the PA catheter will produce artifacts on the monitor screen.	Ensures the ability to see the waveform during insertion and ensures that there are no connection issues or catheter defects before insertion.		
16. While observing the monitor and the markings on the PA catheter (Fig. 58.2), follow these steps: A. Advance the catheter through the introducer until the tip is 15–20 cm from the right internal jugular or left subclavian, and then advance to the superior vena cava into the right atrium. Confirm placement in right atrium from the waveform on the monitor. B. Slowly inflate the balloon with 1.5 mL of air after verifying a right-atrial waveform. C. Advance the catheter through the tricuspid valve into the right ventricle. Assess for the right-ventricular waveform. D. Continue to advance the catheter from the right ventricle through the pulmonic valve into the PA, and assess for the PA waveform. E. Advance the catheter until a PAOP waveform (*a, c, v* waves) is visualized to obtain a PAOP. F. Passively allow the balloon to deflate. G. Observe the waveform change from the PAOP waveform to the PA waveform.	Waveforms and pressure values change while moving from the superior vena cava to the right atrium to the right ventricle to the pulmonary artery and into the wedge position.	If there is any resistance when inflating the balloon, allow the balloon to deflate, advance the catheter another centimeter, and attempt to inflate the balloon again. The catheter should reach the PA after advancing 40–55 cm from the internal jugular vein, 35–55 cm from the subclavian vein, 60 cm from the femoral vein, 70 cm from the right antecubital fossa, and 80 cm from the left antecubital fossa. When inserting the PA catheter into the subclavian vein, have the patient bring his or her ear to the shoulder on the side of the insertion site. This creates a sharp angle between the jugular and subclavian veins and may help prevent misdirection of the catheter into the internal jugular vein. During insertion, monitor the ECG tracing for dysrhythmias. Run a graphic strip of the insertion waveforms. The balloon should only be inflated when advancing the catheter and should always be deflated when the catheter is withdrawn.	
17. Ensure proper placement by wedging the PA catheter again, and print a graphic strip of the waveforms.	Ensures proper placement and accurate readings.	If the PA wedges with less than 1.25 mL of air, the catheter may be too deep.	
18. Extend the sterile catheter sleeve over the catheter, and secure it in place.	Maintains sterility of the PA catheter to allow repositioning of the catheter.[4]	The duration of catheter sterility in the sleeve is unknown. One team of researchers found that the catheter was thought to be sterile up to 4 days.[4] Another team of researchers also studied catheter sterility using the sleeve; they recommend that the PA catheter should not be repositioned after 4 hours. Be cautious not to overtighten the sleeve, pinching the catheter.	

*Level M: Manufacturer's recommendations only.

Procedure	for Performing Pulmonary Artery Catheter Insertion—*Continued*	
Steps	Rationale	Special Considerations
19. Apply an occlusive, sterile dressing, and secure the catheter. Avoid applying adhesive tape or dressing to the sterile catheter sleeve.	Reduces the incidence of infection and prevents dislodgement.	Dressings may be a sterile gauze or a sterile, transparent, semipermeable dressing.[4] Follow institutional standards for application of a chlorhexidine-impregnated sponge (see Procedure 75, Central Venous Catheter Insertion [Assist], Nursing Care and Removal).
20. Note the centimeter marking at the introducer site.	Aids in ensuring placement and troubleshooting.	The tip of the PA catheter may migrate.
21. Obtain a chest radiograph.	Confirms that the catheter tip is positioned in the PA.	
22. Remove sterile gown, drape, and **PE**. Discard used supplies in appropriate receptacles.	Reduces transmission of microorganisms; standard precautions.	
23. **HH**		

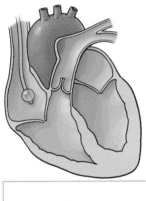

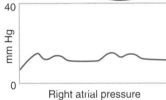

Right atrial pressure

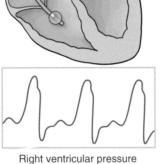

Right ventricular pressure

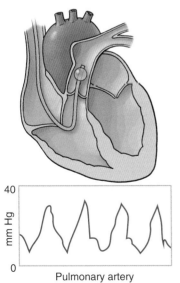

Pulmonary artery

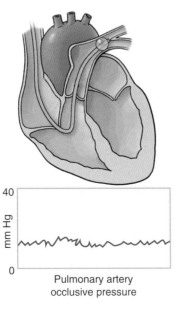

Pulmonary artery
occlusive pressure

Figure 58.2 Pulmonary artery catheter advancing through the heart with appropriate waveforms. *(Modified from Bucher L, Melander S: Critical care nursing, Philadelphia, 1999, Saunders.)*

Expected Outcomes

- Accurate placement of the pulmonary artery catheter
- Adequate and appropriate waveforms
- Ability to obtain accurate information about cardiac pressures
- Evaluation of information to guide diagnosis and/or therapeutic interventions

Unexpected Outcomes[12]

- Pneumothorax or hemothorax
- Infection or sepsis
- Ventricular dysrhythmias
- Misplacement (e.g., hepatic vein)
- Valvular damage
- Vessel wall erosion
- Hemorrhage
- Hematoma
- Pericardial or ventricular rupture
- Venous air embolism
- Cardiac tamponade
- Pulmonary artery infarction
- Pseudoaneurysms
- Catheter-site infection
- Air embolism
- PA rupture
- PA dissection
- PA catheter balloon rupture
- PA catheter knotting
- Heparin-induced thrombocytopenia or thrombosis
- Thromboembolism
- Pain
- Balloon rupture

Patient Monitoring and Care

Steps	Rationale	Reportable Conditions
		These conditions should be reported to the provider if they persist despite nursing interventions.
1. Perform systematic cardiovascular, peripheral vascular, and hemodynamic assessments before and immediately after insertion:		
A. Assess level of consciousness.	Assesses for signs of adequate perfusion; air embolism may present with restlessness; the patient may present with a decreased level of consciousness if the catheter is advanced into the carotid artery.	• Change in level of consciousness
B. Assess vital signs.	Demonstrates response to the procedure and effectiveness of therapies performed.	• Abnormal vital signs
C. Assess postinsertion hemodynamic values: PA systolic pressure, PA diastolic pressure (PADP), RAP, PAOP, CO, CI, SVR, and other parameters as needed.	Obtains baseline data and assesses patient status.	• Abnormal hemodynamic pressures or cardiac parameters
2. Assess the central line insertion site for hematoma or hemorrhage.	If coagulopathies are present, a pressure dressing may be needed.	• Bleeding that does not stop • Hematoma
3. Assess heart and lung sounds after PA catheter insertion.	Abnormal heart or lung sounds may indicate cardiac tamponade, pneumothorax, or hemothorax.	• Diminished or muffled heart sounds • Absent or diminished breath sounds unilaterally

Patient Monitoring and Care —*Continued*

Steps	Rationale	Reportable Conditions
4. Assess the results of the chest radiograph.	Ensures adequate placement in lung zone 3 below the level of the left atrium.	• Abnormal chest radiograph results
5. Monitor for signs and symptoms of cardiac tamponade and air embolism.	Identifies complications.	• Signs or symptoms of cardiac tamponade or air embolism
6. Monitor the centimeter marking at the introducer site.	Aids in determining if the position of the catheter has moved.	• Changes in the external centimeter marking • Abnormal PA waveforms
7. Follow institutional standards for assessing pain. Administer analgesia as prescribed.	Identifies need for pain interventions.	• Continued pain despite pain interventions

Documentation

Documentation should include the following:
- Patient and family education
- Completion of informed consent
- Universal protocol requirements
- Insertion of PA catheter and sheath introducer
- Type and size of catheter placed
- Size of introducer sheath
- PA pressure values on insertion (RAP, right-ventricular systolic and diastolic pressures, PA systolic pressure, PADP, PAOP)
- Graphic strip of insertion
- Insertion site of the PA catheter
- Centimeter mark at the edge of the introducer
- Any difficulties encountered during placement (e.g., ventricular ectopy, new bundle-branch blocks)
- Patient tolerance
- Confirmation of placement (e.g., chest radiograph)
- Initial values after placement of the catheter (PAPs, PAOP, RAP, CO, CI, SVR, PVR, Svo_2)
- Occurrence of unexpected outcomes
- Additional interventions
- Pain assessment, interventions, and effectiveness

References and Additional Readings

For a complete list of references and additional readings for this procedure, scan this QR code with your smartphone, or visit https://www.elsevier.com/__data/assets/pdf_file/0010/1319833/Chapter0058.pdf.

UNIT II

59 Pulmonary Artery Catheter Insertion (Assist) and Pressure Monitoring

Nikki J. Taylor

PURPOSE Pulmonary artery (PA) catheters are used to determine hemodynamic status in critically ill patients.[2,11,21,28] PA catheters provide information about right-sided and left-sided intracardiac pressures and cardiac output.[9] Additional functions available are fiberoptic monitoring of mixed venous oxygen saturation ($S_{V}O_2$),[31] intracardiac pacing,[23] and assessment of right-ventricular volumes and ejection fraction. Hemodynamic information obtained with a PA catheter is used to aid diagnosis and guide therapeutic intervention, including administration of fluids and diuretics and titration of vasoactive and inotropic medications.[5,11,21]

PREREQUISITE NURSING KNOWLEDGE

- Knowledge of the normal cardiovascular and pulmonary anatomy and physiology.
- Basic dysrhythmia recognition and treatment of life-threatening dysrhythmias.
- Knowledge of the principles of sterile technique.
- Advanced cardiac life support (ACLS) knowledge and skills.
- Knowledge of the components of the PA catheter (Fig. 59.1) and the location of the PA catheter within the heart (Fig. 59.2).
- Knowledge of the setup of the hemodynamic monitoring system (see Procedure 60, Single-Pressure and Multiple-Pressure Transducer Systems).
- Understanding of normal hemodynamic values (see Table 65.1).
- The PA catheter contains a proximal injectate lumen port, a PA distal lumen port, a thermistor connector, and a balloon-inflation port with valve. Some catheters also have two infusion ports, right atrial (RA) and right ventricular (RV) lumens that can be used for infusion of medications and intravenous fluids.[12]
- The PA distal lumen is used to monitor systolic, diastolic, and mean pressures in the PA. This lumen also allows for sampling of mixed venous blood. The proximal injectate lumen is used to monitor the RA pressure, inject the solution used to obtain cardiac output (CO), and may be used for infusions of medications or intravenous fluids. The balloon-inflation port is used to advance the PA catheter tip to the wedge position and measure the pulmonary artery occlusion pressure (PAOP).[12,35]
- PAOP may be referred to as *pulmonary artery wedge pressure* or *pulmonary capillary wedge pressure.*
- The PA diastolic pressure and the PAOP are indirect measures of left ventricular (LV) end-diastolic pressure.

Usually, the PAOP is approximately 1 to 4 mm Hg less than the pulmonary artery diastolic pressure (PADP). Because these two pressures are similar, the PADP is commonly followed, which minimizes the frequency of balloon inflation, thus decreasing the potential of balloon rupture and PA trauma.

- Significant differences between the PADP and the PAOP may exist for patients with pulmonary hypertension, chronic obstructive lung disease, acute respiratory distress syndrome, pulmonary embolus, and tachycardia. PADP is not used as a substitute for PAOP in these circumstances.
- See Procedure 58, Pulmonary Artery Catheter Insertion (Perform), for common indications for insertion of a PA catheter.
- Hemodynamic monitoring with a PA catheter has no absolute contraindications, but an assessment of risk versus benefit to the patient should be considered. Relative contraindications to PA catheter insertion include presence of fever, presence of a mechanical tricuspid valve, presence of an endocardial pacemaker, and a coagulopathic state. A patient with left bundle-branch block may develop a right bundle-branch block during PA catheter insertion, resulting in complete heart block.[1,2] In these patients, a temporary pacemaker should be readily available.
- PA pressures may be elevated as a result of PA hypertension, pulmonary disease, mitral valve disease, LV failure, atrial or ventricular left-to-right shunt, pulmonary emboli, or hypervolemia.
- PA pressures may be low due to hypovolemia or low pulmonary vascular resistance (e.g., vasodilation).
- Transduced waveforms that are viewable during insertion include RA, RV, PA, and PA occlusion (PAO; Figs. 59.2 and 59.3).
- The RA and PAO waveforms have *a*, *c*, and *v* waves[8]:
  - ❖ The *a* wave reflects atrial contraction, the *c* wave reflects closure of the atrioventricular valve, and the *v* wave reflects passive filling of the atria during ventricular systole (Figs. 59.4 and 59.5).

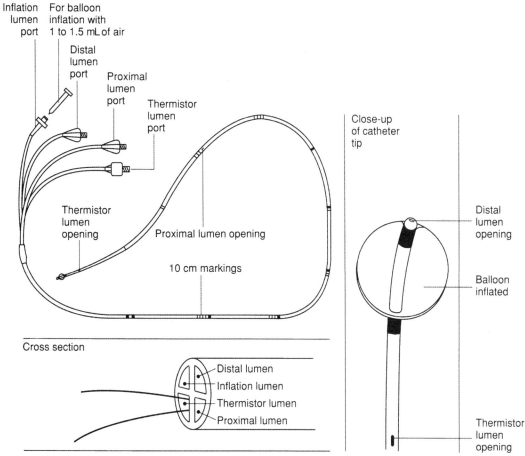

Figure 59.1 Anatomy of the pulmonary artery (PA) catheter. The standard 7.5F thermodilution PA catheter is 110 cm in length and contains four lumens. It is constructed of radiopaque polyvinyl chloride. Black markings are on the catheter in 10-cm increments beginning at the distal end. At the distal end of the catheter is a latex rubber balloon of 1.5-mL capacity, which, when inflated, extends slightly beyond the tip of the catheter without obstructing it. Balloon inflation cushions the tip of the catheter and prevents contact with the right-ventricular wall during insertion. The balloon also acts to float the catheter into position and allows measurement of the pulmonary artery occlusion pressure. The *narrow black bands* represent 10-cm lengths, and the *wide black bands* indicate 50-cm lengths. *(From Visalli F, Evans P: The Swan-Ganz catheter: a program for teaching safe effective use. Nursing 81[11]:1, 1981.)*

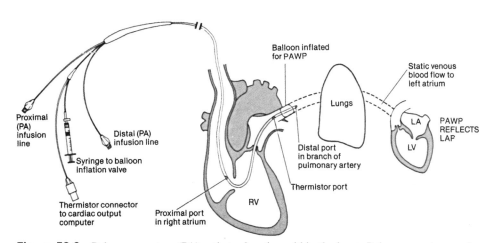

Figure 59.2 Pulmonary artery (PA) catheter location within the heart. Pulmonary artery occlusion pressure (PAOP) is an indirect measure of left-atrial *(LA)* and left-ventricular *(LV)* end-diastolic pressure. Pulmonary artery occlusion pressure (PAOP) is also referred to as *pulmonary artery wedge pressure (PAWP)*. LAP, Left atrial pressure. *(From Kersten LD: Comprehensive respiratory nursing, Philadelphia, 1989, Saunders.)*

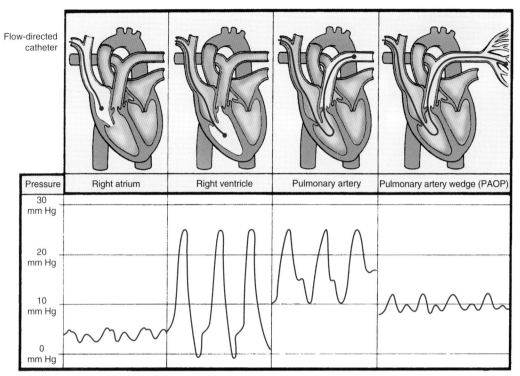

Figure 59.3   Illustration of ECG tracings in relation to pulmonary artery catheter location during insertion *(From Urden, LD, Stacy KM, Lough ME:* Thelan's critical care nursing: diagnosis and management, *ed 4, St. Louis, 2002.)*

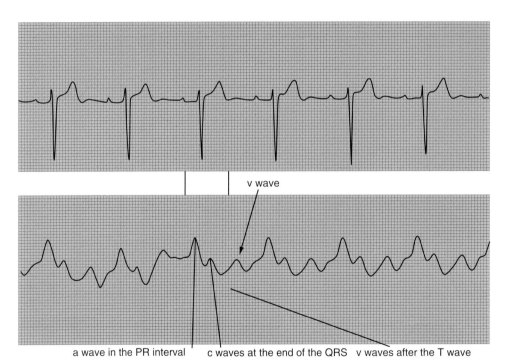

a wave in the PR interval   c waves at the end of the QRS   v waves after the T wave

Figure 59.4   Identification of *a, c,* and *v* waves in the waveform for right-atrial and central venous pressure. Atrial waveforms are characterized by three components: *a, c,* and *v* waves. The *a* wave reflects atrial contraction, the *c* wave reflects closure of the tricuspid valve, and the *v* wave reflects passive filling of the atria. *(From Ahrens TS, Taylor LK:* Hemodynamic waveform analysis, *Philadelphia, 1992, Saunders.)*

ECG

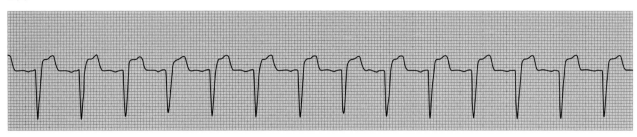

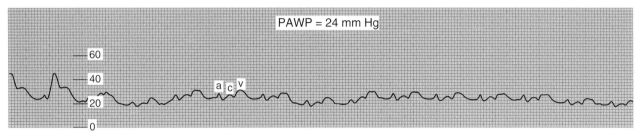

Figure 59.5 Normal pulmonary artery occlusion pressure (PAOP) waveform. Note the delay in the *a, c, and v* waves because of the time needed for the mechanical events to show a pressure change. This waveform is from a spontaneously breathing patient. The *arrow* indicates end-expiration, where the mean of *a* wave pressure is measured. Pulmonary artery occlusion pressure (PAOP) is also referred to as *pulmonary artery wedge pressure (PAWP).*

❖ The *a* wave reflects ventricular filling at end diastole. The mean of the *a* wave is determined by averaging the top and bottom values of the *a* wave.

❖ Elevated *a* and *v* waves may be evident in right atrial pressure (RAP/central venous pressure [CVP]) and in PAOP waveforms. These elevations may occur in patients with cardiac tamponade, constrictive pericardial disease, and hypervolemia.

❖ Elevated *a* waves in the RAP/CVP waveform may occur in patients with pulmonic or tricuspid valve stenosis, RV ischemia or infarction, RV failure, PA hypertension, and atrioventricular (AV) dissociation.

❖ Elevated *a* waves in the PAOP waveform may occur in patients with mitral valve stenosis, acute LV ischemia or infarction, LV failure, and AV dissociation.

❖ Elevated *v* waves in the RAP/CVP waveform may occur in patients with tricuspid valve insufficiency.

❖ Elevated *v* waves in the PAOP waveform may occur in patients with mitral valve insufficiency or a ruptured papillary muscle.

• Insertion and placement verification should occur as follows:

❖ The PA catheter is typically inserted through the subclavian, internal jugular, or femoral vein.[35]

❖ The standard 7.5F PA catheter is 110 cm long and has narrow black markings at 10-cm increments and wide black markings at 50-cm increments (see Fig. 59.1). The catheter should reach the PA after being advanced approximately 40 to 55 cm from the internal jugular vein, 35 to 50 cm from the subclavian vein, and 60 cm from the femoral vein.[12]

❖ Verification of PA catheter position is validated with waveform analysis.[1] Correct catheter position shows a PAO waveform when the balloon is inflated and a PA waveform when the balloon is deflated.

❖ Confirmation of the PA catheter position is also verified with chest radiography.

❖ The PA catheter balloon contains latex, which may cause allergic reactions. Latex-free catheters are available.

EQUIPMENT[2]

• PA catheter (non–heparin-coated PA catheters and latex-free PA catheters are available)
• Percutaneous sheath introducer kit and sterile catheter sleeve
• Pressure modules and cables for interface with the monitor
• Cardiac output cable with a thermistor/injectate sensor and/or continuous CO monitor
• Pressure-transducer system, including flush solution recommended according to institutional standards, a pressure bag or device, pressure tubing with transducers, and flush device (see Procedure 60, Single-Pressure and Multiple-Pressure Transducer Systems)
• Dual-channel recorder
• Sterile normal saline intravenous (IV) solution for flushing of the introducer and catheter infusion ports
• Antiseptic solution (e.g., 2% chlorhexidine-based preparation)
• Head covers, fluid-shield masks, sterile gowns, sterile gloves, nonsterile gloves, and full sterile drapes
• 1% lidocaine without epinephrine
• Sterile basin or cup
• Sterile water or normal saline solution
• Sterile dressing supplies
• Stopcocks (may be included in some pressure-tubing systems)
• Sterile injectable or noninjectable caps
• Leveling device (low-intensity laser or carpenter level)
Additional equipment, to have available as needed, includes the following:
• Fluoroscope[34] or ultrasound machine

UNIT II

- Emergency resuscitation equipment
- Temporary pacing equipment
- Indelible marker
- Transducer holder and IV pole
- 3-mL syringe, slip tip, and Luer-Lok
- Chlorhexidine-impregnated sponge

PATIENT AND FAMILY EDUCATION

- Provide the patient and family with information about the PA catheter, the reason for the PA catheter insertion, an explanation of the equipment, and the opportunity to ask questions.[2] *Rationale:* The patient and family will understand the procedure, why it is needed, and how it will help manage care. Patient and family anxiety may decrease.
- Explain the patient's expected participation during the procedure. *Rationale:* This explanation will encourage patient assistance.

PATIENT ASSESSMENT AND PREPARATION

Patient Assessment

- Determine baseline hemodynamic, cardiovascular, peripheral vascular, and neurovascular status. *Rationale:* Assessment provides data that can be used for comparison with postinsertion assessment data and hemodynamic values.
- Determine the patient's baseline pulmonary status. If the patient is mechanically ventilated, note the type of support, ventilator mode, and presence or absence of positive end-expiratory pressure (PEEP) or continuous positive airway pressure. *Rationale:* The presence of positive pressure mechanical ventilation alters hemodynamic waveforms and pressures.

- Assess the patient's medical history specifically related to problems with venous access sites, cardiac anatomy, and pulmonary anatomy. *Rationale:* Identification of obstructions or disease should be made before the insertion attempt.
- Assess the patient's current laboratory profile, including electrolyte, coagulation, and arterial blood gas results. *Rationale:* Laboratory abnormalities are identified. Baseline coagulation studies are helpful in determination of the risk for bleeding. Electrolyte and arterial blood gas imbalances may increase cardiac irritability.

Patient Preparation

- Verify the correct patient with two identifiers. *Rationale:* Before performing a procedure, the nurse should ensure the correct identification of the patient for the intended intervention.
- Ensure that the patient and family understand the preprocedural teaching and have spoken with the provider placing the catheter. Answer questions as they arise, and reinforce information as needed. *Rationale:* Understanding of previously taught information is evaluated and reinforced.
- Ensure that informed consent has been obtained.[2] *Rationale:* Informed consent protects the rights of the patient and makes a competent decision possible for the patient.
- Perform a preprocedure verification and time out. *Rationale:* This ensures patient safety.
- Validate the patency of the alternate central or peripheral IV access catheter. *Rationale:* Access may be needed for administration of emergency medications or fluids.
- Assist the patient to the supine position.[1] *Rationale:* This position prepares the patient for skin preparation, catheter insertion, and setup of the sterile field.
- Sedate the patient and/or give analgesics as prescribed as needed. *Rationale:* Movement of the patient may inhibit insertion of the PA catheter.

Procedure   for Assisting With Pulmonary Artery Catheter Insertion and Pressure Monitoring

Steps	Rationale	Special Considerations

Assisting with PA Catheter Insertion
1. **HH**
2. Prepare the flush solution for the pressure-transducer systems (see Procedure 60, Single-Pressure and Multiple-Pressure Transducer Systems).
  A. Use an IV bag of normal saline.
  B. Follow institutional standards for using heparinized flush solutions if a heparinized solution is prescribed and not contraindicated. **(Level B*)**
	Heparinized flush solutions may be used to minimize thrombi and fibrin deposits on catheters that might lead to thrombosis or bacterial colonization of the catheter.	Although heparin may prevent thrombosis,[25] it has been associated with thrombocytopenia and other hematological complications.[29] Further research is needed regarding the use of heparin versus normal saline to maintain PA catheter patency.

3. Prime or flush the pressure-transducer systems (see Procedure 60, Single-Pressure and Multiple-Pressure Transducer Systems).	Removes air bubbles. Air bubbles introduced into the patient's circulation can cause air embolism. Air bubbles within the tubing dampen the waveform.	Air is more easily removed from the hemodynamic tubing when the system is not under pressure.

*Level B: Well-designed, controlled studies with results that consistently support a specific action, intervention, or treatment.

Procedure for Assisting With Pulmonary Artery Catheter Insertion and Pressure Monitoring—*Continued*		
Steps	**Rationale**	**Special Considerations**
4. Apply and inflate the pressure bag or device to 300 mm Hg.	Each flush device delivers 1–3 mL/hour to maintain patency of the hemodynamic system.	
5. Connect the pressure cables (RA and PA) to the bedside monitor (see Fig. 60.2).	Connects the pressure-transducer systems to the bedside monitoring system.	
6. Set the scales on the bedside monitor for each anticipated pressure waveform.	Prepares the bedside monitor.	The scale for the RA/CVP pressure commonly is set at 20 mm Hg, and the PA scale commonly is set at 40 mm Hg. Scale settings may vary based on monitoring equipment. The scales can be adjusted if needed after the PA catheter is inserted based on patient pressures.
7. Level the RA (proximal) air-fluid interface (zeroing stopcock) and the PA (distal) air-fluid interface (zeroing stopcock) to the phlebostatic axis (see Figs. 60.7 and 60.9)[1].	The phlebostatic axis approximates the level of the atria and is the reference point for patients in the supine position.	The reference point for the atria changes when the patient is in the lateral position (see Fig. 60.8).
8. Zero the system connected to the PA (distal) lumen and to the RA (proximal) lumen of the PA catheter by turning the stopcock of each system off to the patient, opening it to air, and zeroing the monitoring system (see Procedure 60, Single-Pressure and Multiple-Pressure Transducer Systems). Replace with a new occlusive cap, and turn the stopcocks off to the air-fluid interface.	Prepares each monitoring system so pressures can be obtained during catheter insertion. New sterile caps prevent infection.	
9. 🅷🅷		
10. 🅿🅴		All healthcare personnel involved in the procedure must apply head coverings, fluid-shield masks, and sterile gowns.
11. Assist the provider as needed with opening the packaging of sterile drapes and opening the PA catheter and introducer kits.	Aids in preparing for the procedure.	The patient will be fully draped with exposure of only the insertion site.
12. If inserting a PA catheter with the ability to monitor mixed venous oxygenation,[31] the fiberoptics are calibrated before removal from the package (see Procedure 63, Continuous Venous Oxygen Saturation Monitoring).	Calibrates the system before insertion.	Follow the manufacturer's guidelines for catheter calibration.
13. When the sheath introducer is in place, connect a normal saline IV solution to the infusion port.	Maintains the patency of the sheath introducer infusion port.	
14. Connect the pressure-transducer system to the PA distal and proximal ports of the PA catheter when the provider inserting the PA catheter hands them off to the critical care nurse.	Provides assistance in preparing the catheter.	

Procedure continues on following page

UNIT II

Procedure for Assisting With Pulmonary Artery Catheter Insertion and Pressure Monitoring—*Continued*

Steps	Rationale	Special Considerations
15. Flush the air from the catheter.	Removes air from the pulmonary artery catheter.	Flush additional infusion ports, and attach sterile injectable or noninjectable caps.
16. Observe as provider wiggles the PA catheter (sometimes called *whipping*).[2,26]	The movement of the catheter will be seen on the monitor. This ensures that there are no connection issues or catheter defects before insertion.	
17. The provider will insert the PA catheter through a sterile catheter sleeve (see Procedure 58, Pulmonary Artery Catheter Insertion [Perform]).	Maintains sterility of the PA catheter to allow repositioning of the catheter.[26,35]	Additional research is needed to determine how long the sleeve remains sterile.
18. As insertion begins, continuously monitor and print the electrocardiogram (ECG) and PA distal pressure waveform strip.[1,2]	Provides documentation of RA, RV, and PA pressures during insertion and dysrhythmia occurrence during insertion.	A dual-channel recorder is preferred so the ECG and the PA waveform can be simultaneously recorded.
19. After the tip of the PA catheter is in the right atrium, inflate the balloon with no more than 1.25–1.5 mL of air, and close the gate valve or the stopcock (Fig. 59.6).	The inflated balloon helps to advance the PA catheter through the right side of the heart and into the PA, minimizing the chance of endocardial damage. Closing the gate valve or the stopcock holds air in the balloon during insertion.	The presence of the tip of the catheter in the right atrium is determined by observing the waveform (for RA/CVP waveform with *a*, *c*, and *v* waves) from the catheter's distal lumen during insertion (see Fig. 59.3). Use the syringe from the PA insertion kit. It will not allow more than 1.5 mL of air to be used. Clearly communicate with the provider inserting the catheter[35]: A. If the provider requests, "Inflate the balloon." B. The critical care nurse should respond, "Inflating the balloon" and "Balloon inflated and locked."
20. Observe for RA, RV, PA, and then PAO pressure waveforms (see Fig. 59.3).	Placement in the PA is validated with waveform analysis.	Monitor the ECG tracing as the PA catheter is inserted because ventricular dysrhythmias may result from RV irritability. RV pressures are obtained only during insertion.

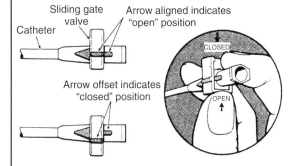

Figure 59.6 Pulmonary artery catheter gate valve. Gate valve in the open position *(top left)*. Gate valve in the closed position *(bottom left)*. *(Courtesy Baxter Edwards Corporation.)*

Procedure	for Assisting With Pulmonary Artery Catheter Insertion and Pressure Monitoring—*Continued*	
Steps	Rationale	Special Considerations
21. Verify that the PA catheter tip is in the proper position. A. When the balloon is deflated, the PA waveform is displayed on the monitor. B. When the balloon is inflated, the PAO waveform is displayed on the monitor.	When the balloon is inflated, the catheter floats from the PA to a smaller pulmonary arteriole. If there is resistance felt as it is reinflating or the waveform shows signs of overwedging, balloon insertion should stop immediately. If the balloon is unable to be fully inflated, this could be a sign that the catheter has passed too far distally and should be deflated and pulled back 1 cm (see Fig. 61.1).	The catheter usually reaches the PA after being advanced approximately 40–55 cm from the internal jugular vein, 35–50 cm from the subclavian vein, and 60 cm from the femoral vein.[26,35] Placement may vary depending on patient size. A chest radiograph is obtained to verify catheter position.
22. After the PA catheter is in place: A. Open the balloon inflation gate valve or stopcock. B. Disconnect the syringe from the balloon-inflation port to passively deflate the balloon. Follow institutional protocols regarding keeping the gate value or stopcock open. Reattach the empty syringe.	The gate valve or stopcock is closed during insertion to retain air in the balloon. The air is then passively released so continuous monitoring of the PA waveform can be performed.	Air is expelled from the syringe, and the empty syringe is reconnected to the balloon inflation valve port. Clearly communicate with the provider inserting the catheter: A. If the provider requests, "Deflate the balloon." B. The critical care nurse should respond, "Deflating the balloon" and "Balloon deflated."
23. Reassess accurate leveling, and secure the pressure transducer system (see Procedure 60, Single-Pressure and Multiple-Pressure Transducer Systems).	Ensures that the air-filled interface (zeroing stopcock) is maintained at the level of the phlebostatic axis. If the air-fluid interface is above the phlebostatic axis, PA pressures are falsely low. If the air-fluid interface is below the phlebostatic axis, PA pressures are falsely high.	Leveling ensures accuracy.[8] The point of the phlebostatic axis should be marked with an indelible marker, especially with use of a pole-mount setup.
24. Zero both the RA and PA pressure transducer systems (see Procedure 60, Single-Pressure and Multiple-Pressure Transducer Systems).	Allows the monitor to use atmospheric pressure as a reference for zero.	
25. Observe the waveform, and perform a dynamic response test (square wave test; see Fig. 53.3).	Determines whether the system is damped. This will ensure that the pressure waveform components are clearly defined and aids in accurate measurement.	The square wave test can be performed by activating and quickly releasing the fast flush. A sharp upstroke should terminate in a flat line at the maximal indicator on the monitor. This should be followed by an immediate rapid downstroke extending below baseline with 1–2 oscillations within 0.12 second and a quick return to baseline.
26. Assist if needed with applying an occlusive, sterile dressing to the insertion site. Be cautious that the sterile sleeve does not come in contact with the sterile dressing (see Procedure 75, Central Venous Catheter Insertion [Assist], Nursing Care, and Removal). If used, confirm that the twist lock is secure on the sterile catheter sleeve but not "over-tight."	Reduces the risk for infection.	Follow institutional standards for application of a chlorhexidine-impregnated sponge (see Procedure 75, Central Venous Catheter Insertion [Assist], Nursing Care, and Removal).

Procedure continues on following page

Procedure	for Assisting With Pulmonary Artery Catheter Insertion and Pressure Monitoring—*Continued*	
Steps	**Rationale**	**Special Considerations**
27. Connect the thermistor connector of the PA catheter to the CO monitor or module (see Procedure 65, Cardiac Output Measurement Techniques [Invasive]).	Allows the core temperature to be monitored and is needed for CO measurement.[8,35]	
28. Document the external centimeter marking of the PA catheter at the introducer exit site.	Identifies the length of the PA catheter inserted and allows for evaluation of PA catheter movement.	If the centimeter marking is not visible at the exit site, measure the distance from the introducer exit site to the nearest visible marking.
29. Set the monitor alarms.	Activates the bedside and central alarm system.	Upper and lower alarm limits are set on the basis of the patient's current clinical status and hemodynamic values.
30. Remove **PE**, and discard used supplies in appropriate receptacles.	Removes and safely discards used supplies.	
31. **HH**		
32. Ensure that the chest radiograph is completed.	Verifies PA catheter positioning.	

Obtaining PA Pressure Measurements
RA/CVP

1. Position the patient in the supine position with the head of the bed from 0 to 45 degrees. **(Level B*)**	Studies have determined that the RA and PA pressures are accurate in this position.[3,6,7,20]	RA and PA pressures may be accurate for patients in the supine position with the head of the bed elevated up to 60 degrees,[7,20,35] but additional studies are needed to support this. Only one study[19] supports the accuracy of hemodynamic values for patients in the lateral positions; other studies do not.[3,13] The majority of studies support the accuracy of hemodynamic monitoring for patients in the prone position.[33] Two studies demonstrated that prone positioning caused an increase in hemodynamic values[27,32]
2. Run a dual-channel strip of the ECG and RA waveform (Fig. 59.7).	RA pressures should be measured from the graphic strip because the effect of ventilation can be identified.	The digital monitor data can be used to measure RA pressure if ventilation does not cause respiratory variation of the RA pressure waveform. Some monitors have the capability of "freeze framing" waveforms. A cursor can be used to measure pressures.

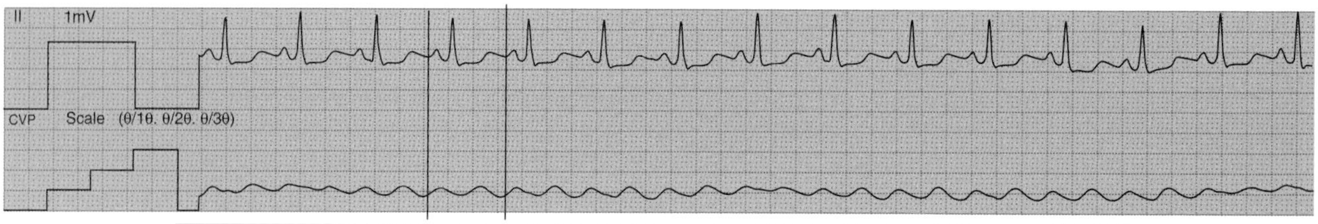

Figure 59.7   Note *vertical lines* drawn from the beginning of the P wave of two of the electrocardiogram complexes down to the right atrial (RA) waveform. The first positive deflection of the RA waveform is the *a* wave; the second positive deflection is the *v* wave. The *c* wave, which would lie between the *a* wave and the *v* wave, is not evident in this strip. *CVP*, Central venous pressure.

*Level B: Well-designed, controlled studies with results that consistently support a specific action, intervention, or treatment.

UNIT II

Procedure	for Assisting With Pulmonary Artery Catheter Insertion and Pressure Monitoring—*Continued*	
Steps	**Rationale**	**Special Considerations**
3. Measure RA pressure at end-expiration.	The effects of intrathoracic pressure on the RAP are minimized at the end-expiration phase of the respiratory cycle.	
4. With the dual-channel recorded strip, draw a vertical line from the beginning of the P wave of one of the ECG complexes down to the RA waveform. Repeat this with the next ECG complex (see Fig. 59.7).	Compares electrical activity with mechanical activity. Usually three waves are present on the RA waveform.	At times, the *c* wave is not present.
5. Align the PR interval with the RA waveform.	The *a* wave correlates with this interval.	
6. Identify the *a* wave.	The *a* wave is seen approximately 80–100 ms after the P wave. The *c* wave follows the *a* wave, and the *v* wave follows the *c* wave.	The *a* wave reflects atrial contraction.[8] The *c* wave reflects closure of the tricuspid valve.[8] The *v* wave reflects passive filling of the atria.[8]
7. Identify the scale setting of the RA waveform on the monitor (Fig. 59.8).	Optimizes the view of the waveform and aids in measurement of the pressure.	The RAP scale commonly is set at 20 mm Hg and may be adjusted to the patient's RAP to optimize the view of the waveform. Scale settings may vary based on monitoring equipment.
8. Measure the mean of the *a* wave to obtain the RAP (see Fig. 59.8).	The *a* wave represents atrial contraction and reflects right ventricular filling at end diastole.	

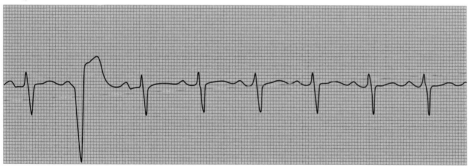

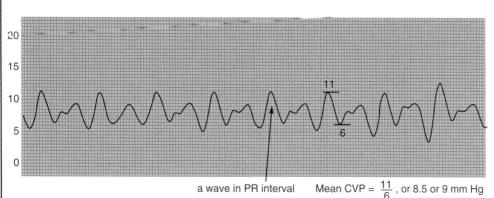

a wave in PR interval   Mean CVP = $\frac{11}{6}$, or 8.5 or 9 mm Hg

Figure 59.8 Obtaining measurements of right-atrial and central venous pressures *(RA/CVP)*. Aligning the *a* wave on the RA/CVP waveform with the PR interval on the electrocardiogram facilitates accurate measurement of RA/CVP at end diastole. *(From Ahrens TS, Taylor LK: Hemodynamic waveform analysis, Philadelphia, 1992, Saunders.)*

Procedure continues on following page

UNIT II

Procedure	for Assisting With Pulmonary Artery Catheter Insertion and Pressure Monitoring—*Continued*	
Steps	**Rationale**	**Special Considerations**

PA Systolic and Diastolic Pressures

1. Position the patient in the supine position with the head of the bed from 0 to 45 degrees. **(Level B*)**	Studies have determined that the RA and PA pressures are accurate in this position.[3,6,7,20]	RA and PA pressures may be accurate for patients in the supine position with the head of the bed elevated up to 60 degrees,[7,20] but additional studies are needed to support this. Only one study[19] supports the accuracy of hemodynamic values for patients in the lateral positions; other studies[14] do not. The majority of the studies[3,13] support the accuracy of hemodynamic monitoring for patients in the prone position, yet two studies showed that prone positioning caused an increase in hemodynamic values.[27,32]
2. Print a dual-channel strip of the ECG and PA waveform (Fig. 59.9).	PA pressures are measured from the graphic strip when respiratory variation of the waveform is noted because the effect of ventilation can be identified.	Some monitors have the capability of "freeze framing" waveforms. A cursor can be used to measure pressures.

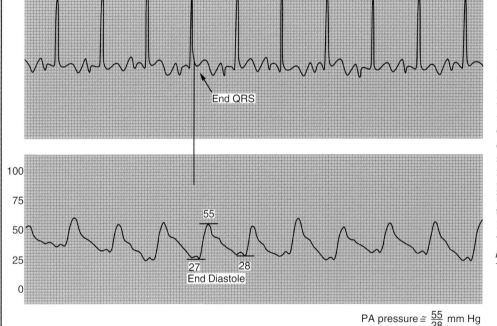

End QRS

100
75
50
25
0

55

27   28
End Diastole

PA pressure $\cong \frac{55}{28}$ mm Hg

Figure 59.9 Obtaining measurements of pressure in the pulmonary artery (PA). For systolic pressure, align the peak of the systolic waveform with the QT interval on the electrocardiogram. For PA diastolic pressure, use the end of the QRS as a marker to detect the PA diastolic phase. Obtain the reading just before the upstroke of the systolic waveform. *(From Ahrens TS, Taylor LK:* Hemodynamic waveform analysis, *Philadelphia, 1992, Saunders.)*

*Level B: Well-designed, controlled studies with results that consistently support a specific action, intervention, or treatment.

Procedure	for Assisting With Pulmonary Artery Catheter Insertion and Pressure Monitoring—*Continued*		
Steps	**Rationale**		**Special Considerations**
3. Measure the PA pressure at end-expiration.	The effects of intrathoracic pressure on the PAP is minimized at the end-expiration phase of the respiratory cycle.		
4. Identify the QT interval on the ECG strip.	Represents ventricular depolarization.		
5. Align the QT interval with the PA waveform.	Allows comparison of cardiac electrical activity with mechanical activity.		
6. Identify the scale setting of the PA waveform on the monitor.	Optimizes the view of the waveform and aids in measurement of the pressure.		The PAP scale commonly is set at 40 mm Hg and may be adjusted to the patient's PAP to optimize the view of the waveform. Scale settings may vary based on monitoring equipment.
7. Measure the PA systolic pressure at the peak of the systolic waveform on the PA waveform (see Fig. 59.9).	Reflects the highest PA systolic pressure.		
8. Align the end of the QRS complex with the PA waveform (see Fig. 59.9).	Compares electrical activity with mechanical activity. The end of the QRS complex correlates with ventricular end-diastolic pressure.		
9. Measure the PA diastolic pressure at the point of the intersection of this line (see Fig. 59.9).	This point occurs just before the upstroke of the systolic pressure.		
PAOP			
1. Position the patient in the supine position with the head of the bed from 0 to 45 degrees. (**Level B***)	Studies have determined that the RA and PA pressures are accurate in this position.[3,6,7,20]		RA and PA pressures may be accurate for patients in the supine position with the head of the bed elevated up to 60 degrees,[7,20] but additional studies are needed to support this. Only one study[19] supports the accuracy of hemodynamic values for patients in the lateral positions; other studies[4,14] do not. The majority of the studies[33] support the accuracy of hemodynamic monitoring for patients in the prone position, but two studies demonstrated that prone positioning caused an increase in hemodynamic values.[27,32]
2. Fill the PA balloon syringe with 1.5 mL of air.	More than 1.5 mL of air may rupture the PA balloon and the pulmonary arteriole.[35]		
3. Connect the PA balloon syringe to the gate valve or stopcock of the balloon port of the PA catheter, and unlock the gate valve (see Fig. 59.6).	This port is designed for balloon air inflation.		
4. Print a dual-channel strip of the ECG and PA waveform.	The PAO pressures are measured from the graphic strip because the effect of ventilation can be identified.		Some monitors have the capability of "freeze framing" waveforms. A cursor can be used to measure pressures.

*Level B: Well-designed, controlled studies with results that consistently support a specific action, intervention, or treatment.

Procedure continues on following page

Procedure	for Assisting With Pulmonary Artery Catheter Insertion and Pressure Monitoring—*Continued*	
Steps	Rationale	Special Considerations
5. Slowly inflate the balloon with air until the PA waveform changes to a PAO waveform (Fig. 59.10).	A slight resistance is usually felt during inflation of the balloon. Only enough air needed to convert the PA waveform to a PAO waveform should be instilled. Thus the entire amount of 1.5 mL of air is not necessarily needed.	Avoid overinflation of the balloon because it can cause pulmonary arteriole infarction or rupture, resulting in potentially life-threatening hemorrhage.[14]
6. Inflate the balloon for no more than 8–15 seconds (2–4 respiratory cycles).[26]	Prolonged inflation of the balloon can cause pulmonary arteriole infarction and/or rupture, with potentially life-threatening hemorrhage.[14]	
7. Disconnect the syringe from the balloon-inflation port to passively deflate the balloon. **(Level M*)**	Allows air to passively escape from the balloon.	Active withdrawal of air from the balloon can weaken the balloon, pull the balloon structure into the inflation lumen, and possibly cause balloon rupture.
8. Observe the monitor to verify the PAO waveform changes back to the PA waveform.	Ensures adequate balloon deflation and safe positioning of the PA catheter for continuous monitoring.[35]	
9. Expel air from the balloon syringe.	The syringe should remain empty when reconnected so accidental balloon inflation does not occur.	

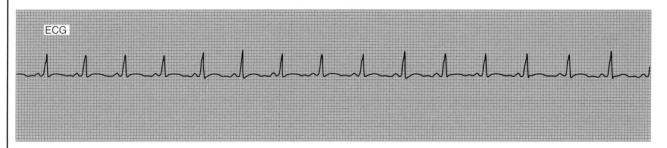

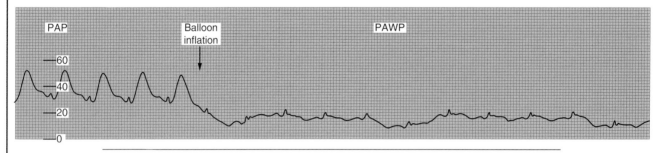

Figure 59.10   Change in pulmonary artery pressure *(PAP)* waveform to pulmonary artery occlusion pressure waveform with balloon inflation. The balloon is inflated while the bedside monitor is observed for change in the waveform. Balloon inflation *(arrow)* in a patient with normal pulmonary artery occlusion pressure. Pulmonary artery occlusion pressure (PAOP) is also referred to as *pulmonary artery wedge pressure (PAWP)*.

*Level M: Manufacturer's recommendations only.

Procedure	for Assisting With Pulmonary Artery Catheter Insertion and Pressure Monitoring—*Continued*	
Steps	Rationale	Special Considerations
10. Reconnect the empty balloon syringe to the balloon-inflation port.	The syringe that is manufactured for the PA catheter should be connected to the PA balloon port to avoid loss of the custom-designed syringe. This syringe can be filled with only 1.5 mL of air, thus serving as a safety feature to minimize the chance of balloon overinflation.	
11. Follow institutional standards regarding keeping the gate valve or the stopcock open.	The most important considerations are that the balloon syringe is attached to the balloon-inflation port, the syringe is empty, and the PA distal waveform reflects a pulmonary artery waveform.	
12. With the dual-channel recorded strip, draw a vertical line from the beginning of the P wave of one of the ECG complexes down to the PAO waveform. Repeat this with the next ECG complex.	Compares cardiac electrical activity with mechanical activity. Two waves (*a* and *v*) to three waves (*a, c,* and *v*) will be present on the PAO waveform.	The *c* waves commonly are not present on PAO waveforms because of the distance the pressure needs to travel back to the transducer.[24]
13. Align the end of a QRS complex of the ECG strip with the PAO waveform (Fig. 59.11).	Aligns the relationship of cardiac electrical activity with mechanical activity.	

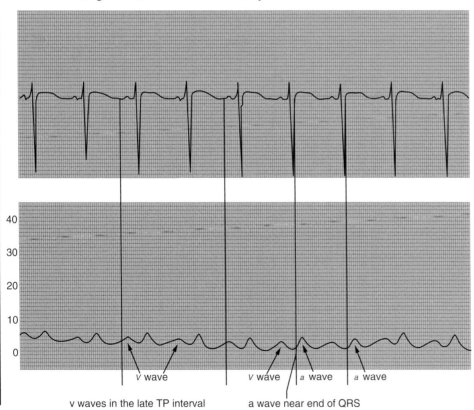

40
30
20
10
0

v wave   *v* wave   / *a* wave   *a* wave

v waves in the late TP interval   a wave near end of QRS

Figure 59.11 Obtaining measurement of the pulmonary artery occlusion pressure (PAOP). For accurate readings, align the *a* wave from the PAO waveform with the end of the QRS on the electrocardiogram at end diastole. Pulmonary artery occlusion pressure (PAOP) is also referred to as *pulmonary artery wedge pressure* (PAWP). (*From Ahrens TS, Taylor LK:* Hemodynamic waveform analysis, *Philadelphia, 1992, Saunders.*)

Procedure continues on following page

Procedure	for Assisting With Pulmonary Artery Catheter Insertion and Pressure Monitoring—*Continued*	

Steps	Rationale	Special Considerations
14. Identify the *a* wave (see Fig. 59.11).	The *a* wave correlates with the end of the QRS complex. The *c* wave follows the *a* wave, and the *v* wave follows the *c* wave.	If only two waves are present, the first wave is the *a* wave, and the second wave is the *v* wave.
15. Identify the scale of the PAO tracing.	Aids in determination of pressure measurement.	The PA scale commonly is set at 40 mm Hg.
16. Measure the mean of the *a* wave to obtain the PAOP (see Fig. 59.5).	The *a* wave represents atrial contraction and reflects LV filling at end diastole.	If PEEP is being used and the PEEP is more than 10 cm H_2O, adjustments in determination of the pressures may be necessary. Follow institutional standards.
17. Compare the PADP with the PAOP.	The PAOP is commonly 1–4 mm Hg less than the PADP. PADPs that correlate with PAOPs represent LV filling pressures.	Significant differences between PADP and PAOP may exist for patients with pulmonary hypertension, chronic obstructive lung disease, acute respiratory distress syndrome, pulmonary embolus, and tachycardia.
18. Follow the PADP if a close correlation is found between the PADP and PAOP.	Considered an accurate measurement of LV filling pressures.	Minimizes the number of times the PA balloon is inflated.
19. Follow the PAOP if >4 mm Hg of difference is found between the PAOP and PADP.	Ensures the accuracy of measurements.	

Measurement of Hemodynamic Pressures at End-Expiration

1. Measure all hemodynamic pressures at end-expiration to ensure accuracy.[12]	Atmospheric and alveolar pressures are approximately equal at end-expiration. Intrathoracic pressure is closest to zero at end-expiration. Measurement of hemodynamic pressures is most accurate at end-expiration because pulmonary pressures have minimal effect on intracardiac pressures.	
2. Determine end-expiration by observing the rise and fall of the chest during breathing and use of printed graphics of hemodynamic, respiratory, capnography, or continuous airway pressure waveforms.	Aids in the determination of the end-expiratory phase of ventilation.	

Determining End-Expiration for the Patient Breathing Spontaneously

1. Record a strip of the PA waveform.	A labeled recording aids in determination of accurate hemodynamic pressure values.	In patients who are breathing spontaneously, the normal inspiratory:expiratory ratio is approximately 1:2.
2. Note that the pressure waveform dips down during the inspiratory phase of spontaneous breathing (Fig. 59.12).	Intrapleural pressure decreases during spontaneous inspiration, and this decrease is reflected by a fall in cardiac pressures.	
3. Note that the pressure waveform elevates during the expiratory phase of breathing (see Fig. 59.12).	At end-expiration, atmospheric and intrathoracic pressures (pleural and alveolar) are equalized; thus cardiac pressures are most accurately reflected.	

Procedure	for Assisting With Pulmonary Artery Catheter Insertion and Pressure Monitoring—*Continued*	
Steps	**Rationale**	**Special Considerations**

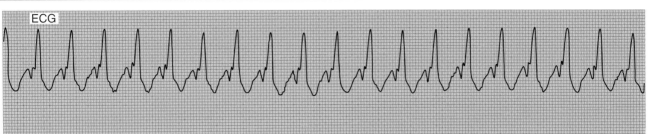

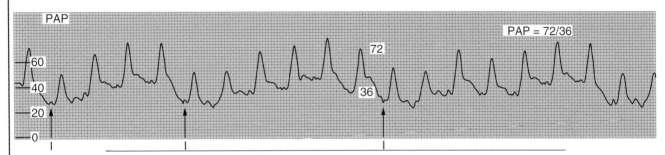

Figure 59.12 Respiratory fluctuations of pulmonary artery pressure (PAP) waveform in a spontaneously breathing patient. The location of inspiration *(I)* is marked on the waveform. The points just before inspiration are end-expiration, where readings are taken.

4. Measure the pressure at the end of the expiratory phase (see Fig. 59.12).	Ensures accurate and consistent pressure measurements.	

Determining End-Expiration for the Patient Receiving Positive Pressure Mechanical Ventilation

1. Record a strip of the PA waveform.	A labeled recording aids in determination of accurate hemodynamic pressure values.	
2. Note that the pressure waveform elevates as a breath is delivered by the ventilator (Fig. 59.13).	As the ventilator delivers a positive pressure breath to the lungs, an increase in intrathoracic pressure results. This increase in intrathoracic pressure causes an increase in cardiac pressures.	
3. Note that the pressure waveform dips down as the breath is exhaled (see Fig. 59.13).	As the mechanical breath is exhaled, intrathoracic pressures decrease, and cardiac pressures are most accurately and consistently measured.	

Determining End-Expiration for the Patient Receiving Intermittent Mandatory Mechanical Ventilation

1. Record a strip of the PA waveform.	A labeled recording aids in determination of accurate hemodynamic pressure monitoring.	
2. If the patient is receiving intermittent mandatory ventilation, measure the pressure during end-expiration.	Aids in accuracy of pressure measurements.	
3. Note that the pressure waveform elevates as a breath is delivered by the ventilator (Fig. 59.14).	As the ventilator delivers a breath to the lungs, an increase in intrathoracic pressure results. This increase in pressure causes an increase in cardiac pressures.	
4. Note that the pressure waveform dips down as the breath is exhaled (see Fig. 59.14).	As the mechanical breath is exhaled, intrathoracic pressure decreases, and cardiac pressures are more accurately reflected.	

Procedure continues on following page

UNIT II

Steps	Rationale	Special Considerations

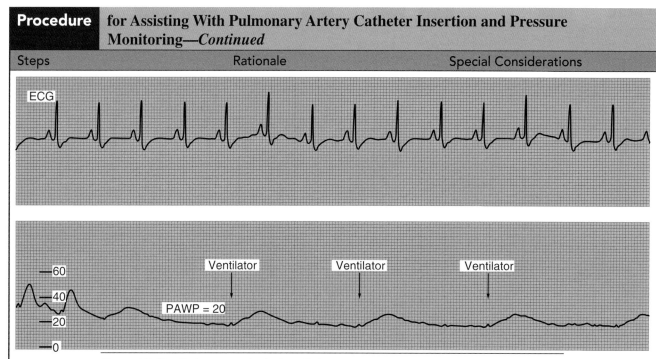

Figure 59.13 Patient on mechanical ventilation (on pressure support–type ventilator) who had no spontaneous respiration because of a neuromuscular-blocking agent (vecuronium). The point of end-expiration is located just before the ventilator artifact. Pulmonary artery occlusion pressure (PAOP) is also referred to as *pulmonary artery wedge pressure (PAWP)*.

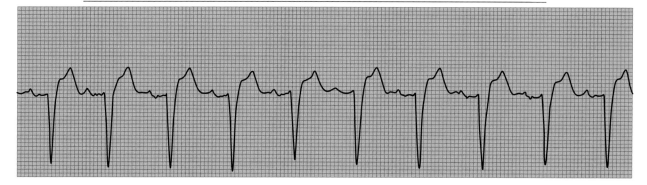

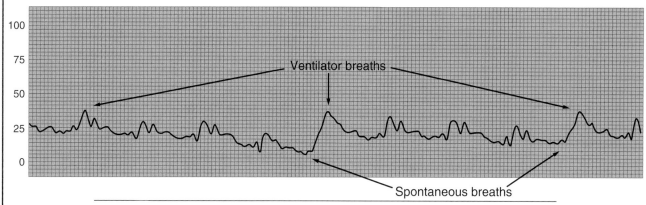

Figure 59.14 Intermittent mandatory ventilation mode of ventilation and the effect on the pulmonary artery waveform. *(From Ahrens TS, Taylor LK:* Hemodynamic waveform analysis, *Philadelphia, 1992, Saunders.)*

| 5. Identify the patient's spontaneous breath (see Fig. 59.14). | This breath may occur just before triggered ventilator breaths. | |
| 6. Determine end-expiration. | Ensures accuracy of measurements. | Airway pressure waveforms can be used to facilitate identification of end-expiration. |

Expected Outcomes

- Accurate placement of the PA catheter
- Adequate and appropriate waveforms
- Ability to obtain accurate cardiac pressure measurements and associated hemodynamic data
- Evaluation of information obtained to guide diagnostic and therapeutic interventions

Unexpected Outcomes[1,2,12,15,23]

- Pneumothorax or hemothorax
- Infection/sepsis
- Ventricular dysrhythmias
- Heart block
- Misplacement
- Hemorrhage
- Hematoma
- Pericardial or ventricular rupture
- Venous air embolism
- Cardiac tamponade
- PA infarction
- PA rupture
- PA catheter balloon rupture
- PA catheter knotting
- Pseudoaneurysm formation
- Heparin-induced thrombocytopenia
- Thrombosis
- Valvular damage
- Pain

Patient Monitoring and Care

Steps	Rationale	Reportable Conditions
		These conditions should be reported to the provider if they persist despite nursing interventions.
1. Recheck transducer leveling whenever patient position changes.	Ensures accurate reference point for the left atrium.	
2. Zero the transducer during initial setup or before insertion if disconnection occurs between the transducer and the monitoring cable, if disconnection occurs between the monitoring cable and the monitor, and when the values obtained do not fit the clinical picture.	Ensures accuracy of the hemodynamic monitoring system.	
3. Place sterile injectable or noninjectable caps on all stopcocks. Replace with new sterile caps whenever the caps are removed.	Stopcocks can be a source of contamination. Stopcocks that are part of the initial setup are packaged with vented caps. Vented caps need to be replaced with sterile injectable or noninjectable caps to maintain a closed system and reduce the risk of contamination and infection.	
4. Monitor the pressure-transducer system (e.g., pressure tubing, transducer, stopcocks) for air, and eliminate air from the system.	Air in the transducer system affects the accuracy of pressure measurements. Air emboli are also potentially fatal.	• Suspected air emboli

UNIT II

Patient Monitoring and Care —*Continued*

Steps	Rationale	Reportable Conditions
5. Continuously monitor hemodynamic waveforms, and obtain hemodynamic values (pulmonary artery systolic pressure, PADP, RAP) hourly and as necessary with condition changes and to evaluate therapy interventions. Follow institutional standards for obtaining hemodynamic values.	Provides for continuous waveform analysis and assessment of patient status.	• Abnormal hemodynamic waveforms or pressures
6. Obtain CO, cardiac index, and systemic vascular resistance and additional parameters after catheter insertion and as necessary per patient condition and interventions.	Monitors patient status and response to therapeutic interventions.	• Abnormal hemodynamic parameters or significant changes in hemodynamic parameters
7. Change the hemodynamic monitoring system (flush solution, pressure tubing, transducers, and stopcocks) every 96 hours. (**Level B***) The flush solution may need to be changed more frequently if near empty of solution.	The Centers for Disease Control and Prevention (CDC), the Infusion Nurses Society,[16,17] and research findings recommend that the hemodynamic flush system can be used safely for 96 hours.[10,25,29] This recommendation is based on research conducted with disposable pressure-monitoring systems used for peripheral and central lines.	
8. Perform a dynamic response test (square wave test) at the start of each shift, with a change of the waveform or after the system is opened to air (see Fig. 53.3).	An optimally damped system provides an accurate waveform.	• Overdamped or underdamped waveforms that cannot be corrected with troubleshooting procedures
9. Label the tubing with the date and time the system was prepared.	Identifies when the system needs to be changed.	
10. Maintain the pressure bag or device at 300 mm Hg.	At 300 mm Hg, each flush device delivers approximately 1–3 mL/hour to maintain patency of the system.	
11. Do not fast flush the distal lumen of the PA catheter for longer than 2 seconds.	PA rupture may occur with prolonged flushing of high-pressure fluid.	• Hemoptysis
12. Never flush the distal lumen of the PA catheter when the balloon is wedged in the pulmonary artery.	Excessive PA pressure may cause PA damage or rupture.	• Hemoptysis
13. Use aseptic technique when withdrawing from or flushing the PA catheter.	Prevents contamination of the system and related infection.	
14. Clear the system, including stopcocks, of all traces of blood after blood withdrawal.	Blood can become a medium for bacterial growth.[10,16,17,25] Clots also may be flushed into the catheter if all blood is not eliminated.	
15. Maintain sterility and integrity of the plastic sleeve covering the PA catheter.	Any tear in the sleeve breaks the sterile barrier, making catheter repositioning no longer possible.	• Defects in the integrity of the plastic sleeve

*Level B: Well-designed, controlled studies with results that consistently support a specific action, intervention, or treatment.

Patient Monitoring and Care —*Continued*

Steps	Rationale	Reportable Conditions
16. Blood products and albumin should never be infused through the PA catheter.	Viscous blood may occlude the catheter. The accuracy of the PA monitoring system may be adversely affected.	
17. IV fluids are never infused via the distal lumen of the PA catheter and are sometimes infused via the proximal lumen of the PA catheter when IV access is necessary.	PA monitoring is not possible, and a life-threatening situation can occur (e.g., undetected wedged PA catheter).	
18. Replace gauze dressings every 2 days and transparent dressings at least every 5–7 days and more frequently as needed.[16,17,25,30] **(Level D*)**	Decreases the risk for infection at the catheter site. The Centers for Disease Control and Prevention (CDC) and the Infusion Nurses Society recommend replacing the dressing when it becomes damp, loosened, or soiled or when inspection of the site is necessary.[17,18,27]	• Signs or symptoms of infection
19. Perform central venous catheter site care (see Procedure 75, Central Venous Catheter Insertion [Assist], Nursing Care, and Removal).	Ensures consistency of dressing change and indicates when the next change will occur.	
20. Print PA waveform strips to place on the patient's chart at the start of each shift and whenever a change in the waveform occurs.	The printed waveform allows assessment of the adequacy of the waveform, the presence of damping, and if respiratory variation is present.	
21. Assess the need for the PA catheter daily. If long-term use of the PA catheter is needed, consider changing the PA catheter every 7 days. **(Level B*)**	The Centers for Disease Control and Prevention (CDC)[25] and research findings[4] recommend that PA catheters do not need to be changed more frequently than every 7 days. There are no specific recommendations regarding routine replacement of PA catheters that need to be in place for >7 days.[25] Guidewire exchanges should not be used routinely. A guidewire exchange should only be used to replace a catheter that is malfunctioning.[25]	• Signs and symptoms of infection at the PA catheter insertion site • Signs and symptoms of sepsis
22. Follow institutional standards for assessing pain. Administer analgesia as prescribed.	Identifies need for pain interventions.	• Continued pain despite pain interventions

*Level B: Well-designed, controlled studies with results that consistently support a specific action, intervention, or treatment.
*Level D: Peer-reviewed professional and organizational standards with the support of clinical study recommendations.

UNIT II

Documentation

Documentation should include the following:
- Patient and family education
- Completion of informed consent
- Universal protocol requirements
- Insertion of the PA catheter
- External centimeter marking of the PA catheter noted at the exit site
- Patient tolerance of the procedure
- Confirmation of PA catheter placement (e.g., waveforms, chest radiograph)
- Date and time of PA catheter site care and dressing change
- Pain assessment, interventions, and effectiveness
- Cardiac rhythm during PA catheter insertion and monitoring
- Site assessment
- PA pressures (RA/CVP, RV [insertion only], PA systolic, diastolic, mean, and PAOP)
- Waveforms (RA/CVP, RV [insertion only], pulmonary artery pressure, PAOP)
- CO/CI and systemic vascular resistance
- Occurrence of unexpected outcomes and interventions

References and Additional Readings

For a complete list of references and additional readings for this procedure, scan this QR code with your smartphone, or visit https://www.elsevier.com/__data/assets/pdf_file/0011/13 19834/Chapter0059.pdf.

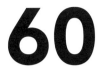

Single-Pressure and Multiple-Pressure Transducer Systems

Janet Regan-Baggs

PURPOSE Single-pressure and multiple-pressure transducer systems provide a catheter-to-monitor interface so intravascular and intracardiac pressures can be measured. The transducer detects a biophysical event and converts it to an electronic signal.

PREREQUISITE NURSING KNOWLEDGE

- Knowledge of the anatomy and physiology of the cardiovascular system.
- Knowledge of the principles of aseptic technique.
- Fluid-filled pressure-monitoring systems used for bedside hemodynamic pressure monitoring are based on the principle that a change in pressure at any point in an unobstructed system can result in similar pressure changes at all other points of the system.
- Pressure transducers detect the pressure waveform generated by ventricular ejection and convert that pressure wave into an electrical signal, which is transmitted to the monitoring equipment for representation as a waveform on the oscilloscope.
- Invasive measurement of intravascular (arterial) pressure requires insertion of a catheter into an artery.
- Invasive measurement of intracardiac (right atrial [RA] and pulmonary artery [PA]) pressures requires insertion of a catheter into the PA.
- Invasive measurement of central venous pressure can be monitored by insertion of a catheter into the internal jugular vein, into the subclavian vein, or via a peripherally inserted central catheter (PICC)[1].
- Alternative sites for pressure monitoring include peripheral veins and the femoral/iliac vein. These sites however require further steps to ensure accuracy.[1]
- A single-pressure transducer system is used to measure pressure from a single catheter (e.g., arterial catheter, central venous; Fig. 60.1).
- A double-pressure transducer system is used to measure pressure from two catheters (e.g., arterial and central venous) or two ports (e.g., PA and RA) from a single catheter (e.g., PA catheter; Fig. 60.2).
- A triple-pressure transducer system is commonly used to measure pressures from the arterial and PA catheters. With this system, arterial pressures, PA pressures, and RA pressures can be obtained (Fig. 60.3).
- For accuracy of the hemodynamic values obtained from any transducer system, leveling, zeroing, and a normal dynamic response are essential.

- All hemodynamic values (PA, RA, and arterial) are referenced to the level of the atria. The external reference point of the atria is the phlebostatic axis.

EQUIPMENT

- Invasive catheter (e.g., arterial, PA, CVC)
- Pressure transducer system, including flush solution recommended according to institutional standards, a pressure bag or device, pressure tubing with transducers, and flush device
- Blood conservation device if using and separate from the transducer system
- Pressure modules and cables for interface with the monitor
- Cardiac output cable with a thermistor/injectate sensor for use with the PA catheter
- Monitoring system (central and bedside monitor)
- Dual-channel recorder
- Sterile injectable and noninjectable caps
- Indelible skin marker
- Leveling device (low-intensity laser or carpenter level)

Additional equipment, to have available as needed, includes the following:
- Heparin (for flush solution if prescribed)
- 3-mL syringe
- Stopcocks (with additional sterile injectable or noninjectable, nonvented caps)
- Foam dressing or hydrocolloid gel pad
- Tape
- Nonsterile gloves
- Transducer holder and intravenous (IV) pole

PATIENT AND FAMILY EDUCATION

- Assess patient and family understanding of hemodynamic monitoring and the reason for its use. ***Rationale:*** Clarification or reinforcement of information is an expressed patient and family need.
- Explain the procedure for hemodynamic monitoring. ***Rationale:*** This information prepares the patient and the family for what to expect and may decrease anxiety.

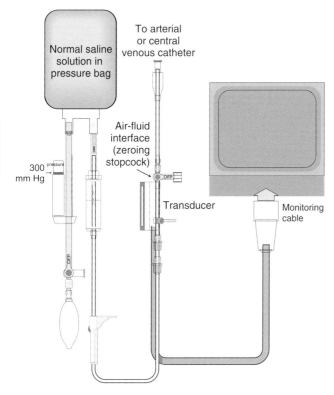

Figure 60.1 Single-pressure transducer system. *(Drawing by Paul W. Schiffmacher, Thomas Jefferson University, Philadelphia, PA.)*

PATIENT ASSESSMENT AND PREPARATION

Patient Assessment

- Assess the patient for conditions that may warrant the use of a hemodynamic monitoring system, including hypotension or hypertension, cardiac failure, cardiogenic shock, cardiac arrest, hemorrhage, respiratory failure, fluid imbalances, oliguria, anuria, and sepsis. ***Rationale:*** Assessment provides data regarding signs and symptoms of hemodynamic instability.
- Obtain the patient's medical history of coagulopathies, use of anticoagulants, vascular abnormalities, cardiac valvular disease, pulmonary hypertension, and peripheral neuropathies. ***Rationale:*** The medical history assists in determining the safety of the procedure and aids in site selection.
- Asses the patient for history of heparin allergy or past medical history of heparin-induced thromboembolism. ***Rationale:*** The medical history aids in determining if a heparinized flush solution should be avoided.

Patient Preparation

- Verify the correct patient with two identifiers. ***Rationale:*** Before performing a procedure, the nurse should ensure the correct identification of the patient for the intended intervention.

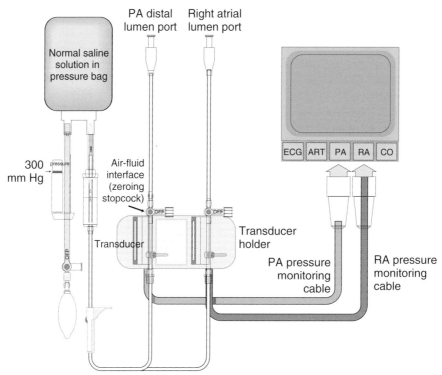

Figure 60.2 Double-pressure transducer system. *ART,* Arterial; *CO,* cardiac output, *ECG,* electrocardiogram; *PA,* pulmonary artery; *RA,* right atrial. *(Drawing by Paul W. Schiffmacher, Thomas Jefferson University, Philadelphia, PA.)*

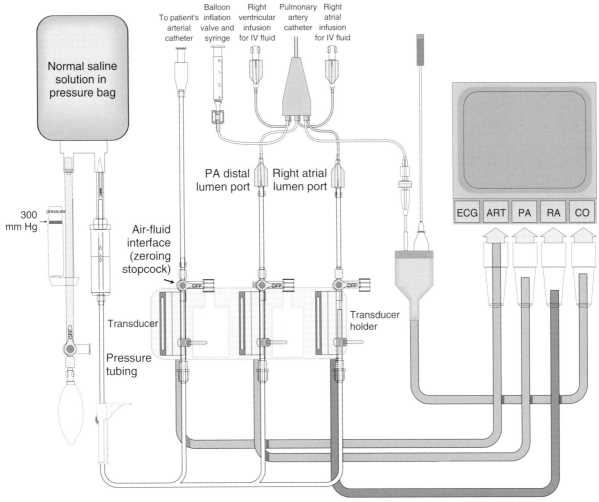

Figure 60.3 Triple-pressure transducer system. *ART,* Arterial; *CO,* cardiac output, *ECG,* electrocardiogram; *PA,* pulmonary artery; *RA,* right atrial. *(Drawing by Paul W. Schiffmacher, Thomas Jefferson University, Philadelphia, PA.)*

- Ensure that the patient and family understand the preprocedural teaching. Answer questions as they arise, and reinforce information as needed. ***Rationale:*** Understanding of previously taught information is evaluated and reinforced.

- Position the patient in the supine position with the head of the bed flat or elevated up to 45 degrees. ***Rationale:*** This positioning prepares the patient for hemodynamic monitoring.

Procedure for Single-Pressure and Multiple-Pressure Transducer Systems		
Steps	Rationale	Special Considerations
Disposable Pressure Transducer System Setup		
1. 🔲		
2. Use an IV bag of normal saline solution. **(Level B*)**	Normal saline solution is preferred. Solutions containing dextrose increase the incidence of infection and should not be used.[16,30,32]	

*Level B: Well-designed, controlled studies with results that consistently support a specific action, intervention, or treatment.

Procedure continues on following page

Procedure	**for Single-Pressure and Multiple-Pressure Transducer Systems—***Continued*	
Steps	**Rationale**	**Special Considerations**
3. Follow institutional standards for adding heparin to the flush solution. **(Level B*)**	Heparinized flush solutions are used to minimize thrombi and fibrin deposits on catheters that might lead to thrombosis or bacterial colonization of the catheter.	Although heparin may prevent thrombosis,[2,13,16,30,32] it has been associated with thrombocytopenia and other hematological complications.[2,32] Studies investigating if arterial catheter patency is affected by the presence of heparin in the flush solution have conflicting findings.[16,32] Further research is needed regarding the use of heparin versus normal saline solution to maintain catheter patency.
4. Label the IV bag, indicating the date and time the solution was hung, the dose of heparin (if used), and your initials.	Identifies the contents of the IV flush bag and identifies when the IV bag needs to be changed.	
5. Open the prepackaged pressure transducer kit with aseptic technique. A. A single-pressure tubing kit can be used for RA or arterial monitoring (see Fig. 60.1). B. A double-pressure tubing kit can be used for PA and RA monitoring (see Fig. 60.2). C. A triple-pressure tubing kit can be used for arterial, PA, and RA monitoring (see Fig. 60.3).	Provides the correct pressure tubing.	Assemble the pressure transducers, pressure tubing, and stopcocks if not preassembled by the manufacturer. Minimize tubing length and number of stopcocks to optimize dynamic response.[25]
6. Add a blood conservation device per institutional guidelines.	Blood conservation devices may reduce iatrogenic anemia, subsequent transfusion, and system contamination.[3,16,26]	Blood conservation devices may negatively affect the dynamic response of the transducer system. Optimize the system, and determine the impact of the addition by performing a square-wave test/dynamic response (Fig. 60.10)[1,3,36]
7. Tighten all connections.	Prepares the system. Tightening the connections prevents air from entering the system and fluid leaks.	
8. Spike the outlet port of the IV solution with the pressure tubing.	Allows access to the IV flush solution.	Separate flush systems are needed if invasive catheters are inserted at different times.
9. Remove air from the flush solution bag.	Reduces bubble formation within tubing and reduces the risk of air entering the system if the bag empties.[25]	
10. Open the roller clamp, and squeeze the drip chamber to fill the chamber half full.	Primes the drip chamber.	Filling the drip chamber at least halfway is important to prevent air bubbles from entering the tubing and allows the nurse to see that the solution is flowing when performing a flush of the invasive line.

*Level B: Well-designed, controlled studies with results that consistently support a specific action, intervention, or treatment.

Procedure	for Single-Pressure and Multiple-Pressure Transducer Systems—*Continued*	
Steps	Rationale	Special Considerations
11. Insert the IV bag into the pressure bag or device on the IV pole. Do not inflate the pressure bag.	Priming the tubing under pressure increases turbulence and may cause air bubbles to enter the tubing.	Air should never be allowed to develop in a hemodynamic system. Air within the system will affect the accuracy of measured values.[25] Micro or macro air emboli can migrate to major organs and present a potentially life-threatening complication.
12. Flush the entire system, including the transducer, stopcocks, pressure tubing, and any additions with the flush solution. A. With the flush device, flush solution from the IV bag through to the tip of the pressure tubing. B. Turn the stopcock off to the patient end of the tubing (Fig. 60.4). C. With the flush device, flush the solution from the IV bag through the stopcock.	Eliminates air from the system.	Vented caps are placed by the manufacturer and permit sterilization of the entire system. These vented caps must be replaced with sterile injectable or noninjectable caps to prevent bacteria and air from entering the system.
D. Replace the vented cap on the stopcock with an injectable or noninjectable cap. E. Open the stopcock to the transducer (Fig. 60.5).	Replace vented caps to reduce the risk of contamination or air entrainment.	Needleless injectable devices or caps may be placed on venous access devices. Avoid placing injectable caps on arterial tubing not intended for injection.[16] *Procedure continues on following page*

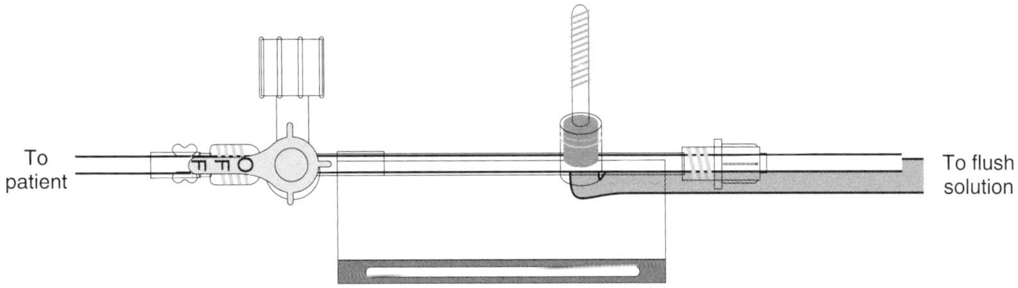

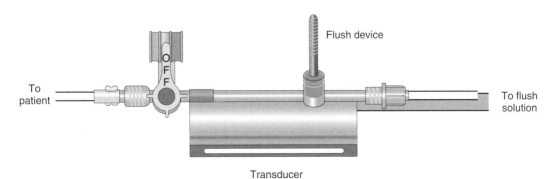

Figure 60.4 Stopcock off to the patient. *(Drawing by Paul W. Schiffmacher, Thomas Jefferson University, Philadelphia, PA.)*

Figure 60.5 Stopcock open to the transducer. *(Drawing by Paul W. Schiffmacher, Thomas Jefferson University, Philadelphia, PA.)*

UNIT II

UNIT II

Procedure	for Single-Pressure and Multiple-Pressure Transducer Systems—*Continued*	
Steps	**Rationale**	**Special Considerations**
13. With use of double-pressure or triple-pressure transducer systems, **repeat Step 12** with each of the pressure transducer systems.	Eliminates air from the systems.	
14. Inflate the pressure bag or device to 300 mm Hg.	Inflating the pressure bag to 300 mm Hg allows approximately 1–3 mL/hour of flush solution to be delivered through the catheter, thus maintaining catheter patency and minimizing clot formation.	
15. With use of a pole mount, insert the transducer into the pole-mount holder (sometimes called a *transducer plate*) (Fig. 60.6).	Secures each transducer.	Place each of the transducers into the space with the correct label (i.e., PA, RA/central venous, or arterial) (see Fig. 60.6). Transducer manufacturers suggest positioning the pressurized flush solution at least 2 feet above the transducer.
16. With sterile technique, connect the end of each transducer tubing to the appropriate catheter port (e.g., PA, RA, arterial).	Allows for monitoring of pressures.	Before assisting with connections, protective equipment must be applied. Ports should be clamped, and the patient should be supine with the head of the bed flat whenever central venous ports are open to air to reduce the risk of air entrainment.[14,16]
17. Remove **PE**, and discard used supplies.		
18. **HH**		
19. Label the pressure tubing and IV solution, indicating the date, time, and your initials.	Identifies when the pressure tubing and IV solution needs to be changed.	Change the pressure transducer system every 96 hours.[16,27]

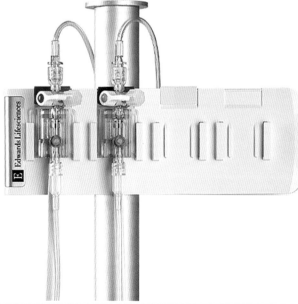

Figure 60.6   Transducers in pole mount. *(Courtesy Edwards Lifesciences, Irvine, CA.)*

Procedure	for Single-Pressure and Multiple-Pressure Transducer Systems—*Continued*	
Steps	Rationale	Special Considerations
Monitor Setup		
1. Turn on the bedside monitor.	Prepares the monitor.	
2. Plug the pressure cables into the appropriate pressure modules in the bedside monitor (see Fig. 60.3).	Necessary for signal transmission to the monitor.	Some monitors are preprogrammed to display the waveform that corresponds to the module for cable insertion (e.g., first position, arterial; second position, pulmonary artery; third position, right atrial).
3. Make a connection between the transducer and the monitor cable.		Confirm that the intended transducer is attached to the correctly labeled monitor module and cable.
4. Confirm that the parameters have turned on, or manually turn on if necessary (e.g., PA, RA, arterial).	Visualizes the correct waveforms.	
5. Set the appropriate scale for the pressure being measured. Ensure that alarms are on and audible.	Necessary for visualization of the complete waveform and to obtain accurate readings. Waveforms vary in amplitude depending on the pressure within the system.	The scale for RA pressure is commonly set at 20 mm Hg. The scale for PA pressure is commonly set at 40 mm Hg. The scale for arterial blood pressure is commonly set at 180 mm Hg. Scales may vary based on monitoring equipment. Scales can be adjusted based on patient pressures.
Leveling the Transducer		
1. 🅷🅷		
2. 🅿🅴		
3. Position the patient in the supine position with the head of the bed from 0 to 45 degrees. **(Level B*)**	Similar positioning may improve the accuracy of identifying the phlebostatic axis and the consistency of serial PAP/PAOP/CVP/RAP measurements. Studies have determined that RA and PA pressures are comparable in multiple positions.[1,4,6-7,9-12,15,17-24, 28-29,33-34]	For patients who are unable to tolerate supine positioning with the head of the bed elevated 0 to 45 degrees, CVP and PA measurements may be obtained with the head of the bed elevated up to 60 degrees. When needed, patients may be in the 20-, 30- or 90-degree lateral or prone position with the head of the bed flat. With each of these positions, the level of the right atrium will be altered from the previously identified phlebostatic axis.[1]
4. Locate the phlebostatic axis for the supine position (Fig. 60.7).	The phlebostatic axis is at approximately the level of the atria and should be used as the reference point for the transducer vent/air-fluid interface.	The reference point for the left-lateral decubitus position is the fourth intercostal space (ICS) at the left parasternal border (Fig. 60.8).[19,33] The reference point for the right-lateral decubitus position is the fourth ICS at the midsternum (see Fig. 60.8).[19,33] Three locations have been used to study the effects of prone positioning on hemodynamic measurements: the mid-axillary line, mid–anterior-posterior diameter, or a point 5 cm vertical distance from the patient's sternal angle. A consistent approach that allows for stabilization (30–60 minutes) after positioning is warranted.[1,6,9,15,23,29]

Procedure continues on following page

Procedure for Single-Pressure and Multiple-Pressure Transducer Systems—*Continued*

Steps	Rationale	Special Considerations

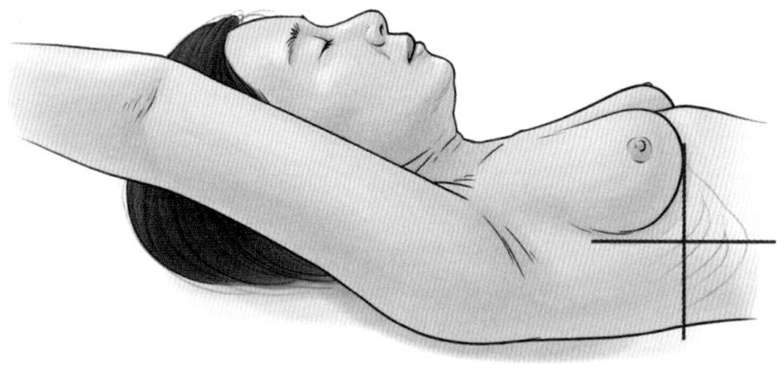

Figure 60.7 Phlebostatic axis in the supine position.

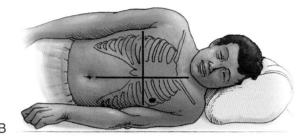

A

B

Figure 60.8 Reference points for the hemodynamic monitoring system for patients in lateral positions. **A,** For the right-lateral position, the reference point is the intersection of the fourth intercostal space and the midsternum. **B,** For the left-lateral position, the reference point is the intersection of the fourth intercostal space and the left-parasternal border. *(From Keckelsen M: Protocols for practice: Hemodynamic monitoring series: Pulmonary artery monitoring, Aliso Viejo, CA, 1997, American Association of Critical-Care Nurses.)*

Steps	Rationale	Special Considerations
A. Identify the fourth ICS on the edge of the sternum. B. Draw an imaginary line along the fourth ICS laterally, along the chest wall. C. Draw a second imaginary line from the axilla downward, midway between the anterior and posterior chest walls. D. The point at which these two lines cross is the level of the phlebostatic axis. E. Mark the point of the phlebostatic axis with an indelible skin marker.	Studies demonstrate inconsistencies in transducer placement among clinicians. Patient position variations may make it even more challenging.[34,35] When the air-fluid interface is lower than the phlebostatic axis, it produces false high-pressure readings. When the air-fluid interface is higher than the phlebostatic axis, it produces false low-pressure readings.	Use a level to align the transducer vent port to the phlebostatic axis after a patient position change. Confirm alignment before pressure measurement.[1,34]
5. Use a leveling device (low-intensity laser or carpenter's level) to align the air-fluid interface with the phlebostatic axis.	Ensures that the zeroing stopcock/air-fluid interface is level with the phlebostatic axis. Leveling to the phlebostatic axis reflects accurate central venous and arterial pressure values.[1,25]	

Pole mount[1,4,31,]**:**
Low-intensity laser:

Procedure	for Single-Pressure and Multiple-Pressure Transducer Systems—*Continued*	
Steps	**Rationale**	**Special Considerations**
A. Place the low-intensity laser leveling device next to the air-fluid interface (zeroing stopcock). B. Point the laser light at the phlebostatic axis. C. Move the pole mount holder up or down until the interface is level with the phlebostatic axis.	Ensures that the air-fluid interface is level with the phlebostatic axis. Leveling to the phlebostatic axis reflects accurate central arterial pressure values.	
Carpenter level: A. Place one end of the carpenter level next to the air-fluid interface (zeroing stopcock). B. Place the other end of the carpenter level at the phlebostatic axis. C. Move the pole-mount holder up or down until the interface is level with the phlebostatic axis (Fig. 60.9).	Ensures that the air-fluid interface is level with the phlebostatic axis. Leveling to the phlebostatic axis reflects accurate central venous and arterial pressure values.	
6. With patient mount: A. Place the pulmonary artery distal/PA air-fluid interface (zeroing stopcock) at the phlebostatic axis.	Ensures that the air-fluid interface is level with the phlebostatic axis. Leveling to the phlebostatic axis reflects accurate central arterial pressure values.	
B. Place the PA proximal (RA) and arterial air-fluid interfaces (zeroing stopcocks) directly next to the pulmonary artery distal/PA air-fluid interface.		Leveling the arterial interface to the tip of an arterial catheter reflects the transmural pressure of a particular point in the arterial tree (e.g., radial artery) and not central arterial pressure.[8,21,25,31]
C. Place a foam dressing or hydrocolloid gel pad between each of the transducers and the patient's skin. D. Secure each of the systems in place with tape.	May prevent device-related pressure injury.[5]	

7. Remove 🔳, and discard.
8. 🔳

Zeroing the Transducer
1. 🔳
2. 🔳

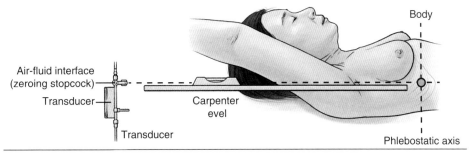

Figure 60.9 Air-fluid interface (zeroing stopcock) is level with the phlebostatic axis using a carpenter level. *(Drawing by Paul W. Schiffmacher, Thomas Jefferson University, Philadelphia, PA.)*

Procedure for Single-Pressure and Multiple-Pressure Transducer Systems—*Continued*

Steps	Rationale	Special Considerations
3. Turn the stopcock off to the patient end of the tubing (see Fig. 60.4).	Prepares the system for the zeroing procedure.	
4. Remove the nonvented cap from the stopcock, opening the stopcock to air.	Allows the monitor to use atmospheric pressure as a reference for zero.	
5. Push and release the zeroing button on the bedside monitor. Observe the digital reading until it displays a value of zero.	The monitor automatically adjusts itself to zero. Zeroing negates the effects of atmospheric pressure.	Some monitors require that the zero be turned and adjusted manually. Some systems also may require calibration. Refer to the manufacturer's guidelines for specific information.
6. Place a new, sterile nonvented cap onto the stopcock.	Maintains sterility.	
7. Turn the stopcock so it is open to the transducer (off to air-fluid interface; see Fig. 60.5).	Permits pressure monitoring and maintains catheter patency.	
8. Observe the waveform and perform a dynamic response test (square-wave test).	Determines whether the system is damped. This will ensure that the pressure waveform components are clearly defined and aid in accurate measurement.	The square-wave test can be performed by activating and quickly releasing the fast flush. A sharp upstroke should terminate in a flat line at the maximal indicator on the monitor. This should be followed by an immediate rapid downstroke extending below baseline with 1–2 oscillations within 0.12 second and a quick return to baseline (see Fig. 60.10).
9. Remove **PE**, and discard used supplies in appropriate receptacles.	Reduces the transmission of microorganisms; standard precautions.	
10. **HH**		

Expected Outcomes

- The pressure-monitoring system is prepared aseptically
- The hemodynamic monitoring system remains closed with secure connections and nonvented caps
- The phlebostatic axis is accurately identified and clearly marked
- The air-fluid interface of the transducer remains leveled to the phlebostatic axis at all times
- The pressure-monitoring system is zeroed at appropriate times

Unexpected Outcomes

- Back bleeding into the transducer system
- Loose connections within the hemodynamic monitoring system
- Stopcocks left open to air without a nonvented cap
- Air bubbles within the system
- Pressure bag inflated to <300 mm Hg

Patient Monitoring and Care

Steps	Rationale	Reportable Conditions
		These conditions should be reported to the provider if they persist despite nursing interventions.
1. Check the IV flush bag every 4 hours and as needed.	Ensures that the IV flush bag contains solution to maintain catheter patency. Some transducer manufacturers recommend maintaining at least a quarter filled flush bag to reduce the risk of air entering the system.	
2. Check that the IV flush bag is maintained at 300 mm Hg every 4 hours and as needed.	Maintains catheter patency.	
3. Change the hemodynamic monitoring system (flush solution, pressure tubing, transducers, and stopcocks) every 96 hours. **(Level B*)** The flush solution may need to be changed more frequently if near empty of solution.	The U.S. Centers for Disease Control and Prevention (CDC)[27] and the Infusion Nurses Society[16] recommend that the hemodynamic flush system can be used safely for up to 96 hours.	
4. If a nonvented cap is removed from a stopcock, it should be replaced with a new sterile injectable or noninjectable cap.	Reduces the risk of infection.	
5. Zero the hemodynamic monitoring system during initial setup or before insertion, after insertion, if disconnection occurs between the transducer and the monitoring cable, if disconnection occurs between the monitoring cable and the monitor, and when the values obtained do not fit the clinical picture. Follow the manufacturer's recommendations for disposable systems.	Ensures the accuracy of the hemodynamic monitoring system.	
6. Perform a dynamic response test (square-wave test) at the start of each shift, with a change of the waveform or when the system has been opened to air (see Fig. 60.10).	An optimally damped system provides an accurate waveform.	Overdamped or underdamped waveforms that cannot be corrected with troubleshooting procedures.
7. Check the hemodynamic monitoring system every 4 hours and any time unexpected pressure measurements are obtained.	Ensures that all connections are tightly secured and that there are no cracks in the system. Ensures that the system is closed with nonvented caps on all stopcocks. Ensures that the system is free from air bubbles and that the transducer remains in the transducer plate and is appropriately leveled.	
8. Set the hemodynamic monitoring system alarms per institutional guidelines.	Provides an immediate alarm for patient-specific high and low pressures.	Report patient physiological changes per institutional standards.

Patient Monitoring and Care

Steps	Rationale	Reportable Conditions

When the fast flush of the continuous flush system is activated and quickly released, a sharp upstroke terminates in a flat line at the maximal indicator on the monitor and hard copy. This is then followed by an immediate rapid downstroke extending below baseline with just 1 or 2 oscillations within 0.12 second (minimal ringing) and a quick return to baseline. The patient's pressure waveform is also clearly defined with all components of the waveform, such as the dicrotic notch on an arterial waveform, clearly visible.

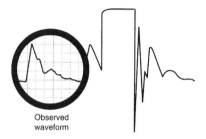

Intervention

A There is no adjustment in the monitoring system required.

The upstroke of the square wave appears somewhat slurred, the waveform does not extend below the baseline after the fast flush and there is no ringing after the flush. The patient's waveform displays a falsely decreased systolic pressure and false high diastolic pressure as well as poorly defined components of the pressure tracing such as a diminished or absent dicrotic notch on arterial waveforms.

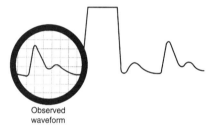

Intervention

To correct for the problem:
1. Check for the presence of blood clots, blood left in the catheter following blood sampling, or air bubbles at any point from the catheter tip to the transducer diaphragm and eliminate these as necessary.
2. Use low compliance (rigid), short (less than 3 to 4 feet) monitoring tubing.
3. Connect all line components securely.
B 4. Check for kinks in the line.

The waveform is characterized by numerous amplified oscillations above and below the baseline following the fast flush. The monitored pressure wave displays false high systolic pressures (overshoot), possibly false low diastolic pressures, and "ringing" artifacts on the waveform.

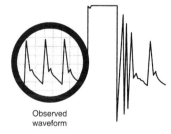

Intervention

To correct the problem, remove all air bubbles (particularly pinpoint air bubbles) in the fluid
C   system, use large-bore, shorter tubing, or use a damping device.

Figure 60.10 Dynamic response test (square-wave test) using the fast flush system. **A,** Optimally damped system. **B,** Overdamped system. **C,** Underdamped system. *(From Darovic GO, Zbilut JP: Fluid-filled monitoring systems. In Hemodynamic monitoring, ed 3. Philadelphia, 2002, Saunders, 122.)*

Documentation

Documentation should include the following:
- Patient and family education
- Date and time of hemodynamic monitoring system preparation
- Hemodynamic monitoring system leveling and zeroing
- Type of flush solution
- Unexpected outcomes
- Additional nursing interventions necessary for troubleshooting
- Hemodynamic values (e.g., ABP, CVP, PAP) as ordered or per institutional policy

References and Additional Readings

For a complete list of references and additional readings for this procedure, scan this QR code with your smartphone, or visit https://www.elsevier.com/__data/assets/pdf_file/0003/1319835/Chapter0060.pdf.

61 Pulmonary Artery Catheter and Pressure Lines, Troubleshooting

Carrie Boom

PURPOSE Troubleshooting of the pulmonary artery (PA) catheter is important to maintain catheter patency, to ensure that data from the PA catheter are accurate, and to prevent the development of catheter-related and patient-related complications.

PREREQUISITE NURSING KNOWLEDGE

- Knowledge of cardiovascular and pulmonary anatomy and physiology.
- An understanding of basic dysrhythmia recognition and treatment of life-threatening dysrhythmias.
- Advanced cardiac life support (ACLS) knowledge and skills
- Knowledge of principles of aseptic technique.
- Understanding of the setup of the hemodynamic monitoring system (see Procedure 60, Single-Pressure and Multiple-Pressure Transducer Systems).
- An understanding of the PA catheter (see Fig. 59.1) and the location of the PA catheter in the heart and pulmonary artery (see Fig. 59.2).
- Pulmonary artery occlusion pressure (PAOP) may be referred to as *pulmonary artery wedge pressure* or *pulmonary capillary wedge pressure* (PCWP).
- After wedging of the PA catheter, air is passively removed by disconnecting the syringe from the balloon-inflation port. Active withdrawal of air from the balloon is avoided because it can weaken the balloon, pull the balloon structure into the inflation lumen, and possibly cause balloon rupture.
- The pulmonary artery diastolic pressure (PADP) and the PAOP are indirect measures of left-ventricular end-diastolic pressure. Usually, the PAOP is approximately 1 to 4 mm Hg less than the PADP. Because these two pressures are similar, the PADP is commonly followed, which minimizes the frequency of balloon inflation, thus decreasing the potential of balloon rupture.
- Differences between the PADP and the PAOP may exist for patients with pulmonary hypertension, chronic obstructive lung disease, adult respiratory distress syndrome, pulmonary embolus, and tachycardia.
- Pulmonary artery pressures (PAPs) may be elevated because of PA hypertension, pulmonary disease, mitral valve disease, left ventricular failure, atrial or ventricular left-to-right shunt, pulmonary emboli, or hypervolemia.
- PAPs may be decreased because of hypovolemia or low pulmonary vascular resistance (e.g., vasodilation).

- The waveforms that occur during insertion should be recognized, including right atrial (RA), right ventricular (RV), PA, and PA occlusion (PAOP; see Fig. 58.2).
- The *a* wave reflects atrial contraction. The *c* wave reflects closure of the atrioventricular valves. The *v* wave reflects passive filling of the atria during ventricular systole (see Figs. 59.4 and 59.5).
- Knowledge of normal hemodynamic values (see Table 65.1).
- Elevated *a* and *v* waves may be evident in RA or central venous pressure (CVP) and in PAOP waveforms. These elevations may occur in patients with cardiac tamponade, constrictive pericardial disease, and hypervolemia.
- Elevated *a* waves in the RA or CVP waveform may occur in patients with pulmonic or tricuspid stenosis, right-ventricular ischemia or infarction, right-ventricular failure, PA hypertension, and atrioventricular dissociation.
- Elevated *a* waves in the PAOP waveform may occur in patients with mitral stenosis, acute left ventricular ischemia or infarction, left ventricular failure, and atrioventricular dissociation.
- Elevated *v* waves in the RA or CVP waveform may occur in patients with tricuspid insufficiency.
- Elevated *v* waves in the PAOP waveform may occur in patients with mitral insufficiency or ruptured papillary muscle.

EQUIPMENT

- Nonsterile gloves
- Syringes (5 or 10 mL)
- Sterile injectable or noninjectable caps
- Sterile 4 × 4 gauze
- Stopcocks
- Needleless blood-sampling access device
- Pressure monitoring cables
- Pressure transducer system, including flush solution recommended according to institutional standards, a pressure bag or device, pressure tubing with transducers, and flush device

Additional equipment, to have available as needed, includes the following:

- Indelible marker (to mark the phlebostatic axis)
- Emergency equipment (code cart)
- Blood-specimen tubes

PATIENT AND FAMILY EDUCATION

- Explain the troubleshooting procedures to the patient and family. *Rationale:* The patient and family are kept informed, and anxiety is reduced.
- Explain the patient's expected participation during the procedure. *Rationale:* This explanation will encourage patient assistance.
- Inform the patient and family of signs and symptoms to report to the critical care nurse, including chest pain, palpitations, new cough, tenderness at the catheter-insertion site, and chills. *Rationale:* The patient is encouraged to report signs of discomfort and potential PA catheter complications.

PATIENT ASSESSMENT AND PREPARATION

Patient Assessment

- Monitor PA waveforms continuously. *Rationale:* The PA catheter may migrate forward into a wedged position, may move back into the right ventricle, or may become dislodged with the catheter tip malpositioned in the RA or central vein.

- Assess the configuration of the PA catheter waveforms. *Rationale:* Thrombus formation at the tip of the catheter lumen or advancement of the catheter in the wedge position may be evidenced by an overdamped waveform.
- Assess the patient's hemodynamic and cardiovascular status. *Rationale:* The patient's clinical assessment should correlate with the PA catheter–derived hemodynamic data.
- Assess the patient and the PA catheter site for signs of infection. *Rationale:* Infection can develop because of the invasive nature of the PA catheter.

Patient Preparation

- Verify the correct patient with two identifiers. *Rationale:* Before performing a procedure, the nurse should ensure the correct identification of the patient for the intended intervention.
- Ensure that the patient understands the preprocedural teaching. Answer questions as they arise, and reinforce information as needed. *Rationale:* Understanding of previously taught information is evaluated and reinforced.
- Determine the patency of the patient's intravenous catheters. *Rationale:* Access may be needed for administration of emergency medications or fluids.

Procedure | for Pulmonary Artery Catheter and Pressure Lines, Troubleshooting

Steps	Rationale	Special Considerations
1. HH		
2. PE		
Troubleshooting a Continuously Wedged Waveform		
1. Identify the wedged waveform (see Fig. 59.5).	Confirms the need for troubleshooting.	Continuous monitoring of the PA waveform is necessary to assess for the presence of the PA waveform. PA catheters should be wedged for no longer than 8–15 seconds (2–4 respiratory cycles) when obtaining a PAOP measurement. The provider should be notified if the overwedged catheter does not float back into the PA. Follow institutional protocols for personnel who can pull back the catheter if the overwedged balloon cannot be corrected immediately. Do not fast flush the device as this may cause PA rupture.
2. Remove the PA balloon inflation syringe, and ensure that the gate valve (see Fig. 59.6) or stopcock is open.	Ensures that air is not trapped within the PA balloon.	
3. Assist the patient in changing position, or if possible, ask the patient to cough.	May help the catheter float out of the wedge position.	Monitor the PA waveform for a change from a PAO waveform to a PA waveform.
4. If troubleshooting is unsuccessful, notify the provider.	Immediate repositioning of the catheter is necessary because prolonged wedging can lead to PA infarction or pulmonary artery hemorrhage.	The critical care nurse may withdraw the PA catheter according to institutional policy.
5. Never flush a wedged PA catheter.	Flushing the catheter in the wedged position may lead to PA rupture and hemorrhage.	

UNIT II

Procedure for Pulmonary Artery Catheter and Pressure Lines, Troubleshooting—*Continued*

Steps	Rationale	Special Considerations

Troubleshooting an Overwedged PA Catheter Balloon

1. Identify an overwedged PA catheter balloon from the PA waveform analysis (Fig. 61.1).	The overwedged PA catheter balloon occurs when the PA catheter balloon is overinflated.	Overinflation of the balloon can cause pulmonary arteriole infarction or rupture, resulting in life-threatening hemorrhage. The provider should be notified if the overwedged catheter does not float back into the PA. Follow institutional protocols for personnel who can pull back the catheter if the overwedged balloon cannot be corrected immediately. Do not fast flush the device as this may cause PA rupture.

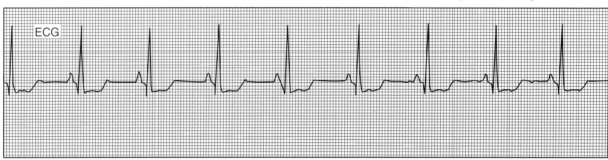

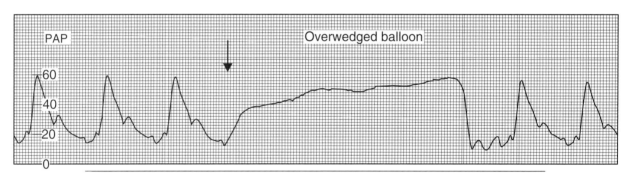

Figure 61.1 Balloon inflation *(arrow)*. Overwedging of the balloon (balloon has been overinflated). The danger of overinflating the balloon is that the pulmonary artery vessel may rupture from the pressure of the balloon. *ECG,* Electrocardiogram; *PAP,* pulmonary artery pressure.

2. Remove the syringe from the gate valve or the stopcock of the PA balloon inflation port.	Facilitates passive removal of air from the PA catheter balloon.	Ensure that the gate valve or stopcock is in the open position (see Fig. 59.6).
3. Note the change in the PA waveform from the overwedged waveform to the PA waveform.	As the balloon deflates, the PA waveform returns.	
4. Fill the syringe with 1.5 mL of air, and connect the syringe to the gate valve or stopcock of the balloon port of the PA catheter. Slowly inflate the balloon with air until the PA waveform changes to a PAOP waveform (see Fig. 59.10), and note the amount of air used.	Determines the amount of air needed to convert the PA waveform to a PAOP waveform.	If a PAOP waveform is achieved with less than 1.5 mL of air, there is an increased risk of spontaneous wedge.

Procedure for Pulmonary Artery Catheter and Pressure Lines, Troubleshooting—*Continued*

Steps	Rationale	Special Considerations
5. Disconnect the syringe from the balloon-inflation port to deflate the balloon, and verify that the PAOP waveform changes back to the PA waveform.	Allows air to passively escape from the balloon.	Active withdrawal of air from the balloon can weaken the balloon, pull the balloon structure into the inflation lumen, and possibly cause balloon rupture.
6. Expel air from the balloon syringe, and reconnect the empty balloon syringe to the balloon-inflation port.	The syringe should remain empty when reconnected so accidental balloon inflation does not occur.	The syringe that is manufactured for the PA catheter should be connected to the PA balloon port to avoid loss of the custom-designed syringe.
7. Follow institutional standards regarding keeping the gate valve or the stopcock open.	The most important considerations are that the balloon syringe is attached to the balloon-inflation port, the syringe is empty, and the PA distal waveform reflects a PA waveform.	Keeping the valve open ensures that no air is trapped in the balloon. Keeping the valve closed adds additional protection from inadvertent syringe manipulation.
8. Note the external centimeter marking of the PA catheter at the introducer exit site.	Identifies whether the PA catheter has migrated forward from the previously documented measurement.	The provider may need to reposition the catheter.
9. Note and record the amount of air needed to wedge the PA catheter.	Prevents overinflation of the PA catheter balloon.	Keeping the valve closed adds additional protection from inadvertent syringe manipulation.

Preventing an Overwedged PA Catheter

1. Fill the syringe with 1.5 mL of air.	Instilling more than 1.5 mL of air may rupture the PA balloon and the pulmonary arteriole.	
2. Connect the PA balloon syringe to the gate valve or stopcock of the balloon-inflation port of the PA catheter.	This port is designed for PA balloon inflation.	The PA balloon syringe is designed so it will not hold more than 1.5 mL of air.
3. Slowly inflate the balloon with air until the PA waveform changes to a PAOP waveform (see Fig. 59.10).	Only instill enough air needed to convert the PA waveform to a PAOP waveform.	If <1.5 mL air is required to obtain a PAOP waveform, there is an increased risk of spontaneous wedge.
4. Inflate the PA balloon for no more than 8–15 seconds (2–4 respiratory cycles).	Avoids prolonged pressure on the pulmonary arteriole.	
5. Disconnect the PA balloon syringe from the balloon-inflation port for passive deflation of the balloon.	Allows air to passively exit from the balloon.	
6. Observe the monitor as the PAOP waveform changes back to the PA waveform.	Ensures adequate balloon deflation.	
7. Expel air from the PA syringe.	The syringe should remain empty when reconnected so accidental balloon inflation does not occur.	
8. Reconnect the empty PA balloon syringe to the balloon inflation port.	Retains the safety syringe.	
9. Follow institutional standards regarding keeping the gate valve or the stopcock open.	The most important considerations are that the balloon syringe is attached to the balloon-inflation port, the syringe is empty, and the PA distal waveform reflects a PA waveform.	Keeping the valve open ensures that no air is trapped in the balloon.

Troubleshooting an Absent Waveform

1. Check to see whether there is a kink in the PA catheter or whether the PA catheter sleeve is overtightened, causing an occlusion.	Kinks may inhibit waveform transmission.	

Procedure continues on following page

UNIT II

Procedure | for Pulmonary Artery Catheter and Pressure Lines, Troubleshooting—*Continued*

Steps	Rationale	Special Considerations
2. Ensure that all connections are tight.	Loose connections allow air into the system and can overdamp or eliminate the waveform.	
3. Ensure that there is fluid in the flush bag and that the pressure on the flush bag or device is delivering 300 mm Hg. The fluid-filled bag under pressure should be a sufficient height above the transducer.	Low pressure may result in a clotted catheter, resulting in loss of the waveform or low pressure in the flush bag.	A square-wave test should not be performed. A clotted catheter under pressure of flush may dislodge clots.
4. Ensure that the roller clamp(s) on the pressure tubing are open.	A clamped pressure line tubing can result in a clotted catheter, resulting in loss of the waveform.	
5. Ensure that the stopcock proximal to the patient is open and the stopcock at the transducer is open (Fig. 61.2).	Stopcocks open to the transducer system allow waveform transmission from the cardiovascular system to the monitor; stopcocks closed to the transducer prevent waveform transmission to the monitor and oscilloscope.	

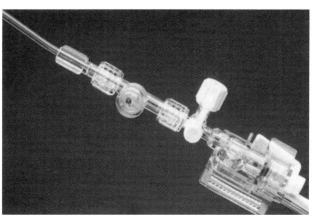

Figure 61.2 The stopcock is open to the transducer. *(From Ahrens TS, Taylor LK: Hemodynamic waveform recognition, Philadelphia, 1993, Saunders.)*

Steps	Rationale	Special Considerations
6. Check that the monitor modules are in the expected positions and labeled correctly.	Necessary for accurately monitoring the correct waveforms.	
7. Check that the cables are in the appropriate pressure modules.	Necessary for signal transmission.	
8. Ensure that the pressure cables are securely plugged into the monitor.	No waveform is transmitted without proper connection.	
9. Ensure that the appropriate monitor parameters are turned on.	Necessary for specific parameter monitoring.	
10. Ensure the appropriate scale has been chosen for pressure being monitored (e.g., 0 to 40–80 mm Hg scale is used for PA monitoring depending on baseline PA systolic pressure).	A smaller scale may cause the waveform to be out of view. A larger scale (e.g., 100 mm Hg) causes the waveform to be smaller and possibly not easily visible on the oscilloscope.	
11. Level and zero the monitoring system (see Procedure 60, Single-Pressure and Multiple-Pressure Transducer Systems).	Ensures accurate setup and function of the monitoring system.	

Procedure for Pulmonary Artery Catheter and Pressure Lines, Troubleshooting—*Continued*		
Steps	Rationale	Special Considerations
12. Aspirate through the stopcock that is closest to the catheter to check for blood return (see Fig. 57.2).	Ensures patency of the PA catheter. Evidence suggests correlation with thrombosed central venous catheter (CVC) and line infection.[3,4]	A clotted/obstructed catheter has no waveform and no blood return when aspirated. The catheter may need to be replaced.
13. Replace the monitoring cable and/or module.	A faulty cable can result in an absent waveform.	If the cable or module is changed, zero the monitoring system.
14. Replace the pressure transducer system.	A faulty transducer can result in an absent waveform.	If the pressure transducer system is changed, zero the new monitoring system.
15. Notify the physician, advanced practice nurse, or other healthcare professional if troubleshooting is unsuccessful.	The catheter may need to be removed or replaced.	
Troubleshooting an Overdamped Waveform		
1. Obtain a monitor strip of the overdamped waveform (Fig. 61.3).	The waveform can be compared with the previous waveforms.	
2. Ensure that all connections are tight.	Loose connections allow air into the system or loss of pressure from the system and can overdamp the waveform.	
3. Ensure that there is fluid in the flush bag and that the pressure on the flush bag or device is set at 300 mm Hg.	Low counterpressure from the flush solution bag results in an overdamped waveform.	
4. Check all tubing for air bubbles. If air exists within the transducer, follow these steps:	Removes air from the system, prevents the air from entering the patient, and ensures accurate monitoring of waveforms.	Check that the IV flush bag and pressure tubing drip chamber contain fluid.
A. Remove the noninjectable cap at the top port of the stopcock, or clean the top of the injectable cap with an antiseptic solution.		
B. Insert a sterile syringe or a blood-sampling access device into the top port of the stopcock or the top of the injectable cap of the stopcock (see Figs. 57.1 and 62.1).		
C. Turn the stopcock off to the patient (see Fig. 57.3).		
D. Fast flush the air from the transducer and system into the syringe, or insert a blood-specimen tube into the blood-sampling access device.		
E. Open the system to the transducer (see Figs. 57.1 and 62.1).		
F. Remove the syringe or the blood-sampling access device from the stopcock.		
G. Zero the hemodynamic monitoring system (see Procedure 60, Single-Pressure and Multiple-Pressure Transducer Systems).		
H. If not using an injectable cap, place a new noninjectable cap on the top port of the stopcock.		
I. Evaluate and then monitor the waveform.		

Procedure continues on following page

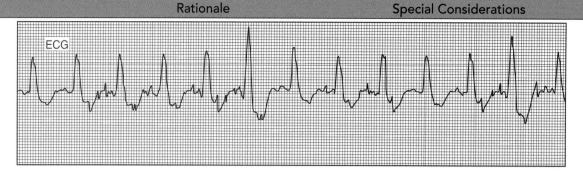

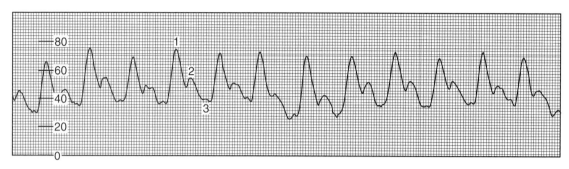

A

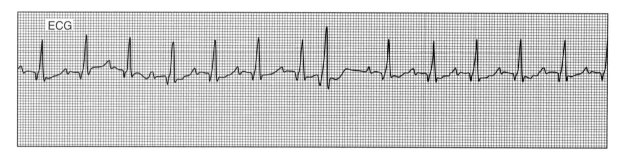

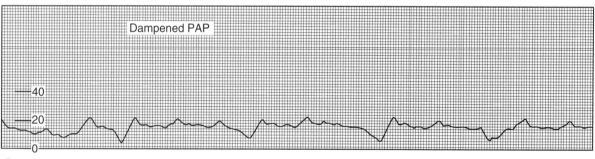

B

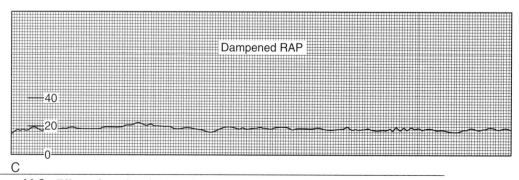

C

Figure 61.3 Effects of overdamping on pulmonary artery pressure *(PAP)* and right-atrial pressure *(RAP)* waveforms. **A,** Normal waveform with elevated pulmonary artery pressures (*1,* systole; *2,* dicrotic notch; *3,* diastole). **B,** Overdamped PAP waveform. **C,** Overdamped RAP waveform. Overdamping of the waveform may result from clots at the catheter tip, catheter against a vessel or the heart wall, air in lines, stopcock partially closed, or a deflated pressure bag. *ECG,* Electrocardiogram.

Procedure	for Pulmonary Artery Catheter and Pressure Lines, Troubleshooting—*Continued*	
Steps	Rationale	Special Considerations

5. If air exists between the pressure bag and a stopcock, follow these steps:
  A. Remove the noninjectable cap at the top port of the stopcock, or clean the top of the injectable cap with an antiseptic solution.
  B. Insert a sterile syringe or a blood-sampling access device into the top port of the stopcock or the top of the injectable cap of the stopcock (see Figs. 57.1 and 62.1).
  C. Turn the stopcock off to the patient (see Fig. 57.3)
  D. Fast flush the air from the transducer and system into the syringe, or insert a blood-specimen tube into the blood-sampling access device.
  E. Open the system to the transducer (see Figs. 57.1 and 62.1).
  F. Remove the syringe or the blood-sampling access device from the stopcock.
  G. If not using an injectable cap, place a new sterile noninjectable cap on the top port of the stopcock.
  H. Evaluate and monitor the PA waveform.

    Removes air from the system, prevents air from entering the patient, and prevents overdamping of the system to ensure accurate monitoring.

6. If the air is between the patient and a stopcock (Fig. 61.4), follow these steps:
  A. Remove the noninjectable cap at the top port of the stopcock, or clean the top of the injectable cap with an antiseptic solution.
  B. Insert a sterile syringe or a blood-sampling access device into the top port of the stopcock or the top of the injectable cap of the stopcock (see Figs. 57.1 and 62.1).
  C. Turn the stopcock off to the flush solution (see Figs. 57.2, 57.4, and 62.2).
  D. Gently pull the air back into the syringe, or insert a blood-specimen tube into the blood-sampling system.
  E. When all of the air is removed, turn the stopcock off to the patient (see Fig. 57.3).
  F. Fast flush the blood from the top port of the stopcock.
  G. Open the system to the transducer (see Figs. 57.2 and 62.1), and flush the line until clear.
  H. Remove the syringe or blood-sampling access device from the stopcock.
  I. Zero the hemodynamic monitoring system (see Procedure 60, Single-Pressure and Multiple-Pressure Transducer Systems).
  J. If not using an injectable cap, place a new sterile noninjectable cap on the top port of the stopcock.
  K. Evaluate and then monitor the pressure waveform.

    Removes air from the system, prevents air from entering the patient, and ensures accurate monitoring of waveforms.

Procedure continues on following page

UNIT II

Procedure	for Pulmonary Artery Catheter and Pressure Lines, Troubleshooting—*Continued*

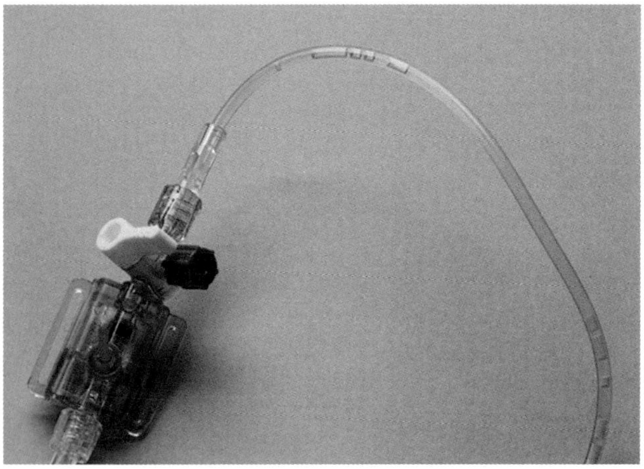

Steps	Rationale	Special Considerations

Figure 61.4   Air between the patient and stopcock. *(Courtesy Edwards Lifesciences, Irvine, CA.)*

7. Aspirate through the stopcock of the catheter to check for adequate blood return.

   A. Remove the noninjectable cap at the top port of the stopcock, or clean the top of the injectable cap with an antiseptic solution.

   B. Connect a 5–10-mL syringe to the stopcock or to the injectable cap.

   C. Turn the stopcock off to the flush solution (see Figs. 57.2, 57.4, and 62.2).

   D. Gently aspirate until blood enters the syringe.

   E. Turn the stopcock open to the transducer (see Figs 57.1 and 62.1).

   F. Fast flush the blood in the tubing back into the patient.

   G. Turn the stopcock off to the patient (see Fig. 57.2), and fast flush the blood from the top port of the stopcock or the injectable cap into the syringe.

   H. Open the stopcock to the transducer (see Figs. 57.1 and 62.1).

   I. Remove the syringe from the top port of the stopcock or the injectable cap.

   J. Zero the hemodynamic monitoring system (see Procedure 60, Single-Pressure and Multiple-Pressure Transducer Systems).

   K. If not using an injectable cap, place a new sterile noninjectable cap on the top of the stopcock.

   L. Evaluate and then monitor the waveform.

Ensures that blood flows easily within the catheter and assesses for the presence of clots.

Procedure for Pulmonary Artery Catheter and Pressure Lines, Troubleshooting—*Continued*		
Steps	**Rationale**	**Special Considerations**
8. Check the transducer for the presence of blood. If blood is present, follow these steps: A. Remove the noninjectable cap at the top port of the stopcock, or clean the top of the injectable cap with an antiseptic solution. B. Turn the stopcock off to the patient (see Fig. 60.4). C. Connect a 5–10-mL syringe to the stopcock or to the injectable cap, or insert a blood-sampling access device. D. Fast flush the blood from the transducer tubing into the syringe, or insert a blood-specimen tube into the injectable access device. E. Remove the syringe or the blood-access device. F. Turn the stopcock open to the transducer (see Fig. 60.5). G. Zero the hemodynamic monitoring system (see Procedure 60). H. If not using an injectable cap, place a new sterile noninjectable cap on the top port of the stopcock. I. Evaluate and monitor the waveform.	Ensures accurate monitoring of waveforms.	If the blood cannot be cleared from the transducer, the transducer system may need to be replaced.
9. Observe the waveform, and perform a dynamic response test (square-wave test) (see Procedure 60, Single-Pressure and Multiple-Pressure Transducer Systems, Fig. 60-10).	Determines whether the system is damped. This will ensure that the pressure waveform components are clearly defined. This aids in accurate measurement.	The square-wave test can be performed by activating and quickly releasing the fast flush. A sharp upstroke should terminate in a flat line at the maximal indicator on the monitor. This should be followed by an immediate rapid downstroke extending below the baseline with 1–2 oscillations within 0.12 second and a quick return to baseline (see Fig. 60.10).
10. Notify the provider if troubleshooting is unsuccessful.	The catheter may need to be removed or replaced.	
Troubleshooting a PA Catheter Waveform in the Right Ventricle		
1. Identify the RV waveform (Fig. 61.5). Note the PA catheter centimeter markings to evaluate if the catheter was pulled back inadvertently.	The RV systolic waveform resembles the PA systolic waveform, however, the RV waveform does not have a dicrotic notch. In addition, the diastolic pressure of the RV waveform is lower than the PADP. The normal PADP is 8–15 mm Hg; the normal RV diastolic pressure is 0–8 mm Hg.	The PA catheter waveform being an RV tracing requires immediate attention. However, a CVP/RAP waveform in the RV may indicate either migration of the catheter (evaluate for damped PA waveform or spontaneous wedge) or may simply be caused by cardiomegaly (Fig. 61.6). If a CVP/RAP migrates into the RV and there are no concerns that the PA catheter has migrated distally, ensure measurement at end-diastole just prior to systolic upstroke (exclude systole entirely).

Procedure continues on following page

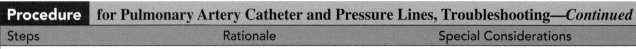

Procedure for Pulmonary Artery Catheter and Pressure Lines, Troubleshooting—*Continued*

Steps	Rationale	Special Considerations

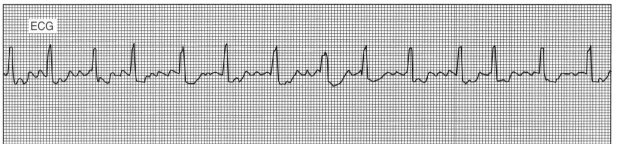

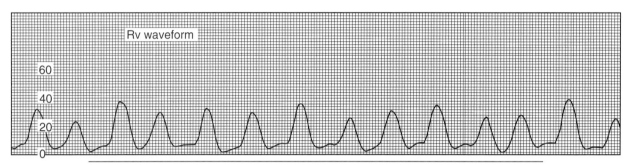

Figure 61.5   Right ventricular pressure *(RVP)* waveform. This waveform was seen coming from the pulmonary artery *(PA; distal)* lumen of a PA catheter. The catheter was coiled in the right ventricle *(RV)*. ECG, Electrocardiogram.

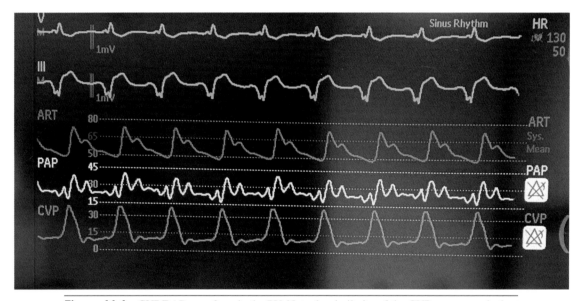

Figure 61.6   CVP/RAP waveform in the RV. Note the similarity of the CVP *v* wave equivalent to PA systolic pressure. This finding may indicate either migration of the catheter (although note no damped PA waveform or evidence of spontaneous wedge) or, as in this case, may simply be caused by cardiomegaly. CVP in this case must be measured at the base of the waveform and is found to be ~10 mm Hg. (Personal photograph.)

Procedure for Pulmonary Artery Catheter and Pressure Lines, Troubleshooting—*Continued*		
Steps	Rationale	Special Considerations
2. Inflate the PA balloon with 1.5 mL of air. Look for a change in the waveform from RV to PA to PAOP (see Fig. 58.2).	The inflated PA balloon cushions the catheter tip and prevents endocardial irritation. The inflated PA balloon may readily float into position in the PA.	The PA catheter tip may cause ventricular dysrhythmias. If the PA balloon is inflated, the ventricular dysrhythmias may decrease because the inflated balloon may cause less irritation of the endocardium. If the balloon remains inflated, continuous monitoring is necessary to identify if the catheter floats into the wedge position. The critical care nurse may also withdraw the catheter until an RA waveform is confirmed or may remove the PA catheter according to institutional policy. The catheter may not advance to the PA and likely will not advance to the PAOP position.
3. Assist the patient with a change of position.	The inflated PA catheter may float into the PA after a position change.	
4. Observe for change in waveform from RV to PA to PAOP (see Fig. 58.2).	Waveform analysis aids identification of the PA catheter position.	The catheter may not advance to the PA and likely will not advance to the wedge position.
5. Remove the syringe from the PA balloon inflation port.	Air passively is released from the PA balloon.	Expel the air from the PA balloon syringe, and then reconnect the empty syringe to the balloon inflation port.
6. Notify the provider to advance the catheter.	Repositioning is likely required if the catheter was pulled back or if it has looped back to the RV. Repositioning may occur either at the bedside or under fluoroscopy.	Follow institutional standards for the personnel trained to advance PA catheters.
7. If the catheter cannot be advanced successfully, it should be pulled back until the distal port of the catheter shows an RAP/CVP waveform.	Avoids ventricular arrhythmia	
8. Observe the PA waveform.	The waveform should return to a PA waveform at the end of repositioning.	
Troubleshooting an Inability to Wedge the PA Catheter		
1. Note the external centimeter marking of the PA catheter at the introducer exit site, and compare this with the most recent documented marking.	Determines whether the catheter has moved from its previous location. Most PA catheters are in the correct position if the external markings of the catheter are between 45 and 55 cm. The PA catheter tip may not be distal enough in the PA to float into the wedge position.	Follow institutional standards for the personnel trained to advance PA catheters.
2. Ensure that the PA balloon is inflated with the maximum 1.5 mL of air.	The full 1.5 mL of air may be necessary to wedge some PA catheters.	Repositioning the patient may aid in changing the position of the catheter and may facilitate successful wedging of the PA catheter.

Procedure continues on following page

Procedure **for Pulmonary Artery Catheter and Pressure Lines, Troubleshooting—*Continued***

Steps	Rationale	Special Considerations
3. Some small amount of resistance should be felt when inflating the PA balloon.	Resistance is present when the PA balloon is intact.	The balloon may rupture because of overinflation, frequent inflations, or repeated aspiration of air from the balloon rather than allowing it to passively deflate. Significant resistance can indicate deep placement of the catheter, and further attempts at inflation should be avoided until troubleshooting resolves the problem.
4. If no resistance is felt or if blood flows back from the balloon lumen, follow these steps: A. Immediately discontinue balloon inflation attempts. B. Remove the syringe. C. Close the gate valve or stopcock. D. Tape the balloon inflation port closed, and label the tape that the balloon should not be used.	If the balloon is ruptured, no resistance is felt during an inflation attempt. Blood may also come back through the balloon lumen.	
5. If the balloon is ruptured or troubleshooting is unsuccessful, notify the advanced practice nurse, physician, or other healthcare provider.	The PA catheter may be removed and/or replaced.	If the PA catheter remains in place, the PADP can be followed if the PADP correlated with the PAOP.
Troubleshooting Unexpected Changes in PAP		
1. Position the patient in the supine position with the head of the bed between 0 and 45 degrees.	Similar positioning may improve the accuracy of identifying the phlebostatic axis and the consistency of serial trending of CVP/RAP.	For patients who are unable to tolerate supine positioning with the head of the bed at 0 to 45 degrees, CVP and PA monitoring may be obtained with the head of the bed elevated up to 60 degrees, with the patient in up to a 90-degree lateral position, or prone after allowing stabilization of 5–15 minutes (or longer for prone positioning).[1] With each of these maneuvers, the level of the right atrium will be altered from the previously identified phlebostatic axis.[2]
2. Ensure that the air-fluid interface (zeroing stopcock) is level with the phlebostatic axis (see Procedure 60).	Ensures accurate pressure measurements. If the air-fluid interface is above the phlebostatic axis, PA pressures are falsely low. If the air-fluid interface is below the phlebostatic axis, PA pressures are falsely high.	
3. Zero the transducer-monitoring system (see Procedure 60, Single-Pressure and Multiple-Pressure Transducer Systems).	Ensures the accuracy of the monitoring system.	
4. Check for air bubbles in the pressure-monitoring system, and eliminate bubbles if present.	Air contributes to an overdamped pressure transducer system, resulting in falsely low pressure measurements.	

Procedure for Pulmonary Artery Catheter and Pressure Lines, Troubleshooting—*Continued*

Steps	Rationale	Special Considerations
5. Trace the entire system from the patient's pressure tubing, transducer, pressure cables, and monitor module interface to ensure accuracy of the system setup.	Misalignment of the monitor module interface, cables, transducers, and/or tubing connections can result in unexpected hemodynamic waveforms and pressure measurements.	Investigate this possibility any time the patient has been recently disconnected from or reconnected to the monitoring system.
6. Assess the patient's hemodynamic parameters, and compare them with assessment data.	Hemodynamic data and assessment data should correlate.	If the hemodynamic data and assessment data do not correlate, review hemodynamic measurement steps for potential sources of inaccuracy.
7. Ensure that vasoactive medications or inhaled pulmonary vasodilators have been correctly titrated, and ensure that there has been no interruption in intended therapies.	Incorrect, decreased, or inadvertently discontinued medications can alter PA pressures.	Evaluate any aerosolization equipment and/or medication delivery system to ensure proper functioning.
8. If the PAP changes and hemodynamic parameters are accurate, administer/ titrate fluids or vasoactive agents as prescribed, and notify the advanced practice nurse or physician.	Hemodynamic data guide therapeutic interventions.	

Troubleshooting Blood Backup Into a PA Catheter or Pressure-Transducer System

Steps	Rationale	Special Considerations
1. Turn the stopcock off to the patient (see Fig. 60.4).	Prevents blood from going into the transducer.	If blood cannot be cleared from the transducer, the transducer may have to be replaced.
2. Ensure that the transducer system is closed, all connections are tight, and all stopcocks are closed to air and have nonvented caps.	Loose connections or open stopcocks cause a decrease in pressure within the fluid-filled system, and blood may exert a back pressure into the pressure tubing.	A crack in the system necessitates replacing the entire monitoring system.
3. Ensure that there is fluid in the flush solution bag and that the pressure on the flush bag or device is delivering 300 mm Hg.	Low pressure from the bag results in blood backup.	
4. Once the source of the problem is located and corrected, flush the entire line to remove blood from the system.	Prevents clot formation within the monitoring system.	
5. Zero the hemodynamic monitoring system (see Procedure 60, Single-Pressure and Multiple-Pressure Transducer Systems).	Ensures accuracy of the monitoring system.	
6. Observe the waveform, and perform a dynamic response test (square-wave test).	Determines whether the system is damped. This will ensure that the pressure waveform components are clearly defined and aids in accurate measurement.	The square-wave test can be performed by activating and quickly releasing the fast flush. A sharp upstroke should terminate in a flat line at the maximal indicator on the monitor. This should be followed by an immediate rapid downstroke extending below baseline with 1–2 oscillations within 0.12 seconds and a quick return to baseline (see Fig. 60.10).
7. Evaluate and monitor the PA waveform.	Ensures presence of the correct waveform, location of PA catheter, and system functioning.	

Procedure continues on following page

UNIT II

Patient Monitoring and Care —*Continued*

Steps	Rationale	Special Considerations
Troubleshooting When the Patient Develops Hemoptysis or Bloody Secretions From the Endotracheal Tube During PA Catheter Monitoring		
1. Notify the provider immediately.	PA perforation with hemorrhage is a potentially lethal complication of PA catheter insertion.	
2. Maintain patency of the airway.	Prevents alterations in ventilation and oxygenation.	Prepare for intubation if the patient is not already intubated.
3. Remain with the patient for monitoring and reassurance.	Reduces anxiety and fear; provides essential assessment.	
4. Be prepared to follow these steps:	Blood loss from the PA can be fatal. Immediate surgical or interventional radiology repair of the PA may be necessary.	
A. Send blood specimens to assess coagulation status and to prepare for blood-product transfusions.		
B. Assist if needed with calling for a chest radiograph.		
C. Prepare the patient for transport to the procedural area/operating room as requested.		
After All Troubleshooting Interventions		
1. Remove **PE**, and discard used supplies.		
2. **HH**		

Expected Outcomes

- Normal pulmonary tissue perfusion
- Absence of PA catheter–related dysrhythmias and other complications
- Absence of signs of PA catheter–related infection
- Absence of discomfort associated with a PA catheter
- Accurate PA waveform, pressure monitoring, and data

Unexpected Outcomes

- PA balloon rupture
- Pulmonary infarction and rupture
- PA catheter–related infection
- Air embolism
- Discomfort at the PA catheter insertion site
- Ventricular tachycardia unresponsive to antidysrhythmic medications

Patient Monitoring and Care

Steps	Rationale	Reportable Conditions
		These conditions should be reported to the provider if they persist despite nursing interventions.
1. The PA waveform should be continuously monitored.	Provides assessment of proper placement of the PA catheter and abnormal waveforms such as PAOP or RV waveforms.	• Abnormal waveforms (e.g., continued PAOP waveform, overwedged and RV waveforms)
2. Pressure alarms should be set and remain on at all times.	Alerts the critical care nurse to pressure changes and to disconnections in the pressure-monitoring system.	• Abnormal hemodynamic values
3. Evaluate the hemodynamic monitoring system and waveform configurations.	Ensures that the system is intact and functioning appropriately.	• Abnormal waveforms
4. Monitor hemodynamic status (e.g., PA, PAOP, RA, cardiac output, cardiac index, systemic vascular resistance).	Guides diagnosis, appropriate therapeutic interventions, and evaluation of therapies.	• Abnormal hemodynamic monitoring values • < 1.5mL required to obtain wedge • Suspected overwedge
5. Assess the hemodynamic waveforms and pressure values before and after troubleshooting.	Identifies that troubleshooting has been successful.	• Unsuccessful troubleshooting attempts • Suspected occluded PA catheter • Suspected continuous wedge
1. Follow institutional standards for assessing pain. Administer analgesia as prescribed.	Identifies need for pain interventions.	• Continued pain despite pain interventions

Documentation

Documentation should include the following:

- Patient and family education
- Troubleshooting intervention and outcome
- Occurrence of unexpected outcomes and interventions
- Pain assessment, interventions, and effectiveness
- Patient tolerance of procedure
- Site assessment
- External centimeter marking of PA catheter noted at exit site

References and Additional Readings

For a complete list of references and additional readings for this procedure, scan this QR code with your smartphone, or visit https://www.elsevier.com/__data/assets/pdf_file/0004/1319836/Chapter0061.pdf

UNIT II

PROCEDURE

62 Blood Sampling From a Pulmonary Artery Catheter

Kathleen M. Cox

PURPOSE To obtain blood from a pulmonary artery (PA) catheter for determination of mixed venous oxygen saturation.

PREREQUISITE NURSING KNOWLEDGE

- Knowledge of anatomy and physiology of the pulmonary and cardiovascular system.
- Understanding principles and can perform sterile and aseptic technique and infection control.
- Physiological gas exchange and acid-base balance.
- Technique for specimen collection and labeling per institutional policy.
- Principles of hemodynamic monitoring.
- Knowledge about the care of patients with PA catheters (see Procedure 59, Pulmonary Artery Catheter Insertion [Assist],) and stopcock manipulation (see Procedure 60, Single-Pressure and Multiple-Pressure Transducer Systems).
- The most frequent blood specimen obtained from the PA is one for mixed venous oxygen saturation (SvO_2) analysis.[6,8]
- SvO_2 measures the oxygen saturation of the venous blood in the PA (see Procedure 63, Continous Venous Oxygen Saturating Monitoring).
- SvO_2 samples may be obtained to calibrate the equipment when continuously monitoring SvO_2 values.[2]
- Routine blood sampling from the PA catheter is not recommended because entry into the sterile system may increase the incidence of catheter-associated infection.[1,3,5]

EQUIPMENT

- Nonsterile gloves
- Goggles or fluid shield face mask
- Antiseptic solution (e.g., 2% chlorhexidine-based solution)
- Needleless blood sampling access device (blood-transfer device)
- Two 10-mL syringes
- Blood-specimen tubes
- Blood gas sampling syringe
- Needleless cap (injectable cap) or nonvented cap (noninjectable cap)
- Laboratory form and specimen label
- Specimen transport bag(s)
  Additional equipment to have available as needed includes the following:
- Additional syringes
- Bag of ice
- Sterile 4 × 4 gauze pad

PATIENT AND FAMILY EDUCATION

- Explain the purpose for blood sampling to the patient and family. *Rationale:* Provision of information helps the patient and family make informed decisions, reduces anxiety, and facilitates cooperation.
- Explain the patient's expected participation during the procedure. *Rationale:* Discussion of the patient's participation supports patient autonomy and sense of control and increases patient cooperation.[1]

PATIENT ASSESSMENT AND PREPARATION

Patient Assessment

- Assess the patient's cardiopulmonary and hemodynamic status, including abnormal lung sounds, respiratory distress, dysrhythmias, decreased mentation, agitation, and skin color changes. *Rationale:* These signs and symptoms could necessitate blood sampling for venous oxygenation.
- Assess for a decrease in cardiac output related to changes in preload, afterload, or contractility. *Rationale:* Mixed venous blood samples are used to evaluate changes in cardiopulmonary function.
- Assess the hemodynamic waveforms. *Rationale:* Determines that the PA catheter is in the proper position in the pulmonary artery.

Patient Preparation

- Verify the correct patient with two identifiers. *Rationale:* Before performing a procedure, the nurse should ensure the correct identification of the patient for the intended intervention.
- Confirm that the patient and family understand the preprocedural teaching by having them verbalize understanding. Clarify key points by reinforcing important information, and answer all questions. *Rationale:* Understanding of previously taught information is evaluated and reinforced.
- Position the patient so the intended blood sampling port is exposed. *Rationale:* Optimal positioning improves the ease of obtaining the blood sample and reduces potential contamination of the port.

Procedure | for Blood Sampling From a Pulmonary Artery Catheter

Steps	Rationale	Special Considerations
1. **HH** HH		
2. **PE** PE		
3. When drawing a mixed venous oxygen (Sv_{O_2}) sample, open the arterial blood gas (ABG) kit and expel the excess air and heparin from the syringe.[4]	Prepares the ABG syringe.	Heparin is usually in powdered form.
4. Temporarily suspend the PA alarms.	Prevents the alarm from sounding because the PA waveform is lost during the blood draw.	
5. PA distal stopcock: A. Remove the nonvented cap (noninjectable cap) from the stopcock of the distal lumen of the PA catheter. *or*	Prepares the line for blood sampling.	
B. Clean the needleless cap (injectable cap) at the top of the stopcock of the distal lumen of the PA catheter with an antiseptic solution, and allow to dry.[1,3] (**Level B***)	Prepares the line for blood sampling and reduces the risk for infection.	Follow institutional standards.
6. Place a sterile syringe or a needleless blood sampling access device (blood-transfer device) into the top port of the stopcock of the distal lumen of the PA catheter (Fig. 62.1).	Prepares for blood sampling.	

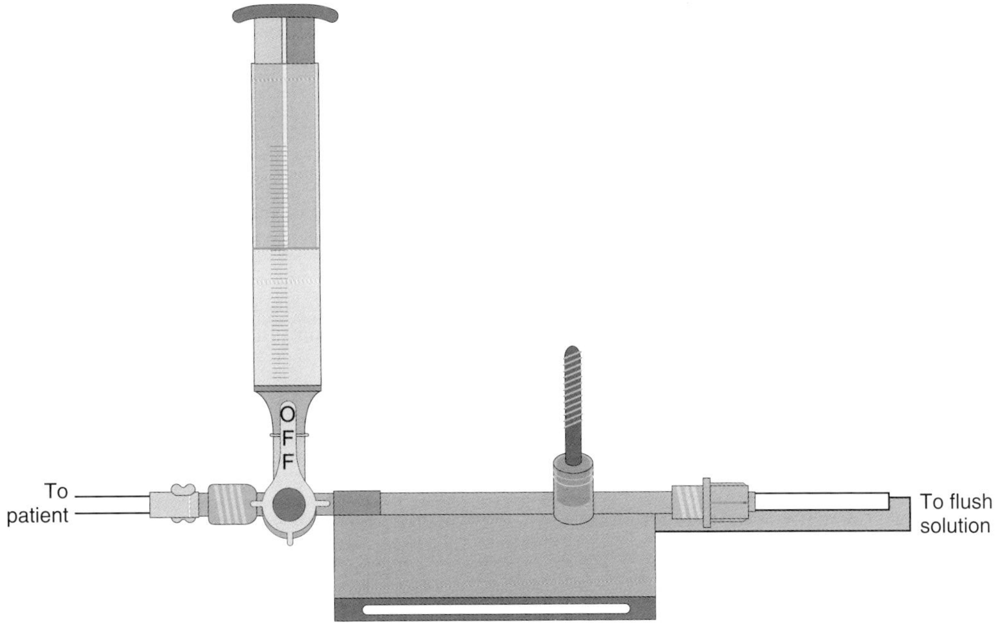

Figure 62.1 A syringe attached to the port of the three-way stopcock. The stopcock is turned "off" to the port of the stopcock. *(Drawing courtesy Paul W. Schiffmacher, Thomas Jefferson University, Philadelphia, PA.)*

To patient — | To flush solution

7. Turn the stopcock off to the flush solution (Fig. 62.2)	The syringe or needleless blood-sampling access device is then in direct contact with the blood in the PA.	

*Level B: Well-designed, controlled studies with results that consistently support a specific action, intervention, or treatment.

Procedure   **for Blood Sampling From a Pulmonary Artery Catheter—*Continued***

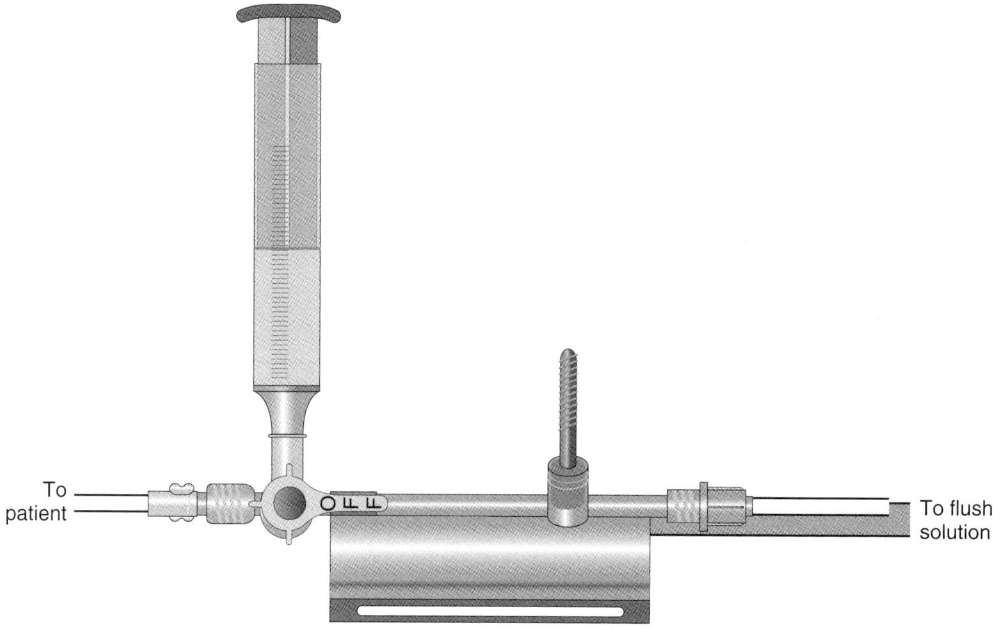

Steps	Rationale	Special Considerations

Figure 62.2 A syringe attached to the port of the three-way stopcock. The stopcock is turned "off" to flush solution. *(Drawing courtesy Paul W. Schiffm-acher, Thomas Jefferson University, Philadelphia, PA.)*

Steps	Rationale	Special Considerations
8. With a syringe, slowly and gently aspirate the discard volume, or, if using a needleless blood-sampling access device, engage the blood specimen tube to obtain the discard volume. **(Level B*)**	Clears the catheter of flush solution. The discard volume includes the dead space (from the tip of the distal lumen to the top port of the stopcock) and the blood diluted by the flush solution (e.g., 3.5 mL).[1,3,7]	If additional laboratory studies are needed, larger discard volumes may be necessary for accurate results.[3,7]
9. Turn the stopcock off to the syringe or the needleless blood-sampling access device (see Fig 62.1).	Stops blood flow and closes the top port of the stopcock.	
10. Remove the syringe or the blood specimen tube, and discard it in the appropriate receptacle.	Removes and safely disposes of the discard.	
11. Insert an ABG syringe into the stopcock, or insert the ABG syringe into the needleless blood-sampling access device.	Prepares for removal of a blood sample.	
12. Turn the stopcock off to the flush system (see Fig. 62.2).	Prepares for blood sampling.	
13. Slowly aspirate the Svo_2 sample (per institutional policy).	Slow aspiration is important to prevent contamination of the mixed venous sample with arterial blood from the pulmonary capillaries, which will falsely elevate the Svo_2 value.[6]	
14. Turn the stopcock off to the syringe or the needleless blood sampling access device (see Fig. 62.1).	Prevents bleeding.	
15. Remove the ABG syringe.	Detaches the specimen.	

*Level B: Well-designed, controlled studies with results that consistently support a specific action, intervention, or treatment.

Procedure continues on following page

Procedure for Blood Sampling From a Pulmonary Artery Catheter—*Continued*

Steps	Rationale	Special Considerations
16. Expel any air bubbles from the ABG syringe, cap the syringe, and place it on ice.	Ensures the accuracy of the Svo_2 results.	
17. Turn the stopcock off to the patient.	Prepares the system.	

18. Fast-flush the remaining blood from the top port of the stopcock:
  A. Remove the nonvented or noninjectable cap.
  B. Flush the blood onto a sterile gauze pad, into a discard syringe, or into a blood specimen tube, and discard the waste into the appropriate receptacle.
	Clears blood from the system.	

19. Turn the stopcock off to the top port of the stopcock (see Fig. 62.1).	Opens the system up for continuous PA pressure monitoring.	Remove the needleless blood-sampling access device if used.
20. Attach a new sterile nonvented cap (noninjectable cap), or clean the needleless cap (injectable cap) with antiseptic solution.	Maintains a closed sterile system.	
21. Flush the remaining blood in the PA catheter back into the patient.	Promotes patency of the PA catheter.	
22. Observe the monitor for return of the PA waveform.	Ensures continuous monitoring of the PA waveform.	
23. Remove PE, **PE** and discard used supplies.	Reduces the transmission of microorganisms; standard precautions.	
24. **HH**		
25. Turn the alarms back on.	Activates the alarm system.	
26. Label the specimen, and place it in a transport bag.	Properly identifies the patient and laboratory tests to be performed.	Confirm identifying information. Label the blood-gas laboratory slip as a mixed venous sample.
27. Send the specimen for analysis.	Needed for ABG analysis.	Follow institutional policy regarding the use of ice for ABG samples.

Expected Outcomes

- Adequate blood sample with minimal blood loss
- PA catheter patency maintained
- Svo_2 value and trends within normal range (60% to 80%)

Unexpected Outcomes

- Inability to obtain Svo_2 sample
- Clotting of the PA catheter
- Arterial sample obtained as a result of rapid withdrawal of blood from the pulmonary capillaries instead of mixed venous oxygen sample for blood-gas analysis

UNIT II

Patient Monitoring and Care

Steps	Rationale	Reportable Conditions
		These conditions should be reported to the provider if they persist despite nursing interventions.
1. Before and after the blood withdrawal, assess and evaluate the PA waveform.	Ensures that the PA catheter is properly positioned.	• Abnormal PA waveforms or values
2. Correlate the Svo_2 results with the measured cardiac output.	Changes in the Svo_2 indicate changes in cardiac output and hemodynamic status.	• Abnormal mixed venous oxygen saturation, preload, afterload, cardiac output, and cardiac index
3. Correlate the Svo_2 results with the clinical assessment data.[6,8]	Svo_2 decreases with: • Increased oxygen consumption • Decreased oxygen delivery Svo_2 increases with: • Decreased tissue oxygen consumption • Increased oxygen delivery	• Fever • Shivering • Seizures • Agitation • Pain • Decreased cardiac output • Decreased hemoglobin • Decreased arterial oxygen saturation • Hypothermia

Documentation

Documentation should include the following:
• Patient and family education
• Time and date of the Svo_2 sample
• Svo_2 results
• Any difficulties with PA catheter blood sampling
• Nursing interventions performed
• Unexpected outcomes

References and Additional Readings

For a complete list of references and additional readings for this procedure, scan this QR code with your smartphone, or visit https://www.elsevier.com/__data/assets/pdf_file/0005/1319837/Chapter0062.pdf

63 Continuous Venous Oxygen Saturation Monitoring

Joni L. Dirks

PURPOSE Venous oxygen saturation monitoring is performed to measure the oxygen saturation of hemoglobin in the venous blood. The value can be obtained either from the pulmonary artery (PA; mixed venous oxygen saturation–Svo_2) or from the superior vena cava (central venous oxygen saturation–$Scvo_2$). Measurement can be performed intermittently with individual blood samples or continuously with a specialized fiberoptic catheter and an associated computer or module. Assessment of venous oxygen saturation provides an indication of the balance between a patient's oxygen delivery and oxygen consumption.

PREREQUISITE NURSING KNOWLEDGE

- Anatomy and physiology of the cardiopulmonary system.
- Physiological principles related to invasive hemodynamic monitoring.
- Technical aspects of central venous catheter (CVC) placement and pressure monitoring (see Procedure 56).
- Technical aspects of pulmonary artery catheter (PAC) placement (see Procedures 58, Pulmonary Artery Catheter Insertion [Perform], and 59, Pulmonary Artery Catheter Insertion [Assist] and Pressure Monitoring) and pressure monitoring (see Procedure 60, Single-Pressure and Multiple-Pressure Transducer Systems).
- Proper technique for obtaining blood samples from a CVC or PAC (see Procedures 57, Blood Sampling From a Central Venous Catheter, and 62, Blood Sampling From a Pulmonary Artery Catheter).
- Physiological concepts of oxygen delivery, oxygen demand, and tissue oxygen consumption.
- Clinically, venous oxygen saturation provides an index of overall oxygen balance because it reflects the dynamic relationship between the patient's oxygen delivery and oxygen consumption. Low venous oxygen saturation has been associated with increased mortality, morbidity, and length of stay in critically ill patients.[2] Early detection of oxygen imbalance can facilitate interventions and evaluation of treatment in high-risk patients.[3,15,17,18]
- Whenever the demand for oxygen exceeds the supply, the body will initiate compensatory mechanisms to increase oxygen delivery (by increasing cardiac output) and increase oxygen extraction at the tissue level.
- In a critically ill patient with limited cardiac output, increased extraction occurs to meet the demand for oxygen at the tissue level. The result is a decreased level of oxygen returning to the heart and a lower Svo_2 or $Scvo_2$ measurement. Many factors can affect the requirements for oxygen and subsequently Svo_2/$Scvo_2$ (Box 63.1).[13,14]
- Svo_2 does not correlate *directly* with any of the determinants of oxygen delivery (i.e., cardiac output, hemoglobin,

and arterial oxygen saturation) or oxygen consumption. Because a critically ill patient is in a dynamic state, Svo_2/$Scvo_2$ must be viewed in light of these changing determinants and considered an index of oxygen balance.[13,14]
- A normal Svo_2 generally is 60% to 80%, and a clinically significant change in Svo_2 (5% to 10%) can be an early indicator of physiological instability.[13,14,20]
- Svo_2 values of less than 60% may result from either inadequate oxygen delivery or excessive oxygen consumption. It should be noted that in sepsis a patient may have a normal or high Svo_2 value, which may indicate impaired cellular function or severe arteriovenous shunting.[7] It is always important to consider the clinical picture along with Svo_2 values.
- The percent of venous oxygen saturation as measured in the PA (Svo_2) is flow weighted and represents a true mixing of all venous blood in the body: inferior vena cava (IVC), superior vena cava (SVC), and coronary sinus.
- PACs are being used less frequently in critically ill patients, so the use of CVCs to measure venous saturation has emerged as an alternative.[4] The percent of venous oxygen saturation as measured in the SVC ($Scvo_2$) reflects the mixing of venous blood from the superior half of the body. It does not include blood from the IVC and coronary sinus.
- $Scvo_2$ and Svo_2 do not correlate absolutely, but trend together in a variety of hemodynamic states.[13] In healthy patients, $Scvo_2$ is slightly lower than Svo_2. In periods of hemodynamic instability, $Scvo_2$ is higher than Svo_2, with a difference that ranges from 5% to 13% resulting from a redistribution of blood flow caused by the various pathophysiologies.[13] Therefore $Scvo_2$ overestimates Svo_2 in shock conditions; a low $Scvo_2$ likely indicates an even lower Svo_2.
- Continuous venous saturation monitoring is performed with a three-component system (Fig. 63.1):
  - A fiberoptic central venous or PA catheter contains two optical filaments that exit at the distal lumen. One filament serves as a sending fiber for the emission of light; the other serves as a receiving fiber for the light reflected back from the blood in the vessel (Fig. 63.2).
  - The optic module houses the light-emitting diodes (LEDs), which transmit various wavelengths of light,

BOX 63.1 Common Conditions and Activities That Affect Venous Oxygen Saturation Values

DECREASED CENTRAL AND MIXED VENOUS OXYGEN SATURATION

Decreased Oxygen Delivery
- Heart failure
- Hypovolemia
- Hemorrhage
- Hypoxemia

Increased Oxygen Consumption
- Fever
- Pain
- Agitation
- Shivering
- Seizures
- Increased work of breathing
- Infection
- Burns
- Numerous nursing procedures (e.g., dressing changes, suctioning, turning, and chest physiotherapy)

INCREASED CENTRAL AND MIXED VENOUS OXYGEN SATURATION

Increased Oxygen Delivery
- Fluid resuscitation
- Inotropic medications
- Blood transfusion
- Oxygen therapy

Decreased Oxygen Consumption
- Hypothermia
- Analgesia
- Sedation
- Pharmacological paralysis
- Cellular dysfunction (shunting, sepsis)
- Mechanical ventilation
- Decreased musculoskeletal activity

and a photodetector, which receives light. The light wavelengths are shone through a blood sample as it travels between the LED and the photodetector. Desaturated hemoglobin, saturated hemoglobin (oxyhemoglobin), and dyshemoglobin (carboxyhemoglobin, methemoglobin) have different light-absorption characteristics. The ratio of hemoglobin to oxyhemoglobin is determined and reported as a percentage value.[5,6,10-12] All patient data, including calibration of saturation values and patient identification information, are stored in this component. This module should not be disconnected from the patient's catheter. If the need to disconnect is unavoidable, refer to the manufacturer's instructions for inputting patient information and reestablishing calibration.

❖ An oximeter computer, either a stand-alone unit or a module for a bedside monitoring system, has a microprocessor that converts the light information from the optic module into an electrical display. This display is updated every few seconds for continuous monitoring. This information may be displayed as a continuous graphic trend, a numeric display, or both, depending on the manufacturer.

- Proper calibration of the monitor and catheter ensures accuracy of venous saturation values. The two types of calibration are in vitro, in which the catheter and optics module are calibrated before insertion, and in vivo, in which the venous saturation value from the system is compared with a laboratory co-oximeter value from a blood sample drawn from the catheter tip. Follow the manufacturer's recommendations for performing calibration procedures. Daily in vivo calibrations are recommended by most manufacturers or when there is concern about the validity of the value.[13] In addition, proper blood sampling techniques from the distal port of the PAC or CVC catheter are necessary for ensuring accurate values for calibration.[5,6]

Reflection spectrophotometry

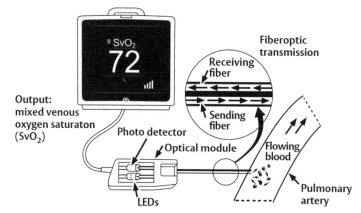

Figure 63.1 Oximetry system with reflectance spectrophotometry. *(From McGee WT, Headley J, Frazier JA, editors: Quick guide to cardiopulmonary care. Irvine, CA, 2018, Edwards Lifesciences Corporation.)*

UNIT II

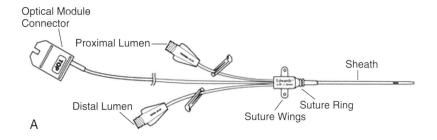

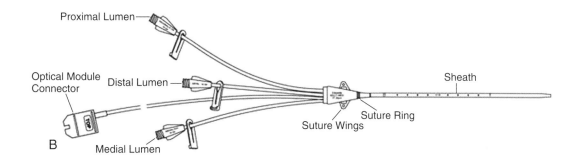

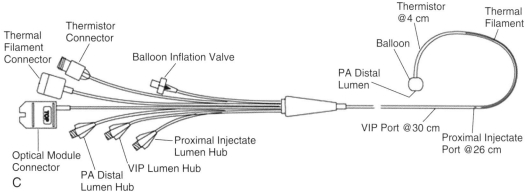

Figure 63.2 Oximetry catheters. **A,** Central venous catheter. **B,** Small French size for pediatric applications. **C,** Pulmonary artery catheter. *(From McGee WT, Headley J, Frazier JA, editors: Quick guide to cardiopulmonary care, Irvine, CA, 2018, Edwards Lifesciences Corporation.)*

EQUIPMENT

- Fiberoptic PAC for SvO_2 (various sizes, 4 to 8F; various lumens; various lengths, 25 to 110 cm)
- Fiberoptic CVC for $ScvO_2$ (various sizes for pediatric to adult use, 4.5 to 8.5F; various lengths, 5 to 20 cm; double or triple lumen) or oximetry PICC (5F, 40 to 55 cm; includes dedicated lumen for light transmission and single or multiple fluid lumens)
- Optic module
- Oximeter computer or bedside monitoring system module
- Equipment required for central venous monitoring or PA catheterization and pressure monitoring

PATIENT AND FAMILY EDUCATION

- Assess patient and family understanding of the clinical benefits of venous oximetry monitoring. *Rationale:* For information to be the most appropriate, assessment of the level of patient and family understanding of the need for $ScvO_2$ or SvO_2 monitoring is important. By explaining the usefulness of SvO_2 monitoring in language that nonmedical personnel can understand, the patient and family are able to ask appropriate questions and understand more clearly the clinical presentation of the patient and implications for further treatment therapies.
- Explain the continuous nature of this monitoring system and the significance of the alarms. *Rationale:* Explanation of the procedure to the patient and family helps alleviate fears and concerns. Additional monitors may produce increased anxiety in the patient and family.

PATIENT ASSESSMENT AND PREPARATION

Patient Assessment

Indications for use of $ScvO_2/SvO_2$ monitoring include the following:[3,13,15,17,19,21]

- High-risk surgery (abdominal, cardiovascular, vascular)
- Acute decompensated heart failure
- Shock
- Sepsis
- Multisystem organ dysfunction

❖ Trauma
❖ Acute respiratory distress syndrome

Patient Preparation

- Verify the correct patient with two identifiers. ***Rationale:*** Before performing a procedure, the nurse should ensure the correct identification of the patient for the intended intervention.
- Answer patient questions as they arise, and reinforce information as needed. ***Rationale:*** This communication evaluates and reinforces understanding of previously taught information.

Procedure	**for Continuous Mixed Venous Oxygen Saturation Monitoring**	
Steps	Rationale	Special Considerations
1. 🄷🄷		
2. 🄿🄴		
3. Assemble necessary equipment and supplies for continuous monitoring.	Ensures that equipment is ready and available for the procedure.	
4. Connect the power cord to the computer, turn on the computer, and observe the system check on the computer screen. (**Level M***)	Allows electronics to warm up; confirms component function.[5,6,10-12]	Some monitors allow toggling between Svo_2, $Scvo_2$, or So_2. Ensure that the proper label is used.[5,6]
5. Input patient height and weight data as per institutional standards.	Allows for calculation of derived hemodynamic parameters.[5,6,12]	This may be done after placement.
6. Connect the optics module to the computer. (**Level M***)	LEDs are housed in an optics module. Approximately 5–10 minutes are needed to warm the light source sufficiently.[5,6,10-12]	Warm-up times may vary by manufacturer and ambient room temperature.
7. Remove the outer wrap of the catheter package, and aseptically peel back the inner wrap portion that covers the optic connector of the catheter. (**Level M***)	Provides access to the inner package; isolates the connector from the catheter tip to maintain sterility during in vitro calibration.[5,6,10-12]	Catheter packaging may vary according to manufacturer. Follow the manufacturer's directions for use to ensure proper handling.
8. Firmly connect the optic connector to the optic module. (**Level M***)	Ensures that connections are tight and properly aligned for light transmission[5,6,10-12]	
9. Perform in vitro calibration or standardization. (**Level M***)	Standardizes or calibrates the light source to the catheter. Calibration is performed before catheter insertion. The catheter tip should be left in the calibration cup or container in the package during in vitro calibration.[5,6,10-12]	Catheter lumens must be dry. Do not flush the catheter before performing this step, or in vitro calibration will be invalid. Patient hemoglobin or hematocrit values may be entered at this point if available, or calibration can be performed using default values.
10. Pull back the remaining wrap covering the catheter package with aseptic technique. (**Level M***)	Prepares the catheter for insertion.[5,6,10-12]	
11. Carefully remove the catheter from the tray with sterile technique. Pull the catheter tip up and out of the calibration cup. (**Level M***)	Prevents transmission of microorganisms; prevents damage to the fiberoptics in the catheter and the balloon of the PA catheter.[5,6,10-12]	Fiberoptics in the catheter and PA catheter balloon are fragile and may be damaged if not handled properly.
12. Attach the pressure tubing, and prime lumens with flush solution (see Procedure 60, Single-Pressure and Multiple-Pressure Transducer Systems).	Enables monitoring of chamber pressures during PAC insertion; maintains patency of lumens.	Refer to institutional standards for use of heparinized flush solution.[14]
13. Perform a preprocedure verification and time out if nonemergent.	Ensures patient safety.	
14. Assist the provider with CVC or PAC site preparation and catheter insertion.	Provides assistance to the provider while the catheter is inserted.	If a PICC is selected for $Scvo_2$ monitoring (Fig. 63.3), insertion may be performed by specially trained RNs.[11]

*Level M: Manufacturer's recommendations only.

Procedure for Continuous Mixed Venous Oxygen Saturation Monitoring—*Continued*

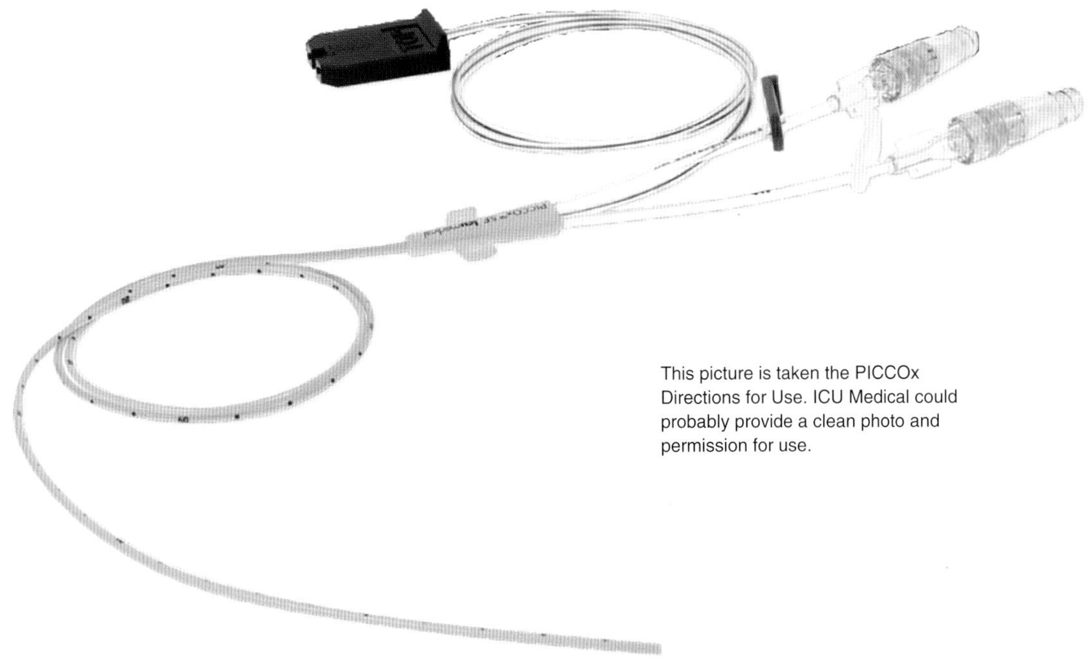

Steps	Rationale	Special Considerations

Figure 63.3 Peripherally inserted central catheter with oximetry (*Courtesy ICU Medical, Inc.*)

Steps	Rationale	Special Considerations
15. Observe PA waveforms during insertion.	Central PAC tip placement is necessary for optimal light reflection.[5,6,12]	Inflation volume of 1.25–1.5 mL is recommended for proper catheter tip placement.[5,6,11] Ensure passive deflation of the balloon before proceeding.
16. Verify adequate light intensity or signal quality on the Svo_2 or $Scvo_2$ monitor after initiating monitoring. **(Level M*)**	Light intensity or signal quality verifies adequate reflection of the light signals from the catheter tip. Troubleshooting should be performed to obtain an adequate signal before recording $Svo_2/Scvo_2$ values.	Signal quality may be compromised if the catheter tip is in contact with the vessel wall or the catheter is kinked.
17. Set high and low alarm limits, and activate alarms. **(Level D*)**	Individualizes alarm settings according to patient baseline.[18] Audible alarms notify the clinician of significant changes in $Scvo_2/Svo_2$ values and trends.	
18. Apply a sterile dressing to the insertion site. **(Level D*)**	Reduces transmission of microorganisms.[16]	Follow institutional standards for central venous catheter dressings.
19. Firmly secure the optic module near the patient. **(Level M*)**	Excessive tension on the catheter or optic module may break the optic fibers.[5,6,10-12]	
20. After calibration and insertion of the catheter, obtain a baseline set of hemodynamic and oxygenation indices.	Provides baseline information for comparison with the patient's response to interventions.	

*Level D: Peer-reviewed professional and organizational standards with the support of clinical study recommendations.
*Level M: Manufacturer's recommendations only.

Procedure continues on following page

UNIT II

Procedure	for Continuous Mixed Venous Oxygen Saturation Monitoring—*Continued*		
Steps	**Rationale**	**Special Considerations**
21. Continuously monitor PA pressure tracings and Svo_2/$Scvo_2$ values. **(Level D*)**	Spontaneous catheter migration may occur after insertion.[1] Position may influence signal quality if the catheter tip is positioned against a vessel wall. Fluids infused through the distal lumen of the CVC (lipids, boluses) may also influence signal quality.[5,6]	If the PAC becomes wedged, the readings may reflect postcapillary arterialized blood, and the Svo_2 value may suddenly increase.[13,14] The PICC $Scvo_2$ catheter has lumens that can be used for pressure monitoring, fluid infusion, or blood draws.[10,11]
22. Obtain catheter-placement confirmation per institutional standards (i.e., chest radiograph).	Provides confirmation of the proper catheter.	

Venous Blood Sampling Skill/in Vivo Calibration

23. ▣ (if independent from catheter placement).		
24. ▣ (if independent from catheter placement).		
25. Draw a venous blood sample from the distal port of the catheter for in vivo calibration (see Procedure 62, Blood Sampling From a Pulmonary Artery Catheter, for mixed venous blood sampling or Procedure 57, Blood Sampling From a Cental Venous Catheter for central venous blood sampling).	In vivo calibration may be necessary to verify the accuracy of the computer and value displayed after insertion of the fiberoptic catheter. Ideally, the patient's hemodynamic and oxygenation status should be stable for optimal calibration.[5,6,10-12]	Mixed venous samples should be drawn from the distal port of the PAC.[13] Central venous samples should be drawn from the distal port of the CVC.[13]
26. Perform a verification or in vivo calibration per manufacturer's instructions or institutional standards. **(Level D*)**	In vivo calibration verifies the accuracy of the $Scvo_2$/Svo_2 being displayed.[5,6,8,10-13] In vivo calibration is required if the catheter was inserted *without* performing preinsertion calibration or if the catheter is disconnected from the optical module. In vivo calibration may also be performed on a routine basis (typically every 24 hours) or whenever the displayed value is in question.[14]	Follow specific recommendations from the manufacturer about the frequency of calibration and specific steps to implement the process. If the value of the Svo_2 measured by the laboratory differs by more than 5% from the value displayed on the monitor, the bedside system should be recalibrated.[13]
27. Ensure that measurement is performed with a laboratory co-oximeter. **(Level D*)**	Co-oximetry measures direct fractional oxyhemoglobin saturation; blood gas analyzers calculate oxygen saturation from measured partial pressure values. A calculated saturation value from a gas analyzer may not correlate with the actual patient value and, if used for calibration, may produce erroneous results.[8,13]	
28. Observe the bedside monitor display for return of the PA/central venous pressure waveform, and resume Svo_2/$Scvo_2$ monitoring. **(Level D*)**	Reconfirms catheter tip placement in the PA/SVC/right atrium.[14]	Proper positioning of the catheter is important for accurate measurement of venous oxygen saturation and to prevent possible complications.[1,14]
29. Dispose of used supplies and equipment.		
30. Remove personal protective equipment. ▣	Reduces the transmission of microorganisms and body secretions; standard precautions.	
31. ▣		

*Level D: Peer-reviewed professional and organizational standards with the support of clinical study recommendations.

Expected Outcomes

- Svo_2 values and trends within normal range (60%–80%)[13,14]
- $Scvo_2$ values and trends greater than 65% to 70%[8,22]
- $Scvo_2$/Svo_2 trends not fluctuating greater than 5% to 10% of baseline value[14]
- Hemodynamic and oxygenation parameters optimal for patient condition

Unexpected Outcomes

- Svo_2 values less than 60% or greater than 80%
- Svo_2 value trends greater than 10% from baseline
- $Scvo_2$ value trends less than 65% to 70%
- Infection from presence of an indwelling PAC or CVC
- PA occlusion, infarction, or rupture

Patient Monitoring and Care

Steps	Rationale	Reportable Conditions
		These conditions should be reported to the provider if they persist despite nursing interventions.
1. Ensure that no kinks or bends are found in the catheter.	Fiber-optics are fragile and can break if not handled carefully. Overtightening of the introducer connector can cause crimping and breakage of the fiberoptics.[5,6,10-13] Subclavian or internal jugular approaches for insertion may cause kinking in the vessel if the vessel is tortuous. Sending and receiving wavelengths may show either a change in light signal or values that do not reflect the patient's status.	• Change in PA waveform or Svo_2 value that does not correlate to patient condition • Changes in RA waveforms or $Scvo_2$ value that do not correlate to patient condition
2. Monitor PA waveforms continuously. **(Level D*)**	Migration of the catheter tip may reflect postcapillary arterialized blood causing an elevation in the Svo_2 value. Uncorrected catheter migration places the patient at risk for PA infarction or rupture.[1,14]	• Permanent wedge waveform
3. Observe Svo_2 value and trends.	Normal Svo_2 values range from 60% to 80%[14]; values outside this range may indicate an imbalance between oxygen delivery and consumption. A value change of greater than 5%–10% may signify a clinically significant change.[14] If the patient's clinical presentation differs from the observed Svo_2 value or trends, recheck the accuracy of the monitoring system.	• Svo_2 values greater than 80% or less than 60%
4. Observe $Scvo_2$ value and trends. **(Level B*)**	$Scvo_2$ values trend with Svo_2. Target values for goal-directed therapy in patients with sepsis and septic shock are no longer recommended, but persistently low values are associated with increased mortality.[9,17]	• $Scvo_2$ values less than 65%

*Level B: Well-designed, controlled studies with results that consistently support a specific action, intervention, or treatment.

Documentation

Documentation should include the following:

- Patient and family education
- $Scvo_2$/Svo_2 whenever the hemodynamic profile is recorded
- Additional oxygenation indices as indicated
- Specific nursing activities (e.g., suctioning, turning the patient, or titrating a vasoactive drug) and the relationship of the event with the continuous trend, especially if the event produces a marked change in the value
- Unexpected outcomes
- Nursing interventions

References and Additional Readings

For a complete list of references and additional readings for this procedure, scan this QR code with your smartphone, or visit https://www.elsevier.com/__data/assets/pdf_file/0006/1319838/Chapter0063.pdf

PROCEDURE

64 Pulmonary Artery Catheter Removal

Nikki J. Taylor

PURPOSE The pulmonary artery catheter is removed when hemodynamic monitoring is no longer clinically indicated, when complications occur (e.g., dysrhythmias, pseudoaneurysms), or when there is risk for infection associated with prolonged use of intravascular catheters.

PREREQUISITE NURSING KNOWLEDGE

- Normal cardiovascular anatomy and physiology.
- Normal values for intracardiac pressures.
- Normal coagulation values.
- Normal waveform configurations for right-atrial pressure, right-ventricular pressure, pulmonary artery pressure, and pulmonary arterial occlusive pressure.
- Venous access routes.
- Principles of aseptic technique.
- Advanced cardiac life support knowledge and skills.
- Potential complications associated with removal of the pulmonary artery (PA) catheter.
- Clinical and technical competence in PA catheter removal.
- The state nurse practice act is important to ensure that removal of a PA catheter is not prohibited.
- Air embolism can occur during removal of the catheter. Air embolism after removal of the catheter is the result of air drawn in along the subcutaneous tract and into the vein. During inspiration, negative intrathoracic pressure is transmitted to the central veins. Any opening external to the body to one of these veins may result in aspiration of air into the central venous system. The pathological effects depend on the volume and rate of air aspirated.
- Indications for the removal of the PA catheter include the following:
  - The patient's condition no longer necessitates hemodynamic monitoring.
  - Complications occur because of the presence of the PA catheter.
  - The patient shows evidence of a catheter-related infection that may be associated with the PA catheter.
- Contraindications to percutaneous removal of the PA catheter include the following[2]:
  - The PA catheter is knotted (observed on chest radiograph).
  - Any additional catheter terminating in the right atrium including permanent pacemaker, temporary transvenous pacemaker, or implantable cardioverter defibrillator (ICD) is present (as the catheter should be removed by a provider).

EQUIPMENT

- 1.5-mL syringe
- Sterile and nonsterile gloves
- Gown
- Fluid-shield face mask or goggles
- 4 × 4 sterile gauze pads
- Central line dressing kit (contents vary by institution)
- Two moisture-proof absorbent pads
- One roll of 2-inch tape

Additional equipment, to have available as needed, includes the following:

- Obturator/cap for introducer catheter port with hemostasis valve
- Additional dressing supplies (e.g., transparent dressing)
- Air occlusive dressing
- Suture removal kit
- Scissors
- Sterile specimen container
- Emergency equipment

PATIENT AND FAMILY EDUCATION

- Explain the procedure and the reason for removal of the catheter. *Rationale:* This explanation provides information and decreases anxiety.
- Explain the importance of patient participation during removal of the catheter. *Rationale:* The explanation ensures patient cooperation and facilitates safe removal of the catheter.
- Instruct the patient and family to report any shortness of breath, bleeding, or discomfort at the insertion site after removal of the catheter. *Rationale:* This identifies patient discomfort and early recognition of complications.

PATIENT ASSESSMENT AND PREPARATION

Patient Assessment

- Assess the electrocardiogram (ECG), vital signs, and neurovascular status of the extremity distal to the catheter insertion site. ***Rationale:*** This assessment serves as baseline data.
- If the introducer will also be removed, assess the current coagulation values of the patient. ***Rationale:*** If the patient has abnormal coagulation study results, hemostasis may be difficult to obtain after the introducer catheter is removed.
- Verify catheter position with waveform analysis or a chest radiograph. ***Rationale:*** This ensures accuracy of catheter position and absence of catheter knotting.
- Determine whether the patient has a permanent pacemaker, temporary transvenous pacemaker, or ICD. ***Rationale:*** PA catheter removal by a critical care nurse is contraindicated in the presence of a permanent pacemaker, temporary transvenous pacemaker, or ICD. Entanglement of the PA catheter and the pacemaker electrodes can occur.
- Assess the integrity of the PA catheter. ***Rationale:*** The PA catheter should be removed by a provider if the integrity of the PA catheter or introducer is compromised (e.g., visible cracks are noted).
- Assess the catheter insertion site for redness, warmth, tenderness, presence of drainage, and presence of bleeding.

Rationale: Signs and symptoms of infection as well as bleeding are assessed.

Patient Preparation

- In collaboration with the provider, determine when the PA catheter should be removed. ***Rationale:*** The invasive catheter is removed when it is no longer indicated.
- Verify the correct patient with two identifiers. ***Rationale:*** Before performing a procedure, the nurse should ensure the correct identification of the patient for the intended intervention.
- Ensure that the patient and family understand the preprocedural teaching. Answer questions as they arise, and reinforce information as needed. ***Rationale:*** Understanding of previously taught information is evaluated and reinforced.
- Place the patient in the supine position with the head of the bed in a slight Trendelenburg position (or flat if the Trendelenburg position is contraindicated or not tolerated by the patient). ***Rationale:*** The patient should be positioned so the catheter exit site is at or below the level of the heart.[9,10] A normal pressure gradient exists between atmospheric air and the central venous compartment that promotes air entry if the compartment is open. The lower the site of entry below the heart, the lower the pressure gradient, thus minimizing the risk of air being drawn in and thus a venous air embolism.

Procedure for Pulmonary Artery Catheter Removal

Steps	Rationale	Special Considerations
1. **HH**		
2. **PE**		All providers, nurses, and other healthcare professionals in the room should wear personal protective equipment including a face mask with eye shield.
3. Transfer or discontinue intravenous (IV) solution and flush solutions.	Prepares the catheter for removal.	Ensure that the patient has the proper alternative IV access to transfer solutions/medications that were administered through the PA catheter before removal. This is also important in the event that emergency medications are required.
4. Place a moisture-proof absorbent pad under the patient's upper torso and another under the PA catheter.	Collects blood and body fluids associated with removal; serves as a receptacle for the contaminated catheter.	

Procedure | for Pulmonary Artery Catheter Removal—*Continued*

Steps	Rationale	Special Considerations
5. Place the patient supine in a slight Trendelenburg position.[5-7,12,14,21] (**Level E***)	Minimizes the risk for venous air embolus. The patient should be positioned so the catheter exit site is at or below the level of the heart.[10-12]	Place the patient flat if the Trendelenburg position is contraindicated, not tolerated by the patient, or a femoral PA catheter will be removed. If the PA catheter is in the femoral vein, extend the patient's leg, and ensure that the groin area is adequately exposed.
6. Have the patient turn his or her head away from the PA catheter and insertion site.	Decreases the risk for contamination.	This step is not needed if a femoral PA catheter is used.
7. Open supplies.	Prepares for removal.	
8. Remove the syringe from the balloon inflation port, ensure that the gate valve or stopcock is in the open position, and observe the PA waveform.	Allows air to passively escape from the balloon and ensures adequate balloon deflation.	Myocardial or valvular tissues can be damaged if the PA catheter is removed with the balloon inflated.
9. Remove the old dressing. Perform site cleansing per institutional protocol.	Prepares for removal.	Signs of local or systemic infection may determine the need to send a culture of the catheter tip.
10. Unlock the sterile catheter sleeve from the introducer catheter.	Prepares for removal.	
11. Discard nonsterile gloves in an appropriate receptacle, perform hand hygiene, and apply sterile gloves.	Removes and safely discards used supplies. Reduces the transmission of microorganisms; standard precautions.	
12. If present, clip the sutures securing the PA catheter.	Frees the PA catheter for removal.	
13. Ask the patient to take a deep breath in and hold it.[12,16-21] (**Level E***)	Minimizes the risk for venous air embolus.	If the patient is receiving positive pressure ventilation, withdraw the catheter during the end of the inspiratory phase of the respiratory cycle or while a breath is delivered via a bag-valve-mask device.
14. While stabilizing the introducer catheter, gently withdraw the PA catheter with a constant, steady motion (Fig. 64.1).	Ensures removal of an intact catheter.	Observe the ECG tracing rhythm and the waveforms from the distal lumen during removal. Dysrhythmias may occur during removal but are usually self-limiting.[1,3,16,18,19] If resistance is met, do not continue to remove the catheter; notify the provider immediately. Resistance may be caused by catheter knotting, kinking, or wedging.

*Level E: Multiple case reports, theory-based evidence from expert opinions, or peer-reviewed professional organizational standards without clinical studies to support recommendations.

Procedure continues on following page

Procedure for Pulmonary Artery Catheter Removal—*Continued*

Steps	Rationale	Special Considerations

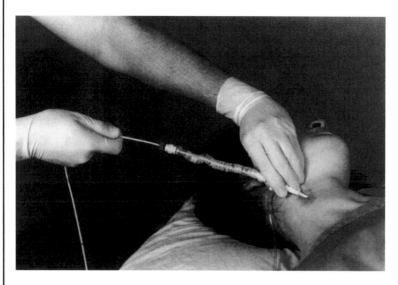

Figure 64.1 While stabilizing the introducer, gently withdraw the pulmonary artery catheter using a constant, steady motion.

Steps	Rationale	Special Considerations
15. Temporarily cover the hemostasis valve with a sterile, gloved finger until the sterile obturator/cap is attached.	The hemostasis valve must be occluded to minimize the risk for air embolus and blood loss.	The introducer may remain in place to provide central venous access.
16. Instruct the patient to exhale as soon as the PA catheter is removed.	Once the catheter is removed, the patient can breathe normally.	
17. Place the PA catheter on the moisture-proof absorbent pad, and inspect it to ensure that the entire catheter was removed.	Allows for assessment of the catheter.	If the catheter tip will be cultured, have another provider assist with cutting the tip with sterile scissors and placing it in a sterile specimen container before placing the PA catheter on the moisture-proof absorbent pad.
18. If the introducer remains in place, perform site care, and apply a sterile dressing to the site per institutional standards.	Decreases the risk for infection at the insertion site.	
19. If the introducer is to be removed, clip the sutures or remove the securing device (see Procedure 75, Central Venous Catheter Insertion [Assist], Nursing Care, and Removal).	Frees the introducer for removal.	
20. Ensure that the patient is still supine in a slight Trendelenburg position.[5-7,12,14,21] **(Level E*)**	Minimizes the risk for venous air embolus. The patient should be positioned so the catheter exit site is at or below the level of the heart.[10-12]	Cases have been reported of venous air embolus occurring after removal of central venous catheters when patients were not in the supine slight Trendelenburg position.

Procedure for Pulmonary Artery Catheter Removal—*Continued*

Steps	Rationale	Special Considerations
21. Ask the patient to take a deep breath in and hold it.[16-21] **(Level E*)**	Minimizes the risk for venous air embolus.	If the patient is receiving positive pressure ventilation, withdraw the catheter during the inspiratory phase of the respiratory cycle or while a breath is delivered via a bag-valve-mask device. If the introducer is in the femoral vein, extend the patient's leg, and ensure that the groin area is adequately exposed.
22. Withdraw the introducer, pulling parallel to the skin and using a steady motion.	Minimizes trauma.	If resistance is met, do not continue to remove the introducer. Notify the provider immediately.
23. As the introducer exits the site, apply pressure with a gauze pad.	Minimizes the risk for venous air embolus and promotes hemostasis.	
24. Instruct the patient to exhale as soon as the introducer is removed.	Once the catheter is removed, the patient can breathe normally.	
25. Lay the introducer on the moisture-proof absorbent pad. Check to be sure that the entire introducer was removed.	Ensures removal of the entire introducer.	If the introducer tip will be cultured, have another provider assist with cutting the tip with sterile scissors and placing it in a sterile specimen container before placing the introducer on the moisture-proof absorbent pad. Routine culturing of tips on removal is not recommended.[10]
26. Continue applying firm, direct pressure over the insertion site with the gauze pad until bleeding has stopped.	Ensures hemostasis.	Because central venous catheters are placed in large veins, 10 minutes may be needed for hemostasis to occur. Pressure may be needed for a longer period if the patient has been receiving anticoagulant therapy or if coagulation study results are abnormal.
27. Apply an occlusive dressing consisting of sterile petroleum-based ointment and sterile gauze, and cover with tape or a transparent semipermeable membrane dressing[6,9,14,16] **(Level E*)**	Decreases the risk for infection at the insertion site and minimizes the risk for venous air embolus.	Mark the dressing with the date, time, and your initials. Indicates when the dressing was placed.
28. Maintain the patient in the supine position for 30 minutes after catheter removal.[9]	May decrease the risk of postprocedure venous air embolism.	
29. Remove **PE**, and discard used supplies in appropriate receptacles.	Reduces the transmission of microorganisms; standard precautions.	
30. **HH**		

*Level E: Multiple case reports, theory-based evidence from expert opinions, or peer-reviewed professional organizational standards without clinical studies to support recommendations.

Expected Outcomes

- The PA catheter is removed
- The introducer may or may not be removed

Unexpected Outcomes

- Dysrhythmias
- Valvular damage
- PA rupture
- Thrombosis
- Venous air emboli
- Uncontrolled bleeding
- Infection
- Inability to percutaneously remove the PA catheter because of knotting or kinking
- Pain
- Broken catheter/fragmentation

Patient Monitoring and Care

Steps	Rationale	Reportable Conditions
		These conditions should be reported to the provider if they persist despite nursing interventions.
1. Assess the need for the PA catheter daily. If long-term use of the PA catheter is needed, consider changing the PA catheter every 7 days. **(Level B*)**	The U.S. Centers for Disease Control and Prevention (CDC)[15] and research findings[4,8] recommend that PA catheters do not need to be changed more frequently than every 7 days. There are no specific recommendations regarding routine replacement of PA catheters that need to be in place for >7 days.[4,6,10] Guidewire exchanges should not be used routinely. A guidewire exchange should only be used to replace a catheter that is malfunctioning.[13]	• Signs and symptoms of infection at the PA catheter insertion site • Signs and symptoms of sepsis
2. Monitor the patient's vital signs, pulse oximetry, and level of consciousness before and after the PA catheter and/or introducer removal.	Provides baseline data and data that identify changes in patient condition.	• Abnormal vital signs • Persistent shortness of breath or tachypnea • Cyanosis or decreased oxygen saturation • Changes in mental status • Signs of acute cardiac ischemia (e.g., chest pain, ECG changes)
3. Monitor the patient's cardiac rate and rhythm during PA catheter withdrawal.	Ventricular dysrhythmias may occur as the PA catheter passes through the right ventricle.	• Ventricular dysrhythmias that occur after the PA catheter is removed
4. Monitor for signs and symptoms of venous air embolus and, if present, immediately place the patient in the left lateral Trendelenburg position.	Venous air embolus is a potentially life-threatening complication. The left lateral Trendelenburg position prevents air from passing into the left side of the heart and traveling to the arterial circulation.	• Respiratory distress • Dyspnea • Coughing • Tachypnea • Altered mental status (agitation, restlessness) • Cyanosis • Gasp reflex • Sucking sound near the site of catheter insertion/air entrainment • Petechiae • Cardiac dysrhythmias • Chest pain • Hypotension

Procedure continues on following page

Steps	Rationale	Reportable Conditions
5. After removal of the introducer, assess the site for signs of bleeding frequently as per institutional protocol.	Bleeding or a hematoma can develop if there is still bleeding from the vessel.	• Bleeding • Hematoma development
6. Remove the dressing, and assess for site closure 24 hours after introducer removal.	Verifies healing and closure of the site.	• Abnormal healing
7. Follow institutional standards for assessing pain. Administer analgesia as prescribed.	Identifies the need for pain interventions.	• Continued pain despite pain interventions

*Level B: Well-designed, controlled studies with results that consistently support a specific action, intervention, or treatment.

Documentation

Documentation should include the following:
• Patient and family education
• Patient assessment before and after removal of the PA catheter
• Patient's response to the procedure
• Pain assessment, interventions, and effectiveness
• Date and time of removal
• Occurrence of unexpected outcomes
• Nursing interventions taken
• Application of an air-occlusive dressing
• Site assessment including a neurovascular assessment if the catheter introducer was removed from an extremity

References and Additional Readings

For a complete list of references and additional readings for this procedure, scan this QR code with your smartphone, or visit https://www.elsevier.com/__data/assets/pdf_file/0005/1357421/Chapter0064.pdf

UNIT II

65 Cardiac Output Measurement Techniques (Invasive)

Susan Scott

PURPOSE Cardiac output (CO) measurements are used to assess and monitor cardiovascular status. CO monitoring can be used in the evaluation of patient responses to various therapies, including fluid management interventions, vasoactive and inotropic medication administration, and mechanical assist devices. CO measurements can be obtained either continuously or intermittently via a pulmonary artery (PA) catheter. They may also be obtained intermittently via the transpulmonary thermodilution method. Cardiac output measurements provide data that may be useful in directing and/or improving the care for critically ill patients with hemodynamic instability.

PREREQUISITE NURSING KNOWLEDGE

- Normal anatomy and physiology of the cardiovascular system and pulmonary system
- Basic dysrhythmia recognition and treatment of life-threatening dysrhythmias.
- Pathophysiological changes associated with structural heart disease (e.g., ventricular dysfunction from myocardial infarction, diastolic or systolic changes, and valve dysfunction).
- Principles of aseptic technique.
- PA catheter (see Fig. 59.1 in Procedure 59, Pulmonary Artery Catheter Insertion [Assist] and Pressure Monitoring), lumens and ports, and the location of the PA catheter in the heart and PA (see Fig. 59.2 in Procedure 59, Pulmonary Artery Catheter Insertion [Assist] and Pressure Monitoring).
- Pressure transducer systems (see Procedure 60, Single-Pressure and Multiple-Pressure Transducer Systems).
- Competence in the use and clinical application of hemodynamic waveforms and values obtained with a PA catheter including assessing normal and abnormal waveforms and values for right atrial pressure (RAP), pulmonary artery pressure (PAP), and pulmonary artery occlusion pressure (PAOP) is needed. PAOP may also be termed *pulmonary artery wedge pressure* (PAWP).
- Vasoactive and inotropic medications and their effects on cardiac function, ventricular function, coronary vessels, and vascular smooth muscles is needed.
- CO is defined as the amount of blood ejected by the left ventricle (LV) per minute and is the product of stroke volume (SV) and heart rate (HR). It is measured in liters per minute.
- Normal CO is 4 to 8 L/min. The four physiological factors that affect CO are preload, afterload, contractility, and heart rate.
- *Stroke volume* is the amount of blood volume ejected from either ventricle per beat. Left ventricular stroke volume is

the difference between left ventricular end-diastolic volume and left ventricular end-systolic volume. Left ventricular stroke volume is normally 60 to 100 mL/contraction. Major factors that influence stroke volume are preload, afterload, and contractility.

- *Right heart preload* refers to the volume in the right ventricle (RV) at the end of diastole, and clinicians assess it indirectly by evaluating the pressure that the volume generates (RAP or central venous pressure [CVP]). Elevations in left heart filling pressures may be accompanied by parallel changes in RAP, especially in patients with left systolic ventricular dysfunction. Other factors that affect RAP are venous return, intravascular volume, vascular capacity, and pulmonary pressure. Right heart preload is increased in right heart failure, right ventricular infarction, tricuspid regurgitation, pulmonary hypertension, and fluid overload. Right heart preload is decreased in hypovolemic states.
- *Left heart preload* refers to the volume in the LV at the end of diastole, and clinicians assess it indirectly by evaluating the pressure that the volume generates (PAOP). When LV preload or end-diastolic volume increases, the muscle fibers are stretched. The increased tension or force of contraction that accompanies an increase in diastolic filling is called the *Frank-Starling law.* According to the Frank-Starling law, the heart adjusts its pumping ability to accommodate various levels of venous return. Note: In patients with advanced chronic LV dysfunction and remodeled hearts (spherical- or globular-shaped LV instead of the normal elliptical-shaped LV), the Frank-Starling law does not apply. In these patients, muscle fibers of the heart are already maximally lengthened; as a result, the heart cannot respond significantly to increased filling or stretch with increased force of contraction.
- *Afterload* refers to the force the ventricular myocardial fibers must overcome to shorten or contract. It is the force that resists contraction. The amount of force the LV must overcome influences the amount of blood ejected into the systemic circulation. Afterload is influenced by peripheral

vascular resistance (the force opposing blood flow within the vessels), systolic blood pressure, systolic stress, and systolic impedance. Peripheral resistance is affected by the length and radius of the blood vessel, arterial blood pressure, and venous constriction or dilation. The systolic force of the heart is increased in conditions that cause vasoconstriction (increased afterload), including aortic stenosis, hypertension, or hyperviscosity of blood (e.g., polycythemia). The systolic force of the heart is decreased in conditions that cause vasodilation or decrease the viscosity of blood (e.g., anemia). Right ventricular afterload is calculated as pulmonary vascular resistance. Left ventricular afterload is calculated as systemic vascular resistance.

- *Contractility* is defined as the ability of the myocardium to contract and eject blood into the pulmonary or systemic vasculature. Contractility is increased by sympathetic neural stimulation, and the release of calcium and norepinephrine is decreased by parasympathetic neural stimulation, acidosis, and hyperkalemia. Contractility and heart rate can be influenced by neural, humoral, and pharmacological factors.
- In addition to stroke volume, CO is affected by heart rate. Normally, nerves of the parasympathetic and sympathetic nervous system regulate heart rate through specialized cardiac electrical cells. Heart rate and rhythm are influenced by neural, humoral, and pharmacological factors. Decreased heart rate can be the result of factors such as increased parasympathetic neural stimulation, decreased sympathetic neural stimulation, or decreased body temperature. Increased heart rate can be triggered by factors that cause catecholamine release, such as hypoxia, hypotension, pain, or anxiety. The more rapid the heart rate, the less time is available for adequate diastolic filling, which can result in a decreased CO. Because multiple factors regulate cardiac performance and affect CO, these factors must be assessed.
- *Cardiac index* adjusts the CO to an individual's body size (square meter of body surface area), making it a more precise measurement than CO.
- Refer to Table 65.1 for normal hemodynamic values and calculations.
- At the bedside, invasive CO measurements may be obtained via a PA catheter or a system composed of both a central venous catheter and a femoral artery catheter; this is referred to as the *transpulmonary thermodilution* (TPTD) method. The TPTD method involves the intermittent injection of a known volume (10 to 20 mL) of cold saline into the superior vena cava via a central venous catheter. An arterial cannula with an integrated thermistor (in the femoral artery) measures the change in blood temperature over time.[12,31]
- When using a PA catheter, CO may be obtained via the intermittent bolus method or the continuous CO method.
- Thermodilution CO via a PA catheter measures right ventricular outflow; therefore, intracardiac right-to-left shunts as well as tricuspid and pulmonic valve insufficiency can result in inaccurate measurements.[3,4,31,47]
- The thermodilution cardiac output (TDCO) method via PA catheter: an injectate solution of a known volume (10 mL) and temperature (room or cold temperature) is injected into

the right atrium (RA) through the proximal port of the PA catheter. The injectate exits the catheter into the RA, where it mixes with blood and flows through the RV to the PA. A thermistor is embedded in the catheter 4 cm from the tip of the PA catheter and detects the change in blood temperature as the blood passes the tip of the catheter in the PA.
- The CO is calculated as the difference in temperatures on a time versus temperature curve.
- The PA catheter has an inline temperature sensor to sense change in temperature over time, which is plotted as a curve and displayed on the bedside monitor screen. CO is mathematically calculated from the area under the curve and is displayed digitally and graphically on the monitor screen. The area under the curve is inversely proportional to the rate of blood flow. Therefore a high CO is associated with a small area under the curve, whereas a low CO is associated with a large area under the curve (Fig. 65.1).
- The thermistor near the distal tip of the catheter detects the temperature change and sends a signal to the CO computer and bedside monitor. The computer calculates the CO with the modified Stewart-Hamilton equation, and the CO number is displayed on the monitor screen. The average result of three to five measurements is used to determine CO.
- Accuracy of TDCO is dependent on adequate mixing of blood and injectate, forward blood flow, steady baseline temperature in the PA, and appropriate procedural technique.[4,24,37] In addition, loss of thermal indicator (heat), respiratory artifact, and hemodynamic instability can cause variability from one injection to another.[24,31,35,38]
- Traditionally cardiac output measurements have been recommended to be performed at end-expiration, though there is research suggesting that this may not be necessary.[25,29,41]
- Commercially available closed-system delivery sets[26] (CO-Set; Edwards Lifesciences, LLC, Irvine, CA) can be used with both cold and room-temperature injectate (Figs. 65.2 and 65.3).
- The continuous cardiac output (CCO) method proceeds as follows:
  - Continuous measurement of CO can be performed without the need for injected fluid.
  - The PA catheter with CCO capability contains a 10-cm thermal filament located close to the injection port (14 to 25 cm from the tip of the catheter, near the proximal lumen port). When a PA catheter is properly placed, the thermal filament section of the catheter is located in the RV. This filament emits a pulsed low heat energy signal in a 30- to 60-second pseudorandom binary (on/off) sequence, which allows blood to be heated and the heat signal adequately processed over time as blood passes through the ventricle. A bedside computer constructs thermodilution curves detected from the pseudorandom heat impulses and measures CO automatically. The computer screen displays digital readings updated every 30 to 60 seconds that reflect the average CO of the preceding 3 to 6 minutes. The CCO eliminates the need for fluid boluses, reduces contamination risk, and provides a continuous CO trend.[2,3,10,38]
  - Because the CCO computer constantly displays and frequently updates the CO, treatment decisions can be

TABLE 65.1 | **Hemodynamic Parameters**

Parameters	Calculations	Normal Value
BSA	Weight (kg) × height (cm) and calculate on nomogram	Varies with size
CO	HR × SV	4–8 L/min
SV	CO × 1000 / HR	60–100 mL/beat
SVI	SV/BSA	30–65 mL/beat/m^2
CI	CO/BSA	2.5–4.5 L/min/m^2
HR		60–100 beats/min
Preload		
CVP or RAP		2–6 mm Hg
LAP		4–12 mm Hg
Pulmonary artery diastolic pressure (PADP)		5–15 mm Hg
pulmonary artery occlusion pressure (PAOP)		4–12 mm Hg
RVEDP		0–8 mm Hg
LVEDP		4–10 mm Hg
Afterload		
SVR	MAP − CVP/RAP × 80/CO	900–1400 dynes/s/cm^{-0}
SVRI	MAP − CVP/RAP × 80/CI	2000–2400 dynes/s/cm^{-0}/m^2
PVR	PAMP − PAOP × 80/CO	100–250 dynes/s/cm^{-0}
PVRI	PAMP − PAOP × 80/CI	255–315 dynes/s/cm^{-5}/m^2
Systolic blood pressure		100–130 mm Hg
Contractility		
EF:		
Left	LVEDV × 100/SV	60%–75%
Right	RVEDV × 100/SV	45%–50%
Stroke work index:		
Left	SVI (MAP − PAOP) × 0.0136	50–62 g·m/m^2/beat
Right	SVI (MAP − CVP) × 0.0136	5–10 g·m/m^2/beat
Pressures:		
MAP	DBP + (SBP − DBP)	70–105 mm Hg
PAMP	PADP + (PASP − PADP)	9–16 mm Hg

BSA, Body surface area; *CI,* cardiac index; *CO,* cardiac output; *CVP,* central venous pressure; *DBP,* diastolic blood pressure; *EF,* ejection fraction; *HR,* heart rate; *LAP,* left atrial pressure; *LVEDV,* left ventricular end-diastolic volume; *LVEDP,* left ventricular end-diastolic pressure; *MAP,* mean arterial pressure; *PADP,* pulmonary artery diastolic pressure; *PAMP,* pulmonary artery mean pressure; *PAOP,* pulmonary artery occlusion pressure; *PASP,* pulmonary artery systolic pressure; *PVR,* pulmonary vascular resistance; *PVRI,* pulmonary vascular resistance index; *RAP,* right atrial pressure; *RVEDP,* right ventricular end-diastolic pressure; *RVEDV,* right ventricular end-diastolic volume; *SBP,* systolic blood pressure; *SV,* stroke volume; *SVI,* stroke volume index; *SVR,* systemic vascular resistance.
Modified from Urden LD, Stacy KM, Lough ME: *Critical care nursing,* ed 8, St. Louis, 2018, Elsevier.

expedited. Derived hemodynamic calculations (e.g., cardiac index, systemic vascular resistance) can be obtained with greater frequency, thereby providing up-to-time information in assessment of response to therapies that affect hemodynamics.[13]

- CCO has been compared with TDCO, transesophageal Doppler scan technique, and aortic transpulmonary technique to determine its precision. Study results all show small bias, limits of agreement, and 95% confidence limits, reflecting that CCO provides accurate measurement of CO and is a reliable method.[1,2,27,36,38,48,59]
- Adequate mixing of blood and indicator (heat) is necessary for accurate CCO measurements. Conditions that prevent appropriate mixing or directional flow of the indicator or blood include intracardiac shunts or tricuspid regurgitation.
- The CCO method is based on the same physiological principle as the TDCO method (indicator-dilution technique).

- The TDCO method uses a bolus of injectate as the indicator for measurement of CO. The CCO method uses heat signals produced by the thermal filament as the indicator. The CCO computer provides a time-averaged rather than instantaneous CO reading. CCO values are influenced by the same principles as TDCO.
- The heated thermal filament has a temperature limit to a maximum of 44°C (111.2°F). When calibrated by the manufacturer, CCO computers produce reliable calculations within a temperature range of 30°C to 40°C (86°F to 104°F) or 31°C to 43°C (87.8°F to 109.4°F). An error message appears if the temperature in the PA is out of range. Follow the manufacturer's guidelines.
- Infusions through proximal lumens should be limited to maintenance of patency of the lumen. Concomitant infusions through the proximal lumen can theoretically affect CCO measurements by altering the PA temperature.

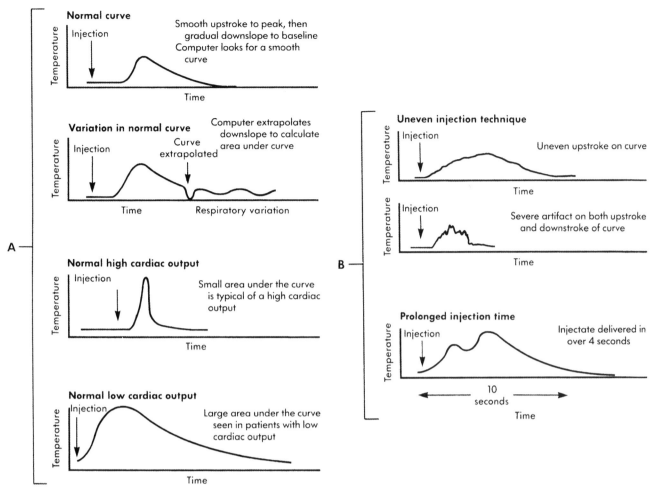

Figure 65.1 **A,** Variations in the normal cardiac output curve seen in certain clinical conditions. **B,** Abnormal cardiac output curves that produce an erroneous cardiac output value. *(From Urden LD, Stacy KM, Lough ME:* Critical care nursing: diagnosis and management, *ed 8, St. Louis, 2018, Mosby.)*

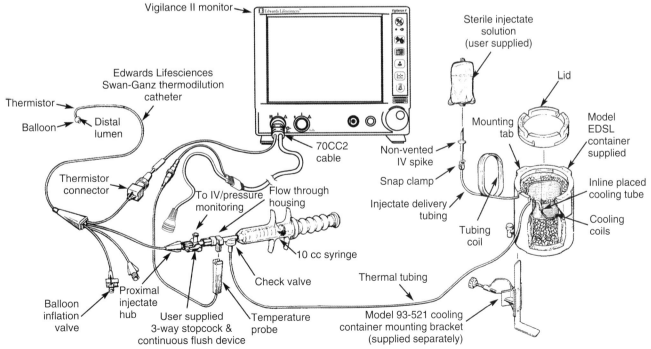

Figure 65.2 Closed injectate delivery system. Cold temperature injectate. *(Courtesy Edwards Lifesciences, LLC, Irvine, CA.)*

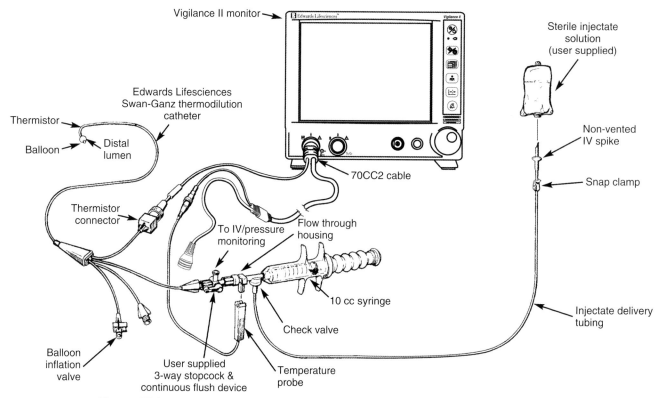

Vigilance II monitor

Sterile injectate solution (user supplied)

Edwards Lifesciences Swan-Ganz thermodilution catheter

Thermistor

Balloon

Distal lumen

Non-vented IV spike

Thermistor connector

70CC2 cable

Snap clamp

To IV/pressure monitoring

Flow through housing

10 cc syringe

Injectate delivery tubing

Check valve

Balloon inflation valve

User supplied 3-way stopcock & continuous flush device

Temperature probe

Figure 65.3   Closed injectate delivery system. Room temperature injectate. *(Courtesy Edwards Lifesciences, LLC, Irvine, CA.)*

Studies have shown that such infusions can cause variations in TDCO measurements.[24,35,56]

- The baseline blood temperature should be constant to ensure accurate readings, so concurrent infusions of fluid through the same line may result in inaccurate readings.[9,19,35]
- Because bolus injections are not needed with the CCO method, the prevalence of user error is theoretically reduced.[18,37]
- The CCO catheter can be used to obtain both CCO and TDCO measurements.
- The CCO does not reflect acute changes in CO values because the updated value on the monitor display is an average of 60 seconds to 3 minutes of data. When monitoring a patient with an unstable condition that is being aggressively treated with medication or other therapies, one should be aware of the delay in data displayed. In those cases, depending on the system used, there may be options for a manual cardiac output to be performed or a STAT CO performed by the system may done.

EQUIPMENT FOR CO VIA PA CATHETER

- Nonsterile gloves
- Cardiac monitor
- Hemodynamic monitoring system (see Procedure 60, Single-Pressure and Multiple-Pressure Transducer Systems)
- PA catheter (in place)
- CO computer or module
- Connecting cables

Additional equipment to have available as needed includes the following:

- Bolus thermodilution
- Injectate temperature probe
- Injectate solution
- 10-mL prefilled syringes (NS or D5W per institutional protocol)
- Injectate solution bag with intravenous (IV) tubing and three-way Luer-lock stopcock
- Closed CO injectate system
- Method to cool the injectate (ice or proprietary device for cold injectate only)
- Nonvented caps for stopcocks

PATIENT AND FAMILY EDUCATION

- Explain the procedure for CO and the reason for its measurement. Include expectations related to sensations during the procedure. (The patient should not experience pain or discomfort.) *Rationale:* Explanation decreases patient and family anxiety. Preparatory information of sensations decreases patient fear of the impending procedure.
- Explain the monitoring equipment involved, the frequency of measurements, and the goals of therapy. *Rationale:* Explanation encourages the patient and family to ask questions and voice specific concerns about the procedure.
- Explain any potential variations in temperature the patient may or may not experience if a cold injectate is used. *Rationale:* This explanation acknowledges the varying physical responses to the injectate and the possible perception of cold solution and may decrease anxiety associated with the procedure.

PATIENT ASSESSMENT AND PREPARATION

Patient Assessment

- Assess the patient's history of medication therapy, including medication allergies, recent bolus therapies, and current medications. *Rationale:* Medications can influence CO measurements.
- Assess the patient's medical history for the presence of coronary artery disease, valvular heart disease, and left or right ventricular dysfunction. *Rationale:* Medical history provides baseline information regarding cardiovascular performance.
- Assess current intracardiac waveforms (e.g., PAP, RAP, PAOP). *Rationale:* This assessment ensures that the PA catheter is positioned properly.
- Assess the patient's vital signs, fluid balance, heart and lung sounds, skin color, temperature, level of consciousness, peripheral pulses, cardiac rate and rhythm, and hemodynamic values. In patients with advanced systolic heart failure, assess for pulsus alternans (alternating strong and weak pulses). *Rationale:* Clinical information provides data regarding blood flow and tissue perfusion. Abnormalities can influence the variability of CO measurements.
- Ensure that no medication is infusing into the proximal port when using the bolus CO method. *Rationale:* The patient will receive a bolus of the medication infusing into the proximal port. This is not an issue with the CCO method.

Patient Preparation

- Verify the correct patient with two identifiers. *Rationale:* Before performing a procedure, the nurse should ensure the correct identification of the patient for the intended intervention.
- Ensure that the patient and family understand preprocedural information. Answer questions as they arise, and reinforce information as needed. *Rationale:* Understanding of previously taught information is evaluated and reinforced.
- Assist the patient to the supine position. *Rationale:* CO measurements are most accurate in the supine position.

Procedure	for Measurement of Cardiac Output With the Closed or Open Thermodilution Method		
Steps	**Rationale**		**Special Considerations**
1. ▮▮			
2. ▮▮			
3. Select the injectate delivery system: open or closed method. (**Level B***)	Both systems are reliable.[31,38,45,49]		A closed system may eliminate cost and time expenditures of individual syringe preparation. The closed system has infection control benefits because of reduced manipulation of the system.[10,39,42]
4. Select cold or room temperature injectate. (**Level B***)	Room temperature injectate may be used for most patients. Research on room temperature versus cold injectate supports the accuracy of either method.[5,8,11,16,28,50,51,54,57]		The acceptable temperature range for cold and room temperature injectate varies by system (manufacturer). Generally, room temperature is 18°C–25°C, and cold is 0–12°C.
5. Select the injectate bolus amount (generally 10 mL). (**Level B***)	An injectate of 10 mL may be used for most patients.[16,35,36,44]		Volumes of 5 mL may necessitate additional injections because of greater variability of individual measurements.[36]
6. Connect the CO cable to the PA catheter.	Prepares the system.		
7. Select the computation constant consistent with the type and size of the PA catheter, injectate volume, and injectate temperature. Confirm the injectate delivery system.	The computation constant is a correction factor determined by the catheter manufacturer that corrects for the gain of indicator (heat) that occurs as the injectate moves through the catheter from the hub of the injectate port to the injection port opening in the RA. The catheter manufacturer provides a table to determine the correct computation constant. The computation constant must be accurate for valid and reliable CO measurements.		Carefully select the correct computation constant for the type and catheter size, injectate volume, and cold or room temperature injectate. Confirm the setting on the CO computer/monitor. Recheck the computation constant before each series of CO measurements. Follow the manufacturer guidelines.

*Level B: Well-designed, controlled studies with results that consistently support a specific action, intervention, or treatment.

Procedure continues on following page

Procedure for Measurement of Cardiac Output With the Closed or Open Thermodilution Method—*Continued*

Steps	Rationale	Special Considerations
8. Connect the CO computer to the power source if it is a stand-alone device, or turn on the CO computer or module.	Supplies the energy source.	
9. Note the temperature of the injectate (on the computer or monitor screen).	The injectate temperature should be at least 10°C less than the patient's core temperature.[15,20,33]	Follow manufacturer's recommendations.
10. Position the patient supine, with the head of the bed elevated no more than 45 degrees. **(Level B*)**	Studies of patients in the supine position with the head of bed flat or elevated up to 45 degrees have not shown significant differences in TDCO measurements.[23,26,30,59] Consistency in patient position may increase stability in consecutive CO readings.	CCO values may be accurate with the patient's head of the bed elevated to 45 degrees.[11,17,22,60] The patient's medical condition and level of instability may determine positioning. Position should be documented and communicated. Consistent positioning when obtaining CO measurements over time decreases measurement variability. CO in patients sitting in a chair may be accurate[46] The lateral recumbent position increases variability in CO measurements and is not recommended.[13,14,60]
11. Verify the position of the PA catheter by assessing both the RA and PA waveforms for proper waveform contours.	Proper positioning of the PA catheter ensures that the distal thermistor is located in the PA. The distal thermistor sensor calculates the time-temperature data. Excessive coiling of the PA catheter in the RA or RV can result in poor positioning of the distal thermistor in relation to the injectate port.[27]	Improper positioning of the PA catheter tip may result in erroneous values.[18,19,27,34]
12. Observe the patient's cardiac rate and rhythm.	A rapid heart rate or dysrhythmias may decrease CO and lead to variability in CO measurements.	
13. If possible, consider restricting infusions delivered through the introducer or other central lines. **(Level C*)**	TDCO measurements obtained during administration of other infusions can cause variability in CO measurements (by as much as 40% higher).[24,35,59]	
14. Remove PE, and discard used supplies.	Reduces the transmission of microorganisms; standard precautions.	
15. HH		

*Level B: Well-designed, controlled studies with results that consistently support a specific action, intervention, or treatment.
*Level C: Qualitative studies, descriptive or correlational studies, integrative reviews, systematic reviews, or randomized controlled trials with inconsistent results.

Procedure for Closed Method of Syringe Preparation and Cardiac Output Determination		
Steps	Rationale	Special Considerations

Follow **Steps 1–13** of the Procedure for Measurement of Cardiac Output With the Closed or Open Thermodilution Method.

Steps	Rationale	Special Considerations
1. ▣▣		
2. ▣▣		
3. Obtain the injectate solution		
4. Aseptically connect the IV tubing to the injectate solution.	Prepares the system.	
5. Hang the IV injectate solution on an IV pole; prime the tubing.	Eliminates air from the tubing.	Injectate is typically normal saline, but 5% dextrose may be used (per institutional protocol)
6. Remove the sterile cap from the proximal lumen of the PA catheter.	Prepares for the injectate connection.	
7. Connect the injectate tubing to the proximal lumen of the PA catheter via a three-way Luer-lock stopcock (see Figs. 65.2 and 65.3).	Connects the injectate solution to the PA catheter.	
8. Connect the injectate syringe to the three-way stopcock (see Figs. 65.2 and 65.3).	The syringe is used for solution injection.	Connect the system so the CO syringe is in a straight line with the PA catheter to decrease resistance with injection of solution. To ensure accurate readings, when using a multiport PA catheter, the proximal port should be used rather than the venous infusion port.[47]
9. Connect the inline temperature probe (see Figs. 65.2 and 65.3).	Measures the injectate temperature.	Verify the temperature.
10. If using cold injectate, set up the cold injectate system (e.g., CO-Set closed injectate system; see Fig. 65.2).	If using cold injectate, cool the injectate solution to 0–12°C (32°F–53°F).	Refer to manufacturer's recommendations. Cold injectate may be proarrhythmic in some patients.[43,55]
11. Turn the stopcock so it is open to the injectate solution (closed to the patient), and withdraw 10 mL of the injectate solution into the syringe.	Prepares for injection.	
12. Turn the stopcock so it is closed to the injectate solution and open to the patient. Support the stopcock with the palm of the nondominant hand to aid in injectate administration.	Minimal handling (<30 seconds) of the syringe is recommended to avoid thermal indicator variation that may introduce error into the CO calculation.[6,9,34]	Syringe holders or automatic injector devices are available for use.
13. Activate the CO computer, and wait for the message to inject.	The CO computer or module must be ready before injection of solution.	Follow manufacturer's guidelines.
14. Before administering the bolus injectate, observe for a steady baseline temperature (e.g., the line before the CO curve begins should be flat without undulations) on the monitor screen (see Fig. 65.1).	An abnormal baseline may increase variability in CO measurements and introduce error.[1]	Patients with advanced systolic heart failure (low ejection fraction) are more susceptible to a wavering initial baseline from unstable PA blood temperature.

Procedure continues on following page

Procedure	for Closed Method of Syringe Preparation and Cardiac Output Determination—*Continued*		
Steps	**Rationale**	**Special Considerations**	
15. Observe the patient's respiratory pattern. Prepare to begin administering the injectate at the same point in the respiratory cycle.	Variations in transthoracic pressure during respiration can affect CO by altering venous return.[25,27,49,53,54] Some literature states that timing of injection with respirations is not necessary.[35] Other literature states that injection should be made at the same point in the respiratory cycle.[27]	Follow institutional standards.	
16. Administer the bolus injectate rapidly and smoothly in 4 seconds or less.	Prolonged injection time may result in false low CO. Rates of 2–4 seconds for injection of 5–10 mL of injectate yield accurate results.[6,17,52]	A prolonged injection time interferes with time and temperature calculations. One respiratory cycle is generally <4 seconds. One ventilation cycle on a ventilator is generally 4 seconds.	
17. Assess the CO curve and value on the monitor screen (see Fig. 65.1).	The CO curve must be a normal curve. A normal curve starts at baseline (baseline must be a straight, flat, nonwavering line) with a smooth upstroke and a gradual downstroke. If the CO curve is not normal, the CO measurement obtained from the injection should be discarded. Abnormal contours of the curve may indicate improper catheter position. An abnormal CO curve may represent technical error.	Normal CO is 4–8 L/min. Abnormal CO curves may also provide information about the patient's clinical condition, such as tricuspid valve regurgitation.	
18. Repeat **Steps 3 to 17** (up 6 times).	Discard all CO measurements that do not have normal CO curves or have wandering baselines.	The device will provide an indicator when the system allows the next measurement.	
19. Determine the CO measurement by calculating the average of three measurements within 10% of a middle (median) value. **(Level E*)**	Determines accurate CO value.[58]		
20. Return the proximal stopcock at the RA lumen to the original position.	Resumes RA monitoring.		
21. Continue infusions delivered through the introducer or other central lines.	Continues therapy.		
22. Observe the PA and RA waveforms on the monitor.	Continues hemodynamic monitoring.		
23. Remove and discard used supplies in appropriate receptacles.	Reduces the transmission of microorganisms; standard precautions.		
24. Determine the hemodynamic calculations.	Assesses cardiac performance and hemodynamic status.	Compare the values with prior values, and determine whether the plan of care requires alterations.	

*Level E: Multiple case reports, theory-based evidence from expert opinions, or peer-reviewed professional organizational standards without clinical studies to support recommendations.

Procedure	**for Open Method of Syringe Preparation and Cardiac Output Determination**	
Steps	Rationale	Special Considerations

Follow **Steps 1–13** of the Procedure for Measurement of Cardiac Output With the Closed or Open Thermodilution Method.

1. ▓HH▓		
2. ▓PE▓		

3. Prepare syringes, or obtain manufactured prefilled syringes for CO determination.
  A. Clean the injectate port of the IV bag (0.9% saline or 5% dextrose per institutional protocol) with an alcohol wipe.
  B. Apply a dispensing port to the bag's injectate port
  C. Aseptically withdraw the injectate solution from the IV bag into three to five 10-mL syringes, and cap securely.
	Prepares the injectate for CO measurements.	Prefilled syringes may decrease variability related to injectate volume. Manufactured prefilled syringes may be stored per manufacturer's recommendations. A solution that is drawn up should be used immediately for CO measurements. A solution that is drawn up in the clinical area (as opposed to under a laminar flow area) and has no preservative should not be stored for later use. A dispensing port negates the use of needles and reduces the incidence of accidental needlesticks.

4. If cold injectate is used: Cool the injectate solution	Injectate can be cooled either using an iced slush or by drawing fluid from an IV bag that has been refrigerated.	Cold injectate is used for transpulmonary thermodilution cardiac output. Cardiac output measurements via a PA catheter is typically room temperature. Place syringes in a bag in the container, not directly into the slush, or use a proprietary device that cools the fluid as it flows through the tubing. Handling of a cold syringe causes warming and hampers validity of CO measurements.[6,9,34] Cold injectate may be proarrhythmic.[43,55]
5. Remove the nonvented cap from the proximal lumen stopcock of the PA catheter.	Prepares the stopcock.	
6. Aseptically connect one of the sterile CO injectate syringes onto the proximal lumen stopcock of the PA catheter.	Reduces the risk of introducing microorganisms into the system.	
7. Turn the stopcock so it is closed to the flush solution and open between the injectate syringe and the patient. Support the stopcock with the palm of the nondominant hand.	Prepares the system for injectate administration.	Minimize handling (<30 seconds)
8. Connect the inline temperature probe (see Figs. 65.2 and 65.3).	Measures the injectate temperature.	
9. Activate the CO computer, and wait for a message to inject.	The CO computer or module must be ready before injection of the solution.	Follow manufacturer's guidelines.
10. Before administering the bolus injectate, observe for a steady baseline temperature (e.g., the line before the CO curve begins should be flat without undulations) on the monitor screen (see Fig. 65.1).	An abnormal baseline may increase variability in CO measurements and introduce error.[1]	Patients with advanced systolic heart failure (low ejection fraction) are more prone to a wavering initial baseline from unstable PA blood temperature.

UNIT II

Procedure continues on following page

Procedure	for Open Method of Syringe Preparation and Cardiac Output Determination—*Continued*	
Steps	**Rationale**	**Special Considerations**
11. Observe the patient's respiratory pattern. Prepare to begin administering the injectate at the same point in the respiratory cycle.	Significant variations in transthoracic pressure during respiration may affect CO by altering venous return.[25,49,53,54] Some literature states that timing of injection with respirations is not necessary.[35] Other literature states that injection should be made at the same point in the respiratory cycle.[27]	Follow institutional standards.
12. Administer the bolus injectate rapidly and smoothly in 4 seconds or less.	Prolonged injection time may result in false low CO. Rates of 2–4 seconds for injection of 5–10 mL of injectate yield accurate results.[6,17,52]	A prolonged injection time interferes with time and temperature calculations.
13. Assess the CO curve and value on the monitor screen (see Fig. 65.1).	The CO curve must be a normal curve. A normal curve starts at baseline (baseline must be a straight, flat, nonwavering line) with a smooth upstroke and a gradual downstroke. If the CO curve is not normal, the reading should be discarded. Abnormal contours of the curve may indicate improper catheter position. An abnormal CO curve may represent technical error.	Normal CO is 4–8 L/min. Abnormal CO curves may also provide information about the patient's clinical condition, such as tricuspid valve regurgitation.[4]
14. Repeat **Steps 6 to 13** (up to six times total)	Obtains CO measurements. Discard all CO measurements that do not have normal CO curves or have wandering baselines.	Asepsis is essential as the stopcock is turned and syringes are exchanged between CO measurements.
15. Determine the CO measurement by calculating the average of three measurements within 10% of a middle (median) value. **(Level E*)**	Determines an accurate CO value.[58]	
16. After the last injectate is completed: A. Turn the right atrial lumen stopcock of the PA catheter so the system is open between the patient and the transducer. B. Aseptically remove the last injectate syringe. C. Place a new, sterile, nonvented cap on the stopcock port.	Closes the system; maintains sterility of the system.	
17. Observe the PA and RA waveforms on the monitor.	Continues hemodynamic monitoring.	
18. Remove and discard used supplies in appropriate receptacles.	Removes and safely discards used supplies.	
19. Determine hemodynamic calculations.	Assesses cardiac performance and hemodynamic status.	Compare values with prior values, and determine whether the plan of care requires alterations.

*Level E: Multiple case reports, theory-based evidence from expert opinions, or peer-reviewed professional organizational standards without clinical studies to support recommendations.

Procedure for Measurement of Cardiac Output With the Continuous Cardiac Output Method		
Steps	Rationale	Special Considerations
1. 🔲		
2. 🔲		
3. Turn on the CO computer or module.	Provides energy.	
4. Connect the CO cable to the PA catheter.	Prepares equipment.	
5. Observe PA waveforms (e.g., RA, PA).	Determines whether the PA catheter is in the correct position.	The thermal filament should float freely in the RV to prevent the loss of indicator (heat) into the cardiac tissue. If the loss of indicator occurs, the CO value is overestimated, giving erroneous readings. Follow manufacturer's guidelines. The device may not measure CO if the PA catheter is malpositioned.
6. Position the patient supine with the head of the bed up to 45 degrees. **(Level C*)**	CCO measurements are most accurate in a supine position, but head-of-bed angle can be varied for comfort, between 0 and 45 degrees.[13,21]	Document body position at the time of hemodynamic data collection.
7. Check the heat signal indicator on the CO computer or module per manufacturer's recommendations.	CCO systems assess the quality of the measured thermal signal. Relationships are in response to thermal noise or signal-to-noise ratio.	CCO monitors provide messages for troubleshooting signal-to-noise ratio interferences. Refer to manufacturer recommendations.
8. Note that the CCO values reflect an average of the preceding 3–6 minutes of data collection.	CCO measurements are averaged over the preceding 3–6 minutes and are not individual measurements.	CCO values are updated every 60 seconds to 3 minutes. Continuous data collection reflects phasic changes in the respiratory cycle. CCO measurements are not timed to the respiratory cycle.
9. When documenting CCO values, also document other hemodynamic findings.	Provides data regarding hemodynamic status.	
10. Compare the CCO value with the patient's current clinical status and hemodynamic findings. **(Level B*)**	CCO is a global assessment parameter and must be appreciated as part of the patient's total hemodynamic profile at a given time.	The CCO method eliminates many of the potential user-related and technique-related errors associated with the intermittent bolus CO method. Research shows clinically acceptable correlation between the TDCO technique and the CCO method in the steady state.[1,2,7,38,40] Future studies are needed to determine efficacy in patients in various phases of acute hemodynamic instability and in specific patient populations. Also, the effects of changes in positioning need to be studied further, especially in patients with structural or functional heart damage.

*Level B: Well-designed, controlled studies with results that consistently support a specific action, intervention, or treatment
*Level C: Qualitative studies, descriptive or correlational studies, integrative reviews, systematic reviews, or randomized controlled trials with inconsistent results.

Procedure continues on following page

UNIT II

Procedure for Measurement of Cardiac Output With the Continuous Cardiac Output Method—*Continued*

Steps	Rationale	Special Considerations
11. Note: The CCO catheter system can be used to obtain intermittent TDCO by following **Steps 1–13** of the Procedure for Measurement of Cardiac Output With the Closed or Open Thermodilution Method, and then follow the steps in either the Procedure for Closed Method of Syringe Preparation and Cardiac Output Determination or the Procedure for Open Method of Syringe Preparation and Cardiac Output Determination.		
12. Remove and discard used supplies in appropriate receptacles.	Removes and safely discards used supplies.	

Expected Outcomes

- Accurate CO measurement are obtained
- Hemodynamic profile and derived parameters are obtained with accuracy, whether through the continuous or intermittent method
- Sterility and patency of the PA catheter is maintained

Unexpected Outcomes

- Inability to accurately measure CO
- Erroneous readings because of technical, equipment, or operator error
- Contamination of the system
- Occlusion of the proximal PA lumen

Patient Monitoring and Care

Steps	Rationale	Reportable Conditions
		These conditions should be reported to the provider if they persist despite nursing interventions.
1. Maintain patency of the PA catheter.	PA catheter patency is essential for accurate monitoring.	• Inability to maintain PA catheter patency
2. Monitor RA and PA waveforms for confirmation of proper catheter position.	Proper placement determines accurate hemodynamic and CO measurement.	• Abnormal RA or PA waveforms or values
3. Maintain the sterility of the PA catheter.	Reduces the risk for catheter-associated infections.	• Fever, site redness, drainage, or symptoms consistent with infection
4. Calculate cardiac index, systemic vascular resistance, and other parameters as prescribed or indicated.	Determines cardiac performance and current hemodynamic status.	• Abnormal cardiac index, systemic vascular resistance, or other hemodynamic values
5. Monitor vital signs and respiratory status hourly and as indicated.	Changes in vital signs or respiratory status may indicate hemodynamic compromise.	• Changes in vital signs • Changes in respiratory status

Patient Monitoring and Care —*Continued*

Steps	Rationale	Reportable Conditions
6. Include the fluid volume used in the TDCO in the patient's total fluid volume intake.	Additional volume given intermittently should be included in the total intake for accurate fluid volume assessment.	• Signs or symptoms of fluid overload (e.g., respiratory distress, crackles, increased PADP or PAOP, elevated jugular venous pressure, new or worsening S3 gallop, worsening edema)
7. Assess the patient's response to therapies.	Hemodynamic monitoring may expedite treatment decisions.	• Significant worsening or improvement in CO and hemodynamic parameters • Pulmonary vascular resistance (PVR) and systemic vascular resistance (SVR)
8. If using a closed system delivery set (CO set), change the system components (tubing, syringe, stopcocks, and IV solution) every 96 hours with the hemodynamic monitoring system (see Procedure 60, Single-Pressure and Multiple-Pressure Transducer Systems).	Reduces the incidence of infection.	

Documentation

Documentation should include the following:
- Patient and family education
- CO, cardiac index, SVR, volume indicators (PAOP and RAP)
- Baseline PA blood temperature
- Continuous or intermittent bolus method
- Volume and temperature of injectate
- Concurrent headrest elevation, vital signs, and hemodynamic measurements
- Titration or administration of medications that affect contractility (e.g., dobutamine, milrinone, dopamine, epinephrine), vascular resistance (e.g., vasoconstrictors such as norepinephrine, vasopressin, phenylephrine), vasodilators (e.g., intravenous nitrates, nitroprusside, nicardipine, or nesiritide), and intravascular volume (e.g., fluids, diuretics)
- Significant medical therapies or nursing interventions that affect CO (e.g., intraaortic balloon pump or ventricular assist device therapies, volume expanders, position changes), vascular resistance, or intravascular volume (e.g., sedation, blood/blood products, headrest elevation, fluid restriction, sodium restriction)
- Unexpected outcomes
- Additional interventions, including psychosocial or emotional/psychiatric interventions that might influence hemodynamic trends

References and Additional Readings

For a complete list of references and additional readings for this procedure, scan this QR code with your smartphone, or visit https://www.elsevier.com/__data/assets/pdf_file/0008/1319840/Chapter0065.pdf

66 Noninvasive Cardiac Output Monitoring

Susan Scott

PURPOSE Noninvasive cardiac output monitoring is a technology that can be used to obtain hemodynamic data on a continuous basis without the use of invasive cardiac output procedure measures.

PREREQUISITE NURSING KNOWLEDGE

- Anatomy and physiology of the cardiovascular system.
- Anatomy and physiology of the vasculature and adjacent structures.
- Understanding of the pathophysiological changes that occur in heart disease and affect flow dynamics.
- Understanding of the hemodynamic effects of vasoactive medications and fluid resuscitation.
- Principles involved in hemodynamic monitoring.[8]
- The appropriateness, criteria, and contraindications of the use of noninvasive cardiac output. A patient who is constantly moving despite cues or even spontaneous movement will provide highly inaccurate numbers. This requires immobility of the patient which may not be feasible for some patients due to toileting, pain, and so on.
- Principles of noninvasive cardiac output monitoring.[6,11,13,14]
- Definitions and norms for cardiac output, cardiac index, systemic vascular resistance, stroke volume, stroke index, preload, afterload, and contractility (see Table 65.1)
- Arterial pressure represents the forcible ejection of blood from the left ventricle into the aorta and out into the arterial system.
- Noninvasive cardiac output methods are easy to use, and there is little if any risk associated with their application.
- Noninvasive cardiac output methods are typically compared with the thermodilution method because this is considered the "gold standard" for determining cardiac output.[6,12]
- The noninvasive methods do not have the same risks associated with invasive methods (e.g., infection, bleeding), though they are not interchangeable when compared to thermodilution cardiac output.[3-5,8,10-12]
- One noninvasive cardiac output method is bioreactance. Skin electrodes are placed on the chest. A signal is sent into and out of the chest via the electrodes. They measure the difference in the amplitude between the input and exiting signals. The output signal received from the chest is affected by fluids in the thorax and by the change in the direction of the impedance caused by the pulsatile flow in the aorta. The bioreactance identifies the change in fluid in the aorta and through a series of calculations obtains the stroke volume and cardiac output.[3,8,9,15] This method has mixed results in the literature but may be used for trending cardiac output in some populations.[1-3,7,9,11]

- Another type of noninvasive device obtains a cardiac output based on arterial pressure pulse contour analysis. It works via an inflatable cuff wrapped around a finger, along with a device that measures the diameter of the artery within the finger using infrared technology.[11] The cuff inflates numerous times each second to keep the blood volume in the finger constant. With each systole, the device senses the increase in diameter of the arteries and inflates the cuff to keep the diameter of the arteries constant. An arterial blood pressure waveform is derived from the adjustments in the finger cuff, and cardiac output is estimated from this waveform.[11] There is evidence to suggest that this method may not be accurate in patients who are morbidly obese,[1] patients with a low ejection fraction,[5] and patients with severe peripheral vasoconstriction or high-dose vasopressors.[14,15] This method has been found to be most accurate in patients with high cardiac output and low systemic vascular resistance index, and the greatest utility of this technology is its trending ability.[3,7,10,16]

EQUIPMENT

- Electrocardiographic (ECG) monitor (i.e., hardwire or telemetry); may also include transport ECG monitor
- ECG lead wires, which may or may not be disposable
- Skin electrodes, gelled and disposable
- Noninvasive cardiac output monitor
- Noninvasive cardiac output cables
- Noninvasive electrodes and probes

Additional equipment, to have available as needed, includes the following:
- Arm board

PATIENT AND FAMILY EDUCATION

- Explain the rationale for noninvasive cardiac output monitoring, including how the reading is displayed at the bedside. *Rationale:* This explanation may decrease patient and family anxiety.
- Explain the standard of care to the patient and family, including application of the monitoring device, alarms, and length of time the technology is expected to be utilized. *Rationale:* This explanation encourages the patient and family to ask questions and voice concerns about the procedure and decreases patient and family anxiety.

- Explain the patient's expected participation during the procedure. *Rationale:* Patient cooperation during use of the device is encouraged.
- Explain the importance of keeping the affected extremity immobile based on the technology utilized. *Rationale:* This explanation helps the patient understand the importance of the device and ensures an accurate waveform.
- Instruct the patient to report any discomfort related to the device. *Rationale:* There should be minimal to no discomfort associated with this technology.

PATIENT ASSESSMENT AND PREPARATION

Patient Assessment

- Obtain the patient's medical history, including any perfusion problems to the upper extremities. *Rationale:* This provides baseline information and may aid in selecting the extremity for monitoring. Decreased perfusion may impair the signal to the selected extremity.
- Assess the patient's vital signs and compliance factors (e.g., age, gender, height, weight). *Rationale:* This assessment provides baseline data and information that must be entered into the noninvasive cardiac output monitor.

Patient Preparation

- Ensure that the patient and family understand the preprocedural teaching. Answer questions as they arise, and reinforce information as needed. *Rationale:* Understanding of previously taught information is evaluated and reinforced.
- Verify the patient with two identifiers. *Rationale:* Before performing a procedure, the nurse should ensure the correct identification of the patient for the intended intervention.

Procedure	for Noninvasive Cardiac Output Monitoring[†]	
Steps	**Rationale**	**Special Considerations**
Noninvasive Cardiac Output Monitoring Using the Bioreactance Method		
1. **HH**		
2. **PE**		
3. Apply the electrodes to the patient based on the manufacturer's instructions. **(Level M*)**	Proper electrode placement is needed for acquisition of accurate hemodynamic data.	Follow the manufacturer's guidelines regarding the proper locations for electrode placement.
4. Turn on the noninvasive cardiac output monitor.	Prepares the equipment.	
5. Input the specific patient data as required by the noninvasive cardiac output monitor **(Level M*)**	The data are used to calculate hemodynamic parameters.	Calibrate and/or recalibrate based on the manufacturer's instructions.
6. Observe the waveforms and data displayed on the monitor. **(Level M*)**	Accurate hemodynamic calculations are dependent on quality input.	Follow the manufacturer's guidelines.
7. Remove **PE**, and discard used supplies.	Reduces the transmission of microorganisms; standard precautions.	
8. **HH**		
Noninvasive Cardiac Output Monitoring Using the Arterial Pressure Contour Analysis Method		
1. **HH**		
2. **PE**		
3. Determine the correct finger cuff size, and apply the cuff to the finger(s) based on the manufacturer's instructions. A. Apply the finger cuff(s) snugly enough so the cuff does not move. **(Level M*)**	Proper application of the pressure cuff is needed for acquisition of accurate hemodynamic data.	Based on the manufacturer, there may be one cuff applied to more than one finger.
4. Attach cables, and stabilize the finger cuffs to the patient's wrist and to the monitoring system.		Based on the manufacturer's instructions

*Level M: Manufacturer's recommendations only.

[†] Procedures will vary based on the specific device and manufacturer. Always follow the manufacturer's recommendations for setup and use.

UNIT II

Procedure   for Noninvasive Cardiac Output Monitoring†—*Continued*

Steps	Rationale	Special Considerations
5. Turn on the noninvasive cardiac output monitor.	Prepares the equipment.	
6. Enter the specific patient data as required by the noninvasive cardiac output monitor (i.e., gender, height, weight, and age). **(Level M*)**	These data are used to calculate hemodynamic data.	Ensure that correct data is entered (i.e. height and weight should not be estimated).
7. Zero/calibrate the system.	Prepares the system.	Based on the manufacturer's instructions. This may include frequent noninvasive blood pressure.
8. Set alarms.	Alerts the nurse to important hemodynamic changes.	
9. Monitor the display screen for signal quality to ensure that data obtained is accurate.	Poor signal may result in inaccurate data.	Based on the manufacturer's instructions
10. To discontinue monitoring, follow the manufacturer's instructions.	Some devices may be damaged if removed while the system is still running.	
11. Remove and discard disposables.	Reduces the transmission of microorganisms; standard precautions.	Ensure that reusable portions are disinfected per the manufacturer's instructions

*Level M: Manufacturer's recommendations only.

Expected Outcomes

- Generation of reliable, continuous hemodynamic data, including cardiac output, cardiac index, stroke volume variation, pulse pressure variation, and systemic vascular resistance.
- Hemodynamic data are incorporated into patient assessment, diagnosis, and therapeutic interventions.

Unexpected Outcomes

- Inability to accurately monitor hemodynamic parameters.
- Hemodynamic data do not reflect clinical presentation.
- Pressure related injury from finger cuffs, skin irritation from bioreactance patches.
- Discomfort from finger cuffs when used for prolonged periods.

Patient Monitoring and Care

Steps	Rationale	Reportable Conditions
		These conditions should be reported to the provider if they persist despite nursing interventions.
1. Continuously monitor heart rate and rhythm.	Provides assessment of patient status.	• Irregular heart rates; patients with irregular heart rhythms are not good candidates for these devices because of irregularities in arterial flow. This will cause extreme vacillations within the hemodynamic profiles displayed. • Dysrhythmias
2. Obtain vital signs per institutional protocols and as needed.	Provides assessment of patient status.	• Irregular heart rates • Abnormal blood pressure • Abnormal respirations • Report hemodynamic values that are not consistent with the patient's clinical picture
3. Obtain cardiac indices as prescribed or as per institutional protocols.	Provides assessment of patient's hemodynamic status.	• Abnormal cardiac output and cardiac index • Abnormal systemic vascular resistance

Documentation

Documentation should include the following:
- Patient and family education
- Peripheral vascular and neurovascular assessment
- Pain assessment, interventions, and effectiveness
- Vital signs, cardiac output, cardiac index, and other hemodynamic parameters
- Unexpected outcomes
- Additional nursing interventions

References and Additional Readings

For a complete list of references and additional readings for this procedure, scan this QR code with your smartphone, or visit https://www.elsevier.com/__data/assets/pdf_file/0009/1319841/Chapter0066.pdf.

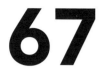 Esophageal Cardiac Output AP Monitoring: Perform

Alexander P. Johnson and Jessica Raymond

PURPOSE Insertion of an esophageal probe for monitoring aortic blood flow is used to assess the hemodynamic condition of critically ill patients. Esophageal cardiac output monitoring or esophageal Doppler monitoring (EDM) uses Doppler ultrasound technology to provide information regarding left ventricular performance and patient fluid status.

PREREQUISITE NURSING KNOWLEDGE

- Cardiovascular anatomy and physiology.
- Anatomy of the upper gastrointestinal tract.
- The appropriateness, criteria, and contraindications of the insertion of an esophageal probe for monitoring aortic blood flow.
- The ability to recognize EDM aortic waveforms by visual display and auditory pitch.
- Normal and associated values of EDM-derived aortic waveforms (Fig. 67.1 and Table 68.1).
- Normal and abnormal waveforms that guide esophageal probe insertion (Fig. 68.1).
- Clinical and technical competence in esophageal probe insertion and esophageal monitoring.
- Clinical and technical competence in understanding esophageal Doppler monitor functions and options.
- Corrected flow time (FTc), peak velocity (PV), and stroke distance (SD) come directly from the Doppler velocity measurements; stroke volume (SV) and cardiac output (CO) are derived using an algorithm generated from patient nomogram information (see Table 68.1).
- The base of the waveform is used as a marker of left ventricular preload and displayed as FTc.
- The waveform height is used as a marker of contractility and is displayed as PV.
- Minute distance (MD) is the distance (cm) moved by the column of blood through the aorta in 1 minute.
- SD is the distance (cm) moved by the column of blood through the aorta in one systolic period. SD is a true representation of SV.
- A narrowed waveform base with decreased FTc may indicate hypovolemia.[2-5]

- A widened waveform base with increased FTc (>360 ms) may indicate response to fluid challenge or hypervolemia.[2-5]
- A reduced waveform height with low PV may indicate left ventricular failure.[2-5]
- An increased waveform height with increased PV may indicate a hyperdynamic state.[2-5]
- A reduced waveform height with a narrow waveform base may indicate elevation in systemic vascular resistance (SVR).[2-5]
- Indications for EDM are as follows:[1,6]
  ❖ Potential status of hypoperfusion (e.g., hypovolemia, cardiogenic shock, hemorrhagic shock, septic shock)
  ❖ Hemodynamic monitoring and evaluation of patients with major organ dysfunction (e.g., renal failure, respiratory failure, liver failure)
  ❖ Differential diagnosis of hypotensive states
  ❖ Aid in the diagnosis of heart failure, cardiogenic shock, papillary muscle rupture, mitral regurgitation, ventricular septal rupture, or cardiac rupture with tamponade
  ❖ Preemptive or resuscitative management of high-risk cardiac patients undergoing surgical procedures during preoperative, intraoperative, and postoperative periods
- Contraindications to EDM include oral or upper gastrointestinal tract anomalies, coagulopathies, coarctation of the aorta, and intraaortic balloon pump therapy.[2,6]
- Proper positioning of the esophageal probe is essential for accurate data collection and waveform monitoring.
- EDM technology utilizes a thin silicone probe, approximately 6 mm in diameter and 90 cm in length.
- Once the patient's age, height, and weight are entered into the monitor, they are programmed into a memory chip within the probe. EDM nomogram limits are as follows:
  ❖ Age: 16 to 99 years
  ❖ Weight: 66 to 330 pounds
  ❖ Height: 59 to 83 inches
- When nomogram limits are surpassed, calculated data such as SVR, SV, stroke volume index (SVI), CO, and cardiac index (CI) are not obtainable. Velocity data such as FTc, PV, SD, and MD will still be measured. Refer to the specific manufacturer's nomogram limits.

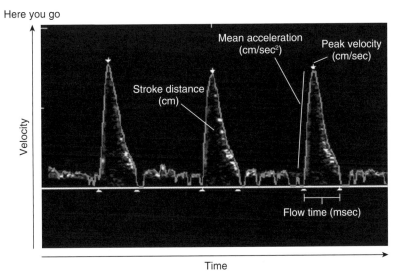

Figure 67.1   The EDM/EDM + waveform. *(From the EDM quick reference guide, with kind permission of Deltex Medical, Greenville, SC.)*

EQUIPMENT

- EDM monitor, patient interface cable, power cord
- EDM probe
- Water-soluble lubricant
- Nonsterile gloves
- Sedative or analgesic

Additional equipment, to have available as needed, includes the following:

- Topical lidocaine
- Tongue blade
- Supportive equipment if conscious sedation is necessary (e.g., oxygen, Ambu bag, suction, oral airway)
- Gown, mask, and goggles or face shield

PATIENT AND FAMILY EDUCATION

- Explain the procedure and the reason for the EDM monitoring. *Rationale:* This explanation increases patient understanding and may decrease patient anxiety.
- Explain that the procedure may stimulate gagging and that sedation may be given to promote comfort. *Rationale:* This explanation prepares the patient and may decrease his or her anxiety.
- Inform the patient of the risks and anticipated benefits of the esophageal monitoring probe. *Rationale:* This allows the patient to make an informed decision.

PATIENT ASSESSMENT AND PREPARATION

Patient Assessment

- Obtain the patient's medical history specifically related to oral or upper gastrointestinal anomalies (e.g., esophageal strictures, varices, oral surgery, trauma, ulcers). *Rationale:* This assesses for contraindications to insertion.

- Assess the patient's hemodynamic, cardiovascular, peripheral vascular, and neurovascular status. *Rationale:* This assessment provides baseline data that can be used for comparison with postinsertion data.
- Assess the patient's respiratory status. If the patient is mechanically ventilated, note the type of support: ventilator-assisted breathing and/or continuous positive airway breathing. *Rationale:* Determines the patient's baseline pulmonary status.
- If the patient currently has respiratory compromise or could develop respiratory compromise with the adjunct of conscious sedation, consider mechanical ventilation. *Rationale:* Protects airway and provides oxygenation. Sedation and/or local anesthesia may be needed for probe insertion and tolerance.
- Assess the patient's current laboratory profile, including electrolyte and coagulation studies. *Rationale:* Baseline coagulation studies are helpful in determining the risk for bleeding. Electrolyte abnormalities may contribute to cardiac irritability.

Patient Preparation

- Verify the correct patient with two identifiers. *Rationale:* Before performing a procedure, the nurse should ensure the correct identification of the patient for the intended intervention.
- Ensure that the patient and family understand the preprocedural teaching. Answer questions as they arise, and reinforce information as needed. *Rationale:* This process evaluates and reinforces the understanding of previously taught information.
- Obtain informed consent. *Rationale:* Informed consent protects the rights of the patient and ensures that he or she can make a competent decision.
- Perform a preprocedure verification and time out. *Rationale:* This ensures patient safety.
- Consider administration of sedation or analgesics. *Rationale:* This decreases the anxiety and gagging that may occur and can enhance probe tolerance.

Procedure for Esophageal Cardiac Output Monitoring: Perform

Steps	Rationale	Special Considerations
1. 🅷🅷		
2. 🅿🅴 Nonsterile gloves, goggles or facesheild, and mask	Prevent transmission of microorganisms.	Similar to PPE required for orogastric or nasograstric tube insertion.
3. Plug the esophageal Doppler monitor into the wall outlet, and turn it on.	Provides the energy source.	
4. Connect the interface cable to the esophageal Doppler monitor.	Prepares the equipment.	
5. Connect the esophageal probe to the interface cable.	Prepares the equipment.	
6. When prompted, enter the patient's age, weight, and height into the esophageal Doppler monitor. A. Turn the control knob to change the values. B. Press the control knob to enter the selected values. C. Push the keypad under the words "accept data." D. If any data are incorrect, press "change data" to return to the nomogram screen and change any data that have been incorrectly entered; then repress the "accept data" keypad. If the probe has been used previously, the patient information will appear on the screen. Probes are reusable by the same patient. (cleansing and storage should be performed according to the institution's policy)	Prepares the monitor. The monitor will confirm data entry and change to the probe focus mode.	Data must be in these ranges: Age: 16–99 years Weight: 66–330 pounds Height: 59–83 inches If a patient's data are outside the nomogram limits, estimated values cannot be obtained, but velocity data are available. Refer to the manufacturer's recommendations for nomograms.
7. Wash hands, and don nonsterile gloves.	Mitigates transmission of microorganisms.	
8. Administer sedation if necessary.	Promotes patient comfort and ability to tolerate the esophageal probe insertion.	The esophageal probe may cause gagging. Topical lidocaine may be used to reduce gagging.
9. Apply a water-based lubricant on 6–10 cm of the distal end of the esophageal probe.	Minimizes mucosal injury and irritation during insertion; facilitates insertion and aids in signal acquisition.	It is important that only water-soluble lubricant be used in probe placement. Oil-soluble lubricant cannot be absorbed through the pulmonary mucosa and may cause respiratory complications if the probe is inadvertently placed in the lungs.
10. Insert the probe orally with the bevel edge toward the hard palate. If possible, insert the probe as early as possible into the patient to create a good mucus bond. This can be done prior to connecting the probe to the monitor.	Begins the insertion process.	Nasal insertion may also be appropriate in select patients if oral insertion is contraindicated. Insertion should never be forced. Forceful insertion can cause mucosal damage to the posterior pharynx or the esophagus.
11. Utilize the depth markings on the esophageal probe to facilitate positioning. There are 3 depth markers on the probe placed at 35, 40 and 45 cm. If the probe is placed in a normal sized adult the signal will be found between marker 1 & 2 when placed orally and 2 & 3 when placed nasally. Generally once in place, the patient's incisors should be between the 35-cm and 40-cm length markings (Fig. 67.2).	Aids in proper probe depth adjustment. Facilitates re-acquisition of the signal for subsequent measurements.	Proper probe depth is essential to obtain optimal aortic signal.

Procedure	for Esophageal Cardiac Output Monitoring: Perform—*Continued*	
Steps	Rationale	Special Considerations

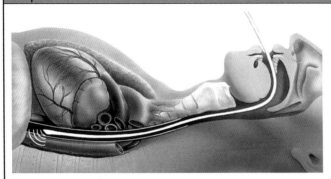

Figure 67.2 EDM location within the thorax. Lateral view of the thorax with the esophageal Doppler in place. The ultrasound beam at the end of the probe *(beveled end)* is directed at the descending thoracic aorta to measure stroke volume and cardiac output. Probe depth is usually 35 to 40 cm at approximately T5–T6. *(From the EDM quick reference guide, with kind permission of Deltex Medical, Greenville, SC.)*

Steps	Rationale	Special Considerations
12. For oral placement insert the probe so that the 2nd depth marker is inserted to the level of the incisors. (Nasal placement the 3rd depth marker placed to the level of the nostril) Rotate the probe slowly through 360 degrees in one direction. Observe the esophageal Doppler monitor, and listen for an auditory signal to establish the optimal descending aortic until the ideal waveform appears and is heard as the sharpest audible pitch. If no waveform is found remove the probe by approximately 1 cm and rotate through 360 degrees in the opposite direction. Do not rotate and change depth at the same time (see Fig. 67.1 and Fig. 68.1). If unable to obtain an aortic waveform, consider that the probe may be in the trachea. If this occurs, remove the probe, and attempt reinsertion.	Enhances the accuracy of the probe insertion.	The ideal waveform has a black center outlined with red and yellow. The sound pitch should be clear and should correspond with the aortic flow pattern noted on the monitor screen. A tall, peaked wave with clear sound suggests good signal characteristics. Adjust the sound volume as needed.
13. Observe the peak velocity display (PVD) on the monitor to assess for the greatest peak velocity achieved. **(Level M*)**	The highest peak velocity is usually associated with the best visual and auditory signal.	Follow the specific manufacturer's recommendations for the PVD (e.g., sharp upstroke with moderately crisp peak to the waveform).
14. Press the filter button to activate the signal artifacts filter when appropriate. **(Level M*)**	Eliminates visual and auditory low-frequency signals (usually due to excess heart valve or wall motion noise).	Follow the specific manufacturer's recommendations for noise filters.
15. Press the auto gain button for optimal amplification of the signal. **(Level M*)**	Optimizes amplification of the waveform.	Follow the specific manufacturer's recommendations for optimal waveform management.
16. Press the range (i.e., scale) button to change the waveform scale. **(Level M*)**	Aids in visualization of the waveform display.	Follow the specific manufacturer's recommendations for optimal waveform visualization.
17. If activation of auto gain does not provide parameter display, press "run" after an optimal signal is obtained. A green line called the *follower* should hug the contour of the waveform. **(Level M*)**	Indicates initiation of monitoring.	A white arrow depicts the beginning and end of systole and the peak velocity of each cycle. Follow the manufacturer's recommendations for beginning the monitoring process.

Procedure continues on following page

UNIT II

Procedure for Esophageal Cardiac Output Monitoring: Perform—*Continued*

Steps	Rationale	Special Considerations
18. Record the displayed data from the top of the EDM screen. **(Level M*)**	SD, PV, and FTc are the main direct measurements. All volumetric other data are calculated from these three measurements along with body surface area.	Follow the specific manufacturer's recommendations for obtaining and recording data.
19. Remove gloves, and discard used supplies.	Reduces the transmission of microorganisms; standard precautions.	
20. 🔲		
21. Compare SV, CI, SD, FTc, and PV values with normal values (see Table 68.1).	Determines hemodynamic status.	

*Level M: Manufacturer's recommendations only.

Expected Outcomes

- Accurate placement of the esophageal probe
- Adequate and appropriate waveforms
- Ability to obtain accurate information regarding hemodynamic parameters
- Evaluation of information obtained to guide therapeutic interventions

Unexpected Outcomes

- Oral, pharyngeal, or esophageal mucosal tears; ulceration; or infection
- Hematoma
- Hemoptysis
- Hemorrhage
- Probe placed into the trachea or bronchus
- Vagal response during insertion or from gagging
- Vomiting or aspiration
- Esophageal-tracheal fistula formation
- Pain

Patient Monitoring and Care

Steps	Rationale	Reportable Conditions
		These conditions should be reported to the provider if they persist despite nursing interventions.
1. Perform systematic cardiovascular and neurological assessments before, during, and after insertion of the probe.	Obtains baseline data and assesses patient status. Assesses for signs of adequate perfusion. Evaluates patient response to the procedure and medications administered.	• Changes in level of consciousness • Changes in vital signs • Abnormal hemodynamic parameters
2. Monitor the patient's mouth for signs of trauma from the probe insertion.	Identifies skin breakdown.	• Redness, ulceration • Swelling, drainage • Foul odor • Bleeding • Skin breakdown
3. Perform oral care per institutional policy[2] while the probe is in place. The esophageal probe may be left in place if tolerated; the probe usually does not require taping to maintain placement.	Oral tubes tend to cause mouth dryness and increase the potential for mucosal breakdown.	• Patient unable to tolerate esophageal probe placement (e.g., inability to relieve gagging, anxiety) • Device-related pressure injuries
4. Follow institutional standards for assessing pain. Administer analgesia as prescribed.	Identifies the need for pain interventions. Promotes patient comfort.	• Unrelieved patient discomfort

---

Patient Monitoring and Care —*Continued*

Steps	Rationale	Reportable Conditions
5. Monitor aortic waveforms while the esophageal probe is in place. Waveforms should be assessed when data collection is needed, such as every hour.	Ensures proper probe placement.	• Abnormal waveforms

Documentation

Documentation should include the following:
- Patient and family education
- Signed informed consent
- Appearance of waveforms
- Sedatives or analgesia administered
- Patient tolerance of the procedure
- Hemodynamic data obtained
- Occurrence of unexpected outcomes
- Nursing interventions taken

References and Additional Readings

For a complete list of references and additional readings for this procedure, scan this QR code with your smartphone, or visit https://www.elsevier.com/__data/assets/pdf_file/0010/1319842/Chapter0067.pdf

68 Esophageal Cardiac Output Monitoring: Assist, Care, and Removal

Alexander P. Johnson and Jessica Raymond

PURPOSE Esophageal Doppler monitoring of aortic blood flow is used to assess the hemodynamic condition of critically ill patients. Esophageal cardiac output or esophageal Doppler monitoring (EDM) uses Doppler ultrasound technology to provide information regarding left ventricular performance and patient fluid status.

PREREQUISITE NURSING KNOWLEDGE

- Cardiovascular anatomy and physiology.
- Anatomy of the upper gastrointestinal tract.
- Recognize the EDM aortic waveforms by visual display and auditory pitch.
- Normal and associated values aortic waveforms (Table 68.1; see Fig. 67.1).
- Additional waveforms that guide esophageal probe insertion (Fig. 68.1).
- Technique and importance of obtaining an optimal signal.
- Clinical and technical competence in understanding the esophageal Doppler monitor functions and options.
- Corrected flow time (FTc), peak velocity (PV), and stroke distance (SD) come directly from the Doppler velocity measurements; stroke volume (SV) and cardiac output (CO) are derived using an algorithm generated from the patient nomogram information (see Table 68.1).
- The base of the waveform is used as a marker of left ventricular preload and displayed as FTc.
- The waveform height is used as a marker of contractility and is displayed as PV.
- Minute distance (MD) is the distance (cm) moved by the column of blood through the aorta in 1 minute.
- SD is the distance (cm) moved by the column of blood through the aorta in one systolic period. SD is a true representation of SV.
- A narrowed waveform base with decreased FTc may indicate hypovolemia.[3-6]
- A widened waveform base with increased FTc (>360 ms) may indicate response to fluid challenge or hypervolemia.
- A reduced waveform height with low PV may indicate left ventricular failure.
- An increased waveform height with increased PV may indicate a hyperdynamic state.
- A reduced waveform height with a narrow waveform base may indicate elevation in systemic vascular resistance (SVR).
- Optimal positioning of the probe is essential for accurate data collection (see Procedure 67, Esophageal Cardiac Output Monitoring: Perform).

- EDM technology uses a thin silicone probe, approximately 6 mm in diameter and 90 cm in length.
- Once the patient's age, height, and weight are entered into the monitor, they are programmed into a memory chip within the probe. EDM nomogram limits are as follows:
  - ❖ Age: 16 to 99 years
  - ❖ Weight: 66 to 330 pounds
  - ❖ Height: 59 to 83 inches
- When nomogram limits are surpassed, calculated data such as SVR, SV, stroke volume index (SVI), CO, and cardiac index (CI) are not obtainable. Velocity data such as FTc, PV, SD, and MD will still be measured. Refer to the specific manufacturer's nomogram limits.

EQUIPMENT

- EDM monitor, patient interface cable, power cord
- EDM probe
- Water-soluble lubricant
- Nonsterile gloves

Additional equipment, to have available as needed, includes the following:

- Topical lidocaine
- Tongue blade
- Supportive equipment if conscious sedation is necessary (e.g., oxygen, Ambu bag, suction, oral airway)
- Gown, mask, and goggles or face shield
- Sedatives or analgesics as necessary

PATIENT AND FAMILY EDUCATION

- Explain the procedure and the reason for the EDM monitoring. *Rationale:* This explanation increases patient understanding and may decrease patient anxiety.
- Explain that the procedure may stimulate gagging and that sedation may be given to promote comfort. *Rationale:* This explanation prepares the patient and may decrease his or her anxiety.
- Explain the monitoring and troubleshooting procedures to the patient and family. *Rationale:* This explanation

TABLE 68.1	Normal Ranges for Measured Parameters Obtained From Esophageal Doppler Monitoring*	
Corrected Flow Time (FTc)	Age	Peak Velocity (PV)[1,2]
330–360 milliseconds	20 years	90–120 cm/sec
	30 years	85–115 cm/sec
	40 years	80–110 cm/sec
	50 years	70–100 cm/sec
	60 years	60–90 cm/sec
	70 years	50–80 cm/sec
	80 years	40–70 cm/sec
	90 years	30–60 cm/sec

*Note: Normal ranges should not be confused with a physiological target. Modified from Singer M: Esophageal Doppler monitoring of aortic blood flow: beat-by-beat cardiac output monitoring. *Int Anesthesiol Clin* 31:99–125, 1993; Gardin JM, Davidson DM, Rohan MK, et al. Relationship between age, body size, gender, and blood pressure and Doppler flow measurements in the aorta and pulmonary artery. *Am Heart J* 113:101–109, 1987.

keeps the patient and family informed and reduces their anxiety.

• Instruct the patient about signs and symptoms to report to the critical care nurse and staff, including oral bleeding, sore throat, and displacement of the probe. ***Rationale:*** This encourages the patient to report changes and problems.

PATIENT ASSESSMENT AND PREPARATION

Patient Assessment

• Assess the patient's hemodynamic, cardiovascular, peripheral vascular, and neurovascular status. ***Rationale:*** This assessment provides baseline data that can be used for comparison with postinsertion data.

• Assess the patient's current laboratory profile, including electrolyte and coagulation studies. ***Rationale:*** Baseline coagulation studies are helpful in determining the risk for bleeding. Electrolyte abnormalities may contribute to cardiac irritability.

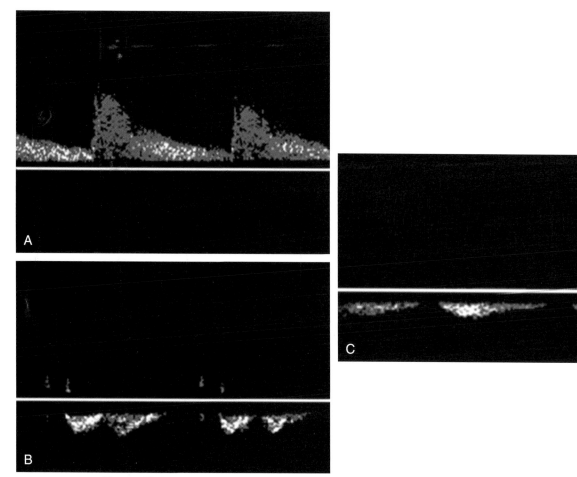

Figure 68.1 Additional waveforms that guide esophageal probe insertion. **A,** Celiac axis: Probe too low. **B,** Intracardiac: Rotate probe. Adjust depth as necessary. **C,** Azygos vein: Correct depth or slightly low. Rotate and/or withdraw probe slightly. *(From the EDM quick reference guide, with kind permission of Deltex Medical, Greenville, SC.)*

Patient Preparation

- Verify the correct patient with two identifiers. ***Rationale:*** Before performing a procedure, the nurse should ensure the correct identification of the patient for the intended intervention.
- Ensure that the patient and family understand the preprocedural information. Answer questions as they arise, and reinforce information as needed. ***Rationale:*** This process evaluates and reinforces understanding of previously taught information.
- Ensure that informed consent was obtained. ***Rationale:*** Informed consent protects the rights of the patient and ensures that he or she can make a competent decision.
- Administer sedation, analgesia, and local anesthetics as prescribed. ***Rationale:*** This may decrease the pain, anxiety and gagging that occurs with probe manipulation.

Procedure	for Esophageal Cardiac Output Monitoring: Assist, Care, and Removal	
Steps	**Rationale**	**Special Considerations**
1. **HH**		
2. Ensure that the esophageal Doppler monitor is plugged into the wall outlet and is turned on.	Provides the energy source.	
3. Ensure that the interface cable is connected to the esophageal Doppler monitor and that the esophageal probe is connected to the interface cable.	Prepares the equipment.	
4. If needed, assist with entering patient information into the esophageal Doppler (i.e., patient's age, weight, and height).	Prepares the monitor. The monitor will confirm data entry and change to the probe focus mode.	Data must be in these ranges: Age: 16–99 years Weight: 66–330 pounds Height: 59–83 inches
If the probe has been used previously, the patient information will appear on the screen. Probes are reusable by the same patient.		If a patient's data are outside the nomogram limits, estimated values cannot be obtained, but velocity data are available.
A. Turn the control knob to change the values.		Refer to the manufacturer's recommendations for nomograms.
B. Press the control knob to enter the selected values.		
C. Push the keypad under the words "accept data." If any data are incorrect, press "change data" to return to the nomogram screen, and change any data that have been incorrectly entered; then repress the "accept data" keypad.		
5. **HH** HH		
6. **PE** PE		
7. Nonsterile gloves, goggles or faceshield, and mask	Prevent transmission of microorganisms.	Similar to PPE required for orogastric or nasograstric tube insertion.
8. Administer sedation, analgesia, and topical anesthetics as prescribed and as needed.	Decreases the patient's anxiety; promotes patient comfort and the ability to tolerate esophageal probe insertion.	The esophageal probe may cause gagging. Topical lidocaine may be used to reduce gagging.
9. Assist, if needed, with probe insertion.	Provides needed assistance and stability of patient's head and neck.	
10. Monitor the patient's response to probe insertion.	Ensures that the patient is able to tolerate the procedure.	
11. Assist as needed with comparing the EDM values to normal values and the patient's baseline values.	Increases and decreases in SD, PV, or FTc depict specific hemodynamic physiology.	Follow the manufacturer's recommendations for normal values and interpretation. Normal values should not be confused with physiological targets (see Table 68.1).

Procedure	for Esophageal Cardiac Output Monitoring: Assist, Care, and Removal—*Continued*	
Steps	Rationale	Special Considerations
12. Administer IV fluids and/or vasoactive agents as prescribed.	Provides interventions to improve cardiac output.	
13. Validate the effectiveness of medical therapy by obtaining values again after the prescribed therapy has been completed.	Values may show the need for therapy adjustments.	It is important that the probe is refocused before each patient assessment, ensuring an optimal signal. Initiate the filter feature to decrease artifact as needed.
14. If prescribed and tolerated by the patient, leave the probe in place throughout therapy adjustments.	Continues monitoring.	A provider may need to adjust the position of the esophageal probe. The probe can also be removed and replaced as needed. Follow institution standards.
15. Remove gloves, and discard used supplies.	Reduces the transmission of microorganisms; standard precautions.	
16. **HH**		
Finding the Maximum Flow		
1. **HH**		
2. **PE**		
3. Adjust the volume control knob on the esophageal Doppler monitor.	Auditory signals are necessary for accurate probe placement.	
4. Grasp the probe gently in one hand.	Manipulates the position of the esophageal probe.	
5. Rotate left and right, and then slowly pull back and insert the probe while listening for the sharpest audible pitch associated with the highest peak velocity.	Facilitates locating the appropriate aortic signal.	A provider may need to adjust the position of the esophageal probe. Follow institution protocol. The esophageal probe should be adjusted until the sharpest aortic waveform possible is obtained in terms of both visual display and audible pitch.
6. Remove gloves, and discard used supplies.	Reduces the transmission of microorganisms; standard precautions.	
7. **HH**		
Troubleshooting the Absence of an Aortic Waveform		
1. **HH**		
2. **PE**		
3. Locate the depth markings to ensure that the probe has not been dislodged. Then consider if the probe has rotated away from the optimal position.	An optimal waveform is obtained when the distance to aortic flow is minimized.	
4. Ensure that the monitor, cable, and probe are all connected appropriately.	Loose connections will distort values.	
5. Readjust the esophageal probe as needed according to the insertional procedure.	Ensures accurate positioning.	A provider may need to adjust the position of the esophageal probe. Follow institution protocols.
6. Remove gloves, and discard used supplies.	Reduces the transmission of microorganisms; standard precautions.	
7. **HH**		

Procedure continues on following page

Procedure for Esophageal Cardiac Output Monitoring: Assist, Care, and Removal—*Continued*

Steps	Rationale	Special Considerations
Removal of the Esophageal Probe		
1. 🅷🅷	Reduces the transmission of microorganisms; standard precautions	A provider may need to remove the esophageal probe. Follow institution protocol.
2. 🅿🅴		
3. Gently pull the esophageal probe from the esophagus and mouth.	Careful removal decreases the possibility of causing mucosal tears.	
4. Place the probe in a clean container, or wrap it for future reuse.	Probes may be used on an intermittent basis for a single patient.	Follow institutional standards for cleansing and storing single-patient reusable probes.
5. Remove gloves, and discard used supplies.	Reduces the transmission of microorganisms; standard precautions.	
6. 🅷🅷		

Expected Outcomes

- Accurate placement of the esophageal probe
- Adequate and appropriate waveforms
- Ability to obtain accurate information regarding hemodynamic parameters
- Evaluation of information obtained to guide therapeutic interventions

Unexpected Outcomes

- Oral, pharyngeal, or esophageal mucosal tears; ulceration; or infection
- Hematoma
- Hemoptysis
- Hemorrhage
- Probe placed into the trachea or bronchus
- Vagal response during insertion or from gagging
- Vomiting or aspiration
- Esophageal-tracheal fistula formation
- Pain

Patient Monitoring and Care

Steps	Rationale	Reportable Conditions
		These conditions should be reported to the provider if they persist despite nursing interventions.
1. Perform systematic cardiovascular and neurological assessments before, during, and after insertion of the probe.	Obtains baseline data and assesses patient status. Assesses for signs of adequate perfusion. Evaluates patient response to the procedure and medications administered.	- Changes in level of consciousness - Changes in vital signs - Abnormal hemodynamic parameters
2. Monitor the EDM waveforms while the esophageal probe is in place.	Provides assessment of proper placement of the probe; normal and abnormal waveforms.	- Abnormal waveforms
3. Monitor hemodynamic status as frequently as prescribed and as needed (e.g., SV, CO, CI, SVR, FTc, PV). Follow institutional standards.	Guides therapy.	- Changes in hemodynamic monitoring values
4. Assess EDM waveforms and values before and after troubleshooting. Assess waveforms when data collection is needed, such as every hour. Follow institutional standards.	Identifies that troubleshooting has been successful.	- Unsuccessful troubleshooting attempts

Patient Monitoring and Care —*Continued*

Steps	Rationale	Reportable Conditions
5. Perform oral care per organizational policy while the probe is in place. The esophageal probe may be left in place if tolerated; the probe usually does not require taping to maintain placement.	Oral tubes tend to cause mouth dryness, which increases the potential for mucosal breakdown.	• Patient unable to tolerate esophageal probe placement (e.g., inability to relieve gagging, anxiety). • Device-related pressure injury
6. Follow institutional standards for assessing pain. Administer analgesia as prescribed.	Identifies the need for pain interventions. Promotes patient comfort.	• Unrelieved patient discomfort

Documentation

Documentation should include the following:
- Patient and family education
- Appearance of waveforms
- Sedatives or analgesia administered
- Hemodynamic data obtained
- Patient tolerance
- Pain
- Site assessment
- Occurrences of unexpected outcomes and interventions

References and Additional Readings

For a complete list of references and additional readings for this procedure, scan this QR code with your smartphone, or visit https://www.elsevier.com/__data/assets/pdf_file/0011/1319843/Chapter0068.pdf

UNIT II

PROCEDURE

69 Femoral Arterial and AP
Venous Sheath Removal

Laura A. Wilson

PURPOSE Arterial and venous sheaths are placed for cardiac catheterizations and interventional procedures. Achieving and maintaining hemostasis after their removal is essential to prevent access site complications.

PREREQUISITE NURSING KNOWLEDGE

- Femoral artery and vein anatomy.
- The technique for the percutaneous approach to the insertion of the arterial and venous sheaths.
- Technical and clinical competence in removal of arterial and venous sheaths.
- Anticoagulation and antiplatelet therapy used during interventional procedures.
- The technology (i.e., activated clotting time [ACT] machine) used to determine the timing of arterial sheath removal and knowledge of the institution's standards regarding the appropriate ACT level before arterial sheath removal.
- The importance of peripheral vascular and neurovascular assessment of the affected extremity (e.g., assessment of the quality and strength of the pulse to be accessed and the pulses distal to the access site, assessment for a bruit).
- The variety of hemostasis options available should include the following:
  - ❖ Manual compression alone or in combination with noninvasive hemostasis pads
  - ❖ Mechanical compression devices
  - ❖ Collagen plug devices
  - ❖ Percutaneous suture-mediated closure devices
  - ❖ Percutaneous staple/clip closure devices
- Collagen plug devices, percutaneous suture-mediated closure devices, and percutaneous staple/clip closure devices are deployed into the artery by the provider at the end of the diagnostic catheterization or interventional procedure.
- Sheath removal can be associated with many complications, including the following:
  - ❖ External bleeding at the site
  - ❖ Internal bleeding (e.g., localized hematoma or retroperitoneal bleed)
  - ❖ Vascular complications (e.g., pseudoaneurysm, arteriovenous fistula, dissection, thrombus, or embolus)

- ❖ Neurovascular complications (sensory or motor changes in the affected extremity)
- ❖ Vasovagal complications

EQUIPMENT

- Cardiac monitoring system
- Blood pressure monitoring system
- Antiseptic solution (e.g., 2% chlorhexidine-based preparation)
- Nonsterile gloves
- Sterile gloves
- Protective eyewear
- Dressing supplies
- 10-mL syringe

Additional equipment, to have available as needed, includes the following:
- Selected hemostasis option (mechanical compression device or noninvasive hemostasis pad)
- Alcohol pads
- Indelible marker
- Selected analgesic and/or sedative as prescribed
- Portable Doppler ultrasound machine
- Suture removal kit
- ACT machine
- Readily available emergency medications (e.g., atropine), additional IV fluids, and resuscitation equipment

PATIENT AND FAMILY EDUCATION

- Explain the procedure to the patient and family. ***Rationale:*** This explanation provides information and may help decrease anxiety and fear. This also encourages the patient to ask questions and voice concerns about the procedure.
- Explain the importance of bed rest, not lifting the head off the pillow, maintaining the head of the bed at no higher than 30 degrees, and keeping the affected extremity straight after the procedure. ***Rationale:*** The patient is prepared for what to expect after the procedure, and patient cooperation is elicited to decrease the risk for bleeding, hematoma, and other vascular complications.

AP This procedure should be performed only by clinicians who have demonstrated competence and are credentialed to perform it. In addition, the procedure must be within the scope of practice defined by their professional licensure, and in accordance with professional practice acts. Physicians, advanced practice nurses, and physician assistants may be credentialed to perform this procedure.

- Explain that the procedure may produce discomfort and that pressure will be felt at the site until hemostasis is achieved. Encourage the patient to report discomfort, and reassure the patient that analgesia and or sedation will be provided. *Rationale:* Explanation prepares the patient for what to expect and allays fears.
- After sheath removal, instruct the patient to report any warm, wet feeling; numbness; or pain at the puncture site. Also, instruct the patient to report any sensory or motor changes in the affected extremity. *Rationale:* This aids in the early recognition of complications and identifies the need for additional pain interventions.

PATIENT ASSESSMENT AND PREPARATION

Patient Assessment

- Assess the patient's medical history for bleeding disorders. *Rationale:* Bleeding disorders may increase the risk for bleeding or vascular complications.
- Assess the patient's platelet count, prothrombin time, international normalized ratio, and partial thromboplastin time before sheath removal. *Rationale:* Laboratory results should be within acceptable limits (per institutional standards) to decrease the risk for bleeding after sheath removal.
- Assess the patient's complete blood count (CBC). *Rationale:* Assessment determines baseline data.
- Assess the patient's ACT before sheath removal. *Rationale:* Results should be within acceptable limits (per institutional standards) to decrease the risk for bleeding after sheath removal.
- Assess the patient's electrocardiographic rhythm and vital signs. *Rationale:* Baseline data are established. Collaborate with the provider if the patient's blood pressure is elevated; elevated blood pressure may need to be treated before sheath removal to achieve and maintain hemostasis.
- Review the documented baseline assessment of the access site before vascular access, including assessment for presence or absence of bruit. *Rationale:* Baseline assessment data are established.
- Assess the extremity distal to the sheath for quality and strength of pulses, color, temperature, sensation, and movement. *Rationale:* Baseline assessment data are established before sheath removal.
- Assess for patency of the intravenous (IV) access, and ensure that more than 500 mL of IV fluid remains in the IV bag or is readily available. *Rationale:* This assessment allows for emergency medication or fluids to be administered if necessary (e.g., vasovagal reaction).

Patient Preparation

- Verify the correct patient with two identifiers. *Rationale:* Before performing a procedure, the nurse should ensure the correct identification of the patient for the intended intervention.
- Ensure that the patient and family understand the preprocedural teaching. Answer questions as they arise, and reinforce information as needed. *Rationale:* Understanding of previously taught information is evaluated and reinforced.
- Verify that provider has placed an order stating when the femoral sheath can be removed. *Rationale:* Before performing a procedure, the nurse should determine the timing of removal of the femoral sheath.
- Mark the distal pulses with an indelible marker. *Rationale:* Marking facilitates the ability to locate pulses after the procedure.
- If a mechanical device is used to maintain pressure, position the device under the patient. *Rationale:* The device is positioned before sheath removal because patient movement must be minimized after sheath removal.

Procedure for Arterial and Venous Sheath Removal

Steps	Rationale	Special Considerations
1. HH		
2. PE		
3. Place a blood pressure cuff on the patient's arm, and obtain the patient's blood pressure.	Establishes a baseline blood pressure before sheath removal.	Monitor the patient's blood pressure frequently as per institutional protocols during arterial sheath removal until hemostasis is achieved. If possible, place the blood pressure cuff on the opposite arm of the IV to allow for uninterrupted flow of IV fluids.
4. Place the head of the bed in the flat position.	Prepares the patient for the procedure, and improves the ability to achieve hemostasis.	
5. Administer analgesia or sedation as prescribed. (**Level B***)	Analgesia and sedation have been shown to reduce the discomfort associated with sheath removal.[4,16,22]	The routine use of subcutaneous lidocaine infiltrated around the catheter site has not been proven to reduce the discomfort associated with sheath removal.[4,11,21,22]

*Level B: Well-designed, controlled studies with results that consistently support a specific action, intervention, or treatment.

UNIT II

Procedure	**for Arterial and Venous Sheath Removal—*Continued***	
Steps	**Rationale**	**Special Considerations**
6. Turn off the arterial catheter alarm.	Monitoring is no longer needed; prevents the alarm from sounding.	
7. Open the suture-removal kit if the sheaths are sutured in place.	Prepares for sheath removal.	
8. If using a noninvasive hemostasis pad in conjunction with manual compression, open the pad using sterile technique.	Prepares for sheath removal and ensures sterility.	
9. Remove the arterial and venous sheath dressing.	Prepares for sheath removal.	
10. Cleanse the arterial and venous sites with an antiseptic solution (e.g., 2% chlorhexidine solution).	Decreases the risk for infection.[15]	Follow institutional protocols.
11. Attach a 10-mL syringe to the blood-sampling port of the stopcock, turn the stopcock off to the flush bag, and gently draw back 5–10 mL of blood into the syringe.	Ensures that there is no clot in the sheath.	Notify the provider if unable to withdraw blood.
12. Remove and discard the nonsterile gloves and used supplies in the appropriate receptacle.	Removes and safely discards used supplies.	
13. 🅷🅷		
14. Apply sterile gloves.	Maintains asepsis.	
15. Remove sutures, if present.	Prepares for sheath removal.	Additional stabilizing devices may be used and removed.
16. Palpate the femoral pulse.	Allows for more accurate positioning of the hemostasis option (manual or mechanical).	
17. Determine the method that will be used to achieve hemostasis. **(Level B*)**	Both manual and mechanical compression devices are effective in achieving hemostasis and reducing the risk of groin complications.[8,10,17,14] Studies comparing arterial closure devices to either manual or mechanical compression are inconclusive regarding the optimal method of arterial closure in terms of vascular complications.[6-10,13,17-20]	Collagen plug devices, percutaneous suture-mediated closure devices, and percutaneous staple/clip closure devices are deployed into the artery by the provider at the end of the catheterization or interventional procedure.
18. Position the hemostasis option (manual or mechanical) 1–2 cm above the site where the arterial sheath enters the skin. (If using a noninvasive hemostasis pad in conjunction with manual pressure, see **Step 21**.) With manual pressure, ensure positioning with the arms straight down, directly over the femoral artery.	The arterial puncture site (arteriotomy) is superior and medial to the skin puncture site because the arterial sheath is inserted at a 45-degree angle. Body weight is used to apply firm pressure.	If the patient is obese or has a large abdomen, a second person may be needed to assist with sheath removal. Adjust the bed height for the comfort of the person holding manual pressure.
19. Simultaneously depress the hemostasis option (manual or mechanical), and gently remove the arterial sheath from the femoral artery during exhalation.	Prevents bleeding. Removing the arterial sheath during the exhalation phase of the respiratory cycle may prevent the patient from "bearing down" during arterial sheath removal.	Never withdraw the sheath if resistance is met. Notify the provider.

*Level B: Well-designed, controlled studies with results that consistently support a specific action, intervention, or treatment.

Procedure | for Arterial and Venous Sheath Removal—*Continued*

Steps	Rationale	Special Considerations
20. Continue to apply firm pressure.	Firm pressure is needed to achieve hemostasis.	The distal pulse may decrease during application of full pressure but should not be completely obliterated. If manual compression is being performed, another person is needed to assess distal perfusion.
A. Maintain manual pressure above the arterial puncture site for approximately 20 minutes or as per institutional protocols.	The length of time needed to achieve hemostasis depends on several factors, including the size of the sheath used; the type of procedure; the use of bivalirudin, heparin, or antiplatelet medications during the procedure; the ACT level at the time of sheath removal; and the patient's anatomy at the femoral insertion site. Patients who are hypertensive or obese may need a longer application of pressure.	Follow institutional protocols.
B. Maintain the mechanical compression device. (**Level M***)	Prevents bleeding.	With use of a mechanical device, set the pressure of the device according to the manufacturer's recommendations and institutional protocols. Tissue damage may occur if prolonged pressure is maintained (i.e., longer than 2–3 hours).[1,8,17] During mechanical compression, monitoring of the arterial puncture site and distal pulses is essential.
21. With use of a noninvasive hemostasis pad in conjunction with manual compression:		Follow the manufacturer's guidelines.
A. Apply manual pressure 1–2 cm proximal to the skin insertion site (see **Step 18**).	The arterial puncture site (arteriotomy) is superior and medial to the skin puncture site because the arterial sheath is inserted at a 45-degree angle.	
B. Place the noninvasive hemostasis pad directly over the puncture site before removing the sheath.	Prevents bleeding	
C. Remove the sheath.	Removes the unneeded catheter.	
D. Reduce the proximal pressure to allow a small amount of blood from the arterial puncture site to moisten the noninvasive hemostasis pad; then quickly reapply the proximal manual pressure. (**Level M***)	Noninvasive hemostasis pads must be moistened to activate the hemostatic mechanism.	
E. Hold firm manual pressure proximal to the skin insertion site and over the noninvasive hemostasis pad at the puncture site.	The arterial puncture site (arteriotomy) is superior and medial to the skin puncture site because the arterial sheath is inserted at a 45-degree angle.	

*Level M: Manufacturer's recommendations only.

Procedure continues on following page

UNIT II

Procedure	for Arterial and Venous Sheath Removal—*Continued*	
Steps	Rationale	Special Considerations
F. Gradually release the proximal pressure after 3–4 minutes; however, pressure should be maintained over the puncture site for at least 10 minutes.	Ensures hemostasis.	The total time of compression depends on the same factors listed for manual compression (see **Step 20A**).
G. Place a new sterile gauze pad over the hemostasis pad and, cover it with a sterile dressing.	Maintains asepsis.	The noninvasive hemostasis pad is left in place for 24 hours.
22. While achieving hemostasis, assess the circulation of the extremity distal to the site of the arterial sheath removal.	Verifies adequate circulation while hemostasis is achieved.	The pulse may decrease during application of full pressure but should not be completely obliterated. If manual compression is being performed, another person is needed to assess distal perfusion.
23. With use of manual compression or mechanical compression, discontinue pressure once hemostasis is achieved.	Pressure is no longer needed.	With use of a mechanical device, follow the manufacturer's recommendations, institutional protocols, or the provider's prescription regarding the gradual reduction of pressure from the device. Notify the provider if unable to achieve hemostasis.
24. When a venous sheath is in place, remove the venous sheath approximately 5–10 minutes after removal of the arterial sheath, and maintain manual pressure over both sites for approximately 10 additional minutes or until hemostasis is achieved.[4,14]	Achieves both arterial and venous hemostasis. The arterial sheath is removed first because pressure must be applied to the arterial site longer than the venous site to achieve hemostasis. In addition, the venous line may be used to give additional IV fluids or medications, if needed (e.g., vasovagal reaction).	Follow the manufacturer's guidelines and institutional standards. Collagen plug devices, percutaneous suture-mediated devices, and percutaneous staple/clip closure devices are not used for venous punctures. If a collagen plug device, a percutaneous suture-mediated device, or a staple/clip closure device is deployed in the arteriotomy immediately after the procedure, the venous sheath must still be removed with manual pressure applied for at least 10 minutes. Noninvasive hemostasis pads may be used in conjunction with manual pressure to achieve hemostasis for venous punctures.
25. After hemostasis is achieved, palpate the area around the arterial site.	Determines whether bleeding or a hematoma has occurred around the arterial site.	If bleeding or a hematoma is noted around the arterial site after hemostasis is achieved, apply manual pressure and notify the provider.
26. Apply a sterile dressing to the arterial and/or venous sites.	Maintains asepsis.	Follow institutional protocols for the type of sterile dressing to be applied (transparent vs. pressure dressing). A sterile transparent dressing allows for easier assessment of the puncture site for bleeding or hematoma formation.
27. Remove **PE** and sterile equipment, and discard used supplies in appropriate receptacles.	Reduces the transmission of microorganisms; standard precautions.	
28. **HH**		

Expected Outcomes

- Arterial and venous sheaths removed with hemostasis achieved
- Adequate peripheral vascular and neurovascular integrity of the extremity distal to the site of sheath removal (positive sensation, movement, capillary refill, color, temperature, pulse)
- No evidence of peripheral vascular or neurovascular complications
- Cardiovascular and hemodynamic stability

Unexpected Outcomes

- Inability to remove the arterial or venous sheaths
- Inability to achieve hemostasis
- Impaired perfusion to the extremity distal to the site of sheath removal
- Impaired motor/sensory status of the extremity distal to the site of sheath removal
- Loss of arterial pulses distal to the site of sheath removal
- Development of a hematoma or new bruit
- Development of a retroperitoneal bleed
- Development of a pseudoaneurysm or arteriovenous fistula
- Vasovagal response during removal of the arterial sheath
- Hemodynamic instability
- Angina or shortness of breath
- Decrease in hemoglobin greater than 2 g compared with preprocedure values
- Unrelieved pain

Patient Monitoring and Care

Steps	Rationale	Reportable Conditions
		These conditions should be reported to the provider if they persist despite nursing interventions.
1. Assess the peripheral vascular and neurovascular status of the affected extremity after removal of the arterial sheath frequently as per institutional protocols.	A thrombus, embolus, or dissection may precipitate changes in peripheral vascular or neurovascular status, necessitating early intervention.	• Change in strength of pulses in the affected extremity (diminished or absent) • Coldness or coolness of the distal extremity • Paresthesia in the affected extremity • Pallor, cyanosis of the affected extremity • Pain in the affected extremity • Decrease in mobility of the affected extremity
2. Obtain vital signs after removal of the arterial sheath frequently as per institutional protocols.	Changes in vital signs may occur because of a vasovagal response or blood loss.	• Abnormal vital signs
3. Assess the puncture site frequently as per institutional protocols, including assessment of presence or absence of bruit.	Detects the presence of bleeding, hematoma, or bruit.	• Bleeding at arterial or venous sites • Hematoma development • New bruit • Pain at the access site
4. Monitor the electrocardiographic data during and after sheath removal.	Detects the presence of dysrhythmias. Bradydysrhythmias are common with vasovagal reactions.	• Dysrhythmias
5. After hemostasis is achieved, the head of the patient's bed can be elevated up to 30 degrees. **(Level B*)**	Minimizes back discomfort and does not increase vascular complications.	• Occurrence of bleeding • Hematoma development • Abnormal vital signs • New bruit • Changes in peripheral vascular or neurovascular status • Back pain not relieved with position changes or analgesics

*Level B: Well-designed, controlled studies with results that consistently support a specific action, intervention, or treatment.

UNIT II

Patient Monitoring and Care —*Continued*

Steps	Rationale	Reportable Conditions
6. Maintain bed rest for 1–6 hours after hemostasis is obtained when manual or mechanical pressure is used as per institutional protocols. **(Level B*)** With collagen plug devices, percutaneous suture-mediated closure devices, percutaneous staple/clip closure devices, and noninvasive hemostasis pads, the bed rest time is decreased to between 1 and 4 hours, depending on the manufacturer's recommendations; follow institutional standards. Maintain bed rest after venous sheath removal as per institutional protocols.	Minimizes back discomfort, minimizes complications of prolonged bed rest, and does not increase vascular complications. Bed rest times vary depending on the size of sheath used; the type of procedure; the use of bivalirudin, heparin, or antiplatelet medications during the procedure; and institutional standards.[2,5,12,14] Patients with venous punctures need less time in bed than those with arterial punctures because the venous system is a lower-pressure system, so the incidence of vascular complications is decreased.	• Occurrence of bleeding • Hematoma development • Abnormal vital signs • New bruit • Changes in peripheral vascular or neurovascular status • Back pain not relieved with position changes or analgesics
7. Follow institutional protocols for assessing pain. Administer analgesia as prescribed, and reassess per institutional protocols.[3]	Identifies the need for pain interventions.	• Continued pain despite pain interventions

*Level B: Well-designed, controlled studies with results that consistently support a specific action, intervention, or treatment.

Documentation

Documentation should include the following:
- Patient and family education
- Date and time of sheath removal
- Site of arterial and venous sheath removal
- Quality of arterial and venous sheaths removed (e.g., intact, cracked)
- Any difficulties with removal
- Patient tolerance of the procedure
- Pain assessment, interventions, and effectiveness
- Any medications administered
- Time hemostasis is obtained
- Method of hemostasis
- Site assessment after hemostasis is obtained, including presence or absence of a bruit
- Heart rate and rhythm, blood pressure, and respiratory rate
- Peripheral vascular and neurovascular checks to the affected extremity
- Occurrence of unexpected outcomes
- Nursing interventions
- Evaluation of any nursing intervention

References and Additional Readings

For a complete list of references and additional readings for this procedure, scan this QR code with your smartphone, or visit https://www.elsevier.com/__data/assets/pdf_file/0003/1319844/Chapter0069.pdf.

PROCEDURE

70 Radial Arterial Sheath Removal

Marie Cassalia

PURPOSE Radial arterial sheaths are placed for cardiac catheterizations and interventional procedures. The radial approach improves patient comfort and decreases bleeding complications. This approach is associated with far lower rates of bleeding and vascular complications compared with the femoral access site.[6] Transradial access (TRA) is also associated with reduced mortality in high-risk patient subgroups, such as those presenting with acute coronary syndrome (ACS).[2] Achieving and maintaining hemostasis after their removal is essential to prevent access-site complications.

PREREQUISITE NURSING KNOWLEDGE

- Radial and ulnar artery anatomy.
- How to perform and interpret a modified Allen's test using plethysmography and oximetry.
- The technique for the percutaneous insertion of the radial artery sheath.
- Peripheral vascular and neurovascular assessment of the affected extremity.
- Radial artery access is sometimes associated with procedure failure (i.e., inability to access the radial artery or advance the catheter), so the femoral site may also be prepared for possible access.
- The radial artery sheath is removed with the use of a radial compression device at the end of the diagnostic or interventional procedure.
- Hemostasis
- Commercially available radial compression devices are available to assist in achieving hemostasis. One device is the TR Band Radial Compression Device (Terumo Medical Corporation, Somerset, NJ) (Fig. 70.1).
- Technical and clinical competence in the removal of the radial compression device.
- Conditions that support the choice for radial access include the presence of bleeding disorders, current anticoagulant use, morbid obesity, and severe peripheral arterial disease.
- Contraindications to a radial approach include an abnormal modified Allen's test (confirmed by the plethysmo-oxymetric test[6] or Barbeau test), absence of a radial pulse, end-stage renal disease with the potential need for a forearm arteriovenous fistula or the presence of a dialysis fistula, small or heavily calcified radial arteries, and severe vasospastic disease such as Raynaud's Disease.
- Complications of radial artery sheath removal include the following[1]:
  - ❖ External bleeding at the site
  - ❖ Internal bleeding (e.g., localized hematoma)
  - ❖ Vascular complications (e.g., radial artery occlusion from thrombus, embolization, dissection, or spasm; pseudoaneurysm; arteriovenous fistula; radial artery perforation)
  - ❖ Neurovascular complications (sensory or motor changes in the affected extremity)
  - ❖ Compartment syndrome
  - ❖ Vascular infection

EQUIPMENT

- Cardiac monitoring system
- Blood pressure monitoring system
- Pulse oximeter sensor with monitor
- Antiseptic solution (e.g., 2% chlorhexidine-based preparation)
- Nonsterile gloves
- Protective eyewear
- Dressing supplies
- Commercially available inflatable bladder-based radial compression device
- 10-mL syringe or syringe supplied with the radial compression device

  Additional equipment, to have available as needed, include the following:
- Alcohol pads
- Selected analgesia and sedative as prescribed
- Portable Doppler ultrasound machine
- Arm board

PATIENT AND FAMILY EDUCATION

- Explain the procedure to the patient and family. ***Rationale***: This explanation provides information and may help decrease anxiety and fear, therefore encouraging the patient and family to ask questions and voice concerns about the procedure.
- Explain the importance of keeping the radial compression device on the affected wrist after the procedure for the prescribed time frame to maintain hemostasis after the procedure. ***Rationale***: The patient is prepared for what to expect after the procedure, and patient cooperation is elicited to decrease the risk for bleeding, hematoma, and other vascular complications.
- Explain that the procedure may produce discomfort and that pressure will be felt at the site until hemostasis is

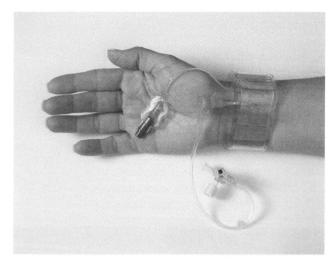

Figure 70.1   TR Band radial compression device. *(Terumo Medical Corporation, Somerset, NJ.)*

achieved. Encourage the patient to report discomfort, and reassure the patient that analgesia will be provided if needed. *Rationale*: Explanation prepares the patient for what to expect and allays fears.

- After radial arterial sheath removal, instruct the patient to report any warm, wet feeling, or pain at the puncture site. Also, instruct the patient to report any sensory or motor changes in the affected extremity. *Rationale*: This aids in the early recognition of complications and identifies the need for additional pain interventions.
- After radial compression device removal, instruct the patient to avoid flexing the wrist (e.g., playing golf, carpentry), lifting more than 5 pounds for 5 to 7 days, and submersion in water for 3 days.[7] Instruct the patient to inform the provider of any loss of sensation, tenderness, sudden color change, tingling of the fingers and hands, redness,

swelling, uncontrolled bleeding, or discharge at the access site.[7] *Rationale*: Explanation prepares the patient for what to expect and aids in recognition of complications.

PATIENT ASSESSMENT AND PREPARATION

Patient Assessment

- Assess the patient's complete blood count, platelet count, prothrombin time, international normalized ratio, and partial thromboplastin time. *Rationale*: Laboratory results should be within acceptable limits (per institutional protocols) to decrease the risk for bleeding after sheath removal.
- Assess the patient's electrocardiographic rhythm and vital signs. *Rationale:* Baseline data are established and determine hemodynamic stability.
- Review the documented baseline assessment of the extremity distal to the sheath for color, temperature, sensation, movement, and pulse oximetry waveform. *Rationale*: Baseline assessment data are established.

Patient Preparation

- Verify the correct patient with two identifiers. *Rationale*: Before performing a procedure, the nurse should ensure the proper identification of the patient for the intended intervention.
- Ensure that the patient and family understand the preprocedural teaching. Answer questions as they arise, and reinforce information as needed. *Rationale*: Understanding of previously taught information is evaluated and reinforced.
- Ensure that the provider has placed an order stating when to begin removing air from the radial compression device. *Rationale*: Before performing a procedure, the nurse should determine when to start removing air from the radial compression device.

Procedure **for Radial Arterial Sheath Removal**		
Steps	Rationale	Special Considerations
1. 🅗🅗		
2. 🅟🅔		
3. At the completion of both diagnostic and interventional procedures, the radial artery compression device is placed around the wrist per the manufacturer's recommendations (see Fig. 77.1).	Mechanical compression is more convenient and uses fewer resources (personnel) than manual compression. Because mechanical compression uses a stable continuous pressure, it may be superior to a manual approach regarding postprocedural access site complications.[3]	There is no need to obtain an activated clotting time because the radial artery is more superficial and easier to compress than the femoral artery.[4]

Procedure for Radial Arterial Sheath Removal—*Continued*		
Steps	Rationale	Special Considerations
4. Using a syringe, a prescribed amount of air is injected into the port to inflate the bladder (per physician preference and manufacturer guidelines) as the radial sheath is removed. Once the sheath is out, air is slowly removed using the syringe until a flash of blood is seen at the radial insertion site. Then another 1–2 cm^3 of air is reinjected into the port.	Enough pressure is applied over the radial arteriotomy site to achieve patent hemostasis or nonocclusive compression.	Some radial compression devices come with a special syringe only used for that specific device. Each compression device has a maximum amount of air that can be injected into the bladder. Do not exceed the manufacturer guidelines for inflation. The patient will leave the procedure room with the compression device in place and the bladder inflated. An arm board may be used to prevent hyperflexion and hyperextension of the wrist.
5. Place a blood pressure cuff on the opposite extremity to obtain the patient's blood pressure.	Avoids an increase in pressure on the affected radial artery.	
6. Place a pulse oximeter sensor on the thumb or index finger of the affected extremity, and observe the waveform on the monitor.[6]	Aids in determining adequate perfusion to the distal digits.	
7. Determine whether an adequate pulse oximetry waveform is present. **(Level B*)**	Patent (nonocclusive) hemostasis allows enough radial artery compression to result in hemostasis.	Complete occlusion of blood flow over the arteriotomy site (e.g., a tight elastic pressure bandage) leads to higher rates of radial artery occlusion and may impede venous return to the hand, leading to swelling and discoloration of the hand or fingers.[5] If the waveform is dampened or absent, release air from the bladder using the syringe, per institutional standards or manufacturer's guidelines, until the waveform returns. If bleeding occurs during this time, reinflate the bladder to achieve hemostasis, and immediately notify the provider.
8. Compress the ulnar artery of the affected extremity. If the waveform continues, blood flow in the radial artery is confirmed.	Absence of the waveform with ulnar artery compression confirms diminished or absent blood flow in the radial artery.	If the waveform is lost with ulnar artery compression, immediately notify the provider.
9. Determine the time the bladder of the radial compression device was inflated in the procedure room and the amount of air that was placed in the bladder.	Establishes baseline information and provides hand-off communication to the next physician, advanced practice nurse, or other healthcare professional for when to begin releasing the air (pressure) from the bladder.	A flowsheet may be used as a communication tool. Air (pressure) is released from the bladder at specific time increments.
10. Maintain the initial bladder compression for the prescribed time. **(Level M*)**	Maintains initial hemostasis.	Follow institutional standards and manufacturer's guidelines for how long to maintain the initial bladder compression before beginning to release air from the bladder. The initial bladder compression may be longer for interventional procedures than for diagnostic procedures based on factors such as the amount of anticoagulation used and the sheath size. The initial bladder compression time may vary from 30 minutes to 2 hours.

*Level B: Well-designed, controlled studies with results that consistently support a specific action, intervention, or treatment.
*Level M: Manufacturer's recommendations only.

Procedure continues on following page

UNIT II

Procedure for Radial Arterial Sheath Removal—*Continued*

Steps	Rationale	Special Considerations
11. If no bleeding is noted, using the syringe, release the prescribed amount of air from the bladder at the specified intervals (e.g., remove 3 cm^3 of air every 15 minutes) until all of the air is removed. **(Level M*)**	Gradually decreases pressure and assesses the progress of hemostasis.	Follow institutional standards and manufacturer guidelines for time intervals and the amount of air to be released. When attaching the syringe to the connector, keep a finger on the plunger so all of the air does not escape at once. Some devices have a safety mechanism to prevent this from occurring.
12. If bleeding occurs at any point during the release of air from the bladder, reinject the specified amount of air (e.g., 3 cm^3) for the specified period (e.g., 15 minutes), and reassess hemostasis. If there is no bleeding after reinflation (e.g., 15 minutes), resume releasing air from the bladder (e.g., 3 cm^3 of air every 15 minutes) according to institutional protocol or manufacturer's guidelines until all of the air is removed from the bladder.	Maintains hemostasis.	Follow the manufacturer guidelines and institutional protocols.
13. When all air is removed from the bladder and hemostasis is obtained, monitor the site for another 5 minutes with the compression device in place.	Determines that hemostasis is maintained.	If bleeding recurs, the bladder can be reinflated with the prescribed amount of air to achieve hemostasis.
14. Carefully remove the radial compression device.	Removes equipment.	
15. Cleanse the area with an antiseptic solution, and apply a dry, sterile dressing.	Maintains asepsis.	Follow institutional protocols.
16. The dressing should not encircle the entire wrist.	Avoids impaired arterial circulation and venous return.	
17. Assess the area.	Determines whether there is any bleeding or hematoma.	If bleeding or hematoma is noted around the arterial site, apply manual pressure, and notify the provider.
18. Remove PE, and discard used supplies in the appropriate receptacles.	Reduces the transmission of microorganisms; follow institutional protocols.	
19. HH		

*Level M: Manufacturer's recommendations only.

Expected Outcomes

- Arterial sheath removed with hemostasis achieved and continued nonocclusive hemostasis during deflation of the radial compression device's air bladder.
- Adequate peripheral vascular and neurovascular integrity of the digits distal to the site of sheath removal (positive sensation, movement, capillary refill, color, temperature, radial and ulnar pulse, good pulse oximeter waveform with the sensor on the thumb or index finger of the affected extremity)
- No evidence of peripheral vascular or neurovascular complications
- Cardiovascular and hemodynamic stability

Unexpected Outcomes

- Inability to achieve hemostasis during deflation of the radial compression device's air bladder
- Impaired perfusion to the digits distal to the site of sheath removal
- Impaired motor/sensory status of the extremity distal to the site of sheath removal
- Loss of the radial or ulnar pulse
- Development of a hematoma or new bruit
- Development of a pseudoaneurysm or arteriovenous fistula
- Development of a dampened or absent pulse oximeter waveform
- Hemodynamic instability
- Unrelieved pain

Patient Monitoring and Care

Steps	Rationale	Reportable Conditions
		These conditions should be reported to the provider if they persist despite nursing interventions.
1. Assess the peripheral vascular and neurovascular status of the affected extremity frequently per institutional protocol while the compression device is in place. After the compression device is removed, assess frequently per institutional protocols.	Changes in peripheral vascular or neurovascular status may indicate radial artery occlusion or other complications.	• Change in strength of radial or ulnar pulse in the affected extremity (diminished or absent) • Coldness or coolness of the distal extremity • Prolonged capillary refill time • Paresthesia in the affected extremity • Pallor, cyanosis of the affected extremity • Pain in the affected extremity • Decreased mobility of the affected extremity • Loss of the pulse oximetry waveform
2. Obtain vital signs after removal of the arterial sheath frequently per institutional protocols.	Determines hemodynamic stability or instability.	• Abnormal vital signs
3. Assess the puncture site every frequently per institutional protocols while the radial compression device is in place. Once it is removed, assess frequently per institutional protocols including assessment of presence or absence of a bruit.	Detects the presence of bleeding, hematoma, or bruit.	• Bleeding at the arterial site • Hematoma development • New bruit
4. Monitor the pulse oximeter waveform (with the sensor on the thumb or forefinger of the affected extremity) after removal of the sheath frequently per institutional protocols.	Dampening or loss of the waveform may indicate radial artery occlusion.	• Dampening or loss of the pulse oximeter waveform
5. Monitor the electrocardiographic data during and after sheath removal.	Detects the presence of dysrhythmias.	• Dysrhythmias
6. The patient may raise the head of the bed to the desired level and may get out of bed with assistance.	Radial artery access does not require prolonged bed rest; therefore the head of the bed can be raised to a level of comfort, and early mobility can be facilitated.	• Occurrence of bleeding • Hematoma development • Abnormal vital signs • New bruit • Changes in peripheral vascular or neurovascular status
7. Follow institutional protocols for assessing pain. Administer analgesia as prescribed.	Identifies need for pain interventions.	• Continued pain despite pain interventions
8. Avoid obtaining blood for laboratory tests, and avoid taking the patient's blood pressure in the affected extremity for 24 hours.	Avoids unnecessary pressure on the affected radial artery to promote healing and to prevent complications.	

Documentation

Documentation should include the following:

- Date and time of sheath removal and initial hemostasis in the procedure room
- Quality of arterial sheath removed (e.g., intact, cracked)
- Any difficulties with sheath removal
- Patient and family education
- Patient tolerance of the procedure
- Pain assessment, interventions, and effectiveness
- Any medications administered
- Any issues during radial compression device deflation (e.g., uncontrolled bleeding)
- Date and time radial compression device is removed
- Evidence of patent hemostasis
- Site assessment after hemostasis obtained and the radial device removed, including the presence or absence of a bruit
- Heart rate and rhythm, blood pressure, and respiratory rate
- Peripheral vascular and neurovascular checks to the affected extremity
- The occurrence of unexpected outcomes
- Nursing interventions
- Evaluation of any nursing intervention

References and Additional Readings

For a complete list of references and additional readings for this procedure, scan this QR code with your smartphone, or visit https://www.elsevier.com/__data/assets/pdf_file/0004/1319845/Chapter0070.pdf.

PROCEDURE

71

Pericardial Catheter Management

Brandi L. Holcomb

PURPOSE Placement of an indwelling pericardial catheter allows for the slow and/or intermittent evacuation of fluid from the pericardial space. An indwelling pericardial catheter also allows for the infusion of medications (e.g., antibiotics or chemotherapeutic agents) into the pericardial space.

PREREQUISITE NURSING KNOWLEDGE

- Anatomy and physiology of the cardiovascular system including an understanding of the principles of cardiac conduction, electrocardiogram (ECG) lead placement, and dysrhythmia interpretation.
- Aseptic technique.
- Advanced cardiac life support (ACLS) knowledge and skills.
- The pericardial space normally contains 20 to 50 mL of fluid.
- Pericardial fluid has electrolyte and protein profiles similar to plasma.
- Pericardial effusion is generally defined as the accumulation of fluid within the pericardial space that exceeds the stretch capacity of the pericardium, generally more than 50 to 100 mL.[6]
- Intrapericardial fluid accumulation can be acute or chronic, therefore it varies in presentation of symptoms. Acute effusions are usually a rapid collection of fluid occurring over minutes to hours and may result in hemodynamic compromise with volumes less than 250 mL.[8] Chronically developing effusions occurring over days to weeks allow for hypertrophy and distention of the fibrous pericardial membrane. Patients with chronic effusions may accumulate greater than or equal to 2000 mL of fluid before exhibiting symptoms of hemodynamic compromise.[8]
- Symptoms of cardiac tamponade are nonspecific, so the diagnosis relies on clinical suspicion and associated signs and symptoms. Acute pericardial effusions are usually a result of trauma, myocardial infarction, or iatrogenic injury, whereas chronic effusions can result from conditions such as bacterial or viral pericarditis, cancer, autoimmune disorders, uremia, and so on.[6] With a decrease in cardiac output, the patient often develops chest pain, dyspnea, tachycardia, tachypnea, pallor, cyanosis, impaired cerebral and renal function, diaphoresis, hypotension, neck vein distention, distant or faint heart sounds, and pulsus paradoxus.[8]
- Pericardiocentesis is an effective treatment for pericardial effusion (see Procedures 37, Pericardiocentesis [Perform] and 38, Pericardiocentesis [Assist]). For chronic or rapidly

accumulating effusions, an indwelling pericardial catheter may be placed for continuous or intermittent drainage of excess fluid.

- The pericardial catheter may be connected to a closed drainage system (Fig. 71.1).
- The pericardial catheter may also be left in place to facilitate the infusion of medications (e.g., antibiotics, chemotherapeutic agents) depending on the patient's clinical manifestations.
- An indwelling catheter should usually be removed within 48 to 72 hours after placement to avoid risk of infection or iatrogenic pericarditis.[7] Depending on the patient's underlying condition, the catheter may be left in place for longer periods to facilitate resolution of pericardial effusion, cardiac tamponade, or infusion of medication.[7] Pericardial catheters should be removed immediately for any signs of infection or an abrupt increase in white blood cell count.[7]

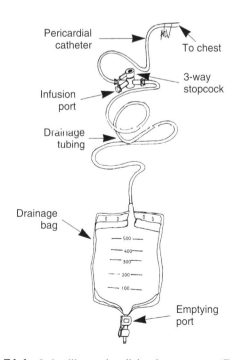

Figure 71.1 Indwelling pericardial catheter system. *(From Hammel WJ: Care of patients with an indwelling pericardial catheter. Crit Care Nurs 18[5]:40–45, 1998.)*

- Pericardial catheters are generally removed when the pericardial drainage decreases to less than 25 to 30 mL for the preceding 24-hour period.[8]
- Extended catheter drainage is associated with a reduction of the reoccurrence of cardiac tamponade compared with a single pericardiocentesis in patients with pericardial effusion related to malignancy.[6]

EQUIPMENT

- Pericardial catheter
- Sterile drapes: 4 small drapes and a full-body drape
- Sterile and nonsterile gloves, gowns, masks, protective eyewear
- Sterile 0.9% normal saline (NS) solution for irrigation and sterile basin
- Sterile syringes: 3-, 5-, 30-, or 60-mL Luer-Lok
- Sterile 1000-mL vacuum bottle available for the initial procedure
- Antiseptic solution (e.g., 2% chlorhexidine-based preparation, alcohol swab)
- Sterile 4 × 4 gauze
- Sterile transparent occlusive dressing
- Adhesive tape
- Sterile three-way Luer-Lok stopcock with nonvented caps and replacement caps
- Drainage tubing
- Pericardial drainage bag

Additional equipment, to have available as needed, includes the following:

- Anticoagulant flush available for dwell if prescribed (i.e., heparin)
- Cytotoxic disposal receptacle (when chemotherapeutic or cytotoxic agents are prescribed; also used to avoid aerosolization of the medication once disconnected from the patient)
- Emergency cart (defibrillator, emergency respiratory equipment, emergency cardiac medications)

PATIENT AND FAMILY EDUCATION

- Explain to the patient and family the reason necessitating the indwelling pericardial catheter (e.g., relief of pressure on the heart). *Rationale:* Communication of pertinent information helps the patient and family understand the procedure and the potential risks and benefits, subsequently reducing anxiety and apprehension.[11]
- Discuss potential discomfort the catheter may cause with inspiration and the insertion site. Reassure the patient and family that pain medication will be prescribed and administered as necessary. *Rationale:* This explanation prepares and informs the patient of the pain-management plan and reassures the patient that pain management is a priority.

- Instruct the patient and family about the patient's risk for recurrent pericardial effusion, describing the potential signs and symptoms (e.g., dyspnea, dull ache or pressure within the chest, dysphagia, cough, tachypnea, hoarseness, hiccups, or nausea).[5,6,8] *Rationale:* Early recognition of signs and symptoms of recurrent pericardial effusion may prompt detection of a potentially life-threatening problem.

PATIENT ASSESSMENT AND PREPARATION

Patient Assessment

- Assess the patient's neurological, cardiovascular, and hemodynamic status including heart rate, cardiac rhythm, heart sounds (S_1, S_2, rubs, murmurs), blood pressure (BP), mean arterial pressure, peripheral pulses, oxygen saturation via pulse oximetry, respiratory status, and if available, pulmonary artery pressures, pulmonary artery occlusion pressure (PAOP), right-atrial pressure (RAP), cardiac output (CO) and cardiac index (CI), and systemic vascular resistance. *Rationale:* Provides baseline data.
- Assess the patient for dyspnea, tachypnea, tachycardia, muffled heart sounds, precordial dullness to percussion, or altered level of consciousness; hypotension (systolic BP <100 mm Hg or decreased from patient's baseline); increased jugular venous pressure/jugular distention; pulsus paradoxus (inspiratory decrease in systolic BP amplitude) greater than 12 to 15 mm Hg; equalization of RAP, PAOP, and pulmonary artery diastolic pressure; and decreased CO/CI.[1,2] *Rationale:* Assessment of these signs and symptoms of possible cardiac tamponade is essential for identification of potential complications and catheter patency.
- Determine the patient's allergy history (e.g., heparin, antiseptic solutions). *Rationale:* This assessment decreases the risk for allergic reactions by avoiding known allergenic products.

Patient Preparation

- Confirm that the patient and family understand the preprocedural teaching by having them verbalize understanding. Clarify key points by reinforcing important information, and answer all questions. *Rationale:* Preprocedural communication provides a framework of patient expectations, enhances cooperation, and reduces anxiety.[2,11]
- Verify the correct patient with two patient-specific identifiers. *Rationale:* The nurse should always ensure the correct identification of the patient for the intended intervention for patient safety.

Procedure	for Pericardial Catheter Management		
Steps	**Rationale**	**Considerations**	

General Management of the Patient With a Pericardial Catheter Without a Drainage System

Steps	Rationale	Considerations
1. **HH**		
2. **PE**		Consider putting a mask on the patient during the actual procedure if the patient is not intubated (in a contained system), especially if the patient has methicillin-resistant *Staphylococcus aureus* (MRSA)-positive results on nasal swab or known colonization.
3. Assist the provider with the pericardiocentesis procedure (see Procedures 37, Pericardiocentesis [Perform], and 38, Pericardiocentesis [Assist]).	Provides assistance as needed.	The pericardial catheter may be inserted in the operating room, in a special procedure environment (e.g., cardiac catheterization laboratory or interventional laboratory), or at the bedside.
4. Ensure that the connections between the pericardial catheter and the stopcock are tight.	Ensures that the integrity of the system is intact.	At the completion of the pericardiocentesis, the stopcock is turned off to the patient, and a sterile nonvented cap is placed on the stopcock port.
5. Observe the pericardial fluid drainage for color, amount, and consistency.	Ensures pericardial catheter patency. The presence of fibrin matrix in the drainage can result in obstruction of the catheter and be problematic for future manual taps.	Pericardial fluid is commonly straw-colored, serous drainage. A two-dimensional (2D) or Doppler echocardiogram can be performed after the pericardiocentesis to assess for reaccumulation of pericardial fluid.[6]
6. Perform catheter site care.	Prevents infection.	
A. **HH**		
B. **PE**		
C. Remove the dressing, and discard it in an appropriate receptacle.	Allows for site assessment and prepares for site care.	
D. Assess the skin surrounding the catheter-insertion site.	Assesses for signs and symptoms of infection.	
E. Remove and discard the nonsterile gloves in an appropriate receptacle.	Maintains aseptic technique.	
F. **HH**		
G. Apply sterile gloves.	Prepares for the procedure.	
H. Cleanse the skin around the pericardial catheter insertion site using a back-and-forth motion while applying friction for 30 seconds with an antiseptic solution (e.g., 2% chlorhexidine-based solution),[2,7] and allow time to dry. **(Level D*)**	Reduces the rate of recolonization of skin microflora. The U.S. Centers for Disease Control and Prevention (CDC) does not have a specific recommendation for care of pericardial catheters or site care.[3]	
I. Ensure that the catheter and stopcock are securely anchored to the chest.	Reduces the possibility of displacement.	

*Level D: Peer-reviewed professional and organizational protocols with the support of clinical study recommendations.

Procedure continues on following page

Procedure for Pericardial Catheter Management—*Continued*		
Steps	Rationale	Considerations
J. Apply a sterile, occlusive dressing over the catheter insertion site. Label the dressing with the date, time, and initials of the person performing the dressing change.	Provides a sterile environment. Identifies the last dressing change.	
K. Remove 🅿🅴, and discard used supplies in the appropriate receptacles.		
L. 🅷🅷		
7. *If pericardial fluid removal is desired,* aspirate pericardial fluid every 4–6 hours as prescribed or as often as clinically indicated through the three-way stopcock using sterile technique.[2]	Removes excess pericardial fluid and relieves symptoms of cardiac tamponade; ensures catheter patency.	Follow institutional protocols regarding personnel permitted to aspirate and flush pericardial catheters (e.g., registered nurses, providers). Consider placing a mask on the patient during the procedure if the patient is not intubated. Pericardial fluid samples may be collected for select diagnostic tests (e.g., protein, glucose, hematocrit, white blood cell count, bacterial or fungal cultures).
A. 🅷🅷		
B. 🅿🅴		
C. Ensure that the stopcock is turned off to the patient, and then remove the nonvented cap from the infusion port of the three-way stopcock.	Prepares for fluid removal.	
D. Clean the infusion port cap at the top of the stopcock with an antiseptic solution for 15 seconds, and allow to dry.[2,3,7]	Decreases the risk for infection.	
E. Attach a sterile, 60-mL Luer-Lok syringe to the three-way stopcock.	Prepares for fluid removal.	
F. Turn the stopcock open to the syringe and patient.	Permits aspiration of fluid.	
G. Gently aspirate pericardial fluid while monitoring patient response.	Gentle removal is necessary to avoid pericardial or myocardial injury.	
H. After completion of the fluid withdrawal, turn the stopcock off to the patient.	Stops pericardial drainage.	
I. Disconnect the specimen syringe from the stopcock.	Removes the specimen.	
J. Connect the flush syringe to the stopcock.	Prepares the equipment for flushing.	
K. Turn the stopcock open to the syringe and patient, and gently flush the pericardial catheter with 2–5 mL of sterile 0.9% NS solution or heparinized saline solution as prescribed.	Clears the pericardial catheter and promotes catheter patency.	Monitor vital signs and the ECG tracing while flushing the pericardial catheter to assess patient response to the procedure; follow institutional protocols for administration of dwell solution.

Procedure for Pericardial Catheter Management—*Continued*		
Steps	Rationale	Considerations
L. Turn the stopcock off to the patient, and disconnect the flush syringe.	Removes equipment.	
M. Carefully place a new sterile nonvented cap on the stopcock.	Maintains a sterile, closed system and reduces the risk of infection.	
N. Measure the amount of drainage.	Records the amount of drainage.	
O. Remove **PE**, and discard used supplies in the appropriate receptacles.		
P. **HH**		
8. *If the pericardial catheter is blocked or obstructed to flow:*		Follow institutional protocols regarding personnel permitted to aspirate and flush pericardial catheters (e.g., registered nurses, providers).
A. **HH**		
B. **PE**		
C. Examine the catheter to determine whether there is an external mechanical cause of the pericardial catheter blockage, and correct if present. Consider the following: i. Kinks in tubing. ii. Tubing may be compressed underneath patient. iii. Turn or reposition patient to facilitate flow.	Relieves mechanical obstruction to flow.	
D. Assess for loose tubing connections and, if loosened, tighten connections.	Ensures an intact drainage system.	
E. Determine correct positioning of the stopcock. If needed, correct the stopcock position.	Facilitates unobstructed fluid drainage.	
F. If the previous steps do not correct the obstruction to flow, do the following: i. Turn the stopcock off to the patient, and remove the cap from the infusion port of the stopcock.	Attempts to relieve the obstruction. Prepares the equipment.	
ii. Clean the infusion port of the stopcock with an antiseptic solution for 15 seconds, and allow to dry.[2,3,7]	Decreases the risk of infection.	
iii. Attach the syringe for the flush, and turn the stopcock open to the patient.	Prepares the equipment.	

Procedure continues on following page

Procedure for Pericardial Catheter Management—*Continued*

Steps	Rationale	Considerations
iv. Turn the stopcock open to the syringe and patient, and gently flush the pericardial catheter with 2–5 mL of sterile 0.9% NS solution or heparinized saline solution as prescribed (use NS if the patient is sensitive to heparin).	Attempts to improve pericardial catheter patency. Heparinized saline solution may be used for a dwell if the drainage tends to be serous or fibrous in consistency.[12]	Monitor vital signs and the ECG tracing to determine patient response while flushing the pericardial catheter. Follow institutional protocols for administration of dwell solution, if prescribed.
v. Gently attempt to aspirate flush solution.	Allows for aspiration of flush solution and pericardial fluid.	Deduct the volume of flush solution from the total volume for accurate measurement of pericardial fluid volume.
vi. Determine whether the pericardial catheter is patent and fluid is draining.	Assesses the proper functioning of the system.	Monitor vital signs and ECG.
vii. If the above measures do not remove the catheter blockage, notify the provider immediately.	Additional interventions are indicated.	
9. *If medications are prescribed for infusion into the pericardium:*		Follow institutional protocols for **PE** when administering cytotoxic or antineoplastic medications. Follow institutional protocols regarding personnel permitted to instill medications into the pericardial space.
A. **HH**		
B. **PE**		
C. Review the prescribed medication, dose, method of delivery, amount, and time for dwell. Assemble the medication, tubing, pump or syringe, and two flush syringes of 0.9% NS (2–5 mL each).[2,3]	Ensures the accuracy of medication administration and prepares the equipment.	
D. Ensure that the stopcock is off to the patient, and remove the cap from the infusion port.	Prepares for the procedure.	
E. Clean the infusion port of the stopcock with an antiseptic solution for 15 seconds, and allow to dry.[2,3,7]	Reduces the risk of infection.	
F. Attach a flush syringe of sterile 0.9% NS, and turn the stopcock open to the patient. Establish patency of the catheter by gentle infusion and withdrawal of 0.9% NS.	Ensures catheter patency.	
G. Turn the stopcock off to the patient, and disconnect the flush syringe.	Removes the equipment.	

UNIT II

Procedure for Pericardial Catheter Management—*Continued*		
Steps	Rationale	Considerations
H. Attach the prescribed medication (either infusion or syringe). With the use of a syringe for delivery, gently instill the medication. If using an infusion pump, set the appropriate medication infusion rate.	Administers the medication as prescribed.	Infusion of the medication may activate signs and symptoms of cardiac tamponade.[9,10] Monitor vital signs and the ECG tracing while infusing the medication to assess patient response.
		If the patient has any abnormal signs or symptoms, stop the infusion and notify the provider.
I. Turn the stopcock off to the patient when the medication delivery is complete.	Stops the medication administration.	
J. Disconnect the tubing or syringe.	Removes the equipment.	
K. Attach a flush syringe of 0.9% NS.	Prepares the equipment.	
L. Turn the stopcock open to the patient, and gently flush the catheter.	Ensures that the medication is completely in the pericardium and none remains in the catheter.	
M. Turn the stopcock off to the patient, and apply a sterile nonvented cap to the infusion port.	Closes and maintains the integrity of the system.	
N. Allow the medication to dwell for the prescribed time.	Allows time for the medication to act.	
O. When the dwell time is complete, remove the infusion port cap. Clean the infusion port of the stopcock with an antiseptic solution for 15 seconds, and allow to dry.[2,3,7] Attach a syringe large enough to retrieve the medication plus the pericardial fluid accumulation.	Prepares the equipment.	
P. Gently withdraw the medication and pericardial drainage.	Removes the medication.	Volume of the retrieved fluid should be equivalent to the volume of medication that was instilled, plus the flush solution and additional pericardial fluid that accumulated during the dwell time.
Q. Turn the stopcock off to the patient, and disconnect the syringe.	Removes the equipment.	
R. Attach a flush syringe of 2–5 mL of 0.9% NS with or without heparin as prescribed.[3,7]	Prepares the equipment.	
S. Turn the stopcock open to the patient, and instill the 0.9% NS or heparin flush.	Clears the pericardial catheter.	
T. Turn the stopcock off to the patient, remove the flush syringe, and apply a sterile nonvented cap to the infusion port.	Closes the pericardial catheter system and maintains the integrity of the closed system.	

Procedure continues on following page

Procedure for Pericardial Catheter Management—*Continued*

Steps	Rationale	Considerations
U. Remove **PE**, and discard used supplies in the appropriate receptacles.		Discard any antineoplastic or cytotoxic agent, tubing, and flush syringes in the designated biohazard receptacle.
V. **HH**		

General Management of the Patient With a Pericardial Catheter Closed Drainage System

Steps	Rationale	Considerations
1. **HH**		
2. **PE**		
3. Assist the provider with the pericardiocentesis (see Procedures 37, Pericardiocentesis [Perform] and 38, Pericardiocentesis [Assist]).	Provides assistance as needed.	The pericardial catheter may be inserted in the operating room, in a special procedure environment (e.g., cardiac catheterization laboratory or interventional laboratory), or at the bedside.
4. Ensure that the connections between the pericardial catheter and the stopcock are tight.	Ensures the integrity of the system.	At the completion of the pericardiocentesis, a nonvented sterile cap is placed on the stopcock port and the stopcock is turned off to the patient or open to drainage as prescribed.
5. Position the drainage-collection receptacle lower than the catheter-insertion point to facilitate drainage, and observe the fluid for color, amount, and consistency.	Ensures pericardial catheter patency. The presence of fibrin matrix in the drainage can obstruct the catheter and be problematic for future manual taps.	Pericardial fluid is commonly straw-colored, serous drainage. A 2D or Doppler echocardiogram can be performed after the pericardiocentesis to assess for reaccumulation of pericardial fluid.[9,10]
6. Perform catheter-site care.	Prevents infection.	Observe the site for any evidence of drainage and notify the provider if present.
A. **HH**		
B. **PE**		
C. Remove the dressing, and discard it in an appropriate receptacle.	Allows for site assessment and prepares for site care.	
D. Assess the skin around the catheter insertion site.	Assesses for signs and symptoms of infection.	
E. Remove and discard the nonsterile gloves in an appropriate receptacle.	Maintains aseptic technique.	
F. **HH**		
G. Apply sterile gloves, and establish a sterile field.	Prepares for the procedure.	
H. Cleanse the skin around the pericardial catheter insertion site using a back-and-forth motion while applying friction for 30 seconds with an antiseptic solution (e.g., 2% chlorhexidine-based solution).[2,3] Allow the antiseptic to remain on the insertion site and to air dry completely.[7] (**Level D***)	Reduces the rate of colonization of skin microflora. The CDC does not have a specific recommendation for care of pericardial catheters or site care.[3]	

*Level D: Peer-reviewed professional and organizational protocols with the support of clinical study recommendations.

Procedure for Pericardial Catheter Management—*Continued*		
Steps	**Rationale**	**Considerations**
I. Determine whether the catheter and stopcock are securely anchored to the chest.	Ensures a secure system and reduces the possibility of displacement.	
J. Apply a sterile, occlusive dressing over the catheter-insertion site. Label the dressing with the date, time and initials of the person performing the dressing change.	Provides a sterile environment. Identifies the last dressing change.	
K. Remove **PE**, and discard used supplies in the appropriate receptacle.		
L. **HH**		
7. *If pericardial fluid removal is desired:* Intermittently or continuously drain the pericardial fluid as prescribed by turning the stopcock off to the infusion port and open between the patient and the drainage bag (see Fig. 71.1).	Removes pericardial fluid.	Follow institutional protocols regarding personnel permitted to aspirate and flush pericardial catheters (e.g., registered nurses, providers).
A. *Intermittent drainage:* If intermittent drainage is prescribed, the stopcock is usually off to the patient and opened every 4–6 hours to drainage or as clinically indicated with Doppler scan or 2D echocardiogram and patient presentation until the accumulation of fluid is resolved (follow the prescribed regimen).		
B. *Continuous drainage:* If continuous drainage is prescribed, the stopcock remains open between the patient and the drainage bag and off to the infusion port (follow the prescribed regimen).		
C. Empty the pericardial drainage bag every 8 hours or sooner if prescribed.	Reduces the possibility of colonization in the bag and the potential reflux of fluid to the patient.	Pericardial fluid samples may be collected for selected diagnostic tests.
i. **HH**		
ii. **PE**		
iii. Turn the stopcock off to the patient.	Reduces the risk of pneumopericardium.	
iv. Open the emptying port of the drainage bag, and drain the pericardial fluid into a receptacle for measurement and waste disposal.	Discards drainage.	

Procedure continues on following page

Procedure for Pericardial Catheter Management—*Continued*

Steps	Rationale	Considerations
v. Close the port, and secure the drainage bag.	Closes and maintains integrity of the system.	
vi. Resume the prescribed drainage mode.	Continues prescribed treatment.	
D. After completion of intermittent fluid drainage, temporarily turn the stopcock off to the patient for the flush procedure.	Prepares for the procedure.	
i. **HH**		
ii. **PE**		
iii. Remove the infusion port cap, clean the infusion port at the top of the stopcock with an antiseptic solution for 15 seconds, and allow to dry.[2,3,7]	Reduces the risk of infection.	
iv. Connect the flush syringe, turn the stopcock open to the syringe and patient, and gently flush the pericardial catheter with 2–5 mL of sterile 0.9% NS solution or heparinized saline solution as prescribed (use NS if the patient is sensitive to heparin).	Clears the pericardial catheter and maintains catheter patency.	
v. Turn the three-way stopcock off to the patient, and disconnect the flush syringe.	Maintains integrity of the closed system and minimizes the risk of pneumopericardium.	
vi. Place a new sterile nonvented cap on the infusion port.	Maintains asepsis.	
vii. Remove **PE**, and discard used supplies in appropriate receptacles.		
viii. **HH**		
8. *If the pericardial catheter is blocked or obstructed to flow:*		Follow institutional protocols regarding personnel permitted to aspirate and flush pericardial catheters (e.g., registered nurses, providers).
A. **HH**		
B. **PE**		
C. Determine whether the drainage system is lower than the insertion point, and reposition if needed.	Facilitates drainage by gravity.	

Procedure	for Pericardial Catheter Management—*Continued*	
Steps	**Rationale**	**Considerations**

D. Examine the catheter to determine whether there is an external mechanical cause of the pericardial catheter blockage, and correct if present. Consider the following:
  i. Kinks in tubing.
  ii. Tubing may be compressed underneath patient.
  iii. Turn or reposition the patient to facilitate flow.
	Relieves mechanical obstruction to flow.	

E. Assess for loose tubing connections, and if loosened, tighten connections.	Ensures intact drainage system.	
F. Determine correct positioning of the stopcock. If needed, correct the stopcock position.	Facilitates unobstructed fluid drainage.	
G. If the previous steps do not correct the obstruction to flow, do the following:		
i. Remove the infusion port cap, clean the infusion port at the top of the stopcock with an antiseptic solution for 15 seconds, and allow to dry.[2,3,7]	Decreases the risk of infection.	
ii. Connect the flush syringe, turn the stopcock open to the syringe and patient, and gently flush the pericardial catheter with 2–5 mL of sterile 0.9% NS solution or heparinized saline solution as prescribed (use NS if the patient is sensitive to heparin).	Attempts to improve pericardial catheter patency. Heparinized saline solution may be used for a dwell if the drainage tends to be serous or fibrous in consistency.[1]	Monitor vital signs and ECG tracing while flushing the pericardial catheter to assess patient response. Follow institutional protocols for administration of dwell solution, if prescribed.
iii. Turn the stopcock off to the infusion port and allow the fluid to passively drain, or turn the stopcock off to the drainage bag and gently attempt to aspirate the flush solution through the attached syringe.	Allows drainage of flush solution and pericardial fluid.	Volume of the drained fluid should be equivalent to the volume of the flush solution and additional accumulated pericardial fluid; deduct the amount of flush used to accurately measure output.
iv. Determine whether the pericardial catheter is draining and patent.	Assesses patency of the system.	

Procedure continues on following page

UNIT II

Procedure for Pericardial Catheter Management—*Continued*		
Steps	Rationale	Considerations
v. If the previous measures are ineffective for drainage but the catheter itself is patent, consider changing the tubing and the drainage bag system.	Ensures integrity of the system and may facilitate drainage.	Ensure the stopcock is off to the patient at the time of the change.
vi. After the tubing/bag change, assess the patency of the system.	Determines whether the system is functioning.	
vii. If these measures do not remove the catheter blockage, notify the provider immediately.	Additional interventions are necessary.	Accumulation of fluid in the pericardium without the possibility of drainage may result in tamponade.
viii. Remove **PE**, and discard used supplies in appropriate receptacles.		
ix. **HH**		
9. *If medications are prescribed for infusion into the pericardium:*		Follow institutional protocols for **PE** when administering cytotoxic or antineoplastic medications. Follow institutional protocols regarding personnel permitted to instill medications into the pericardial .
A. **HH**		
B. **PE**		
C. Review the prescribed medication, dose, method of delivery, amount, and time for dwell. Assemble the medication, tubing, pump or syringe, and two flush syringes of sterile 0.9% NS (2–5 mL each).[3,6]	Ensures the accuracy of medication administration.	
D. Turn the stopcock off to the patient, remove the infusion port cap, clean the infusion port at the top of the stopcock with an antiseptic solution for 15 seconds, and allow to dry.[2,3,7]	Reduces the risk of infection.	
E. Turn the stopcock off to the drainage bag. Attach the prescribed medication (either infusion or syringe).	Prevents inadvertent instillation of medication into the drainage bag.	
F. With the use of a syringe for delivery, gently instill the medication as prescribed. If using an infusion pump, set the appropriate medication-infusion rate. (Patency of the catheter is established by the presence of drainage. If there is a question about catheter patency, follow the flush procedure listed in the medication infusion section of "General Management of the Patient with a Pericardial Catheter without a Drainage System.")	Administers the medication.	Infusion of the medication may activate signs and symptoms of cardiac tamponade.[12] Monitor vital signs and ECG tracing while infusing the medication to assess patient response. If the patient has abnormal signs and symptoms, stop the infusion and notify the provider.

Procedure for Pericardial Catheter Management—*Continued*

Steps	Rationale	Considerations
G. If the medication is to dwell in the pericardial space before reestablishment of pericardial drainage:		
i. Turn the stopcock off to the patient at the completion of the infusion.		
ii. Disconnect the medication syringe or tubing.		
iii. Attach a syringe with 2–5 mL of sterile 0.9% NS flush, and turn the stopcock off to the drainage bag.		
iv. Gently flush the catheter, and turn the stopcock off to the patient for the completion of the dwell time as prescribed.	Ensures that the medication is instilled in the pericardial space and does not lie in the catheter.	
v. Disconnect the syringe and close system with a sterile nonvented cap.		
vi. After the dwell time is complete, turn the stopcock off to the infusion port and open to drainage.	Allows pericardial drainage to resume.	The drain time should allow for all of the medication to exit the pericardium.
vii. Measure the amount of the solution infused and the drainage collected.		The volume of the drained fluid should be equivalent to the volume of the medication instilled, the flush solution, and additional accumulated pericardial fluid; deduct the amount of medication infused and flush used to accurately measure output.
viii. Resume the prescribed drainage mode: continuous or intermittent. If intermittent, follow the prescription for the drain time after infusion.		
a. Once the drain time is completed, clean the infusion port of the stopcock with an antiseptic solution for 15 seconds.[2,3,7]	Reduces the risk for infection.	

Procedure continues on following page

Procedure for Pericardial Catheter Management—*Continued*		
Steps	**Rationale**	**Considerations**
b. Connect the flush syringe, turn the stopcock open to the syringe and patient, and gently flush the pericardial catheter with 2–5 mL of sterile NS solution or heparinized saline solution as prescribed (use NS if the patient is sensitive to heparin).	Maintains pericardial catheter patency.	
c. Turn the stopcock off to the patient until the next time the patient is due for intermittent drainage.	Maintains integrity of the system.	
d. Remove **PE**, and discard used supplies in appropriate receptacles.		
e. **HH**		

*Level D: Peer-reviewed professional and organizational protocols with the support of clinical study recommendations.

Expected Outcomes

- Patent pericardial drainage system
- Resolution of pericardial effusion
- Hemodynamic stability
- Patient free from infection
- Patient free from pain and anxiety
- Medications administered as prescribed

Unexpected Outcomes

- Infection
- Pain
- Catheter obstruction
- Reaccumulation of pericardial fluid
- Cardiac tamponade and hemodynamic instability
- Dysrhythmias
- Cardiac arrest

Patient Monitoring and Care

Steps	Rationale	Reportable Conditions
		These conditions must be reported to the provider if they persist despite nursing interventions.
1. Perform cardiovascular and hemodynamic assessments frequently and as patient condition necessitates, or as prescribed.	Assesses for signs of cardiac tamponade and determines hemodynamic stability.	• Signs of cardiac tamponade: dyspnea, tachypnea, tachycardia, hypotension, increased jugular venous pressure/jugular distension, pulsus paradoxus, muffled heart sounds, precordial dullness to percussion, altered level of consciousness. • Equalization of RAP, PAOP • CI <2.5 L/min/m^2 • Dysrhythmias

Patient Monitoring and Care —*Continued*

Steps	Rationale	Reportable Conditions
2. Assess the patency of the pericardial catheter: A. Without a closed drainage system, as needed or as prescribed. B. With a closed drainage system, as needed or as prescribed.	Pericardial catheter blockage may predispose the patient to excessive accumulation of pericardial fluid that may lead to cardiac tamponade and/or hemodynamic instability.	• Inability to obtain pericardial drainage or cessation of pericardial drainage • Signs and symptoms of cardiac tamponade or hemodynamic instability • Evidence of accumulation of pericardial fluid on Doppler or 2D echocardiography
3. Assess the amount and type of fluid draining from the pericardial catheter.	Provides information regarding the continued need for the catheter and potential problems.	• Change in the amount, color, or consistency of pericardial drainage from patient's baseline
4. Change the pericardial catheter dressing every 24 hours.[2]	Provides an opportunity to assess for signs and symptoms of infection. Infective pericarditis is associated with increased mortality and morbidity rates.[5] The CDC recommends replacing dressings on intravascular catheters when the dressing becomes damp, loosened, or soiled or when inspection of the site is necessary.[3]	• Elevated white blood cell counts • Elevated temperature • Signs and symptoms of infection at the insertion site (e.g., pain, erythema, drainage)
5. If in use, change the pericardial tubing and drainage bag every 72 hours.[2,9]	Reduces the risk of infection.	
6. Follow institutional protocols for assessing pain, and administer analgesia as prescribed.	Identifies need for pain interventions. The patient may experience chest pain or pleuritic-type pain while the pericardial catheter is in place.	• Continued pain despite interventions
7. Identify parameters that demonstrate clinical readiness for removal of the indwelling pericardial catheter.[8,9]	Facilitates early removal of the pericardial catheter and reduces the risk of infection.	• Pericardial drainage <25–30 mL over the previous 24 hours[9] • Hemodynamic stability as evidenced by systolic BP >100 mm Hg, CI >2.5 L/min/m², absence of pulsus paradoxus, no equalization of RAP, PA diastolic pressure, and PAOP • Absence of pericardial effusion on Doppler or 2D echocardiography[9]
8. Identify situations in which the pericardial effusion cannot be resolved with use of pericardial drainage via tap or closed system.[9]	Additional interventions may be needed.	• Hemodynamic instability • Continued pericardial effusion

Procedure continues on following page

UNIT II

Documentation

Documentation should include the following:
- Patient and family education
- Universal protocol requirements
- Patient tolerance of the indwelling pericardial catheter
- Dressing, tubing, and drainage bag changes
- Amount of pericardial drainage each shift, including net volumes when catheter is flushed or medications are infused
- Volumes of injectate or aspirate
- Characteristics of the pericardial drainage: color, consistency, and/or changes
- Hemodynamic status
- Pain assessment, interventions, and effectiveness
- Occurrence of unexpected outcomes/treatments
- Nursing interventions

References and Additional Readings

For a complete list of references and additional readings for this procedure, scan this QR code with your smartphone, or visit https://www.elsevier.com/__data/assets/pdf_file/0005/1319846/Chapter0071.pdf.

72 Transesophageal Echocardiography (Assist)

Marie Woznicki

PURPOSE Transesophageal echocardiography (TEE) offers an alternative approach for obtaining high-quality images of the heart structures that may not be well visualized with a conventional transthoracic echocardiography (TTE) approach. TEE obtains images of the heart from a transducer inside the esophagus. The esophagus lies immediately behind the heart, and clear images of the heart can be obtained with this technology.

PREREQUISITE NURSING KNOWLEDGE

- Knowledge of cardiovascular anatomy and physiology.
- Basic arrhythmia recognition and treatment of life-threatening dysrhythmias.
- Advanced cardiac life support (ACLS) knowledge and skills.
- A topical anesthetic is used in the oropharyngeal area; thus, the patient's gag reflex may be diminished or absent, putting the patient at risk for aspiration.[3]
- It is essential to know the institution's conscious sedation protocols.
- Sedation can put the patient at risk for respiratory depression.[8]
- Transesophageal echocardiography is considered an aerosol-generating procedure; therefore it is imperative to be familiar with the institution's personal protective equipment policies for aerosol-generating procedures.[6]
- A fiberoptic probe with an ultrasound transducer is inserted through the mouth into the esophagus just behind the heart (Fig. 72.1). The transducer located at the tip of the probe sends high-frequency sound waves toward the heart, which return as echoes. The echoes are converted, by computer, into moving images of the heart. The image is displayed on a screen and can be recorded on videotape or compact disk (CD), printed on paper, or sent electronically to a picture-archiving communication system. This test is used to visualize structures of the heart and aorta that may not be seen with a standard TTE and to clarify structures that may be otherwise poorly seen. The test may be performed as an outpatient or inpatient procedure or in the operating room.[3]
- Various modes of echocardiography are used to examine the heart, blood vessels, valve function, and blood flow. The three techniques include the following:
  - ❖ Motion-mode (M-mode) echocardiography: This is a one-dimensional echocardiogram that visualizes time, depth, and intensity. It looks like a tracing instead of a picture of the heart and is used to measure the exact size of the heart chambers.

- ❖ Two-dimensional (2D) echocardiography: This shows the actual shape and motion of the different heart structures. These images represent "slices" of the heart in motion.
  - ❖ Three-dimensional (3D) echocardiography provides added dimensions to the 2D echocardiogram. It provides detailed anatomical assessment of cardiac pathology, chamber volume measurement, and views of heart valves, enabling a better appreciation of the severity and mechanisms of valve diseases.
  - ❖ Doppler echocardiography: This assesses the flow of blood through the heart. The signals that represent blood flow are displayed as a series of black-and-white tracings or color images on the screen.
- A TEE is considered a safe and relatively noninvasive diagnostic technique. However, severe, even life-threatening complications have been reported.[3]
- General indications for TEE are as follows[1-3]:
  - ❖ Evaluation of cardiac and aortic structures and function with inadequate TTE images or in whom diagnostic information is not obtainable by TTE
  - ❖ Rule out clot prechemical and/or electrical cardioversion
  - ❖ Suspected acute thoracic aortic pathology including but not limited to dissection/transection
  - ❖ Evaluation of valvular (mitral) structure and function to assess appropriateness for and to assist with planning of an intervention
  - ❖ Diagnosis of infective endocarditis with a high pretest probability (e.g., *Staphylococcus* bacteremia, fungemia, prosthetic heart valve, or intracardiac device)
  - ❖ Evaluation for cardiovascular source of embolus with no identifiable noncardiac source
  - ❖ Intraoperative cardiac monitoring
  - ❖ Guiding the management of catheter-based intracardiac procedures such as septal defect closure or atrial appendage obliteration and transcatheter valve procedures
  - ❖ Prosthetic valve disorders
- Contraindications to TEE can be divided into absolute and relative. Gastrointestinal (GI) evaluation and clearance should be considered before the procedure.

Transesophageal Echocardiogram (TEE)

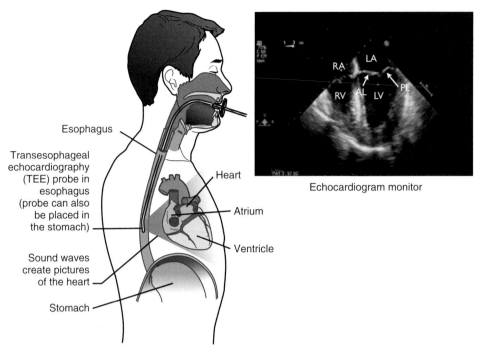

Esophagus

Transesophageal
echocardiography
(TEE) probe in
esophagus
(probe can also
be placed in
the stomach)

Heart

Atrium

Ventricle

Sound waves
create pictures
of the heart

Stomach

Echocardiogram monitor

Figure 72.1 Transesophageal echocardiography *(TEE)* probe inserted through the mouth and into the esophagus just behind the heart.

- Absolute contraindications are as follows[2,3]:
  - Diseases of the throat/esophagus/stomach including but not limited to known obstructive esophageal disease, obstruction, stenosis, tumors, fistulae, or varices
  - Esophageal perforation, laceration
  - A history of esophageal radiation or unresolved esophageal dilation
  - Perforated viscus
  - Dysphagia and odynophagia
  - Active upper GI bleeding
  - Patients who ate within 6 to 8 hours of the study, unless emergent as in aortic dissection or trauma
  - Unwilling patients
  - Inability to obtain intravenous access
- Relative contraindications are as follows[2,3]:
  - Upper GI surgery
  - Recent upper GI bleed
  - History of radiation to neck and mediastinum
  - Barrett's esophagus
  - History of dysphagia
  - Restriction of cervical mobility from severe cervical arthritis
  - Esophageal varices
  - Coagulopathy, thrombocytopenia
  - Active esophagitis
  - Active peptic ulcer disease
  - Loose teeth
- A TEE does not pose a risk for infection. Patients with prosthetic valves do not need antibiotics prescribed before the procedure.[7]

EQUIPMENT

- Transesophageal ultrasound probe
- Echocardiography machine (compatible with the probe)
- Constant low wall suction with connecting tubing and rigid pharyngeal suction-tip catheter
- Protective mask, goggles, nonsterile gloves, and barrier gowns
- Water-soluble lubricant
- Oxygen, with both nasal prongs and mask available
- Topical anesthetic such as lidocaine solution with an administration device (i.e., mucosal atomization device), viscous lidocaine, or benzocaine spray (as prescribed)
- Premedication for sedation and appropriate reversal agents (as prescribed)
- Syringes, blunt needles, and labels for medications
- Antiseptic agents for IV connection cleaning such as alcohol prep pads
- IV insertion kit (if adequate IV access is not in place)
- IV tubing
- One bag (500 mL or 1000 mL) of 0.9% normal saline IV solution
- Syringes of proper size for aspirating and flushing IV access if needed
- Tongue depressor
- Emesis basin
- Flashlight (to assess the oropharyngeal area, especially in the case of trauma)
- Disposable bite guard (with or without a strap to hold it in place)
- Thermometer

- Continuous electrocardiographic monitor
- Continuous pulse oximetry monitor and equipment
- Continuous capnography monitor and tubing (per institutional protocols)
- Automatic blood pressure machine and cuff (with manual blood pressure cuff available for backup use)
- Two pillows, one supporting the neck and one supporting the back, to maintain the side-lying position
- Bags with respective labels for carrying the probe to and from the procedure (institution specific)
- ACLS cart, airway equipment, and medications

Additional equipment, to have available as needed, includes the following:

- Denture cup with patient identification
- Tonsillar forceps and cotton balls with radiopaque string attached (institution specific)
- Methylene blue, if benzocaine spray is used
- Ultrasound gel
- Three-way stopcock and syringes (at least two 10-mL syringes with normal saline flush solution and one 10-mL empty syringe) for the administration of the saline contrast agent if used

PATIENT AND FAMILY EDUCATION

- Assess the patient and family's understanding of the procedure and the indication for therapy. *Rationale:* Information about the procedure increases patient cooperation and decreases patient and family anxiety and apprehension.
- Verify that the patient understands the preparation for the procedure, which includes not having food or nonclear liquids for at least 6 hours and nothing by mouth (NPO) for 2 to 3 hours before the procedure as prescribed.[3,9] Before the test, the patient may take daily medications, with a sip of water, as prescribed or according to institutional standards. *Rationale:* Undigested material in the stomach increases the risk for aspiration. Prescribed medications may be needed.
- Explain that the local anesthetic may make the patient's tongue and throat feel swollen and that he or she may feel unable to swallow. The gag reflex will be inhibited by the local anesthetic and may last approximately 1 hour after administration. They may experience gagging or retching during the numbing process and during the initial passage of the probe. *Rationale:* The explanation may assist in decreasing patient anxiety during the procedure.
- Explain to the patient he or she will be sedated to decrease anxiety, to increase comfort, and for ease in passing the probe. *Rationale:* This information may decrease patient and family anxiety.
- Describe to the patient that he or she will be monitored closely during and after the procedure. *Rationale:* The explanation assists in decreasing patient and family anxiety.
- Explain to the patient he or she will require transportation after the procedure and must be accompanied by a responsible adult if it is performed in an ambulatory setting. *Rationale:* Even short-acting medications may not be metabolized for a few hours, making it unsafe to drive.

PATIENT ASSESSMENT AND PREPARATION

Patient Assessment

- Verify the correct patient with two identifiers. *Rationale:* Before performing a procedure, the nurse should ensure the correct identification of the patient for the intended procedure.
- Assist the physician, advanced practice nurse, or other healthcare professional with assessing the patient's medical history for absolute and relative contraindications for the TEE procedure. *Rationale:* Screening for absolute and relative contraindications for the TEE procedure prevents adverse outcomes.
- Assess the patient's baseline cardiac rhythm. *Rationale:* The patient's rhythm may have converted if the indication for the procedure was an arrhythmia. Passage of a large-bore tube may cause vagal stimulation and bradyarrhythmias.
- Assess the patient's history of medication allergies. *Rationale:* Identifying allergies may avoid an adverse medication reaction.
- Confirm that the patient was NPO for the prescribed length of time. *Rationale:* NPO status for an appropriate period before the procedure allows for gastric emptying and decreases the likelihood of aspiration.
- Assess the patient's medication history.[1] *Rationale:* Frequent use of certain medications (e.g., analgesics and anxiolytics) or illicit drugs and alcohol may affect the patient's response to moderate sedation and the medications.
- Confirm medications the patient has taken within the past 4 hours. *Rationale:* Recent sedative, analgesic, and vasoactive medications may affect the patient's tolerance and response to the medications given during the procedure.
- Assess the patient's height, weight, baseline respiratory, hemodynamic, and neurological status before anesthetizing the posterior pharynx and administering any sedative agents. *Rationale:* Baseline assessment data provide information to use as a comparison for further assessment once medications have been administered.
- Assess the patient's baseline vital signs, oxygen saturation, and if applicable capnography reading. *Rationale:* Close monitoring of vital signs and oxygenation during the procedure and comparison with baseline are essential to assess the patient's tolerance of the procedure.
- Assess the patient's baseline pain characteristics, site, and severity. *Rationale:* Baseline assessment data provide information to use as a comparison during and after the procedure.
- Assess the patient's presedation level of consciousness using an organization-approved scoring system (e.g., Modified Aldrete Score).[3] *Rationale:* Using a scoring system for conscious sedation may prevent oversedation and will establish a baseline for postprocedure comparison.
- Assess the patient for medical problems that contraindicate or increase the risk of conscious sedation. Consider using the American Association of Anesthesiologists' Physical Status Classification Score per institution policy. *Rationale:* Preprocedure screening may find a history or

evidence of difficult intubation, sleep apnea, and complications of sedation or anesthesia.[3]

Patient Preparation

- Verify that the patient and family understand the preprocedural teaching. Answer questions as they arise, and reinforce information as needed. ***Rationale:*** Understanding of previously taught information is evaluated and reinforced. Patient and family anxiety may be decreased.
- Verify that informed consent was obtained, including consent for anesthesia and agitated saline contrast injection, if required. ***Rationale:*** Informed consent is necessary before invasive procedures and the administration of conscious sedation. Informed consent protects the rights of the patient and makes a competent decision possible for the patient; however, in emergency circumstances, time may not allow the form to be signed.
- Instruct the patient to void before the procedure. ***Rationale:*** Voiding before the procedure minimizes disruption of the examination.
- Perform a preprocedure verification and time-out. ***Rationale:*** This ensures patient safety and confirms the correct patient, procedure, and equipment availability.
- Initiate or continue electrocardiographic monitoring, apply an automatic blood pressure cuff (if arterial blood pressure monitoring is not already in place), initiate oxygen saturation monitoring, and, if prescribed, initiate capnography. ***Rationale:*** These measures allow for close cardiovascular and respiratory monitoring during the procedure. Follow organizational practice regarding capnography monitoring.
- Ensure that the ordered IV access is in place and functional, usually a 20-gauge or larger IV. ***Rationale:*** IV access is needed to administer premedication and for possible emergency medications. A 20-gauge or larger IV is needed for the injection of contrast if prescribed.

- Maintain the prescribed IV infusion during the procedure. ***Rationale:*** IV infusion maintenance ensures that the IV is functioning and available should an emergency arise.
- Have the patient remove any dentures or dental prostheses. ***Rationale:*** Dentures may interfere with the safe passage of the transesophageal probe.
- Set up the suction system with the connecting tubing and a rigid pharyngeal suction tip device attached and ready for use. Check for adequate suction vacuum. ***Rationale:*** This setup is necessary for suctioning the patient's oral secretions during the procedure.
- Prepare the prescribed local anesthetics (e.g., benzocaine, viscous lidocaine); sedatives (e.g., midazolam, diazepam); analgesics (e.g., fentanyl, morphine sulfate); reversal agents (e.g., naloxone, flumazenil); medications to decrease salivary secretions as needed; and methylene blue (if benzocaine use is planned).[3] ***Rationale:*** Sedatives and analgesics reduce patient anxiety, promote comfort, facilitate cooperation during the procedure, and decrease myocardial workload. Reversal agents are required for emergencies. Methylene blue is needed to reverse methemoglobinemia if it occurs with the use of benzocaine.[3]
- Have agitated normal saline solution available per organization protocol if prescribed for saline contrast echocardiography (bubble study). ***Rationale:*** The contrast agent enhances the ability to evaluate the cardiac shunt.
- Administer supplemental oxygen as prescribed. ***Rationale:*** Administration of oxygen may be needed to maintain adequate patient oxygenation during the procedure.
- Have atropine available at the bedside. ***Rationale:*** Atropine is necessary if a vagal reaction occurs with the insertion and passage of the transesophageal probe.
- Have an ACLS cart, medications, and airway equipment available at the patient's side.[3] ***Rationale:*** Emergency equipment is necessary to have close by in case an emergency situation arises.

Procedure for Transesophageal Echocardiography (Assist)

Steps	Rationale	Special Considerations
1. **HH**		
2. **PE**		
3. Assist if needed as the provider anesthetizes the patient's posterior pharynx with the topical agent.	Decreases discomfort caused by passage of the probe.	If possible, allow the patient to sit up to increase comfort and decrease anxiety or the feeling of choking.
4. Assist the patient to the left-lateral decubitus position. Use pillows to ensure correct alignment of the patient's spine with the head and body.	The left-lateral decubitus position allows secretions to collect in the dependent areas of the mouth for ease of suctioning and to prevent aspiration in case the patient vomits.	Patients may be examined in the supine position if required by anatomy or hemodynamic stability or if the patient is endotracheally intubated.[3]
5. Reassess vital signs, oxygen saturation, capnography, neurological status, cardiac rhythm, respiratory status, and pain before administration of IV medications for moderate sedation.	Closely monitors the patient and determines whether there are any changes in the patient's condition.	

Procedure for Transesophageal Echocardiography (Assist)—*Continued*		
Steps	**Rationale**	**Special Considerations**
6. Administer IV medication for moderate sedation as prescribed.[3] **(Level D*)**	Allows the patient to cooperate in facilitating passage of the probe during the procedure.	Confirm that the appropriate antagonists are readily available. Continually assess the patient, as they may need additional medication throughout the procedure.
7. Assist the provider as needed with insertion of the probe.		Gag and cough reflexes may be compromised by topical anesthetics, and the patient may vomit as the probe is passed, increasing the risk for aspiration.
A. Prepare to insert a bite guard when directed by the provider.	The bite guard prevents the patient from biting the probe or the fingers of the physician, advanced practice nurse, or other healthcare professional and avoids damage to the teeth and mouth.	
B. Assist the provider as requested with lubrication of the probe and oropharynx and applying ultrasound contact gel or viscous lidocaine to the distal end of the probe.	Lubrication of the probe minimizes mucosal injury and irritation and facilitates the ease of passage of the probe. Contact gel transmits ultrasound signals.	
C. Ask the patient to slightly bend his or her head in a forward flex.	Proper head position eases insertion of the probe into the esophagus.	
D. Alternatively, if needed, assist the provider with the jaw-thrust technique if required to guide the probe insertion.		
E. Encourage the patient to simulate swallowing while the probe is passed if requested by the provider.	The swallowing maneuver causes the epiglottis to close the trachea and directs the probe into the esophagus.	Some providers may not want to draw attention to the throat and will not ask the patient to swallow, but rather will wait for a natural swallow motion to occur and then insert the probe.
F. Suction the oral secretions as needed to ensure patency of the airway.	Removes secretions. This may be needed due to the patient's diminished gag reflex and the inability of the patient to swallow oral secretions.	Manipulation of the probe may cause stimulation of secretions.
G. Provide the patient with reassurance and encouragement to keep the bite guard in place, maintain the required position, hold still without attempts to speak, and focus on his or her breathing pattern.	May decrease patient anxiety and promote patient cooperation.	Some patients may be able to tolerate the procedure without analgesia or anesthesia when encouragement is provided.[3]
8. Provide the provider with updates of the patient's status during the TEE procedure.	Keeps the provider informed of the patient's condition and possible need for additional sedation or analgesics.	
9. Assist with the administration of the saline contrast agent as prescribed and per institutional standards.[3,5]	The administration of saline contrast enhances the view of the cardiac structures and function.	Assist with instructing the patient to perform the Valsalva maneuver, sniffing, or coughing to enhance right-to-left shunting images, if requested by the provider.[5]

*Level D: Peer-reviewed professional and organizational standards with the support of clinical study recommendations.

Procedure continues on following page

Procedure for Transesophageal Echocardiography (Assist)—*Continued*

Steps	Rationale	Special Considerations
10. Assist if needed with removal of the probe.	Provides assistance.	Anesthetics may be less effective at the end of the procedure, increasing the gag and cough reflexes, thus increasing the patient's risk of vomiting as the probe is removed. Using a rigid pharyngeal suction-tip catheter, suction as necessary as the tube is removed to prevent aspiration.
11. Place the probe in an appropriate receptacle for cleaning.	Reduces the transmission of microorganisms and prepares the equipment for sterilization.	
12. Continue assessment and monitoring until the patient returns to baseline as prescribed; follow institutional protocols.	Ensures patient safety.	Keep the patient on the left side with his or her head slightly elevated until the gag, swallow, and cough reflexes are intact.
13. Discard used supplies in appropriate receptacles.	Removes and safely discards used supplies using standard precautions.	
14. ▣▣		

Expected Outcomes

- Clear visualization of cardiac structures and function
- Immediate preliminary diagnosis
- *Note:* Negative study results are helpful in excluding cardiac sources of compromise
- Patent airway
- Acceptable level of comfort with no adverse reactions to sedation or analgesia

Unexpected Outcomes

- Esophageal or gastric perforation
- Esophageal, oropharyngeal, or gastric injury or lacerations
- Oropharyngeal hematoma
- Vasovagal hypotension from esophageal manipulation
- Substernal chest pain
- Temporary dysphagia
- Aspiration
- Respiratory depression
- Hematoma in the oropharynx
- Unresolved hypotension or hypertension
- Arrhythmias, bradycardia, or tachycardia
- Laryngospasm
- Bronchospasm
- Change in neurological status
- Air embolism in patients with right-to-left shunt with use of saline contrast
- Heart failure
- Pain
- Methemoglobinemia

Patient Monitoring and Care

Steps	Rationale	Reportable Conditions
		These conditions should be reported to the provider if they persist despite nursing interventions.

Patient Monitoring and Care —*Continued*

Steps	Rationale	Reportable Conditions
1. Assess and monitor cardiovascular, respiratory, and neurological status at a minimum of 5-minute intervals during and 15-minute intervals after the TEE procedure until the patient's condition returns to baseline, the prescribed parameters (e.g., vital signs within 10% of baseline),[3] and as required by institutional standards.	Changes in vital signs; heart rhythm; capnography values; oxygenation; and neurological, respiratory, and cardiovascular status may indicate complications related to the procedure.	Changes in the following: • Neurological status • Oxygenation • Capnography • Heart rate and rhythm • Blood pressure • Respirations • Cardiovascular status
2. Maintain IV access and infusions as prescribed during and after the procedure.	Maintaining IV access and infusions ensures IV patency in case emergency medications are needed.	
3. Monitor the patient's sedation score using a tool (i.e., Modified Aldrete Score)[3] during and after the procedure following institutional standards.	Determines the patient's response to IV moderate sedation and the need for additional sedation.	• Sedation score outside of prescribed parameters • Worsening sedation score after discontinuation of the sedation
4. Assess pain at a minimum of 5-minute intervals during and 15-minute intervals after the TEE procedure until the patient's condition returns to baseline. Administer analgesia as prescribed.	May indicate a complication of the procedure or identify the need for pain interventions. Mild throat discomfort is common as the topical anesthetic wears off.	• New onset of pain • Unresolved discomfort not relieved after the probe is removed • Unusual throat discomfort
5. Monitor for signs and symptoms of esophageal trauma or perforation.[3,4]	Identifies complications.	• Dysphagia • Odynophagia • Mackler's triad: vomiting, chest pain, and subcutaneous emphysema • Fever • Agitation • Tachycardia • Hypotension • Chest pain • Respiratory distress • Tachypnea • Dyspnea • Pneumothorax • Pleural effusions
6. Monitor for intraprocedural complications or reasons to terminate the TEE early.[3]	Determines the patient's response to the procedure and identifies complications.	• Patient becomes agitated and is unable to cooperate with the procedure • Change in neurological status • Dental or oropharyngeal trauma • Apnea • Hypoxemia • Hypercapnia • New arrhythmia • New hypotension or hypertension • Perforation or subcutaneous emphysema • GI or other bleeding • Chest pain • Benzocaine-induced methemoglobinemia

Procedure continues on following page

Patient Monitoring and Care —*Continued*

Steps	Rationale	Reportable Conditions
7. Monitor patients who received benzocaine for symptoms of methemoglobinemia. Prepare to treat methemoglobinemia with supplemental oxygen and methylene blue solution given by slow IV administration as prescribed.[3]	Severe methemoglobinemia is life threatening.	• Dyspnea • Nausea • Tachycardia • Cyanosis • Decreased pulse oximetry levels
8. Assess the patient for the return of normal pharyngeal function. If the patient is not upright, keep the patient on his or her left side with the head of the bed elevated until the gag, swallow, and cough reflexes are intact.	The topical anesthesia decreases the gag, swallow, and cough reflexes and increases the risk of aspiration.	• Prolonged absence of gag, swallowing, or cough reflexes
9. Offer clear liquids, and gradually progress to solid food after return of pharyngeal function as prescribed.	Topical anesthesia decreases the gag reflex and increases the risk of aspiration.	• Nausea • Vomiting • Stomach discomfort • Increase in odynophagia or dysphagia after 24 hours, may possibly indicate soft tissue or esophageal injury.[3]
10. Ask the patient to repeat his or her understanding of the postprocedural instructions.	Having patients repeat the postprocedural instructions confirms their understanding of what they should and should not do.	• Patient unable to understand postprocedural instructions
11. Ensure the safety of the ambulatory patient. Ensure that vital signs have returned to 10% of baseline before ambulation.[3] Have a family member or friend explain postprocedure education and sign appropriate documents as needed. Advise the patient to refrain from important decisions and driving while the effects anesthetic remain (i.e., for the remainder of the day). Provide the patient with a copy of the written discharge instructions per institutional protocols. Counsel the patient to call the provider if odynophagia or dysphagia persists for 24 hours.[3] Ensure that the patient is accompanied by a responsible adult.	This information is provided to patients who are being discharged.	

Documentation

Documentation should include the following:
- Date and time of procedure
- Initial patient assessment
- Patient and family education
- Preprocedural verifications and time out
- Completion of informed consent form
- Vital signs, pulse oximetry, capnography, neurological status, respiratory status, and pain evaluation immediately before sedation and during and after the procedure
- Establishment and assessment of IV patency

References and Additional Readings

For a complete list of references and additional readings for this procedure, scan this QR code with your smartphone, or visit https://www.elsevier.com/__data/assets/pdf_file/0006/1319847/Chapter0072.pdf.

PROCEDURE

73 Arterial Puncture

Mindy Stites

PURPOSE Arterial puncture is performed to obtain a sample of blood for arterial blood gas (ABG) analysis.

PREREQUISITE NURSING KNOWLEDGE

- An ABG analysis measures the pH and the partial pressure of oxygen and carbon dioxide. ABG samples are also analyzed for oxygen saturation and for bicarbonate values. These analyses are done primarily to evaluate a patient's oxygenation status, acid-base balance, and ventilation. Additional laboratory tests (e.g., electrolytes, ammonia and lactate levels) can be performed on arterial blood samples.
- Indications for ABGs vary and include patients with chronic and acute respiratory disorders (e.g., chronic obstructive pulmonary disease, pneumonia, adult respiratory lung disease) and acute metabolic or shock disorders (e.g., sepsis, post–cardiac arrest, acute kidney injury). ABG analysis frequently is performed on patients in shock, receiving oxygen or mechanical ventilation therapies, or experiencing changes in respiratory therapy or status.
- Principles of aseptic technique.
- Anatomy and physiology of the vasculature and adjacent structures.
- The brachial artery is a continuation of the axillary artery in the upper extremity. It bifurcates just below the elbow (Fig. 73.1). From the bifurcation, the ulnar artery moves down the forearm on the medial side and the radial artery on the lateral side.
- The preferred artery for arterial puncture is the radial artery. Although this artery is smaller than the ulnar artery, it is more superficial and can be stabilized more easily during the procedure. The use of the brachial artery is a safe and reliable alternative site for arterial puncture.
- At times, the femoral artery is used for arterial puncture. The use of this artery can be technically difficult because of the proximity of the artery to the femoral vein (Fig. 73.2).
- Arterial cannulation is considered for patients who need frequent arterial blood samples, continuous arterial pressure monitoring, or evaluation of vasoactive medication therapy (see Procedures 52, Arterial Catheter Insertion [Perform] and 53, Arterial Catheter Insertion [Assist], Care, and Removal).
- The most common complications associated with arterial puncture include pain, vasospasm, hematoma formation, infection, hemorrhage, and neurovascular compromise.[1,4,7,10]

- Site selection proceeds as follows:
  - Use the radial artery as first choice. The radial artery is small and easily stabilized because it passes over a bony groove located at the wrist (see Fig. 73.1).
  - Use the brachial artery as second choice, except in the presence of poor pulsation from shock, obesity, or sclerotic vessel (e.g., because of previous cardiac catheterization). The brachial artery is larger than the radial artery. There is risk of median nerve injury because of its proximity to the brachial artery. Hemostasis after arterial puncture is enhanced by its proximity to bone if the entry point is approximately 1.5 inches above the antecubital fossa (see Fig. 73.1).
  - Use the femoral artery in the case of cardiopulmonary arrest or altered perfusion to the upper extremities. The femoral artery is a large superficial artery located in the groin (see Fig. 73.2). It is easily palpated and punctured. Complications related to femoral artery puncture include hemorrhage and hematoma because bleeding can be difficult to control; inadvertent puncture of the femoral vein because of close proximity to the artery; infection because aseptic technique in the groin area is difficult to maintain; and limb ischemia if the femoral artery is damaged.
- Ultrasound guidance can be used for arterial puncture if the technology is available.[1,7,9,11,12]

EQUIPMENT

- One prepackaged ABG kit that contains the following:
  - One 20- to 25-gauge, 1- to 1.5-inch hypodermic needle (Note: longer needles are needed for brachial and femoral artery puncture)
  - One 1- to 5-mL preheparinized (if available) syringe with a rubber stopper or cap
  - One 1-mL ampule of sodium heparin, 1:1000 concentration (if preheparinized syringe is not available)
  - Two 2 × 2 gauze pads
  - 2% chlorhexidine-based antiseptic solution
  - 70% isopropyl alcohol prep pad
  - One plastic bag (for transport of sample to the laboratory)
  - One adhesive bandage

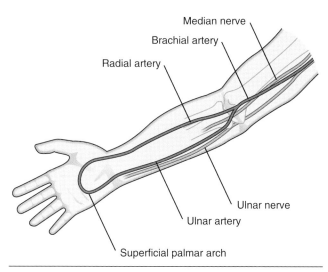

Figure 73.1 Anatomical landmarks for locating the radial and brachial arteries.

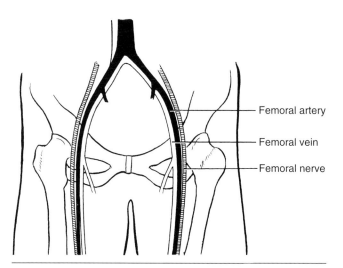

Figure 73.2 Anatomical landmarks for locating the femoral artery.

- Appropriate laboratory form and specimen label
- One pair of nonsterile gloves and eye protection

Additional equipment, to have available as needed, includes the following:
- Small, rolled towel (to support the patient's wrist)
- Sterile gloves
- 1-mL syringe with 25-gauge needle (if lidocaine is used)
- 1% lidocaine (without epinephrine), 1-mL, or eutectic mixture of local anesthetics (EMLA) cream
- Bedside ultrasound machine with vascular probe
- Sterile ultrasound probe cover
- Sterile ultrasound gel

PATIENT AND FAMILY EDUCATION

- Explain the reason for the arterial puncture to the patient and family. *Rationale:* Clarification of information is an expressed patient and family need and helps diminish anxiety, enhance acceptance, and encourage questions.
- Describe the overall steps of the procedure, including the patient's role in the procedure. *Rationale:* This explanation decreases patient anxiety, enhances cooperation, provides an opportunity for the patient to voice concerns, and prevents accidental movement during the procedure.

PATIENT ASSESSMENT AND PREPARATION

Patient Assessment

- Determine the need for arterial cannulation versus puncture. *Rationale:* Repeated arterial punctures increase patient discomfort and the risk for complications.
- Assess for factors that influence ABG measurements, including anxiety, endotracheal suctioning, nebulizer treatment, change in oxygen therapy/ventilator settings, renal replacement therapy, medications and IV fluid composition, patient positioning, body temperature, metabolic rate, and respiratory status. *Rationale:* These conditions or therapies can alter blood gas analysis results.
- Review the patient's current anticoagulation therapy, known blood dyscrasias, and pertinent laboratory values (e.g., platelets, partial thromboplastin time, prothrombin time, and international normalized ratio) before the procedure. *Rationale:* Anticoagulation therapy, blood dyscrasias, or alterations in coagulation studies could prolong hemostasis at the puncture site and increase the risk for hematoma formation or hemorrhage.
- Review the patient's allergy history (e.g., lidocaine, antiseptic solutions, tape). *Rationale:* Assessment decreases the risk for allergic reactions.
- Review the patient's past surgical history (e.g., use of radial artery for coronary artery bypass surgery, fistulas, or shunts). *Rationale:* Arterial puncture should be avoided in extremities affected by these conditions.
- Ascertain the patient's nondominant hand, if possible. *Rationale:* A complication to the nondominant hand may have fewer consequences.

Patient Preparation

- Verify the correct patient with two identifiers. *Rationale:* Before performing a procedure, the nurse should ensure the correct identification of the patient for the intended intervention.
- Ensure that the patient and family understand the preprocedural teaching. Answer questions as they arise, and reinforce information as needed. *Rationale:* Understanding of previously taught information is evaluated and reinforced.
- If the patient is receiving oxygen or mechanical ventilation, check that the current therapy has been underway for at least 20 to 30 minutes before obtaining ABG.[3] *Rationale:* Ensures that the ABG results reflect the intervention/therapy change.
- Position the patient appropriately. *Rationale:* Positioning enhances accessibility to the insertion site and promotes patient comfort.
- Radial artery puncture
  - ❖ Assist the patient to a semirecumbent position. *Rationale:* A position of comfort decreases anxiety and may facilitate respiratory effort.

UNIT II

❖ Hyperextend the wrist. A small rolled towel may be placed under the wrist for support. ***Rationale:*** This action moves the artery closer to the skin surface, making the artery easier to palpate.

❖ Palpate for the presence of a strong radial pulse. ***Rationale:*** Identification and localization of the pulse increases the chance of a successful arterial puncture.

• Brachial artery puncture

❖ Assist the patient to a semi-recumbent position. ***Rationale:*** A position of comfort decreases anxiety and may facilitate respiratory effort.

❖ Supinate the patient's arm. A small pillow may be placed under the arm for support. ***Rationale:*** This action increases accessibility for puncture.

❖ Rotate the patient's arm, and palpate for the presence of a strong brachial pulse. ***Rationale:*** Identification and localization of the pulse increase the chance of a successful arterial puncture.

• Femoral artery puncture

❖ Assist the patient to the supine, straight-leg position with the head of bed as flat as the patient can tolerate. ***Rationale:*** This position provides the best position for localizing the femoral artery pulse.

❖ Palpate for the presence of a strong femoral pulse. ***Rationale:*** Identification and localization of the pulse increase the chance of a successful arterial puncture.

Procedure   for Arterial Puncture

Steps	Rationale	Special Considerations
1. 🄷🄷		
2. Verify blood flow through the radial artery by performing the modified Allen's test (Fig. 73.3) or a Doppler ultrasound examination before the puncture.	Assess the patency of the ulnar artery and an intact superficial palmar arch.	The modified Allen's test does not always ensure adequate flow through the ulnar artery.[2,5,6,8,10] A Doppler ultrasound flow indicator can also be used to further verify blood flow.[1,2,5-8,10-12]

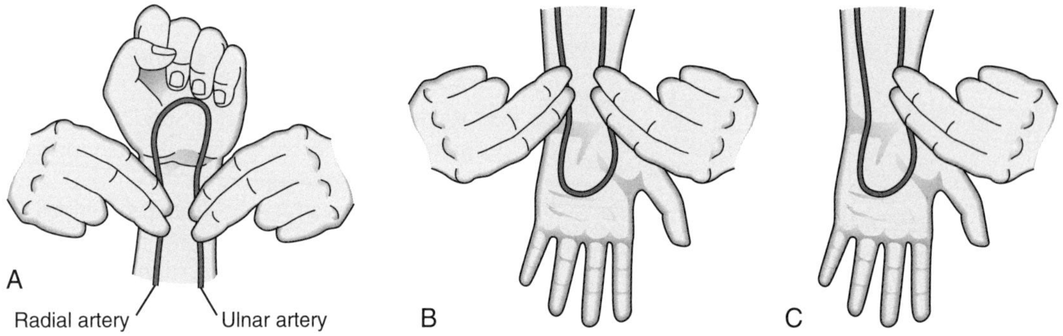

A   Radial artery   Ulnar artery   B   C

Figure 73.3   Modified Allen's test. Elevate the patient's hand, and instruct the patient to open and close the fist several times. **A,** With the patient's fist clenched, simultaneously occlude the radial and ulnar arteries. **B,** Instruct the patient to lower and open the fist. Observe for pallor in the patient's hand. **C,** Release the pressure over the ulnar artery, and observe the hand for the return of color. *(From Bucher L, Melander SD: Critical care nursing, Philadelphia, 1999, Saunders.)*

3. If a preheparinized syringe is not available, heparinize the syringe and needle.	Prevents specimen coagulation.	A small-bore needle is less likely to cause vasospasm of the artery during the procedure.
A. Assemble a 22-gauge needle on the syringe, and prime the entire syringe barrel and needle with heparin as per institutional protocols.	Prepares the syringe.	
B. Expel the heparin from the syringe.	Excess heparin in the syringe can lower the pH and partial pressure of carbon dioxide.	
C. Eliminate any visible air bubbles from the syringe.	Maintains the accuracy of ABG values.	
4. Prepare the site with an antiseptic solution (e.g., 2% chlorhexidine-based preparation).	Limits the introduction of potentially infectious skin flora into the vessel during the puncture.	

Procedure continues on following page

Procedure | **for Arterial Puncture** —*Continued*

Steps	Rationale	Special Considerations
A. Cleanse the site with a back-and-forth motion while applying friction for 30 seconds. B. Allow the antiseptic solution to dry.		
5. Locally anesthetize the puncture site per provider orders and/or institutional protocols.[4,10,13] **(Level C*)**	Provides local anesthesia for arterial puncture.	Most patients report pain during the arterial puncture.[13] Patients have reported reduced pain when a local, intradermal anesthetic agent is used before the arterial puncture.[13]
A. Use a 1-mL syringe with a 25-gauge needle to draw up 0.5 mL of 1% lidocaine without epinephrine.	Minimizes vessel trauma. The absence of epinephrine decreases the risk for peripheral vasoconstriction.	Medications such as lidocaine ointment, amethocaine gel, and EMLA cream may reduce arterial puncture pain.[1,10,13]
B. Aspirate before injecting the local anesthetic.	Determines whether a blood vessel has been inadvertently entered.	
C. Inject intradermally and then with full infiltration around the artery puncture site. Use approximately 0.2–0.3 mL for an adult.	Decreases the incidence of localized pain with injection of all skin layers.	
6. Preset the plunger to the desired sample volume.	Ensures adequate sample volume.	
7. Perform the percutaneous puncture of the selected artery.		Ultrasound technology may be used to assist with insertion.[9]
A. Palpate and stabilize the artery with the index and middle fingers of the nondominant hand.	Increases the likelihood of correctly locating the artery and decreases the chance of vessel rolling.	Use sterile gloves if the site of the artery puncture is palpated after it is antiseptically prepared.
B. With the needle bevel up and the syringe at a 30- to 60-degree angle to the radial or brachial artery, puncture the skin slowly (Figs. 73.4 and 73.5). For a femoral artery puncture, a 60- to 90-degree angle is used (Fig. 73.6).	A slow, gradual approach promotes entry into the artery without inadvertently passing through the posterior wall.	Enter at an angle that is comfortable; certainty of position is more important than angle entry. If too much force is used, the needle may touch the periosteum of the bone and cause considerable pain.

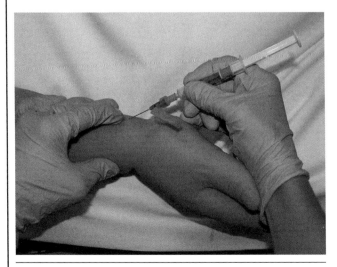

Figure 73.4 Radial artery puncture with the syringe at a 30-degree angle to the artery.

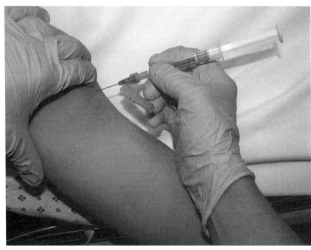

Figure 73.5 Brachial artery puncture with the syringe at a 45-degree angle to the artery.

*Level C: Qualitative studies, descriptive or correlational studies, integrative reviews, systematic reviews, or randomized controlled trials with inconsistent results.

UNIT II

Procedure | for Arterial Puncture —*Continued*

Steps	Rationale	Special Considerations

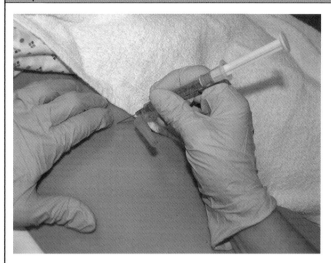

Figure 73.6 Femoral artery puncture with the syringe at a 60-degree angle to the artery.

Steps	Rationale	Special Considerations
C. Observe the syringe for a flashback of blood.	Pulsation of blood into the syringe verifies that the artery has been punctured.	Gentle aspiration may be necessary.
D. If the puncture is unsuccessful, withdraw the needle to just under skin level, angle slightly toward the artery, and readvance. Do not withdraw the needle.	Prevents the necessity of a second puncture and changes the needle angle to facilitate the location of the artery.	Excessive probing of the artery may cause vessel or adjacent nerve injury.
E. Obtain 1 mL of blood.	An ABG analysis requires a minimum of 0.2 mL of blood.	Sample volumes may vary with equipment used. Obtain more than 1 mL of blood for additional laboratory tests, as necessary.
F. Withdraw the needle while stabilizing the barrel of the syringe.	Prevents inadvertent aspiration of air during withdrawal.	Equipment may vary. If a safety guard is available, it should be snapped onto the needle with a one-handed technique by gently pressing the device against a hard surface.
8. Press a gauze pad firmly over the puncture site for several minutes or until hemostasis is established.	Hematomas and hemorrhage can occur if pressure is not applied and maintained correctly. Hematomas can cause circulatory impedance and pain, and they can predispose to infection.	If the patient is receiving anticoagulation therapy or has a bleeding dyscrasia, pressure may need to be applied for as long as 15 minutes.
9. Cover the puncture site with an adhesive bandage once hemostasis is achieved.	Covers the site until healing occurs.	
10. Check the blood sample in the syringe for air bubbles, and express any air bubbles by slowly ejecting the air while covering the syringe tip with a 2 × 2 gauze pad.	Air bubbles can alter the partial pressure of oxygen results.[3,10]	If a safety guard is present, it should be removed and a blood/air filter should be placed on the syringe. Excess air should be evacuated through the blood/air filter.
11. Activate the mechanisms of a safety needle to cover the needle before placing it in the ice cup. In the absence of a safety-engineered device, use a one-hand scoop technique to recap the needle after removal. Gently roll the syringe for 30 seconds.	Prevents leakage of blood and air from entering the sample. Mixes blood and heparin, thus preventing clot formation.	

Procedure continues on following page

Procedure for Arterial Puncture —*Continued*

Steps	Rationale	Special Considerations
12. Remove gloves, and discard used supplies in appropriate receptacles; dispose of needles and other sharp objects in appropriate containers.	Reduces the transmission of microorganisms; standard precautions. Safely removes sharp objects.	
13. 🔲		
14. Label the specimen, and complete the laboratory form. Note the percentage of oxygen therapy, respiratory rate, and ventilator settings, if appropriate, and the patient's temperature and time the specimen was drawn.	Helps the laboratory perform the analysis accurately.	Policies may vary regarding the type of patient information required for laboratory analysis.
15. Expedite the delivery of the sample to the laboratory.	Ideally, the blood gas analysis should be performed within 30 minutes of collection to ensure the accuracy of results.[3,10]	

Expected Outcomes

- The ABG sample is collected correctly such that the accuracy of the results is enhanced
- The puncture site remains free from hematoma, hemorrhage, and infection
- The peripheral vascular and neurovascular systems remain intact (free from complications)
- Alterations in the ABG results are identified and treated accordingly

Unexpected Outcomes

- Pain/severe discomfort during the procedure
- Complications during the puncture or vasospasm
- Complications after the puncture: changes in the color, size, temperature, sensation, movement, or pulse of the extremity used for the arterial puncture; hematoma, hemorrhage, or infection at the puncture site

Patient Monitoring and Care

Steps	Rationale	Special Considerations
		These conditions must be reported to the provider if they persist despite nursing interventions.
1. Observe the puncture site for signs of hemostasis after the procedure.	Postpuncture bleeding can occur in any patient but is more likely to occur in patients with coagulopathies or those who are receiving anticoagulation therapy.	- Bleeding - Hematoma - Changes in vital signs
2. Assess the puncture site and involved extremity for signs of postpuncture complications.	The arterial puncture can result in peripheral vascular and neurovascular compromise of the extremity distal to the puncture site.	- Changes in color, size, temperature, sensation, movement, or pulse in the extremity used for arterial puncture
3. Assess the puncture site for signs or symptoms of infection.	Determines the necessity for further treatment.	- Erythema, warmth, hardness, tenderness, or pain at the puncture site - Presence of purulent drainage from the puncture site
4. Follow institutional standards for assessing pain. Administer analgesia as prescribed.	Identifies the need for pain interventions.	- Pain at the puncture site or in the distal extremity

UNIT II

Documentation

Documentation should include the following:

- Patient and family education
- Arterial site accessed
- Number of attempts
- Local anesthetic used
- Patient's tolerance of the procedure
- Pain assessment and interventions
- Appearance of the site
- Appearance of the limb, color, pulse sensation, movement, capillary refill time, and temperature of the extremity
- Occurrence of unexpected outcomes
- Nursing interventions taken
- Laboratory results

References and Additional Readings

For a complete list of references and additional readings for this procedure, scan this QR code with your smartphone, or visit https://www.elsevier.com/__data/assets/pdf_file/0007/1319848/Chapter0073.pdf.

74 Central Venous Catheter AP Insertion (Perform)

Brandi L. Holcomb

PURPOSE Central venous catheters (CVCs) are inserted for measurement of central venous pressure (CVP) with jugular or subclavian catheter placement. The CVC is generally inserted using either the internal jugular vein (IJ), the subclavian vein (SCV), or the femoral vein site. Clinically useful information can be obtained about right-ventricular preload, cardiovascular status, and fluid balance in patients who do not need pulmonary artery pressure monitoring. Large-bore CVCs allow fluids or blood products to be rapidly infused in the event of acute hemorrhage resulting from trauma or other forms of acute bleeding. CVCs also are placed for infusion of vasoactive medications and to provide access for pulmonary artery catheters and transvenous pacemakers.

PREREQUISITE NURSING KNOWLEDGE

- Normal anatomy and physiology of the cardiovascular system.
- Anatomy and physiology of the vasculature and adjacent structures of the neck, groin, and chest.
- Principles of sterile technique.
- Clinical and technical competence in central line insertion and suturing.
- Competence in chest radiographic interpretation.
- Advanced cardiac life support (ACLS) knowledge and skills.
- Potential complications and associated interventions/consultations for addressing issues.
- Follow guidelines regarding institution credentialing.
- Ultrasonography technique.
- Indications for CVC placement may include the following:
  - Severe blood loss
  - Hemodynamic instability
  - Administration of vesicant irritant medications
  - Administration of total parenteral nutrition
  - Lack of peripheral venous access
  - Assessment of hypovolemia or hypervolemia
  - Monitoring of CVPs
  - Placement of pulmonary artery catheters or placement of transvenous pacemakers
  - Hemodialysis access
- The normal CVP value is 2 to 8 mm Hg.
- The CVP waveform is identical to the right-atrial waveform.[5]
- Interpretation of right-atrial/CVP waveforms including identification of *a, c,* and *v* waves is important. The *a*

wave reflects right-atrial contraction. The *c* wave reflects closure of the tricuspid valve. The *v* wave reflects passive filling of the right atria during right-ventricular systole.

- The CVP provides information regarding right-heart filling pressures and right-ventricular function and volume.[5]
- The CVP is commonly elevated during or after right-ventricular failure, ischemia, or infarction because of decreased compliance of the right ventricle.[5]
- The CVP can be helpful in the determination of hypovolemia. The CVP value is low if the patient is hypovolemic. Venodilation also decreases the CVP value.[5]
- Electrocardiographic monitoring is essential in the accurate interpretation of the CVP value.
- Some contraindications of CVC insertion include anatomical problems, venous obstruction, and coagulopathies. The subclavian site should be avoided in hemodialysis patients and patients with advanced kidney disease to avoid subclavian vein stenosis.[4]
- It is important to weigh the risks and benefits of placing a CVC against the risk for mechanical complications (e.g., pneumothorax, vein laceration, thrombosis, air embolism, misplacement).[4,7]
- A subclavian site is recommended rather than a jugular or femoral site to minimize the risk of infection.[4,5,8]
- The internal jugular site is recommended to minimize catheter cannulation–related risk of injury or trauma.[5,7,8]
- Ultrasound guidance is recommended to place CVCs if the technology is available to reduce the number of cannulation attempts and mechanical complications.[3,4,8,9]
- Regardless of the site selected, complications may occur during or after insertion of a CVC (Table 74.1).

EQUIPMENT

- CVC insertion kit
- CVC of choice (single, dual, or triple lumen) usually supplied with insertion needle, dilator, syringe, and guidewire.

UNIT II

TABLE 74.1   Complications of Central Venous Catheter Insertion

Complication	Clinical Manifestation	Treatment	Prevention

Pneumothorax	• Sudden respiratory distress
	• Chest pain
	• Hypoxia/cyanosis
	• Decreased breath sounds
	• Resonance to percussion
		• Confirmation with chest radiograph
		• Symptomatic treatment
		• Small pneumothorax:
		  • Close monitoring
		  • Daily chest radiograph
		  • O_2
		  • Large pneumothorax:
		  • Chest tube
		  • Cardiopulmonary support
			• Proper patient preparation
			• Sedation as necessary
			• Proper patient positioning
			• Technique and angle of the needle/catheter on insertion
			• Avoidance of multiple passes with the needle
			• Healthcare provider is skilled and experienced in insertion technique
			• Direct visualization with bedside ultrasonography for internal jugular placement

Tension pneumothorax	• Most likely to occur in patients on ventilator support
	• Respiratory distress
	• Rapid clinical deterioration:
	  • Cyanosis
	  • Jugular venous distention (may not be present with severe hypovolemia)
	  • Hypotension
	  • Decreased cardiac output
		• Treatment must be rapid and aggressive
		• Immediate air aspiration followed by chest tube
		• Cardiopulmonary support
			• Proper patient preparation
			• Sedation as necessary
			• Proper patient positioning
			• Reduction of positive end-expiratory pressure to ≤5 cm H_2O at the time of venipuncture
			• Technique and angle of the needle/catheter on insertion
			• Avoidance of multiple passes with the needle
			• Healthcare provider is skilled and experienced in insertion technique
			• Use of peripherally inserted CVC

Delayed pneumothorax	• Slow onset of respiratory symptoms • Subcutaneous emphysema • Persistent pleuritic chest or back pain • Insidious increase in peak airway pressures in ventilated patients	• Confirmation with chest radiograph • Chest tube • Cardiopulmonary support	• Proper patient preparation • Sedation as necessary • Proper patient positioning • Technique and angle of the needle/catheter on insertion • Avoidance of multiple passes with the needle • Healthcare provider is skilled and experienced in insertion technique • Use of peripherally inserted CVC
Hydrothorax hydromediastinum	• Dyspnea • Chest pain • Muffled breath sounds • High glucose level of chest drainage • Low-grade fever	• Stop infusion • Confirmation with chest radiograph • Cardiopulmonary support	• Proper patient preparation • Sedation as necessary • Proper patient positioning • Technique and angle of the needle/catheter on insertion • Avoidance of multiple passes with the needle • Healthcare provider is skilled and experienced in insertion technique • Use of peripherally inserted CVC • Placement of catheter tip in lower superior vena cava • Aspiration of blood before catheter use to confirm vascular placement

TABLE 74.1	Complications of Central Venous Catheter Insertion—cont'd		
Complication	Clinical Manifestation	Treatment	Prevention
Hemothorax	• Respiratory distress • Hypovolemic shock • Hematoma in the neck with jugular insertions	• Confirmation with chest radiograph • Chest tube • Thoracotomy for arterial repair if indicated	• Correction of coagulopathies before insertion • Avoidance of multiple passes with the needle • Evaluation with Doppler scan studies or venogram of suspected thrombosis from prior cannulation before insertion

Arterial puncture/laceration	• Return of bright red blood in the syringe under high pressure
	• Pulsatile blood flow on disconnection of the syringe
	• Arterial waveform/pressures when the catheter is connected to the transducer system
	• Arterial saturation of sample sent for blood gas analysis
	• Deterioration of clinical status:
	  • Hemorrhagic shock
	  • Respiratory distress
	  • Bleeding from the catheter site may or may not be observed
	• Deviation of the trachea with a large hematoma in the neck
	• Hemothorax may be detected on chest radiograph
		• Application of pressure for 3–5 minutes or as needed to promote hemostasis after removal of the needle
		• Elevate the head of the bed if condition is hemodynamically stable
		• Chest tube as indicated
		• Thoracotomy for arterial repair if indicated
			• Correction of coagulopathies before insertion
			• Avoidance of multiple passes with the needle
			• Evaluation with Doppler scan studies or venogram of suspected thrombosis from prior cannulation before insertion
			• Use of small-gauge needle to first locate the vein
			• Direct visualization with bedside ultrasonography for femoral vein placement

Bleeding/hematoma; venous or arterial bleeding	• Bleeding from the insertion site • Hematoma formation not likely to be seen with the subclavian approach • Bleeding may occur internally without visible evidence • Tracheal compression • Respiratory distress • Carotid compression • Pain at the insertion site	• Application of pressure to the insertion site • Thoracotomy for arterial repair • Tracheostomy for tracheal deviation from hematoma • With the femoral approach, manual pressure slightly above the inadvertent arterial puncture site (see Procedure 69, Femoral Artery and Venous Sheath Removal) • If retroperitoneal bleeding occurs, external signs may not be apparent except for signs of hypovolemia. Computed tomography (CT) of the abdomen may be required for diagnosis.	• Correction of coagulopathies before insertion • Avoidance of multiple passes with the needle at venipuncture • Use of a small-gauge needle to first locate the vein • Immediate control of femoral bleeding may prevent large blood loss or hematoma formation
Cardiac dysrhythmias	• Premature atrial complexes • Atrial fibrillation or flutter • Premature ventricular complexes • Supraventricular tachycardia • Ventricular tachycardia • Sudden cardiovascular collapse	• Withdraw the guidewire or catheter from the heart; dysrhythmias should stop if the cause was mechanical in nature • Pharmacological treatment of persistent dysrhythmias	• Avoidance of entry into the heart with the guidewire • Observation of cardiac monitor; tall, peaked P waves can be identified as the catheter tip enters the right atrium

Continued

TABLE 74.1	Complications of Central Venous Catheter Insertion—cont'd		
Complication	Clinical Manifestation	Treatment	Prevention
Air embolism	• Symptoms depend on amount of air drawn in, especially with patients who are spontaneously breathing • Sudden cardiovascular collapse • Tachypnea, apnea, tachycardia • Hypotension, cyanosis, anxiety • Diffuse pulmonary wheezes • "Mill wheel" churning heart murmur • Neurological deficits, paresis, stroke, coma • Cardiac arrest	• Stop airflow • Position the patient on the left side in the Trendelenburg position • Oxygen administration • Air aspiration; transthoracic needle or intracardiac catheter • Cardiopulmonary support	• Adequate hydration status • Head-down tilt or the Trendelenburg position during catheter insertion • Use of small-bore needle for insertion • Application of thumb over needle or catheter hub during ventilation; needle or hub should not be exposed longer than 1 second • Advancement of catheter during positive-pressure cycle in patients on ventilatory support • Avoidance of nicking of catheter with careful suturing technique • Avoidance of catheter exchange from a large-bore catheter (pulmonary artery) to a smaller catheter • Use of Luer-Lok connections • Minimal risk with peripherally inserted CVC
Catheter malposition	• Pain in the ear or neck • Swishing sound in the ear with infusion • Sharp anterior chest pain • Pain in the ipsilateral shoulder blade • Cardiac dysrhythmia • Observation on chest radiograph • Signs or symptoms may be absent • No blood return on aspiration	• Ensure that the bevel of the insertion needle is positioned downward (toward the feet of the patient) before placing the guidewire • Repositioning of the catheter with the guidewire or new venipuncture • Catheter removal	• Proper patient positioning • Avoidance of use of force when advancing the catheter • Use of a guidewire or blunt-tipped stylet
Catheter embolism	• Cardiac dysrhythmias • Chest pain • Dyspnea • Hypotension • Tachycardia • May be clinically silent	• Location of fragment on radiograph • Transvenous retrieval of catheter fragment • Thoracotomy • Interventional radiology retrieval	• Use of "over a guidewire" (Seldinger) insertion technique • Extreme caution with use of through-the-needle catheter designs; never withdraw a catheter through the needle • Use of guidewire or stylet within a catheter that is inserted through a needle
Cardiac tamponade	• Retrosternal or epigastric pain • Dyspnea • Venous engorgement of the face and neck • Restlessness, confusion • Hypotension, paradoxical pulse • Muffled heart sounds • Mediastinal widening • Pleural effusion • Cardiac arrest	• Treatment must be rapid and aggressive • Discontinuation of infusions through the central line • Aspiration through the catheter • Emergency pericardiocentesis • Emergency thoracotomy	• Catheter tip position: Parallel to the walls of the superior vena cava 1–2 cm above the junction of the superior vena cava and right atrium • Use of soft, flexible catheters • Minimal risk with peripherally inserted CVC
Tracheal injury	• Subcutaneous emphysema • Pneumomediastinum • Air trapping between the chest wall and the pleura • Respiratory distress with puncture of endotracheal tube cuff	• Emergency reintubation (for punctured endotracheal tube cuff) • Aspiration of air in mediastinum	• Physician, advanced practice nurse, or other healthcare professional is skilled and experienced in insertion technique • Use of peripherally inserted CVC

TABLE 74.1	Complications of Central Venous Catheter Insertion—cont'd		
Complication	Clinical Manifestation	Treatment	Prevention
Nerve injury	• Patient has tingling/numbness in arm or fingers • Shooting pain down the arm • Paralysis • Diaphragmatic paralysis (phrenic nerve injury)	• Remove catheter if brachial plexus injury is suspected	• Physician, advanced practice nurse, or other healthcare professional is skilled and experienced in insertion technique • Minimal risk with peripherally inserted CVC
Sterile thrombophlebitis	• Potential complication of the peripherally inserted CVC • Redness, tenderness, swelling along the course of the vein • Pain in the upper extremity or shoulder	• Application of heat for 48–72 hours • Removal of catheter	• Strict aseptic technique during catheter insertion • Adequate skin preparation
Pulmonary embolism	• Potential complication of catheter exchange • Often clinically silent • Chest pain, dyspnea, coughing, tachycardia, anxiety, fever	• Spiral chest CT scan • Lung perfusion scan • Cardiopulmonary support with large pulmonary embolism	• Avoidance of catheter exchange in veins with thrombosis

CVC, Central venous catheter.

- Full sterile drapes
- 1% lidocaine without epinephrine
- One 25-gauge ⅝-inch needle
- Large package of 4 × 4 gauze sponges
- Suture kit (hemostat, scissors, needle holder)
- 3-0 or 4-0 nylon suture with curved needle
- Syringes: one 10- to 12-mL syringe; two 3- to 5-mL syringes; two 22-gauge, 1½-inch needles
- Masks, head coverings, goggles (shield and mask combination may be used), sterile gloves, and sterile gowns
- No. 11 scalpel
- Roll of 2-inch tape
- Dressing supplies
- Waterproof pad
- Chlorhexidine-impregnated sponge
- Antiseptic solution (e.g., 2% chlorhexidine-based preparation)
- Nonsterile gloves
- Normal saline flush syringes or 0.9% sodium chloride vials, 10- to 30-mL
- Bedside ultrasound machine with vascular probe
- Sterile ultrasound probe cover

Additional equipment, to have available as needed, includes the following:
- Hemodynamic monitoring system (see Procedure 60, Single-Pressure and Multiple-Pressure Transducer Systems)
- Sutureless catheter securement device
- Intravenous (IV) solution with Luer-Lok administration set for IV infusion
- Luer-Lok extension tubing
- Bedside monitor and oscilloscope with pulse oximetry
- Supplemental oxygen supplies
- Emergency equipment
- Package of alcohol pads or swab sticks
- Package of povidone-iodine pads or swab sticks
- Heparin flushes
- Sterile injectable or noninjectable caps
- Skin protectant pads or swab sticks

PATIENT AND FAMILY EDUCATION

- Explain the need for the CVC insertion, and assess patient and family understanding. *Rationale:* Clarification and understanding of information decrease patient and family anxiety levels.
- Explain the procedure and the time involved. *Rationale:* Explanation increases patient cooperation and decreases patient and family anxiety levels.
- Explain the need for sterile technique and patient positioning and that the patient's face may be covered. *Rationale:* The explanation decreases patient anxiety and elicits cooperation.
- Explain the benefits and potential risks for the procedure. *Rationale:* Information is offered so the patient and/or family can make an informed decision.

PATIENT ASSESSMENT AND PREPARATION

Patient Assessment

- Determine the patient's medical history including neck, chest, and groin surgeries and previous vascular access devices. *Rationale:* Data obtained will assist with site selection.
- Determine the patient's medical history of pneumothorax or emphysema. *Rationale:* Patients with emphysematous lungs may be at increased risk for puncture and pneumothorax, depending on the approach.
- Determine the patient's medical history of anomalous veins. *Rationale:* Patients may have a history of dextrocardia or transposition of the great vessels, which leads to greater difficulty in catheter placement.
- Assess the intended insertion site. *Rationale:* Scar tissue may impede placement of the catheter. Permanent pacemakers or implantable cardioverter defibrillators may

preclude placement. Previous surgery and previous placement of a CVC may cause a thrombus to be present, or there may be stenosis of a vessel.

- Assess the patient's neurological, cardiac, and pulmonary status. *Rationale:* Aids in determining whether the patient can tolerate the Trendelenburg position.
- Assess vital signs and pulse oximetry. *Rationale:* Baseline data enable rapid identification of changes.
- Assess electrolyte levels (e.g., potassium, magnesium, calcium). *Rationale:* Electrolyte abnormalities may increase cardiac irritability.
- Assess for a coagulopathic state, and determine whether the patient has recently received anticoagulant or thrombolytic therapy. *Rationale:* These patients are more likely to have complications related to bleeding. Therefore site selection and the need/ability to provide interventions before insertion of the CVC can be determined prospectively.[6]

Patient Preparation

- Verify the correct patient with two identifiers. *Rationale:* This increases patient safety by ensuring correct identification of the patient for the intended intervention.

- Ensure that the patient and family understand the preprocedural teaching. Answer questions as they arise, and reinforce information as needed. *Rationale:* Understanding of previously taught information is evaluated and reinforced.
- Obtain informed consent. *Rationale:* Informed consent protects the rights of the patient and makes a competent decision possible for the patient; however, in emergency circumstances, time may not allow for this form to be signed.
- Perform a preprocedural verification and time out, *Rationale:* This ensures patient safety.
- Prescribe sedation or analgesics as needed. *Rationale:* The patient may need sedation or analgesics to promote comfort and to ensure adequate cooperation and appropriate placement.
- Place an order for patient restraints, and apply if needed. *Rationale:* In patients with cognitive impairment, restraints may be needed to ensure maintenance of patient positioning and equipment and access site sterility. During the procedure, restlessness and an altered level of consciousness may represent a pneumothorax, hypoxia, or placement in the carotid artery.

Procedure for Performing Central Venous Catheter Insertion

Steps	Rationale	Special Considerations
1. Review indications, contraindications, and potential complications.	Enables appropriate site selection and preprocedural intervention if needed.	
2. Obtain ultrasound equipment if time is available to determine the most appropriate approach.	Prepares equipment.	Assistance may be needed from radiology.
3. HH		
4. PE		All providers and other healthcare professionals in the room should wear protective equipment including head coverings and masks.[4] Persons inserting the catheter or assisting should use face shields or goggles.
5. Place a waterproof pad beneath the site to be accessed.	Avoids soiling of bed linens.	
6. Assist the patient to a position that will optimize access to the site selected.	Proper positioning increases vessel access and optimizes comfort of the patient and physician, advanced practice nurse, or other healthcare professional throughout the process.	
7. Determine the anatomy of the access site. (**Level E***)	Helps ensure proper placement of the CVC and guides the area to be prepped.[4,7]	Ultrasound guidance to place CVCs (if the technology is available) should be used to reduce the number of attempts and complications.[4,7,8]

*Level E: Multiple case reports, theory-based evidence from expert opinions, or peer-reviewed professional organizational standards without clinical studies to support recommendations.

Procedure	for Performing Central Venous Catheter Insertion—*Continued*	
Steps	**Rationale**	**Special Considerations**
8. Prepare skin with an antiseptic solution (e.g., 2% chlorhexidine-based preparation).[5,4,7] **(Level A*)** A. Subclavian vein: scrub from the shoulder to the contralateral nipple line and the neck to the nipple line (Fig. 74.1A). B. Internal jugular vein: scrub midclavicle to the opposite border of the sternum and from the ear to a few inches above the nipple (see Fig. 74.1B). C. Femoral vein: scrub the anterior and medial surface of the proximal thigh to the inguinal ligament.	Limits the introduction of potentially infectious skin flora into the vessel during the puncture.	If there is a contraindication to chlorhexidine, tincture of iodine, an iodophor, or 70% alcohol can be used as alternatives.[4]

*Level A: Meta-analysis of quantitative studies or metasynthesis of qualitative studies with results that consistently support a specific action, intervention, or treatment (including systematic review of randomized controlled trials).

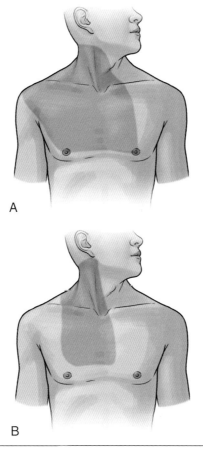

A

B

Figure 74.1 Area of skin preparation for central venous catheter insertions. **A,** Subclavian insertion: scrub from the shoulder to the contralateral nipple line and the neck to the nipple line. **B,** Jugular insertion: scrub mid-clavicle to the opposite border of the sternum and from the ear to a few inches above the nipple. *(Courtesy SureDesign.)*

Procedure continues on following page

Procedure	for Performing Central Venous Catheter Insertion—*Continued*	
Steps	Rationale	Special Considerations
9. Discard used supplies, perform hand hygiene, and apply a sterile gown and gloves.	Minimizes the risk of infection and maintains standard and sterile precautions.	
10. Place the full drape over the patient with exposure of only the insertion site.	Prepares a sterile field.	All physicians, advanced practice nurses, and other healthcare professionals in the room should wear protective equipment including head coverings and masks.[4]
11. Ask the critical care nurse or provider assisting to open the CVC insertion kit, and drop the sterile items onto the sterile field.	Maintains aseptic technique and prepares the work area.	
12. Check landmarks again for the intended catheter insertion site.	Ensures proper placement of the catheter.	

Site Specific: Internal Jugular Vein (Fig. 74.2)
See **steps 1–12** above.

1. Locate the carotid artery.	Helps prevent placing the catheter in the carotid artery.	Ultrasound guidance to place CVCs (if the technology is available) should be used to reduce the number of attempts and complications.[4,7,8]

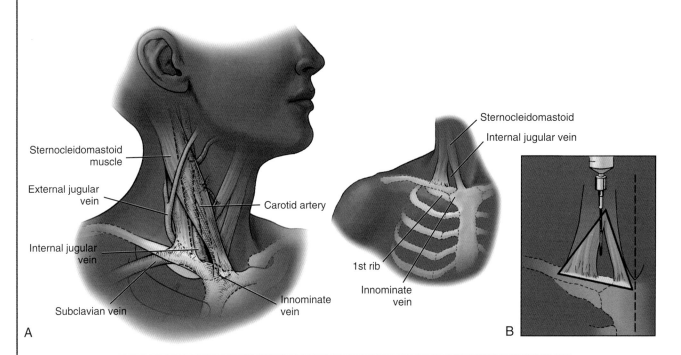

Figure 74.2 Anatomy of the jugular vein. **A,** Anatomy of the internal jugular vein showing its lower location within the triangle formed by the sternocleidomastoid muscle and the clavicle. **B,** Triangle drawn over the clavicle and sternal and clavicular portions of the sternocleidomastoid muscle is centered over the internal jugular vein *(inset). (From Dailey EK, Schroeder JS:* Techniques in bedside hemodynamic monitoring, *St. Louis, 1994, Mosby and redrawn from Daily PO, Griepp RB, Shumway NE: Percutaneous internal jugular vein cannulation.* Arch Surg *101:534–536, 1970. Copyright 1970, American Medical Association.)*

Procedure for Performing Central Venous Catheter Insertion—*Continued*

Steps	Rationale	Special Considerations
2. Identify the jugular vein, and mark it if necessary.	Identifies the intended insertion site.	Localization of the vessel may occur with palpation; however, real-time ultrasound should be utilized with the internal jugular approach if equipment and a trained physician, advanced practice nurse, or other healthcare professional are available.[9]
3. Instruct the patient to turn his or her head slightly away from the insertion site.	Helps identify the landmarks.	Ensure that there are no contraindications to neck mobility. If there are no contraindications to neck mobility, the critical care nurse or another provider assisting with the procedure may need to assist the patient to turn his or her head.
4. Ensure that the patient is in the Trendelenburg position (i.e., 15–25 degrees).[1,2] **(Level E*)**	Minimizes the risk for venous air embolus by increasing the pressure in the large veins above atmospheric pressure, thus reducing the risk of air aspiration. The patient should be positioned so the intended puncture site is at or below the level of the heart.[1,2]	Most patients can tolerate Trendelenburg positioning, but intracranial, respiratory, or cardiac compromise may occur. Therefore evaluation for the need for alternative sites and close monitoring are necessary.
5. Identify the internal jugular vein from the triangle between the medial aspect of the clavicle, the medial aspect of the sternal head, and the lateral head of the sternocleidomastoid muscle (see Fig. 74.2).	A high entry can be made from a posterior approach, a lateral approach, an anterior approach, or a central approach.	The midanterior approach may be preferred in an obese patient. The posterior approach may present a slightly higher risk. The internal jugular vein is 3–4 cm above the medial clavicle and 1–3 cm within the lateral border of the sternocleidomastoid muscle.
6. Administer an anesthetic: A. Attach a 3- or 5-mL syringe with 2 or 3 mL of 1% lidocaine (without epinephrine) to an 18-gauge needle. B. Align the needle with the syringe parallel to the medial border of the clavicular head of the sternocleidomastoid muscle. C. Aim at a 30-degree angle to the frontal plane over the internal jugular vein, toward the ipsilateral nipple. D. Instill the lidocaine.	Promotes patient comfort during the procedure. Helps anesthetize below the subcutaneous tissue.	
7. Prepare the catheter: A. Place sterile injectable or noninjectable caps. B. Flush the catheter and ports with normal saline.	Removes air from the catheter and prepares for insertion.	

*Level E: Multiple case reports, theory-based evidence from expert opinions, or peer-reviewed professional organizational standards without clinical studies to support recommendations.

Procedure continues on following page

UNIT II

Procedure	for Performing Central Venous Catheter Insertion—*Continued*	
Steps	**Rationale**	**Special Considerations**
8. Place the sterile probe over the ultrasound equipment, and locate the vessel.	Maintains sterility.	Another clinician or provider in sterile attire may assist with this step.[8]
9. Use the Seldinger technique for placement of the catheter (Fig. 74.3).	This technique is the preferred method of CVC placement; it uses a dilator and guidewire.	
A. Puncture the skin, and advance the needle while maintaining slight negative pressure within the syringe until free-flowing blood is obtained.	Slight negative pressure helps ensure placement into the vein and decreases the risk for air embolism and pneumothorax. Without slight negative pressure, penetration into the vein will go unrecognized.	Insert at a 45-degree angle to prevent pneumothorax. Avoiding a too-lateral or too-deep needle insertion can reduce the risk for pneumothorax. Lateral movement of an inserted needle can lacerate vessels and should not be done.

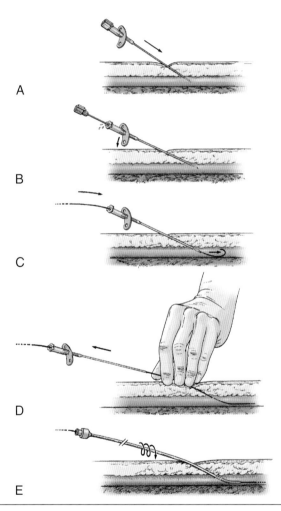

A

B

C

D

E

Figure 74.3 Basic procedure for the Seldinger technique. **A,** The vessel is punctured with the needle at a 30- to 40-degree angle. **B,** The stylet is removed, and free blood flow is observed; the angle of the needle is then reduced. **C,** The flexible tip of the guidewire is passed through the needle into the vessel. **D,** The needle is removed over the wire while firm pressure is applied at the site. **E,** The tip of the catheter or sheath is passed over the wire and advanced into the vessel with a rotating motion. *(From Dailey EK, Schroeder JS: Techniques in bedside hemodynamic monitoring, St. Louis, 1994, Mosby.)*

Procedure for Performing Central Venous Catheter Insertion—*Continued*

Steps	Rationale	Special Considerations
B. After a free flow of blood is returned, turn the bevel to the 3 o'clock position. Once in the vein, have the patient hold his or her breath while the syringe is detached and insert the soft-tipped guidewire 20–25 cm through the needle.	A free flow of blood indicates that a vessel has been entered.	When preparing the syringe and needle, line the bevel up with the numbers on the syringe so you know where the bevel is regardless of how the syringe is manipulated during placement.
C. Remove the needle.		
D. Wipe the guidewire with the sterile 4 × 4 gauze.	Wiping the guidewire dry may ease manipulation.	The guidewire should always pass easily without resistance.
E. Instruct the patient to breathe normally.		
10. With a No. 11 blade, knife edge up, make a small (2- to 3-mm) stab wound at the insertion site.	Eases insertion of the dilator through the skin.	
11. Insert the dilator through the skin, over the guidewire, until 10–15 cm of wire extends beyond the dilator, then remove the dilator while maintaining the position of the guidewire.	The dilator enlarges the subcutaneous tissue and vessel, easing insertion of the catheter and preventing formation of a false channel.	Control of the guidewire should be always maintained to avoid wire embolization.
12. Advance the catheter over the guidewire until 10–15 cm of the guidewire extends beyond the catheter, and then remove the guidewire.	Places the catheter.	Cover the needle hub between manipulations to avoid air embolization.
13. Suture the catheter in place.	Secures the catheter.	A sutureless catheter-securing device may be used to stabilize the CVC.
14. Apply an occlusive, sterile dressing.	Reduces the risk for infection.	Consider use of a chlorhexidine-impregnated sponge dressing.[4,7] Follow institutional protocols.
15. Return the patient to a neutral, or head-up, position.	Promotes comfort.	
16. Assess lung sounds and peak airway pressures (in ventilated patients), and obtain a chest radiograph.	Assesses for placement and complications.	The radiograph must be read before utilization of the catheter for administration of IV fluid and medications.[5,7]
17. Remove **PE**, and discard used supplies in appropriate receptacles.	Reduces the transmission of microorganisms and minimizes exposure to contaminated sharps.	
18. **HH**		

Specific Site: Subclavian Vein (Fig. 74.4)
See **steps 1–12** above.

1. Identify the junction of the middle and medial thirds of the clavicle. The needle insertion should be 1–2 cm laterally.	Identifies the landmarks for catheter placement.	Access from the right side is preferred to avoid inadvertent puncture of the thoracic duct.
2. Depress the area 1–2 cm beneath the junction with the thumb of the nondominant hand and the index finger 2 cm above the sternal notch.	Helps identify the landmarks.	To avoid the subclavian artery, select a puncture site away from the most lateral course of the vein, and do not aim too posteriorly.

Procedure continues on following page

Procedure | **for Performing Central Venous Catheter Insertion—*Continued***

Steps	Rationale	Special Considerations

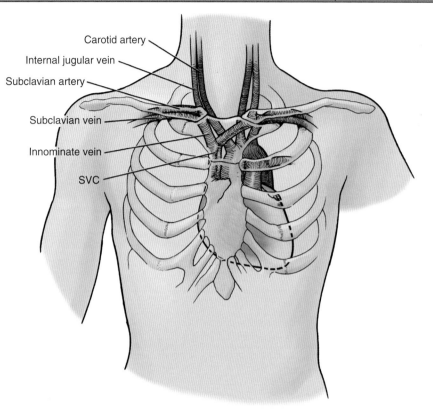

Figure 74.4   Anatomical location of the subclavian vein and surrounding structures. The subclavian vein joins the internal jugular vein to become the innominate vein at about the manubrioclavicular junction. The innominate vein becomes the superior vena cava (SVC) at about the level of the mid-manubrium. *(From Dailey EK, Schroeder JS: Techniques in bedside hemodynamic monitoring, St. Louis, 1994, Mosby.)*

Steps	Rationale	Special Considerations
3. Identify the subclavian vein.	May aid in identifying the intended insertion site.	Utilization of real-time ultrasound should be considered with the subclavian approach if equipment and a trained provider is available.[9]
4. Instruct the patient to turn his or her head away from the insertion site.	Helps identify the landmarks.	Ensure that there are no contraindications to neck mobility. If there are none, the critical care nurse or provider assisting with the procedure may need to assist the patient to turn his or her head.
5. Position the patient for optimal vein access. A. Ensure that the patient is in the Trendelenburg position (i.e., 15–25 degrees). B. Adduct the patient's arms. C. Consider placing a rolled towel between the patient's shoulder blades.	Minimizes the risk for venous air embolus by increasing pressure in the large veins above atmospheric pressure, thus reducing the risk of air aspiration. The patient should be positioned so the intended puncture site is at or below the level of the heart.[1,2]	Most patients can tolerate Trendelenburg positioning, but intracranial, respiratory, or cardiac compromise may occur. Therefore evaluation for the need for alternative sites and close monitoring are necessary.

Procedure **for Performing Central Venous Catheter Insertion—*Continued***

Steps	Rationale	Special Considerations
6. Administer a local anesthetic. A. Attach a 3- or 5-mL syringe with 2 or 3 mL of 1% lidocaine (without epinephrine) to an 18-gauge needle. B. Inject the lidocaine into the area surrounding the intended insertion site.	Promotes patient comfort during the procedure. Helps anesthetize below the subcutaneous tissue.	
7. Prepare the catheter: A. Flush the catheter and ports with normal saline. B. Place sterile injectable or noninjectable caps.	Removes air from the catheter and prepares for insertion.	
8. Place the sterile probe over the ultrasound equipment, and locate the vessel.	Maintains sterility.	Another provider or other healthcare professional in sterile attire may assist with this step.[8]
9. Use the Seldinger technique for placement of the catheter (see Fig. 74.3). A. Insert the needle under the clavicle, and "walk down" until it slips below the clavicle and enters the vein while maintaining negative pressure within the syringe until free-flowing blood is returned (Fig. 74.5).	This technique is the preferred method of CVC placement; it uses a dilator and guidewire. Slight negative pressure helps ensure placement into the vein and decreases the risk for air embolism and pneumothorax. Without slight negative pressure, penetration into the vein will go unrecognized.	Insert at a 45-degree angle to prevent pneumothorax. Avoiding a too-lateral or too-deep needle insertion can reduce the risk for pneumothorax. Lateral movement of an inserted needle can lacerate vessels and should not be done.
B. After a free flow of blood is returned, have the patient hold his or her breath while the syringe is detached, and insert the soft-tipped guidewire 20–25 cm through the needle under constant manual control. C. Remove the needle. D. Wipe the guidewire with the sterile 4 × 4 gauze. E. Instruct the patient to breathe normally.	A free flow of blood indicates that a vessel has been entered. Wiping the guidewire dry may ease manipulation.	
10. With a No. 11 blade, knife edge up, make a small (2- to 3-mm) stab wound at the insertion site.	Eases the insertion of the dilator through the skin.	
11. Insert the dilator through the skin, over the guidewire, advancing under the clavicle until 20–25 cm of wire extends beyond the dilator, then remove the dilator while maintaining the position of the guidewire.	The dilator enlarges the subcutaneous tissue and vessel, easing insertion of the catheter and preventing formation of a false channel.	Control of the guidewire should be always maintained to avoid wire embolization.
12. Advance the catheter over the guidewire until 20–25 cm of the guidewire extends beyond the catheter, and then remove the guidewire.	Places the catheter.	Cover the needle hub between manipulations to avoid air embolization.

Procedure continues on following page

Procedure for Performing Central Venous Catheter Insertion —*Continued*

Steps	Rationale	Special Considerations

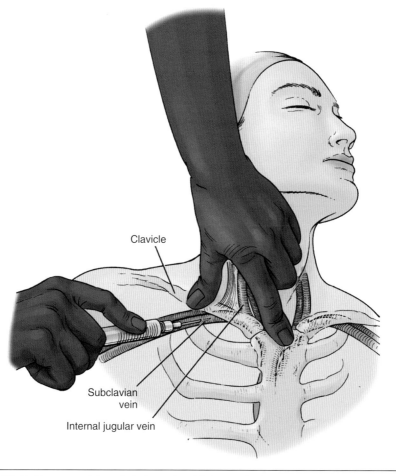

Clavicle

Subclavian
vein

Internal jugular vein

Figure 74.5   Puncture of the subclavian vein with the needle inserted beneath the middle third of the clavicle at a 20- to 30-degree angle aiming medially. *(From Dailey EK, Schroeder JS: Techniques in bedside hemodynamic monitoring, St. Louis, 1994, Mosby.)*

Steps	Rationale	Special Considerations
13. Suture the catheter in place.	Secures the catheter.	A sutureless catheter-securing device may be used to stabilize the CVC.
14. Apply an occlusive, sterile dressing to the site (see Procedure 66, Noninvasive Cardiac Output Monitoring).	Provides a sterile environment.	Consider use of a chlorhexidine-impregnated sponge dressing.[4,7] Follow institutional standards.
15. Return the patient to a neutral or head-up position.	Promotes comfort.	
16. Assess lung sounds and peak airway pressures (in ventilated patients), and obtain a chest radiograph.	Assesses for placement and complications.	The radiograph must be read before utilization of the catheter for administration of IV fluid and medications.[5,7]
17. Remove **PE**, and discard used supplies in appropriate receptacles.	Reduces the transmission of microorganisms and minimizes exposure to contaminated sharps.	
18. **HH**		

Specific Site: Femoral Vein (see Fig. 74.2)
See **steps 1–12** above.

1. Assist the patient to the supine, flat position with the intended leg extended.	Prepares for the procedure.	

Procedure for Performing Central Venous Catheter Insertion —*Continued*

Steps	Rationale	Special Considerations
2. Locate the femoral artery, and mark it if necessary.	Identifies the intended insertion site.	Localization of the vessel may occur with palpation; however, real-time ultrasound should be utilized with the femoral approach if equipment and a trained physician, advanced practice nurse, or other healthcare professional are available.[4,7-9]
3. Administer a local anesthetic. A. Attach a 3- or 5-mL syringe with 2 or 3 mL of 1% lidocaine (without epinephrine) to an 18-gauge needle. B. Inject the lidocaine into the area surrounding the intended insertion site.	Promotes patient comfort during the procedure. Helps anesthetize below the subcutaneous tissue.	
4. Prepare the catheter: A. Flush the catheter and ports with normal saline. B. Place sterile injectable or noninjectable caps.	Removes air from the catheter and prepares for insertion.	
5. Place the sterile probe over the ultrasound equipment, and locate the vessel.	Maintains sterility.	Another clinician or provider in sterile attire may assist with this step.[8]
6. Use the Seldinger technique for placement of the catheter (see Fig. 74.3). A. Insert the needle at a 20- to 30-degree angle 1–2 cm inferior to the inguinal ligament and just medial to the femoral artery. Maintain slight, continuous, negative pressure during insertion, and advance the needle until free-flowing blood is returned. B. After a free flow of blood is returned, detach the syringe, and insert the soft-tipped guidewire 25 cm under constant manual control. C. Remove the needle. D. Wipe the guidewire with the sterile 4 × 4 gauze.	This technique is the preferred method of CVC placement; it uses a dilator and guidewire. Slight negative pressure helps ensure placement into the vein. Without slight negative pressure, penetration into the vein will go unrecognized. A free flow of blood indicates that a vessel has been entered. Wiping the guidewire dry may ease manipulation.	Lateral movement of an inserted needle can lacerate vessels and should not be done.
7. With a No. 11 blade, knife edge up, make a small (2- to 3-mm) stab wound at the insertion site.	Eases insertion of the dilator through the skin.	
8. Insert the dilator through the skin, over the guidewire, until 25 cm of wire extends beyond the dilator, and then remove the dilator while maintaining the position of the guidewire.	The dilator enlarges the subcutaneous tissue and vessel, easing insertion of the catheter and preventing formation of a false channel.	Control of the guidewire should be always maintained to avoid wire embolization.
9. Advance the catheter over the guidewire until 25 cm of the guidewire extends beyond the catheter, and then remove the guidewire.	Places the catheter.	

Procedure continues on following page

Procedure for Performing Central Venous Catheter Insertion —*Continued*

Steps	Rationale	Special Considerations
10. Suture the catheter in place.	Secures the catheter.	A sutureless catheter-securing device may be used to stabilize the CVC.
11. Apply an occlusive, sterile dressing to the site.	Decreases the risk for infection.	Consider use of a chlorhexidine-impregnated sponge dressing.[4,7] Follow institutional protocols.
12. Return the patient to a neutral position with the head of the bed slightly elevated.	Facilitates comfort.	
13. Obtain an x-ray.	Assesses for placement and complications.	The radiograph must be read before utilization of the catheter for administration of IV fluid and medications.[5,7]
14. Remove **PE**, and discard used supplies in appropriate receptacles.	Reduces the transmission of microorganisms and minimizes exposure to contaminated sharps.	
15. **HH**		

Expected Outcomes

- Successful placement of the CVC
- If infusing IV solution, the solution infuses without problems
- The *a, c,* and *v* waves are identified if hemodynamic monitoring is used
- CVP measurements are obtained

Unexpected Outcomes

- Failure to place the catheter
- Arterial puncture
- Catheter embolization
- Vascular injury
- Pain or discomfort during the insertion procedure
- Pneumothorax, tension pneumothorax, hemothorax, or chylothorax
- Nerve injury
- Sterile thrombophlebitis
- Infection
- Cardiac dysrhythmias
- Malposition
- Inadvertent lymphatic or thoracic duct perforation
- Hemorrhage
- Hematoma
- Venous air embolism
- Cardiac tamponade

Patient Monitoring and Care

Steps	Rationale	Reportable Conditions
		These conditions should be reported to the provider if they persist despite nursing interventions.
1. Perform respiratory, cardiovascular, peripheral vascular, and hemodynamic assessments immediately before and after the procedure and as the patient's condition necessitates.	Determines whether signs or symptoms of complications are present, for example, an air embolism may present with restlessness.	- Abnormal level of consciousness - Abnormal vital signs - Abnormal waveforms or pressures - Declining oxygen saturation - Increasing peak airway pressures in patients receiving mechanical ventilation.

Patient Monitoring and Care —*Continued*

Steps	Rationale	Reportable Conditions
2. If the catheter was placed for CVP measurement, assess the waveform.	Ensures that the catheter is in the proper location for monitoring. Allows assessment of *a, c,* and *v* waves and measurement of pressure.	• Abrupt and sustained changes in CVP • Abnormal waveform
3. Assess the insertion site for presence of a hematoma or hemorrhage.	Determines the presence of complications.	• Bleeding that does not stop • Hematoma or expanding hematoma
4. Assess heart and lung sounds before and after the procedure.	Abnormal heart or lung sounds may indicate cardiac tamponade, pneumothorax, chylothorax, or hemothorax.	• Diminished or muffled heart sounds • Absent or diminished breath sounds unilaterally
5. Assess the results of the chest radiograph.	Ensures accurate placement and may aid in identification of complications.	• Abnormal radiograph results
6. Monitor for signs of complications.	May decrease mortality and morbidity if recognized early.	• Signs and symptoms of complications
7. Follow institutional standards for assessing pain. Prescribe analgesia as needed.	Identifies the need for pain interventions.	• Continued pain despite pain interventions
8. If signs and symptoms of venous air embolus are present, immediately place the patient in the left-lateral Trendelenburg position. **(Level E*)**	Venous air embolus is a potentially life-threatening complication. The left-lateral Trendelenburg position prevents air from passing into the left side of the heart and traveling into the arterial circulation.[1,2]	• Respiratory distress • Dyspnea • Coughing • Tachypnea • Altered mental status (agitation, restlessness) • Cyanosis • Gasp reflex • Sucking sound near the site of the catheter insertion/air entrainment • Petechiae • Cardiac dysrhythmias • Chest pain • Hypotension

*Level E: Multiple case reports, theory-based evidence from expert opinions, or peer-reviewed professional organizational standards without clinical studies to support recommendations.

Documentation

Documentation should include the following:
• Patient and family education
• Completion of informed consent
• Preprocedural verifications and time out
• Insertion of the CVC
• Insertion site of the CVC
• Date and time of procedure
• Catheter type
• Lumen size
• Right-atrial pressure and CVP waveform in the event of pressure monitoring
• Centimeter marking at the skin
• Patient response to the procedure
• Pain assessment, interventions, and effectiveness
• Confirmation of placement (e.g., chest radiograph)
• Occurrence of unexpected outcomes
• Additional nursing interventions

References and Additional Readings

For a complete list of references and additional readings for this procedure, scan this QR code with your smartphone, or visit https://www.elsevier.com/__data/assets/pdf_file/0008/1319849/Chapter0074.pdf.

75 Central Venous Catheter Insertion (Assist), Nursing Care and Removal

Emily R. Leiter and Karen L. Johnson

PURPOSE Central venous catheters (CVCs) are inserted for measurement of hemodynamic parameters, administration of fluids, and infusion of vasoactive medications. CVCs also are placed to provide access for pulmonary artery catheters and transvenous pacemakers. The CVC is generally inserted via the internal jugular vein (IJ), the subclavian vein (SCV), or the femoral vein site. Site care of the CVC allows for assessment and care of the catheter insertion site to prevent central-line–associated bloodstream infections (CLABSIs). To minimize the risk of infection, the use of CVC care includes performing hand hygiene, ensuring maximum sterile barrier precautions during insertion, using chlorhexidine as a skin disinfectant, avoiding the use of femoral site insertion, and removing the CVC as soon as possible.[6]

PREREQUISITE NURSING KNOWLEDGE

- Normal anatomy and physiology of the vasculature and cardiovascular system.
- Principles of aseptic technique.
- Advanced cardiac life support (ACLS) knowledge and skills.
- Indications for CVC placement may include the following:
  - ❖ Assessment of central venous pressure (CVP) for fluid volume status (hypovolemia or hypervolemia) (see Procedure 56, Central Venous/Right Atrial Pressure Monitoring)
  - ❖ Placement of a pulmonary artery catheter (see Procedure 59, Pulmonary Artery Catheter Insertion [Assist] and Pressure Monitoring) or a transvenous pacemaker (see Procedure 46, Temporary Transvenous and Epicardial Pacing)
  - ❖ Hemodialysis access
  - ❖ Blood sampling (see Procedure 57, Blood Sampling From a Central Venous Catheter)
  - ❖ Administration of vesicant irritant medications that should not be administered in a peripheral vein
  - ❖ Inability to obtain peripheral venous access or when the duration of IV therapy is greater than 7 days[8]
  - ❖ Administration of total parenteral nutrition
- Some contraindications of CVC insertion include anatomical problems, venous obstruction, and coagulopathies. The subclavian site should be avoided in hemodialysis patients and patients with advanced kidney disease to avoid subclavian vein stenosis.[8]
- It is important to weigh the risks and benefits of placing a CVC against the risk for mechanical complications (e.g., pneumothorax, vein laceration, thrombosis, air embolism, misplacement).[8-10]
- A subclavian site is recommended rather than a jugular or femoral site to minimize the risk of infection.[8,13,15]

- Ultrasound guidance is recommended to place CVCs if the technology is available to reduce the number of cannulation attempts and mechanical complications.[7,8,13,15]
- Regardless of the site selected, complications may occur during or after insertion of a CVC (see Table 74.1).
- The CVP provides information regarding right-heart filling pressures and right-ventricular function and volume.[15]
- The CVP is commonly elevated during or after right-ventricular failure, ischemia, or infarction because of decreased compliance of the right ventricle.[15]
- The CVP can be helpful in the determination of hypovolemia. The CVP value is low if the patient is hypovolemic.
- Signs and symptoms of catheter-related infection. Bloodstream infections related to the use of CVCs are associated with increased morbidity, increased risk of morbidity and mortality, and associated healthcare costs.
- The catheter insertion site should be monitored daily by palpation through a dressing to discern tenderness and by inspection if a transparent dressing is used. Gauze and opaque dressings should not be removed if the patient has no clinical signs of infection. If the patient has local tenderness or other signs of infection, an opaque dressing should be removed and the site inspected visually.[8]
- Knowledge of the state nurse practice act is important because some states do not allow removal of the CVC to be performed by a registered nurse.
- Clinical and technical competence in CVC removal.
- Potential complications associated with the removal of the CVC. An air embolism can occur during or after removal of the catheter as a result of air drawn in along the subcutaneous tract and into the vein. During inspiration, negative intrathoracic pressure is transmitted to the central veins. Any opening external to the body to one of these veins may result in aspiration of air into the central venous system. The pathological effects

depend on the volume and rate of air aspirated. Signs and symptoms include respiratory distress, agitation, cyanosis, gasp reflex, sucking sound, hypotension, petechiae, cardiac dysrhythmias, altered mental status, and cardiac arrest.

EQUIPMENT

- Insertion equipment (see Procedure 74, Central Venous Catheter Insertion [Perform])
- Catheter care:
  - ❖ Fluid-shield face mask or goggles
  - ❖ Nonsterile and sterile gloves
  - ❖ Prepackaged sterile dressing kit or supplies as listed below
  - ❖ Antiseptic solution (e.g., 2% chlorhexidine-based preparation)
  - ❖ Securement device (used with nonsutured CVCs)
  - ❖ Chlorhexidine gluconate–impregnated sponge
- Catheter removal
  - ❖ Gowns, sterile and nonsterile gloves
  - ❖ Antiseptic solution (e.g., 2% chlorhexidine-based preparation)
  - ❖ 4 × 4 gauze pads
  - ❖ Petroleum-based ointment
  - ❖ One roll of 2-inch tape
  - ❖ Two moisture-proof absorbent pads

Additional equipment, to have available as needed, includes the following:

- ❖ Dressing supplies (e.g., semipermeable transparent dressing)
- ❖ Sterile scissors
- ❖ Sterile specimen container (needed if a culture of the catheter tip will be obtained)
- ❖ Suture removal kit
- ❖ Emergency equipment

PATIENT AND FAMILY EDUCATION

- Explain the need for the CVC insertion, and assess patient and family understanding. *Rationale:* Clarification and understanding of information decrease patient and family anxiety.
- Explain the need for sterile technique, patient positioning, and that the patient's face will be covered during insertion and CVC site care. *Rationale:* Clarification and understanding of information decrease patient and family anxiety.
- Explain the procedure to the patient and family and the reason for catheter removal. *Rationale:* This explanation provides information and decreases anxiety.
- Explain the importance of patient participation during catheter removal. *Rationale:* This explanation ensures patient cooperation and facilitates safe removal of the catheter.
- Instruct the patient and family to report any signs and symptoms of shortness of breath, bleeding, or discomfort at the catheter removal site. *Rationale:* Identifies patient discomfort and early recognition of complications.

PATIENT ASSESSMENT AND PREPARATION

Patient Assessment

- Before insertion or catheter removal, assess the patient's neurological, cardiac, and pulmonary status. *Rationale:* Some patients may not tolerate the supine or Trendelenburg position for extended periods because of increased intracranial pressure or cardiopulmonary compromise.
- Assess vital signs and pulse oximetry before insertion. *Rationale:* Baseline data can be compared with data obtained during and after the procedure.
- Before insertion and removal, assess for a coagulopathic state, and determine whether the patient has recently received anticoagulant or thrombolytic therapy. *Rationale:* These patients are more likely to have complications related to bleeding. If the patient has abnormal coagulation study results, hemostasis may be difficult to obtain. Abnormal coagulation results should be discussed with the provider before catheter insertion and removal.
- During catheter care, assess the catheter site for redness, warmth, tenderness, or presence of drainage. *Rationale:* Determines whether signs or symptoms of infection are present.

Patient Preparation

- Before insertion or removal
  - ❖ Verify the correct patient with two identifiers. *Rationale:* This increases patient safety by ensuring correct identification of the patient for the intended intervention.
  - ❖ Ensure that the patient and family understand the preprocedural teaching. Answer questions as they arise, and reinforce information as needed. *Rationale*: Understanding of previously taught information is evaluated and reinforced.
- Before insertion
  - ❖ Ensure that informed consent has been obtained. *Rationale*: Informed consent protects the rights of the patient and makes a competent decision possible for the patient; however, in emergency circumstances, time may not allow for consent to be signed.
  - ❖ Assist in performing a preprocedural verification and time out, if nonemergent. *Rationale:* This ensures patient safety.
  - ❖ Administer sedation or analgesics as prescribed and as needed. *Rationale:* The patient may need sedation or analgesics to promote comfort and to ensure adequate cooperation and appropriate placement.
  - ❖ Depending on the site selected and the patient's body habitus, specific positioning may be needed (e.g., for the subclavian vein, assist with placing a towel posteriorly between the shoulder blades). *Rationale:* Specific positioning techniques for each site assists with optimal vessel access.
- Before catheter care
  - ❖ If the patient is receiving mechanical ventilation, assess the patient's need for suctioning before providing catheter care. Femoral catheter sites must be inspected for

potential contamination from urine or stool. ***Rationale:*** This reduces the risk for catheter site contamination by secretions or excretions.

- Before catheter removal
  - ❖ In collaboration with the provider, determine when the CVC should be removed. ***Rationale:*** The invasive catheter is removed when it is no longer indicated.
  - ❖ In collaboration with the provider, determine whether the catheter's tip will be cultured. ***Rationale:*** This discussion determines if additional supplies may be needed.

❖ Place the patient in the supine position with the head of the bed in a slight Trendelenburg position (or flat if the Trendelenburg position is contraindicated or not tolerated by the patient). ***Rationale:*** The patient should be positioned so the catheter exit site is at or below the level of the heart. A normal pressure gradient exists between atmospheric air and the central venous compartment that promotes air entry if the compartment is open. The lower the entry site below the heart, the lower the pressure gradient, therefore minimizing the risk of air being drawn in and leading to a potential venous air embolism.

Procedure for Assisting With Central Venous Catheter Insertion		
Steps	**Rationale**	**Special Considerations**
1. HH		
2. PE		All providers and other healthcare professionals in the room should wear personal protective equipment, including a head covering and a mask.[6,8]
3. Prepare the IV volution or flush solution.	Prepares the infusion system.	
4. Place the IV tubing, or flush the entire pressure-transducer system if pressure monitoring is anticipated (see Procedure 60, Single-Pressure and Multiple-Pressure Transducer Systems).	Removes air bubbles. Air bubbles introduced into the patient's circulation can cause air embolisms. Air bubbles within the tubing dampen the waveform and can alter pressure results.	
5. Apply pressure and maintain pressure in the pressure bag or device at 300 mm Hg.	Each flush device delivers 1–3 mL/hour to maintain patency of the hemodynamic system.	
6. Place a moisture-proof pad under the patient's back.	Avoids soiling of the bed.	
7. Assist with patient positioning as needed.	Proper positioning increases vessel access and optimizes comfort of the patient.	
8. If needed, remove gloves, wash hands, and apply a sterile gown and gloves. Assist as needed with preparation of the skin with an antiseptic solution (e.g., 2% chlorhexidine-based preparation).[8] (**Level A***)(See Procedure 74, Central Venous Catheter Insertion [Perform], Figure 74.1A and B.)	Limits introduction of potentially infectious skin flora into the vessel during the puncture.	If there is a contraindication to chlorhexidine, tincture of iodine, an iodophor, or 70% alcohol can be used as alternatives.[5]
9. While the provider completes the skin preparation, ensure patient comfort by explaining what is happening at the time. A. Application of the antiseptic is cold and wet. B. Injection of the local anesthetic may burn or sting as the tissue is infiltrated.		

Procedure continues on following page

Procedure for Assisting With Central Venous Catheter Insertion—*Continued*		
Steps	Rationale	Special Considerations
10. Assist as needed with applying a full drape to the patient with exposure of only the insertion site.	Minimizes the risk of infection; maintains aseptic and sterile precautions.	
11. Assist as needed with placement of the sterile ultrasound probe cover.		
12. Place the bed in the Trendelenburg position (15–20 degrees).	Minimizes the risk for venous air embolus by increasing the pressure in the large veins above atmospheric pressure, thus reducing the risk of air aspiration. The patient should be positioned so the intended puncture site is at or below the level of the heart.[2,3]	Most patients can tolerate the Trendelenburg position, but intracranial, respiratory, or cardiac compromise can occur. Therefore evaluation for the need for alternative sites and close monitoring are necessary.
13. Monitor the heart rate, respiratory rate and rhythm, pulse oximetry, intracranial pressure, and any patient response to the procedure.	Assessment may indicate occurrence of intolerance or complications (see Table 74.1).	
14. Observe the cardiac monitor while the guidewire and catheter are advanced, and inform the provider immediately if a dysrhythmia occurs.	Advancement of the guidewire or catheter into the heart may induce cardiac dysrhythmias.	
15. Once the catheter is placed and blood return is ensured, assist if needed with flushing the lumen(s) with normal saline.	Maintains catheter patency.	
16. Assist as needed with applying a sterile, occlusive dressing. Follow institutional protocols.	Reduces the risk of infection.	A sutureless catheter-securing device may be used to stabilize the CVC.
17. If using hemodynamic monitoring, connect the hemodynamic monitoring tubing to the catheter. Level and zero (see Procedure 60, Single-Pressure and Multiple-Pressure Transducer Systems).		
18. Reposition the patient in a comfortable position.		
19. Assess lung sounds and peak airway pressures (if ventilated) and if assistance is needed with obtaining a chest radiograph as prescribed.	Assesses for placement complications.	The chest radiograph must be read and interpreted by a provider before using the catheter for administration of IV fluids and medications.
20. Remove **PE**, and discard used supplies in appropriate receptacles.	Reduces the transmission of microorganisms; standard precautions.	
21. **HH**		

Procedure for Central Venous Catheter Site Care		
Steps	Rationale	Special Considerations
1. **HH**		
2. **PE**		
3. Prepare supplies and equipment.		
4. Position the patient so the CVC site is easily accessible.		If the CVC is in the femoral vein, extend the patient's leg, and ensure that the groin area is adequately exposed while maintaining patient privacy and comfort.
5. If performing site care on an internal jugular or subclavian catheter, have the patient turn their head away from the catheter insertion site.	Decreases the risk for site contamination.	
6. Apply a face mask.		
7. Remove and discard the CVC dressing. Remove securement device if present.		
8. Inspect the catheter, insertion site, and surrounding skin.	Assesses for signs of infection, catheter dislodgment, and leakage or loose sutures.	
9. Remove and discard gloves in the appropriate receptacle.		
10. **HH**		
11. Apply sterile gloves.		
12. Cleanse the skin, catheter and stabilizing device with 2% chlorhexidine-based preparation.[1,5,8,14] (**Level A***)		Follow institutional protocols.
13. Apply a new stabilization device if applicable.		
14. Apply a sterile air occlusive dressing to the site, following institutional protocols.		When CLASI is an issue, despite all other measures in place and adhered to, medication-impregnated dressings, such as chlorhexidine impregnated dressings, should be used to reduce CLABSI.[6,14]
15. Remove **PE**, and discard used supplies in appropriate receptacles.		
16. Document the date and time of the dressing change of the external dressing.		
17. **HH**		

UNIT II

Procedure | for Central Venous Catheter Removal

Steps	Rationale	Special Considerations
1. 🅷🅷		
2. 🅿🅴		All providers and other healthcare professionals in the room should wear personal protective equipment, including a face mask.
3. Transfer or discontinue the IV solution.	Prepares the catheter for removal and ensures that IV fluids are infusing in another site.	
4. Open the sterile scissors or suture removal kit and sterile gauze pads.	Prepares supplies for use.	
5. Place a moisture-proof absorbent pad under the patient's upper torso and another one close to the catheter site.	Collects blood and body fluids associated with removal; serves as a receptacle for the contaminated catheter.	
6. Place the patient supine in a slight Trendelenburg position.[2,4,11]	Minimizes the risk for venous air embolus by increasing the pressure in the large veins above atmospheric pressure, thus reducing the risk of air aspiration. The patient should be positioned so the catheter exit site is at or below the level of the heart.	Place the patient flat if the Trendelenburg position is contraindicated or not tolerated by the patient or a femoral CVC will be removed. If the CVC is in the femoral vein, extend the patient's leg, and ensure that the groin area is adequately exposed. Cases have been reported of venous air embolus occurring after removing a CVC when patients were not in a supine, slight Trendelenburg position.
7. Have the patient turn their head away from the catheter site (if removing an internal jugular or subclavian catheter).	Decreases the risk of contamination.	This step is not needed if a femoral catheter is removed.
8. Remove the catheter dressing and discard.	Prepares for removal.	
9. Remove the nonsterile gloves, perform hand hygiene, and apply a pair of sterile gloves.	Decreases the risk of contamination.	
10. Remove the securing device or, if present, cut sutures and gently pull the sutures through the skin.	Allows for removal of the catheter.	Ensure that the entire suture is removed. Retained sutures can form epithelialized tracts that can lead to infection.
11. Ask the patient to take a deep breath in and hold it if removing an internal jugular or subclavian catheter.	Minimizes the risk for venous air embolus.	If the patient is receiving positive pressure ventilation, withdraw the catheter during the inspiratory phase of the respiratory cycle or when a breath is delivered via a bag-valve-mask device.
12. Withdraw the catheter, pulling parallel to the skin and using a steady motion.	Minimizes trauma.	If resistance is met, do not continue to remove the catheter. Notify the provider immediately.
13. As the catheter exits the site, apply pressure with a gauze pad.	Minimizes the risk for venous air embolus and promotes hemostasis.	The distal end of a multi-lumen catheter should be removed quickly because the exposed proximal and medial openings could permit air entry.

Procedure   for Central Venous Catheter Removal—*Continued*

Steps	Rationale	Special Considerations
14. Instruct the patient to exhale after the catheter is removed.	Once the catheter is removed, the patient can breathe naturally.	
15. Lay the catheter on the moisture-proof absorbent pad. Check to be sure that the entire catheter was removed.	Ensures removal of the entire catheter.	If the introducer tip will be cultured, have another provider assist with cutting the tip with sterile scissors and placing it in a sterile specimen container before placing the catheter on the moisture-proof absorbent pad. Routine culturing of tips on removal is not recommended.[5]
16. Continue applying firm, direct pressure over the insertion site with the gauze pad until the bleeding has stopped.	Ensures hemostasis.	Because CVCs are placed in large veins, hemostasis may take up to 10 minutes to occur. Pressure may be needed for a longer period if the patient has been receiving anticoagulant therapy or if coagulation studies are abnormal.
17. Apply an occlusive dressing, consisting of sterile petroleum-based ointment and sterile gauze, and cover it with tape or a transparent semipermeable membrane dressing.[2,3,5,11]	Decreases the risk of infection at the insertion site and minimizes the risk for venous air embolus.	Label the dressing with the date, time, and your initials.
18. Maintain the patient in the supine position for 30 minutes after catheter removal.[5]	May decrease the risk of postprocedure venous air embolism.	
19. Remove **PE**, and discard used supplies in appropriate receptacles.	Reduces the transmission of microorganisms; standard precautions.	
20. **HH**		

*Level E: Multiple case reports, theory-based evidence from expert opinions, or peer-reviewed professional organizational standards without clinical studies to support recommendations.

Procedure continues on following page

UNIT II

Expected Outcomes

- CVC insertion
  - Successful placement of CVC
  - The *a, c,* and *v* waves are identified if hemodynamic monitoring
  - Chest radiograph is interpreted as being in the correct position, and there are no complications from insertion
- CVC site care
  - Dressing remains dry, sterile, and intact
  - Catheter site remains free from infection
  - Catheter remains in place without dislodgment
- CVC removal
  - The catheter is removed intact
  - Hemostasis is achieved at the catheter site

Unexpected Outcomes

- CVC insertion
  - Failure to place catheter
  - Arterial puncture
  - Catheter embolization
  - Vascular injury
  - Pain or discomfort during the insertion procedure
  - Pneumothorax, tension pneumothorax, hemothorax, or chylothorax
  - Nerve injury
  - Sterile thrombophlebitis
  - Infection
  - Cardiac dysrhythmias
  - Malposition
  - Inadvertent lymphatic or thoracic duct perforation
  - Hemorrhage
  - Hematoma
  - Venous air embolism
  - Cardiac tamponade
- CVC site care
  - Catheter-associated bloodstream infection
  - Infection at the insertion site
  - Accidental removal or dislodgment of the catheter
  - Impaired skin integrity under the dressing
- CVC removal
  - Inability to remove the catheter
  - Catheter not removed intact
  - Venous air emboli
  - Persistent bleeding
  - Hematoma
  - Infection
  - Broken catheter/fragmentation
  - Pain

Central Venous Catheter Insertion (Assist): Patient Monitoring and Care

Steps	Rationale	Reportable Conditions
		These conditions should be reported to the provider if they persist despite nursing interventions.
1. Assess the patient's vital signs, pulse oximetry, and level of consciousness before and after the CVC is removed.	Provides baseline data and data that identify changes in patient condition; allows for immediate interventions.	• Abnormal vital signs • Shortness of breath or tachypnea • Cyanosis or decreased oxygen saturation • Changes in mental status
2. If the catheter was placed for CVP measurement, assess the waveform.	Ensures that the catheter is in the proper location for monitoring. Allows assessment of *a, c,* and *v* waves and measurement of pressure.	• Abrupt and sustained changes in CVP • Abnormal waveform
3. Observe the catheter site for bleeding or hematoma frequently after insertion, per institutional protocol	Postinsertion bleeding may occur in a patient with coagulopathies or arterial punctures, with multiple attempts at vein access, or with the use of through-the-needle introducer designs for insertion.	• Bleeding that does not stop • Hematoma or expanding hematoma

Central Venous Catheter Insertion (Assist): Patient Monitoring and Care—*Continued*

Steps	Rationale	Reportable Conditions
4. Assess heart and lung sounds after the procedure.	Abnormal heart or lung sounds may indicate cardiac tamponade, pneumothorax, chylothorax, or hemothorax.	• Diminished or muffled heart sounds • Absent or diminished breath sounds unilaterally • Continued pain despite interventions
5. Follow institutional protocols for assessing pain; administer analgesia as prescribed.		
6. If signs and symptoms of venous air embolus are present, immediately place the patient in the left-lateral Trendelenburg position. **(Level E*)**	Venous air embolus is a potentially life-threatening complication. The left-lateral Trendelenburg position prevents air from passing into the left side of the heart and traveling into the arterial circulation.[5]	• Respiratory distress • Dyspnea • Coughing • Tachypnea • Altered mental status (agitation, restlessness) • Cyanosis • Gasp reflex • Sucking sound near the site of the catheter insertion/air entrainment • Petechiae • Cardiac dysrhythmias • Chest pain • Hypotension

Central Venous Catheter Site Care: Patient Monitoring and Care

Steps	Rationale	Reportable Conditions
		These conditions should be reported to the provider if they persist despite nursing interventions.
1. Assess the catheter site daily and as needed by palpation through an intact dressing.	If there is tenderness at the insertion site, fever without obvious source, or other signs and symptoms of a local or bloodstream infection, the dressing should be removed to allow thorough examination of the skin.[8]	Signs and symptoms of infection at the catheter insertion site
2. Replace dressings per institutional protocol.		

Central Venous Catheter Removal: Patient Monitoring and Care

Steps	Rationale	Reportable Conditions
		These conditions should be reported to the provider if they persist despite nursing interventions.
1. Assess the patient's vital signs, pulse oximetry, and level of consciousness before and after the CVC is removed.	Provides baseline data and data that identify changes in patient condition.	• Abnormal vital signs • Shortness of breath or tachypnea • Cyanosis or decreased oxygen saturation • Changes in mental status

Procedure continues on following page

Steps	Rationale	Reportable Conditions
2. If signs and symptoms of venous air embolus are present, immediately place the patient in the left-lateral Trendelenburg position.	Venous air embolus is a potentially life-threatening complication. The left-lateral Trendelenburg position prevents air from passing into the heart's left side and traveling into the arterial circulation.	• Respiratory distress • Dyspnea • Coughing • Tachypnea • Altered mental status (agitation, restlessness) • Cyanosis • Gasp reflex • Sucking sound near the site of catheter insertion/air entrainment • Petechiae • Chest pain • Cardiac dysrhythmias • Hypotension
3. After removing the CVC, assess the site for signs of bleeding as per institutional protocol.	Bleeding or a hematoma can develop if there is still bleeding from the vessel.	• Bleeding • Hematoma development
4. Remove the dressing and assess for site closure 24 hours after CVC removal.	Verifies healing and closure of the site.	• Abnormal healing
5. Daily assess the need for the CVC. If long-term use of the CVC is needed, frequently reassess the necessity of the line. **(Level C*)**	The U.S. Centers for Disease Control and Prevention (CDC) Guidelines do not have specific recommendations regarding routine replacement of CVCs.[8] There is some evidence that CVCs do not need to be changed more frequently than every 7 days.[3] There are no specific recommendations regarding routine replacement of CVCs that must be in place for greater than 7 days.[12] Guidewire exchanges should not be used routinely; they should only be used to replace a catheter that is malfunctioning.[8]	• Signs and symptoms of infection at the CVC catheter insertion site • Signs and symptoms of sepsis

*Level C: Qualitative studies, descriptive or correlational studies, integrative reviews, systematic reviews, or randomized controlled trials with inconsistent results.

Documentation

Post–CVC insertion documentation should include the following:
- Patient and family education
- Universal protocol requirements
- Catheter location
- Medications administered
- Right atrial waveform if monitored
- Centimeter marking at the skin
- Patient response to the procedure
- Pain assessment, interventions, and effectiveness
- Fluids administered
- Type of dressing applied
- Occurrence of unexpected outcomes
- Additional nursing interventions

CVC site care documentation should include the following:
- Patient and family education
- Date and time of dressing change
- Assessment of the catheter site
- Type of dressing applied
- Unexpected outcomes
- Additional interventions

CVC removal documentation should include the following:
- Patient and family education
- Date and time of catheter removal
- Site assessment and aseptic technique
- Pain assessment, interventions, and effectiveness
- Application of air occlusive dressing
- Patient tolerance of the procedure
- Unexpected outcomes and interventions

References and Additional Readings

For a complete list of references and additional readings for this procedure, scan this QR code with your smartphone, or visit https://www.elsevier.com/__data/assets/pdf_file/0009/1319850/Chapter0075.pdf.

UNIT II

76 Implantable Venous Access Device: Access, Deaccess, and Care

Shu Wang

PURPOSE Implantable venous access devices or ports are surgically placed and used for delivery of medications, including cytotoxic agents, parenteral solutions, blood products, and for blood sampling for patients who need long-term venous access.

PREREQUISITE NURSING KNOWLEDGE

- Understanding of the implantable venous access device, including the septum and outer borders.
- Anatomy of the venous system.
- Principles of medication delivery. Intermittent use necessitates flushing with normal saline (NS) solution after each use and instillation of heparin as prescribed when the medication infusion is completed.
- Principles of aseptic and sterile techniques is necessary.
- Consequences of infiltration of a vesicant substance.
- There are single- and double-lumen ports. All ports are designed with a portal body and a catheter. The portal body contains a septum and reservoir, which is made of plastic, titanium, polysulfone, or a combination.[4] A slim tube or catheter is connected to the reservoir, which is covered by a disc 2 to 3 cm in width (Figs. 76.1 and 76.2). Provided a noncoring needle is used to access the septum, the septum is capable of resealing when deaccessed. The internal catheter is connected to the patient's venous system and may consist of either silicone or polyurethane.[2,3,5,11]
- Implanted vascular access ports are accessed using a noncoring safety needle. A noncoring needle allows for repeated access of the venous device without damage to the silicone core.
- The noncoring needle chosen should be of optimal length (0.5 to 2 inches), with the most commonly used gauge being 19 to 22.[3,4] Patients with increased subcutaneous tissue may need a longer needle for access. Too short a needle may cause the flanges to press against the skin surrounding the portal chamber, leading to patient discomfort and possibly resulting in damage to the skin overlying the venous access device. Too long a needle may result in a rocking motion that can cause discomfort, possible

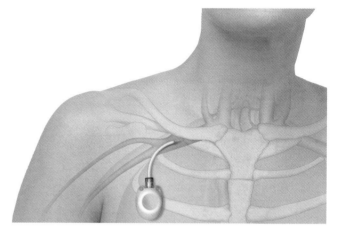

Figure 76.1 Port placement. *(Courtesy Bard Corporation, Murry Hill, NJ.)*

migration out of the portal septum, or damage to the integrity of the septum, impairing it for further use.

- Implantable power ports allow for venous access and the ability for power-injected contrast-enhanced computed tomography (CECT) scans.[10] If the patient has a power-injectable port, the noncoring needle set used must be labeled as power injectable compatible.

EQUIPMENT

- Nonsterile gloves
- Sterile gloves
- Mask
- Noncoring needle, winged with 90-degree angle and extension tubing (ensure that the appropriate size and length of needle is used; also confirm that the port is a power port if being used for power injection and that the correct noncoring needle is being used for access)[3,4]
- Dressing supplies
- Antiseptic solution (e.g., 2% chlorhexidine–based solution, 10% betadine solution and 70% alcohol solution)
- Two 10-mL syringes
- Luer-Lok vial access device
- Needleless injection cap
- Single-use 30-mL vial of NS

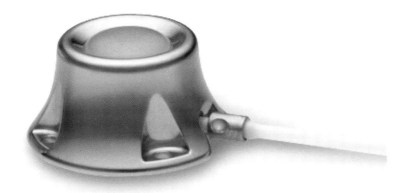

Figure 76.2 PORT-A-CATH reservoir with self-sealing septum and catheter. *(Courtesy Smiths Medical ASD, Inc., St. Paul, MN.)*

- ½-inch Steri-Strips or stabilization device
- Heparin flush, 100 units/mL concentration, if deaccessing
- Central venous catheter dressing change kit

Additional equipment, to have available as needed, includes the following:

- Topical anesthetic if prescribed eutectic mixture of local anesthetics (EMLA) cream containing 1% lidocaine
- Supplies for obtaining blood samples for laboratory analysis
- Needleless blood sampling access device

PATIENT AND FAMILY EDUCATION

- Assess patient and family readiness to learn, and identify factors that affect learning. *Rationale:* Assessment allows the nurse to individualize teaching and maximize understanding.
- Provide information about the type of implantable venous access device placed and the methods used for accessing and deaccessing it. *Rationale:* Information assists the patient and family in understanding the procedure and decreases patient and family anxiety.
- Encourage the patient to carry a card describing the type of port implanted. *Rationale:* This provides important information that may be needed by other physicians, advanced practice nurses, and other healthcare professionals.
- Explain the patient's role during the procedure and expected outcomes. *Rationale:* The patient is able to participate in care, and cooperation is encouraged.
- Explain the anticipated sensations during the access procedure and infusion of therapies. *Rationale:* Explanation allows the patient to alert the physician, advanced practice nurse, or other healthcare professional to unusual or unexpected sensations.
- Explain site care, signs and symptoms of infection, and infiltration. *Rationale:* Explanation enables the patient and family to participate in care, and the patient is encouraged to report untoward events to physicians, advanced practice nurses, and other healthcare professionals.

PATIENT ASSESSMENT AND PREPARATION

Patient Assessment

- Review the patient's medical history specifically related to the type of port, problems with device implantation, complications with previous access, and allergies to antiseptic solutions. *Rationale:* Baseline data are provided.
- Obtain the patient's vital signs. *Rationale:* Baseline data are provided.
- Review the patient's current laboratory status, including coagulation results. *Rationale:* Baseline coagulation studies are helpful in determining the risk for bleeding. If results are abnormal, consult with the patient's physician or advanced practice nurse before accessing the device.[4,10]
- Determine if the patient has a power port by palpating the top of the port to identify three palpations (bumps) on the septum, arranged in a triangle. Also, palpate the sides of the port to identify if the device is in the shape of a triangle.[10,11] *Rationale:* Determines the type of device in place and guides the use of the correct noncoring needle set.

Patient Preparation

- Verify the correct patient with two identifiers. *Rationale:* Before performing a procedure, the nurse should ensure the correct identification of the patient for the intended intervention.
- Ensure that the patient and family understand the preprocedural teaching. Answer questions as they arise, and reinforce information as needed. *Rationale:* Understanding of previously taught information is evaluated and reinforced.
- Assist the patient to the supine position with the head of the bed elevated up to a 30-degree angle. *Rationale:* Positioning prepares the patient and allows optimal access to the implanted venous access device.

Procedure for Implantable Venous Access Device: Access, Deaccess, and Care

Steps	Rationale	Special Considerations
Accessing an Implantable Venous Access Device		
1. **HH**		
2. **PE**		
3. Remove the patient's gown away from the venous access device.	Optimizes the viewing area and ensure aseptic field.	
4. Assess the venous access device: A. Palpate the subcutaneous tissue to determine the borders of the access device.[4,10] B. Palpate the venous access device borders, and locate the septum and the center of the septum. **(Level M*)**	Allows for identification of the type of port that was implanted and whether the port is single or double lumen.	
5. Assess the site for signs and symptoms of infection or other complications (e.g., erythema, induration, pain, or tenderness at the site).	Minimizes the risk of accessing an infected area.	Before accessing, examine the chest for complications, including evidence of thrombosis (veins of ipsilateral chest and neck), erythema, swelling, or tenderness, which may indicate system leakage or infection. A radiograph is recommended if leakage is suspected.[1,10]
6. Discard gloves in the appropriate receptacle.	Removes and safely discards used supplies.	
7. **HH**		
8. Carefully open the central venous catheter dressing kit with the sterile inner surface of the wrap.	Maintains asepsis and prepares supplies. Creates a sterile field.	Disinfect the table as needed. Venous access devices have the lowest risk for catheter-related blood system infections, provided that aseptic and sterile techniques are used throughout care delivery.[3,4,6,8] The kit should include sterile gloves and masks.
9. Prepare supplies A. With sterile technique, remove the wrapper from two 10-mL syringes, and place them on the sterile field. B. Remove the packaging, and place the winged or safety-noncoring needle with extension tubing, needleless injection cap, and Steri-Strips or stabilization device on the sterile field.	Places equipment within reach during the procedure. Maintains the sterility of the procedure.	If prefilled saline syringes are provided in a sterile package, they can be placed onto the field. Eliminate Steps 9-11.
10. Remove the cap from the NS vial; wipe the top of the NS vial with an alcohol wipe, and allow it to dry.	Reduces microorganisms.	

*Level M: Manufacturer's recommendations only.

Procedure continues on following page

Procedure	for Implantable Venous Access Device: Access, Deaccess, and Care—*Continued*	
Steps	**Rationale**	**Special Considerations**
11. Prepare additional supplies: A. Put on a face mask. B. Put a sterile glove on your dominant hand. C. With a sterile gloved hand, pick up a sterile 10-mL syringe. D. With the nonsterile hand, pick up the NS vial. E. Use the sterile gloved hand to withdraw 10 mL of NS solution, touching only the sterile syringe. F. Repeat the above to fill the second sterile syringe with 10 mL of saline. G. As described previously, use the sterile gloved hand to withdraw 10 mL of NS.	Prepares for the procedure.	
12. Apply the remaining sterile glove.	Maintains asepsis.	
13. With sterile technique A. Attach the needleless injection cap to the extension tubing on the noncoring needle. B. Attach the 10-mL NS syringe to the needleless cap. C. Prime the tubing with NS solution away from the sterile field.	Prepares the equipment. Removes air from the extension tubing, preventing possible air embolism.	
14. Retain the priming syringe on the needleless cap, and return the primed equipment to the sterile field.		
15. Cleanse the implanted venous access device site or port with 2% chlorhexidine-based antiseptic solution. Cleanse the site using a back-and-forth motion while applying friction for 30 seconds. Allow the antiseptic to remain on the insertion site and to dry completely before catheter insertion.[3,4,5,8,10] **(Level D*)**	Reduces the risk of infection.	Administer topical anesthetic if prescribed to reduce discomfort.[4]
16. Pick up the noncoring needle with the NS syringe attached with the dominant hand, and remove the protective cap.		
17. Use the nondominant hand to stabilize the borders of the venous access device.		
18. Triangulate the venous access device between the thumb and first two fingers of the nondominant hand (Fig. 76.3).	Stabilizes the venous access device within the chest wall and prevents slippage. Protects the provider, or other healthcare professional from a potential needle injury.	

*Level D: Peer-reviewed professional and organizational standards with the support of clinical study recommendations.

UNIT II

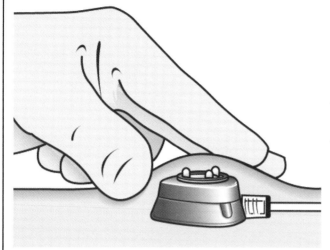

Figure 76.3 Triangulating the PowerPort Implanted Port with the nondominant hand. *(Courtesy Bard Corporation.)*

19. With the dominant hand, firmly grasp the protective cap or wings of the noncoring needle, and insert it firmly into the center of the port septum at a 90-degree angle perpendicular to the skin surface (Fig. 76.4).

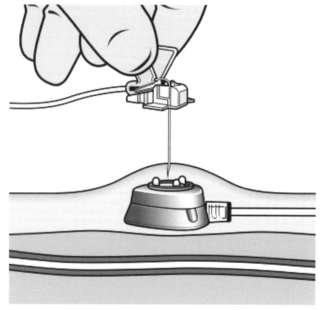

Figure 76.4 Needle access of the PowerPort Implanted Port with a noncoring PowerLoc Needle. *(Courtesy Bard Corporation.)*

20. Advance the needle through the skin and septum until reaching the base of the portal reservoir when you feel portal backing (Fig. 76.5).

With use of a noncoring safety needle, grasp the vertical fin between the thumb and middle finger and press downward with the index finger.[4,5,10]

Procedure continues on following page

Procedure for Implantable Venous Access Device: Access, Deaccess, and Care—*Continued*		
Steps	**Rationale**	**Special Considerations**

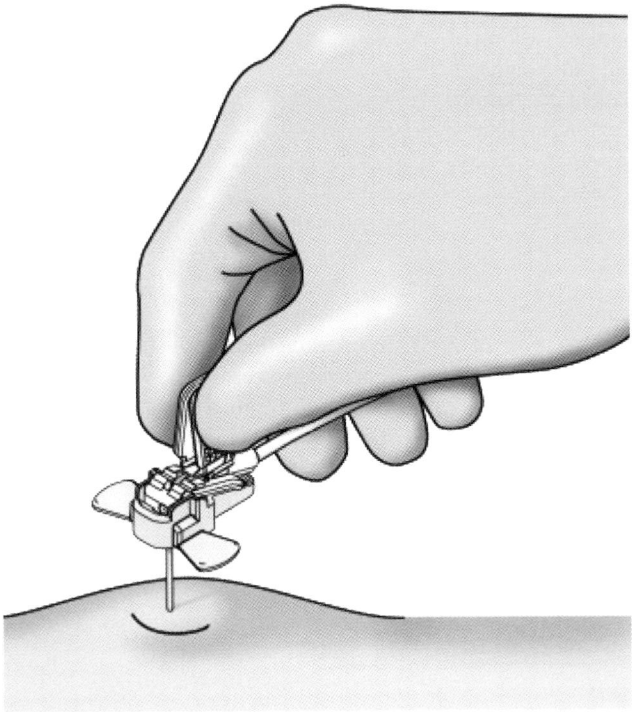

Figure 76.5 The noncoring PowerLoc Needle is inserted until the base of the port reservoir is felt. *(Courtesy Bard Corporation.)*

Steps	Rationale	Special Considerations
21. Note that resistance is felt as the needle reaches the base of the reservoir.		Once the septum is punctured, avoid tilting or rocking the needle, which may cause fluid leakage or damage to the system.[2]
22. Aspirate blood to check for patency, and then flush the venous access device with 5 mL of NS solution.	Determines the patency of the venous access device.	Avoid use of syringes with less than a 10-mL volume for flushing or administration of infusate. Smaller syringes exert pressure exceeding 40 psi and may cause catheter rupture or fragmentation with possible embolization.[2,10]
23. Observe the skin surrounding the noncoring needle for leakage of fluid or infiltration at the access site.	Assesses for potential access problems.	
24. Gently aspirate blood to check for patency, and then flush with the remaining 5 mL of NS.	Verifies placement.	If a blood return is not evident, gently flush with the push-pull method and reposition the patient. If a blood return is still not evident, continue the access procedure and apply a dressing to minimize the risk of infection. Contact the patient's physician or advance practice nurse. Administer a lytic agent and obtain a radiographic or dye shadow study as prescribed.[1]
25. Position the wings flush with the patient's skin.	Anchoring minimizes discomfort for the patient.	

UNIT II

Procedure | for Implantable Venous Access Device: Access, Deaccess, and Care—*Continued*

Steps	Rationale	Special Considerations
26. Stabilize the needle by attaching Steri-Strips in a cross or star pattern over the wings of the noncoring needle, or use of the stabilizing device as per protocol.	Stabilizes the needle inserted in the septal core and minimizes rocking of the needle, which can cause damage to the septum and patient discomfort. Also, minimizes needle movement in the septum, thereby ensuring integrity of the septal core for future use.	Follow institutional protocols.
27. Apply a sterile, occlusive dressing.	Maintains asepsis.	A gauze dressing is preferred if oozing or blood seepage occurs at the insertion site.
28. Label the dressing with the date, time of cannulation, needle gauge and length, and initial.	Provides important clinical information.	If the accessed device is not to be used immediately, flush it with heparin as prescribed.
29. Initiate continuous or intermittent infusion.	Begins therapy.	Attach intravenous (IV) tubing to the catheter hub for continuous infusion or injection cap for intermittent infusions.
30. Remove **PE**, and discard used supplies in appropriate receptacles.	Removes and safely discards used supplies.	
31. **HH**		

Deaccessing an Implantable Venous Access Device

1. **HH**		
2. **PE**		
3. Ensure good blood return before deaccessing the implantable venous access device. When ready, flush the venous access device with 20 mL of NS, followed by heparin flush as prescribed (e.g., 5 mL of 100 units/mL heparin).[5,7]	Prepares and optimizes catheter patency while not in use.	
4. Loosen the transparent or gauze dressing and Steri-Strips or the stabilization device from the site.	Facilitates removal.	
5. Use the thumb and forefinger of the dominant hand to grasp the dressing and the Steri-Strips or the stabilization device along with the winged flanges of the needle.	Prepares for needle removal.	
6. With the nondominant hand, apply gentle stabilizing pressure to the venous access device while removing the needle by pulling straight up and out in a firm, continuous motion.	Minimizes patient discomfort and ensures controlled withdrawal of a sharp object.	With use of a noncoring safety needle, grasp the horizontal flanges securely, pull up, and squeeze the flanges together. The flanges fold together, forcing the needle inside the locked wings and covering the needle. The wings will lock in place.
7. Assess the site for redness or drainage.	Identifies possible complications.	
8. Discard the noncoring needle in a designated container.	Safely removes sharp objects.	
9. Apply a dressing to the site if oozing occurs.	Provides absorption.	
10. Remove **PE**, and discard supplies in appropriate receptacles.	Removes and safely discards used supplies.	
11. **HH**		

Procedure continues on following page

Procedure	for Implantable Venous Access Device: Access, Deaccess, and Care—*Continued*	
Steps	**Rationale**	**Special Considerations**

Obtaining a Blood Specimen From an Implantable Venous Access Device

Steps	Rationale	Special Considerations
1. 🅷🅷		
2. 🅿🅴		
3. If present, shut off the IV infusion, and disconnect the IV tubing from the extension tubing on the noncoring needle.	Maintains asepsis.	
4. Place a sterile cap on the end of the IV tubing.	Maintains asepsis.	
5. Thoroughly cleanse the injection cap with an alcohol wipe, and allow it to dry. Do not remove the cap.[3-5,9,10] **(Level D*)**	Minimizes infection and exposure of the provider, or other healthcare professional to blood and body fluids.[2]	
6. Attach a 10-mL syringe with NS, and flush the venous access device.	Clears the catheter of medication or IV fluid.	
7. Attach a new sterile 10-mL syringe or a needleless blood sampling access device.	Prepares supplies.	
8. Determine the appropriate discard volume. **(Level E*)**	Clears the catheter of solution. The discard volume includes the dead space and the blood diluted by the flush solution. Portal reservoirs average 0.5 mL volume; catheters average 0.6 mL for single-lumen systems.[7] Recommendations are that at least three times the dead space be withdrawn.[7] Discard 5–10 mL of blood.[4,7]	Blood for coagulation tests should not be withdrawn through a heparinized catheter if the results will be used to monitor anticoagulant therapy or to determine whether a patient has a coagulopathy. Blood specimens should be redrawn peripherally when results are abnormal.[2] Follow institutional protocols.
9. Gently aspirate the discard volume into the syringe, or engage a blood specimen tube into the needleless blood sampling access device to obtain the discard volume and allow the tube to passively fill.[4,5]	Withdraws the discard.	Minimizes needlestick injury and exposure to blood and decreases infection risk to the patient by reducing the incidence of opening the catheter system.
10. Remove the discard syringe or the blood specimen tube.	Prepares for blood sampling.	
11. Insert a new syringe into the injection cap, or place a new blood specimen tube into the needleless blood sampling access device.	Prepares for removal of the specimen sample.	
12. Slowly and gently aspirate blood, or engage the blood specimen tube into the needleless blood sampling access device.	Obtains the blood specimen.	
13. Remove the syringe or the blood specimen tube.	Removes the specimen.	
14. After the blood specimen is obtained, flush the port with 10–20 mL of NS.[4,7]	Clears blood from the system.	Flush with an additional 10–20 mL of NS if the blood does not clear completely from the extension tubing.
15. Clamp the extension tubing.		

*Level D: Peer-reviewed professional and organizational standards with the support of clinical study recommendations.

*Level E: Multiple case reports, theory-based evidence from expert opinions, or peer-reviewed professional organizational standards without clinical studies to support recommendations.

Procedure for Implantable Venous Access Device: Access, Deaccess, and Care—*Continued*

Steps	Rationale	Special Considerations
16. Replace a new injection cap with strict aseptic technique.	Reduces infection.	Ensure using alcohol wipes to thoroughly clean the hub before attaching the new injection cap.
17. Reconnect the IV, and continue the infusion.	Resumes therapy.	If the IV infusion is completed, administer heparin as prescribed.
18. Remove **PE**, and discard used supplies in appropriate receptacles.	Removes and safely discards used supplies.	
19. **HH**		
20. Label the specimen(s) and the laboratory form.	Properly identifies the patient and laboratory tests to be performed.	
21. Send the laboratory specimen(s) for analysis.	Expedites determination of laboratory results.	

Expected Outcomes

- Site without redness, pain, or tenderness
- Venous access device is stable
- Venous access device is accessed without difficulty
- Venous access device flushes easily without evidence of resistance or infiltration
- No evidence of leakage at the septal site
- Blood specimens are obtained as prescribed
- Venous access device is deaccessed without difficulty

Unexpected Outcomes

- Port reddened, tender, or painful on palpation
- Skin erosion
- Implanted device unstable in the chest wall with palpation
- Catheter migration
- Catheter "pinch-off" (compression of catheter between the clavicle and the first rib)
- Portal body inversion or "twiddler's syndrome"
- Patient describes burning sensation in the subcutaneous tissue with flushing or infusion
- Sluggish or no blood return with aspiration
- Evidence of leakage of flush solution at the septal site
- Patient describes pain at the site, chest, ear, or shoulder with flushing
- Signs or symptoms of local or systemic infection
- Swollen neck or arm[2,9]

Patient Monitoring and Care

Steps	Rationale	Reportable Conditions
		These conditions should be reported to the provider if they persist despite nursing interventions.
1. During IV infusions, assess the venous access device for patency and signs of infiltration every 4 hours and as needed.	Determines adequate functioning of the venous access device.	Signs or symptoms of infiltration at the venous access site
2. Replace gauze dressings every 2 days and transparent dressings at least every 7 days.[3,8,9] Follow institutional protocols. **(Level D*)**	Decreases the risk for infection at the catheter site. The dressing should be changed if it becomes damp, loosened, or soiled or when inspection of the site is necessary.[3,8]	Signs or symptoms of infection
3. Follow institutional protocols for assessing and managing pain.	Identifies the need for pain interventions.	Continued pain despite pain interventions

*Level D: Peer-reviewed professional and organizational standards with the support of clinical study recommendations.

Procedure continues on following page

Patient Monitoring and Care —*Continued*

Steps	Rationale	Reportable Conditions
4. Follow-up care for deaccessed device includes reaccessing the device to administer monthly flush with 5 mL of 100 units of heparin as prescribed.[7,8,10]	Maintains catheter patency.	
5. Assess for signs and symptoms of infection.	Determines the presence of infection.	Redness, pain, or drainage at the site; fever, elevated white blood cell count

Documentation

Documentation should include the following:
- Assessment of the site before accessing and deaccessing the port
- Location and cannulation of the device
- Needle length and gauge
- Appearance of blood return before, during, and after infusion
- Date and time of therapy administration
- Specimens obtained and sent for analysis
- Laboratory results
- Pain assessment, interventions, and effectiveness
- Unexpected outcomes
- Additional interventions
- Patient's response to the procedure and therapy
- Education of the patient and family regarding the procedure and therapies administered

References and Additional Readings

For a complete list of references and additional readings for this procedure, scan this QR code with your smartphone, or visit https://www.elsevier.com/__data/assets/pdf_file/0010/1319851/Chapter0076.pdf.

UNIT II

77 Peripherally Inserted Central Catheter and Midline Catheters AP

Kathleen M. Cox

PURPOSE Peripherally inserted central catheters (PICCs) are used to deliver central venous therapy to provide venous access for patients who require infusates that are not peripherally compatible (e.g., vesicants, irritants). Midline catheters specifically are used to provide venous access for patients who have limited peripheral venous access and who require intravenous (IV) therapy for approximately 2 weeks. Both midline catheters and PICCs can be considered for patients requiring IV therapy beyond 7 days and up to approximately 2 weeks for a midline catheter. PICCs are generally recommended for patients who need long-term therapy up to and beyond 30 days.[2,4,6,7] PICCs can be used for all types of infusion therapy including chemotherapy, total parenteral nutrition, analgesia, blood products, intermittent inotropic medications, and long-term antibiotics.

PREREQUISITE NURSING KNOWLEDGE

- Successful completion of specialized education in ultrasound-guided midline or peripherally inserted central catheter (PICC) insertion utilizing a modified Seldinger technique and demonstrated competency.[1,6] In addition, opportunities to demonstrate clinical competency on a regular basis (e.g., yearly) may be needed.
- Principles of sterile technique.
- Anatomy and physiology of the vasculature and adjacent structures in the upper extremity, neck, and chest.
- Assessment of upper-extremity venous access using ultrasound.
- A patient receiving a PICC or midline catheter should have a peripheral vein that can accommodate a 22-gauge microintroducer needle to perform the modified Seldinger technique. The smallest device in the largest vein allows for maximal hemodilution of the infusate and minimizes the risk of phlebitis and thrombosis.[4,6] The catheter-to-vein ratio should be 45% or less.
- The basilic, medial cubital, cephalic, and brachial veins should be considered for cannulation with a PICC or midline catheter (Fig. 77.1). The basilic vein is the larger vessel and is the vein of choice for insertion of a PICC/midline catheter. The brachial vein is the second choice because of its close proximity to the brachial artery

and nerve structures. The cephalic vein has been associated with an increased risk of thrombosis. Patient preference for arm selection (e.g., nondominant hand, lifestyle, activity restrictions, ability to care for the catheter) should be considered with selection of the insertion site.[2,6] Once inserted, the PICC is advanced to the lower segment of the superior vena cava at or near the cavoatrial junction.[6,7] Midline catheters do not enter the central vasculature. The catheter tip for the midline is located at or near the level of the axilla and below the level of the shoulder.[2]

- Patient indications for the insertion of a PICC are not limited to inpatient therapies. A PICC is also placed for patients who require intravenous (IV) therapy in the home setting for chronic heart failure, cancer treatment, chronic pain management, nutritional support, fluid replacement (e.g., hyperemesis gravidarum) and long-term antibiotics.[2]
- PICCs or midlines may be preferred over percutaneously inserted central venous catheters for patients with trauma of the chest (e.g., burns) or certain pulmonary disorders (e.g., chronic obstructive pulmonary disease, cystic fibrosis).[2] PICCs/midline catheters eliminate the risks associated with insertion of percutaneously inserted central venous catheters in the neck or chest (e.g., pneumothorax).[2]
- PICCs and midlines are contraindicated in patients with sclerotic veins, chronic kidney disease stages 4 and 5, lymphedema, mastectomy with lymph node dissection, arteriovenous graft, fistula, radial artery surgery, or extremities affected by cerebral vascular accident. Other access devices may be a better choice in patients with altered upper extremity skin integrity or upper extremity fractures in whom PICC/midline complications could compromise wound healing.

AP This procedure should be performed only by clinicians who have demonstrated competence and are credentialed to perform it. In addition, the procedure must be within the scope of practice defined by their professional licensure, and in accordance with professional practice acts. Physicians, advanced practice nurses, and physician assistants may be credentialed to perform this procedure.

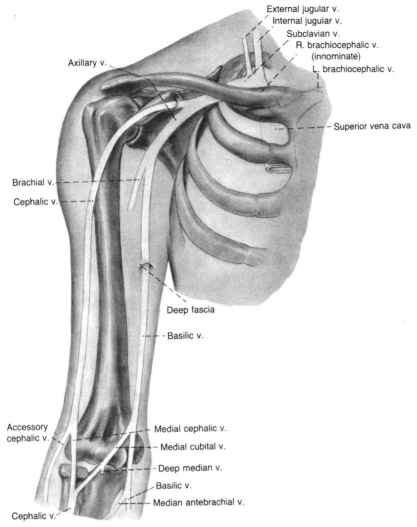

Figure 77.1   Location of the veins of the right shoulder and upper arm. *(From Jacob SW, Francone CA: Elements of anatomy and physiology, ed 2, Philadelphia, 1989, Saunders.)*

- The most common complications associated with PICCs and midline catheters are phlebitis, thrombosis, and catheter occlusion.[2,4,6,7]
- A variety of PICCs and midline catheters are available for use. PICCs/midline catheters are flexible catheters that are made of silicone or polyurethane. Catheter diameters range from 2F to 6F, and the catheter length ranges from 40 cm to 65 cm. For adults, 4F to 5F catheters that are 60 cm in length are typical.
- PICCs are available as single-lumen, double-lumen, and triple-lumen catheters, with and without valves. Midline catheters are available as single-lumen or double-lumen catheters.
- Some PICCs are designed to handle power injections (e.g., contrast media for computed tomographic scans). Although some midlines are also labeled for power injection, there is still some question whether the midline tip placement is deep enough to accommodate the hypertonicity of contrast fluid effectively. This decision will depend on the patient, the clinical situation, and the provider's familiarity with the procedure.[2]
- A PICC or midline catheter can be inserted with or without the use of a modified Seldinger technique. When a

modified Seldinger technique is used, venous access is achieved with a small-gauge (20- or 22-gauge) peripheral IV catheter. Once the IV catheter is inserted, the stylet is removed and the guidewire is threaded through the IV catheter. The IV catheter is then removed, and the dilator/introducer is inserted over the guidewire. The dilator and guidewire are removed, leaving the introducer in the vein to allow for passage of the PICC or midline catheter into the vein. Once the PICC/midline catheter is in place, the introducer is removed. Care must be taken with the use of a guidewire. Although advancement of the introducer is enhanced by the firmness provided by the guidewire, the guidewire can inadvertently traumatize the vessel.
- There are alternate PICC and midline placement techniques, and the manufacturer's guidelines should be followed.
- A variety of safety-engineered introducers are available and should be used to reduce the risk for blood exposure and needlestick injury.[4,6]
- PICCs and midline catheters can be placed at the patient's bedside, in interventional radiology, or in specialized rooms dedicated for PICC/midline insertions.

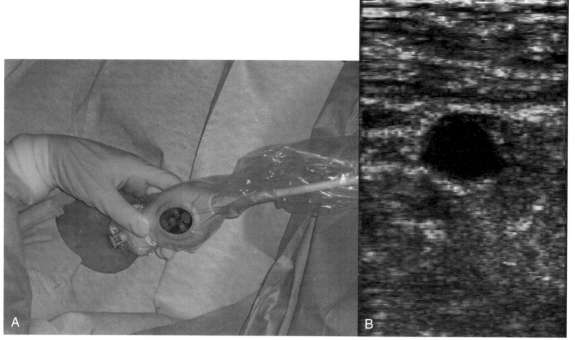

Figure 77.2   Use of ultrasound technology to assist with vein location. **A,** The ultrasound scan probe is positioned over the insertion site. **B,** Depiction of ultrasound scan–assisted catheter insertion. *(Courtesy Bard Access Systems, Salt Lake City, UT.)*

- Ultrasound guidance is recommended to place PICCs and midline catheters if the technology is available. Ultrasound guidance is associated with improvement in insertion success rates, reduced number of needle punctures, and decreased insertion complication rates.[4]
- Ultrasound technology can be used to assist with vein assessment and PICC/midline catheter insertion (Fig. 77.2). Tip-locating technology using ECG and Doppler can be utilized to further assist the clinician in confirming tip location in the superior vena cava. The catheter tip for the midline is located at or near the level of the axilla and below the level of the shoulder.[5]
- Longitudinal or transverse views can be used when placing the PICC or midline catheter with ultrasound guidance. The needle tip should remain in view at all times. If the tip of the needle cannot be visualized, the probe, not the needle, should be moved to reestablish visibility.[4,5]

EQUIPMENT

- Catheter-insertion kit
- PICC or midline catheter of choice
- Single-use tourniquet
- Sterile and nonsterile measuring tape
- Waterproof underpad/linen saver
- Sterile gown
- Head cover
- Mask
- Goggles or eye protection
- Two pairs of nonpowdered sterile gloves
- Sterile drapes and towels, including one fenestrated full barrier drape
- Antiseptic solution (e.g., 2% chlorhexidine-based preparation)

- 10-mL vial of heparin (concentration and use per institutional standards)
- 30-mL vial of normal saline (NS) solution
- Needleless connector with/without short extension tubing
- One to three 10-mL, 20-gauge, 1-inch needle syringes (blunt needles recommended), depending on the number of lumens
- Sterile 4 × 4 gauze pads or sponges
- Sterile 2 × 2 gauze pads or sponges
- Sterile, transparent, semipermeable dressing
- Bedside ultrasound machine with vascular probe
- Sterile ultrasound probe cover
- Sterile ultrasound gel
- Catheter securement device

Additional equipment, to have available as needed, includes the following:

- One 1-mL, 25-gauge, ⅝-inch needle syringe (if intradermal lidocaine is used)
- 1% lidocaine without epinephrine or 1 to 2 mL of eutectic mixture of local anesthetics (EMLA) cream (optional)

PATIENT AND FAMILY EDUCATION

- Explain the reason for the PICC/midline catheter insertion, the benefits and risks associated with placement, and the alternatives to PICC/midline catheter placement. *Rationale:* Clarification of information is an expressed patient need and helps diminish anxiety, enhance acceptance, and encourage questions.
- Describe the major steps of the procedure, including the patient's role in the procedure. *Rationale:* Explanation decreases patient anxiety, enhances cooperation, provides an opportunity for the patient to voice concerns, and

UNIT II

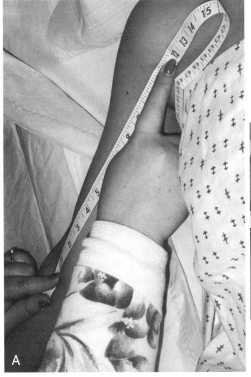
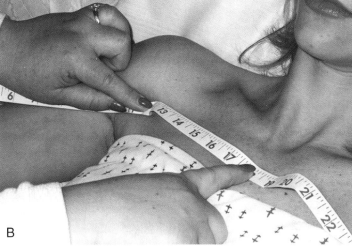

Figure 77.3   Measurement of the catheter length for placement in the superior vena cava. **A,** First, measure the distance from the selected insertion site to the shoulder. **B,** Continue measuring from the shoulder to the sternal notch, and add 3 inches (7.5 cm) to this number.

prevents accidental contamination of the sterile field and equipment.

- Instruct the patient and family to refuse injections, venipuncture, and blood pressure measurements on the arm with the PICC/midline catheter. ***Rationale:*** The risk for catheter-related complications and catheter damage is minimized.
- Provide appropriate patient and family discharge education regarding the care and maintenance of the PICC/ midline catheter if the patient will be discharged with the PICC/midline catheter in place. ***Rationale:*** Education reduces the risk for catheter-related complications from lack of knowledge and skills needed to care for the PICC/ midline catheter after discharge.

PATIENT ASSESSMENT AND PREPARATION

Patient Assessment

- Assess the patient's medical history for mastectomy, fistula, shunt, CVA, or radial artery surgery. ***Rationale:*** PICC/midline catheter insertion should be avoided in extremities affected by these conditions to preserve veins for future needs and because the risk for complications is increased.
- Obtain the patient's baseline vital signs and cardiac rhythm. ***Rationale:*** Cardiac dysrhythmias can occur if the catheter is advanced into the heart. Baseline data facilitate the identification of clinical problems and the efficacy of interventions.
- Assess the vasculature of the proposed extremity for appropriate vessel size, round shape, normal path, and

compressibility. These assessments should be performed without a tourniquet to establish the appropriate vein-to-catheter ratio and to ensure adequate blood flow around the catheter in situ. ***Rationale:*** Placing a catheter in a healthy vein with adequate blood flow around the catheter will optimize catheter function and decrease the risk of thrombosis.

- Determine the patient's allergy history (e.g., lidocaine, heparin, EMLA cream, antiseptic solutions, tape, latex). ***Rationale:*** Assessment decreases the risk for allergic reactions with avoidance of known allergenic products.

Patient Preparation

- Verify the correct patient with two identifiers. ***Rationale:*** Before performing a procedure, the nurse should ensure the correct identification of the patient for the intended intervention.
- Ensure that the patient and family understand the preprocedural teaching. Answer questions as they arise, and reinforce information as needed. ***Rationale:*** Understanding of previously taught information is evaluated and reinforced.
- Ensure that informed consent has been obtained. ***Rationale:*** Informed consent protects the rights of the patient and allows the patient to make a competent decision.
- Perform a preprocedure verification and time out. ***Rationale:*** Ensures patient safety.
- Assist the patient to the supine position with the head of the bed elevated. ***Rationale:*** Ensures patient comfort.
- For PICC placement in the superior vena cava, use the nonsterile measuring tape to measure the distance from the selected insertion site to the shoulder (Fig. 77.3A) and from the shoulder to the sternal notch (see Fig. 77.3B). Add 3 inches (7.5 cm, or the measured distance from the

sternal notch to the third intercostal space) to this number for catheter placement in the superior vena cava. ***Rationale:*** Accurate measurement ensures proper tip position in the distal portion of the superior vena cava at the cavoatrial junction and determines the length of the catheter to be inserted.

- For midline catheter placement in the axillary vein with the tip ideally near the midclavicular line, select a puncture site within the ~7 cm "green zone" in the upper arm (~4 cm below the axilla and ~2 cm above the antecubital space). The choice of a 20- or 25-cm midline catheter is based on the planned puncture site and the catheter length that would locate the tip nearest the midclavicular line.[3,5] ***Rationale:*** Accurate measurement ensures proper tip position in the midaxillary area and determines the length of the catheter to be inserted.
- Measure the mid–upper arm circumference of the selected extremity. ***Rationale:*** Measurement provides a baseline

for evaluation of suspected thrombosis after PICC or midline insertion. Increases of greater than 2 cm over baseline may be indicative of venous thrombosis. A diagnostic ultrasound scan should be obtained.

- Stabilize the position of the arm with a towel or pillow. ***Rationale:*** Stabilization increases patient comfort, secures the work area, and facilitates access to the selected vein.
- Instruct the patient on proper head positioning. The head is positioned to the contralateral side (away from the insertion site) throughout the procedure, except when the PICC is advanced from the axillary vein to the superior vena cava. At this point, the patient is instructed to position his or her head toward the ipsilateral side (toward the insertion site) with the chin dropped to the shoulder. This maneuver is not necessary when inserting a midline. ***Rationale:*** Proper positioning limits the risk for the catheter being inadvertently directed into the jugular vein when placing a PICC.

Procedure for Peripherally Inserted Central Catheter and Midline

Steps	Rationale	Special Considerations
1. Obtain ultrasound equipment.	Prepares equipment.	Assistance may be needed from radiology.
2. **HH**		
3. **PE**		
4. Place a waterproof pad under the selected arm.	Avoids soiling of bed linens.	
5. Determine the anatomy of the access site. **(Level E*)**	Helps ensure proper placement of the PICC or midline and guides the area to be prepped.[4,6]	
6. Wash the insertion area with soap and water.	Prepares insertion site.	
7. Discard used supplies, and remove gloves.	Removes and safely discards used supplies.	
8. **HH**		
9. With the measuring tape, perform the preinsertion anatomic measurements (see Fig. 77.3).	Catheters are provided at various lengths.	This can be guided by ultrasound. Make a note of the required catheter length.
10. Position the tourniquet high on the upper extremity, near the axilla, but do not constrict venous blood flow at this time.	Placement high on the extremity avoids contamination of the sterile field.	
11. Open the PICC/midline catheter insertion tray, and drop the remaining sterile items onto the sterile field.	Maintains aseptic technique; prepares the work area, including procurement of all necessary equipment; avoids interruption of the procedure and contamination of the work area.	
12. **HH**		
13. Apply a sterile gown and sterile gloves.	PICC/midline insertion is a sterile procedure.	Personnel protective equipment (e.g., head cover, mask, goggles) is needed as well as sterile equipment. Blood splashing may occur with the use of guidewires, stylets, and breakaway or peel-away introducers.

*Level E: Multiple case reports, theory-based evidence from expert opinions, or peer-reviewed professional organizational protocols without clinical studies to support recommendations.

Procedure continues on following page

UNIT II

Procedure for Peripherally Inserted Central Catheter and Midline—*Continued*

Steps	Rationale	Special Considerations
14. Prepare the catheter according to the manufacturer's recommendations.	Each manufacturer recommends a specific preparation protocol for each type of catheter.	
15. Fill the 10-mL syringe with NS. Add the needleless connector to the short extension tubing, and prime it with NS. Leave the syringe attached.	Prepares the system.	If inserting a double-lumen or triple-lumen catheter, prime the additional lumen(s) of the catheter with NS.

16. Prepare the site with a 2% chlorhexidine-based antiseptic solution.[4,6,8]
  A. Cleanse the site with a back-and-forth motion while applying friction for 30 seconds.
  B. Allow the antiseptic to remain on the insertion site and to air-dry completely before catheter insertion.[4,6,8] **(Level D*)**
	Limits the introduction of potentially infectious skin flora into the vessel during the puncture.	

17. Discard gloves in the appropriate receptacle.	Removes and safely discards used supplies.	
18. 🅷🅷		
19. Apply the tourniquet snugly, approximately 6 inches (15 cm) near the axilla well outside of the sterile field.	Provides vasodilation of the vein for venipuncture.	Constriction should effectively cause venous distention without arterial occlusion.
20. 🅷🅷		
21. Apply a new pair of sterile gloves.	PICC/midline insertion is a sterile procedure.	
22. Instruct the patient to lift his or her arm; place a sterile drape underneath and the fenestrated drape over the entire patient, leaving the venipuncture site exposed. Place a sterile 4 × 4 gauze pad over the tourniquet.	Maintains the sterile field and facilitates aseptic technique.	Ultrasound scan technology can be used to assist with catheter insertion (see Fig. 77.2).
23. Instruct the patient to turn his or her head away from the insertion site.	Prevents contamination of the field by organisms from the patient's respiratory tract.	If the patient is not intubated ensure the patient has on a mask.
24. Inject a skin weal of approximately 0.5 mL of 1% lidocaine without epinephrine at or adjacent to the venipuncture site. **(Level B*)**	Provides local anesthesia for venipuncture with large-gauge needles and introducers. Local anesthesia should be administered with insertion of a PICC or midline.[2,4,6,7]	Patients report less pain when a local anesthetic agent is used before venipuncture.[2,3] Lidocaine may produce stinging, burning, obscuring of the vein, or venospasm. The use of EMLA (a topical anesthetic cream) before venipuncture has been researched.[2] If it is used, manufacturer's recommendations should be followed.
25. Perform the venipuncture according to catheter design and manufacturer's instructions.	Catheters vary according to design and introducing techniques.	Relocate the intended vein with the ultrasound probe and use the ultrasound images to guide the insertion process.[2,4,5,6]

*Level B: Well-designed, controlled studies with results that consistently support a specific action, intervention, or treatment.
*Level D: Peer-reviewed professional and organizational protocols with the support of clinical study recommendations.

Procedure	for Peripherally Inserted Central Catheter and Midline—*Continued*	
Steps	**Rationale**	**Special Considerations**
26. Perform the modified Seldinger technique (Fig. 77.4). A. Insert a microintroducer needle or cannula, and observe for blood return in the flashback chamber (see Fig. 77.4, *1*). B. Advance the floppy tipped guidewire 2 to 4 inches (5–10 cm) through the needle or cannula (see Fig. 77.4, *2*).[6] C. Remove the needle or cannula back over the guidewire, and insert the dilator/introducer over the guidewire (see Fig. 77.4, *4*). D. Gently advance the dilator/ introducer until the tip is well within the lumen of the vein (see Fig. 77.4, *5*). E. Remove the guidewire and then the dilator leaving the introducer in place (see Fig. 77.4, *6*). F. Insert the PICC approximately 6–8 inches (15–20 cm); for midline, insert approximately 10–15 cm.	Use of a guidewire enhances the advancement of the dilator/ introducer. Establishes venous access.	Place a finger over the opening of the catheter to limit blood loss and risk for air embolism (see Fig. 77.4, *2*). If unable to access the vein, the procedure should be terminated and an alternate access site selected. A small dermatotomy or nick in the skin using a sterile scalpel adjacent to the guidewire may facilitate the advancement of the dilator/ introducer (see Fig. 77.4, *3*). If a scalpel is not provided in the PICC insertion kit, a No. 11 blade should be used. Place a finger over the opening of the introducer to limit blood loss and the risk for air embolism (see Fig. 77.4, *6*). Sterile forceps may be used to insert the catheter into the introducer and advance the catheter into the vein (see Fig. 77.4, *7*).
27. Release the tourniquet with sterile technique (e.g., with a sterile 4 × 4 gauze pad).	The tourniquet may inhibit catheter advancement.	
28. Instruct the patient to turn his or her head toward the cannulated arm and to drop his or her chin to the chest. This maneuver is not necessary with a midline insertion. The midline should be advanced until the hub is against the skin.	Changes the angle of the jugular vein and decreases the potential for malpositioning of the catheter in the jugular vein.	
29. Advance the remainder of the catheter until approximately 4 inches (10 cm) remain while observing the heart rate and rhythm.	Cardiac dysrhythmias may occur if the catheter is advanced into the heart.	Never advance the catheter if resistance is felt. Excessive pushing could lead to perforation of the vein, catheter malposition, or pericardial perforation.
30. Instruct the patient to return his or her head to the contralateral side (away from the insertion site).	Prevents contamination of the field by organisms from the patient's respiratory tract.	
31. Pull the introducer out of the vein and away from the insertion site, and remove it (see Fig. 77.4, *8* and *9*).	The introducer sheath should remain in place until the catheter is properly positioned.	Methods of removing the introducer vary according to the manufacturer.

Procedure continues on following page

Procedure	for Peripherally Inserted Central Catheter and Midline—*Continued*	
Steps	Rationale	Special Considerations

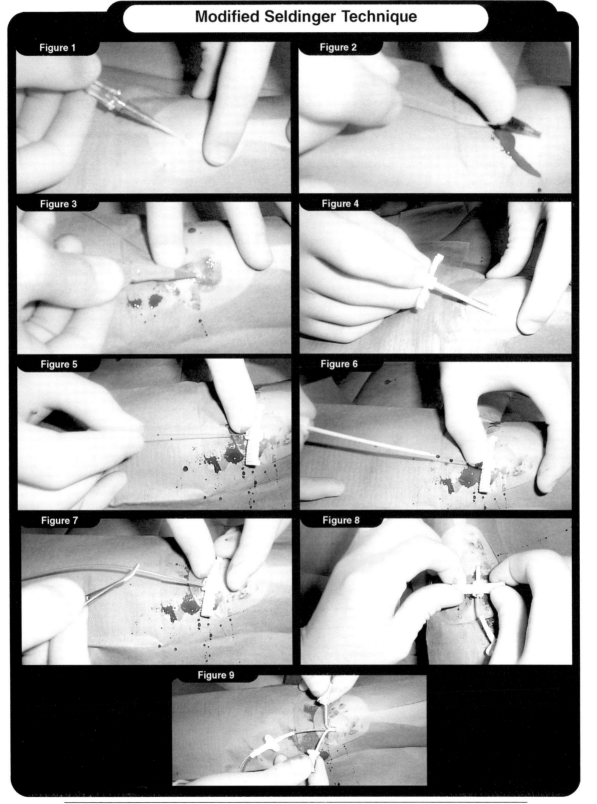

Figure 77.4 Modified Seldinger technique. *1*, Insertion of the peripheral intravenous catheter. *2*, Advancement of the guidewire through the catheter. *3*, Small skin nick to facilitate the advancement of the dilator/introducer. *4*, Insertion of the dilator/introducer over the guidewire. *5*, Advancement of the dilator/introducer. *6*, Removal of the dilator and guidewire. *7*, Insertion of the catheter using sterile forceps. *8*, Removal of the introducer. *9*, Introducer peeled apart and removed. *(Courtesy Bard Access Systems, Salt Lake City, UT.)*

UNIT II

Procedure	for Peripherally Inserted Central Catheter and Midline—*Continued*	
Steps	Rationale	Special Considerations
32. Measure the length of the catheter remaining outside the skin and reposition, if necessary, to the predetermined length. Approximately 1 inch (2.5 cm) of the catheter should remain externally.	Ensures proper catheter tip position.	The catheter should be advanced to the zero mark. Optimally, no more than 2 cm should remain external to the insertion site.
33. Attach the primed extension tubing (with injection port) to the catheter; aspirate for evidence of blood, and flush with NS with use of a push/pause technique.	Use of extension tubing provides easier access to the catheter and reduces local trauma at the insertion site. Aspiration affirms patency of the catheter. The push/pause technique during flushing optimizes catheter long-term patency.[4,6]	Most PICCs have their own extension sets and only require a needleless connector.
34. Inject the recommended amount and concentration of heparin as prescribed into the catheter, clamp the extension tubing, and remove the syringe. Repeat the procedure with use of a double-lumen or triple-lumen catheter.	Maintains catheter patency and prevents backflow of blood in the catheter.	Recommendations vary regarding the use, amount, and concentration of heparin to maintain catheter patency. Refer to manufacturer's recommendation or institutional protocols. Contraindicated in persons with known allergies to heparin.
35. Secure the catheter at the insertion site by applying a catheter securement device (Fig. 77.5).	Prevents inward or outward migration of the catheter.	Follow institutional protocols.

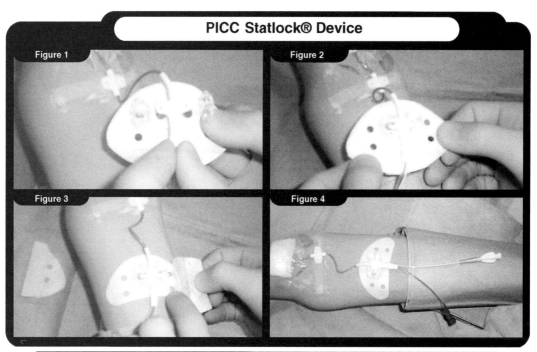

Figure 77.5   PICC Statlock device. *1*, Insertion of the wings of the PICC onto the device. *2*, Placement of the device on the forearm. *3*, Application of the sterile, transparent, semipermeable dressing over the device. *4*, Device properly secured. (*Courtesy Bard Access Systems, Salt Lake City UT.*)

Procedure continues on following page

Procedure for Peripherally Inserted Central Catheter and Midline—*Continued*

Steps	Rationale	Special Considerations
36. Apply a dressing. A. If bleeding is noted, cover the insertion site with a sterile 2 × 2 gauze pad, and then cover the site with a sterile, transparent, semipermeable dressing. B. If there is no bleeding, omit the gauze, apply a chlorhexidine-impregnated gel dressing or sponge to the site, and then cover it with a sterile transparent semipermeable membrane dressing.[1,6]	Decreases catheter-related infections.	A 2 × 2 gauze can be folded and placed immediately below the insertion site to act as a "wick" for any drainage in the first 24 hours. If the chlorhexidine impregnated sponge or gel dressing is applied at the insertion site, the dressing can remain for 7 days before changing.
37. Remove **PE** and sterile equipment, and discard used supplies in appropriate receptacles.	Reduces the transmission of microorganisms; Standard Precautions.	Ensure that sharp objects are safely removed.
38. **HH**		
39. Prepare the patient for a chest radiograph to determine the tip location if a tip-locating technology was not used.	Confirms placement of the catheter tip and detects any complications.	Some PICCs or midlines require contrast media for good visualization. Infusions should not be initiated until the catheter tip placement is confirmed.

Expected Outcomes

- The PICC tip is positioned in the distal portion of the superior vena cava at the cavoatrial junction; the midline tip is positioned near the midclavicular line.
- The PICC or midline remains patent.
- The insertion site and upper extremity remain free from phlebitis and thrombophlebitis.
- The insertion site, catheter, and systemic circulation remain free from infection.

Unexpected Outcomes

- Pain or discomfort during the procedure
- Complications on insertion, such as cardiac dysrhythmias, pericardial tamponade, air embolism, catheter embolism, arterial puncture, and nerve (brachial plexus) injury
- Complications after insertion, such as phlebitis, thrombophlebitis, thrombosis, infection (e.g., insertion site, catheter, systemic), and infiltration

Patient Monitoring and Care

Steps	Rationale	Reportable Conditions
		These conditions should be reported to the provider if they persist despite nursing interventions.
1. Observe the patient for signs or symptoms of cardiac dysrhythmias and pericardial tamponade during the procedure. If cardiac dysrhythmias occur, pull the catheter back, and reassess the patient.	Cardiac dysrhythmias may occur if the catheter is advanced into the heart. Pericardial tamponade may occur if the catheter penetrates the atrium.	• Cardiac dysrhythmias • Hemodynamic instability (changes in vital signs, level of consciousness, peripheral pulses, narrow pulse pressure, jugular venous distention)
2. Assess the patient, and obtain the chest radiographic report confirming proper catheter tip placement before initiating any intravenous solutions.	Ensures accurate catheter tip placement and aids in identification of potentially life-threatening complications.	• Abnormal chest radiographic report • Change in lung sounds • Chest pain • Respiratory distress

Patient Monitoring and Care —*Continued*

Steps	Rationale	Reportable Conditions
3. Observe the dressing and insertion site every 30 minutes for the first 4 hours after insertion.	Postinsertion bleeding may occur in patients with coagulopathies or with arterial punctures, multiple attempts at venipuncture, or use of the through-the-needle introducer design for insertion.	• Excessive bleeding • Hematoma
4. Assess the insertion site and upper extremity every shift for signs and symptoms of phlebitis, thrombophlebitis, or infiltration.	Mechanical phlebitis is the most common complication within the first 72 hours after insertion. Thrombophlebitis may occur at any time after catheter insertion.	• Pain along the vein • Edema at the puncture site • Erythema • Ipsilateral swelling of the arm, neck, or face • Venous occlusion (changes in arm circumference >2 cm from baseline) • Infiltration
5. Assess the catheter for venous blood return and patency before initiating infusions. A. Cleanse the extension tubing with 70% isopropyl alcohol or alcohol-based chlorhexidine used for medical devices. Allow to dry. B. Connect a 10-mL syringe filled with 10 mL of NS to the extension tubing. C. Release the clamp, and aspirate slowly to verify blood return. D. Flush with 10 mL of NS (with a push/pause technique), and then administer the infusion.	Verifies the position of the catheter in the vascular space and patency before initiation of infusions.	• Catheter occlusion (failure to obtain blood return on aspiration or resistance to irrigation)
6. Assess the catheter for dislodgment or migration by measuring the length of the external catheter.	The catheter may no longer be properly positioned if the length of the external catheter is longer or shorter than the length measured at the time of insertion.	• Change in external catheter length • Catheter occlusion • Cardiac dysrhythmias • Pain or burning during infusions • Palpation of the catheter in the internal jugular vein • Palpation of a coiled catheter • Infiltration
7. If there was insertional bleeding, the initial dressing should be left in place for 24 hours. After this: A. Assess the insertion site and upper forearm while performing a sterile dressing change. B. Transparent, semipermeable dressings should be changed at least weekly.[1] C. Sterile gauze dressings should be changed every 48 hours.[1,6] D. Dressings should be changed if they become damp, loosened, or visibly soiled.[1] **(Level D*)**	Policies may vary regarding the type of dressing and frequency of dressing changes after the initial dressing change.	• Redness, warmth, hardness, tenderness, pain, or swelling at the insertion site • Presence of purulent drainage from the insertion site • Local rash or pustules

*Level D: Peer-reviewed professional and organizational standards with the support of clinical study recommendations.

Procedure continues on following page

Patient Monitoring and Care —*Continued*

Steps	Rationale	Reportable Conditions
8. Monitor the insertion site and patient for signs and symptoms of local or systemic infection.	The incidence of infection related to the catheter may result from failure to maintain asepsis during insertion, failure to comply with dressing change protocols, immunosuppression, frequent access to the catheter, and long-term use of a single IV access site.	• Redness, warmth, hardness, tenderness, pain, or swelling at the insertion site • Presence of purulent drainage from the insertion site • Local rash or pustules • Fever, chills, or elevated white blood cell count • Nausea and vomiting
9. Avoid measuring blood pressure, performing venipuncture, or administering injections in the extremity with a PICC or midline catheter. Follow institutional protocols regarding placing a sign at the patient bedside regarding avoiding use of the extremity with the PICC or midline catheter.	Minimizes the risk for catheter-related complications and catheter damage.	
10. Follow institutional protocols for assessing pain. Administer analgesia as prescribed.	Identifies the need for pain interventions.	• Continued pain despite pain interventions

Documentation

Documentation should include the following:
- Patient and family education
- Completion of informed consent
- Preprocedure verification and time out
- Known allergies
- Mid–upper arm circumference
- Date and time of the procedure
- Catheter type, size, and length, including the length of catheter remaining outside the insertion site
- Type and amount of local anesthetic (if used)
- Location of the PICC or midline catheter insertion site and the vein accessed
- The method of securing the catheter
- Confirmation of catheter tip placement
- Problems encountered during or after the procedure or nursing interventions
- Patient tolerance of the procedure
- Pain assessment, interventions, and effectiveness
- Vital signs and cardiac rhythm
- Assessment of the insertion site

References and Additional Readings

For a complete list of references and additional readings for this procedure, scan this QR code with your smartphone, or visit https://www.elsevier.com/__data/assets/pdf_file/0011/1319852/Chapter0077.pdf.

78 Use of a Massive Infusion Device and a Pressure Infuser Bag

Debra Valdivieso

PURPOSE A massive infusion device is used to rapidly replace depleted intravascular volume in a critically ill patient. The infuser can simultaneously warm fluids and/or blood products and infuse them at rates up to 30,000 mL/hour. The ability to warm the fluids helps prevent and treat hypothermia, which will, in turn, minimize the risk of coagulopathy. Indications to use this device include patients with severe hemorrhage, as seen in trauma, gastrointestinal bleeding, intraoperative or postoperative bleeding, septic shock, and burns. The device utilizes specialized tubing that has the ability to expand during pressure, accommodating the rapid infusion rate and warming ability of the device.

PREREQUISITE NURSING KNOWLEDGE

- Aseptic technique and principles of fluid resuscitation and blood transfusion.[17]
- Massive transfusion is the transfusion of plasma to packed red blood cells (PRBCs) in a 1:1 ratio typically consisting of greater than 10 units of PRBCs within a 24-hour period.[5,7-11,17]
- Early implementation of massive transfusion protocols utilizing predetermined ratios are implemented to facilitate adherence to hemostatic protocols in resuscitation.[2,4,5,10,20]
- Acute coagulopathy is the result of hypothermia, acidosis, ongoing bleeding, and dilution and decreased activity of clotting factors. Hypothermia, acidosis, and coagulopathy are known as the trauma triad of death, occurring in 25% to 30% of trauma patients.[5,8,10-13,20]
- The early implementation of platelet administration must also be included in massive transfusion protocols. Previous doctrine maintained that platelets should not be administered through a fluid warmer, but newer research has found that platelet function is not decreased when transfused through a fluid warmer.[13,15,20]
- Acute coagulopathy can be recognized early by laboratory tests such as international normalized ratio (INR), activated partial thromboplastin time (aPTT), platelet counts, fibrinogen levels, and thromboelastography (TEG).[2,4,9,11,17]
- Hypothermia is commonly caused by the initial injury and subsequent treatment modalities. Decreased coagulation protease activity and impaired platelet function occur when core temperatures are reduced from 36°C to 33°C.[4,11]
- Measures to prevent and treat hypothermia include solar blankets, heated blankets, warmed blood products and fluids, continuous arteriovenous rewarming, and cardiopulmonary bypass, used in extreme cases of hypothermia (see Procedure 124, Thermoregulation: Heating, Cooling, and Targeted Temperature Management).
- When large volumes of IV fluids are being infused into patients, the fluids must be warmed to prevent hypothermia. Although institutions vary in what constitutes large volumes, a good rule of thumb is to institute fluid rewarming measures when more than 2 L of fluid are required in less than 1 hour.
- Current resuscitation strategies, known as *damage control resuscitation* (DCR), focus on rapid hemorrhage control, early recognition and correction of acute coagulopathy, permissive hypotension, minimization of crystalloid, and early initiation of fresh-frozen plasma (FFP) in a ratio of 1:1 with PRBCs. DCR is the standard of care and is incorporated into clinical practice guidelines.[2,9-12]
- Uncontrolled hemorrhage and the associated complications account for approximately 40% of trauma-related deaths.[11]
- Goals of therapy are to stop the bleeding, actively rewarm the patient, and administer blood products early to reverse coagulopathy, facilitate clot formation, and restore oxygenated blood–carrying capacity to vital organs. Blood products can be more rapidly infused when hemodiluted with compatible crystalloids.[1,2,4,5,9,11,17,18]
- Ongoing assessment to evaluate for transfusion-related complications include transfusion-related lung injury (TRALI), transfusion-associated circulatory overload (TACO), increased leukocyte adhesion and reperfusion injury, acute tubular necrosis, hypothermia, hypokalemia, hypocalcemia, hemolytic and allergic reactions, and air embolism.[2,17]
- Use of a rapid infusion device, such as the Level 1 Fast Flow Fluid Warmer or the Belmont Rapid Infuser (Figs. 78.1 and 78.2), can warm and infuse fluids at rates from 2.5 to 1000 mL/hour for the Belmont and 75 to 30,000 mL/hour for the Level 1 Fast Flow Fluid Warmer. The

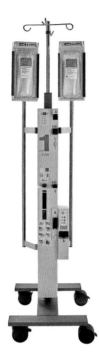

Figure 78.1   Level 1 Fast Flow Fluid Warmer. *(© 2022 Copyright ICU Medical Inc. or its Affiliates. All rights reserved.)*

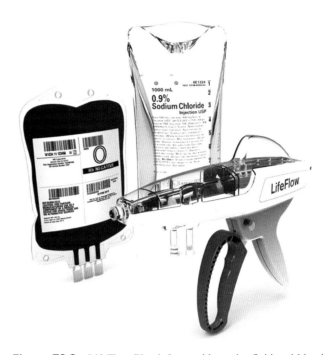

Figure 78.3   LifeFlow Plus infuser with carrier fluid and blood product. *(Courtesy 410 Medical, Durham, NC.)*

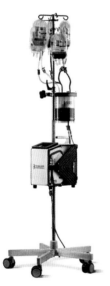

Figure 78.2   Belmont Rapid Infuser. *(Courtesy Belmont Medical Technologies, Billerica, MA.)*

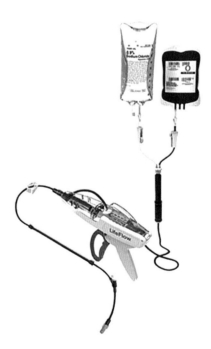

Figure 78.4   LifeFlow Plus image with blood tubing connected. *(Courtesy 410 Medical, Durham, NC.)*

tubing is made of soft plastic that expands to allow rapid infusion of fluids under pressure. Some rapid infusers include automated pressure chambers to compress intravenous (IV) bags. They allow for fast and easy bag changes and can accommodate both 1-L IV bags and 500-mL blood product bags. Pressure is maintained at a constant 300 mm Hg and is turned on and off via a simple toggle switch at the top of each pressure chamber. Older infusers simply have an IV pole from which to hang fluids and/or blood products, and separate pressure infuser bags must be used. Most facilities have readily available pressure bags, which is also an option for rapid infusion. Ensure

that the 500-mL bag is utilized for blood products. Newer, handheld devices, such as The LifeFlow and LifeFlow Plus (410 Medical, Inc., Durham, NC), allow for rapid infusion of fluids or blood products without a pressure bag (Figs. 78.3 and 78.4). Usually, multiple IVs are used, including peripheral and central sites. Venous access may also be obtained surgically via a venous cut-down of the basilic or saphenous veins when peripheral access cannot be obtained.[19]

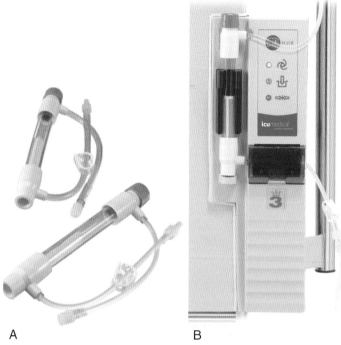

Figure 78.5 **A,** Rapid infuser filters. **B,** Insertion of the filter in the Level 1 Fast Flow Fluid Warmer with the clamp open. (*© 2022 Copyright ICU Medical Inc. or its Affiliates. All rights reserved.*)

- Both crystalloid and colloid IV solutions are used for resuscitating patients who are hypovolemic with hemodynamically unstable conditions. Crystalloids directly increase intravascular volume. Colloids expand plasma volume by pulling interstitial fluid back into the vascular space via osmosis. Numerous crystalloid and colloid preparations are available in isotonic, hypotonic, and hypertonic preparations. Crystalloids most commonly used in aggressive fluid resuscitation are 0.9% normal saline (NS) and lactated Ringer's (LR) solutions.
- The use of colloids such as albumin, dextran, and hetastarch allows the effective restoration of intravascular volume with smaller amounts of fluid; however, these colloids coat red blood cells (RBCs) and platelets, which may result in type and cross-match difficulties and clotting problems. Even slight overresuscitation with colloids increases the risk for fluid overload and pulmonary edema.[6,19]
- Blood and blood products are natural colloids used to replace lost blood and restore coagulation factors. In the patient with significant ongoing hemorrhage, infusion of blood and clotting factors is critical to restoring intravascular volume. Type O-negative blood is the universal donor for all patients and can be given in extreme emergencies before the completion of typing and cross-matching. PRBCs and whole blood are used to replace oxygen-carrying components; FFP, platelets, and cryoprecipitate are used to replace essential clotting factors.[4,12]

EQUIPMENT

- Rapid infuser (see Fig. 78.1) or handheld infusion device (see Figs. 78.2 and 78.3)
- Disposable fluid administration sets

- Replaceable filter with gas vent (Fig. 78.5)
- Blood administration set
- Pressure infuser bag (if appropriate)
- IV pole
- IV fluids or blood products as prescribed
- Sterile or distilled water for the warmer
- Nonsterile gloves
- Fluid shield face mask or goggles
- Antiseptic solution (e.g., 2% chlorhexidine-based preparation)

Additional equipment, to have available as needed, includes the following:
- Emergency equipment
- Indwelling urinary catheter
- Supplies for blood gas sampling

PATIENT AND FAMILY EDUCATION

- Explain the need for the rapid infusion of fluids, the purpose of warming fluids, and how the equipment operates. ***Rationale:*** Patient and family anxiety about unfamiliar equipment at the bedside may be decreased.
- Explain that prevention of hypothermia will be a priority. ***Rationale:*** This explanation prepares the patient and family for what to expect.

PATIENT ASSESSMENT AND PREPARATION

Patient Assessment

- Assess blood pressure, heart rate, respiratory rate, peripheral pulses, and level of consciousness. ***Rationale:***

Assessment is necessary to determine the severity of the patient's volume depletion and shock. It also provides baseline data.

- Assess temperature using a bladder probe or pulmonary artery catheter. ***Rationale:*** Assessment is necessary to assess for the development of hypothermia while large volumes of fluids are infused. Core temperatures most accurately reflect true body temperature.
- Assess patient history, including precipitating events, surgical and medical interventions, and history of cardiac problems. ***Rationale:*** Potential or actual need for massive fluid resuscitation and the risk for fluid overload are identified.
- Assess hemodynamic parameters, including baseline central venous pressure (CVP) and, if available, pulmonary artery pressure (PAP), pulmonary artery occlusion pressure (PAOP), cardiac output (CO) and cardiac index (CI), systemic vascular resistance (SVR), and mixed venous oxygen saturation (Svo_2). Assessment of right ventricular ejection fraction, oxygen delivery and consumption, and oxygen extraction ratio should also be included if the technology is available. ***Rationale:*** Baseline information is provided about the patient's preload, afterload, and cardiac contractility.
- Assess laboratory values to include arterial blood gases, serum electrolytes, serum lactate, base deficit, hemoglobin, hematocrit, and coagulation studies. ***Rationale:*** Baseline oxygenation, presence of metabolic acidosis, severity of ongoing hemorrhage, and severity of coagulopathy are determined so the need for intervention and the effectiveness of interventions can be determined.
- Assess patency of multiple large-bore IV sites. ***Rationale:*** Multiple sites are often necessary to infuse enough fluids and blood products to support the patient's vital signs. Extra sites, in addition to those used for rapid infusion, should be kept patent in case one of the other sites becomes nonfunctional or is accidently pulled out. The infusion of medications should take place through one of these extra sites, rather than through the same IV as blood or blood products.

Patient Preparation

- Verify the correct patient with two identifiers. ***Rationale:*** Before performing a procedure, the nurse should ensure the correct identification of the patient for the intended intervention.
- Ensure that informed consent has been obtained. ***Rationale:*** Informed consent protects the rights of the patient and makes a competent decision possible for the patient.

- Ensure that the patient and family understand the need and purpose for rapid infusion. Answer questions as they arise, and reinforce information as needed. ***Rationale:*** Understanding of previously taught information is evaluated and reinforced.
- Place additional peripheral IV sites. ***Rationale:*** Aggressive fluid resuscitation requires additional IV access besides the one site being used with the rapid infuser. Backup IV sites can be used if other sites infiltrate or become dislodged; extra sites may also be used to infuse medications, such as vasopressors, that should be kept separate from rapid infusion lines. Ideal sites for large IV catheter access are the antecubital fossa, saphenous veins, and the veins of the forearm and upper arm.
- Assist the physician or advanced practice nurse with placement of the central venous catheter and/or a pulmonary artery catheter. ***Rationale:*** This placement allows for the assessment of volume status before and after infusion of fluids and blood products. It also allows for assessment of core temperature with the pulmonary artery catheter thermistor and provides central venous access in the event vasoactive medications are needed.
- Place an automatic blood pressure monitor on the patient's arm that is not being infused with the rapid infusion device. Set it to check blood pressure every 5 minutes. ***Rationale:*** Assessment of the patient's hemodynamics and response to fluid replacement is provided. This is typically used temporarily until an arterial catheter is inserted by the physician or advanced practice nurse.
- Assist the provider with placement of an arterial line. ***Rationale:*** Placement allows for continuous assessment of the blood pressure during resuscitation and provides convenient access for blood sampling.
- Obtain a blood sample for type and cross-match, per facility protocol. Some facilities require two tubes to be sent if a large volume of blood is expected to be transfused. ***Rationale:*** This action prepares for blood transfusion.
- Obtain baseline hematocrit, chemistry panel, and coagulation studies. Repeat, as prescribed, every 15 to 60 minutes until hemorrhage is controlled. ***Rationale:*** These studies guide replacement of blood products and essential electrolytes.
- Place an indwelling urinary catheter as prescribed. ***Rationale:*** Patients who need aggressive fluid resuscitation should have an indwelling urinary catheter placed to determine volume status and end-organ perfusion.
- Cover the patient with warm cotton blankets or a warm-air blanket. Cover the patient's head with a warmed blanket, a towel, forced air warming device, or an aluminum cap. ***Rationale:*** Additional heat loss is minimized.

UNIT II

Procedure | for Use of a Massive Infusion Device

Steps	Rationale	Special Considerations
1. HH		
2. PE		
3. Verify the IV fluids and blood products prescribed.	Determines products and amounts to be infused.	The provider will prescribe the volume and type of additional IV fluids and blood products, and laboratory studies. Follow institutional protocols for performing pretransfusion blood verification.
4. Set the fluid temperature.	Warming fluids helps prevent hypothermia.[4,5]	
5. Turn on the device.	Allows the system to warm before moving fluid through the warming chamber.	Follow the manufacturer's guidelines for setup of each device.
6. Open the Y-set fluid administration package provided by the manufacturer. Close all clamps.	Prevents accidental spillage of blood or fluid. Prevents the flow of fluid through the circuit before the machine is warmed.	
7. Spike the fluid or blood with both sides of the Y-set.	Allows for a smooth transition from an empty bag to the next bag.	
8. Hang fluid and/or blood products on the small hooks inside the rapid infuser pressure chambers, leaving the chamber doors open (see Fig. 78.1), or place the fluid and/or blood products in separate pressure infuser bags.	Clearing the tubing of air is easier if the tubing is primed while the bags are still unpressurized.	Autotransfusion bags do not fit into the pressure chambers. Caution must be maintained so air is not pushed through the tubing and into the patient causing an air embolism. Follow institutional protocols regarding removal of air from infusion bags.
9. Push the bottom end of the heat exchanger rod firmly into the bottom socket, and snap the heat exchanger into the guide (see Fig. 78.2).	The bottom of the heat exchanger must be firmly placed, or it will not fit into the top socket.	
10. Slide the top socket up, and place the top end of the exchanger into the placement tract.	Locks the warming chamber into place at both the top and bottom sockets.	
11. Slide the top heat exchanger socket down over the heat exchanger tube until the pole latch clicks into place.	Secures the heat exchanger.	
12. Snap the gas vent filter into the holder on the lower portion of the pole assembly with the orange end up.	Filters air and blood clots from the tubing.	Only fits into the machine one way because the tubing is not long enough to be placed incorrectly.
13. Squeeze the drip chambers so they are half full.	Minimizes entrapment of bubbles in the tubing. Allows visualization of the drip chamber so the drip rate can be assessed.	
14. Open the clamp on one side of the Y-set.	Ensure that only one side of the Y-tubing is open during priming; otherwise, fluid will be pumped from one bag to the other and not through the tubing.	
15. Remove the male Luer-Lok cap at the end of the IV tubing; open the clamps.	Does not prime unless the end cap has been removed.	

Procedure	for Use of a Massive Infusion Device—*Continued*	
Steps	Rationale	Special Considerations
16. Remove the filter from its holder, and invert it. Prime the tubing; close the roller clamp. Turn the filter back over, and replace it in its holder.	Prevents entrapment of large amounts of air.	
17. Tap the filter or air eliminator against the cabinet several times. Monitor the fluid line for bubbles during use.	Releases any residual trapped air.	Never administer fluids if air bubbles are found between the filter chamber and the patient connection. Run IV fluid into the trash container to rid tubing of any residual air. When no more bubbles are observed leaving the gas vent filter, all of the air has been vented from the filter or air eliminator.
18. Open the roller clamp partially, and slowly infuse fluid.	Infusing slowly allows for assessment of any air bubbles. The air filter eliminates bubbles in the tubing.	If unable to clear the line of air and more than ¼ inch of air is present at the top of the filter, replace the filter.
19. Replace the male Luer-Lok cap at the end of the tubing; close the clamps.	Maintains asepsis of the tubing.	
20. Close the pressure chamber doors, and latch.	Prepares the fluid bags for pressurization when the machines are turned on and the pressure switch is activated.	Be certain that the latch is secure before the chamber is pressurized.
21. Perform all function and alarm checks per the manufacturer instructions.	Validates proper equipment function.	
22. Wait for the temperature readout to reach the operating temperature of 41°C.	Prevents hypothermia by ensuring that the chamber is warm before fluids are run through it and into the patient.	
23. Flip the toggle switch at the top of the pressure chamber to "on/+," or inflate the separate pressure bags.	Pressurizes the chambers.	The pressure automatically inflates to 300 mm Hg. Fluids infuse via gravity flow without being pressurized; however, high flow rates cannot be achieved unless the pressure bags are inflated.
24. Cleanse the injection site with antiseptic solution.[3,16] (**Level B***)	Reduces the risk for infection.	Follow institutional protocols. Chlorhexidine and povidone-iodine solutions may be more effective than alcohol in reducing external microbial contamination.[3]
25. Connect the distal end of the tubing to the IV. It is not recommended to use a needleless connector adaptor on the patient line during massive transfusion.[1]	Prepares for the infusion. Needleless connectors decrease the time required to deliver the blood product via the massive transfusion device.[1]	
26. Open the roller clamp to infuse the fluid and/or blood products.	Fluids or blood products now infuse under pressure.	It is best to infuse one side at a time, especially when blood products are infusing, to prevent mixing of fluids and blood products. The pressure system is designed to leave a small volume remaining to prevent air emboli.

*Level B: Well-designed, controlled studies with results that consistently support a specific action, intervention, or treatment.

Procedure continues on following page

Procedure for Use of a Massive Infusion Device—*Continued*		
Steps	Rationale	Special Considerations
27. Set the rate by gradually opening the clamp.	Fluids and/or blood products given via rapid infusers are administered as boluses over short periods; roller clamps are usually left wide open until the bolus is complete.	If a slower bolus is desired, adjust the roller clamp to decrease the flow of fluid.
Changing the Bags		
1. Close the top clamp on the side of the Y-connector with the empty fluid and or blood products bag.	Prevents air from entering the tubing.	Follow the manufacturer's guidelines for changing infusion bags for each device.
2. Open the clamp on the side of the Y-connector with the full fluid and/or blood products bag; infuse the fluid.	Keeping one side of the Y-connector spiked with fluid/and or blood products ready to infuse is helpful when patients have severely unstable conditions and need immediate boluses of fluid.	
3. Turn the "on/+" switch above the pressure chamber to the "off" position, and remove the empty bag.	Releases pressure from the pressure chamber.	
4. Replace the empty fluid/and or blood products bag with a full one.	The next bag of IV fluid and/or blood products must be ready to infuse to avoid delays in infusion in case the patient's blood pressure falls precipitously.	
5. Close the pressure chamber door and latch; flip the control switch above the pressure chamber to "on/+."	Repressurizes the chamber.	
Replacing the Filter or Air Eliminator		
1. Close the clamps on the disposable fluid administration set just proximal to the filter and between the filter and the patient connection.	The filter should be replaced after 3 hours of use, after 4 units of blood, or if the fluid rate slows because of clotting.	Follow the manufacturer's guidelines for replacing the filter or air eliminator for each device.
2. Remove the old filter or air eliminator from the holder, and place the new filter or air eliminator in the holder.	Keep the old filter or air eliminator connected to the disposable fluid administration set until ready to change to the new one. Minimizes the potential for contaminating exposed tubing ends.	
3. Disconnect the old filter or air eliminator at the upper Luer-Lok, and connect the tubing to the new filter.	Prepares for placement of new equipment.	
4. Disconnect the patient line Luer-Lok from the old filter or air eliminator, and connect it to the new one.	Prepares for placement of new equipment.	
5. Open the clamp just proximal to the filter or air eliminator to restart the fluid. Invert the filter until completely filled with fluid, and then turn it back to the proper position and replace in the holder. Open the clamp between the filter and the patient connection.	Infusion of the fluid resumes.	

Procedure | for Use of a Massive Infusion Device—*Continued*

Steps	Rationale	Special Considerations
6. Remove the filter or air eliminator from the holder, and tap until all bubbles are eliminated; reinsert it. Check the patient line for bubbles before opening the roller clamp.	Facilitates removal of bubbles.	If air bubbles are present, disconnect the tubing from the patient, and infuse into the trash container until the line is clear of air. Reconnect to the patient, and resume the infusion. If the alarm sounds after setup, check to ensure that the filter is properly snapped into place.
Troubleshooting Alarms		
1. If the alarm sounds and the disposable light is illuminated, check to be sure the disposable tubing set is properly placed in the machine.	The system will not run if the disposable tubing is not completely set into the machine.	The tubing set can become inadvertently dislodged. Follow the manufacturer's guidelines for troubleshooting alarms for each device.
2. If the alarm sounds and the water level light is illuminated, check the water level in the chamber, and replace as needed with sterile or distilled water.	The system will not run if the water level is too low.	
3. If the system alarms "overtemp," turn off the machine, and use a different rapid infuser.	Fluids inadequately warmed will contribute to hypothermia. Fluids overly warmed will contribute to hemolysis of RBCs.	Notify biomedical engineering of the problem.
Transporting a Patient With a Rapid Infuser		
1. Turn off the rapid infuser.	If the infuser is still on when the administration set is removed from its holder, water will spurt out of the warming chamber and aluminum tube.	Follow the manufacturer's guidelines for each device to transport a patient with a rapid infuser.
2. Remove the disposable administration set from its holder on the infuser, and place it in the bed alongside the patient or hang it on the transport IV pole.	The rapid infusers described here do not operate on a battery. Fluids infuse via gravity, or separate pressure infuser bags can be used.	Fluids run briskly via gravity drainage. If pressure is still necessary to infuse fluids, separate pressure infuser bags must be used as long as the machine is not plugged in. Interventions to minimize heat loss must be in place while the infuser is not plugged in. An aluminum head covering, warmed cotton blankets, and warm-air blankets help prevent heat loss. Removing the administration set from the machine and transporting the patient separately from the infuser is less awkward and minimizes the risk for pulling out the IV lines during transport.
3. Plug the infuser into an electric outlet once you reach the intended destination.	Establishes a power source.	
4. Return the administration set into the infuser. Turn on the machine. Return fluid bags to the pressure chambers.	The infuser is now ready to repressurize the chambers and warm the fluid. Any bubbles are eliminated by the filter.	If bubbles are not removed and more than ¼ inch of air is at the top of the filter, the filter must be replaced.
5. Remove **PE**, and discard used supplies in the appropriate receptacle.	Safely discards used supplies.	
6. **HH**		

UNIT II

UNIT II

Procedure   for a Pressure Infuser Bag or Handheld Device

Steps	Rationale	Special Considerations
1. ▣ HH		
2. ▣ PE		
3. Obtain and set up the IV fluid or blood component system.	The infusion system should be assembled before inserting the IV fluid or blood product into the pressure infuser bag or handheld device.	If administering blood products, follow institutional protocols for performing pretransfusion blood verification.
4. Cleanse the injection site with antiseptic solution.[4,16] **(Level B*)**	Reduces the risk for infection.	Follow institutional protocols. Chlorhexidine and povidone-iodine solutions may be more effective than alcohol in reducing external microbial contamination.[4,16]
5. If administering a blood component, piggyback the blood tubing into the 0.9% NS solution, or connect it directly into the IV line.	Allows the transfusion to proceed.	Follow institutional protocols for use of 0.9% NS solution as the primary IV fluid line. FFP and platelets should be given directly into the IV line. Do not piggyback them.
6. Open the roller clamp on the tubing.	Allows the infusion to proceed.	The rate of the infusion is dependent on the amount of pressure applied to the unit, not the position of the roller clamp. If using a handheld device, the rate of administration is dependent on the speed at which the user squeezes the handle and on individual patient need and vascular access gauge. The LifeFlow Plus can deliver 1 unit of blood or 500 mL fluid in less than 3 minutes.
7. Place the unit of blood or IV fluid through the mesh or plastic cover of the deflated pressure infuser bag so the entire bag to be infused remains within the mesh or plastic panel. For handheld device, skip to **step 11**.	Allows pressure to be evenly applied.	Do not allow the top of the bag to be infused appear above the mesh or plastic covering because this interferes with flow. Ensure the correct size pressure infuser bag for the volume to be infused (500-mL or 1-L size).
8. Secure the bag to be infused in place with a Velcro strap, or hang it on the hook in the pressure infuser bag. Hang the infuser bag on the IV pole.	Prevents the bag to be infused from slipping out of the bag when hung from the IV pole.	A standard sphygmomanometer cuff should never be used to administer large-volume transfusions because it does not exert uniform pressure on all parts of the component container.
9. Inflate the pressure infuser bag to achieve the desired rate of flow.	The pressure of the infuser bag is used to adjust flow, not the position of the roller clamp.	The pressure should not exceed 300 mm Hg to avoid damaging RBCs, rupturing the IV or blood bag, dislodging the IV catheter, or injuring the vein. The patient may have discomfort in an extremity if a peripheral catheter is used; if appropriate, decrease the pressure to maintain patient comfort.

*Level B: Well-designed, controlled studies with results that consistently support a specific action, intervention, or treatment.

Procedure for a Pressure Infuser Bag or Handheld Device—*Continued*

Steps	Rationale	Special Considerations
10. When the infusion is complete, deflate the pressure infuser bag.	Slows the infusion.	
11. If infusing blood, close the roller clamp to the blood component, and flush the primary infusion tubing with 0.9% NS solution if used as the primary IV line.	Allows the patient to receive blood sequestered in the tubing.	
12. When the infusion is complete, disconnect the IV fluid, NS solution, or blood tubing from the IV line.	Completes infusion; standard precautions.	
13. Remove gloves, and discard used supplies in an appropriate receptacle.	Safely discards used supplies.	The blood container and administration set should be handled as hazardous waste.

Expected Outcomes

- Patient's blood pressure and heart rate return to baseline
- Patient's core temperature remains above 36°C
- CVP, PAP, PAOP, CO, CI, and SVR reflect return of euvolemia and hemodynamic stability
- IV sites remain patent
- Rapid flow of blood components
- Urine output at least 0.5 mL/kg/hour

Unexpected Outcomes

- Blood pressure remains below baseline despite multiple liters of fluid and blood products
- Core temperature falls below 36°C, so more aggressive rewarming interventions become necessary
- Hypothermia-induced coagulopathy develops as the temperature falls below 35°C
- Inability to restore normal intravascular status occurs, as seen by CVP <6, PAOP <6, CO <4 L/min, CI <2 L/min/m^2, or SVR >1500 dynes/sec
  - Infiltration of IV site
  - Clotting of rapid infuser filter
  - Anuria or oliguria with urinary output <0.5 mL/kg/hour
  - Patient discomfort

Patient Monitoring and Care

Steps	Rationale	Reportable Conditions
		These conditions should be reported to the provider if they persist despite nursing interventions.
1. Monitor the patient's vital signs frequently per institutional protocols. As the patient's condition becomes more stable, assessment of vital signs may be performed less frequently per institutional protocols.	Determines the severity of shock, responsiveness to fluids and blood products, and the need for additional fluids.	• Systolic blood pressure below 90 mm Hg despite fluid administration • Abnormal vital signs

Procedure continues on following page

Patient Monitoring and Care —*Continued*

Steps	Rationale	Reportable Conditions
2. Assess the patient's core temperature frequently per institutional protocols. (**Level E***)	Patients who are in severe shock have impaired thermogenesis. This, in combination with the infusion of inadequately warmed fluids and/or blood products, leads to hypothermia. Hypothermia-induced coagulopathies begin at a core temperature of 35°C and exacerbate any hemorrhage already occurring. In addition, severe physiological complications from hypothermia, such as cardiovascular instability, electrolyte changes, urine concentration problems, and shifts in the oxygen-hemoglobin dissociation curve, affect the patient's ability to respond to physiological stress. Prevention of hypothermia is a critical goal for patients undergoing massive fluid resuscitation.[6-8]	• Worsening hypothermia or unrelieved hypothermia
3. Assess the integrity of IV sites frequently per institutional protocols.	IV sites under pressure are at higher risk for infiltration. In addition, lines can be inadvertently pulled out during radiographic filming, turning, and other aspects of patient care during a massive resuscitation. Multiple IV sites are recommended to be available at all times in the event an IV infiltrates or is discontinued.	• Infiltrated IV sites • Problems obtaining IV sites
4. Assess hemodynamic parameters frequently per institutional protocols.	Determines intravascular volume status and responsiveness to interventions. Patients may still be inadequately resuscitated even though vital signs, urine output, and hemodynamic parameters have returned to normal. A complete clinical picture (including laboratory tests in conjunction with vital signs, urine output, and hemodynamic parameters) is the best way to determine whether a patient has been adequately resuscitated.[13]	• Abnormal hemodynamic parameters • Abnormal trends in hemodynamic monitoring
5. Assess urine output frequently per institutional protocols.	Urine output is an assessment of end-organ perfusion. If little or no urine is produced, it is assumed that the kidneys are not being perfused; therefore other major viscera are also probably not being adequately perfused. Trauma to the urinary tract may interfere with accurate assessment of urine output because clots may block urine drainage, and laceration to ureters may result in extravasation of urine into the peritoneum.	• Urine output <0.5 mL/kg/hour

*Level E: Multiple case reports, theory-based evidence from expert opinions, or peer-reviewed professional organizational protocols without clinical studies to support recommendations.

Patient Monitoring and Care —*Continued*

Steps	Rationale	Reportable Conditions
6. Obtain hemoglobin, hematocrit, and coagulation studies as prescribed. These are usually measured soon after transfusion of blood; follow institutional protocols.	Determines the presence of ongoing blood loss and coagulopathy.[8]	• Abnormal hemoglobin, hematocrit, and coagulation results
7. Obtain arterial blood gases base deficit and lactic acid as prescribed and indicated.	Determines the persistence of metabolic acidosis and identifies the need for additional interventions to improve perfusion to major organs.[13]	• Abnormal laboratory results
8. Obtain electrolytes as prescribed.	• Patients undergoing large-volume resuscitation are at risk for hypokalemia, hypomagnesemia, hypocalcemia, and hypophosphatemia.	• Abnormal laboratory results
9. Monitor the patient for signs and symptoms of a transfusion reaction. If a transfusion reaction is suspected, stop the transfusion, and follow institutional protocols for suspected transfusion reaction.	Blood component replacement therapy constitutes the infusion of a foreign substance into the recipient.	• Signs and symptoms of a transfusion reaction.
10. Follow institutional protocols for assessing pain. Administer analgesia as prescribed.	Identifies the need for pain interventions.	• Continued pain despite pain interventions

Documentation

Documentation should include the following:

- Patient and family education
- Completion of informed consent
- Rationale for use of the rapid infuser
- Blood pressure, heart rate, respiratory rate, lung sounds, and peripheral pulses throughout the resuscitation
- The patient's core temperature while the rapid infusers are used
- Hemodynamic parameters, including CVP, PAP, PAOP, CO, CI, and SVR
- Urine output, estimated blood loss, and other measured output
- Laboratory results, including arterial blood gases, hematocrit, hemoglobin, electrolytes, base deficit, and lactic acid
- Appearance of IV sites
- IV insertions
- Total IV fluids and blood products in intake and output record
- Unexpected outcomes
- Additional interventions
- Pain assessment, interventions, and effectiveness

References and Additional Readings

For a complete list of references and additional readings for this procedure, scan this QR code with your smartphone, or visit https://www.elsevier.com/__data/assets/pdf_file/0003/1319853/Chapter0078.pdf.

PROCEDURE

79 Intraosseous Access

Marci Ebberts

PURPOSE Intraosseous (IO) access refers to placing a specialized hollow-core needle through the skin and bone and entering the intermedullary space to access the bloodstream. This procedure is warranted in the acute setting when intravenous (IV) access is not feasible by conventional means and vascular access is essential for critical conditions requiring timely access. IO access may be used for administration of fluid and or medications and to collect essential critical laboratory diagnostics.

PREREQUISITE NURSING KNOWLEDGE

- National and international leading healthcare organizations including the American Heart Association (AHA),[14] Emergency Nurses Association (ENA),[6] American Association of Critical Care Nurses (AACN),[4] International Committee on Resuscitation,[7] and Association of EMS Physicians have concluded that IV and IO administration are comparable and predictable in drug delivery, the pharmacological effects are equal, and in the setting of failed intravenous access, intraosseous access should be the first alternative.
- Pre-hospital personnel, hospital physicians, and advanced practice providers and nurses may insert, maintain, and remove IO devices after receiving appropriate training.[5,8] As with all healthcare providers in clinical practice, safety and competence in addition to the clinician's professional discipline scope of practice, regulatory boards, educational preparation along with clinical experience and institutional guidelines including policies and procedures should always be consulted prior to IO utilization.
- Failed or delayed vascular access remains a substantial problem while caring for patients in need of life-saving treatment. IO is a safe and effective procedure for critically ill adults who require emergent vascular access. IO access is warranted when vascular access is absent or difficult to obtain and in emergent, acute, or critical medically necessary situations.[13]
- When peripheral cannulation is unsuccessful and essential vascular access is required in conditions such as cardiopulmonary arrest, major trauma, shock, or when peripheral vascular collapse is present, IO access is essential and appropriate. IO access is applicable and warranted in patients with life-threatening status asthmaticus, edema, and burns and in obese patients in whom vascular access may be impaired.
- The IO route should be the first alternative to peripheral IV when peripheral access cannot be obtained and emergent vascular access is necessary. There are instances when IO access should be the first attempted vascular access, such as in prehospital pediatric trauma cases[17] or in patients with known limited vascular access.[8]

- The IO route should always be considered a bridge to more definitive vascular access and should not be maintained longer than 24 hours because of an increased risk of complications.[5,8]
- There are multiple IO access devices available, and they can be categorized as manual, impact driven, or power drills/drivers. Manual devices are inserted using only the force of the clinician's hand to drive a hollow steel needle with removable trocar. Impact-driven devices use a spring-loaded needle, which when deployed, rapidly punctures the bony cortex to arrive in the intramedullary space. Handheld power drills are battery operated and insert the IO with a rotational force. Each of these has advantages and disadvantages, and the manufacturer's recommendations for use should be followed.
- The available IO access sites for adult patients depend on the specific device as well as the manufacturer's guidelines relevant to the patient's physical and clinical presentation. When medications and fluids are introduced into the medullary canal, they flow through the vascular plexi directly into the vascular system allowing for a predictable and measurable therapeutic response equal to that of traditional (IV) infusion.[8]
- Available IO access sites, depending on the specific device and following each manufacturer's guidelines, include the following:
  - ❖ Sternum (manubrium): 1 to 1.5 cm below the sternal notch
  - ❖ Proximal humerus: greater tubercle
  - ❖ Proximal tibia: 1 to 2 cm medial and inferior to the tibial tuberosity (on the flat portion of the tibia)
  - ❖ Distal tibia: 2 cm proximal to the medial malleolus
  - ❖ Distal femur: 1 cm proximal to the patella (with the leg in a straight position), and 1 to 2 cm medially.[5]
  - ❖ The proximal humerus may be the preferred site due to faster medication absorption, less pain, and fast infusion rates,[1] although the proximal tibia may be more easily accessible.[8] Manufacturer's guidelines for individual IO devices may advise order of preferred site selection.
  - ❖ Sternal access provides faster infusion compared with long bones.[11,17] Not all IO devices are recommended for use in the sternum, and the use of a specific

adaptor may be required depending on the manufacturer's guidelines.

❖ Contraindications for IO insertion include a fracture to the same bone or a previous IO attempt in the same bone within the previous 48 hours.[8]

❖ Infusion of blood and blood products is safe and effective through IO access, without concern for hemolysis.[2] There may be indications, including the need for massive transfusions, to obtain two IO access sites for double the rate of infusion.[16]

❖ Flow rates of peripherally inserted IV catheters are far faster than can be achieved with IO catheters, but the IO route may be superior given the difficulty accessing a peripheral vein during hypovolemia.[17] IO catheter insertion is significantly faster than central venous access.[3] When treating hypovolemic shock, faster flow rates through the IO may be achieved by using a pneumatic infusion bag set to 300 mm Hg or using a three-way stopcock and manual pressure from a 50-mL syringe.[17]

❖ IO blood can be used for many laboratory tests including typing and screening, electrolyte values, chemistries, blood gas values, drug levels, and hemoglobin levels. The first aspirate does not need to be discarded.[5]

❖ Potassium values from an IO sample may be higher than those from a venous sample.[9]
  ○ IO samples may be used for point-of-care testing.[9]
  ○ Once definitive IV access is obtained, laboratory tests should be repeated.[5]

• The onset of action for medications is similar to that of IV medications, and no drugs or fluids are absolutely contraindicated for IO use.[12]

• IO access is acceptable for IV contrast administration for advanced imaging.[10,15]

• All resuscitation medications, isotonic fluids, and blood products may be given via the IO route.[14]

• Medications administered via the IO route should be followed by a 5- to 10-mL flush of normal saline solution (2 to 5 mL for pediatrics).[5] Resistance to the manual flush will be felt but does *not* indicate incorrect placement. If swelling or infiltration is observed, remove the device and attempt IO access in another bone.[5]

• Complications of IO access include extravasation, which could lead to compartment syndrome, osteomyelitis, fracture, fat and air embolism, and infection.[1] In pediatrics, the additional potential complication of epiphyseal plate necrosis can be avoided by ensuring that the IO is attempted away from the epiphyseal plate.[5]

• Relative contraindications to IO access include infection at the access site, artificial joint replacement at the insertion site,[17] inability to locate landmarks,[5] and bone disorders such as osteoporosis and osteogenesis imperfecta.[1]

EQUIPMENT

• Nonsterile gloves
• Antiseptic solution (e.g., 2% chlorhexidine-based preparation)
• IO insertion device (follow the manufacturer's guidelines for information that may be age or weight based)
• Tape
• IV tubing and extension tubing
• Isotonic crystalloid fluid, as prescribed
• Two 5- to 10-mL syringes
• Prescribed medications
• Pressure bag for IV solution
• Dressing supplies

Additional equipment, to have available as needed, includes the following:
• Blood-specimen tubes
• 1% or 2% preservative-free lidocaine without epinephrine
• Three-way stopcock
• Sterile 2 × 2 gauze pads

PATIENT AND FAMILY EDUCATION

• If the clinical situation permits, explain to the patient and family the reason for the IO access. ***Rationale:*** Clarification

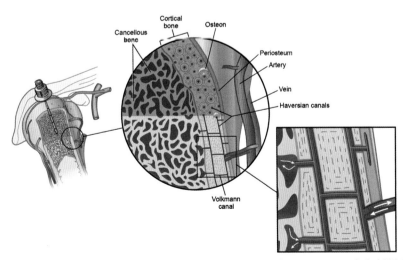

Figure 79.1 Intraosseous circulation. (*Image courtesy of Teleflex Incorporated. © 2023 Teleflex Incorporated. All rights reserved.*)

of information is an expressed patient need and helps diminish anxiety, enhance acceptance, and encourage questions.
- Describe the major steps of the procedure, including the patient's role in the procedure. ***Rationale:*** Explanation decreases patient anxiety, enhances cooperation, provides an opportunity for the patient to voice concerns, and prevents inadvertent contamination of the sterile field and equipment.
- Explain the expected outcomes of the procedure. ***Rationale:*** Explanation reduces anxiety and clarifies the duration and goals of IO access.

PATIENT ASSESSMENT AND PREPARATION

Patient Assessment

- Assess the patient for fractures or infections at the insertion site, for previous bone surgeries at the site, and for a history of osteoporosis or fractures of the target bone. ***Rationale:*** An alternate site should be accessed to avoid possible complications associated with the previous conditions.

- Obtain the patient's baseline vital signs and cardiac rhythm. ***Rationale:*** Baseline data facilitate the identification of clinical problems and identify the urgency of obtaining IO access.
- If possible, determine the patient's allergy history (e.g., lidocaine, antiseptic solutions). ***Rationale:*** This assessment decreases the risk for allergic reactions by avoiding known allergenic products.

Patient Preparation

- Verify the correct patient with two identifiers. ***Rationale:*** Before performing a procedure, the nurse should ensure the correct identification of the patient for the intended intervention.
- Ensure that the patient and family understand the preprocedural teaching. Answer questions as they arise, and reinforce information as needed. ***Rationale:*** Understanding of previously taught information is evaluated and reinforced.
- Perform a preprocedure verification and time out, if nonemergent. ***Rationale:*** Ensures patient safety.

Procedure | for Intraosseous Access

Steps	Rationale	Special Considerations
1. **HH**		
2. **PE**		
3. Assist the patient to a position of comfort for access of the appropriate insertion site.	Prepares the patient for the procedure and allows for optimal visualization.	
4. Palpate the intended insertion site, palpating both margins of the bone if possible.	Guides IO device placement; ensures central penetration of the bone	Each IO manufacturer has instructions for preferred sites for the specific device.
A. Proximal tibia:		
i. Identify the tibial tuberosity.		
ii. Move 2 cm medially and 1 cm proximally.		
B. Distal tibia:		
i. Identify the medial malleolus.		
ii. Move two cm proximally at the midline of the medial aspect of the leg.		
C. Sternum (for use with specifically designed devices):	The manubrium, 1 cm below the sternal notch, is the ideal location for the sternal IO.	
i. Identify the sternal notch.		
ii. Align the target patch with the sternal notch according to the manufacturer's directions		

Procedure	for Intraosseous Access—*Continued*	
Steps	**Rationale**	**Special Considerations**
D. Humerus: i. Position the patient with the arm internally rotated to identify the greater tubercle. ii. Move 1 cm lateral from the greater tubercle. E. Distal femur: i. With the patient's leg straight, locate the patella. ii. Move 1 cm proximal and 1–2 cm medial.	This position protects the bicep tendon and the upper extremity nerves while protruding the greater tubercle for easier identification.	
5. Cleanse the intended site and surrounding area with antiseptic solution (e.g., 2% chlorhexidine-based preparation).	Limits the introduction of potentially infectious skin flora into the insertion site.	
6. Stabilize the insertion site with the nondominant hand.	Maintains proper positioning	Ensure that the nondominant hand is NOT in line with IO placement to prevent inadvertent injury.
7. Deploy the device according to the manufacturer's recommendations and the training completed.	Different mechanisms (manual, drill, or impact) require different procedural steps. Specific steps for the device chosen should be followed.	
8. Secure the IO catheter or needle as recommended by the manufacturer. **(Level M*)**	Prevents the needle from moving.	
9. Apply a sterile, occlusive dressing.	Promotes a sterile environment.	
10. Remove the stylet, if required by manufacturer, and attach extension tubing to the hub of the IO device.	Allows access to the intramedullary space. A syringe should not be attached directly to the hub of the IO due to the risk of dislodgement.	
11. Confirm placement: A. Ensure stability of the device in the bone. B. Aspirate blood or marrow. C. Flush the needle with 10 mL of normal saline solution.	Verifies needle placement in the marrow cavity.	Follow institutional protocols. If blood specimens are needed, attach a 5-mL syringe and aspirate bone marrow and blood from the site.[1,12] Aspiration of marrow may occlude the IO device with bone. Lack of marrow aspirate does not indicate improper placement.[8] Resistance to the manual flush will be felt but does *not* indicate incorrect placement. If swelling or infiltration is observed, remove the device and attempt IO access in another bone.
12. If the patient is alert, slowly (over 60 seconds)[17] infuse lidocaine (without epinephrine) into the IO device as prescribed. Wait 2 minutes before flushing the device.	Promotes comfort. Allows lidocaine to take effect.	The infusion of fluids and medications can be painful to the conscious patient.
13. Secure the tubing, and tape it to the patient's skin.	Secures the tubing system.	Care should be taken when positioning and transferring the patient to avoid dislodgment of the IO device.

*Level M: Manufacturer's recommendations only.

Procedure continues on following page

UNIT II

Procedure for Intraosseous Access—*Continued*

Steps	Rationale	Special Considerations
14. Infuse IV fluids with a pressure bag or manual pressure.	IO lines often need pressure to ensure adequate flow.	The resistance of fluid flow through an IO may exceed the pressure limits on infusion pumps.
15. Observe for swelling of the tissue surrounding the insertion site	Identifies extravasation.	
16. Administer prescribed medications via the IO device, and follow each medication with a 5- to 10-mL normal saline solution flush as prescribed.[15] **(Level E*)**	Following medications with a saline solution flush ensures delivery of medication into the marrow cavity and blood vessels.	Resistance to the manual flush will be felt but does *not* indicate incorrect placement. If swelling or infiltration is observed, remove the device, and attempt IO access in another bone.[13,17]
17. Remove **PE**, and discard used supplies in appropriate receptacles.	Removes and safely discards used supplies.	
18. **HH**		

Procedure for Removal of the Intraosseous Access

Steps	Rationale	Special Considerations
1. **HH**		
2. **PE**		
3. Replace the IO site within 24 hours or as soon as venous access is obtained.	IO access is a temporary access site.	For minimization of the risk of complications, the IO device should be removed as soon as alternate vascular access is obtained or within 24 hours.
4. Follow the manufacturer's guidelines for removal. Some devices require a twisting motion to remove, and others pull directly out. Do not rock the device or apply alternating lateral pressure to remove it. **(Level M*)**	IO device is no longer needed. Rocking the device can increase the diameter of the insertion site and cause damage.	Follow the manufacturer's guidelines.
5. Apply an occlusive, sterile dressing to the site.	Promotes a sterile environment.	
6. Remove **PE**, and discard used supplies in appropriate receptacles.	Reduces the transmission of microorganisms; standard precautions. Safely removes sharp objects.	
7. **HH**		

*Level E: Multiple case reports, theory-based evidence from expert opinions, or peer-reviewed professional organizational protocols without clinical studies to support recommendations.
*Level M: Manufacturer's recommendations only.

Expected Outcomes

- Access to venous circulation for the administration of medications and fluids
- The IO line remains patent
- The tip of the IO needle lies in the marrow cavity
- The insertion site, catheter, and systemic circulation remain free from infection

Unexpected Outcomes

- Inability to infuse medications or fluids
- Infection
- Extravasation
- Complications such as compartment syndrome, fractures, osteomyelitis, and necrosis

Patient Monitoring and Care

Steps	Rationale	Reportable Conditions
		These conditions should be reported to the provider if they persist despite nursing interventions.
1. Observe for signs and symptoms of infection.	Identifies possible complications.	• Edema around the site • Pain, tenderness, or erythema around the site • Drainage from the site • Increased temperature • Elevated white blood cell count
2. Observe the IO insertion site for signs and symptoms of extravasation or compartment syndrome.	A misplaced device or excessive movement after insertion may lead to a leakage of fluids outside of the marrow cavity and can impair circulation to the extremity.	• Increased circumference of the extremity • Increased pain in the extremity • Change in extremity sensation, color, temperature, or pulses
3. Follow institutional protocols for assessing pain. Administer analgesia as prescribed.	Identifies the need for pain interventions.	• Continued pain despite pain interventions

Documentation

Documentation should include the following:
- Patient and family education
- Preprocedure verification and time out
- Site of insertion
- Number of IO insertion attempts
- Sites of previous IO insertion attempts
- Brand of the IO device inserted and, if appropriate, manufacturer's needle description
- Confirmation of IO needle placement
- Date and time of insertion
- Type and amount of anesthetic used
- Assessment of insertion site
- Method of securing the IO needle in place
- Problems encountered during or after the procedure
- Pain assessment, interventions, and effectiveness
- Vital signs and cardiac rhythm
- Date and time the IO device is removed
- Assessment of the site after the IO device is removed

References and Additional Readings

For a complete list of references and additional readings for this procedure, scan this QR code with your smartphone, or visit https://www.elsevier.com/__data/assets/pdf_file/0004/1319854/Chapter0079.pdf

PROCEDURE

80

Peripheral Nerve Stimulation: Train-of-Four Monitoring

Elizabeth P. Gunter

PURPOSE   A peripheral nerve stimulator (PNS) is used when a neuromuscular-blocking agent (NMBA) is administered to assess nerve-impulse transmission at the neuromuscular junction of select skeletal muscles.

PREQUISITE NURSING KNOWLEDGE

- A PNS is used in conjunction with the administration of an NMBA to block skeletal muscle activity.
- NMBAs are given in the intensive care unit along with sedatives and opioids, most commonly to facilitate mechanical ventilation in patients with severe lung injury. NMBAs are also used to assist with the management of increased intracranial pressure after a head injury; for severe muscle spasms associated with seizures, tetanus, and drug overdose; to reduce intraabdominal hypertension; and in hypothermia protocols to reduce overt shivering post–cardiac arrest.[1,6]
- NMBAs do not affect sensation or level of consciousness. Because NMBAs lack amnesic, sedative, and analgesic properties, sedatives and analgesics should *always* be given concurrently to alleviate discomfort and anxiety from unintentional patient awareness of blocked muscle activity. Sedatives and analgesics must be initiated *before* NMBAs because neuromuscular blockade hinders the assessment of anxiety and pain.[2]
- Numerous medications, such as aminoglycosides and other antibiotics, beta blockers, calcium channel blockers, corticosteroids, antiemetics, statins, and anesthetics alter the metabolism and efficacy of NMBAs.[5] Additionally, conditions such as acidosis, various electrolyte imbalances, diabetes, and obesity can also alter the effects of neuromuscular-blocking agents. Thus the level of blockade is subject to variation, which necessitates vigilant monitoring via nursing assessment and a PNS before titration of the NMBA.[5,6]
- The muscle twitch response to a small electrical stimulus delivered by the PNS corresponds to an estimated number of nerve receptors blocked by the NMBA and assists the clinician in the assessment and titration of the medication dosage. The level of blockade is estimated by observing the muscle twitch after stimulating the appropriate nerve with a small electrical current delivered by the PNS.
- The train-of-four (TOF) method of stimulation is most commonly used for ongoing monitoring of NMBA use. After delivery of four successive stimulating currents to a select peripheral nerve with the PNS, the clinician will observe four muscle twitches if there is an absence of significant neuromuscular blockade. The four twitches signify that fewer than 75% of the neuromuscular junction receptors are blocked. Three twitches correspond to approximately 75% blockade, and two to one twitches in response to four stimulating currents correlate with approximately 80% to 90% blockade of the receptors.[8] One to two twitches is the recommended level of block, although the appropriate level has not yet been determined through research in the critically ill population.[1] Absence of twitches may indicate that 100% of receptors are blocked, which exceeds the desired level of blockade (Table 80.1).[8]

- The stimulating current is measured in milliamperes (mA). The typical range required to stimulate a peripheral nerve and elicit a muscle twitch is 20 to 50 mA, although increasing the current to 70 or 80 mA may be necessary, especially in the obese patient.[5]
- Some stimulators do not indicate the mA. Instead, digital or dialed numbers ranging from 1 to 10 represent the range of mA from 20 to 80 mA. With use of these instruments, the usual setting is 2 to 5, although a setting of 10 is sometimes necessary. Other stimulators (with and without digital displays) automatically adjust the voltage output relative to resistance and deliver the current accordingly.[4]
- The ulnar nerve in the wrist is recommended for testing, although the facial and the posterior tibial nerves may also be used. Once a site is selected for testing the TOF response, the same site should be used throughout treatment to ensure consistency.[8]
- Peripheral nerve monitoring is used in conjunction with the assessment of clinical goals. ***Clinical decisions should never be made solely on the basis of the TOF twitch response.***[6]
- Titration of the drugs based on clinical assessment and muscle twitch response guides the clinician to provide a sufficient level of blockade without overshooting the goal. Overshooting the level of blockade with use of excessive doses of NMBAs is of special concern in the critically ill patient because it may predispose the patient to prolonged paralysis and muscle weakness.[3,7] Monitoring with a PNS during the administration of NMBAs results in the use of less medication, hastens recovery of spontaneous ventilation, and accelerates restoration of neuromuscular transmission (NMT), which is necessary for resumption of muscle activity.[9] Although some patients have severe

TABLE 80.1	Train-of-Four Stimulation as a Correlation of Blocked Nerve Receptors[8]
TOF Twitches/Stimulus	Percent of Receptors Blocked (Approximate)
0/4	100%
1/4	90%
2/4	75%–80%
3/4	75%
4/4	<75%

TOF, Train-of-four.

From Smetana KS, Roe NA, Doepker BA, Jones GM: Review of continuous infusion neuromuscular blocking agents in the adult intensive care unit. *Crit Care Nurs Q* 40(4):323-343, 2017.

muscle weakness after neuromuscular blockade, peripheral nerve monitoring during NMBA therapy facilitates prompt recovery of NMT when therapy is terminated.[8,9]

EQUIPMENT

- PNS
- Two pre-gelled electrode pads (typically, the same pads that are used for electrocardiography monitoring)
- Two lead wires packaged with the PNS
- Alcohol pads for skin degreasing and cleansing
- Additional equipment to have available as needed includes the following:
  - A bipolar touch stimulator probe may be substituted for the pre-gelled electrodes and lead wires
  - Scissors or clippers if hair removal is necessary

PATIENT AND FAMILY EDUCATION

- If time permits, assess the patient's and family's level of understanding about the condition and rationale for the procedure. *Rationale:* This assessment identifies the patient's and family's knowledge deficits concerning the patient's condition, the procedure, the expected benefits, and the potential risks. It also allows time for questions to clarify information and voice concerns. Education decreases patient anxiety and enhances cooperation.
- Explain the procedure and the reason for the procedure if the clinical situation permits. If not, explain the procedure and reason for the administration of NMBAs after they have been initiated. *Rationale:* This education enhances patient and family understanding and decreases anxiety.
- Describe the equipment to be used. *Rationale:* This description may decrease anxiety.
- Reassure the patient and family that medications for sedation and analgesia are provided throughout this therapy so the patient is comfortable while paralyzed. Also explain that patient comfort and safety will be maintained via repositioning, application of lubricating eye drops, and other measures to promote mucosal and skin integrity. *Rationale:* Reassurance that appropriate care will be provided during NMBA therapy reduces anxiety.
- Describe the experience of the stimuli as a slight prickly sensation. *Rationale:* The use of sensation descriptors may reduce anxiety.
- Explain that the electrodes require periodic changing, which feels like removing an adhesive-backed bandage. *Rationale:* This explanation may decrease anxiety.

PATIENT ASSESSMENT AND PREPARATION

Patient Assessment

- Verify the correct patient with two identifiers. *Rationale:* Before performing a procedure, the nurse should ensure the correct identification of the patient for the intended intervention.
- Assess the patient for the best location for electrode placement. Consider criteria such as edema, fat, hair, diaphoresis, wounds, dressings, and arterial and venous catheters. *Rationale:* This assessment improves conduction of stimulating current through dermal tissue.
- Assess the patient for history or presence of hemiplegia, hemiparesis, or peripheral neuropathy. *Rationale:* Motor response to nerve stimulation of the affected limb may be diminished; receptors may be resistant to NMBAs and lead to excess doses.[9]
- Assess whether burns are present or topical ointments are being used. *Rationale:* In patients with burns or topical ointments, for whom electrode adherence is difficult, a bipolar touch probe may be more effective than the electrode pads and lead wires. Poor electrode adherence interferes with conduction of the stimulating current.

Patient Preparation

- Ensure that the patient and family understand the preprocedural teaching. Answer questions as they arise, and reinforce information as needed. *Rationale:* Evaluates and reinforces understanding of previously taught information.
- Clip hair at the electrode placement sites if necessary. *Rationale:* This action improves electrode contact, which facilitates current flow to the nerve.
- Cleanse the skin, and degrease the skin with alcohol. *Rationale:* Cleansing improves electrode contact, which facilitates current flow to the nerve.
- Apply the electrodes, and test the TOF response to determine the adequacy of the location before initiating NMBA administration. In an emergent situation, testing the TOF response before NMBA administration may not be possible. *Rationale:* Testing improves the reliability of the interpretation of the TOF response.
- Whenever possible, determine the supramaximal stimulation (SMS) level before initiating an NMBA. The SMS is the level at which additional stimulating current elicits no further increase in the intensity of the four twitches. In an emergent situation, determination of the SMS level before NMBA administration may not be possible. *Rationale:* This determination helps establish adequate stimulating current and improves the reliability of testing.

Procedures for Peripheral Nerve Stimulators

Steps	Rationale	Special Considerations
Testing the Ulnar Nerve 1. **HH** 2. **PE** 3. Extend the patient's arm, palm up, in a relaxed position; cleanse it with an alcohol pad (Fig. 80.1).	The ulnar nerve is superficial and easy to locate; degreasing increases conduction.	
4. Before applying electrodes, mark the electrode placement sites with an indelible marker.	Marking the placement of the electrodes ensures site consistency when electrodes are changed.	
5. Apply two pre-gelled electrodes over the path of the ulnar nerve (see Fig. 80.1). Place the distal electrode on the skin at the flexor crease on the ulnar surface of the wrist, as close to the nerve as possible. Place the second electrode approximately 1–2 cm proximal to the first, parallel to the flexor carpi ulnaris tendon. **(Level E*)**	Enables stimulation of the ulnar nerve. Skin resistance causes the greatest impediment to current flow, which can be reduced through clean, dry skin and secure electrodes. The electrode gel enhances conduction. Maintaining the electrodes as close as possible in alignment with the nerve minimizes artifact from direct muscle stimulation.[9]	Ensure that the patient's wrist is clean and dry.
6. Use caution in selecting the site of the electrode placement to avoid direct stimulation of the muscle rather than the nerve. **(Level E*)**	Direct muscle stimulation elicits a response similar to the TOF, which makes evaluation of blocked nerve-impulse transmission difficult.	In patients with hemiplegia, place the electrodes on the unaffected limb because resistance to NMBAs on the affected side may lead to excess doses.[9] In patients with limbs immobilized from orthopedic casts, use the unaffected limb because possible resistance to some NMBAs on the affected limb may lead to excess doses.[5]

*Level E: Multiple case reports, theory-based evidence from expert opinions, or peer-reviewed professional organizational standards without clinical studies to support recommendations.

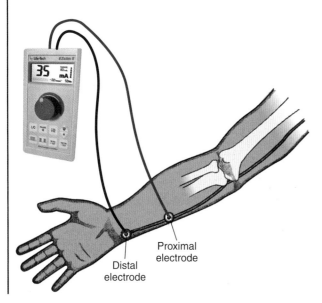

Figure 80.1   Placement of electrodes along the ulnar nerve.

Procedure continues on following page

UNIT III

Procedures for Peripheral Nerve Stimulators—*Continued*

Steps	Rationale	Special Considerations
7. Plug the lead wires into the PNS, matching the negative (black) and positive (red) leads to the black and red connection sites.	Necessary for the conduction of electrical current.	
8. Attach the lead wires to the electrodes. Connect the negative (black) lead to the distal electrode over the crease in the palmar aspect of the wrist. Connect the positive (red) lead to the proximal electrode.	Prepares the equipment.	
9. Turn on the PNS, and select the current determined by the SMS or, if not performed, a low current (10–20 mA is typical).	Excessive current results in overstimulation and can cause repetitive nerve firing.	Patients with diabetes mellitus may need higher stimulating current than patients without diabetes because of impaired motor nerve fibers and nerve endings.[5,9]
10. Depress the TOF key; through tactile assessment, determine twitching of the thumb, and count the number of twitches. Do not count finger movements, only the thumb.	Finger movements result from direct muscle stimulation. The quality of the twitches may be subtle and decrease in amplitude with increasing edema; detection with tactile methods increases sensitivity and accuracy.	Placing the operator's hand over the fingers helps reduce interpretation of artifactual movement. Use the dominant hand for tactile assessment because it may more accurately detect the TOF response.
11. Maintain a consistent current with each stimulation.	Increases reliability and validity in the quality of the twitch response.	
12. Discard used supplies, and remove 🅿🅴.		
13. 🅷🅷		
Testing the Facial Nerve		
1. 🅷🅷		
2. 🅿🅴		
3. Before applying electrodes, mark the electrode placement sites with indelible marker.	Marking the placement of the electrodes ensures site consistency when electrodes are changed.	
4. Place one electrode on the face at the outer canthus of the eye and the second electrode approximately 2 cm below, parallel with the tragus of the ear (Fig. 80.2).	Stimulates the facial nerve. Maintaining the electrodes as close as possible in alignment with the nerve minimizes artifact from direct muscle stimulation.[9]	Ensure that the patient's face is clean and dry. When wounds, edema, invasive lines, and other factors interfere with ulnar nerve testing, the facial or posterior tibial nerves may be substituted. The risk for direct muscle stimulation is greater, however, with resulting underestimation of blockade. Also, the alternate nerves correlate less well with blockade of the diaphragm.[1] **(Level C*)**

*Level C: Qualitative studies, descriptive or correlational studies, integrative reviews, systematic reviews, or randomized controlled trials with inconsistent results.

UNIT III

Procedures for Peripheral Nerve Stimulators—*Continued*

Steps	Rationale	Special Considerations

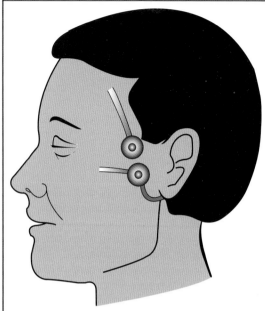

Figure 80.2   Placement of electrodes along the facial nerve.

5. Plug the lead wires into the PNS, matching the black and red leads to the black and red connection sites.

Necessary for conduction of the electrical current.

6. Attach the lead wires to the electrodes. Connect the negative (black) lead to the distal electrode at the tragus of the ear. Connect the positive (red) lead to the proximal electrode at the outer canthus of the eye.

Prepares the equipment.

7. Turn on the PNS, and select the current determined by the SMS or, if not performed, a low current (10–20 mA is typical).

Excessive current results in overstimulation and can cause repetitive nerve firing.

8. Depress the TOF key; through tactile assessment, determine twitching of the muscle above the eyebrow, and count the number of twitches.

Determines the neuromuscular blockade at the junction between a branch of the facial nerve and orbicularis muscle.

9. Discard used supplies, and remove **PE**.

9. **HH**

Testing the Posterior Tibial Nerve
   1. **HH**
   2. **PE**
   3. Before applying electrodes, mark the electrode placement sites with indelible marker.

Ensures site consistency when electrodes are changed.

   4. Place one electrode approximately 2 cm posterior to the medial malleolus (Fig. 80.3). **(Level E)***

Stimulates the posterior tibial nerve. Maintaining the electrodes as close as possible in alignment with the nerve minimizes artifact from direct muscle stimulation.[9]

Ensure that the patient's skin is clean and dry.

*Level E: Multiple case reports, theory-based evidence from expert opinions, or peer-reviewed professional organizational standards without clinical studies to support recommendations.

Procedure continues on following page

Procedures for Peripheral Nerve Stimulators—*Continued*

Steps	Rationale	Special Considerations

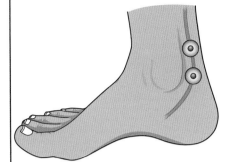

Figure 80.3 Placement of electrodes along the posterior tibial nerve.

Steps	Rationale	Special Considerations
5. Place the second electrode approximately 2 cm above the first (see Fig. 80.3).	Maintaining the electrodes as close as possible in alignment with the nerve minimizes artifact from direct muscle stimulation.[9]	
6. Plug the lead wires into the PNS, matching the black and red leads to the black and red connection sites.	Necessary for conduction of the electrical current.	
7. Attach the lead wires to the electrodes. Connect the negative (black) lead to the distal electrode 2 cm posterior to the medial malleolus. Connect the positive (red) lead to the proximal electrode 2 cm above the medial malleolus.	Prepares the equipment.	
8. Turn on the PNS, and select the current determined by the SMS or, if not performed, a low current (10–20 mA is typical).	Excessive current results in overstimulation and can cause repetitive nerve firing.	
9. Depress the TOF key; through tactile assessment of plantarflexion of the great toe, count the number of twitches.	Determines the neuromuscular blockade at the junction between the posterior tibial nerve and the flexor hallucis brevis muscle.	
10. Discard used supplies, and remove **PE**.		
11. **HH**		

Determining the Supramaximal Stimulation

Steps	Rationale	Special Considerations
1. **HH**		
2. **PE**		
3. Beginning at 5 mA, increase the milliamperes in increments of 5 mA until four twitches are observed.	Uses the lowest level necessary to elicit the twitches.	
4. Note the amount of current (in milliamperes) that corresponds to four vigorous twitches. Administer one to two more TOF stimuli to confirm the response. This current level is then used in TOF testing for that site.	If no increase in intensity of the muscle twitch is found when the milliamperes are increased, the SMS is the level at which four vigorous twitches were observed.	For example, if a strong response is observed at 30 mA, raise the current to 35 mA. If no increase is seen in intensity of the twitch, the SMS is 30 mA. If an increase is seen, raise the milliamperes to 40 mA. If an additional increase is seen in twitch intensity, raise it to 45 mA. If the intensity shows no further increase, the SMS is 40 mA.

UNIT III

Procedures **for Peripheral Nerve Stimulators—*Continued***

Determining the Train-of-Four Response During Neuromuscular-Blocking Drug Infusion

1. **HH**
2. **PE**
3. Retest the TOF 10–15 minutes after a bolus dose or when continuous infusion of NMBA is given/initiated/changed. | Evaluates the level of blockade provided. | Always assess electrode condition and placement before testing.
4. If more than one twitch occurs and neuromuscular blockade is unsatisfactory for clinical goals, increase the infusion rate as prescribed or according to hospital protocol, and retest in 10–15 minutes. | Signifies that less than 85%–90% of receptors are blocked.
5. Retest every 4–8 hours, or per hospital protocol, after a clinically stable and satisfactory level of blockade is achieved. | Evaluates the level of blockade and avoids underestimation and overestimation of blockade.
6. Discard supplies, and remove **PE**.
7. **HH**

Troubleshooting With Zero Twitches

1. **HH**
2. **PE**
3. Change the electrodes, and ensure that the patient's skin is clean and dry. **(Level E*)** | Drying of the gel or poor contact from moisture or soiling compromises conduction.[6]
4. Check the lead connections and the PNS for mechanical failure, and change the battery if needed. **(Level E*)** | Low battery voltage is a common cause of PNS malfunction.
5. Increase the stimulating current. **(Level E*)** | The current may be inadequate to stimulate the nerve, especially for increasingly edematous patients.[9]
6. Retest another nerve (the other ulnar nerve or facial or posterior tibial nerves). | Avoids overestimating the level of blockade with false zero-twitch responses.
7. If no other explanations are found for a zero response, check the NMBA infusion for the rate, dose, and concentration. Reduce the infusion rate of the NMBA as prescribed or according to hospital protocol. **(Level E*)** | Excessive neuromuscular blockade produces absence of a twitch response and, if allowed to persist, may contribute to prolonged paralysis or severe weakness.[7] Peripheral hypothermia may cause a decrease in twitch response and may require a decrease in NMBA by 80%.[9]
8. Discard supplies, and remove **PE**.
9. **HH**

---

*Level E: Multiple case reports, theory-based evidence from expert opinions, or peer-reviewed professional organizational standards without clinical studies to support recommendations.

Procedure continues on following page

Expected Outcomes

- Slight discomfort during the TOF test
- The muscles of the thumb twitch, rather than the fingers, when the ulnar nerve is stimulated
- The twitch response approximates the number of blocked peripheral nerve receptors. For example, four twitches before initiating the NMBA infusion and one to two twitches when a desired level of blockade is achieved as described in Table 80.1
- The NMBA dosage is titrated according to both the TOF test and assessment of clinical goals
- Resumption of four twitches occurs within an appropriate time frame when the NMBA is discontinued

Unexpected Outcomes

- Moderate to severe discomfort from the TOF test
- Impaired skin integrity when the electrodes are removed
- The fingers twitch when the ulnar nerve is stimulated as a result of artifact; if the thumb does not twitch, this signifies direct muscle rather than ulnar nerve stimulation
- Resumption of four twitches does not occur within an appropriate time frame after discontinuation of NMBA

Patient Monitoring and Care

Steps	Rationale	Reportable Conditions
		These conditions should be reported to the provider if they persist despite nursing interventions.
1. Cleanse and thoroughly dry the skin before applying the electrodes.	Improves electrode adherence.	
2. Change the electrodes every 24 hours or whenever they are loose or when the gel becomes dry.	Optimizes conduction of the stimulating current. Also assists with decreasing the risk for skin breakdown from the adhesive on the electrodes. Use caution when removing the old electrodes so as not to disrupt skin integrity.	• Skin breakdown
3. Select the most accessible site with the smallest degree of edema and hair and with no wounds, catheters, or dressings that impede accurate electrode placement over the selected nerve.	Facilitates ease in testing, electrode adherence, and the conduction of current.	
4. Never use the Single Twitch, Tetany, or Double Burst settings, if available on the PNS. (**Level E***)	These methods are designed for profound neuromuscular blockade and may cause extreme discomfort.[4]	
5. Assess the patient's oxygenation and ventilation, neurological function, and tissue perfusion before increasing the rate of the NMBA infusion.	The patient may have subtle movement of the extremities with an acceptable TOF response. Clinical decisions should never be made solely on TOF test results.	• Excessive patient movement despite acceptable TOF • Change in vital signs • Decreased oxygenation (e.g., measured via arterial blood gas or pulse oximetry) • Change in neurological function • Cardiac dysrhythmias or change in patient condition
6. Extreme caution must be exercised to prevent the PNS lead wires from contacting an external pacing catheter or pacing lead wires.	Direct electrical current can be conducted from the PNS through the pacing wires to the heart.	

*Level E: Multiple case reports, theory-based evidence from expert opinions, or peer-reviewed professional organizational standards without clinical studies to support recommendations.

UNIT III

Patient Monitoring and Care —*Continued*

Steps	Rationale	Reportable Conditions
7. Perform the TOF testing every 4–8 hours during NMBA infusion after the patient's condition is clinically stable and a satisfactory level of neuromuscular blockade is achieved, or per institutional policy.	Determines an effective dose of NMBA.	• Abnormal TOF results
8. Consider objective methods of sedation monitoring, such as EEG signal processing (see Procedure 82, EEG Monitoring Assist and Nursing Care, or evoked potentials, during NMBA therapy.[6] **(Level E*)**	Muscle paralysis during NMBA therapy hinders sedation assessment with subjective instruments.	
9. Remove the electrodes, lead wires, and PNS from the patient for magnetic resonance imaging or exposure to any magnetic field.	Metal objects are attracted to the magnetic field.	
10. Follow institutional standards for assessing pain. Administer analgesia as prescribed.	Identifies the need for pain interventions.	• Continued pain despite pain interventions

*Level E: Multiple case reports, theory-based evidence from expert opinions, or peer-reviewed professional organizational standards without clinical studies to support recommendations.

Documentation

Documentation should include the following:
- Patient and family education
- The time, baseline SMS milliamperes, most recent milliamperes, TOF twitch response, and nerve site tested
- The TOF response as $0/4$, $1/4$, $2/4$, $3/4$, or $4/4$
- Dosage of NMBA
- Assessment data (e.g., neurological, pulmonary, cardiovascular)
- Unexpected outcomes
- Troubleshooting attempts
- Additional interventions
- Pain assessment, interventions, and effectiveness

References and Additional Readings

For a complete list of references and additional readings for this procedure, scan this QR code with your smartphone, or visit https://www.elsevier.com/__data/assets/pdf_file/0005/1319855/Chapter0080.pdf

81

Noninvasive Brain Tissue Monitoring: Near-Infrared Cerebral Spectroscopy

Amanda Virginia

PURPOSE Tissue oxygen saturation can be measured using near-infrared spectroscopy (NIRS) to provide a continuous noninvasive measurement of cerebral oximetry based on light transmission and absorption from an applied sensor. NIRS quantifies cerebral oxygenation, as it correlates with cerebral perfusion, based on similar principles utilized by pulse oximetry. The clinical application of NIRS has expanded from cardiac surgery to utilization in the critical care setting.[10]

PREREQUISITE NURSING KNOWLEDGE

- Knowledge of cerebral oxygen supply and demand as indicators of brain homeostasis.
  - Cerebral autoregulation allows cerebral blood flow (CBF) to remain constant despite variations in mean arterial pressure between 50 and 150 mm Hg. Because of high metabolic demands and an inability to store oxygen, the brain is dependent on consistent blood flow for oxygen supply.[15] Noninvasive brain tissue monitoring, such as cerebral oximetry, may guide treatment plans as it correlates with cerebral blood flow.[14]
  - Carbon dioxide (CO_2) directly modulates CBF. An increase in CO_2 results in vasodilation and may thereby increase CBF.[13] The partial pressure of arterial oxygen (Pao_2) indirectly affects cerebral circulation. A decrease in Pao_2 leads to vasodilation and may result in a marked increase in CBF.
  - Cerebral metabolic rate of oxygen ($CMRo_2$) is the rate of oxygen consumption by the brain. The brain consumes approximately 20% of total body oxygen.[4]
  - Cerebral oxygen saturation (Sto_2) represents the percent of oxygen remaining after demand. Cerebral oximetry is determined by the amount of light scattering to the sensor after spectral absorption in the tissue. Most of the NIRS radiation samples nonpulsatile venous blood (75%), which differs from pulse oximetry, which monitors arterial circulation to measure arterial oxygen saturation (Sao_2).[3,16]
  - Cerebral desaturations can lead to prolonged mechanical ventilation, cognitive dysfunction, increased length of hospital stay, and other sequelae.[5] The development of noninvasive technology, such as NIRS, provides a direct measurement of cerebral tissue oxygenation for interpretation and management.
- NIRS measures real-time changes in regional oxygen supply and demand, allowing for early intervention and optimization of patient outcomes.[8]

- Absorption of light by tissues is wavelength dependent, and near-infrared radiation falls within the region of 700 to 1000 nm.[10,16] At these wavelengths, oxygenated hemoglobin and deoxygenated hemoglobin have varying spectral absorptions. The difference in their light absorption is measured and calculated as the tissue's oxygen extraction. Using a modified Beer-Lambert equation, the NIRS monitor displays this as a tissue oxygen saturation (Sto_2).[10,15]
  - The light travels through skin, subcutaneous tissue, bone, cerebrospinal fluid, and tissue. The depth of the light transmission is one-third the distance between the light source and detector, which varies based on the sensor and monitor utilized.[15] An adhesive sensor composed of a light source and two detectors measures both shallow and deep signals to estimate oxygen saturation of the targeted tissue (Fig. 81.1).[5,8]
  - In cerebral oximetry monitoring, the NIRS sensors are placed on the forehead and provide a transcutaneous measurement of tissue oxygenation in the cerebral cortex (Fig. 81.2).[5] Placement of the sensors should be at least 3 cm superior to the orbital border to avoid the frontal sinus, which can alter the depth of light penetration (Fig. 81.3).[5,11] The sensors can emit light to a depth that can sample the tissue oxygenation in the cerebral cortex, which is susceptible to changes in $CMRo_2$ and CBF.[2] A normal range of cerebral Sto_2 is 60% to 80%.
  - A decline in Sto_2 may be treated by increasing CBF and oxygen availability through clinical interventions such as increasing carbon dioxide, increasing cardiac output, increasing hemoglobin, increasing oxygen content, and decreasing metabolic demands.
  - Cerebral oximetry limitations may include varying skull thickness or amounts of cerebrospinal fluid, epidural or subdural hematoma, extracerebral signals, and pharmacological impact on systemic hemodynamics.[7]
  - NIRS signal quality may be altered as a result of interference with ambient light, signal loss during long recordings, improper sensor placement, or poor contact

with the skin.[9] Depending on the manufacturer of the monitoring device, skin pigmentation can also impair StO_2 readings.[2]

- NIRS monitors utilize a proprietary algorithm to produce a value of cerebral oxygenation. The monitoring devices employ varying radiation wavelengths, light sources, and distances between the detectors, making the data trends specific to the applied sensors (see Fig. 81.3).[3,5,12] Absolute NIRS monitors utilize four or more wavelengths, whereas trending NIRS monitors only use two wavelengths.
  - ❖ The LED light source emits five broad-spectrum wavelengths to account for anatomical differences among patients, such as skin pigmentation and melanin (see Fig. 81.2).[5]
  - ❖ The LED light penetrates approximately 2 to 2.5 cm to reach the cerebral cortex tissue for precise measurements

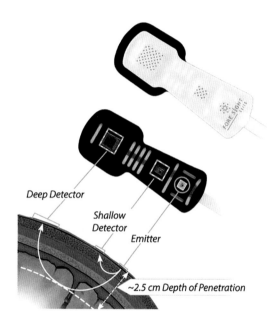

Figure 81.1 Adhesive sensor composed of a light source and two detectors used to estimate oxygen saturation of the targeted tissue. *(Courtesy Edwards Lifesciences, Irvine, CA.)*

of cerebral oximetry +/– 3%. Light penetration can vary depending on the manufacturer.

- NIRS is well appreciated for its clinical applications in the perioperative arena. Intraoperative cerebral NIRS is utilized for cardiovascular and thoracic surgeries, pediatric cardiac congenital surgery, electrophysiology procedures, and more.[2-3,10] Its emerging applications in the critical care setting have recently expanded and are aimed at maintaining adequate oxygen delivery to tissues for the prevention of end-organ injury.
  - ❖ Neurological examinations are relied on to assess brain perfusion, but newer technologies such as NIRS can provide continuous, noninvasive, objective data to guide interventions.[16] NIRS produces values that correlate with jugular venous oxygen saturation, brain tissue oxygen tension, and CT perfusion.[17]
  - ❖ Throughout the first 24 hours of critical illness, therapeutic management of the partial pressure of carbon dioxide ($PaCO_2$), heart rate, and hemoglobin concentration can produce a significant impact on oxygen delivery to brain tissue.[16]
  - ❖ Increased age is associated with cognitive impairment and cardiovascular disease. Hypertension, diabetes, and cigarette smoking are risk factors that compromise cerebral perfusion and worsen cognitive function. Monitoring of cerebral oximetry can improve neurological outcomes, prevent postoperative cognitive dysfunction, reduce the risk of cerebral ischemia, and reduce mortality.[2,5,15] Additionally, low cerebral tissue oxygenation is associated with delirium in the critical care setting.[1,16,17]
  - ❖ The utilization of cerebral NIRS monitoring has increased, particularly in pediatric intensive care units. Early diagnosis of shock, cerebral circulatory arrest, and indicators of low cardiac output after cardiac surgery can help guide the postoperative management of pediatric congenital cardiac surgery.[8,10]
  - ❖ Alternate clinical applications of NIRS for measurement of tissue oximetry:
    - ○ Resuscitation in hemorrhagic or septic shock[10]
    - ○ Resuscitation for extracorporeal life support[11]

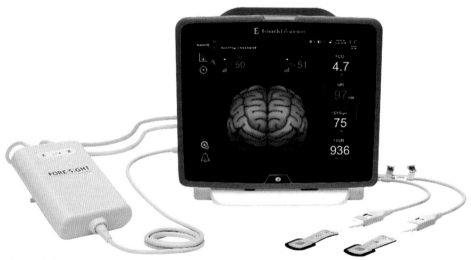

Figure 81.2 Near-infrared spectroscopy (NIRS) sensors connected to a monitor that displays tissue oxygenation as a percent. *(Courtesy Edwards Lifesciences, Irvine, CA.)*

○ Neurological outcomes after cardiac arrest with a return of spontaneous circulation[15]
○ Somatic tissue oxygenation at sites such as the abdomen, flank, and muscle
○ Monitoring for distal limb ischemia as a complication of femoral cannulation

EQUIPMENT[5,6]

- Nonsterile gloves
- Monitor and cables
- Sensor
- Alcohol prep

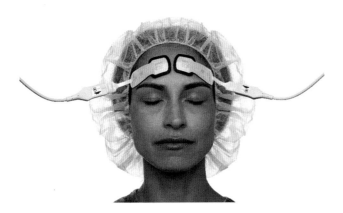

Figure 81.3 Proper placement of the sensors 3 cm above the orbital border. *(Courtesy Edwards Lifesciences, Irvine, CA.)*

PATIENT AND FAMILY EDUCATION

- Explain the purpose of NIRS monitoring to the patient and family. *Rationale:* NIRS is an adhesive sensor that provides the percent of brain tissue oxygenation to detect early changes in oxygen supply or demand for the prevention of worsening cardiovascular or neurological outcomes.[3,8]
- Explain that cerebral tissue oximetry monitoring (Sto_2) is a regional assessment that aids in patient management and guides the need for further evaluations. *Rationale:* This prepares the family that cerebral oximetry is part of a much broader assessment of cerebral perfusion and hemodynamic status.
- Explain that audible alarms facilitate notification of abrupt changes in cerebral oximetry below a determined value. *Rationale:* This teaches the patient and family that a false alarm may occur in certain circumstances. Early detection of significant decreases or increases in cerebral oximetry allow for prompt interventions to optimize patient management.

PATIENT ASSESSMENT AND PREPARATION

Patient Assessment (Figs. 81.4 and 81.5)

- Assess the patient's neurological status. *Rationale:* A baseline assessment will allow the nurse to correlate cerebral tissue oxygenation (Sto_2) with neurological status.[8]

Cerebral oximetry (StO_2) physio-relationship graphic

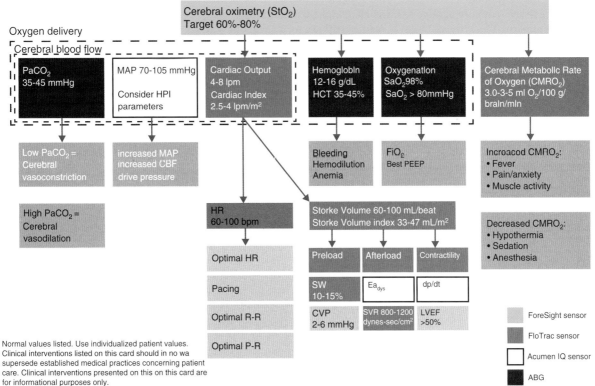

Figure 81.4 Graphic representation of how partial pressure of carbon dioxide *(Paco2)*, mean arterial pressure *(MAP)*, cardiac output *(CO)*, hemoglobin, arterial oxygen saturation *(Sao2)*, and cerebral metabolic rate of oxygen (CMRo2) can affect cerebral oximetry. *(Courtesy Edwards Lifesciences, Irvine, CA.)*

UNIT III

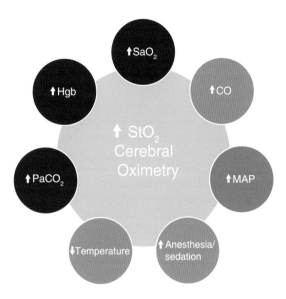

Figure 81.5 Interventions that increase cerebral oxygenation. *(Courtesy Edwards Lifesciences, Irvine, CA.)*

- Assess the patient's ventilation and oxygenation. ***Rationale:*** A baseline assessment of the fractioned of inspired oxygen (Fio_2), positive end-expiratory pressure (PEEP), minute ventilation (MV), end-tidal carbon dioxide ($ETco_2$), and arterial blood gas (ABG) will assist with optimization of Sto_2.

- Assess the patient's cerebral perfusion pressure by identifying the MAP and intracranial pressure. Monitor heart rate and cardiac output when available. Obtain and review hemoglobin laboratory results. ***Rationale:*** Assessment of hemodynamic status can identify factors that can affect baseline Sto_2 values.

Patient Preparation

- Verify correct patient with two identifiers. Rationale: Before performing a procedure, the nurse should ensure the correct identification of the patient for the intended intervention.

- Identify and confirm that a monitor, cables, and sensors are available. Cleanse the patient's skin with alcohol, and allow it to dry. For cerebral NIRS, the sensors will be placed on the forehead. For measurement of tissue oxygenation in alternate locations, assess if the skin requires shaving to remove excess hair. Rationale: The skin should be clean and free from hair to eliminate interference with the light source and sensors.

Procedure for Near-Infrared Cerebral Oximetry[5,6]

Steps	Rationale	Special Considerations
1. **HH**		
2. **PE**		
3. Connect the plug into an outlet, and turn on the monitor.	The battery pack has a limited backup power source.	Battery life is displayed on the monitor.
4. Slide the tissue oximetry module into the monitor.	The HemoSphere monitoring platform allows for viewing of both tissue oximetry and hemodynamics on the same monitor.	
5. Connect the cables to the module.	The module has two ports to connect the cable. Port A will illuminate green, and Port B will illuminate blue.	Two cables can be connected to the module to monitor additional sites of oxygenation. The LED illuminates which cable is connected to which port.
6. On the HemoSphere monitor, select New Patient or Continue Same Patient.	Enter patient data including Patient ID, age, gender, height, and weight.	Sto_2 will work in either invasive or noninvasive mode.
7. Open the sensor package, and remove the protective lining. Apply the sensor on the left and ride side of the forehead using midline as a reference.	Place the sensor close to the hairline or at least 3 cm above the orbit border. Avoid placing the sensor over hair, tattoos, skin breakdown, edema, or open wounds.	Selection of sensor sizes: • Large sensor: >40 kg • Medium sensor: >3kg • Small sensor: <8 kg • Nonadhesive small sensor: <8 kg
8. Connect the sensor to the cable, and pad any pressure points at the connection.	When connecting the cable into the port (A or B) and channel (1 or 2), take note if the sensor location does not correlate with the actual placement.	
9. Set up the display to show to correct sensor location.	Click on the patient figure, and then make sure to select the correct port and channel. Choose from a variety of sensor locations along with the correct monitoring mode (adult or pediatric).	Pediatric mode accounts for the differences between neonates, infants, children, and adults.

UNIT III

Procedure for Near-Infrared Cerebral Oximetry[5,6]—Continued

Steps	Rationale	Special Considerations
10. The monitor tile displays the StO_2 along with other parameters.	On the top from left to right: sensor location, channel selected, hemodynamic parameter being displayed, and reference value. On the bottom right, there is a signal quality indicator.	If all four bars of the signal quality indicator are displayed, the signal is optimal. If three bars are displayed, the signal is moderately compromised.
11. Touch the StO_2 tile on the monitor, select the sensor location, and choose the skin check reminder at the appropriate interval.	Skin checks should be completed every 12 hours with critical care assessments.	Assess the skin surrounding the sensor, and remove/replace as necessary.

Expected Outcomes

- Sensor has an optimal signal quality indicator.
- Monitoring begins immediately and baseline references are recorded with initial placement.
- StO_2 baseline is within normal range 60%–80% for both the left and right sensors.
- Early detection of decreases in StO_2 or significant trends (>20%) away from the baseline.
- Interventions aimed to return the StO_2 to baseline or improve cerebral tissue oxygenation.

Unexpected Outcomes

- Cerebral oximetry declined 20% from baseline with or without change in neurological assessment.
- Cerebral desaturation events of less than 55% for greater than 3 min.
- No improvement in StO_2 in response to interventions or improvements in cardiovascular or respiratory status.
- Skin breakdown from the sensor or pressure from the cable.
- Signal quality indicator less than 4 with correct placement of cerebral oximetry sensors and minimal interference.

Patient Monitoring and Care

Steps	Rationale	Reportable Conditions
		These conditions should be reported to the provider if they persist despite nursing interventions.
1. Assess the patient's baseline neurological function and cerebral tissue oximetry (StO_2) values immediately after the procedure.[10]	NIRS is a noninvasive monitor of oxygen supply and demand. Assessment of the cerebral cortex StO_2 is one part of the overall status of the patient. A normal StO_2 range is 60%–80% (Fig. 81.6).	- Baseline StO_2 values outside the normal range.
2. Evaluate the StO_2 values every hour along with neurological assessment.	Close monitoring of StO_2 values will identify trends that might not trigger audible alarms. Sustained trends deviating from baseline should be monitored closely and correlated with the patient's neurological status.	- Follow institutional standards for reporting StO_2 changes from baseline. - A decline of 20% from baseline value or sustained values less than 60%.[8]
3. Perform a skin assessment every 4 hours and sensor placement.	Place padding under the connection between the sensor and cable if it creates a pressure point or skin breakdown. Verify that the sensor has not migrated and is still adhering to the forehead.	- Skin breakdown or pressure points at the location of the sensor and cables.

Procedure continues on following page

Patient Monitoring and Care —*Continued*

Steps	Rationale	Reportable Conditions

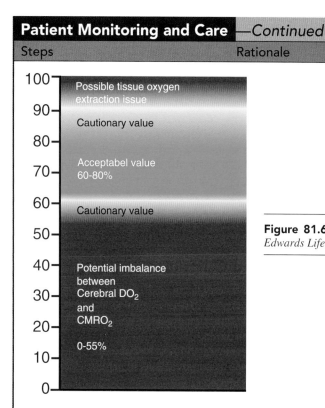

Figure 81.6 The normal range for cerebral oximetry is 60% to 80%. *(Courtesy Edwards Lifesciences, Irvine, CA.)*

Documentation

Documentation should include the following:
- Patient and family education
- Location of sensors
- Sensor site assessment
- Baseline tissue oximetry (Sto_2)
- Hourly Sto_2 values
- Fraction of inspired oxygen (Fio_2)
- Minute ventilation (MV)
- Pulse oximetry (Spo_2)
- Mean arterial pressure (MAP)
- Recent cardiac output (if available)
- Recent hemoglobin (if available)
- Recent arterial blood gas (if available)
- Continued trends away from baseline
- Decrease of 20% from baseline value
- Sustained values less than 60%
- Nursing interventions

References and Additional Readings

For a complete list of references and additional readings for this procedure, scan this QR code with your smartphone, or visit https://www.elsevier.com/__data/assets/pdf_file/0006/1319856/Chapter0081.pdf

82 EEG Monitoring Assist and Nursing Care

Brooke Wagner

PURPOSE Electroencephalography (EEG) is a graphical measurement of the electrical activity within the brain. EEG is used to evaluate changes in neurological structures and functions. Routine EEG can be used to evaluate abnormal events and diagnose seizures, continuous EEG can be used to monitor the effectiveness of neurological treatments, diagnose and localize seizures, and stereotactic EEG (SEEG) can be used to localize seizure foci before surgical resection.

PREREQUISITE NURSING KNOWLEDGE

- Knowledge of neuroanatomy and physiology.
- EEG measures excitatory and inhibitory changes in post-synaptic membrane potentials. Waveforms represent the synchronized electrical activity of a large cortical area.[7,8,10]
- Indications for EEG are as follows:
  - Diagnosis of nonconvulsive seizures, nonconvulsive status epilepticus, and seizure mimics[4,5,8,10]
  - Assessment of treatment efficacy for seizures and status epilepticus[4,5,8,10]
  - Evaluation of impaired consciousness with or without a previous seizure or brain injury[4,5,8,10]
  - Evaluation of encephalopathy after a severe brain injury for purposes of prognostication[4,5,8,10]
  - Monitoring high-risk patients when undergoing neuromuscular blockade, sedation, or an induced coma[4,5,10]
  - Continuous video monitoring correlates EEG recordings to behavioral or clinical changes[5,6]
  - Stereotactic and subdural EEG localizes seizure foci, maps areas of functional brain tissue, and are used to plan surgical resection of the focus[9,10]
- Types of electrodes
  - For routine EEG, metal disks or cups (Fig. 82.1) are applied using conductive paste. The electrodes are made of gold, silver, silver chloride, tin, or platinum.[4,6,8]
  - Continuous EEG often uses cups adhered with collodion. A hole in the cup allows for refilling of the conductive gel.[4,6,8]
  - MRI- and CT-compatible electrodes are plastic with impregnated carbon or silver. If the patient needs frequent imaging, these electrodes may reduce skin breakdown and time off the EEG monitor, since they do not need to be removed or reapplied.[4,6,8]
  - Subdural grids and strips (SDGs) (Fig. 82.2) are stainless steel or platinum disks embedded in a synthetic material and are made in various shapes and sizes. The electrodes are placed on the cortex through a burr hole or open craniotomy.[10]

- Depth electrodes (SEEG) are flexible leads placed in the brain parenchyma stereotactically with robotic assistance. Leads may differ in length and number of contacts.[9,10]
- Scalp electrodes are positioned according the International 10-20 Electrode Placement System. Sixteen to 21 electrodes are placed, and each is labeled alphanumerically. The letters correspond to the lobes of the brain: frontal (F), parietal (P), temporal (T), occipital (O), and central (C) areas. Odd numbers are on the left, and even numbers are on the right.[1,4,6,8,10]
- A montage is a standardized layout of electrode pairs, or channels, on a monitor (Fig. 82.3). The longitudinal bipolar montage, or "double banana," displays 16 channels for interpretation[6,8,10].
- On average, 10 depth electrodes are placed, but there are no standard SEEG montages because placement locations and number of contact leads vary.[9]
- Many factors affect EEG recordings. Cranial structures between the cortex and the electrode resist the measurement of electrical signals. Metabolic changes and pharmaceuticals may potentiate or impair the ability to generate action potentials.[5,10]
- In many cases, interpretation of EEG waveforms is currently outside the scope of nursing, however familiarity with common waveforms may improve identification of artifact or seizure activity.[3,4,7,8]
  - Alpha waveforms
    - Hz 8 to 13
    - Seen in the parietal, occipital and posterior temporal regions
    - Best seen when patients are awake but resting and are affected by opening and closing the eyes
    - Associated with level of consciousness.
    - Affected by medications such as phenytoin and valproic acid.
  - Beta waveforms
  - Hz 14 to 30
  - Seen in the frontal regions
  - Affected by drowsiness, barbiturates, and benzodiazepines

- Reduced amplitude on one side indicates a pathological change such as stroke or tumor
- Delta waveforms
  - Hz 0.1 to <4
  - Seen in the posterior regions
  - Associated with sleep and hyperexcitable states
  - Affected by structural lesions
- Theta waveforms
  - Hz 4 to <8
  - Seen in the temporal and thalamic regions
  - Affected by structural lesions
  - Occur more frequently in children and adolescents
- Routine EEGs may last 30 to 60 minutes, while continuous or SEEG may last days to weeks.[4,6,7,10]
- Routine EEGs may take place in a neurodiagnostic laboratory or at the bedside. CEEG or SEEG usually occur in the ICU or an epilepsy monitoring unit.[3]
- Seizures are excessive abnormal and synchronous discharges that cause changes in neurological function and behavior.[10]

- Status epilepticus is a seizure lasting longer than 5 minutes or the occurrence of two consecutive seizures without the return of baseline neurological function between each seizure.[7,10]
- The assessment of a seizing patient includes the following[7,8,10]:
  - Vital signs and autonomic changes such as apnea, flushing, or tachycardia
  - Level of consciousness and mental status
  - Eye fluttering, blinking, staring, nystagmus, and gaze preference
  - Motor movements within the face, limbs or trunk on one side or both. Note any twitching, jerking, tremors, posturing, rhythmic movements, or loss of tone.
  - Automatisms including chewing, lip smacking, or picking
  - Incontinence of the bowel or bladder
  - Time of onset, duration, and progression of the seizure
  - Convulsive seizures may become nonconvulsive with only subtle clinical signs indicating ongoing epileptic activity

EQUIPMENT

- Clean gloves
- Pillow, neck roll, or cushion for positioning
- Safety equipment such as pads for side rails, lap belt, and floor mats
- Emergency equipment such as wall suction, oxygen, nasal cannula, and code cart
- Shampoo or other skin and hair cleanser
- Towels
- EEG electrodes
- EKG electrode
- Sleeve to protect electrode wires
- EEG monitor and cables, hardwired or portable
- Camera, hardwired or portable
- Alarm button

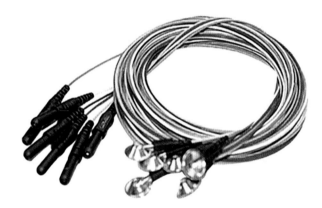

Figure 82.1   Electroencephalography (EEG) electrode lead cups. *(Courtesy Cadwell.)*

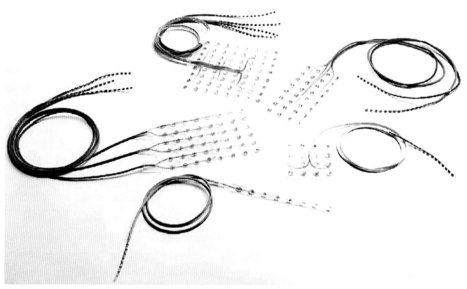

Figure 82.2   Subdural grid/strip electrodes. *(Courtesy of PMT Corporation.)*

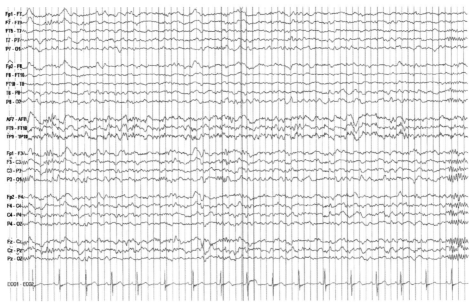

Figure 82.3 16-channel electroencephalography (EEG) display.

- Tape measure
- Marking pen
- Skin prep solution
- Cotton-tipped applicators
- Cotton balls
- Tongue depressor
- Gauze or pads for skin protection
- Headwrap made of stretchable or mesh gauze roll or tubular retainer net
- Tape, breathable
- Conductive paste, adhesion gel, and collodion
- Syringes, per institutional guidelines
- Acetone for collodion removal
- Foam peel and stick electrodes

PATIENT AND FAMILY EDUCATION

- Assess the patient's and family's understanding of the purpose of EEG. *Rationale:* Explanation may decrease patient and family anxiety.
- Explain the procedure to the patient and family including the potential for photic stimulation, hyperventilation, and sleep deprivation. Orient to the equipment including the EEG monitor, camera, strobe light, and other personnel.[3,8] *Rationale:* Facilitates patient cooperation during the procedure.
- Reassure the patient and family that the electrodes can only record waveform and cannot stimulate or shock the patient. *Rationale:* Knowledge and information may lessen anxiety. Anxiety can change EEG waveforms.[10]
- Teach the patient and family about the importance of maintaining electrode adhesion and to refrain from pulling, scratching the head, removing the headwrap, or changing position without coordinated movement of electrode cables. Staff assistance is needed for ambulation and some changes in position.[9] *Rationale:* Prepares the patient

and family for what to expect and decreases the risk of dislodging electrodes.

- Encourage the patient and family's role in using the alarm button and reporting any symptoms of a seizure.[6] *Rationale:* Early recognition and treatment of seizures and status epilepticus is associated with more favorable patient outcomes.[4,5]
- Explain the importance of reporting skin irritation, itching, pain, and any drainage. *Rationale:* Reporting of symptoms ensures appropriate and timely assessment and intervention if needed.[2,4,5,7]

PATIENT ASSESSMENT AND PREPARATION

Patient Assessment

- Obtain the patient's history, current medications, time of the last dose, and overall medication compliance. *Rationale:* Baseline data are provided and identifies the potential risk for seizures.[5,8]
- Review the patient's seizure history including the clinical presentation of prior seizures, auras, triggers, duration, and postictal state. *Rationale:* Baseline data are established.[7]
- Obtain a neurological assessment including vital signs, level of consciousness, mental status, cranial nerves, motor, and sensation. *Rationale:* Enables the nurse to identify any changes that may occur, especially the onset or continuation of a seizure.[6,9]
- Assess the patient's scalp for breakdown, surgical wounds, neuromonitoring devices, or other scalp lesions. *Rationale:* Baseline data are provided.[2,6,7]

Patient Preparation

- Verify the correct patient with two identifiers. *Rationale:* Before performing a procedure, the nurse should ensure

the correct identification of the patient for the intended intervention.
- Ensure that the patient's hair is clean without oils, creams, or hairsprays.[6] *Rationale:* Electrodes will better adhere to the scalp and conduct EEG waveforms.
- Ensure that the patient has followed instructions for sleep deprivation, holding prescribed medications, and

caffeine consumption and has not taken additional sedating medication.[3,7,8] *Rationale:* Sleep deprivation and holding prescriptions may be necessary to better classify EEG waveforms while caffeine and sedating medications impair them.

Procedure	**EEG Monitoring Assist and Nursing Care**	
Steps	Rationale	Special Considerations
1. Assist the neurodiagnostic technician or other neurological personnel to obtain equipment as needed.	Equipment may be portable, hardwired (epilepsy monitoring unit), stored on the unit, or in the neurodiagnostic laboratory.	
2. **HH**		
3. **PE**		
4. Initiate seizure precautions per institutional standards. Precautions may include padded side rails, floor mats, lap belts, suction, and other equipment.[7] **(Level E*)**	Ensures a safe environment if the patient has a seizure.	
5. Collaborate to identify the appropriate type of EEG electrodes to apply.	The duration of the EEG, the patient's ability to mobilize, and skin fragility affect EEG electrode choice. SDGs and SEEG electrodes are placed stereotactically in an operating room by a physician.[9,10] **(Level D*)**	Paste is more appropriate for routine EEGs and immobile patients, while collodion is recommended for long-term monitoring and highly mobile patients.[8] **(Level D*)** Flat electrodes and thin wires are preferable to cups and thicker wires if patients have fragile skin.[2] **(Level E*)** CT- or MRI- compatible electrodes are preferred if the patient needs frequent imaging.[2,4,6] **(Level D*)**
6. Collaborate to identify monitoring devices, surgical incisions, or other scalp lesions to avoid during placement.	Electrodes should only be placed on intact skin. They are adjusted bilaterally to obtain symmetric waveforms.[4,6] **(Level D*)**	
7. Assist with positioning the patient as needed.	The patient may need to be in the lateral position to place temporal or occipital leads.	

Procedure	EEG Monitoring Assist and Nursing Care—*Continued*	
Steps	**Rationale**	**Special Considerations**
8. Assist with placement of electrodes as needed. Follow institutional standards. A. The side of a cotton swab or a gauze-wrapped finger should be used to apply a skin preparation solution to the scalp.[2] **(Level E*)** B. Add conductive medium to the cup or disk electrode head, and place it against the scalp. Do not press. Add gauze or a pad under the electrode hub. C. Place collodion or tape over the electrode. D. If cups are adhered with collodion, fill the cup with conductive gel. E. Wrap the head with gauze or a net. Two fingers should fit beneath the wrap. If taped in place, do not put tape over an electrode. F. Do not use scissors to cut the gauze. G. Apply the electrode sleeve. H. If immobile, place a neck roll or small cushion to offload the head.	Institutional standards may dictate neurodiagnostic personnel who can apply electrodes.[6] **(Level D*)** Reduces irritation between the scalp and the electrode.[2] **(Level E*)** Reduces risk for pressure injuries. Keeps the electrode in place. Gel is required for waveform conduction. Prevents rubbing and dislodgement of electrodes. Prevents pressure injury. May cut through an electrode wire.[9] **(Level E*)** Prevents dislodgement and tangling of wires. Prevents pressure injury.[2] **(Level E*)**	Blunt-tip needle use is discouraged because they may abrade the skin within the cup.[2] **(Level E*)** Nets allow for better visibility, airflow, and access to electrodes.[2] **(Level E*)** Obtain a wound consult for specialty cushions.[2] **(Level E*)**
9. Assist with stimulating the patient as needed.	The nurse may be more familiar with the level of stimulation needed to elicit a response from obtunded or sedated patients.	
10. For continuous, video, or stereotactic EEG, follow institutional standards and collaborate regarding: A. Assessing the quality of waveforms across all channels, video camera positioning, functionality of audio or intercom, and functionality of the alarm button. B. Ensuring that cables connecting EEG leads to the wall are untangled and long enough to reach the bathroom.[9] **(Level E*)**	Institutional standards may only allow neurodiagnostic personnel to troubleshoot electrodes and other EEG equipment.[6] **(Level D*)** Ensures EEG waveforms and channels have a high-quality waveform. Prevents electrodes from becoming loose or dislodged.	Neurodiagnostic personnel are often not available 24 hours a day. SDGs and SEEG electrodes cannot be replaced at the bedside.[9,10] **(Level D*)**

Procedure continues on following page

Procedure EEG Monitoring Assist and Nursing Care—*Continued*		
Steps	Rationale	Special Considerations

11. Assist as needed with the removal of EEG electrodes.
    A. The paste becomes soft after applying a warm towel for 1 to 2 minutes.[6] **(Level D*)**
    B. Use a cotton ball and acetone to remove collodion.
    C. Complete a neurological assessment after removal of SEEG electrodes.[9] **(Level E*)**
	Institutional standards may only allow neurodiagnostic personnel to remove electrodes.[6] **(Level D*)** Acetone can dissolve tubing and plastics such as those used for ECMO and ventricular drains.[6] **(Level D*)** SDGs and SEEG electrodes may cause hemorrhaging during removal.[9] **(Level E*)**	SDGs and SEEG electrodes may only be removed by a physician at the bedside or in the operating room.[9] **(Level D*)**

12. Wash the remaining paste or collodion from the scalp.[2] **(Level E*)**	Improves the ability to assess the scalp.	Acetone is irritating to the eyes, mucous membranes, and skin.[9] **(Level D*)**
13. Assess the scalp for infection, bleeding, and breakdown.[4,6,7,9,10] **(Level D*)**	Identifies complications.	
14. PE Discard supplies and PPE in appropriate receptacles.	Removes and safely discards used supplies; safely removes sharp objects.	
15. HH		

Expected Outcomes

- Clear EEG waveforms displayed
- Prompt identification of abnormal waveforms
- Scalp and electrode insertion sites are clean and dry
- No change or deterioration in neurological assessment

Unexpected Outcomes

- Dislodged electrodes
- Inability to obtain EEG
- Scalp or intracranial infection
- Intracranial hemorrhage or cerebral edema
- Cerebrospinal fluid (CSF) leak
- Untreated seizures or status epilepticus

Patient Monitoring and Care

Steps	Rationale	Reportable Conditions
		These conditions should be reported to the provider if they persist despite nursing interventions.
1. Maintain seizure precautions.[7] **(Level E*)**	Ensures a safe environment if the patient has a seizure.	
2. Assess the neurological status as warranted by institutional guidelines.	A change in neurological status could indicate seizure, hemorrhage, or intracranial infection.[5,7,9,10] **(Level D*)**	Signs and symptoms of seizures, status epilepticus, or nonconvulsive status epilepticus.
3. Assess the headwrap and electrodes for loose or dislodged electrodes twice a day.[6] **(Level D*)** Unless trained, do not remove head wraps covering SEEG electrodes.[9] **(Level E*)**	Ensures that EEG waveforms and channels have a high-quality waveform. Electrodes are carefully wrapped and looped within the gauze by the provider.	If only neurodiagnostic personnel may troubleshoot electrodes, notify of loose headwraps, lose or disconnected electrodes, and poor-quality waveforms.[8]
4. If allowed to troubleshoot per institutional guidelines, reapply scalp electrodes by reapplying paste, refilling the cup with gel, and/or repositioning the electrode.[4] **(Level D*)**	Ensures that EEG waveforms and channels have a high-quality waveform.	Loose headwraps, loose or disconnected electrodes, and poor-quality waveforms despite interventions.[8,9]

Patient Monitoring and Care —*Continued*

Steps	Rationale	Reportable Conditions
5. If able to visualize the scalp, assess the skin and electrode sites for signs of infection, breakdown, bleeding, and CSF leak twice a day or as warranted by institutional guidelines.[2,4,6,7,9,10] **(Level D*)**	Identifies complications. Consult wound care as needed.[2] **(Level E*)**	Redness, rash, itching, warmth, swelling, drainage, purulence, pressure injuries, bleeding, or CSF leak.[2,4,6,7,9,10]
6. Frequently rotate and use a small cushion or neck roll for positioning[2,4] **(Level D*)**	Prevents breakdown by applying less pressure to the head and electrodes.	
7. If used, assess whether the video camera is focused and able to see the whole patient. Adjust the lighting in the room as needed.[6] **(Level D*)** Per institutional standards, adjust the camera.[6] **(Level D*)**	Signs and symptoms of seizures may include subtle twitching of the eyes or extremities.[7,10]	Camera is not focused or the whole patient is not visible.
8. Ensure that the cables connecting the EEG leads to the wall are untangled and long enough to reach the bathroom.[9] **(Level E*)**	Prevents dislodgement of electrodes.	Dislodgment of electrodes or poor-quality waveforms.
9. In case of emergency, disconnect electrodes according to institutional guidelines.	Quickly removing paste, collodion, SDGs, and SEEG electrodes may result in skin breakdown, abrasions, hemorrhage, CSF leaks, or death.[9,10] **(Level D*)**	Rationale for emergent disconnection. Neurological assessment changes. Skin breakdown or abrasions. Bleeding or CSF leakage from the scalp or SDG or SEEG insertion sites.
10. Mark clinical events for review per institutional guidelines[6] **(Level D*)** A. Annotate the EEG record if trained. B. Record activities in the medical record. C. Complete the activity log kept at the bedside.	Allows the electroencephalographer to determine if abnormal EEG findings are pathophysiological or caused by routine care such as turning, bathing, or eating.[6] **(Level D*)**	Signs and symptoms of seizures, status epilepticus, or nonconvulsive status epilepticus. Inability to manage a seizure despite interventions.
11. Document all medications per institutional guidelines.[6] **(Level D*)**	Allows the electroencephalographer to determine the effect of pharmaceuticals on EEG findings.[6]	
12. Monitor the patient for headache or discomfort. Follow institutional guidelines for assessing pain.	Patients may experience pain after surgical placement of SDGs or SEEG electrodes.[9] **(Level E*)** A headache may also indicate an intracranial hemorrhage or infection.[9,10] **(Level D*)**	Inability to manage pain. Persistent headache despite interventions.[9,10]
13. Monitor the patient for neurological assessment changes. If a seizure occurs, follow institutional guidelines or administer prescribed medications.	Patients undergoing EEGs are at risk for seizures, especially when removed from medications for the purposes of classifying seizures or identifying a focus for surgical resection.[9,10] **(Level D*)**	Signs and symptoms of seizures, status epilepticus, or nonconvulsive status epilepticus. Inability to manage a seizure despite interventions.

Procedure continues on following page

Documentation

Documentation should include the following:

- Date and time of routine EEG
- Date and time electrodes were applied for continuous EEG
- Date and time continuous or stereotactic electrodes were removed
- Presence of artifact or loose electrodes
- Notification of proper personnel for electrode maintenance
- Notification of physician for any complications
- Safety precautions initiated and maintained
- Neurological assessment findings
- Seizure assessment if needed
- Integumentary assessment findings
- CSF leak color and amount
- Consultation for wound care

References and Additional Readings

For a complete list of references and additional readings for this procedure, scan this QR code with your smartphone, or visit https://www.elsevier.com/__data/assets/pdf_file/0007/1319857/Chapter0082.pdf.

83 Signal Processed Electroencephalography

Malissa Mulkey

PURPOSE Signal processed electroencephalography (spEEG) devices and sensors acquire electroencephalography (EEG) signals that can be processed using computer algorithms. Although there are several types of signal processed devices with ongoing development and emerging technology, some examples include the Bispectral Index (BIS), Sedline, Ceribell, and Emotiv's EPOC (Figs. 83.1 to 83.3).

These portable bedside spEEG devices may provide real-time appraisal of brain wave activity during therapeutic interventions when visual clues of cerebral function are limited or disappear.[9] Processed EEG–derived parameters can be used to assess level of consciousness and brain arousal state(s) in critically ill patients as well as patient responses to sedative, hypnotic, and anesthetic agents.[19,16,1] Thorough neurological assessment and judicious interpretation spEEG data and other available parameters may provide early indication of progressive brain injury and inform care decisions.[2,12,3] Goals of care should be known and communicated clearly among all members of the multidisciplinary team before initiation of clinical care, treatment, or interventions.

A comprehensive clinical assessment for establishing therapeutic goals and endpoints should be integrated within the plan of care and modified as appropriate based on patient condition.

PREREQUISITE NURSING KNOWLEDGE

- Although there are a wide variety of uses for spEEG, some common uses include diagnosis and monitoring of neurological and psychiatric disorders such as seizures, sleep stages, level of arousal, and response to treatment and interventions.[6]
- Cerebral physiology, including how brain physiology is altered consequent to metabolic and/or structural injury as well as central nervous system (CNS) depressants.[17,15]
- Cerebral injury and hypoperfusion (hemodynamic stability, global neurological injury, severe hypoxemia) are related to direct alterations in cerebral metabolic stability.[10]
- Monitoring parameters (central vs. peripheral nervous system).
- Interrelationship between the electrical activity of the brain and cerebral metabolism.
- Factors that affect cerebral metabolism and EEG activity.
- EEG activity reflects brain physiology and requires successive, energy-using steps. These steps include electrical impulse discharge at the thalamus, impulse transmission to the cerebral cortex, presynaptic neurotransmitter release, and postsynaptic neurotransmitter uptake.[9,8]
- Evaluation of EEG waveforms complements CNS evaluation in context with information obtained through the clinical neurological assessment.[9,13]

- EEG-based monitoring:
  - ❖ EEG tracings are obtained and recorded through the application of scalp electrodes.
  - ❖ Electrical activity that occurs between a pair of electrodes is captured to compose a single channel or waveform.
- Electrical activity in the brain is then displayed and recorded on a monitor.[5]
- Multiple processing steps are applied to raw EEG waveform data to evaluate: frequency, amplitude, regularity, degree of organization, paroxysmal features, focal abnormalities, and waveform characteristics.
- Typical EEG waveforms and frequencies include the following:
  - ❖ Gamma (30 to 80 Hz): Thought to occur during modulation of sensory input and internal processes such as working memory and attention.
  - ❖ Beta (12 to 30 Hz): Normally seen when a patient is alert or anxious with eyes open. Accentuated by sedative-hypnotic drugs, especially benzodiazepines. May be reduced or absent in the setting of cortical damage.
  - ❖ Alpha (8 to 12 Hz): Primary rhythm seen when an individual is relaxed with eyes closed.
  - ❖ Theta (4 to 8 Hz): Normal in children up to 13 years of age and during sleep. Abnormal in awake adults. Frequently seen in the presence of diffuse or generalized disorders.
  - ❖ Delta (<4 Hz): Normal in infants or adults during sleep stages 3 and 4. May be seen with diffuse or generalized disorders.

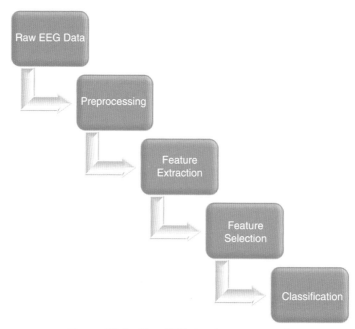

Figure 83.1   How EEG signals are processed.

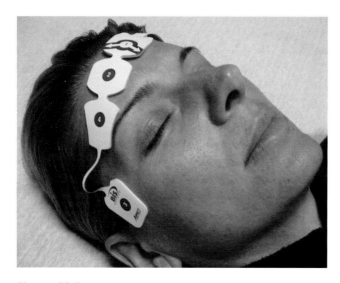

Figure 83.2   BIS sensor in place illustrating anatomical landmarks for optimal sensor placement. The BIS Extend sensor in place. The sensor may be placed on the right or left side. *Circle 1* is positioned at the center of the forehead approximately 2 inches (5 cm) above the nose. *Circle 4* is placed directly above and parallel to the eyebrow. *Circle 3* is placed on the temple area between the hairline and the outer canthus of the eye. *Circle 2* is placed between *Circles 1 and 4* on the patient's forehead.

- EEG recordings do not discriminate the electrical signals they receive. Activity that does not originate in the cerebral cortex is considered artifact. Examples include eye movements, sweating, electrodes that do not have good skin contact, and electrical activity from bedside monitors and beds.
    - In spEEG, the signal is filtered and digitalized to remove artifacts (low-frequency and high-frequency) and aid in evaluating cortical activity.[7,13]
- Regardless of the type of EEG monitoring, sensors or electrodes are placed on the patient's head in a predetermined arrangement or montage. The number of electrodes is determined by manufacturer design and purpose for monitoring.
- Initial monitoring and setup of the sensor and equipment includes appropriate setup and configuration of monitoring systems and integration with other critical care patient monitoring systems.[18]
- Understanding of the effects of temperature extremes (hypothermia vs. hyperthermia) on brain physiology.[4]
- Any clinical state or drug therapy affecting cerebral metabolism may be reflected in EEG waveforms.[18,14]
- Indications and contraindications of specific medication classes should be understood.
- Information derived from monitoring may be used to guide sedative, hypnotic, and metabolic suppression and analgesic therapies.[11,20,14]

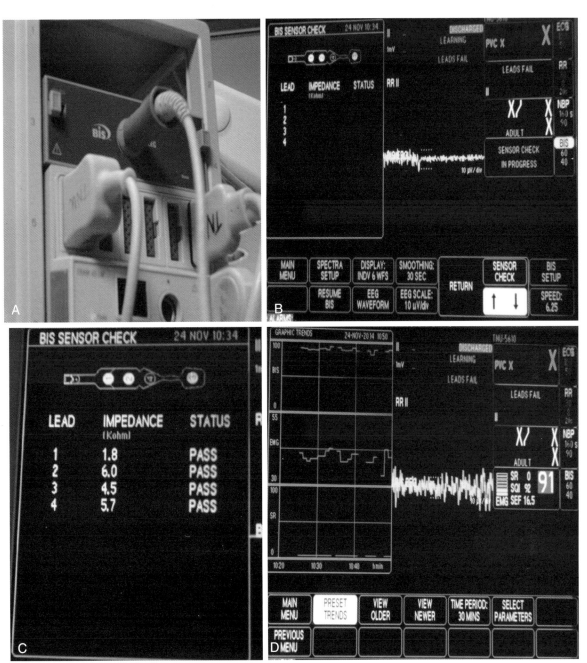

Figure 83.3   Illustration of setup and configuration of BIS monitoring within General Electric (GE) critical care monitoring system. **A,** Placement of BIS module within the bedside monitor to establish availability of the parameter. **B,** Initial EEG signal and monitor start-up with initial BIS sensor impedance check. In this setup screen, smoothing rate, sensor check, EEG sweep speed, and additional options for BIS setup may be determined. **C,** Satisfactory completion of sensor check on all electrodes with impedances within acceptable parameters for acquisition of EEG data. **D,** Completion of sensor check, availability of single-channel EEG tracing (EEG tracing at 6.25 mm/sec sweep speed), SQI indicating adequate signal for BIS determination, EMG and BIS value (91). Graphic trending *(BIS, EMG, SR)* available by selecting parameters and time indices. This may be utilized for observing data over time and in response to therapies alterations in clinical state such as shivering during therapeutic hypothermia. BIS technology is licensed to multiple patient monitoring vendors. This illustration using GE monitors is one of multiple options available.

COMMON MONITORS

Device	Bispectral Index	Sedline	Ceribell	EPOC
Sensor locations	Frontal; unilateral or bilateral	Frontal; bilateral	All lobes (frontal, temporal, parietal, and occipital) circumferential	Frontal; parietal bilateral
Number of channels (waveforms)	1 or 4	4	8	14
Battery life	45 minutes	4 hours	10 hours	12 hours
Weight (g)	1588	1647	400	116

EQUIPMENT

- EEG monitoring device (or module if using system integrated with the bedside monitor).
- Electrode housed sensor(s)
- Detachable power cord
- Alcohol pads
- Gauze pads
- Nonsterile gloves

Additional equipment, to have available as needed, includes the following:

- Soap and water
- Emergency equipment

PATIENT AND FAMILY EDUCATION

- Assess factors that affect the patient's (if still awake) and family's readiness to learn. *Rationale:* Teaching is individualized to specific patient and family needs.
- Explain the purpose of EEG monitoring, including content regarding specific information obtained, how it may be used, and an explanation of the equipment. *Rationale:* The patient (if still awake) and family may experience less anxiety and have increased understanding of the patient equipment at the bedside.
- Explain to the patient and family what will happen with the initiation of monitoring (skin preparation, placement of electrodes/sensors, moderate pressure for electrode contact). *Rationale:* This explanation prepares the patient and family for events associated with initiation of EEG monitoring and also provides an opportunity to reinforce preprocedural teaching and assess level of understanding.
- Although rare, some patients may have mild skin irritation develop in the area in contact with the sensor. This irritation typically resolves within 1 hour after sensor removal. *Rationale:* The patient and family are prepared for the

possible minor issue with sensor application and the possible need for removal or repositioning of the sensor.
- Explain that monitoring and electrode placement pose no risk to the patient beyond that of mild skin irritation (in rare instances) and that no discomfort will be experienced as part of the monitoring procedure. *Rationale:* Anxiety may be decreased.

PATIENT ASSESSMENT AND PREPARATION

Patient Assessment

- Assess the patient's level of sedation, responsiveness, and arousal. *Rationale:* Baseline data are provided.
- In collaboration with the multidisciplinary team, establish overall goals and endpoints of therapy. *Rationale:* A coordinated plan is established with integration of the EEG data into decision-making regarding the patient's current plan of care.
- Assess the skin at the intended sites for sensor placement. *Rationale:* This provides baseline information regarding the patient's skin.
- Assess the patient's neurological status. *Rationale:* Baseline data are provided. EEG data may reflect significant neurological injury, which must be determined before initiation of monitoring. If possible, obtain baseline EEG data before initiating therapies and or interventions.

Patient Preparation

- Verify the correct patient with two identifiers. *Rationale:* Before performing a procedure, the nurse should ensure the correct identification of the patient for the intended intervention.
- Determine anatomical landmarks for the sensor placement. *Rationale:* Landmarks provide for accurate placement of sensors.

Procedure   for Monitoring

Steps	Rationale	Special Considerations
1. Connect the power cord to the monitor, and plug it into the electrical wall outlet.	Prepares the equipment.	Equipment may vary because a stand-alone monitor or a module may be used that is incorporated into the bedside monitoring system.
2. Connect the monitoring system and related cable (s) to the monitor (if applicable).	Prepares the equipment.	
3. Turn on the monitor, and observe as a system check is run. **(Level M*)**	The system initiates a self-test to ensure that the equipment and connections are operating effectively.	If a hardware problem exists, remove from care area, and refer to the operator manual. If needed, remove the device from service, and refer to biomedical engineering.
4. Cleanse the intended sensor area with alcohol pads, and dry with gauze. **(Level M*)**	A thorough skin preparation removes debris and oily residue from the skin and facilitates optimal electrical contact for EEG data acquisition.	Mild soap and water is an acceptable alternative. Ensure that the skin is dry before applying the sensors.
5. 🅷🅷		
6. 🅿🅴		
7. Apply the EEG sensor(s) to the patient's head a. Whole-brain spEEG will require sensors over the entire scalp. b. Frontal lobe spEEG may require only a single unilateral sensor. c. See manufacturer's recommendations in the user manual for device-specific sensor locations.	Ensures consistency of the anatomical location for sensor placement and optimizes the electrical contact between the monitoring system and the skin for facilitation of EEG data acquisition. EEG data acquisition begins shortly after optimal connection is established between the patient and the monitoring system.	The conductive parts of the electrodes, sensor, or connectors should not contact other conductive parts of the monitoring system. Data acquisition begins when impedances are acceptable. If electrodes(s) show high impedance, repeat pressing of electrodes to optimize electrical contact. If significant artifact is present, move the device and cables away from sources of external electrical or mechanical artifact. Sources of artifact include fluid or forced-air warming systems, ventricular assist devices, high-frequency ventilation, suction, pacemakers, and oscillating mattresses. In the event such as high impedance or sensor removal, repreparation and sensor replacement may be necessary.
8. Ensure that all connections are connected.	Connects the sensor, cable, and device.	
9. Secure the cables and device, and maintain in an easily accessible location near the patient's head (e.g., patient's pillow or sheet), avoiding close proximity to sources of mechanical or electrical interference.	Placing the device and cables close to the patient's head minimizes the vulnerability of the EEG signal to interference from other electronic equipment or patient care devices.	
10. Set up the monitor based on the manufacturer's recommendations in the user manual to select the specific monitor settings, including event markers and display type. **(Level M*)**	Settings such as event markers and display type should be consistent with specific device capability, facility protocols, and provider-specific orders.	

*Level M: Manufacturer's recommendations only.

Procedure continues on following page

UNIT III

Procedure for Monitoring—*Continued*

Steps	Rationale	Special Considerations
11. When the monitor settings have been adjusted to a specific patient, data collection can begin.	Data collection can proceed after all preparatory steps and monitor settings are completed appropriately. This ensures optimal electrical contact between the patient and the monitoring system and optimal electrical safety. In addition, confirmation of display settings and secondary parameters at the outset of monitoring effectively tailors the monitor display and data acquisition to the specific patient.	
12. Observe the monitor display for: A. High impedance alarm/ notification. If displayed, press each electrode again to optimize electrical contact. Remove the sensor, cleanse the skin, and place a new sensor if necessary.	Data acquisition begins when impedances are acceptable.	A sensor check is initiated automatically during the system start-up.
B. Artifact: If artifact is present, move the digital signal converter away from sources of external electrical or mechanical artifact.	Artifact may result from use of fluid or forced-air warming systems, ventricular assist devices, high-frequency ventilation, suction, pacemakers, and oscillating mattresses.	
13. When monitoring is discontinued, remove electrodes/ sensors from the patient, and turn off the device.		
14. Disconnect sensors from the device. Discard used supplies in an appropriate receptacle.	Removes and safely discards used supplies.	
15. 🄷🄷		

*Level C: Qualitative studies, descriptive or correlational studies, integrative reviews, systematic reviews, or randomized controlled trials with inconsistent results.

Expected Outcomes

- Optimal placement of the sensors consistent with anatomical landmarks and manufacturer's recommendations.
- Skin remaining intact in the area of the sensor placement.
- Data acquisition and display after monitor setup and completion of self-test.
- Optimal EEG data acquisition with minimal or no artifact.
- Clear EEG waveform visible on the monitor display.
- EEG data is effective in providing feedback on the state of the brain and responses to treatment and/or intervention.

Unexpected Outcomes

- Skin irritation in the area of the sensor placement.
- Suboptimal EEG signal acquisition such that a clear waveform and treatment responses can be identified.
- Device values or sounds do not correlate with clinical assessment or respond inconsistently to treatments and interventions.

Patient Monitoring and Care

Steps	Rationale	Reportable Conditions
		These conditions should be reported to the provider if they persist despite nursing interventions.
1. Follow institutional standards for assessing the patient.	Identifies the need for interventions.	• Not meeting protocol or provider prescribed parameters.
2. Assess the skin condition in the area of the sensor placement.	Ensures that the skin is intact.	• Altered skin integrity or irritation after sensor placement
3. Maintain the device in close proximity to the patient's head.	Decreases the vulnerability of the EEG signals to electrical interference from other sources.	
4. Monitor values and secondary parameters as determined by goals of care, clinical status, and response to interventions.	Identifies trends in values and secondary parameters.	• EEG values and/or parameters are not consistent with clinical assessment or condition.
5. Identify goals or endpoints of therapy at the beginning of monitoring.	Improves patient outcomes with an organized, evidence-based approach to care.	• Not progressing toward achievement of goals or endpoint of therapy
6. Change the sensor per manufacturer's recommendations, at least every 24 hours or more frequently as needed (e.g., diaphoresis, loose electrodes).	Maintains optimal electrical contact between the patient and the monitoring system.	
7. Observe the EEG channel as determined by the patient's clinical state and therapeutic interventions. A significant decrease in EEG amplitude and/ or frequency may become visible and reportable.	The EEG amplitude and frequency change is based on the patient's clinical state, evolving injury, and medication therapy. The EEG also (under normal conditions) changes in response to varying levels and types of stimulation. In most conditions, electrocardiographic (ECG) artifact is not visible in an EEG waveform. ECG artifact visible in the EEG channel may indicate significant EEG suppression.	• A decrease in EEG frequency or amplitude may indicate neurological injury. Or critical pathology and warrant further evaluation with neuroimaging diagnostic EEG or clinical examination
8. Observe the EEG data, values, and parameters in response to stimulation.	An EEG that is unresponsive to stimulation may indicate neurological injury and possibly poor prognosis.	• Significant ECG artifact in the EEG channel

Documentation

Documentation should include the following:
- Goals and endpoints of monitoring and therapy
- Family education regarding EEG monitoring
- Clinical assessment
- EEG values, parameters, and quality of signal at the start of monitoring and with changes or titration of therapy
- EEG values, parameters, and quality of signal recording in the patient medical record at least hourly and more frequently as indicated
- Occurrence of skin irritation at the site of the sensor placement with action taken
- Unexpected outcomes and interventions
- Sudden changes in values or waveforms independent of obvious clinical changes or alterations in therapy

UNIT III

References and Additional Readings

For a complete list of references and additional readings for this procedure, scan this QR code with your smartphone, or visit: https://www.elsevier.com/__data/assets/pdf_file/0008/1319858/Chapter0083.pdf

PROCEDURE

84

Brain Tissue Oxygen Monitoring: Insertion (Assist), Nursing Care, and Troubleshooting

Megan T. Moyer

PURPOSE The purpose of brain tissue oxygen monitoring is end-organ preservation to support a meaningful recovery for patients with, or at high risk of, cerebral ischemia and/or hypoxia. It is used for measurement and continuous monitoring of regional brain tissue oxygenation for prevention and detection of secondary brain injury. Monitoring of brain tissue oxygen provides important information relative to the delivery of oxygen to cerebral tissue of the injured brain. Growing evidence suggests that clinical care informed by brain tissue oxygen monitoring may lead to improved clinical outcomes.

PREREQUISITE NURSING KNOWLEDGE

- Knowledge of neuroanatomy and physiology, specifically intracranial dynamics.
- Knowledge of sterile and aseptic technique.
- Incorporated as an adjunct monitor of trends in concert with concurrent neurological multimodality monitoring parameters (intracranial pressure [ICP], cerebral perfusion pressure [CPP], systemic jugular venous oxygen [$SjvO_2$], cerebral microdialysis), brain tissue oxygen monitoring reflects the oxygenation of cerebral tissue local to the sensor placement.[2,4,7,8,10,14,15,17]
- Each of the devices described in this chapter denotes partial pressure of the brain tissue differently, for example $PbtO_2$, $PbrO_2$, $PtiO_2$, tiO_2, PtO_2. For the remainder of the text in this procedure, brain oxygen will be referred to as $PbtO_2$. The tables that represent the individual devices will denote the nomenclature adopted by that manufacturer.
- In institutions where $SjvO_2$ is used as a monitoring parameter, the difference between $SjvO_2$ measurements and $PbtO_2$ values must be noted. $SjvO_2$ is a measure of the oxygen contained in the blood draining from the cerebral venous sinuses into the jugular bulb (a measure of global brain oxygenation), whereas $PbtO_2$ measures regional (local to the catheter placement in the cerebral white matter) brain tissue oxygenation. $SjvO_2$ monitoring accuracy can be influenced by poor sampling technique, positioning, and clot formation on the catheter, making this method of monitoring less reliable than $PbtO_2$ monitoring. A normal $SjvO_2$ range is between 55% and 75%, making cerebral ischemia any number less than 55%. The choice of monitoring device depends on the patient's pathology.[1,7,8,17]

- Cellular death is preceded by a cascade of events following low brain oxygen levels that result in anaerobic metabolism, lactic acid accumulation, and release of excitatory neurotransmitters causing neurotoxicity.[7,11]
- A brain tissue oxygen probe may be inserted into the brain parenchyma through an intracranial bolt or tunneled.[5,7,16,17]
- $PbtO_2$ monitoring provides information that reflects brain tissue oxygen levels associated with cerebral oxygen demand and systemic oxygen delivery, therefore identifying cerebral ischemia.[2,3,6,12,7,17]
- $PbtO_2$ values are relative within an individual and vary depending on a range of factors including precondition, duration, location, tissue condition, and sensor type. Establishing and following the patient's cerebral oxygen trends provides the physicians, advanced practice nurses, and other healthcare professionals with information that will aid in the assessment and treatment of cerebral hypoxia and prevention of further secondary brain damage. Brain hypoxia is associated with increased mortality and poor outcome.[2,6,10,12,13,17]
- Indications for $PbtO_2$ monitoring include patients at risk for secondary injury from cerebral edema. Conditions most likely to cause cerebral edema include severe traumatic brain injury (TBI), aneurysmal and traumatic subarachnoid hemorrhage, brain tumor, stroke, and any condition that increases ICP.[2,3,6,12,17]

Relative contraindications for $PbtO_2$ monitoring and needle insertion into the body include coagulopathy, anticoagulation therapy, insertion site infection, and/or susceptibility to infections or infected tissue. A platelet count of less than 50,000 is considered a contraindication. This value may differ according to different hospital protocols. Blood coagulation must be carefully monitored during therapeutic hypothermia, hepatic coma, or other conditions that impair blood coagulation.[5,16]

Pbto$_2$ probes are safe with computed tomography (CT). Consult the manufacturer's guidelines for magnetic resonance imaging specificity by probe.[5,16]

- Cerebral oxygen data are accurate and reliable when the Pbto$_2$ probe is located in the deep white matter of the brain, the location where oxygen availability is most stable.[7,13]
- Insertion depth affects the cerebral blood flow values obtained due to values differing between the cerebral cortex and subcortical white matter.[7,13]
- Parameters such as ICP and brain tissue temperature can be measured immediately at the time of probe placement, but accurate Pbto$_2$ values may be delayed up to 2 hours because time is needed for the brain tissue to settle after the microtrauma caused by probe and catheter placement.[5,7,16]
- Pbto$_2$ monitoring has been demonstrated to be safe and effective in both clinical and laboratory settings.[6,7]
- The normal range for Pbto$_2$ values is between 20 and 35 mm Hg.[7,8] Treatment goals usually aim to keep Pbto$_2$ ≥20 mm Hg.
- A Pbto$_2$ <20 mm Hg is when an intervention should be considered because of potentially compromised brain oxygen. A Pbto$_2$ of <15 mm Hg represents impending brain hypoxia.[7-11]
- A Pbto$_2$ <10 mm Hg is directly associated with increased lactate and glutamate, severe disability, poor outcome at discharge, and death.[11]
- A Pbto$_2$ <5 mm Hg is indicative of increased cerebral levels of glutamate, glycerol, or the lactate/pyruvate ratio, indicating a critical level of brain tissue oxygen.[11,16]
- Brain tissue oxygen values can be used to manage potential cerebral hypoxia. Clinical interventions can be aimed at increasing oxygen delivery or decreasing cerebral oxygen demand, including but not limited to ventilator manipulation, CPP augmentation, sedation, head repositioning, intravenous fluid boluses, airway suctioning, and blood transfusions. Simultaneously increasing the number of Pbto$_2$ interventions has been shown to worsen the time to correcting Pbto$_2$; instead, implementing one intervention at a time may have a better impact.[2,3,12]
- Decreases in Pbto$_2$ values occur when cerebral blood flow or cerebral oxygen delivery is inadequate or states of increased metabolic demands exist, indicating the potential for secondary brain injury. Pbto$_2$ can detect subtle changes that can lead to the early identification of cerebral hypoxia and ischemia.[6,9] Table 84.1 outlines interventions for increased or decreased Pbto$_2$.
- Increases in Pbto$_2$ values denote decreased oxygen uptake by cerebral cells that may be caused by states of increased oxygen delivery or decreased oxygen utilization.[9]
- Manufacturers' recommendations suggest device placement should not exceed 5 days to continue to receive accurate measurement.[5,16]
- The provider placing the probe device determines the catheter placement location after review of the CT scan and after consideration of the most appropriate monitoring area based on diagnosis, pathology, and technical feasibility, avoiding areas of infarct or hematoma.[9] Placement of the probe may be ipsilateral or contralateral to the pathology.

- ❖ Placement may be near a lesion when the clinical goal is to monitor oxygen availability to damaged but salvageable tissue.
- ❖ If a patient has a subarachnoid hemorrhage, the probe may be placed in the area of the brain expected to develop vasospasm. Placement is determined by the distribution of subarachnoid blood on CT scan and by aneurysm location.
- When interpreting the Pbto$_2$ data, the clinician should be aware of the catheter probe location.[13]
- Neurological outcome and Pbto$_2$ may be affected by the location of the probe.[8,13]
- Evidence and consensus based recommendations include the following:
  - ❖ Several observational studies suggest improved outcome with additional Pbto$_2$-directed care compared with intracranial pressure (ICP) and cerebral perfusion pressure (CPP) management only.[7,12]
  - ❖ Treatment strategies have historically been studied in isolation; therefore almost no high-level evidence exists regarding relative efficacy, sequential ordering, or combination of management strategies for acute brain injury.[7,12]
  - ❖ The Brain Oxygen Optimization in Severe Traumatic Brain Injury Phase 2 Clinical Trial (BOOSt-2)[12]
    - ○ The Brain Oxygen Optimization in Severe Traumatic Brain Injury (BOOSt-2) clinical trial represented one of the first targeted TBI management trials that was precision medicine and not treating TBI as a uniform diagnosis. The BOOSt-2 trial was designed as a two-arm single-blind prospective randomized multicenter phase 2 trial assessing safety and efficacy of a management protocol optimizing Pbto$_2$ following severe TBI. Subjects ($n = 119$) 18 to 70 years of age were enrolled from October 2009 to March 2014 ($n = 62$ ICP only; $n = 57$ ICP + Pbto$_2$).
    - ○ Brain tissue oxygen monitoring was initiated an average of 9.05 hours from time of injury. TheBOOSt-2 trial was stopped early by the Independent Medical Monitor Data and Safety Monitoring Committee (DSMC) because of successful demonstration of the primary outcome. The BOOSt-2 study obtained the following data for a definitive Phase 3 study: physiological efficacy, feasibility of implementing a complex management protocol at multiple centers, and confirming nonutility (or clinical effectiveness) of Pbto$_2$-directed interventions. The use of multimodal monitoring with Pbto$_2$-directed care compared with ICP and CPP management only in severe TBI management reduced the brain tissue hypoxia trend toward lower mortality and more favorable outcomes.
    - ○ Enrolled subjects were followed up in 6 months by an evaluator for a Glasgow Outcome Scale Extended (GOS-E). Mortality was 34% in the control group compared with 25% in the intervention group. In the intervention group, 11% more had a favorable outcome, and more than twice as many patients achieved the highest outcome in GOS-E (GOS-E 8/ Upper good recovery).
  - ❖ The Seattle International Severe Traumatic Brain Injury Consensus Conference (SIBICC)[3]

TABLE 84.1	Management of Increased or Decreased Pbto$_2$ Values

Decreased Pbto$_2$ Values

Increased oxygen demand	Increased ICP	Treat the increased ICP with osmotic diuretics, cerebrospinal fluid drainage, sedation (e.g., barbiturates, propofol), craniotomy.
	Pain	Administer analgesics.
	Shivering	Rewarm, if needed, or administer agents to stop shivering (e.g., Demerol, Thorazine, paralytic agents). If a cooling device in use, perform skin counterwarming.
	Agitation	Administer sedation agents.
	Seizures	Administer benzodiazepines and adjunct anticonvulsant agents.
	Fever	Treat the underlying cause of the fever, initiate a cooling device if needed, and administer antipyretic agents.
Decreased oxygen delivery	Hypotension	Administer isotonic fluids (normal saline or hypertonic saline solution) or vasopressors.
	Hypovolemia	Administer isotonic fluids (normal saline or hypertonic saline solution), blood replacement.
	Anemia	Administer blood-replacement products.
	Hypoxia	Rule out pneumothorax or artificial airway obstruction. Increase Fio$_2$, PEEP, and interventions to mobilize pulmonary secretions and maximize pulmonary function.

Increased Pbto$_2$ Values

Increased oxygen delivery	Hyperdynamic (elevated ICP)	Consider sedation agents, temperature management, and/or positioning to treat elevated ICP.
Decreased oxygen demand	Hypothermia	Rewarm to achieve normothermia or mild hypothermia as prescribed for management of cerebral metabolism.
	Sedatives	Decrease sedation, anesthesia, or paralysis as prescribed.
	Anesthesia	
	Neuromuscular blockade agents	

Fio$_2$, Fraction of inspired oxygen; *ICP*, intracranial pressure; *Pbto$_2$*, brain oxygen; *PEEP*, positive end-expiratory pressure.

- SIBICC is a consensus statement to assist clinicians managing severe TBI patients monitored with both brain oxygen and intracranial pressure (ICP) monitoring based on a Delphi-method (class III evidence) consensus approach. The SIBICC recommendations were published as two different products; the first presented management of patients with ICP monitoring only, and the second algorithm was based on combined monitoring of ICP and Pbto$_2$.

- The consensus working group agreed that Pbto$_2$ monitoring should be the second monitored variable after ICP monitoring.
- Currently, two brain tissue oxygen-monitoring systems are available: the Integra Licox monitor and the RAUMEDIC Neurovent-PTO. Both are invasive monitors that provide continuous direct Pbto$_2$ monitoring.[5,7,16]

CATEGORY	The RAUMEDIC NEUROVENT-PTO Monitor[16]	The Licox Pto$_2$ Monitor (Fig. 84.1) and Licox CMP Monitor (Fig. 84.2)[5]
Parameters	One catheter, three parameters (ICP, temperature, and oxygen)	Two catheters, three parameters (one, ICP; two, oxygen and temperature)
Oxygen measurement	Fiberoptic*: uses oxygen quenching to measure oxygen partial pressure	Modified Clark Cell Electrode: A sensor that is able to measure the dissolved oxygen concentration in liquid. It consists of two electrodes surrounded by an electrolyte solution and covered by an oxygen-permeable membrane. As oxygen crosses the membrane, it is consumed in a chemical reaction that generates a small electrical current between the electrodes.
Measurement range	22 mm^2 (90 degrees around the sensing area)	18 mm^2 (360 degrees circumferentially around the sensing area). Sensing area is 5 mm from the catheter tip.

CATEGORY	The RAUMEDIC NEUROVENT-PTO Monitor[16]	The Licox Pto_2 Monitor (Fig. 84.1) and Licox CMP Monitor (Fig. 84.2)[5]
Insertion method	Bolt or tunnel	Bolt or tunnel
Catheter and probe storage	Room temperature	Temperature, 2°C to 10°C; humidity, 25% to 80%; relative humidity, noncondensing.
Temperature accuracy	±0.1°C	±0.2°C

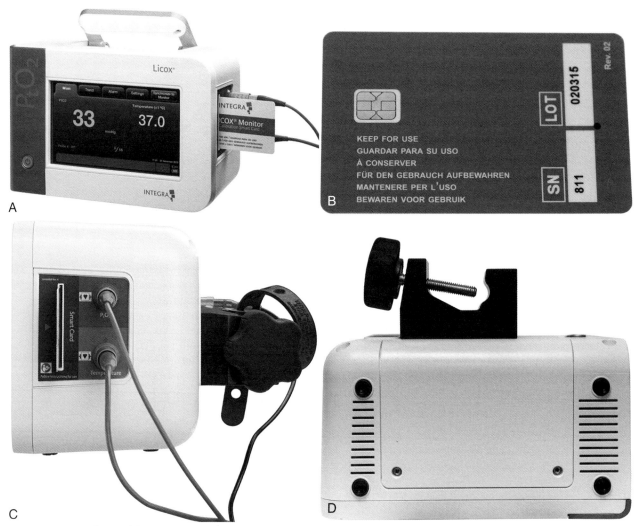

Figure 84.1   **A,** The Integra Licox Pto2 Monitor with card inserted into slot. **B,** Smart card. **C,** The Integra Licox Pto2 Monitor right panel. **D,** The Integra Licox Pto2 Monitor back panel.

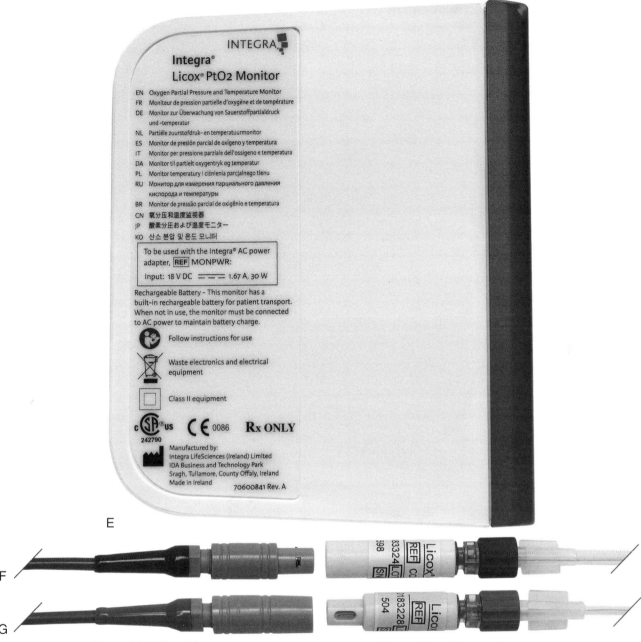

Figure 84.1, Cont'd **E,** The Integra Licox Pto2 Monitor left panel. **F** and **G,** Connecting the Pto₂ probe and temperature probe to their probe cables. *(Courtesy Integra Neurosciences, Plainsboro, NJ.)*

PATIENT AND FAMILY EDUCATION

- Assess patient or family understanding of the purpose of Pbto₂ monitoring. Most patients who need brain tissue oxygen monitoring have an altered level of consciousness with a score of 8 or less on the Glasgow Coma Scale; education is then directed toward the family. *Rationale:* Understanding may reduce anxiety and stress, stimulates requests for clarification or additional information, and increases awareness of the goals, duration, and expectations of the monitoring system.
- Explain the insertion process, patient monitoring, and care involving the Pbto₂ monitoring system. *Rationale:* Explanation may alleviate anxiety and stress and stimulates requests for clarification or additional information.
- Explain the expected outcomes of the Pbto₂ system. *Rationale:* Explanation may decrease patient and family anxiety and stress by increasing awareness of Pbto₂ monitoring duration and therapy goals.

PATIENT ASSESSMENT AND PREPARATION

Patient Assessment

- Assess the patient's neurological status. *Rationale:* Performing a baseline neurological assessment enables the

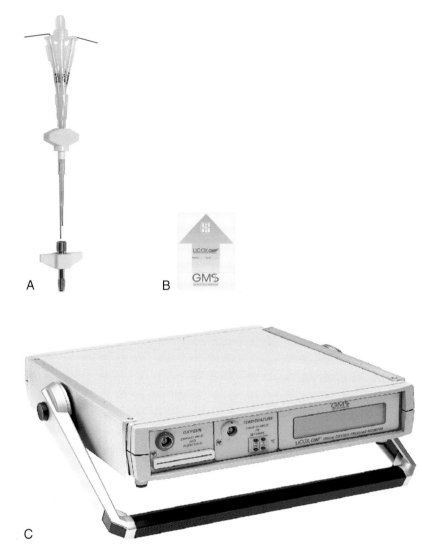

Figure 84.2   **A,** Model IM3 triple-lumen introducer. **B,** Smart card where calibration data for the oxygen probe is electronically stored. **C,** Licox CMP monitor, AC 3.1. *(Courtesy Integra Neurosciences, Plainsboro, NJ.)*

nurse to identify changes that may occur as a result of the Pbto$_2$ probe insertion.

- Assess the patient for signs or symptoms of local infection at the intended insertion location. ***Rationale:*** Evidence of local infection is a contraindication to brain tissue oxygen catheter placement.
- Obtain and review coagulation laboratory results (e.g., complete blood count, platelet count, prothrombin time, partial thromboplastin time, bleeding time, international normalized ratio) as prescribed. ***Rationale:*** Assessment identifies the patient's risk for bleeding.

Patient Preparation

- Verify the correct patient with two identifiers. ***Rationale:*** Before performing a procedure, the nurse should ensure the correct identification of the patient for the intended intervention.
- Ensure that the patient and family understand the preprocedural teaching. Answer questions as they arise, and reinforce information as needed. Most patients who need brain tissue oxygen monitoring are in an altered level of

consciousness with a Glasgow Coma Scale score of 8 or less. ***Rationale:*** Previously taught information is evaluated and reinforced.

- Ensure that informed consent has been obtained. ***Rationale:*** Informed consent protects the rights of the patient and makes a competent decision possible for the patient; however, in emergency circumstances, time may not allow for the consent form to be signed.
- Participate in a preprocedural verification and time out. ***Rationale:*** This ensures patient safety.
- Administer sedation or analgesia as prescribed before beginning the insertion procedure. ***Rationale:*** Sedation or analgesia facilitates the insertion process.
- Assist the patient to the semi-Fowler's position with the head in the neutral position and the head of the bed elevated 30 to 45 degrees. ***Rationale:*** Patients who are candidates for brain tissue oxygen monitoring may have increased ICP. Elevating the head of the bed and placing the head in the neutral position act to decrease ICP by enhancing jugular venous outflow and provide for optimal insertion accessibility.

EQUIPMENT

For the RAUMEDIC Neurovent-PTO Monitoring System

- Sterile gown, sterile drapes, sterile gloves, caps, face masks with eye shield
- Shave preparation kit
- Antiseptic solution
- EASY logO Monitor and connecting fiberoptic, yellow, blue, gray, and red cables
- NEUROVENT-PTO catheter (1)
- RAUMEDIC BOLT KIT PTO
- RAUMEDIC DRILL KIT CH5
- Cranial access kit (use the hand drill, not the drill bit)
- 4 × 4 gauze (2)
- Large Tegaderm (2)
- Arm board folded in half (1)
- 2-inch tape

For the Integra Licox Pto$_2$ Monitor

- Sterile gowns, sterile drapes, sterile gloves, nonsterile gloves, caps, goggles, and face masks

- Shave preparation kit
- Antiseptic solution
- Pbto$_2$ monitor (see Fig. 84.1A) or module
- Connecting cables
- Cranial access tray; use the drill, but use the Licox bit in the Licox kit
- Pbto$_2$ probe
- Scalpel
- Dressing supplies, including 4 × 4 gauze and tape
- Sterile dry gauze; may be placed at the insertion site

Additional equipment to have available as needed includes the following:
- An intravenous (IV) arm board may be used to stabilize the monitor probe and cable
- Intracranial bolt system
- Extra transparent and soft-cloth adhesive dressing or a dry, sterile occlusive dressing
- A compatible fiberoptic ICP catheter may be inserted through the intracranial bolt system as well and will require a separate monitor to measure ICP.

Procedure	for Brain Tissue Oxygen Monitoring for the Integra Licox Pto$_2$ Monitor: Insertion (Assist) and Care		
Steps	**Rationale**	**Special Considerations**	
1. **HH**			
2. Plug the monitor power cord into an AC power outlet.	Provides the power source.	On the back of the monitor, attach the red connector end of the AC power cord into the red port labeled "Input 18V." Insert the plug end of the AC power adapter into an AC wall outlet.	
3. Attach the cables (e.g., oxygen cable, temperature cable) to the Pbto$_2$ monitor.	Prepares the equipment.	Refer to the manufacturer's guidelines as needed. Monitors and cables may be color-coded.	
4. Turn on the monitor. On the front of the monitor, press the power button. Once the button illuminates, the Integra logo will appear on the touch screen for a few seconds before initiating the setup process.	Prepares the monitor.		
5. After the setup process completes, listen for a 1-second startup tone.	Verifies that audio alarms are functioning correctly; verifies that the monitor's screen displays the main panel.	There is a short beep when the monitor is first turned on; this is not the 1-second startup tone.	
6. Wash hands, and apply goggles or masks with face shields, caps, and gowns, and assist with the sterile procedure.	Prepares for a sterile procedure.		
7. Assist as needed with site preparation (e.g., shave preparation and cleansing with antiseptic solution).	Prepares for a sterile procedure.	Antiseptic solution choice should be determined by institutional policy. Use of povidone-iodine versus chlorhexidine is controversial. The antiseptic solution should be allowed to dry before the initial incision is made.[9] Studies suggest chlorhexidine is neurotoxic.[9]	

Procedure continues on following page

UNIT III

Procedure	for Brain Tissue Oxygen Monitoring for the Integra Licox Pto$_2$ Monitor: Insertion (Assist) and Care—*Continued*		
Steps	Rationale	Special Considerations
8. Assist as needed in draping the head, neck, and chest of the patient.	Prepares a sterile environment for the insertion process.	
9. Assist as needed with opening the sterile trays and probes.	Facilitates efficiency of the insertion process.	
10. Insert the calibration card for calibration of the monitor unique to each Pbto$_2$ probe.[5] **(Level M*)**	The Licox monitor requires insertion of a calibration card, referred to as the *smart card,* which has numbers on it that match those on the oxygen probe that is being inserted. This card is placed into a card slot located on the right side of the monitor by aligning the arrow on the card with the arrow on the monitor. The calibration card can only be used with the probe that has the same numbers on it and is included in the same packaging (see Fig. 84.1A–G).	Do not discard Pto$_2$ probe packaging before removing the smart card. Each card contains calibration data specific to that that probe. Inserting a new smart card during the recording of trend data will reset the trend data. Only use the smart card supplied with the Pbto$_2$ probe. If the calibration card is lost, another corresponding Pbto$_2$ probe and smart card must be used.
11. Assist as needed with insertion of an intracranial bolt (see Procedure 87, Intracranial Pressure Monitoring, Nursing Care, Troubleshooting, and Removal).	May be inserted before Pto$_2$ probe insertion.	Use the bit from the Licox kit. It is critical for dural opening to assure accurate parenchymal probe placement.
12. Assist as needed with insertion of the oxygen probe and temperature probe.	Facilitates the insertion process.	The oxygen probe and temperature probe may be separate (triple-lumen bolt system) or may be combined (double-lumen bolt system). The additional lumen is for the ICP probe.
13. Connect the oxygen and temperature probes to the monitor cables.	Prepares for monitoring.	
14. Observe the temperature and Pbto$_2$ values.	Initiates monitoring. The temperature values should be accurate; however, time is needed for the brain tissue to settle after the microtrauma caused by catheter placement.	
15. If possible, use a cable to transfer the values from the Pbto$_2$ monitor to the bedside monitor. Set the upper and lower alarm limits.	Allows integration of the monitoring systems. The currently available brain tissue oxygen monitoring system does not have an alarm system. Integrating the monitoring system with the bedside monitor allows (1) a larger display of the numeric values and (2) audible upper and lower alarm limits.	Refer to monitor guidelines for specific information.
16. After the system has been placed, assist with placing a sterile, occlusive dressing at the insertion point.	Prevents contamination of the insertion site by microorganisms and protects the site.	A dressing (formed with dry sterile gauze) provides a base to secure the device to an arm board or other securing method.
17. Secure the Pbto$_2$ monitor cables with two anchor points to avoid tension on the Pbto$_2$ and ICP probes.		

*Level M: Manufacturer's recommendations only.

Procedure	for Brain Tissue Oxygen Monitoring for the Integra Licox Pto₂ Monitor: Insertion (Assist) and Care—*Continued*	

Steps	Rationale	Special Considerations
A. Anchor the cables at the patient's head and at the shoulder.	The monitoring cables need to be secured so no tension or disruption of the device occurs at the insertion site.	
B. Secure the cables so they do not get entangled in the side rails and do not touch the floor.	Supports the entire mechanism.	One method to secure the monitor cables is as follows: A. Place an IV arm board or stability anchor to a conical gauze dressing where the device and cables can be secured. B. Anchor the cables from the patient's head to the shoulder in place with a transparent or soft-cloth adhesive dressing. The first tension point is directly on the patient's head where the dressing is anchored to the skin at the point of insertion. The second tension point is at the patient's shoulder. C. Place rolled towels under the secured system.
C. Allow enough slack to accommodate the patient movement and turning.	Prevents gravity drag and tension on the cables and the device.	
18. Discard used supplies in appropriate receptacles.	Removes and safely discards used supplies. Safely removes sharp objects.	
19. 🅷🅷		
Connecting a Single Pto₂ Probe		
1. Connect the Pbto₂ probe cable to the monitor.	Allows integration of the monitoring systems.	Refer to the manufacturer's recommendations in the monitor guidelines for specific information.
2. Insert the Pbto₂ probe's smart card into the monitor.	Prepares the equipment.	Each bedside monitor may have its own unique labels for parameters that are being added (e.g., brain oxygen).
3. Insert the Pbto₂ probe into the patient and connect the probe to the monitor.	Prepares the equipment.	Depending on hospital protocol, you may insert the Pbto₂ probe into the patient either before or after connecting the Pbto₂ probe to the monitor. The purpose of connecting the Pbto₂ probe to the monitor before implantation is to verify the functionality of the probe before clinical use.
4. Allow stabilization time for microtrauma.	Prepares the monitor to adjust to measurements obtained on insertion and the continuous monitoring.	This normally applies to the first 30 minutes after insertion, and the Pbto₂ values may not display optimal information about tissue oxygenation due to tissue injury during insertion of the probe.

Procedure continues on following page

UNIT III

UNIT III

Procedure	for Brain Tissue Oxygen Monitoring for the Integra Licox Pto₂ Monitor: Insertion (Assist) and Care—*Continued*		
Steps	**Rationale**	**Special Considerations**
5. Enter the tissue temperature compensation value manually. A. Enter the tissue temperature compensation that will be used during Pbto₂ measurements. B. On the temperature manual panel, adjust the manual temperature input arrows to the designated temperature to the nearest whole number.	The calculations for Pbto₂ measurements require tissue temperature compensation. If the clinician is not measuring the tissue temperature with a probe, the temperature must be entered manually. Make sure to check the patient's temperature either hourly or before recording the Pbto₂ value for intervention. If any changes in temperature occur, use the manual temperature input arrows to specify the new temperature value accordingly.	

Connecting a Single Pbto₂ Probe With a Single Temperature Probe

1. Connect the Pbto₂ probe cable to the monitor.	Prepares the monitor.	On the monitor's right side, connect the large plug of the blue Pbto₂ probe cable into the blue port labeled "Pbto₂."
2. Connect the temperature probe cable to the monitor.	Prepares the equipment/cables connection to the monitor.	On the monitor's right side, connect the green temperature probe cable to the green port labeled "Temperature."
3. Insert the Pbto₂ probe's smart card to the monitor.	Prepares the monitor.	On the monitor's right side, insert the smart card slot by aligning the arrow on the card with the arrow on the label.
4. Insert the Pbto₂ and temperature probes to the patient, and connect the probes to the monitor.	Prepares the equipment/cables connection to the monitor.	Depending on hospital protocol, you may insert the Pto₂ probe and temperature probe into the patient either before or after connecting the two probes to the monitor.
5. Allow stabilization time for microtrauma.	Prepares the monitor to adjust to measurements obtained on insertion and the continuous monitoring.	This normally applies to the first 20 minutes after insertion, and the Pbto₂ values may not display optimal information about tissue oxygenation due to tissue injury during insertion of the probe.
6. Check Pbto₂ and temperature values.	Initiates monitoring. The temperature values should be accurate.	When using a temperature probe, the temperature measurement being continuously reported by the monitor, with an accuracy of ±1°C, will be applied to the calculation for Pbto₂ measurements.

*Level M: Manufacturer's recommendations only.

Procedure **for Brain Tissue Oxygen Monitoring for the Integra Licox CMP Monitor: Insertion (Assist) and Care**

Steps	Rationale	Special Considerations
1. 🅷🅷		
2. Plug the Pbto$_2$ monitor power cord into an AC wall outlet.	Provides the power source.	
3. Attach the cables (e.g., oxygen cable, temperature cable) to the Pbto$_2$ monitor.	Prepares the equipment.	Refer to the manufacturer's guidelines as needed. Monitors and cables may be color-coded.
4. 🅷🅷		
5. Apply goggles or masks with face shields, caps, gowns, and sterile gloves.	Prepares for a sterile procedure.	
6. Assist as needed with site preparation (e.g., shave preparation and cleansing with antiseptic solution).	Prepares for a sterile procedure.	Antiseptic solution choice should be determined by institutional policy. Use of povidone-iodine versus chlorhexidine is controversial. The antiseptic solution should be allowed to dry before performing the initial incision. Studies suggest chlorhexidine is neurotoxic.[9]
7. Assist as needed in draping the head, neck, and chest of the patient.	Prepares a sterile environment for the insertion process.	
8. Assist as needed with opening the sterile trays and probes.	Facilitates efficiency of the insertion process.	
9. Turn on the Pbto$_2$ monitor.	Prepares the monitor.	
10. Insert the calibration card for calibration of the monitor unique to each Pbto$_2$ probe.	The Licox monitor requires insertion of a calibration card, referred to as the *smart card,* which has numbers on it that match those on the oxygen probe that is being inserted. This card is placed into a card slot located on the front of the monitor. The calibration card can only be used with the probe that has the same numbers on it and is included in the same packaging (see Fig. 84.1A–G).	If the calibration card is lost, another corresponding Pbto$_2$ probe and smart card must be used.
11. Assist as needed with insertion of an intracranial bolt (see Procedure 87, Intracranial Pressure Monitoring, Nursing Care, Troubleshooting, and Removal).	May be inserted before Pbto$_2$ probe insertion.	
12. Assist as needed with insertion of the oxygen probe and temperature probe.	Facilitates the insertion process.	The oxygen probe and temperature probe may be separate (triple-lumen bolt system) or may be combined (double-lumen bolt system). The additional lumen is for the ICP probe.
13. Connect the oxygen and temperature probes to the monitor cables.	Prepares for monitoring.	
14. Observe the temperature and Pbto$_2$ values.	Initiates monitoring. The temperature values should be accurate; however, time is needed for the brain tissue to settle after the microtrauma caused by catheter placement.	

Procedure continues on following page

Procedure	for Brain Tissue Oxygen Monitoring for the Integra Licox CMP Monitor: Insertion (Assist) and Care—*Continued*	
Steps	**Rationale**	**Special Considerations**
15. If possible, use a cable to transfer the values from the Pbto$_2$ monitor to the bedside monitor. Set the upper and lower alarm limits.	Allows integration of the monitoring systems. The currently available brain tissue oxygen monitoring system does not have an alarm system. Integrating the monitoring system with the bedside monitor allows (1) a larger display of the numeric values and (2) audible upper and lower alarm limits.	Refer to the manufacturer's recommendations in the monitor guidelines for specific information.
16. After the system has been placed, apply a sterile occlusive dressing at the insertion point.	Prevents contamination of the insertion site by microorganisms and protects the site.	A dressing (formed with dry sterile gauze) provides a base to secure the device to an arm board or other securing method.
17. Secure the Pbto$_2$ monitor cables with two points of tension to avoid tension on the Pbto$_2$ and ICP probes.		
A. Anchor the cables at the patient's head and at the shoulder.	The monitoring cables must be secured so no tension or disruption of the device occurs at the insertion site.	
B. Secure the cables so they do not become entangled in the side rails and do not touch the floor.	Supports the entire mechanism.	One method to secure the monitor cables is as follows: A. Place an IV arm board or stability anchor to a conical gauze dressing where the device and cables can be secured. B. Anchor the cables from the patient's head to the shoulder in place with a transparent or soft-cloth adhesive dressing. The first tension point is directly on the patient's head where the dressing is anchored to the skin at the point of insertion. The second tension point is at the patient's shoulder. C. Place rolled towels under the secured system.
C. Allow enough slack to accommodate patient movement and turning.	Prevents gravity drag and tension on the cables and the device.	
18. Discard used supplies in appropriate receptacles.	Removes and safely discards used supplies. Safely removes sharp objects.	
19. 🅷🅷 **Linking to a Bedside Monitor**		
1. Connect the brain oxygen monitor to the bedside monitor with the attached cable.	Allows integration of the monitoring systems.	Refer to the manufacturer's recommendations in the monitor guidelines for specific information.
2. Select a pressure module, and label the parameter. A waveform need not be displayed, only a numeric display.	Prepares the equipment.	Each bedside monitor may have its own unique labels for parameters that are being added (e.g., brain oxygen).

Procedure for Brain Tissue Oxygen Monitoring for the Integra Licox CMP Monitor: Insertion (Assist) and Care—*Continued*

Steps	Rationale	Special Considerations
3. Manually adjust the temperature on the front of the monitor to the established number of degrees Celsius determined by the institution.	Prepares the equipment.	Follow institutional guidelines. If a separate brain temperature probe or combined brain tissue oxygen and brain temperature probe is not in use, the temperature on the front of the monitor must be adjusted manually every hour to equal the patient's core temperature for accurate determination of the $Pbto_2$.
4. Disconnect the blue and green cables from the brain oxygen monitor.	Prepares the equipment.	
5. Select the designated pressure module, and zero the bedside monitor.	Prepares the equipment.	
6. Plug the blue and green cables back into the front of the brain oxygen monitor.	Allows integration of the monitoring systems.	
7. Note the difference between the brain oxygen monitor reading and the bedside monitor reading.	Confirms that data on the brain oxygen monitor accurately correlate with the bedside monitor.	
8. Readings should be within 1 mm Hg when the blue and green cables are connected to the Licox system at the head of the patient and after the brain tissue has had time to settle (20–120 minutes) after Licox insertion.	Confirms that data on the brain oxygen monitor accurately correlate with the bedside monitor.	Monitoring of $Pbto_2$ values may be delayed as long as 2 hours because time is needed for the brain tissue to settle after the microtrauma caused by probe placement.

Procedure for Brain Tissue Oxygen Monitoring for the RAUMEDIC NEUROVENT-PTO Monitor: Insertion (Assist) and Care

Procedure	Rationale	Special Considerations
1. ▣		
2. Attach the cables to the RAUMEDIC EASY logO (fiberoptic cable to Po_2 port, yellow cable P/T port, gray out ICP, blue out Po_2, red power) (Fig. 84.3).	Prepares the equipment.	
3. Plug the EASY logO monitor power cord into an AC wall outlet.	Provides a power source.	
4. ▣		
5. ▣		
6. Assist as needed with site preparation, opening of sterile trays, draping of the head and neck, and so on.	Prepares for a sterile procedure.	
7. Assist as needed with insertion of the RAUMEDIC bolt (see BOLT Kit PTO IFU) (Fig. 84.4).	Facilitates insertion.	Keep screwing in tool (wrench) for physician, advanced practice nurse, or other healthcare professional to remove bolt when therapy is no longer needed.

Procedure continues on following page

Procedure for Brain Tissue Oxygen Monitoring for the RAUMEDIC NEUROVENT-PTO Monitor: Insertion (Assist) and Care—*Continued*

Procedure	Rationale	Special Considerations

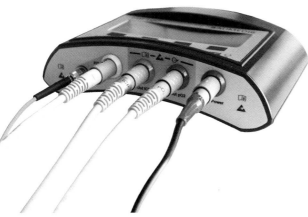

Figure 84.3   *(Courtesy Raumedic Inc., Mills River, NC.)*

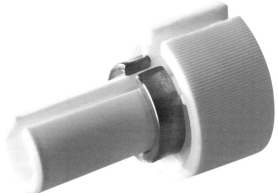

Figure 84.4   *(Courtesy Raumedic Inc., Mills River, NC.)*

8. Assist the physician, advanced practice nurse, or other healthcare professional as needed during insertion of the pressure/temperature/oxygen catheter (see NEUROVENT-PTO catheter IFU) (Fig. 84.5).

Facilitates insertion of a catheter by the physician, advanced practice nurse, or other healthcare professional.

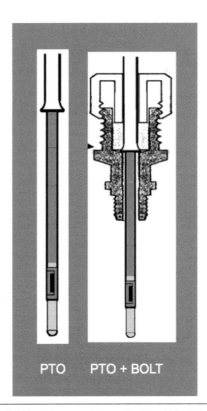

PTO   PTO + BOLT

Figure 84.5   *(Courtesy Raumedic Inc., Mills River, NC.)*

Procedure **for Brain Tissue Oxygen Monitoring for the RAUMEDIC NEUROVENT-PTO Monitor: Insertion (Assist) and Care—*Continued***

Procedure	Rationale	Special Considerations
9. Connect the PTO catheter to the monitor cables (see Fig. 84.7). A. Fiberoptic connection on PTO catheter to Cable LWL (fiberoptic) (Figs. 84.6 and 84.7). B. Blue plug on PTO catheter connects to Cable PTO: gold dot to gold dot (Fig. 84.8).	Prepares for monitoring.	
10. Observe ICP, temperature, and Pbto$_2$ values.	Initiates monitoring. The temperature and ICP values should be accurate; however, a dwell time is needed (up to 2 hours) for accurate Pbto$_2$ monitoring as it is necessary for the brain tissue to settle after microtrauma caused by catheter placement.	You may document Pbto$_2$ during this time with a comment: "dwell time."
11. After the system has been placed, apply a sterile occlusive dressing at the insertion point.	Maintains a sterile environment to prevent infection.	
12. Discard used supplies.		
13. 🅷🅷		

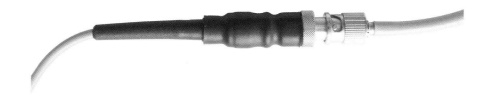

Figure 84.6 *(Courtesy Raumedic Inc., Mills River, NC.)*

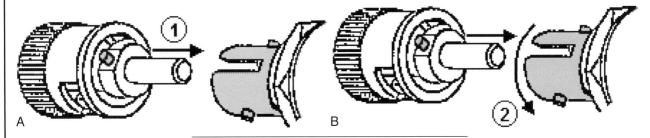

Figure 84.7 *(Courtesy Raumedic Inc., Mills River, NC.)*

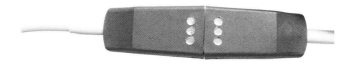

Figure 84.8 *(Courtesy Raumedic Inc., Mills River, NC.)*

Procedure continues on following page

UNIT III

Procedure	for Brain Tissue Oxygen Monitoring for the RAUMEDIC NEUROVENT-PTO Monitor: Insertion (Assist) and Care—*Continued*	
Procedure	Rationale	Special Considerations

Linking to the Bedside Monitor

Procedure	Rationale	Special Considerations
1. Connect the EASY logO to the pressure ports on the bedside monitor using the gray out ICP and blue out Pbto$_2$ cable.	Allows integration of the monitoring systems.	
2. Select the pressure port labels on the bedside monitor for ICP and Pbto$_2$. For Pbto$_2$, a waveform does not need to be displayed; only a value needs to be displayed. Set the alarm parameter from 20 mm Hg to 40 mm Hg or as prescribed.	Prepares the equipment and establishes alarm parameters for monitoring.	
3. To have ICP and Pbto$_2$ values on the bedside monitor, select "Menu."	Prepares the equipment to integrate with bedside monitoring systems.	
4. Select "OUT."	Allows integration of the monitoring systems.	
5. Once the cables have been connected to the bedside monitor, press "OK."	Allows integration of the monitoring systems.	
6. Zero the bedside monitor for both ICP and Pbto$_2$ pressure ports. When zero appears on the bedside monitor, press "OK."	Prepares the bedside monitor.	
7. Checking the sensitivity: when 20 mm Hg is displayed on the bedside monitor, press "OK."	Allows integration of the monitoring systems.	
8. It is not necessary to rezero the bedside monitor daily. It is only necessary when the EASY logO is disconnected and then reconnected to the bedside monitor.	Monitoring has a stable signal.	It is only necessary to rezero after patient transport.

Preparing the RAUMEDIC NEUROVENT-PTO ICP Monitoring for Transport

Procedure	Rationale	Special Considerations
1. Disconnect the PTO catheter from the EASY logO, leaving all cables attached to the EASY logO. Attach the catheter (blue plug, gold dot to gold dot) to the transport cable that has the NPS2 (Fig. 84.9).	Oxygen is not monitored during transport.	Do not allow cables to drag or rest on the floor to prevent accidental removal of the catheter.
2. Plug the NPS2 into the pressure port on the transport monitor.	Provides a connection to the transport monitor.	
3. Press and continue holding the blue zero button on the NPS2, and then press "zero ICP" on the transport monitor. Continue holding the blue button until zero is on the transport monitor.	Allows integration of monitoring systems.	
4. Upon return to the patient's bedside, attach the PTO catheter to the EASY logo, and follow the OUT procedure of the EASY logO to get ICP and Pbto$_2$ values onto the bedside monitor.	Allows integration of monitoring systems for continued monitoring.	

Procedure	for Brain Tissue Oxygen Monitoring for the RAUMEDIC NEUROVENT-PTO Monitor: Insertion (Assist) and Care—*Continued*	
Procedure	**Rationale**	**Special Considerations**

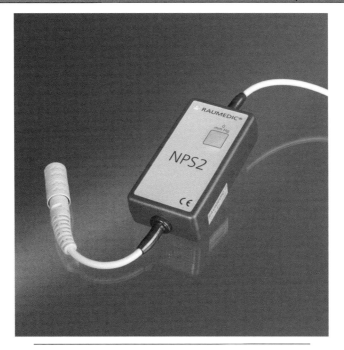

Figure 84.9   *(Courtesy Raumedic Inc., Mills River, NC.)*

Troubleshooting the RAUMEDIC NEUROVENT-PTO

Catheter Implantation Migration

Procedure	Rationale	Special Considerations
1. Assess for catheter placement. The catheter pulls easily out of the bolt when implanted. The physician, advanced practice nurse, or other healthcare professional will ensure that the catheter is fully inserted and tighten the fixing cap (see Fig. 84.2A).	Ensures correct catheter insertion and no dislodgement of the catheter after placement.	Questionable data or data inconsistent with patient presentation suggest that the catheter may be dislodged.

Catheter Connections to Easy Logo Monitor Disconnections

Procedure	Rationale	Special Considerations
1. Error: Cable PTO cable not connected to the catheter. Connect Cable PTO blue plug, gold dot to gold dot. Make sure Cable PTO is connected to the yellow socket on EASY logO.	Ensures correct cable connections and that connections are secure.	
2. Error: Cable LWL (fiberoptic) not connected/locked to PTO catheter.	Ensures correct cable connection and locking the cable tightly to prevent disconnection.	Avoid forceful locking of cables because it may result in cable breakage.
3. Questionable O_2 value Clean inside Cable LWL (fiberoptic) connection to remove dust.	Ensures that the cable is clean and has a good connection with the catheter.	Critically assess oxygen values with patient assessment. Evaluate clinical indications for increased/decreased $Pbto_2$.

Procedure continues on following page

Patient Monitoring and Care —*Continued*

Procedure	Rationale	Special Considerations
Troubleshooting Pbto$_2$ Monitoring Systems		

1. Perform an oxygen challenge test as prescribed.[7,8]
   A. Place the ventilator fraction of inspired oxygen (Fio$_2$) setting on 1.0 (100% oxygen) for 2–5 minutes.
   B. Observe the monitor; an accurate probe will show an increase in Pbto$_2$.
   C. If no response to the increased Fio$_2$ is seen, inform the physician because a head CT scan may be prescribed to confirm correct probe placement. **(Level D*)**
	After the brain tissue has had time to settle from the initial insertion, an oxygen challenge is performed, particularly if the Pbto$_2$ reading is unexpectedly low or a question of probe accuracy exists.[8,9]	Follow the manufacturer's guidelines for error codes that are specific to the Pbto$_2$monitoring system.
		 Institutional standards vary for the length of time an oxygen challenge test is performed. The physician, advanced practice nurse, or other healthcare professional may order a head CT scan after insertion to check catheter placement. Follow hospital-specific guidelines.

2. Assess if an electrical disturbance has occurred.	Strong electromagnetic disturbances can result in Pbto$_2$ measurement errors. Errors can continue for a few seconds after the disturbance.	These disturbances may occur when a high-frequency scalpel or cautery is used or during cardioversion.
3. Assess the cable for damage.	If the probe cable or the extension cable is damaged, it is an electrical hazard, the measured values can be incorrect, or the measurement can be interrupted.	Replace damaged cables.
4. Avoid changes in the temperature of the temperature probe connector:	The temperature measurement may be inaccurate if the connector of the temperature probe is subjected to significant changes in temperature or if the temperature of the connector is beyond the defined range of 18° to 30°C.	
A. Avoid holding the temperature probe connector.	If the probe connector is held with a warm hand, the temperature measurement may be inaccurate until it is released.	
B. Protect the temperature probe connector from direct sunlight or warming devices. **(Level M*)**	Warming of the connector can cause inaccurate temperature readings.	
Removal of the Brain Tissue Oxygen Monitoring System		
1. **HH**		
2. **PE**		
3. Position the patient in the semi-Fowler's position.	Facilitates the procedure.	
4. Turn off the monitor.	Facilitates the removal process.	
5. Assist with removal of the dressing.	Prepares for removal of the catheter.	
6. Assist the physician, advanced practice nurse, or other healthcare professional as needed with removal of monitoring probes.	The physician, advanced practice nurse, or other healthcare professional will remove the catheter and may request assistance.	
7. Apply an occlusive sterile dressing to the site.	Reduces the risk of infection.	Assess for signs of infection, bleeding, and cerebrospinal fluid leakage.
8. Discard used supplies in appropriate receptacles.	Removes and safely discards used supplies.	
9. **HH**		

*Level D: Peer-reviewed professional and organizational standards with the support of clinical study recommendations.
*Level M: Manufacturer's recommendations only.

Expected Outcomes

- Pbto$_2$ probe is placed in the correct position
- Monitoring is able to begin after brain tissue has had time to settle (20 minutes to 2 hours)
- Pbto$_2$ value is between 20 and 35 mm Hg or as determined by the provider to be an acceptable value for the individual patient
- Accurate and reliable Pbto$_2$ monitoring
- Early detection of cerebral hypoxia
- Immediate intervention and management of compromised cerebral oxygenation hypoxia

Unexpected Outcomes

- Pbto$_2$ reading low, with no response to oxygen challenge
- Signs and symptoms of infection
- Hematoma from placement
- Worsened neurological assessment

UNIT III

Patient Monitoring and Care

Steps	Rationale	Reportable Conditions
		These conditions should be reported to the provider if they persist despite nursing interventions.
1. Assess the patient's baseline neurological status, vital signs, and ICP every 15 minutes and more frequently if necessary during and immediately after the procedure.	Provides assessment of patient status before and during the procedure.	• Changes in neurological status • Changes in vital signs • Changes in ICP and CPP
2. Perform an oxygen challenge test as prescribed. A. Place the ventilator Fio$_2$ setting on 1.0 for 2–5 minutes. B. An accurate probe shows an increase in Pbto$_2$.[1,6] (**Level C***)	After the brain tissue has had time to settle from the initial insertion, perform an oxygen challenge, particularly if the Pbto$_2$ reading is unexpectedly low or a question exists of probe accuracy, reliability, or validity.	• Lack of variation response to oxygen challenge • Oxygen challenge tests confirm correct placement of the probe as well as probe functioning
3. Obtain the patient's temperature every 1–2 hours or as prescribed.	Provides a comparison of cerebral and body temperatures. Although the temperature measurements do not correlate exactly, a parallel trend should be seen.	• Abnormal temperatures
4. Maintain the Pbto$_2$ value between 20 and 35 mm Hg or as prescribed.[6,9] (**Level D***)	Represents normal values.	• Elevated Pbto$_2$ values • Decreased Pbto$_2$ values
5. Follow institutional standards for assessing pain. Administer analgesia as prescribed.	Identifies the need for pain interventions.	• Continued pain despite pain interventions

*Level C: Qualitative studies, descriptive or correlational studies, integrative reviews, systematic reviews, or randomized controlled trials with inconsistent results.
*Level D: Peer-reviewed professional and organizational standards with the support of clinical study recommendations.

UNIT III

Documentation

Documentation should include the following:
- After placement of the Pbto$_2$ monitor:
  - Patient and family education
  - Preprocedure verification and time out
  - Completion of informed consent
  - Insertion of the Pbto$_2$ probe
  - Patient tolerance of the procedure
  - Site assessment (mark the Pbto$_2$ probe where it exits the bolt to serve as a visual indicator of movement)
  - Neurological assessments
  - Hourly values, including Pbto$_2$, brain tissue temperature, and neurological multimodality monitoring in use (e.g., ICP, CPP, Sjvo$_2$)
  - Occurrence of unexpected outcomes and interventions
  - Pain assessment, interventions, and effectiveness

References and Additional Readings

For a complete list of references and additional readings for this procedure, scan this QR code with your smartphone, or visit https://www.elsevier.com/__data/assets/pdf_file/0009/1319859/Chapter0084.pdf.

85 Cerebral Blood Flow Monitoring

Tracey M. Berlin

PURPOSE Adequate cerebral blood flow (CBF) is essential for the delivery of oxygen and glucose to brain tissue and for maintenance of normal cerebral metabolic processes. CBF monitoring is performed in the patient with acute brain injury for quantitative measurement and continuous monitoring of regional brain perfusion. Monitoring of regional CBF using thermal diffusion flowmetry (TDF) provides important information related to the delivery of nutrients to brain tissue, autoregulatory status, and cerebral vasoreactivity.

PREREQUISITE NURSING KNOWLEDGE

- Neuroanatomy and physiology, specifically intracranial dynamics.
- Sterile and aseptic technique.
- Concepts of CBF
  - ❖ Although representing only 2% of our body tissues, the brain receives 15% of total cardiac output, accounting for nearly 20% of total body oxygen consumption and 25% of glucose utilization.[1-4]
  - ❖ Adequate CBF ensures proper delivery of energy substrates and oxygen and is essential for brain function and viability. If CBF falls below a certain threshold and oxygen extraction has been maximized, metabolic and electrical functions may deteriorate leading to ischemia, infarction, and irreversible brain damage.[2,3,5-7]
  - ❖ CBF measurement is based on the Fick principle: the quantity of a substance taken up by an organ is equal to the blood flow through that organ multiplied by the difference of the arterial and venous concentrations.[2,8]
- Benefits of CBF monitoring
  - ❖ Used as an adjunct monitor of trends along with other neurological parameters (intracranial pressure [ICP], cerebral perfusion pressure [CPP], and brain tissue oxygen [PbtO$_2$]), intracranial CBF monitoring provides a direct measurement of regional cerebral perfusion and can provide the opportunity to diagnose and to correct insufficient CBF before deficits in tissue oxygenation and metabolism are recognized.[7,9]
- Indications for CBF monitoring
  - ❖ Measurement of CBF is relevant in conditions in which alterations in CBF may lead to cerebral ischemia and infarction. Indications include patients at risk for secondary brain injury, including severe traumatic brain injury (TBI), aneurysmal and traumatic subarachnoid hemorrhage (SAH), brain tumor, stroke, and any condition that potentially alters CBF.[5,6,10]
- CBF values

- ❖ Although CBF may vary depending on metabolic demand and factors that affect vasoreactivity (such as partial pressures of oxygen [PaO$_2$] and carbon dioxide [PaCO$_2$]), the average global CBF in adults is approximately 50 mL/100 g/min. The normal range for CBF in white matter is 18 to 35 mL/100 g/min. In gray, more metabolically active cortical tissue, CBF is higher, ranging from 70 to 80 mL/100 g/min.[2-4]
- ❖ CBF exceeding the amount of blood required for metabolism is referred to as *hyperemia* (typically values above 55 mL/100 g/min). This may be a physiological response as the brain attempts to perfuse injured tissue or when the delivery of blood to the brain exceeds demand. Hyperemia may result in increased ICP as a result of vascular congestion[3,4,8] (Table 85.1).
- ❖ *Ischemia* is defined as a decrease in blood flow below the level necessary to sustain normal cellular structure and function. Electrical and neurological dysfunction occur when CBF falls below 18 to 20 mL/100 g/min, indicating a state of ischemia. Although CBF between 10 and 20 mL/100 g/min may be tolerated for minutes to hours before infarction, CBF of less than 10 mL/100 g/min leads to cellular membrane failure, neuronal death, and rapid transition to infarction (5 mL/100 g/min)[1,4,10,11] (see Table 85.1).
- ❖ Ischemia can be global, as seen in severe hypoperfusion caused by cardiac arrest or intracranial hypertension. Ischemia can also be focal, as seen in occlusion of an intracranial vessel by embolism or thrombus, but may not lead to irreversible damage if adequate collateral blood flow is present.[1,4,11]
- CBF and surrogate measurement techniques
  - ❖ CPP is a surrogate variable for direct measurement of CBF and is the calculated difference between mean arterial pressure (MAP) and ICP; (CPP = MAP − ICP). The ideal CPP threshold for optimal CBF has not been clearly defined but is suggested in literature to be 60 to 70 mm Hg.[8,12,13]
  - ❖ Although widely used as diagnostic and research tools, imaging modalities such as perfusion computed

tomography (CT), perfusion-weighted magnetic resonance imaging (MRI), positron emission tomography (PET), single-photon emission computed tomography

(SPECT), and Xenon flow computed tomography (XeCT) do not provide continuous data for clinical monitoring[8,13] (Table 85.2).

❖ Oxygen monitoring technologies, such as monitoring of brain tissue oxygen, jugular venous bulb oximetry, and near-infrared spectroscopy (NIRS) represent surrogate measures reflecting the quality of flow and oxygen delivery.[2,8]

❖ Laser Doppler flowmetry is an invasive technology that measures the velocity of red blood cells within the capillaries to provide data about cortical CBF.[10]

❖ Transcranial Doppler (TCD) monitoring measures blood flow velocities of the major vascular branches of the brain. TCD monitoring is a noninvasive ultrasound technology that measures blood flow velocity to assess vasospasm severity, location of intracranial stenosis, occlusions, or emboli and to monitor hemodynamic changes associated with impaired intracranial perfusion. TCD velocities may be elevated secondary to increased blood volume or decreased vessel caliber with no effect on local CBF. By measuring blood flow velocity, TCD provides an indirect measure of CBF, but it is best used in conjunction with other parameters for making treatment decisions.[2,8,10,14]

- Regional CBF (rCBF) monitoring with TDF
  ❖ rCBF measurements reflect a local area. Significant variation of CBF occurs in different locations within one hemisphere as well as between hemispheres.[10]

  ❖ Currently only one direct regional CBF monitor using TDF is available for clinical use (from Hemedex, Inc., Cambridge, MA) (Figs. 85.1 and 85.2).

  ❖ TDF, based on the mathematical separation of the thermal conductive and the perfusion components of thermal diffusion in brain tissue, allows for continuous quantitative measurement of rCBF at the patient bedside. TDF provides absolute values of CBF expressed as mL/100 g/min and has been validated by comparison with XeCT[2,6,7,10,13,14] (see Table 85.2).

  ❖ TDF is used following TBI and SAH to detect changes in rCBF and to monitor response to therapy. Following aneurysmal SAH, TDF allows for detection and

TABLE 85.1   Global Cerebral Blood Flow (CBF) Thresholds in Adults

CBF (mL/100 g/min)	Threshold	Consequences
>55–60	Hyperemia	Hyperemia Possible increased ICP due to vascular congestion
30–55	Average CBF	Normal cellular structure and function
20–30	Neurological function	Start of neurological symptoms Altered mental status
16–20	Ischemic threshold Electrical failure	Isoelectric electroencephalogram Loss of evoked potentials Loss of consciousness
10–16	Ionic pump failure	Na+ and K+ pump failure Cytotoxic edema Conversion to anaerobic metabolism
<10	Metabolic failure	Complete metabolic failure Compromise of cellular membrane integrity Neuronal death

*Changes occur sooner when global CBF is compromised compared with regional changes in CBF. Tissue infarction is related not only to quantity of CBF but to the duration of decreased perfusion.[11]

CBF, Cerebral blood flow.

Modified from Malloy R, March K: Intracranial dynamics. In Bader MK, Littlejohns L, Olson DM, editors: *AANN core curriculum for neuroscience nursing,* ed 6, Chicago, 2016, American Association of Neuroscience Nurses, 57–62; Zacharia B, Connolly E: Principles of cerebral metabolism and blood flow. In Le Roux P, Levine J, Kofke W, editors: *Monitoring in neurocritical care.* Philadelphia, 2013, Elsevier, 2–7; Miller C, Armonda R. Monitoring of cerebral blood flow and ischemia in the critically ill. *Neurocrit Care* 21:S121–S128, 2014.

TABLE 85.2   Technologies Available for Measuring Cerebral Blood Flow

Technology	Area of Measurement	Data Type	Pros/Cons
Xenon-enhanced computed tomography	Global	Quantitative	• Useful, comprehensive data
Single-photon emission computed tomography	Global	Quantitative	• Expensive
Positron emission tomography	Global	Quantitative	• Requires patient transport
Computed tomography and magnetic resonance perfusion	Global	Qualitative	• Radiation exposure
Angiography	Global	Qualitative	• Episodic, nontrendable data
Computed tomography angiography	Global	Qualitative	• Qualitative data cannot be used to establish threshold levels of perfusion for treatment decisions.
Functional magnetic resonance imaging	Global	Qualitative	
Laser Doppler flowmetry	Regional	Qualitative	
Thermal diffusion flowmetry	Regional	Quantitative	• Real-time, continuous data at the bedside • Absolute, quantitative data • Can be used to set thresholds for treatment decisions.

Courtesy Hemedex, Inc., Cambridge, MA.

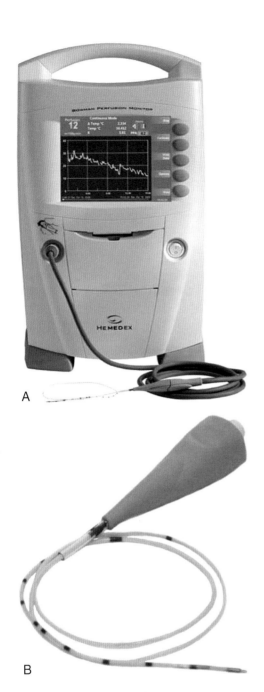

Figure 85.1 **A,** Bowman Perfusion Monitor. **B,** Thermal diffusion probe used to measure cerebral blood flow. *(Courtesy Hemedex, Inc., Waltham, MA.)*

monitoring of decreases in CBF due to cerebral vasospasm[2,6,10] (Fig. 85.3). TDF may also prove useful in the prediction of epileptic seizures by detecting accompanying alterations in cerebral blood flow.[15]

❖ TDF aids in assessing cerebral autoregulation, which plays a significant role in the pathophysiology of TBI, SAH, and ischemic stroke. With intact autoregulation, arterial diameter can increase or decrease (cerebrovascular resistance) to actively control CBF and maintain constant flow over a range of CPPs. Cerebral autoregulation protects the brain from fluctuations in CPP that may cause either hypoperfusion or hyperperfusion.[1-3,8,12,16,17] Associated with a poorer outcome,

impaired autoregulation may make the brain more vulnerable to increased ICP during times of hypertension and to secondary ischemic injury during times of hypotension.[2,3,10,16]

❖ TDF allows the assessment of cerebrovascular reactivity to $Paco_2$ changes and can be of great utility to target moderate hyperventilation, particularly in patients with altered cerebral autoregulation. Hypercapnia and the resulting decrease in extracellular pH causes vasodilation and increased CBF, while hypocapnia leads to vasoconstriction and decreased CBF.[4,6]

❖ rCBF monitoring allows for continuous and direct assessment of CBF. The combination of CBF and cerebrovascular autoregulation has the potential to distinguish between elevations of ICP associated with ischemia or hyperemia, assess the effects of therapeutic interventions, and personalize CPP management to avoid ischemia[7,13] (Fig. 85.4).

• Concepts of TDF and perfusion monitor operation

❖ TDF is an invasive procedure requiring insertion of a perfusion probe into brain tissue either through an intracranial bolt or by tunneling. The perfusion probe is inserted 2.5 to 3.0 cm into white matter and connected to the perfusion monitor via an umbilical cord/cable.[1,9,15,18] (Figs. 85.1 and 85.5).

❖ Perfusion probes are safe with CT but *not* currently with MRI. The probe is currently approved for 10 days of single-patient use. The monitor stores 15 days of data. Data can be downloaded for long-term storage and analysis or integrated with other data management platforms.[18]

❖ Placement of the probe may be ipsilateral or contralateral to the pathology, most commonly in the nondominant frontal lobe, and is determined by the provider based on region of interest, avoiding areas of infarct or hematoma.[9]

❖ A thermistor at the distal tip of the probe heats surrounding brain tissue $\approx 2°C$ to $3°C$ above baseline tissue temperature (measured by a more proximal thermistor) (Fig. 85.6). The power dissipated by the heated thermistor provides a measure of the tissue's ability to carry heat by thermal conduction in the tissue and by thermal convection caused by tissue blood flow.[2,13,14,18,19] Therefore the greater the blood flow, the higher the thermal dissipation and the greater the power required to maintain the temperature elevation. CBF is measured and displayed on the monitor as a perfusion value of mL/100 g/min.[18]

❖ To prevent thermal injury to brain tissue, the probe tip will not heat beyond a safety threshold. Clinically, perfusion will not be measurable if the patient's brain tissue temperature is $\geq 39.5°C$.[2,18]

❖ For accuracy, the perfusion probe must be placed into white matter in an area not affected by cardiac-induced vessel pulsatility that could introduce artifact. A perfusion monitor feature, the probe placement assistant (PPA), quantifies mechanical displacement related to local pulsatility that may affect the measurement.[9] Pulsatility values, represented by PPA, should be low (between 0 and 2.0) and displayed on the screen in a

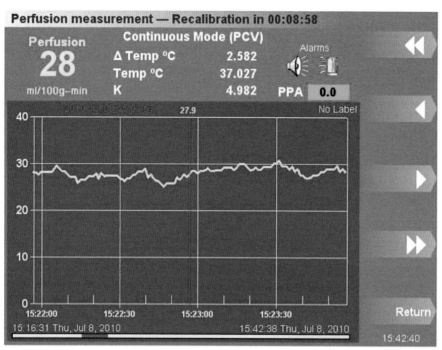

Figure 85.2 Screenshot from the Bowman Perfusion Monitor showing a graphic trend and numeric display of normal cerebral blood flow (perfusion) in white matter. The K value shows normal thermal conductivity (4.8 to 5.9), and the Probe Placement Assistant *(PPA)* shows low probe pulsatility (PPA is 0.0 and *green*). Brain temperature (temp °C) and the temperature difference between the active and passive thermistors (Δ temp °C) are also displayed. *(Courtesy Hemedex, Inc., Waltham, MA.)*

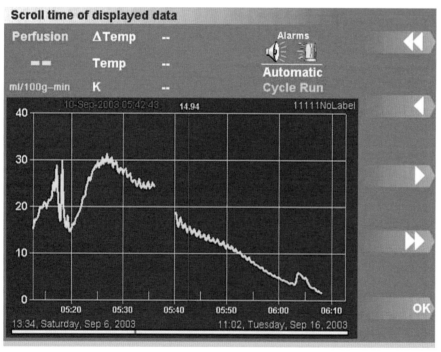

Figure 85.3 Screenshot from the Bowman Perfusion Monitor showing a graphic trend of declining cerebral blood flow in a patient developing vasospasm after aneurysmal subarachnoid hemorrhage. The gap in data from 05:35 to 05:40 represents a normal period of automatic recalibration. Vasospasm was later confirmed by angiography. *(Courtesy Hemedex, Inc., Waltham, MA.)*

green indicator box. As pulsatility rises, values of 2.1 to 5.0 are displayed in a yellow indicator box; values of 5.1 to 10.0 are displayed in a red indicator box, suggesting an unstable thermal field and inaccurate data.

A perfusion measurement will not be displayed if the PPA is red (>5.0).[18]

❖ Thermal conductivity of brain tissue varies with the amount of water content (edema) in the brain.[19] In

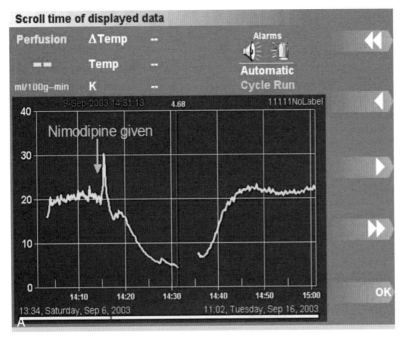

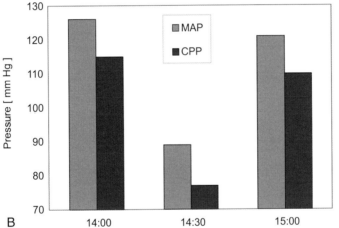

Figure 85.4 **A,** Screenshot from the Bowman Perfusion Monitor showing a graphic trend of declining and subsequent recovery of cerebral blood flow (CBF) in a patient who received a routine dose of nimodipine. This medication is frequently used as the standard of care for prevention of vasospasm after aneurysmal subarachnoid hemorrhage. The sharp increase in CBF just after the time of nimodipine administration represents a motion spike when the patient was repositioned. The gap in data, occurring when CBF was at its lowest, represents a period of recalibration as the Bowman Perfusion Monitor verifies the drastic change in perfusion. **B,** The graph shows this patient's mean arterial pressure *(MAP)* and cerebral perfusion pressure *(CPP)* in the corresponding timeframes. The decline and recovery of CBF that mirrors the decline and recovery of MAP and CPP indicate a loss of cerebral autoregulation. *(Courtesy Hemedex, Inc., Cambridge, MA.)*

normal white matter, thermal conductivity (displayed on the monitor as the K value) is 4.8 to 5.2. If the K value is higher than 5.9 (the upper limit for damaged tissue), it indicates that the probe is positioned in a ventricle or an area of cerebral edema. A low K value (less than 4.8) indicates that the probe is dislodged outside of the brain parenchyma.[18]

❖ The perfusion monitor has three phases: (1) temperature stabilization—establishes baseline tissue temperature and ensures tissue has returned to baseline since previous measurement; (2) calibration—calculation of the K value and PPA; and (3) perfusion measurement. All phases occur automatically when the probe

and cable are connected and also during automatic recalibration periods, which occur every 30 minutes (default)[18] (Fig. 85.7).

❖ The rCBF monitor has several built-in quality-control measures, including periodic recalibration, to ensure the validity and accuracy of real-time measurements.[9]

❖ Limitations to TDF monitoring include the following: loss of perfusion calculations during periodic recalibration (may require 6 to 7 minutes); pulsatility or movement-induced artifact; patient fever above 39.5°C; probe displacement; and lack of global information because of small volume of tissue being monitored.[6,8,13,17,19]

UNIT III

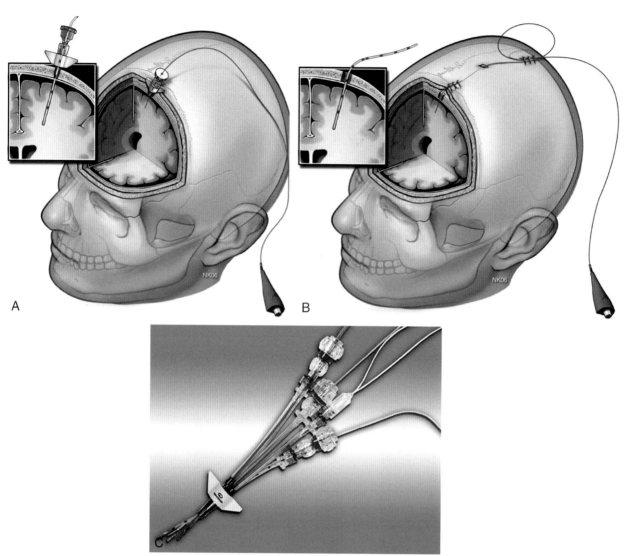

A

B

C

Figure 85.5   Illustrations of placement options for the thermal diffusion probe. **A,** Placement of the probe through a single lumen bolt. Hemedex recommends bolting. **B,** Tunneling of the probe. **C,** Image of the Quad Lumen Bolt for placement of the perfusion probe along with three additional probes/catheters for intracranial monitoring. One, two, and four lumen bolts are available. *(Courtesy Hemedex, Inc., Waltham, MA.)*

EQUIPMENT

- Cranial access kit
- Cranial bolt kit (if using to secure the probe)
- Thermal diffusion probe
- Bowman perfusion monitor with cables
- Sterile gloves and drapes
- Masks, caps, and nonsterile gloves
- Sterile surgical pen (typically included in the cranial access kit)
- Sterile dressing supplies

  Additional equipment to have available as needed includes the following:
- Bedside table
- IV pole

PATIENT AND FAMILY EDUCATION

- Assess patient and family understanding of the purpose of cerebral blood flow/perfusion monitoring. Most patients who need cerebral perfusion monitoring have an altered level of consciousness with a Glasgow Coma Score of 8 or less, so education is typically directed toward the family. *Rationale:* Understanding may reduce anxiety and stress, stimulate requests for clarification or additional information, and increase awareness of the goals, duration, and expectations of the monitoring system.
- Explain the insertion process, patient monitoring, and care involved with CBF monitoring. *Rationale:* Explanation may alleviate anxiety and stress and stimulates requests for clarification or additional information.

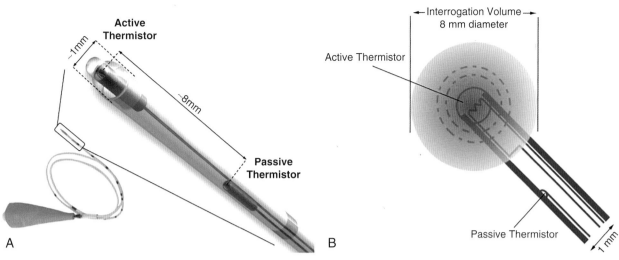

Figure 85.6 Illustrations of the thermal diffusion probe showing (**A**) the active (distal) thermistor that heats brain tissue and measures cerebral blood flow along with (**B**) the passive (proximal) thermistor that measures baseline tissue temperature.

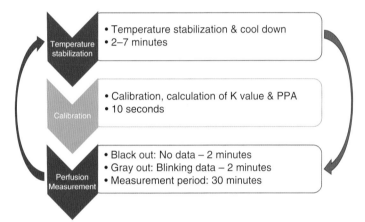

Figure 85.7 Three phases of the perfusion measurement cycle.

PATIENT ASSESSMENT AND PREPARATION

Patient Assessment

- Assess the patient's neurological status. ***Rationale:*** Performing a baseline neurological assessment enables the nurse to identify changes that may occur as a result of probe insertion.
- Assess the patient for signs or symptoms of local infection at the intended insertion location. ***Rationale:*** Evidence of local infection is a contraindication to probe insertion.
- Obtain and review coagulation laboratory results (e.g., complete blood count, platelet count, prothrombin time, partial thromboplastin time, bleeding time, and international normalized ratio). ***Rationale:*** Assessment identifies the patient's risk for bleeding.
- Assess the patient's temperature, and initiate measures according to provider orders to reduce fever. ***Rationale:*** TDF technology will not provide perfusion values while the patient's baseline brain temperature exceeds 39.5°C.

Patient Preparation

- Verify the correct patient with two identifiers. ***Rationale:*** Before performing a procedure, the nurse should ensure the correct identification of the patient for the intended intervention.
- Ensure that the patient and family understand the procedure. Answer questions as they arise, and reinforce information as needed. Most patients who need CBF monitoring have an altered level of consciousness. ***Rationale:*** Information previously taught is evaluated and reinforced.
- Ensure that informed consent has been obtained. ***Rationale:*** Informed consent protects the rights of the patient and makes a competent decision possible for the patient. However, in emergency circumstances, time may not allow for the consent form to be signed.
- Perform a preprocedure verification and time out. ***Rationale:*** Ensures patient safety.
- Administer sedation and/or analgesia as prescribed before beginning the insertion procedure. ***Rationale:*** Sedation and/or analgesia facilitate the insertion process.
- Assist the patient to the semi-Fowler's position (head of the bed elevated 30 to 45 degrees) with the head in a neutral position. ***Rationale:*** Patients who are candidates for CBF monitoring may have increased ICP. Elevating the head of the bed and placing the head in the neutral position decreases intracranial pressure by enhancing jugular venous outflow and provides optimal accessibility for probe insertion.

Procedure	for Cerebral Blood Flow Monitoring: Insertion (Assist), Care, Troubleshooting, and Removal		
Steps	Rationale	Special Considerations	
1. **HH** and **PE**			
2. Place the perfusion monitor near the head of the bed, either on a flat surface or mounted on a sturdy pole.	Secures the monitor and allows the monitor cable to reach the patient's head.		
3. Plug the power cord into an AC wall outlet.	Provides the power source.		
4. Attach the cable (umbilical cord) to the perfusion monitor.	Prepares the equipment.	The cable connection has a twist collar for proper alignment and connection.	
5. Turn on the perfusion monitor using the toggle switch on the right front of the monitor.	Prepares the monitor.		
6. **HH** Apply appropriate sterile and nonsterile barriers	Prepares for the sterile procedure.		
7. Assist as needed with site preparation (e.g., shave preparation, cleansing with antiseptic solution), sterile draping, and opening of sterile packages.	Prepares for the sterile procedure.	Antiseptic solution choice should be determined by institutional policy. The antiseptic solution should be allowed to dry before the initial incision.	
8. Assist as needed with insertion of an intracranial bolt (see manufacturer recommendations in the "Information For Use" [IFU] document).	Bolt system must be inserted before the probe.	The provider must use the drill bit provided in the bolt kit (not the one provided with the drill) to ensure the proper size hole to accommodate the bolt. The provider must be sure to fully incise the dura for correct placement of the probe into brain tissue.	
9. Assist as needed with insertion of the perfusion probe (see manufacturer IFU).	Facilitates the insertion process.	Consult the manufacturer IFU for information on proper depth markings to ensure accurate probe placement.	
10. Connect the perfusion probe to the perfusion monitor cable/umbilical cord.	Initiates monitoring.	Blue connectors must be completely dry. Moisture in the connection will disrupt monitoring.	
11. Observe the message bar on the perfusion monitor screen. If directed to, press the Start button (top soft blue button) to begin monitoring.	Initiates monitoring.	The message bar indicates the current phase of monitoring and displays error messages.	
12. Observe the monitor through the first full cycle of temperature stabilization, calibration, and perfusion calculation. Take note of the initial brain temperature, K value, and PPA. **(Level M*)**	Ensures adequacy of probe placement if the K value is 4.8–5.9 and if the PPA is close to zero.	The full cycle takes 6–7 minutes. The provider should remain at the bedside in sterile attire until the cycle is complete. This allows the opportunity for repositioning of the probe to achieve better placement if necessary.	
13. Assist as needed to mark and secure the probe.	Allows visualization of the insertion level and immediate detection if the probe migrates.	A sterile surgical pen should be used to mark the probe where it exits the bolt.	
14. Secure the probe and cable with two points of tension: tape the probe to the bolt lumen, and anchor the cable to the shoulder.	Prevents entanglement and tension at the insertion site.	Use the provided cable clip to secure the cable to the patient's gown taking care to avoid contact with or pressure on the patient's skin.	
15. Assist as needed with applying a sterile dressing to the insertion site according to hospital protocol.	Protects the insertion site and prevents contamination.		

Procedure for Cerebral Blood Flow Monitoring: Insertion (Assist), Care, Troubleshooting, and Removal—*Continued*		
Steps	**Rationale**	**Special Considerations**
16. Discard used supplies in appropriate receptacles.	Removes and safely discards supplies and sharp objects.	
17. 🖐		
18. Ensure that a CT scan is obtained as prescribed.	A CT scan is recommended to assess probe placement.	A CT scan also helps detect possible complications from insertion (e.g., hemorrhage).
Care of the Perfusion Probe and Monitor		
1. 🖐 and 🖐		
2. Visually inspect the probe and insertion site dressing with each neurological assessment. A. Note the probe marking where it exits the bolt. B. Check the security of the probe at the insertion site. C. Ensure that the cable remains taped to the patient's shoulder. D. Assess the insertion site for signs of drainage, redness, or swelling.[10]	Alerts the caregiver to potential problems with the probe or insertion site.	Notify the provider if the probe has moved or if there are signs of infection at the insertion site.
3. Assess the perfusion trends on the monitor screen, and correlate the trends with neurological examinations, patient activity, and treatments (e.g., medications).	Allows correlation of perfusion with clinical condition/treatments and helps individualize care.	If autoregulation is altered, treatments and medications that affect blood pressure (e.g., nimodipine) may affect cerebral perfusion.
4. Note regular gaps in data (lasting 6–7 minutes) representing temperature stabilization and probe recalibration.	Probe periodically assesses the tissue environment and characteristics to ensure accurate data.	The default recalibration period is every 30 minutes. This can be changed using the Options soft button on the monitor and changing the Perfusion Period.
5. Patient transport: A. Disconnect the probe from the cable. B. Pause monitoring by pushing the Stop button (top blue soft button). C. Resume monitoring on return by reconnecting the probe and cable and then pressing the same button (now labeled Start).	Pauses monitoring for patient transport.	The probe is CT compatible but *not* MRI compatible. The monitor is typically left behind for transport. However, some providers wish to monitor perfusion during surgery or other procedures, such as angiography. The monitor will recalibrate each time the probe is disconnected and reconnected.
Troubleshooting the Monitor		
1. 🖐 and 🖐		
2. If the screen is blank, check the On/Off switch and the power supply.	Ensures power to the monitor.	The perfusion monitor does not have a battery and must be connected to an AC outlet for power.
3. Look for a paper printout of an error code from the front of the monitor.	Perfusion monitor provides report of monitoring errors.	
4. Check the status bar at the top of the monitor screen for a message. **(Level M*)**	Indicates possible reasons for data disruption.	

Procedure continues on following page

UNIT III

Procedure	for Cerebral Blood Flow Monitoring: Insertion (Assist), Care, Troubleshooting, and Removal—*Continued*		
Steps	**Rationale**	**Special Considerations**
5. Assess the insertion site for security of the probe—the exit mark, tightness of compression cap, and so on. Note the K value and PPA.	Provides information about possible probe movement and slippage from the bolt.	If the probe has moved, the monitor will have difficulty with temperature stabilization and may display a high PPA. A low K value may indicate that the probe has become dislodged. A delta temperature >1°C (when the probe is not heating) indicates that the probe is placed too superficially. Because sterility cannot be ensured, the probe should not be reinserted if it has become dislodged.
6. Assess the patient's brain temperature reading on the perfusion monitor screen. The probe will not heat, and perfusion will not be calculated if the brain temperature is ≥39.5°C.	Ensures that an active thermistor will not heat brain tissue above a safety threshold.	Once brain temperature is below 39.5°C, the perfusion probe will resume normal operation.
7. Assess patient activity. The probe is sensitive to relative probe-brain tissue motion and may not provide accurate readings if the patient is restless or if the probe is not secured.	Limited patient movement reduces motion artifact by reducing relative probe-brain tissue motion.	
8. Assess the probe/cable connection for moisture.	A dry probe/cable connection is required for proper monitor function. **(Level M*)**	Allow to air-dry, or apply a source of warm dry air to facilitate drying.
9. Assess whether the cable is damaged; if so, replace the cable.	If the probe cable is damaged, values can be incorrect, or measurement can be interrupted.	Take care when inserting or removing the cable from the monitor—do not pull/push the cable straight in or out. The cable has a twist collar to ensure a secure connection to the monitor.
Removal of the Probe		
1. 🅷🅷 and 🅿🅴		
2. Position the patient in the semi-Fowler's position.	Prepares the patient for device removal.	
3. Turn off the monitor.	Facilitates device removal.	If the message bar indicates that data storage is full, notify your supervisor. The perfusion monitor stores 15 days of data. Data will need to be uploaded to the Hemedex web manager (or other data platform) or deleted for additional data storage to occur.
4. Assist as needed with removal of the dressing, perfusion probe, and bolt system.	Facilitates device removal.	If multiple probes have been inserted into the bolt system, it is important to remove the probes before removing the bolt to prevent injury to brain tissue with the twisting action of bolt removal.
5. Assist if needed with applying an occlusive sterile dressing to the site, according to hospital policy.	Reduces the risk for infection.	Assess for signs of bleeding, cerebrospinal fluid (CSF) leak, and signs and symptoms of infection.
6. Discard used supplies appropriately.	Removes and safely discards used supplies.	The probe(s) and bolt are disposable; the cable and monitor are not.
7. 🅷🅷		
8. Clean monitor, cable, and power cord according to hospital protocol.	Disinfects equipment and prepares it for use on the next patient.	
🅿🅴		

Expected Outcomes

- Perfusion probe is placed in the correct position as evidenced by:
  - K value is 4.8–5.9
  - PPA box appears "green" with a pulsatility index (PI) of 0–2
  - CT scan verifies proper probe position and no evidence of hemorrhage or hematoma
- Monitoring and data display commence with first perfusion cycle
- Perfusion values are acceptable:
  - Perfusion in white matter is between 18 and 50 mL/100 g/min or as indicated by patient condition
- Detection and monitoring of low perfusion states
- Detection and monitoring of hyperemia
- Assessment of treatment effects (e.g., medications) on perfusion
- Immediate intervention and management of compromised CBF
- Ability to individualize patient care by maintaining adequate perfusion according to cerebral metabolic demand
- No adverse events (e.g., hemorrhage, infection) as a result of monitoring

Unexpected Outcomes

- Perfusion probe not placed correctly as evidenced by poor visualization on CT scan
  - K value <4.8 (not in tissue) or >5.9 (in a ventricle or area of edema)
  - PPA box appears "red" with a PI of 5.0–10
- Perfusion values in white matter are <18 mL/100 g/min or >50 mL/100 g/min
- Failure to identify low perfusion or high perfusion conditions
- Inability to adequately perfuse the brain according to metabolic demand
- Adverse events such as hemorrhage or infection occur
- Patient unable to tolerate procedure and monitoring related to pain

Patient Monitoring and Care

Steps	Rationale	Reportable Conditions
		These conditions should be reported to the provider if they persist despite nursing interventions.
1. Assess the patient's baseline neurological status, vital signs, ICP, and CPP every 15 minutes (more frequently if necessary) during and immediately after the procedure, and then hourly or according to institutional standards.	Provides assessment of patient status before, during, and after the procedure.	• Changes in neurological status • Changes in vital signs • Changes in ICP and CPP
2. Maintain perfusion values between 18 and 50 mL/100 g/min or as prescribed.	Represents normal values.	• Decreased perfusion values • Increased perfusion values • Perfusion values that change in response to patient activity or treatment (e.g., a decrease in perfusion following medication administration or adjustment of mechanical ventilator settings)
3. In states of low perfusion, assess for and treat factors that may increase demand for blood flow (pain, fever, agitation, shivering, and seizure) and/or decrease delivery of flow (cardiac issues, bradycardia, hypotension, particularly during loss of cerebral autoregulation, hypovolemia, hypocapnia, and vasoconstriction).[3-5,10] **(Level D*)**	Provides assessment of factors that may reduce CBF.	• Uncontrolled pain/agitation • Fever • Shivering • Seizure • Bradycardia • Hypotension • Hypovolemia • Hypocapnia
4. In states of high perfusion, assess for and treat factors that may decrease the demand for CBF (hypothermia, sedation, paralysis, and anesthesia) and/or increase the delivery of flow (hypervolemia, hypercapnia/vasodilation).[3-5,10] **(Level D*)**	Provides assessment of factors that may increase CBF.	• Hypothermia • Excessive sedation • Hypervolemia • Hypercapnia

*Level D: Peer-reviewed professional and organizational standards with the support of clinical study recommendations.

Documentation

Documentation should include the following:
- Patient and family education
- Preprocedure verifications and time out
- Completion of informed consent
- Insertion of the CBF probe
- Patient tolerance of the procedure
- Insertion site assessment
- Neurological assessments
- Hourly values, including perfusion, K-value, PPA, perfusion temperature, along with other hemodynamic parameters and neurological parameters (e.g., ICP, CPP, Pbto2, $ETco_2$)
- Occurrence of unexpected outcomes and interventions
- Pain assessment, interventions, and effectiveness

References and Additional Readings

For a complete list of references and additional readings for this procedure, scan this QR code with your smartphone, or visit https://www.elsevier.com/__data/assets/pdf_file/0010/1319860/Chapter0085.pdf

86

Cerebral Microdialysis

Thomas Hagerty

PURPOSE Microdialysis is a minimally invasive technique for continuous sampling of the interstitial fluid of tissues and organs; it can be used in cerebral tissue to analyze chemical markers of metabolism and ischemia such as glucose, pyruvate, and lactate as well as markers of cell damage such as glutamate and glycerol.[1,2,11,18,19,21,22] Cerebral microdialysis improves the understanding of energy metabolism and may provide early warning signs of ischemia in patients with traumatic brain injury or subarachnoid hemorrhage.[1,2,20,21] It is a monitoring tool and not a treatment like hemodialysis and should only be used to supplement other advanced neuromonitoring technologies.[7,12]

PREREQUISITE NURSING KNOWLEDGE

- Fundamental understanding of neuroanatomy and physiology.[5]
- Understanding of hypoxia and/or ischemia of the brain.[10]
- Understanding of the technology used for analyzing microdialysis samples (see Fig. 86.5, the ISCUSflex Microdialysis Analyzer).[12,18]
- Understanding of the microdialysis catheter positioning within the brain because positioning can influence sample results. In patients with diffuse disease, the catheter is placed in the subcortical matter of the right frontal cortex. In patients with aneurysmal subarachnoid hemorrhage, the catheter is placed in the frontal watershed ipsilateral to the aneurysm, or in the region of the brain determined to be at greatest risk for developing ischemia and secondary damage.[8,19,21,22]
- Knowledge of cerebral perfusion pressure (CPP). CPP provides the blood flow necessary to meet the metabolic needs of the injured brain and to avoid the exacerbation of ischemic insults.[9,14,16]
- Knowledge of cerebral autoregulation. Cerebral autoregulation is the ability of the brain's arteries and arterioles to constrict and dilate to provide the brain with constant, normal blood flow. In neurologically compromised patients, the brain's autoregulation abilities may become impaired and interfere with perfusion.[4]
- The microdialysis system is composed of the cerebral microdialysis catheter (Fig. 86.1), sterile microdialysis CNS perfusion fluid (Fig. 86.2), perfusion syringe (see Fig. 86.2), and before perfusion pump (Fig. 86.3), microvials (Fig. 86.4), and the tissue fluid chemistry analyzer (e.g., ISCUSflex tissue chemistry analyzer) (Fig. 86.5). The microdialysis catheter has a semipermeable distal end membrane. It is placed into brain tissue through a bolt or burr hole or is implanted during an open craniotomy. The microdialysis catheter is attached to a syringe filled with sterile perfusion fluid (see Fig. 86.2). The syringe is placed in a battery-operated pump that is calibrated to pump the perfusion fluid through the catheter at a rate of

0.3 µL/min (see Fig. 86.3). Tiny amounts of cerebral fluid, called *microdialysate,* pass from brain tissue through the catheter's semipermeable membrane and are collected with the perfusion fluid in a microvial attached to the catheter. The vial is then placed in a point-of-care (POC) analyzer of the chemical substrates (see Fig. 86.5).[7,11,18,19,22]

- The analyzer can accommodate multiple vials, allowing testing on multiple patients at the same time.[11,19,22]
- Normal glucose: 1.7 ± 0.9 mmol/L. The biochemical markers of metabolism and ischemia are reflected in glucose and oxygen as the main components of cell energy. Glucose is broken down to pyruvate during glycolysis. When oxygen is available, pyruvate goes through the citric acid cycle, generating high production of adenosine triphosphate (ATP). During ischemia, a lack of oxygen and glucose results in the conversion of pyruvate to lactate during anaerobic metabolism. Glucose is a primary source of energy to the brain and is an important marker of changes in brain metabolism. Cerebral glucose levels account for approximately two-thirds of systemic glucose.[7,11,19,22]
- Normal pyruvate: 166 ± 47 µm. Pyruvate and lactate reflect cell metabolism. Pyruvate decreases with inadequate glucose supply.[7,11,19,20,22,]
- Normal lactate: 2.9 ± 0.9 µm. Lactate increases with ischemia. During ischemia, a lack of oxygen and glucose results in anaerobic metabolism, reduced levels of pyruvate, and increased levels of lactate. Lactate alone is insufficient as a marker of brain ischemia.[7,11,19,20,22]
- Normal lactate/pyruvate ratio (LPR): 23 ± 4 µm. Ischemia is defined by the combined criteria of LPR >40 and glucose <0.2 mmol/L. The LPR reflects anaerobic metabolism and increases with ischemia. The LPR is a good indicator of ischemic and hypoxic conditions as well as possible mitochondrial damage.[7,11,19,20,22]
- Normal glycerol: 20 to 50 µm. The biochemical markers of cellular damage are reflected in glycerol and glutamate. Glycerol reflects cell injury and lysis and is a marker of cell membrane function. Levels increase when cells do not have sufficient energy to maintain homeostasis.[7,19,22]
- Normal glutamate: 10 µm. Glutamate is an early indirect marker of cell damage and reflects cell membrane breakdown. It increases with ischemia.[7,19,22]

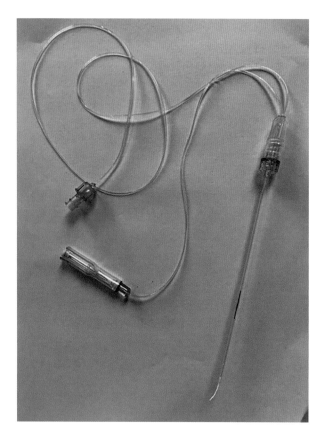

Figure 86.1   Cerebral microdialysis catheter.

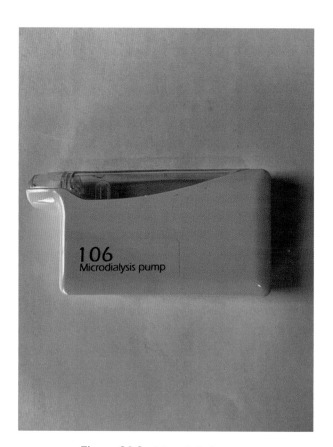

Figure 86.3   Microdialysis pump.

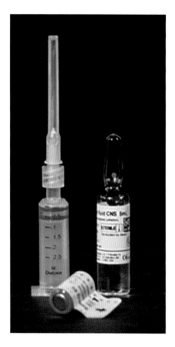

Figure 86.2   Microdialysis pump kit, including perfusion syringe, pump battery, and sterile microdialysis perfusion fluid.

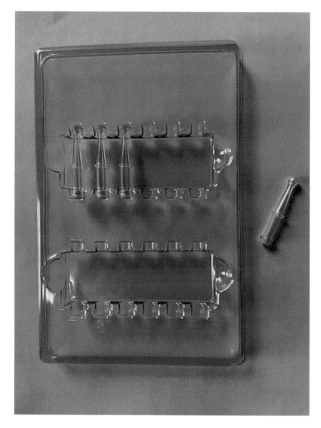

Figure 86.4   Microvials and microvial storage rack.

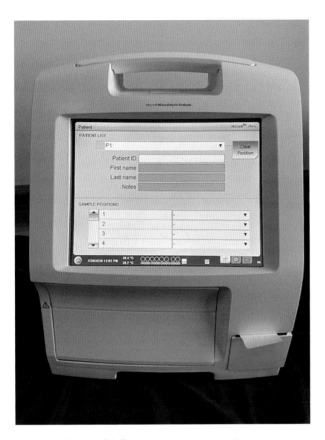

Figure 86.5 Tissue chemistry analyzer.

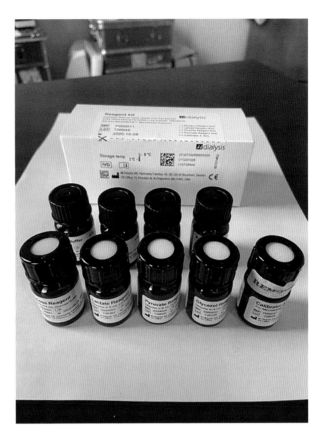

Figure 86.6 Reagents.

- Along with continuous sampling of the interstitial fluid chemistry of the brain tissue, repeated assessment of the patient's neurological status and other multimodality parameters provides focused information for markers of ischemia and cell damage.[4,7,9,12-14,16]

EQUIPMENT

- Sterile gowns, sterile drapes, sterile gloves, nonsterile gloves, caps, gloves, and face masks
- Shave preparation kit
- Antiseptic solution
- Brain microdialysis catheter or microdialysis bolt catheter (see Fig. 86.1)
- Cranial access tray
- Scalpel
- Dressing supplies, including 4 × 4 gauze
- Sterile dressing supplies
- Microdialysis Analyzer (see Fig. 86.5)
- Microdialysis pump (see Fig. 86.3)
- Artificial CSF fluid (see Fig. 86.2)
- Batteries (2 × 3 volt) (see Fig. 86.2)
- Microvials (see Fig. 86.4)
- Microvial racks (see Fig. 86.4)
- Pump syringe (see Fig. 86.2)
- Perfusion fluid (see Fig. 86.2)
- Reagents (Fig. 86.6)

Additional equipment, to have available as needed, includes the following:
- Bedside table

PATIENT AND FAMILY EDUCATION

- Assess patient and family understanding of complex brain injuries that require close monitoring of multiple parameters in hopes of preventing secondary brain injuries. *Rationale:* This assessment may help identify patient and family educational needs.[15,19]
- Explain to the patient and family that the procedure may be performed in the intensive care unit (ICU). *Rationale:* This may reduce patient and family anxiety.[19]
- Explain the basic principles of cerebral metabolites. *Rationale:* This information may answer patient and family questions and reduce anxiety.[19]
- Explain the insertion of the brain microdialysis catheter and the region of the brain where the catheter will be inserted (e.g., at-risk penumbra). *Rationale:* Explain that monitoring areas of the brain may provide crucial information about the biochemistry of the brain and how seriously brain cells are affected by injury to the brain.[19]
- Explain the use of the equipment (see Fig. 86.5). *Rationale:* Explaining how the samples from the brain are transferred to the microdialysis analyzer may allay fears and reduce anxiety regarding the equipment utilized.[19]
- Explain to the patient and family that continual assessment of the patient's neurological status along with continuous sampling of the interstitial fluid chemistry of the brain tissue will be completed hourly and as needed. *Rationale:* Use of microdialysis neurointensive care is focused on tissue ischemia and cell damage and requires frequent assessment and sampling.[19]

PATIENT ASSESSMENT AND PREPARATION

Patient Assessment

- Assess the patient's neurological status. ***Rationale:*** Performing a baseline neurological assessment enables the nurse to identify changes that may have occurred because of the insertion of the microdialysis catheter.[6]
- Assess the patient for signs or symptoms of local infection at the intended insertion location. ***Rationale:*** Evidence of local infection is a contraindication to microdialysis catheter insertion.[6]

Patient Preparation

- Verify the correct patient with two identifiers. ***Rationale:*** Before performing a procedure, the nurse should ensure the correct identification of the patient for the intended intervention.[17]
- Perform a preprocedure verification and time out. ***Rationale:*** This ensures patient safety.[17]
- Ensure that informed consent has been obtained. ***Rationale:*** Informed consent protects the rights of the patient and makes a competent decision possible for the patient; however, in emergency circumstances, time may not allow for the consent form to be signed.[17]
- Administer preprocedural analgesia or sedation as prescribed. ***Rationale:*** The patient must have relief from pain and remain still during microdialysis catheter insertion.[6]

Procedure	for Performing Cerebral Microdialysis	
Steps	Rationale	Special Considerations
1. **HH**		
2. **PE**	Sterile procedure in which the provider dons full sterile PE, face mask, and eye protection or disposable face shield. The critical care nurse will don a surgical hat, face mask, and droplet shield or disposable face shield.[3]	
3. The microdialysis catheter may be introduced through an existing intracranial bolt system or be surgically placed. If not using an intracranial bolt system, the provider will insert the microdialysis catheter into brain tissue and secure the catheter to the scalp.	Placing the catheter through an existing intracranial bolt system must be a sterile procedure if performed at the bedside. The patient may also be taken to the operating room for surgery with removal of the bone flap and placement of the catheter under visual inspection.	This is surgical procedure that is most optimally completed in an operating room. Typically a dressing is not required at the catheter insertion site.
4. If using an intracranial bolted catheter, the critical care nurse supports and monitors the patient during the procedure per institutional protocols. A. The provider will place the bolt and secure it to the skull. B. The provider will insert the catheter into the intracranial bolt or designated microdialysis port/lumen and fix the catheter at the Luer-Lok connector.	The sterile, single-use microdialysis bolt catheter (see Fig. 86.1) is designed for implantation in brain tissue through an intracranial access device that is fixed to the skull. Tightening the compression screw will help secure the catheter.	The intracranial catheter may be inserted in the ICU or the operating room. The catheter is location sensitive. Data will differ depending on the proximity of the catheter to the area of injury. Typically a dressing is not required at the catheter insertion site.
5. Ensure that once the catheter is placed, a brain computed tomography (CT) scan is obtained as prescribed.	Determines the position of the catheter in relation to the tissue pathology.	

Steps	Rationale	Special Considerations
Procedure for Performing Cerebral Microdialysis—*Continued*		
6. Fill and connect the syringe. Once the microdialysis catheter is implanted and the wound is closed, the critical care nurse will perform the following: A. Fill the microdialysis syringe with 2.5 mL of artificial CSF perfusion fluid (ensure that there are no air bubbles). B. Connect the syringe to the catheter.	The artificial CSF perfusion fluid (no more than 2.5 mL) primes the tubing/system (see Fig. 86.2).	Use only the artificial CSF provided by the manufacturer.
7. Prepare the pump: A. Place the syringe in the microdialysis pump with the tip first and the piston second. B. Place the battery in the pump. C. Close the lid, which will start a flush sequence. A blinking light on the syringe pump indicates the stage in the pump sequence. D. Secure the pump near the patient's head.	Prepares the system. The pump is a small battery-driven pump with a flow of 0.3 µL/min (see Fig. 86.3). It is the size of a deck of cards. Closing the lid starts a flush sequence that removes all air from the tubing and the catheter and initiates the microdialysis process. Anchoring the pump with tape prevents accidental dislodgement.	The pump is portable, small, and lightweight and is self-controlled with LED function signals. The battery will need to be changed after 5 days of use (or with every new patient).
8. Place a microvial in the vial holder of the catheter: A. Discard the first vial after 30–60 minutes. B. Place a new vial in the holder to collect the first sample for analysis.	Discard the first sample because it is diluted by the flush solution. The microvial is the collection vial for the interstitial fluid (see Fig. 86.4).	If there is no fluid in the microvial, check the pump's flashing diodes for malfunction. Check the battery, and make sure that: (a) the pump lid is closed, (b) there is perfusion fluid in the syringe, and (c) the catheter tubing is not kinked. If the problem persists, open and close the lid of the pump to initiate a flush.
9. Prepare the system. Refer to the user manual of the microdialysis analyzer for detailed instructions on: A. How to start the microdialysis analyzer. B. Loading rinsing fluid. C. Preparing and loading reagents and control samples. D. Registering the patient in the analyzer. E. Adding a new patient: select an empty patient position, and add the patient's name.	Prepares the system for sample analysis and correct patient identification of samples analyzed.	
10. Prepare the reagents: glucose, lactate, pyruvate, glycerol, and glutamate. A. Mix the solution and powder of each reagent (respectively). B. Mix the solution and powder by first opening the vial with powder. C. Remove and discard the stopper. D. Mix the powder and liquid of each reagent together. E. Set each one aside as the other four reagents are mixed. F. Load into the analyzer in the specified position per the user manual.	Prepares the equipment.	Allow up to an hour for the analyzer to calibrate the new reagents and run the controls. Follow all point-of-care and clinical laboratory regulations. Reagents and perfusion fluid must be replaced every 5 days.

Procedure continues on following page

Procedure for Performing Cerebral Microdialysis—*Continued*

Steps	Rationale	Special Considerations
11. Analyze the microdialysis samples.	Results appear in about 8 minutes.	It is not necessary to reactivate the pump when microvials are removed.
A. Change the microvial every 60 minutes or as prescribed.	Generally, samples are run every hour.[19] Samples may be run more frequently as indicated by changes in the patient's condition; samples can be run every 10 minutes if necessary.	
B. Remove the microvial from the microvial holder of the catheter, and insert a new microvial into the microvial holder of the catheter.	Prepares the equipment.	Data are not provided continuously in real time. Clinicians should monitor trends to detect deterioration in patient brain chemistry.
C. Choose the position of the vial for a specified patient position by adding a catheter name at the preferred vial position in the lower menu of the patient screen.	Prepares the equipment.	Up to 16 different vial positions are available for one patient.
12. Discard used supplies in appropriate receptacles.		
13. 🅷🅷		

Expected Outcomes

- Optimal placement of microdialysis catheter will be confirmed by CT scan.[19]
- Information about trends in brain chemistry will be obtained; this information can assist in delivery of targeted therapy for prevention of secondary ischemic injury.[4,7,9,12-14,16,21]
- Changes in brain chemistry will be noted and treated prior to the appearance of clinical signs and symptoms indicative of secondary damage.[4,7,9,12-14,16,21]
- The effects of clinical therapies (e.g., strict versus relaxed glycemic control) on brain metabolism will be evaluated continuously.[4,7,9,12-14,16,21]

Unexpected Outcomes

- Poor quality data obtained due to suboptimal microdialysis catheter placement (e.g., in dead tissue).
- Theoretical risk of meningitis or ventriculitis caused by microdialysis catheter placement (there do not appear to be any published reports of this).

Patient Monitoring and Care

Steps	Rationale	Reportable Conditions
		These conditions should be reported to the provider if they persist despite nursing interventions.
1. Assess the patient's neurological status frequently per institutional protocols if neurological changes are noted.	Provides continual neurological assessment and the ability to note changes.	• Worsening of level of consciousness (LOC) • Increase in intracranial pressure (ICP) • Decrease in CPP • Decrease in pupillary reactivity and response to stimuli • Alteration of blood pressure and heart rate suggestive of brain stem herniation

Patient Monitoring and Care —*Continued*

Steps	Rationale	Reportable Conditions
2. Monitor the cerebral microdialysis trends (results have at minimum a 1-hour lag time).	Provides trending data and allows assessment of changes that may result from: (a) worsening disease process, (b) procedures, (c) medication adjustments, (d) change in patient position, and (d) change in patient care needs. Evaluates changes in CPP, blood glucose levels, and oxygen saturation against changes in tissue chemistry.	• Changes to lactate-pyruvate ratio (LPR) after medication changes or mobility • Abnormal trends in LPR • Neurological changes such as change in LOC, ICP, CPP, pupil response, response to stimuli, blood pressure, and heart rate that suggest compromise in neurological function • Alert the provider if the chemical condition of the tissue changes, especially when levels and trends are out of normal range
3. Assess the catheter site every 4 hours or more often if indicated per institutional protocol. **(Level D*)**	Provides an opportunity to assess the placement of the catheter and for signs and symptoms of infection.	• Redness or swelling at the catheter site • Leakage around the microdialysis catheter • Catheter dislodgement

*Level D: Peer-reviewed professional and organizational standards with the support of clinical study recommendations.

Documentation

Documentation should include the following:
- Date and time of catheter insertion, reagent activation, loading of the syringe pump, loading of batteries in the pump, and registration of patient data into the analyzer
- All elements of preprocedural verification and time out were met.[17]
- Glucose, lactate, pyruvate, glycerol, and glutamate levels every hour or as prescribed by the physician.[7,12,19]
- Patient and family education[15,19]
- Insertion site assessment[19]
- Hourly vital signs, laboratory values, hemodynamic monitoring (per institutional protocol)
- Assessment of pain and response to pain medication[6]
- Sedation levels[6]
- Neurological assessments[5,10]
- Patient tolerance of the procedure[6]

References and Additional Readings

For a complete list of references and additional readings for this procedure, scan this QR code with your smartphone, or visit https://www.elsevier.com/__data/assets/pdf_file/0011/1319861/Chapter0086.pdf.

87 Intracranial Pressure Monitoring, Nursing Care, Troubleshooting, and Removal

Michael S. Rogers

PURPOSE Intraventricular catheters, when attached to a transducer and external drain system, form an external ventricular drain (EVD) that monitors intracranial pressure (ICP) and allows for the drainage of cerebrospinal fluid (CSF). This device can be used to monitor ICP intermittently or continuously and drain CSF intermittently or continuously in the presence of cranial pathology.

PREREQUISITE NURSING KNOWLEDGE

- Principles of aseptic and sterile technique
- Fundamental knowledge of neuroanatomy and physiology
- The Monro-Kellie doctrine describes three components that comprise the intracranial contents: brain, blood, and CSF. ICP is a result of the dynamic relationship between the pressure exerted by these three components.[14] Normal ICP ranges from 0 to 15 mm Hg. Sustained ICPs of greater than 20 mm Hg are generally considered neurological emergencies.[14]
- Providers commonly insert ventricular or intraparenchymal catheters to measure ICP. Ventricular catheters allow for the drainage of CSF as an intervention to lower ICP. Intraparenchymal catheters do not allow for the drainage of CSF.
- CSF is a clear colorless liquid of low specific gravity with no red blood cells and few white blood cells (<5000 per microliter). CSF is secreted at the rate of 20 to 25 mL/hour[11] by the choroid plexus in the lateral ventricles of the cerebral hemispheres. From the lateral ventricles, CSF drains into the foramen of Monro, the intraventricular foramina, and into the third ventricle adjacent to the thalamus. From the third ventricle, CSF flows down via the aqueduct of Sylvius into the fourth ventricle at the pons and medulla, then into the subarachnoid space and spinal column. CSF is absorbed by the arachnoid villi (also known as *arachnoid granulations*), where it drains into the venous system to be returned to the heart. Approximately 150 mL of CSF circulates within the CSF pathways of the brain and spinal subarachnoid space at any given time.[11]
- Cerebral autoregulation is the intrinsic ability of the cerebral vessels to constrict and dilate as needed to maintain adequate cerebral perfusion. Cerebral autoregulation is impaired with brain injury, and cerebral blood flow becomes passively dependent on the systemic blood flow. The cerebral blood vessels are no longer able to react to maintain perfusion in response to a change in blood pressure.[8,9,17]

- Cerebral perfusion pressure (CPP) is a derived mathematic calculation that indirectly reflects the adequacy of cerebral blood flow. The CPP is calculated by subtracting the ICP from the mean arterial pressure (MAP); thus CPP = MAP − ICP. The normal CPP range for adults is approximately 60 to 100 mm Hg. The optimal CPP for a given patient and clinical condition is not entirely known and may require individualized CPP parameters reflective of the neuropathology and brain perfusion needs. ICP and CPP should be managed concomitantly and in conjunction with other clinical indicators. Research continues regarding the relationship between cerebral blood flow and CPP.
- Elevated ICP is likely with the following medical diagnoses; therefore ICP monitoring is indicated.[5,13]
  - ❖ Traumatic brain injury (TBI)
  - ❖ Intracranial hemorrhage
  - ❖ Subarachnoid hemorrhage (SAH), aneurysmal or traumatic
  - ❖ Large-territory ischemic stroke
  - ❖ Hydrocephalus
  - ❖ Fulminant hepatic failure with encephalopathy
  - ❖ Meningitis
  - ❖ Intracranial cysts
- CSF drainage is likely indicated as a component of ICP management for the following[1]:
  - ❖ Acute hydrocephalus
  - ❖ Ventriculoperitoneal shunt (VPS) failure
  - ❖ SAH
  - ❖ Intraparenchymal hemorrhage
  - ❖ TBI
  - ❖ Postoperative craniotomy
  - ❖ Meningitis
- The ventricular catheter connected to a graduated burette and paired with an external strain gauge transducer (or internal fiberoptic transducer at the tip of the catheter) forms an EVD. EVDs are highly accurate in monitoring ICP and allow for CSF drainage as an intervention.[2,3,5] These catheters typically terminate at the foramen of Monro in the cerebral ventricular system. A fiberoptic catheter passed through a bolt in the skull also provides

quality ICP monitoring but cannot be used for CSF drainage. These fiberoptic catheters may be placed in the epidural, subdural, subarachnoid, ventricular, and intraparenchymal spaces.[2,3,5,13]

- Fiberoptic ventricular catheters and fiberoptic intraparenchymal catheters must be calibrated to atmospheric pressure or "zeroed" before insertion.
- The normal ICP waveform is pulsatile and has three peaks: P_1, P_2, and P_3 (Fig. 87.1), known as the percussive wave, tidal wave, and dicrotic wave, respectively.[14] In a compliant brain, the amplitude of P_1 is the greatest amplitude, with subsequent P_2 and P_3 waves progressively decreasing in amplitude. P_1 is thought to reflect arterial pulsation; P_2 represents intracranial compliance, and P_3 has been described as choroid plexus or venous in origin. In a brain with decreased compliance in the presence of elevated ICP, the amplitude of P_2 may exceed P_1 (Fig. 87.2).
- During ICP elevations, pathological (Lundberg) waveform trends include *a, b,* and *c* waves. The *a* waves, also referred to as *plateau waves,* are associated with ICP values of 50 to 100 mm Hg and last 5 to 20 minutes. The *a* waves (Fig. 87.3) are associated with increased cerebrovascular volume due to vasodilation and resolve with vasomotor stimulation of the brainstem. The *b* waves (Fig. 87.4) are associated with ICP values of 20 to 50 mm Hg, last 30 seconds to 2 minutes, and could be caused by vasodilation secondary to fluctuating $Paco_2$. The *c* waves (Fig. 87.5) are more sinusoidal, can occur within normal ICP range, and likely represent normal interactions with cardiac and pulmonary cycles.[7,18]
- Management of acute brain injury is aimed at decreasing secondary brain injury from increased intracranial pressure, decreased CPP, impaired autoregulation, hypotension, hypoxemia, cerebral ischemia, hypercarbia, hyperthermia, hypoglycemia, hyperglycemia, seizures, or abnormalities in cerebral blood flow. Interventions include blood pressure management, decreased environmental stimuli, elevation of the head of the bed, alignment of the head and neck in a straight position to promote venous drainage, avoidance of constrictive devices about the neck that might impede arterial flow to the brain and venous drainage from the brain, seizure prophylaxis, glucose control, and attaining and maintaining normothermia without shivering.[7,13,14]
- In addition to CSF drainage, management of increased ICP frequently requires the use of certain pharmacological agents to lessen intracranial pressure, including sedation and analgesia, osmotic diuretics, hypertonic saline, neuromuscular blockade, and barbiturates. In the case of barbiturate coma, continuous electroencephalographic (EEG) monitoring (or EEG-based consciousness/sedation monitoring) for burst suppression is necessary to achieve the desired decrease in cerebral oxygen consumption and electrical stimuli. Additional strategies include decompressive craniectomy and hemispherectomy.[1,13]

EQUIPMENT

- Sterile supplies (caps, masks, sterile drapes, gloves, and gowns)

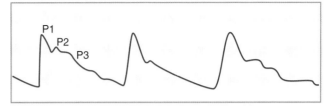

Normal Compliance

Figure 87.1 Components of the intracranial pressure waveform: P_1, P_2, and P_3.

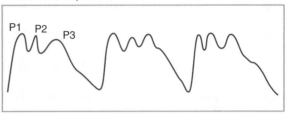

Reduced Compliance

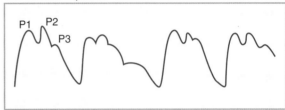

Increased Amplitude

Figure 87.2 Example of intracranial pressure waveforms with P_2 elevation indicating decreased cerebral compliance.

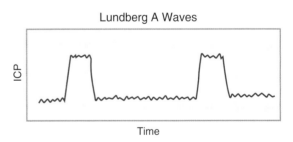

Lundberg A Waves

Figure 87.3 *a* or plateau waves. *ICP,* Intracranial pressure.

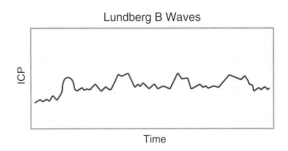

Lundberg B Waves

Figure 87.4 *b* waves. *ICP,* Intracranial pressure.

UNIT III

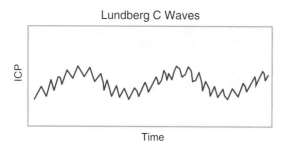

Figure 87.5   c waves. *ICP,* Intracranial pressure.

- Goggles, face shield, or eye protection
- Cranial access tray with drill (for the provider)
- Ventricular catheter (for the provider)
- Local anesthetic (for the provider)
- Cautery as required by institutional standards (for the provider)
- Razor or clippers for depilatory preparation (per institutional protocol)
- Pressure monitor tubing kit (including pressure tubing, transducer, three-way stopcock, or flushless transducer with stopcock)
- Preservative-free normal saline solution[17]
- Nonvented sterile caps
- External drainage system (including tubing, graduated burette, and drainage bag)
- Pressure monitoring cable and module
- Sterile syringes
- Skin/site preparation with antiseptic solution (per institutional policy)
- Sutures or staples (for the provider)
- Sterile dressing (per institutional policy)
- Tape
- Laboratory forms and specimen labels (for CSF specimens)
- CSF specimen tubes (for collection of CSF)
- Leveling device (e.g., carpenter's, laser, or line level)
- Intravenous (IV) pole
- If utilizing fiberoptic catheter with internal transducer:
  - ❖ Stand-alone monitor (for interpretation of fiberoptic data)
  - ❖ Preamp connector cable (connects catheter to stand-alone monitor)
  - ❖ Monitoring cable (connects stand-alone monitor to bedside monitor)

PATIENT AND FAMILY EDUCATION

- Explain the procedure to the patient and family. This procedure may be performed at the bedside and require the patient to be sedated, paralyzed, and/or intubated. *Rationale:* This preserves the ethical principles of informed consent, veracity, and autonomy by providing complete information around the procedure, which empowers the patient and family to decide the direction of their care.[19] Furthermore, patient cooperation during cranial access is of utmost importance for optimal positioning of the catheter and reducing the risk of further injury. The patient and family should be aware that the patient may need to be intubated to maintain a patent airway, ensure adequate oxygenation, and maintain a normal ICP and an adequate CPP.
- Explain the need for safety precautions, such as head of bed elevation, risks associated with overdrainage/underdrainage of CSF, and protection of the catheter insertion site (e.g., from touching with contaminated hands, pulling at the catheter). *Rationale:* Teaching may prevent adverse events during ICP monitoring, ensure accuracy of ICP readings, and reduce the risk of ventriculitis.[6]
- Assess the patient and family for understanding of ICP pressure monitoring. *Rationale:* Knowledge and information may lessen anxiety.
- Explain the family's role in maintenance of an optimal ICP with limitation of patient stimulation, especially during periods of ICP elevations (decreased noise, decreased tactile stimulation, and low lighting). *Rationale:* Environmental factors and nursing interventions affect ICP. Knowledge and information can prevent adverse events, may lessen anxiety, and provides expectations around potential complications.
- Explain the waveforms on the bedside monitor and how CSF diversion, catheter occlusion, and so on impact waveform morphology. Delineate the differences between continuous and intermittent CSF drainage as prescribed. *Rationale:* As a member of the care team, the patient and family can add additional vigilance to ICP management. This explanation presents to the patient and family a more realistic expectation of the events to come.

PATIENT ASSESSMENT AND PREPARATION

Patient Assessment

- Assess for allergies. *Rationale:* Insertion of an external ventricular catheter requires the use of an antiseptic to cleanse the site, local anesthetic, and possibly systemic analgesia and sedation. External ventricular catheters may be impregnated with antibiotics (e.g., clindamycin, rifampin, or minocycline), or systemic antibiotics may be given periprocedurally or prophylactically. Assessment minimizes the risk of allergic reaction.
- Obtain a baseline assessment to include level of consciousness (LOC), mental status, pupil assessment (with pupillometry, if possible), motor capability, sensation, cranial nerves, language, speech, and vital signs. *Rationale:* A baseline neurological assessment enables the nurse to identify changes that may occur during or as a result of the intraventricular/fiberoptic catheter placement.[5]
- Obtain the patient's medical and surgical history to include use of aspirin; use of anticoagulants; prior craniotomies; and the presence of aneurysm clips, embolic materials, permanent balloon occlusions, detachable coils, or a ventriculoperitoneal shunt. *Rationale:* The information obtained determines and guides future treatment based on the neurological examination results and evidence from radiology and angiography.
- Assess the patient's current laboratory profile, including complete blood count, platelet count, prothrombin time, international normalized ratio, and partial thromboplastin

time. ***Rationale:*** Baseline coagulation studies determine the risk for bleeding during intraventricular catheter insertion.[4]

PATIENT PREPARATION

- Verify the correct patient with two identifiers. ***Rationale:*** Before performing a procedure, the nurse should ensure the correct identification of the patient for the intended intervention.
- Ensure that informed consent has been obtained. ***Rationale:*** Informed consent protects the rights of the patient and makes a competent decision possible for the patient;

however, in emergency circumstances, time may not allow for the consent form to be signed.
- Perform a preprocedure verification and time out. ***Rationale:*** This ensures patient safety and reduces error.
- Assess for patency of IV access, and administer preprocedural analgesia or sedation as prescribed. ***Rationale:*** The patient must remain still during catheter insertion. Analgesia and sedation can also assist in lowering ICP.
- Assist the patient to the supine position with the head of the bed at 30 to 45 degrees and the neck in a midline, neutral position. ***Rationale:*** This position provides access for intraventricular/fiberoptic catheter insertion and enhances jugular venous outflow, contributing to possible reduction in ICP.[14]

Procedure	Intracranial Pressure Monitoring and Cerebrospinal Fluid Drainage	
Steps	Rationale	Special Considerations

External Ventricular Drain (EVD) System Assembly

1. HH		
2. PE	Ensures sterile technique	
3. With aseptic technique, flush through the pressure tubing and drainage system with preservative-free saline solution,[17] turning the stopcocks as needed to prime the entire system. Inspect for air bubbles, and flush until removed. When complete, close the stopcock toward the syringe to prevent air entering the system. Remove the syringe, and replace it with a sterile nonvented cap.	Prepares the drainage system for use; flushes air from the system. If air is left in the tubing, it may alter the numeric value or prevent the flow of CSF.[13,15,17]	Use of a syringe filled with sterile, preservative-free normal saline solution to prime the EVD system tubing rather than a bag of flush solution lessens the risk of flush solution being administered through the ventricular catheter into the brain. In addition, the use of a flushless transducer at the zero reference on the drainage system eliminates lengthy tubing that may dampen the waveform (Fig. 87.6).

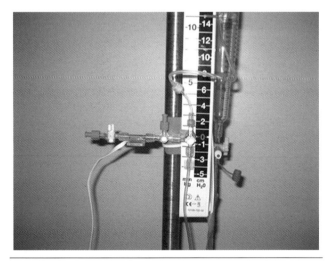

Figure 87.6 External ventricular drainage system with flushless transducer at zero reference level. *(Courtesy Integra Lifesciences Corporation, Plainsboro, NJ.)*

Procedure	Intracranial Pressure Monitoring and Cerebrospinal Fluid Drainage—*Continued*	
Steps	Rationale	Special Considerations
4. Connect the end of the EVD drainage system tubing to the distal stopcock of the pressure monitor tubing (see Fig. 87.6) if not already included in the drainage system. Tighten all connections.[10,13]	Ensures that the system is secure and is a sterile closed system.	
5. Close the clamp or stopcock between the graduated burette and the drainage collection bag (Fig. 87.7).	Ensures the ability to measure hourly drainage in the drip chamber.	

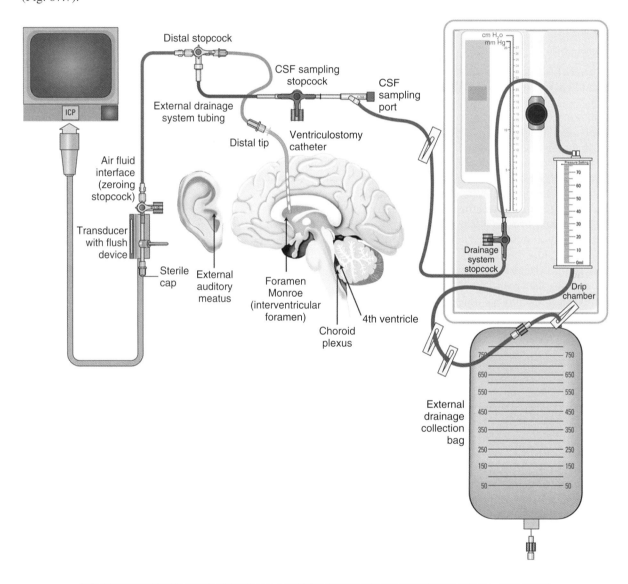

Figure 87.7   External ventricular drainage system. *CSF,* Cerebrospinal fluid. *(Drawing courtesy Paul Schiffmacher, Thomas Jefferson University, Philadelphia, PA.)*

Procedure continues on following page

Procedure | **Intracranial Pressure Monitoring and Cerebrospinal Fluid Drainage—*Continued***

Steps	Rationale	Special Considerations
6. Replace all vented caps with nonvented caps.	Vented caps are used by the manufacturer to permit sterilization of the entire system. These caps must be replaced with sterile nonvented caps to prevent bacteria and air from entering the system.	
7. After flushing the pressure monitor tubing and the external ventricular drainage system tubing, turn the distal stopcock off to the distal tip of the pressure monitor tubing (Fig. 87.8).	The stopcock in this position readies the entire system for connection to the ventriculostomy catheter and prevents flow of fluid into the graduated burette.	

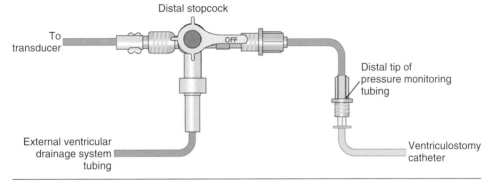

Figure 87.8 Distal stopcock turned off to the distal tip of the pressure monitor tubing. *(Drawing courtesy Paul Schiffmacher, Thomas Jefferson University, Philadelphia, PA.)*

Steps	Rationale	Special Considerations
8. Position the reference level of the drip chamber as prescribed (usually in cm H$_2$O)	The relationship of the reference level of the graduated burette to the anatomical reference point alters the rate of CSF drainage.	The reference level of the drip chamber may need to be adjusted after insertion of the ventricular catheter and the initial ICP is obtained. The reference level is individualized for each patient based on etiology, pathophysiology, management strategies, and patient response.
9. Discard used supplies.	Removes and safely discards used supplies.	
10. **HH**		

Assisting the Provider With Insertion of an Intraventricular Catheter

1. **HH**		
2. **PE** (per institutional policy)		
3. Place the patient in the supine position with the head of the bed elevated for ventricular catheter placement.	Facilitates insertion of the catheter.	Administer sedation and analgesia as prescribed, and monitor the patient per institutional standards for procedural sedation monitoring.
4. Assist as needed with antiseptic preparation of the insertion site.	Reduces the transmission of microorganisms into the ventricles.	Antiseptic agents vary with institutional policies. The choice of povidone iodine versus chlorhexidine as an antiseptic agent is controversial.[6] Both should be allowed to dry completely.

UNIT III

Procedure Intracranial Pressure Monitoring and Cerebrospinal Fluid Drainage—*Continued*		
Steps	**Rationale**	**Special Considerations**
5. For insertion of a fiberoptic ventricular catheter with an internal transducer, calibrate to atmospheric pressure (zero) per the manufacturer's guidelines before the provider inserts the catheter.	Fiberoptic catheters (ventricular or parenchymal) require calibration to atmospheric pressure before insertion. This process must be done before provider insertion and ensures accuracy of the ICP measurement once inserted.	See the procedure "Calibrating to Atmospheric Pressure ("Zeroing") the Transducer (Fiberoptic/Internal Transducer)" below.
6. Connect the drainage/monitoring system to the external tip of the catheter after it is inserted.	Establishes the drainage system.	Observe for initiation of CSF drainage, and obtain an opening ICP.
7. Assist as needed with application of a sterile, occlusive dressing or per institutional standards. Secure the catheter to minimize manipulation and the risk of inadvertent removal.[6,17]	Reduces the risk of infection[6,13]	
8. Label the EVD system visibly and distinctly to differentiate from the intravenous tubing.	Avoids accidental instillation of intravenous medications via the intrathecal route.[6]	
9. Discard supplies.		
10. 🅷🅷		
Connecting the EVD Transducer to the Bedside Monitor		
1. 🅷🅷		
2. 🅿🅴		
3. Turn on the bedside monitor.		
4. Attach a pressure cable into the appropriate pressure module or port in the bedside monitor (see Fig. 87.6).	The signal is transmitted to the bedside monitor so measurements may be converted to waveforms for display and nurse adjudication.	
5. Attach the pressure cable to the transducer connection (attached to the primed pressure tubing of the drainage system).	Ensures the connection from the transducer to the bedside monitor.	
6. Turn on the ICP parameter.	Visualizes the correct waveform.	
7. Set the appropriate scale for the measured pressure.	It is necessary to visualize the complete waveform and to obtain corresponding numerical values. Waveforms vary in amplitude, depending on the pressure within the system.	The normal ICP for an adult is within the range of 0–15 mm Hg.[14,17] Elevated ICPs outside of this range will require adjustment of scale to visualize and properly adjudicate the complete waveform for accuracy.
8. Set the monitor alarm limits for ICP and CPP.	Goals for ICP management are individualized for each patient based on etiology, pathophysiology, and management strategies.	
9. 🅷🅷		
Leveling the Transducer		
1. 🅷🅷		
2. 🅿🅴		
3. Position the patient in the supine position with the head of the bed elevated as prescribed by the provider.[15,17]	Prepares the patient.	The head of the bed is usually placed at 30 degrees to aid in increasing venous return.[11,17]

Procedure continues on following page

Procedure	Intracranial Pressure Monitoring and Cerebrospinal Fluid Drainage—*Continued*	
Steps	Rationale	Special Considerations
4. Place the transducer at the level of the external auditory meatus (see Fig. 87.6).	The external auditory meatus approximates the level of the foramen of Monro (intraventricular foramen).[13,17] Ensure the proper CSF drainage amount to prevent ventricular collapse and possible herniation.[13,15,17]	Some institutions use the tragus or a line drawn from the outer canthus of the eye.[17] Follow institutional policy.
5. Discard supplies.		
6. ▢▢		

Calibrating to Atmospheric Pressure ("Zeroing") the Transducer (External Transducer)

1. ▢▢		
2. ▢▢		
3. Turn the transducer stopcock off to the patient.	Prepares the system for the zeroing procedure.	
4. If indicated for the drainage/ monitoring system in use: remove the nonvented cap from the stopcock, thus opening the stopcock to air.	Sets the atmospheric pressure as a zero reference point.	Some drainage systems may not require removing a cap but simply adjusting the drip chamber to 0 cm H_2O or 0 mm Hg during zeroing and retuning the drip chamber to the level prescribed after the bedside monitor displays a "0" digital value. Follow the catheter manufacturer guidelines and institutional standards.
5. Push and release the zeroing button on the bedside monitor. Observe the digital reading until it displays a value of zero.	Ensures that the monitor has successfully established a zero reference point. Zeroing negates the effects of atmospheric pressure.	Some monitors require that the zero be turned and adjusted manually.
6. Place a new, sterile, nonvented cap on the stopcock.	Maintains sterility.	
7. Turn the stopcock so it is open to the transducer. Observe the ICP waveform and the corresponding numerical value.	Permits pressure monitoring.	
8. Discard used supplies.		
9. ▢▢		

Calibrating to Atmospheric Pressure ("Zeroing") the Transducer (Fiberoptic/Internal Transducer)

1. ▢▢		
2. ▢▢		
3. Ensure that the preamp cable connects the catheter to the stand-alone monitor.	Prepares the system. The catheter is zeroed before insertion and is never rezeroed.	
4. Follow the manufacturer's instructions for zeroing the catheter before insertion.	Sets the atmospheric pressure as a zero reference point. Zeroing negates the effects of atmospheric pressure.	
5. After catheter placement, follow the manufacturer's instructions for the "synchronize to the monitor" interface.	Ensures accurate fiberoptic data at the bedside monitor and allows printing of the ICP tracing.	Ensure the proper CSF drainage amount to prevent ventricular collapse and possible herniation.[14]
6. Place the zero reference at the appropriate external anatomical landmark of the external ventricular drainage device (see Fig. 87.7).		Some institutions use the tragus or a line drawn from the outer canthus of the eye. Follow institutional policy.
7. ▢▢		

UNIT III

Procedure	Intracranial Pressure Monitoring and Cerebrospinal Fluid Drainage—*Continued*

Steps	Rationale	Special Considerations

Monitoring Intracranial Pressure (Continuous Drainage, Intermittent Monitoring)

1. HH
2. PE

Steps	Rationale	Special Considerations
3. Ensure that the head of the bed is at 30 to 45 degrees, the transducer is at the level of the external auditory meatus (or institutional anatomical landmark), and the graduated burette is at the prescribed level.	Allows for accurate and consistent monitoring of the ICP and reduces the risk for overdrainage or underdrainage of CSF. An example of the prescribed level of the graduated burette is 10 cm H_2O above the external auditory meatus.	If continuous drainage is prescribed, the risk of overdrainage of CSF is increased. Unpredicted patient movement and unmonitored ICPs during continuous drainage are some of the potential risks. Bed control locks and bedside monitor parameter alarms can mitigate but not eliminate risk. Continuous drainage is associated with greater risk than intermittent drainage. Excessive drainage may cause overdrainage and a possible collapse of the ventricles, resulting in tearing of the bridging veins of the brain and causing a subdural hematoma.[13,17]
4. Turn the transducer stopcock off to the graduated burette (see Fig. 87.8).	Decreases artifact from simultaneous drainage. Allows for accurate monitoring of ICP by ensuring an uninterrupted fluid column from the patient to the transducer. To obtain an accurate ICP, the stopcock must be turned off to the drain with the catheter open to the transducer only.	Fiberoptic ventricular catheters with internal transducers do not require a turn of the stopcock for accurate measurement.
5. Observe and adjudicate the ICP waveform and value displayed for at least 5 minutes.[12,16]	Provides a value for ongoing assessment. Allows complete analysis of the ICP waveform as the waveform and numeric value of the ICP must be given time to stabilize. The waveform and numeric value of the ICP should correspond.	The normal ICP waveform has at least three distinct pressure oscillations or peaks. These are referred to as P_1, P_2, and P_3 (see Fig. 87.1).[14] Changes in waveform morphology can be attributed to changing intracranial dynamics, compliance of surrounding brain, or obstruction with a clot, tissue, or protein.[7,17,18]
6. Monitor and record ICP (value and waveform) and CPP as prescribed.	Assesses the ICP waveform and values and the CPP value.	Deviations in ICP and CPP may require immediate intervention and should be reported to the provider.[9] Note any changes in CSF flow.
7. Assess, monitor, and record the quantity and quality of CSF output.	Changes in baseline quality and quantity of CSF may require future interventions.	Decreased CSF output could indicate previous overdrainage, ventricular collapse, or catheter obstruction. Increased CSF output could indicate current overdrainage and lead to risk of complications. Changes in quality of CSF could indicate rebleeding or infection.
8. Ensure that the transducer and graduated burette are at the prescribed levels. Resume continuous CSF drainage by turning the transducer stopcock off to the transducer (open to the graduated burette and patient).	Allows for continuous CSF drainage.	If not using a fiberoptic ventricular catheter, opening the transducer stopcock to continuous drainage prevents accurate ICP monitoring during CSF drainage.

Procedure continues on following page

Procedure	**Intracranial Pressure Monitoring and Cerebrospinal Fluid Drainage—*Continued***	
Steps	Rationale	Special Considerations

9. PE
10. HH

Monitoring Intracranial Pressure (Continuous Monitoring, Intermittent Drainage)

1. HH
2. PE

3. Ensure that the head of the bed is 30 to 45 degrees, the transducer is level with the external auditory meatus (or institutional anatomical landmark), and the stopcock is turned off to the graduated burette.	Allows for accurate and consistent monitoring of the ICP and reduces risk for overdrainage or underdrainage of CSF. To obtain an accurate ICP, the stopcock must be turned off to the graduated burette with the catheter open to the transducer only.	Fiberoptic ventricular catheters with internal transducers do not require a turn of the stopcock for accurate measurement.
4. Observe and adjudicate the ICP waveform and value displayed.	Provides a value for ongoing assessment. Allows complete analysis of the ICP waveform as the waveform and numeric value of the ICP. The waveform and numeric value of the ICP should correspond.	Incongruous ICP values and waveforms should not be validated as accurate.
5. Compare the ICP value with the ICP parameter prescribed by the provider. Evaluate if prescribed measures are needed to maintain ICPs below the prescribed parameter.	CSF diversion may be necessary to maintain an ICP below the prescribed parameter if positioning is not successfully managing elevated ICP. For example, if the provider prescribes the ICP to be maintained at <15 mm Hg, drainage of CSF will be initiated if the patient's ICP is >15 mm Hg.	Assess the patency of the system when applicable by lowering the system briefly to assess for CSF dripping into the burette (then return to the ordered anatomical landmark).
6. If indicated, drain the prescribed amount of CSF by turning the transducer stopcock off to the transducer (Fig. 87.9).	Allows the flow of CSF from the ventricles. Draining the prescribed amount mitigates overdrainage of the ventricles.	Never leave a draining EVD unattended. Excessive drainage may cause overdrainage and a possible collapse of the ventricles, resulting in tearing of the bridging veins of the brain and causing a subdural hematoma.

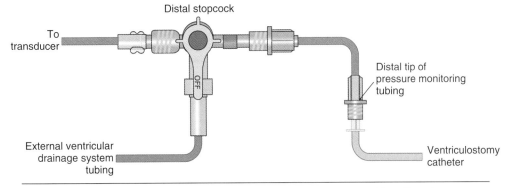

Figure 87.9 Distal stopcock turned off to the external drainage system tubing. (*Drawing courtesy Paul Schiffmacher, Thomas Jefferson University, Philadelphia, PA.*)

UNIT III

UNIT III

Procedure Intracranial Pressure Monitoring and Cerebrospinal Fluid Drainage—*Continued*		
Steps	**Rationale**	**Special Considerations**
7. When drainage is completed, turn the distal stopcock off to the graduated burette (see Fig. 87.8). Record the amount of CSF drained and the postdrainage ICP value.	Check the ICP value to determine whether the parameter is met.	If unable to achieve the prescribed CSF drainage amount, notify the provider.
8. If the ICP parameter is not met after prescribed CSF drainage, contact the provider for additional orders.	CSF drainage alone may not adequately lower ICP. Additional sedation or provider intervention may be necessary.	
9. **PE**		
10. **HH**		
CSF Sampling		
1. **HH**		
2. **PE**		
3. Verify the provider order from for a CSF sample, including laboratory test type and frequency.	Provider orders ensure the necessary institutional steps to successfully process the CSF sample.	If a comparison of serum glucose and CSF glucose is prescribed, a serum glucose sample should be obtained at the same time as the CSF sampling. Normal CSF glucose is two-thirds of blood glucose.[11]
4. Obtain the supplies for sterile CSF sampling as outlined in institutional policies. Open the packaging before donning sterile gloves.	Prepares for the nursing procedure.	
5. Apply the mask with face shield and sterile gloves.	Reduces the transmission of microorganisms and body fluids; standard precautions.	
6. Cleanse the CSF sampling port with an antiseptic solution per institutional policy. Allow the solution to dry.	Reduces the transmission of microorganisms into the ventricles.	
7. Turn the transducer stopcock off to the transducer, and turn the stopcock to the drainage bag under the graduated burette off to the drainage bag (Fig. 87.10).	Allows for direct sampling of CSF while reducing potential contamination or complications.	

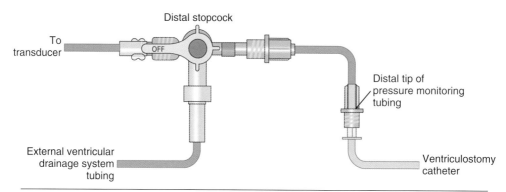

Figure 87.10   Distal stopcock turned off to the transducer. *(Drawing courtesy Paul Schiffmacher, Thomas Jefferson University, Philadelphia, PA.)*

Procedure continues on following page

Patient Monitoring and Care —*Continued*

Steps	Rationale	Special Considerations
8. Slowly withdraw the amount of CSF sample needed by institution from the designated sampling port, and transfer each into a specimen tube. If resistance is met during aspiration, do not continue and notify the provider. Include the sampling amount in the hourly CSF output charting.	Obtains the prescribed sample.	Follow institutional standards for differentiating culture and Gram stain samples from other CSF laboratory testing (e.g., glucose, cell count).
9. Turn the distal stopcock to resume monitoring or resume drainage as prescribed.	Continues monitoring or drainage as prescribed.	
10. Label the CSF specimen tubes in the room, and send them to the laboratory for analysis.	Ensures accurate patient results and prepares the specimen for analysis.	
11. Discard used supplies.	Removes and safely discards used supplies.	
12. 🄿🄴		
13. 🄷🄷		

Expected Outcomes

- Aseptic drainage system
- Accurate and reliable ICP monitoring, CPP calculation, and assessment of cerebral compliance
- Maintenance of ICP within the range of 0 to 15 mm Hg or as prescribed
- Early detection of elevated ICP trends
- Management of increased ICP and decreased CPP
- Protection of cerebral perfusion with maintenance of CPP within prescribed parameters
- Improvement or stabilization of neurological function

Unexpected Outcomes

- CSF infection
- CSF leakage
- Air within the drainage system
- Dislodgment or occlusion of the interventricular/fiberoptic catheter
- Dislodging of the fiberoptic bolt
- Pneumocephalus
- Cerebral hemorrhage
- Sequelae of sustained increased ICP and decreased CPP: cerebral infarction, herniation, and brain death

Patient Monitoring and Care

Steps	Rationale	Reportable Conditions
		These conditions should be reported to the provider if they persist despite nursing interventions.
1. Assess neurological status and vital signs of the patient per provider order or institutional policy.	Evaluates the patient's response to the procedure and trends changes in status. Provides clinical confirmation of and correlation with the monitored ICP data.	• Changes in neurological status • Abnormal vital signs or significant changes in vital sign trends
2. Assess the patient for pain and agitation per institutional standards, and administer medications as prescribed.	Identifies the need for pain interventions, maintains safety around the EVD, and serves as an element of ICP management. Upholds the ethical principle of beneficence.[19]	• Disproportionate change in level of consciousness or pain refractory to analgesia

UNIT III

UNIT III

Patient Monitoring and Care —*Continued*		
Steps	**Rationale**	**Reportable Conditions**
3. Monitor and record each of the following parameters as prescribed: A. ICP (value and waveform) B. CPP C. CSF drainage (amount, color, clarity) and patency of the system.	Assesses the components of neurological status. Provides anticipatory data based on trends. CPP parameters should be individualized to meet the patient's perfusion needs.	• Any gradual or sudden sustained increase in ICP, with or without accompanying neurological changes • Inability to maintain CPP within prescribed parameters • Lack of drainage in the presence of significantly increased ICP requires immediate reporting to the provider; this may indicate an occlusion of the catheter[13,17] or persistent contact of the CSF catheter with the ventricular wall. • Changes in CSF color to bright red with increased output could indicate new-onset bleeding. Changes in CSF clarity or viscosity could indicate infection.
4. If continuous drainage is used, record and monitor CSF output every 1–2 hours. If continuous monitoring with intermittent drainage is ordered, record and monitor CSF output as needed.	Ensures accurate measuring of CSF output necessary to maintain ICP within the provider-established parameter.	• CSF drainage outside of prescribed volume parameters (both high and low parameters) • ICP goal not met after CSF drainage
5. Zero the transducer: A. During the initial setup (or before insertion) B. When connections become dislodged C. When the values do not fit the clinical picture	Ensures accuracy of ICP monitoring.	• Values that do not fit the clinical picture
6. Clamp the EVD during position changes.	Minimizes the risk for underdrainage or overdrainage.	• CSF drainage outside of prescribed volume parameters (both high and low parameters)
7. Maintain the reference level of the transducer and the graduated burette as prescribed.	The relationship of the reference for CSF drainage and ICP monitoring level of the drip chamber to the anatomical reference point alters the rate of CSF drainage.	• Any erroneous ICP values recorded from an unleveled transducer.
8. Maintain the head of the bed at 30 degrees or at the level prescribed by the provider. Maintain neutral head alignment.	Enables venous return to the heart, effectively lowering ICP.	• Elevated ICP despite proper head alignment, head elevation, and prescribed CSF drainage
9. Assess the patency of the drainage system.	Ensures that the catheter is able to drain CSF when needed and that ICP values are accurate since a solid fluid column between the patient and the transducer is necessary for measurement accuracy.	• Lack of drainage or sluggish drainage. The provider may need to irrigate the catheter to reestablish patency. Other maneuvers may include turning or stimulating a cough. Some institutional policies allow the critical care nurse to irrigate the catheter with a limited amount of preservative-free saline solution. Follow institutional standards.
10. Check the system every hour and as needed.	Ensures integrity of the system and absence of air. Aspect of safety surveillance in patient care.	• New drainage system is needed so they can connect the new system to the ventricular catheter.

Procedure continues on following page

Patient Monitoring and Care —*Continued*

Steps	Rationale	Reportable Conditions
11. Set the bedside monitor alarm parameters to correspond with the ICP and CPP goals established by the provider.	Provides an immediate alarm for high and low ICP pressures, which can indicate dangerous patient conditions such as elevated ICP and disconnection of the drainage system, respectively.	• ICP and CPP values sustained outside of provider-established parameters
12. Change the dressing at the catheter insertion site per institutional standards.	Maintains sterility and provides an opportunity for insertion site assessment.[6,17]	• Signs/symptoms of infection, swelling or leaking at the insertion site, or loosened sutures
13. Provide a safe environment to prevent inadvertent dislodgement of the intraventricular/fiberoptic catheter through appropriate catheter positioning and safety measures as needed.	Inadvertent dislodgement of the catheter must be avoided because it can result in pneumocephalus, excessive CSF drainage, ventriculitis, or other patient injury.	• Dislodged ventricular catheter, abnormal ICP value, or abnormal ICP waveform
14. Change the drainage bag and drainage system as needed by institutional standards.	Maintains an intact and closed drainage system.	• Disconnection or need to connect a new drainage system to the ventricular catheter

Documentation

Documentation should include the following:
- Procedural documentation per institutional standards
- Patient and family education
- Initial opening ICP and CPP
- Hourly ICP and CPP[9]
- Analysis of waveform[13,17] with each ICP value recorded
- Nursing interventions used to treat ICP or CPP deviations and outcomes
- Level of the graduated burette and anatomical landmark for zeroing
- Patency of drainage system
- CSF output every 1 to 2 hours or amount drained intermittently[17]
- Description of CSF to include amount, clarity, and color
- Insertion site assessment
- Neurological assessment
- Site care and change of drainage system or bag
- Pain assessment, interventions, and evaluation

References and Additional Readings

For a complete list of references and additional readings for this procedure, scan this QR code with your smartphone, or visit https://www.elsevier.com/__data/assets/pdf_file/0003/1319862/Chapter 0087.pdf.

PROCEDURE

88

Lumbar Puncture (Perform) AP

Faith Newton Good

PURPOSE A lumbar puncture (LP) is performed for access to the subarachnoid space to obtain a cerebrospinal fluid (CSF) sample, measure CSF pressure, drain CSF, infuse medications or contrast agents, and/or place a CSF drainage catheter.[1,3,4,7]

PREREQUISITE NURSING KNOWLEDGE

- Knowledge of neuroanatomy and physiology of the vertebral column, spinal meninges, and CSF circulation, including the location of the lumbar cistern.
- Technical and clinical competence in performing LP.
- Knowledge of sterile technique.
- The presence of meningeal irritation caused by either infectious meningitis or subarachnoid hemorrhage may promote discomfort when the patient is placed in the flexed, lateral decubitus position for the LP.[4-6,21]
- Computed tomography (CT) scan or magnetic resonance imaging supersedes the routine use of LP for many diagnoses.[6,8,22,32]
- Indications for LP include the following[5,6,22,32]:
    - Differential diagnosis of subarachnoid hemorrhage, central nervous system infection, central nervous system autoimmune processes, demyelinating or inflammatory diseases, and some malignant diseases.
    - Therapeutic treatment of hydrocephalus, CSF fistulas, and pseudotumor cerebri.
    - Medication or contrast material administration into the subarachnoid space (e.g., shunt infections or chemotherapy for leukemias involving cerebrospinal involvement).
    - Prevention or management of spontaneous, traumatic, or surgical CSF infections to allow any tears in the dura mater to heal by reducing moisture and pressure at the site of the tear and may be placed before, during, or after surgery.
    - Management of ICP instead of or with an external ventricular drain to drain CSF and remove blood from the subarachnoid space, which may lessen aneurysmal subarachnoid hemorrhage vasospasm.
- Contraindications for LP include the following[4,22,32,33]:
    - Physiological disturbances such as known or suspected intracranial mass or elevated ICP, noncommunicating hydrocephalus, superficial skin infection localized to the site of entry, or congenital spine abnormality.
    - Brain herniation may occur after punctures in the presence of an intracranial mass lesion (e.g., posterior fossa tumors) or increased ICP. A computed tomographic (CT) scan before lumbar puncture subarachnoid catheter insertion to confirm discernible basal cisterns and absence of a mass lesion may lesson the risk of herniation.
    - Platelet count <50,000/mm[4]
    - International normalized ratio >1.5
    - Anticoagulation therapy (e.g., heparin, warfarin)
- Normal CSF values include the following[22,25,27,32]:
    - Opening pressure, 0 to 15 mm Hg
    - White blood cell count, <5/mm
    - Glucose, 60% to 70% of serum blood glucose
    - Protein, 15 to 45 mg/dL
    - Clear colorless appearance
    - Negative culture results
- Recommended CSF tests include the following[22,25,28,32]:
    - Tube #1: Biochemistry:
        - Glucose
        - Protein
        - Protein electrophoresis (if clinically indicated)
    - Tube #2: Bacteriology:
        - Gram stain
        - Bacterial culture
        - Fungal culture (if clinically indicated); requires larger volume
        - Tuberculosis culture (if clinically indicated); requires larger volume
    - Tube #3: Hematology:
        - Cell count
        - Differential
    - Tube #4: Optional studies as indicated:
        - Venereal disease research laboratory test
        - Oligoclonal bands
        - Myelin protein
        - Cytology

AP This procedure should be performed only by clinicians who have demonstrated competence and are credentialed to perform it. In addition, the procedure must be within the scope of practice defined by their professional licensure, and in accordance with professional practice acts. Physicians, advanced practice nurses, and physician assistants may be credentialed to perform this procedure.

EQUIPMENT

- Sterile gloves, caps, masks with eye shields or goggles, and sterile gowns
- Sterile drapes
- Sterile gauze pads

- Antiseptic solution
- Fenestrated drape
- Manometer with three-way stopcock
- Lidocaine, 1% to 2% (without epinephrine)
- 3- to 5-mL syringe
- 20-, 22-, and 25-gauge needles
- 18-, 20-, or 22-gauge spinal needles
- Four numbered capped test tubes
- Adhesive strip or sterile dressing supplies
- Specimen labels
- Laboratory forms
- Glucometer/phlebotomy equipment for serum or whole blood glucose
- Lumbar tray (may contain many of the aforementioned supplies)

Additional equipment to have available as needed includes the following:

- Rolled towels or small pillows to support the patient during positioning
- Alcohol pads or swab sticks
- Two overbed tables (one for the sterile field; one to position the patient, if necessary)

PATIENT AND FAMILY EDUCATION

- Explain the purpose of the LP procedure to the patient and family. *Rationale:* Explanation may decrease patient and family anxiety.
- Explain the need for the patient to remain still and quiet in the lateral decubitus position with the neck, knees, and hips flexed (knees to chest); the axis of the hips vertical; the back close to the edge of the bed; the head of the bed flat; and no more than one pillow under the head (see Figs. 95.1 and 96.1). If the LP is not successful in this position or the patient cannot tolerate this position, explain that the patient may also be positioned leaning over a bedside table or stand.[6,23,26,28] *Rationale:* Patient cooperation during the examination is elicited; the intervertebral space widens in these positions, facilitating entry of the spinal needle into the subarachnoid space.[3,4,6,7]
- Explain that the procedure may produce some discomfort and that local anesthesia will be injected to minimize pain. Also, explain that the patient may receive some mild analgesic and anxiolytic agents as prescribed and needed. *Rationale:* The patient and family are prepared for what to expect.
- Explain that the patient may find it helpful to lie flat for 1 to 4 hours after the LP. *Rationale:* A flat position may promote dural closure; the position was previously thought to reduce the possibility of postprocedure headache, but studies suggest it is not helpful in the prevention of a headache after the procedure.[1,6,15,29]

PATIENT ASSESSMENT AND PREPARATION

Patient Assessment

- Note any pertinent patient history. *Rationale:* An LP is performed to assist with the diagnosis and management of

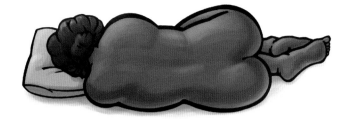

Figure 88.1   The lateral decubitus position appropriate for lumbar puncture. The patient flexes the neck, hips, and knees, and the knees are drawn up tightly to the chest. This increases the intraspinous space for facilitation of needle insertion.

a number of neurological disease processes (see previous indications for LP).

- Obtain a baseline neurological assessment, including assessment for increased ICP, before performing the LP. *Rationale:* Increased ICP during the LP may place the patient at risk for a downward shift in intracranial contents (brain herniation) when the pressure is suddenly released from the lumbar subarachnoid space.[4,22,28,32]
- Assess for coagulopathies, active treatment with heparin, warfarin, or other antiplatelet/anticoagulant medications; local skin infections in close proximity to the site; or pertinent medication allergies. *Rationale:* This assessment identifies potential risks for bleeding, infection, and allergic reactions.[3-6]
- Assess the patient's ability to cooperate with the procedure. *Rationale:* Sudden, uncontrolled movement may result in needle displacement with associated injury or need for reinsertion.
- Identify through history and clinical examination vertebral column deformities or tissue scarring that may interfere with the ability to successfully carry out the procedure. *Rationale:* Scoliosis, lumbar surgery with fusion, and repeated LP procedures may interfere with successful cannulation of the subarachnoid space.[4,26]
- Assess for signs and symptoms of meningeal irritation, which include the following. *Rationale:* A baseline assessment of neurological function is established before the introduction of the needle into the subarachnoid space.
  - ❖ Nuchal rigidity
  - ❖ Photophobia
  - ❖ Brudzinski's or Kernig's sign
  - ❖ Fever
  - ❖ Headache
  - ❖ Nausea or vomiting
  - ❖ Nystagmus

Patient Preparation

- Verify the correct patient with two identifiers. *Rationale:* Before performing a procedure, the nurse should ensure the correct identification of the patient for the intended intervention.
- Ensure that the patient and family understand the preprocedural teaching. Answer questions as they arise, and reinforce information as needed. *Rationale:* Understanding of previously taught information is evaluated and reinforced.

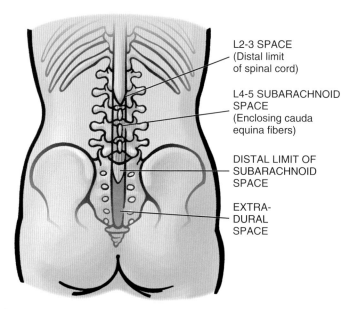

Figure 88.2 The body of the spinal cord ends at L2–L3. The region from L2-L3 through the coccygeal spine encloses the cauda equina (a bundle of lumbar and sacral nerve roots) within the subarachnoid space. It is this area that is appropriate for lumbar puncture.

- Obtain informed consent.[18] **Rationale:** Informed consent protects the rights of the patient and makes competent decision making possible for the patient; however, in emergency circumstances, time may not allow for the consent form to be signed.
- Perform a preprocedure verification and time out, if non-emergent. **Rationale:** Ensures patient safety.

- Obtain the patient's history of allergic reactions. **Rationale:** History can rule out an allergy to lidocaine, the antiseptic solution, and the analgesia or sedation.
- Prescribe an analgesic medication and/or an anxiolytic medication. **Rationale:** These medications may be needed to promote comfort and to decrease anxiety so positioning can be achieved during the procedure.

Procedure for Lumbar Puncture (Perform)

Steps	Rationale	Special Considerations
1. HH		
2. PE		
3. Position or assist with positioning the patient in the lateral recumbent position near the side of the bed with the neck, hips, and knees flexed (knees to chest), the head of the bed flat, and no more than one small pillow under the head (Figs. 88.1 and 88.2). Ask the critical care nurse to assist the patient in attaining and maintaining the position. The nurse should place an arm behind the patient's head and then the other arm around the knees.	The intervertebral space widens in this position, facilitating entry of the spinal needle into the subarachnoid space.	If the LP is not successful in this position or the patient cannot tolerate this position, the patient may also be positioned leaning over a bedside table or stand.[4,23,27,29] Consider performing the LP with fluoroscopy if the patient is morbidly obese or has vertebral column deformities.

Procedure continues on following page

Procedure for Lumbar Puncture (Perform)—*Continued*

Steps	Rationale	Special Considerations
4. With the patient in the lateral decubitus position for examination, identify the intervertebral spaces of L3–L4, L4–L5, and L5–S1; the L3–L4 intervertebral space is level with the top of the iliac crests (see Fig. 88.2).[4,22] **(Level E*)**	The LP is performed below the level of the conus medullaris, which ends at the L1–L2 interspace in the adult. The most common site used for an LP is the L4–L5 intervertebral space, but the L3–L4 or the L5–S1 interspace may be used when cannulation of the L4–L5 interspace is not possible.[5,6,22,31]	An imaginary vertical line is drawn in the midline through the spinous processes between the two iliac crests. A second line is imagined horizontally at the top of the iliac crests and across the spinous processes by the healthcare provider. These lines should intersect the L3–L4 area, and the puncture can be performed at the L3–L4, L4–L5, or L5–S1 interspace.[4,5]
5. Remove ■■, wash hands, and apply sterile gowns and gloves.	Minimizes the risk of infection; maintains sterile precautions.	
6. Set up a sterile field on the bedside stand. A. Preassemble the manometer, attaching the three-way stopcock; set it to the side. B. Open the test tubes, and place them in order of use in the tray slots. C. Draw approximately 3 mL of 1% lidocaine with a 20-gauge needle. Change to a 25-gauge needle for a superficial injection; change to a 22-gauge, 1.5-inch needle for a deeper injection.[4,6,8,32]	Prepares equipment for use in the procedure.	Have the critical care nurse or assistant prepare the numbered labels for the test tubes; ensure that the tubes are labeled in the order in which they are filled to facilitate laboratory differentiation of a traumatic tap versus a subarachnoid hemorrhage.[4,24]
7. Cleanse the skin over the L4–L5 puncture site, including one intervertebral space above and below the site with the antiseptic solution.[11,14,19,21] **(Level C*)**	Reduces transmission of microorganisms and minimizes the risk of infection.	The choice of povidone-iodine or chlorhexidine as an antiseptic agent is controversial. Both should be allowed to dry completely. Some practitioners have found chlorhexidine to be safe in practice,[29] although other studies have suggested that chlorhexidine is neurotoxic.[11,21] Emerging evidence suggests that antibiotic resistance is a growing concern to aseptic chlorhexidine use.[13]
8. Drape the patient with exposure of the insertion site.	Minimizes the risk of infection; maintains sterile precautions.	
9. Administer a local anesthetic with a 25-gauge needle, raising a wheal in the skin. Inject a small amount into the posterior spinous region with a 22-gauge needle.[6,32]	Reduces discomfort associated with needle insertion.	

*Level C: Qualitative studies, descriptive or correlational studies, integrative reviews, systematic reviews, or randomized controlled trials with inconsistent results.

*Level E: Multiple case reports, theory-based evidence from expert opinions, or peer-reviewed professional organizational standards without clinical studies to support recommendations

UNIT III

UNIT III

Procedure | for Lumbar Puncture (Perform)—*Continued*

Steps	Rationale	Special Considerations
10. Insert a 22-, 20-, or 18-gauge spinal needle bevel up[9] through the skin into the intervertebral space of L4–L5, with the needle at an angle of 15 degrees cephalad, aiming toward the umbilicus and level with the sagittal midplane of the body.[4,22] **(Level E*)**	Facilitates passage of the needle between intervertebral spaces toward the dura mater. The use of a smaller atraumatic spinal needle has been associated with a reduced rate of post-LP headache and a lower rate of return to hospital for further intervention for postprocedure headache.[9,10,16,17,33,20]	If bone is encountered on needle insertion, pull back slightly, correct the angle to between 15 and 40 degrees cephalad, and reinsert.[5,6,32] Use the interspace above (L3–L4) or below (L5–S1) the original L4–L5 insertion site if difficulty with advancement of the needle is encountered despite correction of the insertion angle.[4,5] Variations in anatomical configuration of the vertebral column, a history of vertebral column surgery, or repeat LPs may necessitate needle insertion at a different level.[4]
11. Once the needle has been advanced approximately 3–4 cm, withdraw the stylet, and check the hub for CSF. If CSF is not present, replace the stylet and advance slightly. Once CSF is draining, advance the needle another 1–2 mm.[4,22] **(Level E*)**	In most adults, a 3- to 4-cm insertion depth is sufficient to enter the subarachnoid space.	A "popping" sensation is often associated with penetration of the dura mater.[4,6,22]
12. Attach the stopcock of the manometer to the needle. Have the patient straighten his or her legs and relax his or her position. Measure the opening pressure, and note the color of the fluid in the manometer.[4,22] **(Level E*)**	Flexing the legs or straining to maintain a position may artificially elevate CSF pressure.[4,8,22] Opening pressure or normal CSF pressure measurements taken at the lumbar area range from 0–20 cm H_2O (0–15 mm Hg or 50–150 mm H_2O).	If the patient was sitting on the side of the bed leaning over the bedside table for the LP, have the patient lie down on his or her side for the CSF pressure measurement.[5]
13. Consider performing the Queckenstedt test. A. If not contraindicated and within institutional policy. Ask the nurse to simultaneously compress the jugular veins for 10 seconds. B. Watch for a change in subarachnoid CSF pressure on the manometer.[6,21]	The Queckenstedt test is used if an obstruction in the spinal subarachnoid space is suspected. A normal response indicates that the pathway between the skull and the lumbar needle is patent. This maneuver is contraindicated in patients with known or suspected elevated ICP; a sudden release of CSF pressure distally can result in herniation.[6,22]	The Queckenstedt test is contraindicated in patients with increased ICP.[6,22] Normal findings reflect a sharp increase in spinal subarachnoid CSF pressure on compression of the jugular veins; on release, pressure returns to precompression levels. A lack of change in CSF pressure indicates an obstruction of CSF flow.

*Level E: Multiple case reports, theory-based evidence from expert opinions, or peer-reviewed professional organizational standards without clinical studies to support recommendations.

Procedure continues on following page

Procedure for Lumbar Puncture (Perform)—*Continued*

Steps	Rationale	Special Considerations

14. Obtain laboratory samples:
  A. Position the first test tube over the stopcock port.
  B. Turn the stopcock, and drain CSF from the manometer into the first test tube.
  C. Continue filling tubes from the hub of the spinal needle; a minimum of 1–2 mL CSF should be collected in each of the first three test tubes. The second and fourth tubes may require up to 8 mL of CSF depending on the tests ordered (e.g., fungal or tuberculosis testing).[5,6]
  D. Return the stopcock to the "off" position, and discard the manometer.
	By draining CSF from the manometer into the test tubes, the CSF volume withdrawn is minimized.[4,6] Allows for progressive clearing of CSF blood in the case of a traumatic tap.[5,6,28,32]	In subarachnoid hemorrhage, CSF with the same consistency of blood is drained in all four test tubes. In the case of a traumatic tap, progressive clearing of bloody CSF occurs as drainage continues. Also, the supernatant of centrifuged CSF should be clear if the tap was traumatic and xanthochromic if blood has been present for several hours and has undergone hemolysis.[5,6,28,32]

15. Cover the opening of the needle with a sterile gloved finger. Replace the stylet, and withdraw the needle.[1,4,8] **(Level E*)**	Covering the opening of the needle with a sterile gloved finger reduces contamination by microorganisms. Replacing the stylet before withdrawing the needle prevents unnecessary CSF loss and facilitates needle withdrawal without traction on the spinal nerve roots. Reinsertion of the stylet before withdrawal of the spinal needle has also been associated with a reduced incidence rate of post-LP headaches.[7,9,16,33]	Minimizes postprocedure headache.[1,3,4]
16. Apply an occlusive sterile dressing to the puncture site.	Decreases the incidence of infection.	
17. Place the patient in the supine or prone position immediately after the procedure.[1,6] **(Level E*)**	In the supine position, the patient's weight acts as site pressure. In the prone position, the increased abdominal pressure transmits pressure to the site.[30] Some physicians, advanced practice nurses, and other healthcare professionals advocate placing the patient in the supine or prone position for 1–4 hours.[1,2,6]	Whether either the prone or supine position facilitates closure of the dura mater after the LP remains unclear. Neither position has been shown to prevent post–dural puncture headache.[1,4,5,30]
18. Label and send specimens to the laboratory. If there is no same-day serum glucose measurement, consider obtaining a serum glucose sample.	Obtains CSF analysis and assists with the differential diagnosis.[5,22,28,32]	Hyperglycemia or hypoglycemia affects CSF glucose values and can interfere with interpretation of results.[6,22,28,32]
19. Discard used supplies in appropriate receptacles.	Removes and safely discards used supplies; safely removes sharp objects.	
20. **HH**		

---

*Level C: Qualitative studies, descriptive or correlational studies, integrative reviews, systematic reviews, or randomized controlled trials with inconsistent results.

*Level E: Multiple case reports, theory-based evidence from expert opinions, or peer-reviewed professional organizational standards without clinical studies to support recommendations.

Expected Outcomes

- No change in neurological status after the procedure
- Determination of the characteristics of the CSF that supports establishment of the diagnosis
- Recommendation for definitive treatment that promotes restoration of health or optimal functional status
- Postsprocedure headache may occur in up to 70% of patients undergoing LP and is usually self-limiting[9,10,16,22]; the incidence of headache may be reduced with the use of smaller-gauge atraumatic spinal needles and reinsertion of the stylet before the needle is withdrawn.[4,7,16,17,20,22,33] Postmortem studies show that conventional needles cause lacerations that remain open, which can lead to CSF leakage, whereas atraumatic needles are less likely to create persistent perforations that facilitate further CSF loss.[12,20]

Unexpected Outcomes

- In cases of a supratentorial mass or severely elevated ICP, a shift in intracranial contents (brain herniation) may be promoted by the sudden decrease in pressure incurred with LP[4,6,22,28]
- Injury of the periosteum or spinal ligaments may produce local back pain[6,30]
- Infectious meningitis may result from an improper technique that produces contamination[5,6,21,22]
- Traumatic taps may result from inadvertent puncture of the spinal venous plexuses; usually this is a self-limiting process, but it may result in a hematoma in patients with bleeding disorders[4-6,32]
- Transient lower-extremity pain may occur from irritation of a spinal nerve[6,32]
- Persistent CSF leak from the puncture site associated with nonclosure of the dura[4,15]
- Inability to obtain a CSF specimen because of healthcare provider skill level, patient intolerance of the procedure, pathological blockage of CSF flow, or aberrant anatomy[4]
- Persistent headache despite interventions[4,15-17]

Patient Monitoring and Care

Steps	Rationale	Reportable Conditions
		These conditions should be reported to the provider if they persist despite nursing interventions.
1. Monitor the patient's neurological status, including the development of a change in level of consciousness, pupil size and reactivity, new onset of pain, motor weakness, or numbness in the lower extremities, and the patient's procedural tolerance throughout and after the procedure.	Changes in neurological status may be related to sudden intracranial decompression with brain herniation or local irritation of a spinal nerve by the needle or hematoma formation at the puncture site.[3-5,21]	• Deterioration in neurological status • Transient lower-extremity motor or sensory changes associated with spinal nerve irritation or hematoma formation
2. Monitor for postprocedure headache.	Headache occurs in up to 70% of patients after LP.[9,10,30,32]	• Intractable postprocedure headache • Drainage from the LP site
3. Monitor for drainage from the puncture site.	Persistent drainage may indicate an unresolved CSF leak.[1,22,30]	• Dural tear that necessitates a patch or closure • Spinal hematoma that necessitates emergent surgical evacuation
4. Monitor the patient's neurological status at a minimum of every 4 hours for 24 hours after the LP.	Lower extremity motor or sensory changes may indicate a hematoma at the puncture site.[22]	
5. Monitor the effectiveness of measures taken to prevent or treat postprocedure headache.[16]	Determines level of comfort.	• Unrelieved headache
6. Follow institutional standards for assessing pain. Consider administration of a mild analgesic agent, and encourage the patient to remain supine or prone until the headache improves.	Additional treatment measures may be necessary to manage postprocedure headache.[27] Although recent studies do not support either the prone or supine position to prevent post–dural puncture headache, lying in one of these positions may relieve the headache.[1,7,9,15,33]	• Intractable postprocedure headache • Dural tear that necessitates patch or closure.[10,14,30,31]

Procedure continues on following page

Documentation

Documentation should include the following:
- Patient and family education
- Completion of informed consent
- Preprocedure verifications and time out
- Performance of the procedure, significant findings, CSF appearance, and opening pressure
- Amount of CSF removed
- Patient tolerance of the procedure
- Change in neurological status associated with the procedure
- CSF specimens obtained
- Pain assessment, interventions, and effectiveness
- Unexpected outcomes
- Additional interventions

References and Additional Readings

For a complete list of references and additional readings for this procedure, scan this QR code with your smartphone, or visit https://www.elsevier.com/__data/assets/pdf_file/0004/1319863/Chapter0088.pdf.

UNIT III

89 Lumbar Puncture (Assist) and Nursing Care

Sarah R. Martha

PURPOSE A lumbar puncture (LP) is performed for access to the subarachnoid space to obtain a cerebrospinal fluid (CSF) sample, measure CSF pressure, drain CSF, infuse medications or contrast agents, and/or place a lumbar drainage catheter.[2,4,10,18]

PREREQUISITE NURSING KNOWLEDGE

- Knowledge of neuroanatomy and physiology of the vertebral column, spinal meninges, spinal cord, nerve roots, CSF circulation, and intracranial and intraspinal dynamics.
- Knowledge of aseptic techniques.
- LP is usually performed at L3–L4 or L4–L5 in an adult to obtain a CSF sample.[12,37,39]
- Normal intraspinal pressure in the adult is 5 to 20 cm H_2O and usually corresponds with intracranial pressure (ICP). Intraspinal pressure is considered elevated pressure when it is greater than 25 cm H_2O. Intraspinal pressure may be influenced by several factors including edema and positioning.[16,28]

Indications for LP include the following:
- Differential diagnosis of subarachnoid hemorrhage, central nervous system infection, central nervous system autoimmune processes, demyelinating or inflammatory diseases, and some malignant diseases.[12,15,35]
- Therapeutic treatment of hydrocephalus, CSF fistulas, and pseudotumor cerebri.[15,39,49]
- Medication or contrast material administration into the subarachnoid space (e.g., shunt infections or chemotherapy for leukemias involving cerebrospinal involvement).[15,39,49]
- Access to the subarachnoid space for placement of a lumbar subarachnoid drain.[15,39,49]
- Prevention or management of spontaneous, traumatic, or surgical CSF fistulas to allow any tears in the dura mater to heal by reducing moisture and pressure at the site of the tear and may be placed before, during, or after surgery.[7,8,14,19,21,43]
- Management of communicating hydrocephalus related to intraventricular, intracerebral hemorrhage.[19,26]
- Reduction of ICP and management of patients with traumatic brain injury.[5]
- Management of patients with meningitis.[27,41,42]
- Perioperative management of intraspinal pressure during and after thoracoabdominal aortic aneurysmal repair to provide adequate room in the intraspinal space to accommodate spinal cord edema and to improve impaired spinal cord perfusion related to spinal cord edema.
- Management of ICP instead of or with an external ventricular drain to drain CSF and remove blood from the

subarachnoid space, which may lessen aneurysmal subarachnoid hemorrhage vasospasm.[24,25,28-30,40,46]

Contraindications for LP include the following:
- Physiological disturbances such as known or suspected intracranial mass or elevated ICP, noncommunicating hydrocephalus, superficial skin infection localized to the site of entry, or congenital spine abnormality.[15,39,49] Brain herniation may occur after punctures in the presence of an intracranial mass lesion (e.g. posterior fossa tumors), intraspinal mass (e.g., intramedullary), or increased ICP.[10,39] Midline mass effect. A computed tomographic (CT) scan before lumbar subarachnoid catheter insertion to confirm discernible basal cisterns and absence of a mass lesion may lessen the risk of herniation.[2,12,48]
- The patient is coagulopathic, receiving anticoagulation, or thrombocytopenic. If CSF analysis is necessary, the patient may need pretreatment with fresh-frozen plasma, platelets, cryoprecipitate, or the specific factor needed to correct a hematological abnormality.[15,39,49]
- Caution should be taken when patients have a suspected aneurysmal subarachnoid hemorrhage or complete spinal blocks. In such cases, an LP may be performed if the computed tomographic (CT) scan of the patient's head does not indicate signs of increased ICP, such as significant cerebral swelling, hematoma, intracranial tissue shifts, or herniation.[15,39,49]

PATIENT POSITIONING

- Optimal positioning is required to avoid the risk for a dry tap or an unsuccessful puncture attempt. Proper positioning for LP widens the interspinous process space and facilitates the passage of the needle.[4,10,17]
- The preferred positioning for LP is the lateral decubitus with the neck, hips, and knees flexed (knees to chest); the axis of the hips vertical; the back close to the edge of the bed; the head of the bed flat; and no more than a small pillow under the head (Fig. 89.1).
- If the LP is not successful in this position or the patient cannot tolerate this position, the patient may also be positioned sitting on the side of the bed, leaning over a bedside table or stand.[44,47,49]
- LPs may also be performed with fluoroscopy, ultrasound, or computed tomography (CT) for patients who are morbidly obese, patients with spinal deformities, or older adults.[12,45]

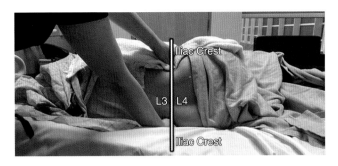

Figure 89.1 The appropriate lateral decubitus position for lumbar puncture. *(From Ellenby MS et al. Lumbar puncture. New England Journal of Medicine 2006;355[13]:e12.)*

Repeated puncture attempts increase the risk for infection, postpuncture headache, and patient discomfort.[10,39]

EQUIPMENT

- Sterile gloves, surgical caps, masks with eye shield, and sterile surgical gowns
- Sterile drapes, sterile towels
- Sterile gauze pads
- Antiseptic solution
- Fenestrated drape
- Manometer with a three-way stopcock
- Lidocaine, 1% to 2% (without epinephrine)
- 3- to 5-mL syringe
- 20-, 22-, and 25-gauge needles
- 20-, 22- and 25- gauge spinal needles
- Sterile suture with needle
- Adhesive strip or sterile dressing supplies (e.g., sterile occlusive dressing)
- Tape (1- and 2-inch rolls)
- Sterile, preservative-free normal saline solution (vial, bag, or prefilled syringe)
- Four consecutively numbered, capped test tubes
- Specimen labels
- Laboratory forms
- Glucometer/phlebotomy supplies for concurrent testing of serum or whole-blood glucose
- Sterile CSF drainage system (tubing, collection bag)
  Additional equipment to have available as needed includes the following:
- Alcohol pads or swab sticks
- Two overbed tables (one for the sterile field; one to position the patient, if necessary)
- Rolled towels or small pillows to support the patient during positioning

PATIENT AND FAMILY EDUCATION

- Provide developmentally and culturally appropriate education based on the desire for knowledge, readiness to learn, and neurological state. *Rationale:* Patient involvement improves compliance during and after the LP procedure and establishes a partnership.
- Explain the purpose of the procedure and the risks, benefits, and complications associated with the procedure to the patient and family. *Rationale:* Understanding of the procedure is reinforced and may decrease anxiety.
- Explain the LP insertion, equipment, monitoring, and care to the patient and family. *Rationale:* Knowledge of expectations can minimize anxiety and encourage questions regarding goals, duration, and expected outcomes of the procedure.
- Explain positioning requirements for the LP and length of time of the procedure. *Rationale:* Cooperation with positioning requirements facilitates the procedure.
- Explain that the nurse will help with position changes to protect the lumbar drainage device. *Rationale:* The patient knows expectations. This will also decrease the risk of overdrainage, which can result in subdural hematoma or sixth nerve palsy.
- Explain that the procedure may cause some mild discomfort. The patient will receive local anesthesia and may also receive some mild analgesia and an anxiolytic. *Rationale:* The patient knows expectations, and anxiety can be reduced.

PATIENT ASSESSMENT AND PREPARATION

Patient Assessment

- Verify the correct patient with two identifiers. *Rationale:* Before performing the LP procedure, the nurse should ensure the correct identity of the patient for the intended LP procedure.
- Ensure that consent is obtained.[34] *Rationale:* Consent protects the rights of the patient and makes competent decision making possible for the patient. In emergency circumstances, time may not allow for consent to be obtained.
- Assess the patient's neurological status. *Rationale:* Establish baseline patient data, including level of consciousness, pupil size and reactivity, sensory and motor function in the upper and lower extremities, vital signs, and bowel and bladder function.
- Assess for signs and symptoms of increased ICP. *Rationale:* Increased ICP during the LP may place the patient at risk for a downward shift in intracranial contents (brain herniation) when the pressure is suddenly released from the lumbar subarachnoid space.
- Assess the patient's current laboratory profile for evidence of a coagulopathy or increased risk of bleeding (e.g., complete blood count, platelets, partial thromboplastin time, prothrombin time, and international normalized ratio). *Rationale:* Baseline values are established. This will determine whether any contraindications are present. Coagulation study results determine the risk for bleeding during and after LP insertion.[25,32,40]
- Review the patient's current medications. *Rationale:* This will determine whether any contraindications are present. Recent anticoagulants or antiplatelet agents may increase the risk of bleeding during and after lumbar subarachnoid catheter insertion.
- Assess for signs and symptoms of meningeal irritation, including the following:
  - Nuchal rigidity
  - Photophobia

❖ Brudzinski's sign (flexion of the knee in response to flexion of the neck)
❖ Kernig's sign (pain in the hamstrings on extension of the knee with the hip at 90-degree flexion)
❖ Fever
❖ Headache
❖ Nausea or vomiting
❖ Nystagmus
• *Rationale*: Baseline neurological function is established before introduction of a needle into the lumbar subarachnoid space.
• Assess for allergies to local anesthetic, antiseptic, and any analgesic or sedative medications. *Rationale:* Risk of allergic reaction is decreased.[4,10,15]

PATIENT PREPARATION

• Administer preprocedural analgesia or sedation as prescribed. *Rationale:* The patient must be correctly positioned and immobile during lumbar subarachnoid catheter insertion and may need sedation or analgesia to tolerate the procedure.
• Administer preprocedural antibiotics as prescribed. *Rationale:* Prophylactic intravenous antibiotics may reduce the risk of infection for patients who are at high risk. Prophylactic antibiotics are not recommended for all patients.
• Perform a preprocedural verification and time out, if nonemergent. *Rationale:* Ensures patient safety; Joint Commission's Universal Protocol for Invasive and Surgical Procedures.

Procedure for Lumbar Puncture (Assist)

Steps	Rationale	Special Considerations
1. HH		Check latest coagulation laboratory tests. Ensure that the patient is not on a heparin drip. This will decrease the risk of bleeding and complications.
2. PE		Practitioners and other healthcare professionals involved in the procedure must apply goggles or masks with face shields, surgical caps, sterile gowns, and sterile gloves.
3. If pressure monitoring is prescribed, assemble a fluid-filled transducer with stopcock and nonvented cap. Using sterile technique, flush the external standalone transducer with sterile, preservative-free normal saline solution.[32] (**Level E***)	Facilitates monitoring after catheter insertion. Preservative in normal saline solution may cause cortical necrosis.[32]	Do not attach a pressurized intravenous fluid bag to the transducer.
4. Using sterile technique, assemble and flush the sterile CSF drainage system compatible with the lumbar subarachnoid catheter device with sterile, preservative-free normal saline solution. Ensure that the filter located at the top of the drainage chamber does not become wet during priming because this will affect drainage.[19,28] (**Level E***)	Prepares the equipment.	Priming the lumbar drainage system with sterile, preservative-free normal saline solution before connecting the system to the lumbar catheter is recommended.[19] Follow institutional standards. It is of note that some physicians prefer and are trained to allow CSF to flush the system once the drain is connected to the catheter.[32]
5. Attach the fluid-filled transducer to the CSF drainage system.	Prepares the equipment.	The transducer may be attached to the CSF drainage system before either is primed, and the transducer may be flushed at the same time the CSF drainage system is primed. Ensure that the cable part of the transducer is facing away from the drainage system.
6. Connect the fluid-filled transducer to the pressure cable and bedside monitor.	Facilitates insertion and immediate lumbar subarachnoid CSF pressure monitoring on insertion.	Ensure that the waveform chosen for CSF monitoring is read on the "mean" setting.
7. Set the reference line of the drip chamber at the level of the transducer, which is typically at zero reference. (Figs. 89.2 and 89.3).	Prepares the CSF drainage system for use.	

*Level E: Multiple case reports, theory-based evidence from expert opinions, or peer-reviewed professional organizational standards without clinical studies to support recommendations.

Procedure continues on following page

Procedure for Lumbar Puncture (Assist)—*Continued*

Steps	Rationale	Special Considerations

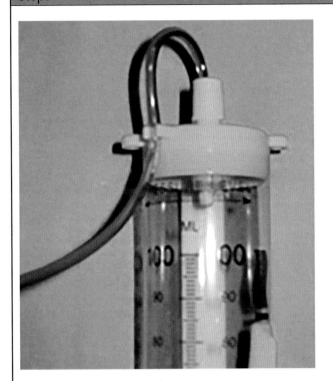

Figure 89.2 Drip chamber at the level of the transducer and the external auditory meatus.

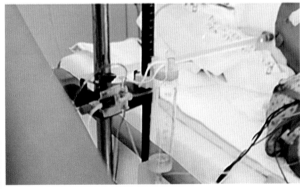

Figure 89.3 Top of the drip chamber with a reference line.

Steps	Rationale	Special Considerations
8. Level the transducer and the zero reference to the anatomic reference point of the patient as prescribed or as per institutional standards.[46] (see Fig. 89.2) **(Level E*)**	Ensures accurate readings on which to base therapy.	The anatomic reference point will be determined by the practitioner and may be the external auditory meatus, shoulder height, or the level of catheter insertion.
9. To zero the system before attaching to the patient, turn the stopcock off to the patient port, remove the nonvented cap on the stopcock, and zero the monitoring system at the anatomic reference point. Replace the sterile nonvented cap. Follow manufacturer's directions. **(Level M*)**	Allows the monitor to use atmospheric pressure as a reference for zero.	The membrane at the top of the drip chamber may allow zeroing without opening the fluid-coupled system to air.

*Level E: Multiple case reports, theory-based evidence from expert opinions, or peer-reviewed professional organizational standards without clinical studies to support recommendations.
*Level M: Manufacturer's recommendations only.

Procedure for Lumbar Puncture (Assist)—*Continued*

Steps	Rationale	Special Considerations
10. Position the reference level of the drip chamber as prescribed.	The relationship of the reference level of the drip chamber to the anatomic reference point alters the rate of CSF drainage.	
11. Assist the patient to the lateral decubitus (side-lying) position, near the side of the bed with the neck, hips, and knees flexed (knees to chest). The head of the bed should be flat, and no more than one small pillow should be under the patient's head (see Fig. 89.1).[10,11,19,39] **(Level E*)**	The intervertebral space widens in this position, facilitating entry of the spinal needle into the lumbar subarachnoid space.	If difficulty is encountered, an alternative position is to have the patient sit on the edge of the bed, leaning over a bedside table. This allows for easier location of midline structures (Fig. 89.4).[11,19,38]

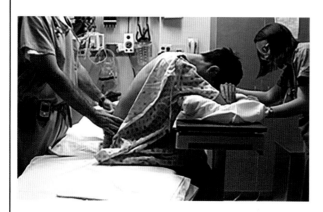

Figure 89.4   Sitting position for lumbar puncture. *(From Roberts JR, Custalow CB, Thomsen TW, editors:* Roberts and Hedges' clinical procedures in emergency medicine and acute care, *ed 7, Philadelphia, 2019, Elsevier.)*

Steps	Rationale	Special Considerations
12. Assist as needed with skin preparation with antiseptic solution.[14,22,23,35,36] **(Level C*)**	Minimizes the risk for infection and protects the insertion site from contamination.	The choice of povidone-iodine or chlorhexidine as an antiseptic agent is controversial. Both should be allowed to dry completely. Studies suggest chlorhexidine may be neurotoxic.[32,36]
13. Assist as needed with draping the patient with sterile sheets and opening sterile trays.	Provides a sterile field for the procedure. Prepares for lumbar catheter insertion.	
14. Provide supplies as needed during catheter insertion.	Facilitates insertion.	Surgeons may insert the lumbar catheter during surgery.
15. Once the needle is in place, instruct the patient to relax and breathe normally and to avoid holding his or her breath. Assist the patient to straighten the legs when indicated by the provider.[12,37] **(Level E*)**	Increased muscle tension or intrathoracic pressure resulting from patients holding their breath may falsely elevate CSF pressure.[12,37] Leg flexion can increase intrathoracic pressure and falsely elevate CSF pressure.[12,37]	

*Level C: Qualitative studies, descriptive or correlational studies, integrative reviews, systematic reviews, or randomized controlled trials with inconsistent results.
*Level E: Multiple case reports, theory-based evidence from expert opinions, or peer-reviewed professional organizational standards without clinical studies to support recommendations.

Procedure for Lumbar Puncture (Assist)—*Continued*

Steps	Rationale	Special Considerations
16. With aseptic technique, assist with holding the manometer in place when it is attached to the spinal needle via a three-way stopcock.	Secures the position of the manometer.	
17. Assist with obtaining the CSF pressure measurement.	Opening pressure or normal CSF pressure measurements taken at the lumbar area range from 5–20 cm H_2O.	The meniscus should show minimal fluctuation related to pulse and respiration. The opening pressure in a traumatic tap is within normal limits unlike the opening pressure in patients with subarachnoid hemorrhage and meningitis.
18. Note the opening CSF pressure (initial), color, and clarity.	Provides baseline data.	
19. Assist with the collection of CSF specimens as needed: A. Assist with stabilizing the manometer with one hand. B. Assist with the handoff of each tube as needed (if not placed upright and in order in the LP tray). Tighten the cap of each tube. C. Label each tube with the patient's name, type of specimen, and the order in which the specimen was collected.	Obtains needed CSF specimens.	
20. Assist with application of an occlusive sterile dressing to the lumbar catheter insertion site.	Reduces contamination and infection of the insertion site.	
21. Secure the lumbar catheter with tape, taking care not to alter the catheter position.	Reduces the potential for lumbar catheter dislodgment.	Some institutions prefer a transparent occlusive dressing to provide visualization of the lumbar catheter insertion site.
22. Attach the CSF drainage system to the lumbar catheter.		
23. Assist the patient to a position of comfort.[3] **(Level C*)**	There is limited evidence to support placing the patient in the prone or supine position. Neither the supine nor prone position has been shown to prevent post–dural puncture headache.	In the supine position, the patient's weight acts as site pressure. In the prone position, the increased abdominal pressure transmits pressure to the site. Some clinicians advocate placing the patient in the supine or prone position for 1–4 hours.
24. If the intraspinal pressure is to be monitored, turn the stopcock off to the patient, and zero the transducer.	Ensures accurate data on which to base therapy.	
25. If intraspinal pressure is to be monitored, observe the waveform morphology, and measure CSF pressure (see also Procedure 87, Intracranial Pressure Monitoring, Nursing Care, Troubleshooting, and Removal).	Provides initial baseline data. Confirms correct placement of the lumbar catheter.	Lumbar CSF pressure waveform data are similar to ICP waveform data. Research supports maintenance of an intraspinal pressure of less than 10 mm Hg after thoracic abdominal aortic resection.[13,20,28]

*Level C: Qualitative studies, descriptive or correlational studies, integrative reviews, systematic reviews, or randomized controlled trials with inconsistent results.

UNIT III

UNIT III

Procedure   for Lumbar Puncture (Assist)—*Continued*

Steps	Rationale	Special Considerations
26. Position the head of the bed as prescribed. Reassess the level of the transducer, zero reference, and level line of the drip chamber. Relevel and rezero as needed. Observe the rate of drainage.	Prevents overdrainage or underdrainage of CSF.	Follow institutional standards and practitioner's orders (e.g., drain based on volume, level, or specific pressure). The hourly drainage amount is generally 10–20 mL/hour.[39,46] Follow orders regarding when to notify the physician regarding troubleshooting and overdraining.
27. Turn the stopcock to continuously monitor with intermittent drainage or to intermittently monitor with continuous drainage. Set alarm limits. Follow institutional standards and physician orders.	The stopcock must be turned off to the drain to obtain an accurate intraspinal pressure.	Set alarms if continuously monitoring to minimize underdrainage or overdrainage.[14]
28. Discard used supplies in an appropriate receptacle.	Removes and safely discards used supplies and personal protective equipment (PPE).	
29. **HH**		
30. Send the specimens to the laboratory.	Ensures that specimens are sent for laboratory analysis.	
31. Document the procedure in the patient's medical record		

LP Troubleshooting

Steps	Rationale	Special Considerations
1. **HH**		
2. **PE**		
3. If the CSF waveform is dampened: A. Assess the integrity of the lumbar catheter device, and correct problems if possible. B. Assess the monitoring system for disconnections, and reconnect the system if needed. C. Assess the level of the transducer, the zero-reference point, and the reference line on the drip chamber for the correct position, and readjust the position and rezero if needed (see Figs 89.2 and 89.3). D. Assess the lumbar drain site.	Damping of the waveform can indicate lumbar catheter occlusion or risk for lumbar catheter displacement. Loose connections may cause dampened waveforms and increase the risk for infection. Loose cables and connecting devices may contribute to mechanical failure.[32] The membrane at the top of the drip chamber may allow zeroing without opening the fluid-coupled system to air. However, one-way valves in the drainage system may affect calibration. If the membrane becomes wet, it may no longer permit accurate readings, and the drip chamber must be changed. The lumbar drain might have migrated or have been pulled accidently.	Lumbar catheter occlusion may result from precipitate in the CSF. Changing the drip chamber involves changing the entire CSF drainage system. Responsibility for changing the CSF drainage system varies among institutions and may not be a nursing responsibility in most institutions. Notify the practitioner for assistance as needed. Notify the practitioner of a broken, dislodged, or disconnected lumbar catheter.
4. Assess for sudden absence of the pressure waveform or significant changes in pressure measurements without an apparent clinical cause. A. Ensure that connections are tight. B. Ensure that leveling is correct. C. Rezero the system.	Ensures accurate measurement of CSF pressure.[46]	Notify the practitioner if a reversible cause cannot be identified. The CSF drainage system or the lumbar catheter may need to be replaced because of lumbar catheter dislodgment or blockage.

Procedure continues on following page

LP Troubleshooting —*Continued*

Steps	Rationale	Special Considerations
5. Assess the flow of CSF through the drainage system by briefly lowering the drip chamber.	Avoids increases in CSF pressure caused by equipment malfunction.[46]	Flushing or changing the system may be necessary. Follow institutional standards as to who is responsible for flushing the system.
6. Discard used supplies in an appropriate receptacle.	Removes and safely discards used supplies and personal protective equipment (PPE).	
7. [HH]		

LP Removal

Steps	Rationale	Special Considerations
1. [HH]		Check the latest coagulation laboratory works. Ensure that the patient is not on heparin drip.
2. [PE]		Comply with universal precautions; personal protective equipment including eye protection should be worn.
3. Assist as needed with removal of the lumbar catheter.	Facilitates lumbar catheter removal.	Culture the lumbar catheter tip as prescribed.
4. Apply a sterile occlusive dressing.	Reduces the risk of infection and contamination.	
5. Discard used supplies in an appropriate receptacle.	Removes and safely discards used supplies.	
6. [HH]		
7. Continue to assess the patient's neurological status and dressing after removal of the lumbar catheter for CSF leak.	Removal of the lumbar catheter may result in neurological deterioration related to increased CSF pressure. CSF leak may indicate increased CSF pressure.[1,9]	

Patient Monitoring and Care

Steps	Rationale	Reportable Conditions
1. Continue monitoring the patient's neurological status and vital signs per practitioner orders and institutional policy. A. Level of consciousness B. Pupillary changes C. Sensation D. Motor function of lower extremities E. Bowel and bladder function F. Comfort level (headache)	Neurological status changes may result from irritation of spinal nerves associated with lumbar catheter placement,[6,28,31] spinal cord damage related to thoracoabdominal aneurysm repair,[6,9,19,28,46] subdural hematoma formation, brain herniation, or tension pneumocranium resulting from overdrainage of CSF.[1,25,29,36] Pain or abnormal sensation radiating down one or both legs may result from spinal nerve irritation, which may necessitate a change in patient or needle position. Respiratory depression or an altered level of consciousness may result from brain herniation or analgesia and sedation.	*These conditions should be reported to the provider if they persist despite nursing interventions.* • Change in level of consciousness • Pupillary changes • Change in sensation of upper and lower extremities • Change in motor function of upper and lower extremities • Changes in bowel and bladder function • Changes in vital signs • Respiratory depression • Headache
2. Follow institutional standards for assessing pain. Administer analgesia as prescribed.	Identifies need for pain interventions.	• Continued pain despite pain interventions

UNIT III

Patient Monitoring and Care —*Continued*

Steps	Rationale	Reportable Conditions
3. Assess the lumbar CSF waveform and pressure, and the color, clarity, and amount of CSF drainage every hour or as prescribed.	Ensures accurate measurement of CSF pressure and monitoring.[31,46]	• Changes in CSF pressure • Changes in amount and/or color of CSF drainage • Changes in CSF waveform morphology • Abnormal CSF pressure
4. Maintain CSF pressure and drainage as prescribed.	In the management of intraspinal pressure after abdominal aortic aneurysm repair, a CSF pressure of <5 mm Hg is recommended.[28,31]	
5. Assess the integrity of the lumbar catheter and drainage device at least hourly.	Determines accurate functioning of the system.	• Loose connections or other openings in the catheter system
6. Zero the monitoring system with insertion, disconnection, or position changes according to institutional standards.	Ensures accuracy of the monitored data.	• Dampened or no waveform after zeroing the monitoring system
7. Assess the insertion site and change the dressing when loose or soiled. Follow institutional standards for dressing changes.	Maintaining an occlusive dressing reduces the risk of infection. Persistent drainage may indicate an unresolved CSF leak.	• Signs or symptoms of infection • Significant drainage at the lumbar catheter insertion site
9. Monitor patient mobility as prescribed to avoid over-drainage or under drain-age.[14,19,25]	Patients may be permitted to sit or ambulate with specific guidelines for placement or clamping of the drainage system.	• Overdrainage or underdrainage with mobility restrictions • Headache
10. Prevent dislodgment of the lumbar catheter through ongoing patient education. Ensure that the lumbar catheter and drainage device are secured. Provide sedation and analgesia as prescribed.	Lumbar catheter dislodgment may result in excessive drainage of CSF.	• Dislodged lumbar catheter
11. Change the CSF pressure monitoring and drainage systems aseptically according to institutional standards.	Reduces the risk of infection.	• Dislodged lumbar catheter • Loose connections or other openings in the catheter system
12. Obtain or assist with obtaining CSF specimens as prescribed by accessing the sampling port on the CSF drainage system with strict aseptic techniques. Follow institutional standards.	Limited data exist to guide or support decisions on the necessary frequency of routine CSF sampling from lumbar catheters.[36]	• Elevated white blood cell (WBC) count in CSF fluid • Elevated protein in CSF fluid • Decreased glucose in CSF fluid • Positive Gram stain • Positive culture and sensitivity • Elevated CSF cytokines (interleukin-6 [IL-6]) may predict bacterial infection earlier than elevated WBC count, elevated protein, or decreased glucose.[41,42]
13. Administer antibiotics as prescribed.	Currently, insufficient data are available to guide or support routine prophylactic antibiotic therapy.[14,19,35]	
14. If overdrainage is suspected, clamp the drain, lower the head of the bed,[7,19,23,25,36] and assess neurological status. (**Level E***)	The patient may be at increased risk of herniation with overdrainage.	• Change in neurological status and vital signs • Overdrainage • Notify the physician to report a change of condition and to receive further orders.

Expected Outcomes

- LP completed
- CSF samples obtained
- Patient's vital signs and level of consciousness stable before, during, and after the procedure
- No change or deterioration in neurological status after the procedure
- Accurate and reliable CSF pressure monitoring
- CSF pressure within the range of 5 to 20 cm H_2O
- Early detection and management of elevated CSF pressure through CSF drainage[1,22,46]
- Resolution of any CSF leak[21,36]
- Puncture site clean and dry
- No headache, neck stiffness, local pain at puncture site, leg spasms, or elevated temperature related to the procedure
- Monitor CSF chemistry, cytology physiology
- Drain subarachnoid hematoma blood from CSF per physician specification; this may decrease risk of vasospasms.[25,29,30]

Unexpected Outcomes

- Significant change in vital signs (respiratory changes, bradycardia, and increased systolic blood pressure)
- Change or deterioration in neurological status or signs of brain herniation, including decreased level of consciousness, pupillary changes, and motor or sensory impairment, and change in vital signs.[10,39,47]
- Bladder or bowel dysfunction[13,19,20,28]
- Abnormal CSF results
- Inability to obtain CSF sample
- Inability to complete procedure (e.g., dislodgment or occlusion of the lumbar catheter)
- Meningitis as evidence by prolonged headache, stiff neck, photophobia, and an acute increase in temperature related to the procedure[15,38,39]
- Excessive drainage at the puncture site[33]
- Persistent headache or low back pain despite interventions
- New and persistent symptoms of pain, numbness, tingling, weakness, or paralysis in the lower extremities[10,15]
- Spinal hematoma or paraspinal abscess[10,15]
- Implantation of epidermoid tumors[15]
- Vasovagal syncope
- Seizure

Documentation

Documentation should include the following:

- Completion of informed consent
- Preprocedural verifications and time out
- Insertion site assessment
- Insertion of the lumbar catheter, including opening CSF pressure, and any difficulties or abnormalities
- Patient tolerance of the procedure
- CSF description (e.g., clarity, color, characteristics)
- Specimens sent to the laboratory for analysis
- CSF laboratory results
- Hourly measurement of CSF pressure and amount of drainage
- Neurological, cardiovascular, and respiratory assessment
- Vital signs
- Waveform tracing at insertion and with continuous monitoring according to institutional standards
- Description of expected and unexpected outcomes
- Nursing interventions used to treat elevated CSF pressure
- Education
- Pain assessment, interventions, and management
- Sedation assessment and management (if sedation was administered)

References and Additional Readings

For a complete list of references and additional readings for this procedure, scan this QR code with your smartphone, or visit https://www.elsevier.com/__data/assets/pdf_file/0005/1319864/Chapter0089.pdf

PROCEDURE

90

Pupillometer

John Bazil

PURPOSE The pupillometer is a handheld device used to provide an objective measurement of the pupillary light reflex (PLR). Subjective assessment of the PLR is not reliable.[4,10] Automated infrared pupillometry (AIP) provides a reliable measurement of one pupil at a time.[18] After obtaining paired PLR measurements of both pupils, the device displays data that allow for comparison of pupillary size and reactivity.

PREREQUISITE NURSING KNOWLEDGE

- A fundamental understanding of the neuroanatomy and function of the optic cranial nerve (CN II) and the oculomotor cranial nerve (CN III) provides clinical correlates for interpreting the outcome of readings obtained with the pupillometer.[3]
  - ❖ The pupil is an opening in the center of the iris of the eye. Light passes through the pupil to the lens, where images are reversed before going through the vitreous humor to the rods and cones embedded throughout the retina.
  - ❖ Images are then converted into electrical signals that travel along the optic cranial nerve (CN II) to the optic chiasm, optic tracts, and lateral geniculate nucleus, where the images are sorted and then relayed to the visual cortex in the occipital lobe.
  - ❖ The size and shape of the pupil determine the amount of light that can enter the eye. The intrinsic muscles in the iris (sphincter pupillae and dilator pupillae) control the size and shape of the eye. The PLR is a brisk, protective mechanism (reflex) that triggers the intrinsic muscles in the iris to contract and thereby decrease the size of the pupil and reduce the amount of light reaching the retina. Testing the PLR evaluates components of both CN II and CN III (Fig. 90.1).[14] The electrical signal created from light entering the eye travels along CN II (afferent) to the Edinger-Westphal nucleus and triggers an efferent signal to travel along CN III from the Edinger-Westphal nucleus to the intrinsic muscles of both eyes. Thus a normal response to light entering either eye is bilateral pupil constriction.[14]
  - ❖ Proper equipment assembly of the pupillometer requires attaching an aseptic SmartGuard to the device with the knowledge that each one is assigned to and linked with a single patient. The Neurological Pupil index (NPi) is based on a collection of pupil measurements conducted in a healthy control population.[2] All variables representing the pupil dynamics were used to create a multidimensional, normative model. These variables are the maximum pupil diameter, constricted

pupil diameter after light exposure (fully constricted), percent change (% CH) in diameter, latency (LAT), constriction velocity (average [CV] and maximum [MCV]), and dilation velocity (DV) (Fig. 90.2). The NPi quantifies the difference between the patient measurement and the normative model. An NPi ≥3 indicates that the pupil measurement falls within the boundaries of the NPi model and is defined as normal. An NPi <3 means the reflex falls outside the boundaries and is defined as abnormal. An NPi <3 may reflect increased intracranial pressure.[13,16]

- ❖ Additional values obtained using AIP include: size (measured in mm) reflecting the pupil size at baseline; latency (measured in hundredths of a second) reflecting the time from light stimulus to initial response; constriction velocity (measured in mm/sec) reflecting the speed at which the pupil constricts; minimum size (mm) reflecting the size of the fully constricted pupil; and dilation velocity (mm/sec) reflecting the speed at which the pupil returns to baseline size after constriction.[6]
- ❖ Neither the eye color nor the presence of cataracts influences the PLR when assessed using AIP.[1]

EQUIPMENT

- Nonsterile gloves
- Pupillometer (Fig. 90.3A)
- Pupillometer charging station (see Fig. 90.3A)
- Pupillometer SmartGuard (see Fig. 90.3B)

Optional Equipment

- Barcode scanner (to scan patient ID such as QR code)
- SmartGuard RFID Reader (to integrate data into the electronic medical record (EMR)

PATIENT AND FAMILY EDUCATION

- Explain the purpose of serial neurological assessments to the patient and family. ***Rationale:*** The pupillary examination is a key assessment element performed during serial neurological examinations.

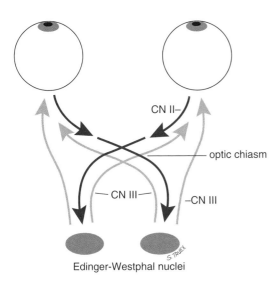

Figure 90.1 CN II and CN III pathways to Edinger-Westphal nuclei.

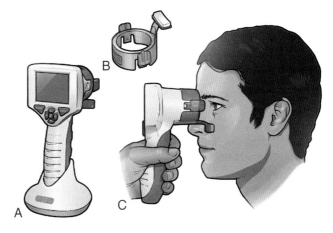

Figure 90.3 NPi-200 Pupillometer shown in docking (A) and with SmartGuard (B) attached and being held in proper position (C) with the pad of the SmartGuard on the zygomatic process (cheekbone).

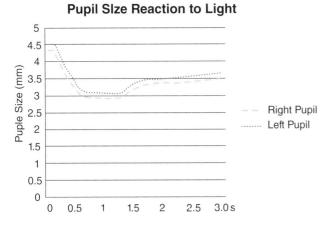

Figure 90.2 Graphic representation of the pupillary light reflex and variables used to calculate the NPi for the left and right pupils.

- Provide education that the pupillometer will be used to evaluate the PLR. *Rationale:* Assessing the PLR is a standard component of the neurological examination. However, the patient and family may be unfamiliar with automated pupil assessment.
- Provide patient and family teaching regarding how the pupillary examination will be completed. *Rationale:* Prepares the patient/family for the proximity of the device to the face and the light stimulus.

PATIENT ASSESSMENT AND PREPARATION

Patient Assessment

- Assess patient and family understanding of information. *Rationale:* Provides an opportunity to clarify information, answer questions, and possibly reduce fear and anxiety associated with a device being used near the face and eyes.
- Assess the patient's ability to maintain eye opening. *Rationale:* The patient must maintain eye opening. If the patient is unable to maintain eye opening during the examination, the practitioner will be required to manually lift the eyelid and keep the eye open during the examination.
- If the patient is conscious, determine whether photophobia is present. *Rationale:* Patients with photophobia will benefit from instructions and warning that a bright light will be used to assess their pupil reactivity.

Patient Preparation

- Verify the correct patient with two identifiers. *Rationale:* Before performing a procedure, the nurse should ensure the correct identification of the patient for the intended intervention. Each SmartGuard is assigned to one patient.
- Identify and confirm that the correct SmartGuard is available. *Rationale:* To reduce the risk of cross-contamination, a separate reusable SmartGuard is used for each patient. The SmartGuard should remain with the patient.

UNIT III

Procedure for Automated Pupillometer Use

Steps	Rationale	Special Considerations
1. 🔲		
2. 🔲		
3. Remove the pupillometer from the charging station.	Prepares the equipment.	Charges the battery of the pupillometer.
4. If the device is not on the charging station, it may be in sleep mode or powered off. A. If the device is in sleep mode, restore power by pressing and holding the UP arrow for approximately 3 seconds to turn on the device.	The device goes into sleep mode when out of the charging station and idle for >5 minutes.	
5. Obtain the patient SmartGuard.	SmartGuard is single-patient multiuse device.	
6. Connect the SmartGuard to the pupillometer (see Fig. 90.3A).	The pupillometer device must be connected to a SmartGuard to obtain a reading.	Gently squeeze the SmartGuard side tabs to position it onto the pupillometer. You will hear an audible click as the SmartGuard engages the device.
7. For a new patient or new SmartGuard: After attaching the SmartGuard, choose either "Manual" or "Barcode Scanner" to enter the patient ID and program the SmartGuard for a specific patient.	The SmartGuard is for single-patient use; scanning the SmartGuard pairs/links the SmartGuard to an individual patient.	Follow hospital protocol for the patient ID (e.g., medical record number).
8. Confirm that the patient is the correct patient. Then choose "Accept" or "Reject" (if re-entry of correct ID is needed).	Verifies that the SmartGuard has been correctly paired with the patient.	Once the ID has been verified, the screen will display a "Ready to scan" message.
9. Determine whether the patient is able to follow commands. A. For awake and cooperative patients, begin with **Step 8.** B. For unresponsive patients, begin with **Step 9.**	The patient who is awake and cooperative will be asked to participate in the examination. If the patient is unresponsive or uncooperative, the examiner will need to maintain the patient's eye open throughout the examination (approximately 3–5 seconds).	
10. For an awake, cooperative patient: Instruct the patient to open eyes wide and focus on a distant point (at least 6 feet away).	Focusing on nearby objects will cause a reflexive pupillary dilation.	
11. For an unresponsive or uncooperative patient: Open the patient's eye by gently lifting the upper eyelid with your finger or thumb. Ensure that the eye is open enough to see the entire pupil.	The entire pupil must be visible for the pupillometer to obtain an accurate reading.	Inability to raise the eyelid is a reportable condition (e.g., periorbital edema).
12. Holding the pupillometer at a 90-degree angle to the patient's eye, place the pad of the SmartGuard against the patient's left or right zygomatic process (cheekbone; see Fig. 90.3C).	The ideal position to hold the pupillometer is at a right angle to the patient's axis of vision. Minimize tilting of the device.	

Procedure continues on following page

Procedure for Automated Pupillometer Use—*Continued*

Steps	Rationale	Special Considerations
13. Target the left or right pupil by pressing and holding either the RIGHT or LEFT button (depending on which eye you are examining). A. Look at the display screen on the pupilometer. B. Ensure that there is a green circle around the pupil.	This step ensures that the pupillometer has located and targeted the pupil for accurate measurement.	Press LEFT when examining OS, and press RIGHT when examining OD. The choice to start with OS or OD is arbitrary; practitioners should consider asking patients which eye they prefer to start with.
14. Release the button, and hold the pupillometer steady in place until the results screen appears (approximately 3 seconds).	The pupillometer will capture the resting size of the pupil, emit a light stimulus, and then video-record the entire PLR.	
15. Ensure that reading was obtained. A red "Rescan" message indicates a measurement error. Repeat the scan for that eye if this message appears.	Looking at the results screen before scanning the other pupil allows determination of the quality of scan and the need to possibly repeat the measurement.	"Rescan" errors may occur if the device cannot capture the entire PLR or the device is moved before measurement is complete.
16. Scan the other eye using **Steps 11–13.**	Provides systematic evaluation of both eyes.	
17. Document the assessment. A. To upload results directly to the EMR: Remove the SmartGuard, and place it on the SmartGuard RFID Reader.* B. To manually document, note the pupil size and NPi for each eye.		*The SmartGuard Reader is an optional device.
18. Report abnormal findings to the appropriate provider.	Alerts the provider to a potential change in patient condition.	Abnormal findings can be verified by a repeat scan.
19. Remove and store the SmartGuard.	The SmartGuard is a patient-specific device and should not be used with other patients.	Store in a clean (nonsterile), dry location.
20. Clean/disinfect the pupillometer according to manufacturer's recommendations using solutions with up to 70% isopropyl alcohol. Ensure that the device is dry before returning it to the charging station.	The charging pins on the bottom of the device must be dry to prevent corrosion and failure of the battery to charge properly.	Please refer to the manufacturer's IFU for additional cleaning instructions.
21. Dock the pupillometer in the charging station.	The pupillometer charges when seated correctly in the charging station.	Ensure that the charging station is plugged into an electrical source.
22. Discard used supplies.		
23. 🅷🅷		

Expected Outcomes

- Accurate and reliable monitoring of the pupil size and the NPi for each pupil (OS and OD)[9,18]
- The NPi will be ≥3.0 in both eyes
- Early detection of changes in intracranial pathology associated with oculomotor nerve function[8,11-13,17]

Unexpected Outcomes

- Inability to measure pupil response with pupillometer (e.g., periorbital edema, scleral edema, cataract, prosthetic eye)
- Nonreactive pupil
- NPi of <3.0 (indicative of abnormal pupillary response)
- Right-to-left NPi difference ≥0.7
- Unequal pupil size before light stimulus (anisocoria)[5,7]

UNIT III

Patient Monitoring and Care

Steps	Rationale	Reportable Conditions
		These conditions should be reported to the provider if they persist despite nursing interventions.
1. Assess the pupils with each serial neurological examination.[15]	Pupillary examination is considered a normal and vital component of the neurological examination.	• Changes in pupillary reaction noted from pervious examination
2. Note the waveform for each pupil.	Similar shape waveform indicates equal responsiveness of OS and OD pupils.	• Nonreactive pupils • Unequal pupils or abnormal waveform
3. Note NPi value.	Normal is ≥3.0.	• NPi <3.0
4. Document the findings.		• Abnormal values
5. Report any abnormal values or significant changes of the pupils to the appropriate provider.	Changes in pupillary reactivity should be correlated over time.	• Abnormal values (NPi <3.0)

Documentation

Documentation should include the following:
• Document findings for each eye
• Date and time of examination
• Initial pupil diameter (size)
• NPi
• Inability to obtain an examination. If unable to obtain an examination, document the reason (e.g., periorbital edema, uncooperative patient)
• Comparison of left/right symmetry
• Some institutions document additional data provided by the device (e.g., latency, % change in size, constriction velocity, and dilation velocity)

References and Additional Readings

For a complete list of references and additional readings for this procedure, scan this QR code with your smartphone, or visit https://www.elsevier.com/__data/assets/pdf_file/0006/1319865/Chapter0090.pdf.

PROCEDURE

91

Cervical Traction and Stabilization: Assist and Nursing Care

Cara Diaz Lomangino

PURPOSE Cervical traction is used in a variety of cases to decompress the spinal cord and/or realign and stabilize the cervical spine. Once cervical traction has been established, the nurse cares for the patient who is immobilized on complete bed rest. Traction must be maintained on a continuous basis until realignment and stabilization with surgical management or orthoses are attained or healing is completed. Stabilization with orthosis (halo device) maintains realignment and immobilization of the cervical spine to allow spinal fractures and supportive structures to heal properly while allowing the patient to mobilize and be off bed rest.

PREREQUISITE NURSING KNOWLEDGE

- Knowledge about the anatomy and physiology of the spinal column, the anatomy of the cervical vertebrae, the spinal cord, the cervical spinal nerves, and the areas of peripheral innervation including dermatomal distribution (Fig. 91.1). In addition, it is important that the nurse understands the pathophysiology and manifestations of spinal cord injury, including ascending edema, spinal shock, and neurogenic shock.[9]
- Observe the patient for signs of motor function decline, normal signs of neurogenic and spinal shock, and interventions required if necessary.[10]
- For traction patients: continuously monitor the patient for changes in motor and sensory function during and after the procedure.
- Knowledge of the neuroanatomy of the facial nerves near the pin site entry points and characteristics of the skull bone and anatomy of weak portions of the skull (Fig. 91.2).
- Continuously assess for changes in respiration during the procedure, and continue to monitor while the patient is in traction.[1,7]
- Cervical spine traction is provided to realign and immobilize the cervical spine when it has become unstable as a result of a cervical spine fracture, malalignment or dislocation caused by trauma or disease, degenerative processes, or spinal surgery.[5,11] After initial medical stabilization and assessment of baseline neurological function, cervical skeletal traction with the tongs or halo ring can be applied to realign the cervical spine.[6] Generally, it is a precursor to definitive stabilization surgery. Occasionally, chronic disease may necessitate long-term cervical traction for a period of weeks to attain realignment and immobilization

to stabilize the spine.[11] The definitive method used to treat cervical fractures depends on the injury classification and provider or institutional preference.

- Tongs consist of a body with one pin attached at each end. The pins are applied to the outer table of the skull on both sides of the temporal bone. Cervical tongs are available in a variety of types, such as Codman, Crutchfield, Gardner-Wells, Symmetry, and PMT (Fig. 91.3) tongs. Generally, titanium instrumentation is used. However, the exact device chosen is at the discretion of the MD/NP/Surgeon.
  - ❖ Two holes are made in the outer table of the skull with a twist drill, and the pins are inserted and tightened until there is a firm fit.[9]
  - ❖ PMT tongs (see Fig. 91.2A), for example, are inserted by placing the razor-sharp pin edges to the prepared areas of the scalp and tightening the screws until the spring-loaded mechanism indicates that the correct pressure has been achieved. To decrease the possibility of tong displacement, all types of pins are well seated into the outer table of the skull and angled inward to keep neutral positioning. Variations of alignment may be made by the provider depending on degree of malalignment.[6]
  - ❖ Tongs are made of stainless steel or a graphite body with titanium pins. The graphite body with titanium pins is compatible with magnetic resonance imaging (MRI).
- Once the tongs are in place, traction can be applied with the use of a rope-and-pulley system or a cable and alignment bracket (Fig. 91.4). Weights are added gradually and followed with radiographic imaging. The physician, advanced practice nurse, or other healthcare professional uses serial radiographs of the cervical spine after each weight increase to assist in determining the optimal amount of traction (measured in pounds) needed to provide optimal alignment. Excessive traction may result in stretching of the spinal cord and subsequent damage, paralysis, and even death.

However, studies have shown that up to one-third of the patient's weight and up to 140 lb has been safe.[3,6,11]

- Cervical traction also may be applied with a halo ring device instead of tongs. This is a stainless steel or graphite ring that is attached to the skull by four stabilizing pins (two anterior and two posterolateral (Fig. 91.5). The halo ring may be chosen over the traction tong if the plan includes a halo vest for definitive treatment. Skull pins can be made of stainless steel, titanium, or ceramic material. Pins are threaded through holes in the ring and then screwed into the outer table of the skull with a torque wrench to limit pounds of pressure applied to the skull and prevent fracturing of the outer table. Traction can be applied using the same concept as the tongs. In cases of halo vest placement, after desired alignment of the cervical spine is achieved, the spine is secured in place by attaching the ring to a body vest or a custom-molded body jacket (see Fig. 91.5). The patient then is able to ambulate out of bed while the head and neck remain immobile.

- Contraindications to using a halo vest include skull fracture, sepsis, head injury, chest injury, and advanced age in most circumstances.[4,13,15] It maintains excellent immobilization of the cervical spine, particularly at the cervicothoracic junction and upper cervical spine.

EQUIPMENT

- Tongs or halo ring
- Consent forms
- Specific type of tongs to be used or the halo ring with insertion pins
- Torque wrench or breakaway torque drivers

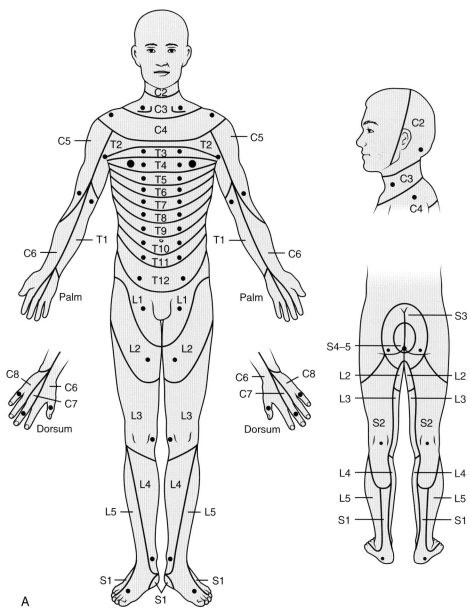

Figure 91.1   A–B, American Spinal Injury Association (ASIA) examination scale with dermatomal distribution. *(American Spinal Injury Association: International Standards for Neurological Classification of Spinal Cord Injury, revised 2019; Richmond, VA.)*

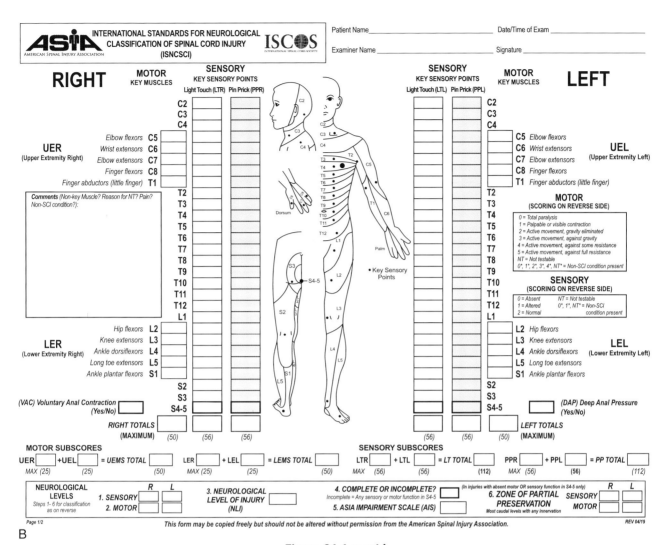

Figure 91.1 cont'd

B

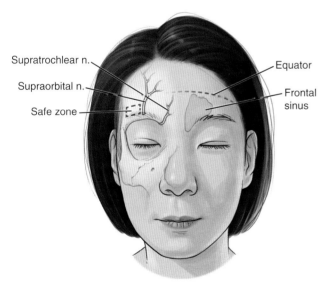

Figure 91.2 Correct tong placement is to the outer two-thirds of the brow below the equator to avoid nerves and vessels. Placement of halo pins and ring. The anterior pins are placed anterolaterally 1 cm above the orbital ridge. This "safe zone" avoids the temporalis muscle laterally and an orbital nerve plexus and frontal sinus medially.

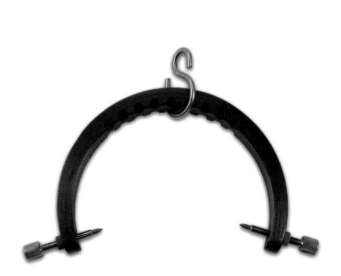

Figure 91.3 Examples of halo traction tongs and halo ring and vest *(Courtesy of PMT Corporation.)*

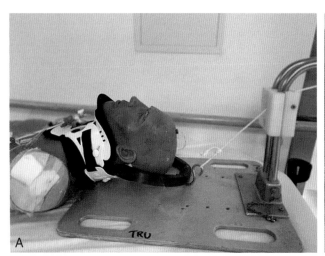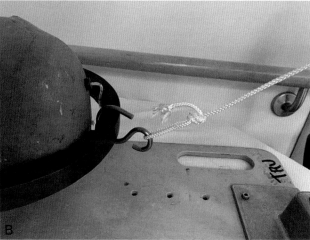

Figure 91.4   **A–B,** Correct setup of traction with weights using PMT traction tongs.

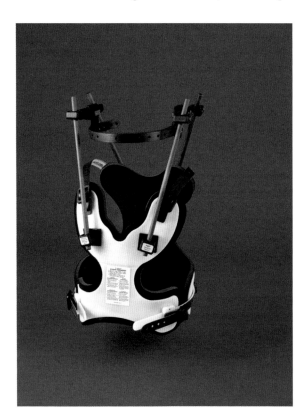

Figure 91.5   PMT halo and vest. *(Courtesy of PMT Corporation.)*

- Local anesthetic: lidocaine, 1% to 2% (with or without epinephrine, depending on the preference of the physician, advanced practice nurse, or other healthcare professional)
- Pain medication or benzodiazepine as ordered by the provider
- Needles (18- and 23-gauge)
- Sterile and nonsterile gloves
- Razor/clippers
- Gowns, masks, and eye shields
- Antiseptic solution
- Sterile sponges
- Sterile drill and bits (for insertion of Crutchfield and Vinke tongs)

- Rope and traction assembly and weights
- S and C hooks for traction tong or traction bail
  Additional equipment to have available as needed includes the following:
- Emergency equipment, C-arm or O-arm for radiographs during weight application, lead (these items are usually obtained by the providers)

PATIENT AND FAMILY EDUCATION

- Explain the procedure and the reason for cervical traction. Clarify any information as needed, and answer all questions by patient or family. Discuss the use of any special equipment, such as a special bed, that may be needed. *Rationale:* Patient and family anxiety is decreased.
- Explain the patient's role in assisting with insertion of the tongs. The nonintubated patient should communicate with the team during traction if he or she feels any changes in sensation, new or worsening pain, or new or worsening change in motor function. *Rationale:* Explanation elicits patient cooperation and facilitates safe insertion.
- Explain that the procedure can be uncomfortable when the incisions are made but that an anesthetic will be administered by the physician, advanced practice nurse, or other healthcare professional. *Rationale:* This information prepares the patient for what to expect.
- Explain what will happen after the procedure including duration of traction or final plan/duration for halo/vest placement *Rationale:* This information prepares the patient for what to expect.

PATIENT ASSESSMENT AND PREPARATION

Patient Assessment

- Conduct a complete neurological assessment that includes evaluation of cranial nerve function, motor strength of major muscles, sensation (usually an American Spinal Injury Association [ASIA] examination), and deep tendon reflexes (biceps, triceps, patella, and Achilles). ***Rationale:*** Baseline data are provided for comparison of postinsertion assessments to quickly determine the presence of neurological compromise or extension of spinal cord injury.

- Assess the patient's vital signs. ***Rationale:*** Baseline data are provided for comparison with assessments after insertion.
- Assess the patient's respiratory pattern, and auscultate lung sounds. Note the use of accessory respiratory muscles and any signs or symptoms of dyspnea. ***Rationale:*** Baseline data are established to determine any compromise to respiratory function as a result of the procedure.
- Inspect the scalp for abrasions, lacerations, or sites of infection. ***Rationale:*** Any potential sites of infection that may contraindicate the insertion of a cervical fixation device into the infected area are identified.
- Assess the level of pain or discomfort and anxiety. ***Rationale:*** Assessment establishes data for decision making regarding the need for analgesia or anxiolytics for comfort and cooperation during the insertion procedure.
- Assess for any allergies to an antiseptic agent, local anesthetic, or analgesia and anxiolytics. ***Rationale:*** Review of medication allergies before administration of a new medication decreases the chances of an allergic reaction.
- Assess for any contraindications to a halo as stated earlier (i.e., infection, skull fracture, open abdomen, open scalp wounds, or advanced age). ***Rationale:*** Ensures appropriate patient selection.

Patient Preparation

- Ensure that the patient and family understand the preprocedural teaching. Answer questions as they arise, and reinforce information as needed. ***Rationale:*** Understanding of previously taught information is evaluated and reinforced.
- Verify the correct patient with two identifiers. ***Rationale:*** Before performing a procedure, the nurse should ensure the correct identification of the patient for the intended intervention.
- Ensure that informed consent has been obtained. ***Rationale:*** Informed consent protects the rights of the patient and makes a competent decision possible for the patient.
- Perform a preprocedure verification and time out, if nonemergent. A time out (per institutional practice) should be performed before placement of cervical tongs or a halo ring and traction. ***Rationale:*** Ensures patient safety.
- Ensure that the head of the bed is flat and that the patient's head is in a neutral position by whatever approved means (e.g., hard/rigid collar) have been instituted. ***Rationale:*** This measure prevents movement of the neck, which may increase the risk of injury or extension of spinal cord injury. Providers will change the angle at their discretion, but the initial positioning should be a neutral spine.[6]

Procedure	for Assisting With Application of Cervical Traction and Stabilization with a Halo Ring or Tongs		
Steps	**Rationale**		**Special Considerations**
1. Obtain a bed with an orthopedic traction frame, weights, and/or rope and pulley system attached to the bed.	Traction must be ready to reduce the potential for movement of the head and neck.		May require assistance from other departments; therefore plan ahead to coordinate.
2. **HH**			If performing in the operating room, use appropriate procedures for scrubbing in.
3. **PE**			All healthcare personnel involved in the procedure must apply personal protective and sterile attire (e.g., fluid shield masks, eye shields, gowns, and sterile gloves).
4. Assist the physician, advanced practice nurse, or other healthcare professional with the tong or halo ring insertion:	Facilitates the procedure.		Because of the high risk for extension of cervical injury, this procedure usually is performed by a neurosurgeon, who can respond rapidly if neurological deterioration becomes evident.
A. Assist as needed with preparation of the pin sites (clipping a small area of scalp hair if indicated and cleansing with antiseptic solution).	Clipping the hair may prevent it from being trapped when the pins are inserted. Cleansing decreases skin surface bacteria.		
B. Assist if needed with draping the patient, leaving insertion sites exposed.	Aids in maintaining sterility.		

Procedure continues on following page

UNIT III

Procedure for Assisting With Application of Cervical Traction and Stabilization with a Halo Ring or Tongs—*Continued*		
Steps	Rationale	Special Considerations
C. Assist as needed with local anesthesia administration.	Decreases patient discomfort during pin insertion.	
D. Stabilize the patient's head and neck during the procedure.	Maintains alignment of the cervical spine and provides support to injured areas.	Cervical stabilization can be maintained with the use of a rigid collar or other devices that prevent head rotation and neck flexion or extension. A soft collar is not considered a stabilizing device. Utmost care must be taken to prevent head and neck flexion or extension. Be prepared for the possibility of respiratory insufficiency, respiratory arrest, hypotension, bradycardia, or cardiac arrest.
E. Carefully follow institutional policies regarding manual cervical spine immobilization.	Institutional policies may provide strict guidelines for the nursing role in manual cervical spine immobilization during traction placement.	Follow institutional policy for confirmatory radiographic studies following the procedure.
5. Monitor the patient for changes in respiratory function, neurogenic shock, spinal shock, changes in motor function, and changes in sensation and pain or swallowing.[2]	Identifies evidence of untoward effects or complications related to the procedure and identifies the need for analgesia.	In addition to untoward effects, the patient may need additional reassurance, support, sedation, and analgesia.
6. Follow hospital policy for pin site care (see Procedure 92, Pin Site and Vest Care).	Maintains asepsis.	Pin site care should be done daily, and the family should be taught the procedure if the patient is being discharged in a halo device.
7. Assist with application and connection to traction as needed.	Aids in a safe and smooth transition to weight application.	Wait for instructions from provider, and repeat back before manipulating the weight.
A. Maintain the patient's head in a neutral position.[6]	Ensures accurate and safe use of the traction.	Certain cases may require manipulation of the angle to achieve the desired spine alignment.[6,11]
B. Assist if needed with the application of prescribed weights.	Assists with moving weights so the provider can maintain alignment.	
C. Ensure that weights are unobstructed and hanging freely.	Ensures the safe use of equipment and maintains the principles of traction.	Once alignment is achieved, the provider may decrease to a "maintenance" weight if the patient will be in traction for a prolonged time.
8. Discard used supplies in an appropriate receptacle.	Removes and safely discards used supplies.	
9. **HH**		

Expected Outcomes

- Tong or halo ring device inserted correctly with no complications or fractures
- Head and neck immobilized to allow for alignment, stabilization, and healing of fractures
- Prescribed amount of weight applied to tongs or halo without movement of tongs/ring
- Traction weights unobstructed and hanging freely
- Improved or stable neurological function (motor and sensory)
- Patient discomfort minimized

Unexpected Outcomes

- Slippage of tongs or halo pins[14]
- Extension or deterioration of neurological deficits or spinal cord injury
- Respiratory compromise or arrest
- Hypotensive episode, bradycardia, cardiac arrest
- Pain
- Bleeding at pin site

Patient Monitoring and Care

Steps	Rationale	Reportable Conditions
		These conditions should be reported to the provider if they persist despite nursing interventions.
1. Assess neurological status every 5 minutes during the procedure, including assessment of level of consciousness, movement in arms and legs, sensation, mastication, and eyelid closure.[2]	Facilitates early recognition of neurological deterioration.	• Any deterioration or extension of baseline neurological function • Increased or new loss of sensation • New or worsening decrease in motor strength
2. Assess respiratory function (respiratory rate, pulse oximetry, lung sounds) before, during, and after the procedure.	Allows for early identification of hypoxia or respiratory distress from neurological deterioration or other potential complications such as aspiration or sedation. A decrease in peripheral oxygen saturation may be an early indicator of respiratory compromise.	• Changes in respiratory function (e.g., decrease in oxygen saturation [SaO_2], increase in end-tidal carbon dioxide [$EtCO_2$]; increase or decrease in respiratory rate, abnormal lung sounds) • Oversedation
3. Assess for neurogenic shock.	Neurogenic shock can occur rapidly and requires prompt intervention.	• Hypotension • Bradycardia • Decreased vascular tone • Hypoxia • Poikilothermia • Unrelieved anxiety
4. Provide emotional support and reassurance to the patient during the procedure.	Decreases anxiety and facilitates patient cooperation.[12]	
5. Monitor pin sites for hemostasis immediately after the procedure and for the next few hours or as indicated by institutional policy.	The scalp is vascular, and continued bleeding may occur at the pin sites that requires assessment and cleansing.	• Unresolved bleeding
6. Check the security of the traction, bed frame, and bed.	The traction frame is attached to the bed and must be secure. Assess the integrity of the traction every 4 hours and as needed.	• Break in the integrity of the traction equipment or the bed frame
7. Maintain the patient's head flat on the bed, and ensure that the bed is flat. The head of the bed frame may be on shock blocks or placed in the reverse Trendelenburg position to provide countertraction.	The head must be flat on the bed to maintain a neutral position. Countertraction is often provided to prevent the patient from being pulled toward the top of the bed. Reposition the patient using the log rolling technique every 2 hours.	• Neck or head out of neutral alignment

Procedure continues on following page

UNIT III

Patient Monitoring and Care —*Continued*

Steps	Rationale	Reportable Conditions
8. If the knot on the traction rope nears the pulley or the wire band nears the bracket, several physicians, advanced practice nurses, or other healthcare professionals may slowly pull the patient down in bed. The patient should never be pulled up in the bed, or traction will be released. Do not remove the weights to move the patient toward the foot of the bed.	The knot of the traction rope must not be resting against the pulley for effective traction. The cover over the wire and bracket alignment device must not be against the alignment screw (head of the bed) for effective traction.	• Evidence of loss of effective traction
9. If cervical traction is lost for whatever reason (e.g., the loop in traction rope holding the weights slips or the pins dislodge), maintain manual cervical spine immobilization, place the patient in a hard/rigid cervical collar, and notify the physician, advanced practice nurse, or other healthcare professional. Elicit the patient's cooperation to minimize extraneous movement.	Immediate intervention is needed to immobilize the patient's head and neck. Reassess motor and sensory function after changing weights or position.	• Changes in motor and/or sensory assessment • Changes in respiratory effort, signs of respiratory distress • Evidence of loss of effective traction
10. Prepare the patient for a bedside confirmatory radiograph of the cervical spine immediately after insertion and application of weights and as prescribed by the physician, advanced practice nurse, or other healthcare professional.	A radiograph is taken to verify alignment of the cervical spine.	• Abnormal radiographic results
11. If additional weights are added or removed by the physician, advanced practice nurse, or other healthcare professional in an attempt to realign the cervical spine, increase the frequency of neurological checks. Expect more frequent cervical radiographs or MRIs to verify alignment.	Monitors for possible risk of secondary spinal cord injury.	• Changes in motor and/or sensory assessment • Changes in respiratory effort, signs of respiratory distress
12. Follow institutional standards for assessing pain. Administer analgesia as prescribed.	Identifies the need for pain interventions.	• Continued pain despite pain interventions

Documentation

Documentation should include the following:
- Patient and family education
- Completion of informed consent
- Preprocedure verifications and time out
- Type of cervical traction applied
- Date and time traction applied
- Local anesthetic used
- Sedation and analgesia used
- Amount of weight applied to the traction
- Weights hanging freely
- Pins secure
- Appearance of pin-insertion site and care[8]
- Ongoing comprehensive assessment data and action taken for abnormal response
- Verification of proper functioning and security of traction equipment
- Documentation of radiographic confirmation of alignment
- Occurrence of unexpected outcomes
- Patient response to care[12]
- Additional interventions
- Pain assessment, interventions, and effectiveness

References and Additional Readings

For a complete list of references and additional readings for this procedure, scan this QR code with your smartphone, or visit https://www.elsevier.com/__data/assets/pdf_file/0007/1319866/Chapter0091.pdf

92 Pin Site and Vest Care

Cara Diaz Lomangino

PURPOSE The halo crown and superstructure (vest) are used to immobilize the upper cervical spine for a variety of reasons including trauma, degenerative diseases, or malalignment. The purpose of this chapter is to review how to care for the parts of the halo including pin site and vest care to prevent any complications during use.

PREREQUISITE NURSING KNOWLEDGE

- Neuroanatomy and physiology of the cervical spine— including the spinal column, vertebrae, the spinal cord, and spinal nerves with their areas of innervation.
- Neuroanatomy of the facial nerves near the pin site entry points and characteristics of the skull bone and anatomy of weak portions of the skull.
- The halo ring and vest may be used as a primary definitive treatment to stabilize the cervical spine, before surgery to reduce spine deformity, or after surgery as an adjunct to interval cervical fixation.
- Components of the halo-vest device, including the halo ring and pins, anterior and posterior posts, vest screws, front and back panels of the vest, and shoulder and side buckles as well as how to use the wrench or torque driver and how to quickly dismantle the vest in case of emergency.
- The nurse must be confident to teach the family how to care for the vest/pin sites at home as many patients discharge to home in the device. This includes emergency removal in the event of choking or cardiac arrest and personal hygiene while in the vest.[9]
- Knowledge about how to access the patient's anterior chest to administer cardiopulmonary resuscitation (CPR) if cardiac arrest occurs. Refer to information from the manufacturer of the halo vest for specific information on emergency access to the chest. (Some vests have a hinged closure like PMT, so the vest can be lifted up at the hinge to allow quick access to the chest). Other vests are not hinged and require a wrench to release the front stabilizing bars to access the chest or airway. *The wrench must be available at all times and, depending on institutional policy, may be maintained on the front of the vest for instant access to the chest.* If the patient needs defibrillation, avoid touching the bars of the traction with the defibrillator.
- Signs and symptoms of new injury or extension of spinal cord injury and the needed interventions.[8]
- Indications for halo use in the patient and the risks and signs of halo failure including "snaking," mobility of any part of the device, and signs of infection.[6,7,10,11]
- The nurse must be familiar with the specific manufacturer in use at the institution as wrenches, pins, and torque drivers may be different (e.g., PMT, Bremer).
- When the vest is not in use, direct traction may be applied to the halo ring device with a rope- and-pulley system and

weights (see Procedure 91, Cervical Traction and Stabilization: Assist and Nursing Care). Patients with a halo ring, pins, and traction applied with weights are cared for similarly to patients in cervical traction with tongs (see Procedure 91, Cervical Traction and Stabilization: Assist and Nursing Care).
- When alignment of the cervical spine is achieved, long-term immobilization of the spine can be achieved by attaching the ring to the body vest, which allows for mobility/discharge and independent living of the patient and is why pin care teaching is so vital[9,10] (Fig 92.1).
- Proper management and monitoring of a patient in a halo-vest device can prevent minor complications that could lead to more serious morbidity and mortality.[1,3,10]

EQUIPMENT

- Halo device (in place; see Procedure 91, Cervical Traction and Stabilization: Assist and Nursing Care)
- Soap and a basin of warm water
- Washcloth and towel
- Nonsterile gloves
- Saline gauze
- Vest liner if replacing (either sheepskin or Coolmax Liner [PMT]) (Fig. 92.2)
- Emergency wrench or torque driver

PATIENT AND FAMILY EDUCATION

- Describe turning, positioning, and skin care procedures before performing them. *Rationale:* Patient and family anxiety is decreased.
- Explain to the patient and family that the halo vest's side panels should only be opened as prescribed by the physician, advanced practice nurse, or other healthcare professional and according to the manufacturer's guidelines. If the side panels are opened, the patient must be flat and supine.[1,4,9,11] *Rationale:* Integrity of the halo-vest device and alignment of the spine is maintained.
- Because the halo vest limits movement of the head, patients must be taught to scan the environment for objects in their path that could lead to falls, including how to safely walk up and down stairs. *Rationale:* Patient safety and independence are maintained. The halo vest changes the center of gravity and limits movement, thus requiring adaptations for performing activities of daily living (ADLs).

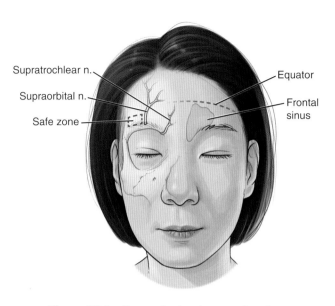

Figure 92.1   Proper pin site placement location.

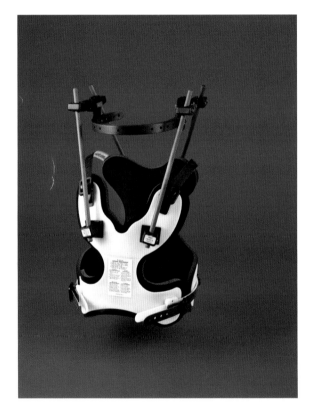

Figure 92.2 PMT Cool-liner vest. *(Courtesy of PMT Corporation.)*

- If the patient is ambulatory, explain modifications in meeting basic needs such as bathing, toileting, eating, dressing, ambulation precautions, and safety needs.[9] *Rationale:* Self-care skills and awareness of special safety precautions are developed.
- For patients who will be discharged home wearing a halo-vest device, begin a comprehensive teaching program with the patient and family. *Rationale:* The patient and family are prepared for care in the home environment.[9,11]

- Explain to the patient and family that the patient cannot be turned with the struts (posts) of the halo-vest device. *Rationale:* The patient and family are prepared for care in the home environment.
- Explain that driving, riding a motorcycle or bicycle, and operating machinery are unsafe with a halo-vest device. *Rationale:* Patients recognize limited activities.
- Explain that the pins of the halo transmit vibration and cold sensation to the patient's skull. *Rationale:* The patient and family are alerted to possible sensations during ADLs.
- Explain that if the patient hears "clicking" or "popping," the screws may be loose, and the patient should contact the physician immediately.[10,11] Inform the patient and family not to adjust the pins in the skull. Family members may be taught how to tighten the halo washers and bolts with the wrench before discharge as prescribed. *Rationale:* The patient and family are prepared for care in the home and can identify when emergency care may be needed.
- Explain that if the patient has any decline in neurological function (i.e., decreased or abnormal sensory function, decline in motor ability, or increased pain), the physician should be contacted immediately. *Rationale:* Decline in neurological function may indicate extension of spinal cord injury and the need for immediate interventions.
- Educate the family on signs and symptoms of infection at pin sites and the snaking motion of the head. Teach the patient and family that the patient should not be able to nod "yes" or to shake their head "no." This would indicate that the halo is loose.[10] *Rationale:* The patient and family are prepared to watch for signs threatening integrity of the device and alignment.

PATIENT ASSESSMENT AND PREPARATION

Patient Assessment

- Perform a complete neurological assessment (Box 92.1). *Rationale:* This assessment provides baseline data.
- Assess skin integrity along the patient's scalp.[6,7] *Rationale:* This assessment ensures that there is no skin breakdown near the screws and does not requiring manipulating the halo.
- Assess for difficulty swallowing and risk for aspiration.[2] *Rationale:* Assessment identifies a patient at high risk and the need to modify oral intake.
- Assess the skin at the edges of the vest and where the vest may overlap for redness or abrasion, especially over bony prominences. *Rationale:* Skin irritation related to the halo-vest device is identified.
- Check the fit of the vest for tightness or looseness. *Rationale:* The need for change or modification of the vest is identified. Patient weight loss and position changes (sitting to standing) may contribute to vest looseness.[10,11]
- Check the halo vest for loose straps or screws, dirt, odor, or evidence of the need to repair or replace the vest. *Rationale:* The vest may need to be repaired or the liner changed.

BOX 92.1   Muscle Strength Grading Scale

0/5–No detectable muscle contraction
1/5–Weak muscle contraction observed or palpated without active
    movement
2/5–Active movement of body part when effect of gravity is eliminated
3/5–Active movement of body part against gravity
4/5–Active movement of body part against gravity with some resistance
5/5–Active movement of body part against gravity with full resistance
    (normal muscle strength)

From Stewart-Amidei C: Assessment. In Bader MK, Littlejohns LR, Olson DM, editors:
AANN Core curriculum for neuroscience nursing, ed 6, Glenview, 2016, American
Association of Neuroscience Nurses, 63-96.

- Ensure that the emergency wrench is in the packet and/or attached to the vest. ***Rationale:*** This allows for emergent removal if necessary.
- Ensure that all pins, screws, bolts, and washers are intact on the device; no stripping has occurred; and no pieces are missing. ***Rationale:*** Tight connections are necessary to

ensure stabilization of the device for effective immobilization of the spine.

Patient Preparation

- Ensure that the patient and family understand the preprocedural information. Answer questions as they arise, and reinforce information as needed. ***Rationale:*** Understanding of previously taught information is evaluated and reinforced.
- Verify the correct patient with two identifiers. ***Rationale:*** Before performing a procedure, the nurse should ensure the correct identification of the patient for the intended intervention.
- Assist patients, as they lie supine in a neutral position, with proper body alignment for the purpose of halo vest liner change and routine skin care. ***Rationale:*** Patients are kept safely in alignment and accessible for inspection.
- Observe the sides and back of the vest and adjacent skin with the patient standing, if possible. ***Rationale:*** Observation provides an opportunity to inspect all areas in which the skin and vest come in contact.

Procedure   for Halo Ring and Vest Care

Steps	Rationale	Special Considerations
1. **HH**		
2. **PE**		
3. If unbuckling is prescribed for vest care, position the patient flat on their back, and unbuckle the vest while maintaining cervical alignment[1] **(Level E*)**	Gains access to the underlying skin.	Review the manufacturer's recommendations with regard to vest care. Follow institutional policy with regard to vest care.
4. Assess the patient's skin.	Determines skin integrity.	Insensate patients may be more vulnerable to skin breakdown. The halo vest should fit snugly but not cause skin breakdown or discomfort over pressure areas. The fit of the halo and the liner is checked daily. The sheepskin or liner should be smooth and without wrinkles and extend to the edges of the vest to protect the skin from abrasions. The sternum, ribs, scapulae, and clavicle areas are especially at high risk for skin breakdown.
5. Bathe the skin with soap and water. Minimize moisture to avoid wetting the liner of the vest. If unbuckling the vest is not recommended by the manufacturer or institutional policy, pass a damp, thin towel between the skin and liner, reaching all skin surfaces.	Cleanses the skin. Allows for skin assessment.	Dry the skin thoroughly, and avoid excessive lotion or powder; these are not good for the liner.

Procedure for Halo Ring and Vest Care—*Continued*

Steps	Rationale	Special Considerations
6. Auscultate lung sounds.	Identifies adventitious breath sounds.	Lung sounds may be decreased at the bases in patients with poor diaphragm and intercostal muscle function.
7. Perform anterior and posterior chest physiotherapy, if indicated.	May enhance secretion maintenance and facilitate airway clearance.	A slight decrease in vital capacity related to vest placement may be seen.
8. Rebuckle the vest. (**Level E***)	Maintains cervical immobilization.	Ensure that the buckle is secured for proper fit without restricting breathing when the patient sits upright.
9. To cleanse the back of the patient, turn the patient to the side without using the struts of the halo, keep the head of the bed flat, and **repeat Steps 3–8.** (**Level E***)	Facilitates assessment of the back of the body.	While the back is exposed, it is a good time to check the tightness of the posterior screws/struts of the halo.
10. If prescribed, change or assist with changing the anterior sheepskin or liner as needed.	Provides comfort and cleanliness and protects the skin.	Follow institutional standards for liner change. The anterior portion of the liner may require frequent changes because of secretions or drainage from a tracheostomy or from spills during eating.[2] Protect the liner during meals, and use towels and plastic when washing the hair to minimize the need for frequent liner changes.
A. Place the patient supine with the head of the bed flat.	Provides support and alignment.	
B. Unbuckle one side strap on the vest while maintaining cervical spine alignment and immobilization.	Provides access to the sheepskin.	
C. Roll the soiled liner on the unbuckled portion of the anterior vest to the center of the vest to facilitate removal of the sheepskin.	Simplifies the liner change.	
D. Match half the clean liner to the corresponding portion of the anterior vest, and roll the remainder to the center of the vest.		
E. Buckle the side strap of the vest.	Maintains cervical immobilization.	
F. Unbuckle the other side strap, and remove the remainder of the soiled liner.		
G. Unroll the clean liner, and match to the corresponding Velcro strips on the vest.		
H. Buckle the side strap.		
11. Change or assist with changing the posterior sheepskin liner as needed:	Promotes comfort and protects the skin.	Follow institutional standards for liner change.

Procedure continues on following page

UNIT III

Procedure for Halo Ring and Vest Care—*Continued*

Steps	Rationale	Special Considerations
A. Position the patient with the head of the bed flat and the patient turned to the side-lying position. Alternately, the patient can be turned prone, with a pillow under the chest and a pillow under the head, if the patient's respiratory status tolerates this position.	Provides support and protects the skin.	
B. Unbuckle one side strap of the halo vest while maintaining cervical spine alignment and immobilization.	Provides support and alignment.	
C. Roll the soiled liner on the unbuckled portion of the posterior vest to the center of the vest to facilitate removal of sheepskin.	Simplifies the liner change.	
D. Match half the clean liner to the corresponding portion of the posterior vest, and roll the remainder to the center of the vest.	Provides comfort and protects the skin.	
E. Buckle the side strap of the vest.	Maintains cervical immobilization.	
F. Roll the patient to the opposite side.	Maintains cervical spine alignment.	
G. Unbuckle the side strap on the vest while maintaining cervical spine alignment and immobilization. Remove the remainder of the soiled liner.	Accesses the opposite side of the liner.	
H. Unroll the clean liner, and match to the corresponding Velcro strips on the vest.	Secures the liner in place.	
I. Buckle the side strap.	Maintains cervical immobilization.	
12. Daily or every shift pin site care.	Keeps pin sites clean and prevents infection.[5,7,9]	Patients with long hair will get caught in screw threads. Keep hair clipped short if the halo will be on long term.
13. Using sterile gauze or cotton tip applicators and normal saline or iodine solution gently cleanse around pin sites removing any exudate or scabs.[5,6,7] **(Level A*)**	Keeps pin sites clean of infection and irritation.	Check institutional policy for the preferred cleansing solution; more research is needed for identifying a superior strategy.[6,7]

*Level A Meta-analysis of quantitative studies or metasynthesis of qualitative studies with results that consistently support a specific action, intervention, or treatment (including systematic review of randomized controlled trials).

*Level E Multiple case reports, theory-based evidence from expert opinions, or peer-reviewed professional organizational standards without clinical studies to support recommendations.

Expected Outcomes

- Cervical alignment is maintained
- The underlying skin remains intact and free from irritation
- The vest is functional, fits well, and is clean and odorless
- The pin sites are clean
- Mobility and sensation are maintained if the patient is neurologically intact
- The patient's safety and comfort is maintained

Unexpected Outcomes

- Loose pins[6,7]
- Pin site infection, osteomyelitis, or intracranial abscess[5,7,9]
- Poor fit (too loose or too tight) of halo vest or body jacket
- Skin breakdown or irritation under or around the vest
- Persistent spinal instability and loss of vertebral alignment[10,11]
- New or worsened injury to the spinal cord caused by spine mobility
- New or additional loss of neurological function
- Orthostatic hypotension
- Respiratory distress
- Injury from fall during ambulation with a halo vest

Patient Monitoring and Care

Steps	Rationale	Reportable Conditions
		These conditions should be reported to the provider if they persist despite nursing interventions.
1. Assess motor and sensory function immediately after application of the halo vest and every 2–4 hours per institutional standards.	Determines neurological status.	• Any deterioration from baseline neurological function (e.g., loss of more dermatomal sensation; decrease in motor strength)
2. Monitor for dyspnea, hypoxia, or decreasing tidal volumes (monitor pulse oximetry, and measure tidal volumes).	Assesses for hypoxia or respiratory distress from extension of neurological dysfunction or compromised respiratory function from vest constriction. A decrease in oxygen saturation or a decrease in tidal volume may be early indicators of respiratory compromise and risk for pneumonia or mortality.	• Decreased oxygen saturation • Decreased tidal volumes from baseline • Dyspnea
3. Follow institutional standards for assessing pain. Administer analgesia as prescribed.	Identifies the need for pain interventions.	• Continued pain despite pain interventions
4. Monitor for dysphagia.[2]	Dysphagia is a possible side effect of cervical immobilization with a halo vest and can be associated with altered nutritional status and aspiration or risk for pneumonia.	• Dysphagia
5. Check the fit of the vest, especially if the patient has lost or gained a significant amount of weight.	The vest may be too big if significant weight loss occurs or too small if improperly fitted originally or if the patient gains weight.	• Inability to securely fit the vest
6. At least once each shift, observe the skin at the edges of the vest and where the vest may overlap. Replace the vest liner if it is wet or soiled.	Promotes comfort and skin integrity.	• Skin irritation noted; the liner is wet or dirty and needs replacement • Call the physician to replace the liner per institutional standards
7. Wash exposed skin with warm water and soap; rinse well and dry. Be careful not to wet the liner.	Maintains cleanliness of the skin and protects the liner.	• Any assistance needed with the liner replacement

Procedure continues on following page

UNIT III

Patient Monitoring and Care —*Continued*

Steps	Rationale	Reportable Conditions
8. Monitor pin sites daily or every shift.	Monitors pin sites and prevents infection.	• Evidence of infection
9. Check the integrity of the halo, pins, struts, and vest.[9]	Provides for safe use of equipment and appropriate therapy.	• Any break in integrity of the equipment
10. Move the patient and the halo vest as a unit to avoid pressure that may dislodge the pins. Never use the anterior or posterior struts (posts) that attach the halo to the vest for moving a patient.	Prevents dislodgment of pins and injury.	• Evidence of dislodgment of the pins or halo
11. Support the patient with pillows when positioning the patient in the proper body alignment.	Provides comfort of the halo-vest device. A pillow behind the patient's head decreases the patient's sensation of being suspended.	• Evidence of dislodgment of the pins or halo
12. Discuss possible changes in body image related to the halo-vest device; provide emotional support.[9]	A dramatic change in body image occurs with the wearing of the halo-vest device and must be acknowledged.	• Maladaptation to altered body image
13. Discuss safety in ambulation and fall prevention (e.g., scanning with eyes to compensate for inability to move head; walking more slowly). Consider recommendation of a physical therapy consult.	Because of the immobilization of the head and neck, the patient is at risk for falls.	• Patient instability
14. Follow manufacturer's recommendations and institutional policies for obtaining immediate access to the chest in the event of an emergency. A wrench must be at the bedside or attached to the vest at all times, and staff must be aware of how to access the halo vest in an emergency. (**Level M***)	Supports basic safety procedures.	• Hemodynamic instability necessitating opening the vest

*Level M: Manufacturer's recommendations only.

Documentation

Documentation should include the following:
- Patient and family education
- Date, time, and which vest/pin care was completed
- Skin and pin assessment
- Integrity of the vest including any loose screws or bolts
- Neurological (motor/sensory assessment) and pulmonary assessment (tidal volume, pulse oximetry)
- Liner changes as needed
- Date and time of chest physiotherapy performed
- Occurrence of unexpected outcomes
- Patient response to care
- Additional interventions
- Pain assessment, interventions, and effectiveness

References and Additional Readings

For a complete list of references and additional readings for this procedure, scan this QR code with your smartphone, or visit https://www.elsevier.com/__data/assets/pdf_file/0008/1319867/Chapter0092.pdf .

UNIT III

PROCEDURE

93

Epidural Catheters: Insertion (Assist) and Pain Management

Andrea Barron

PURPOSE Epidural catheters are used to provide regional anesthesia and analgesia by delivering medications directly into the epidural space surrounding the spinal cord. Insertion of an epidural catheter is a sterile procedure that is performed by a team of healthcare providers and allows for continuous, intermittent, or patient-controlled medication administration.

PREREQUISITE NURSING KNOWLEDGE

- State boards of nursing and individual institutions that perform epidural therapy may have detailed guidelines and policies involving the insertion and management of epidural catheters. Healthcare providers should abide by the state guidelines and institutional policies.
- Aseptic technique involves the practices of preventing microbial contamination and is sometimes referred to as *clean technique.* Sterile technique involves the practices of maintaining the environment to reduce the chance of microbial contamination to as low as possible.[2,17]
- Epidural catheter insertion and continuing epidural therapy should be under the supervision of a nurse anesthetist, anesthesiologist, or acute pain service provider to ensure positive patient outcomes.[1,6]
- The spinal cord and brain are covered by three membranes, collectively called the *meninges.* The outer layer is the dura mater, the middle layer is the arachnoid mater, and the inner layer is the pia mater. The epidural space lies between the dura mater and the bone and ligaments of the spinal canal (Fig. 93.1) and contains fat, blood vessels, connective tissue, and spinal nerve roots.[4,14,16,21]
- Epidural catheters can be used effectively for short-term (e.g., acute, obstetrical, postoperative, trauma) or long-term (e.g., chronic, advanced cancer) pain management. Medications administered via an epidural catheter may be given with a continuous, intermittent (bolus) or with a patient-controlled epidural anesthesia (PCEA) pump system.[4,9,14,19,21]
- Epidural analgesia provides a number of well-documented advantages in the postoperative period, including decreased morbidity and mortality, attenuation of the surgical/trauma stress response, improved pain relief, earlier extubation, less sedation, decreased incidence of pulmonary complications, earlier return of bowel function, decreased incidence of deep venous thrombosis, earlier

ambulation, earlier discharge from high-acuity units, and potentially shorter hospital stays.[1,4,9]
- A variety of medication options can be administered via epidural catheter, including local anesthetics, opiates, mixtures of local anesthetics and opiates, α_2-adrenergic agonists, and other agents.[4,6,9,16,21]
- The pharmacology of medications administered for analgesia via epidural catheter, including side effects and duration of action, must be understood. Nurses should be familiar with the psychosocial and physiological implications for the appropriate treatment of pain and the consequences of undertreatment of acute pain.[4,9]
- Opioids used for neuraxial analgesia include fentanyl, sufentanil, morphine, and hydromorphone.[16] Fentanyl and sufentanil are lipophilic opioids that can have a more rapid onset and a shorter duration than morphine and hydromorphone, which are hydrophilic.[8,9]
- All opioids administered via epidural catheter can cause respiratory depression, sedation, nausea, vomiting, pruritus, and urinary retention.[1,4,8,9,16,21] The lowest efficacious dose of opioids should be administered to minimize the risk of adverse effects.

EQUIPMENT

- One epidural catheter kit or the following supplies[4,14,21]:
  - One 25-gauge,⅝-inch (0.5 × 16 mm) injection needle
  - One 23-gauge, 1¼-inch (0.6 × 30 mm) injection needle
  - One 18-gauge, 1½-inch (1.2 × 40 mm) injection needle
  - One 5-mL locking-tip syringe
  - One 20-mL locking-tip syringe
  - One locking tip loss-of-resistance syringe
  - One 18-gauge, 3¼-inch (1.3 × 80 mm) epidural needle
  - One 0.45 × 0.85–inch epidural catheter
- One introducer stabilizing catheter guide
- One Luer-lock catheter
- One 0.2-μm Luer-lock catheter connector
- One epidural flat filter
- Topical skin antiseptic, as ordered

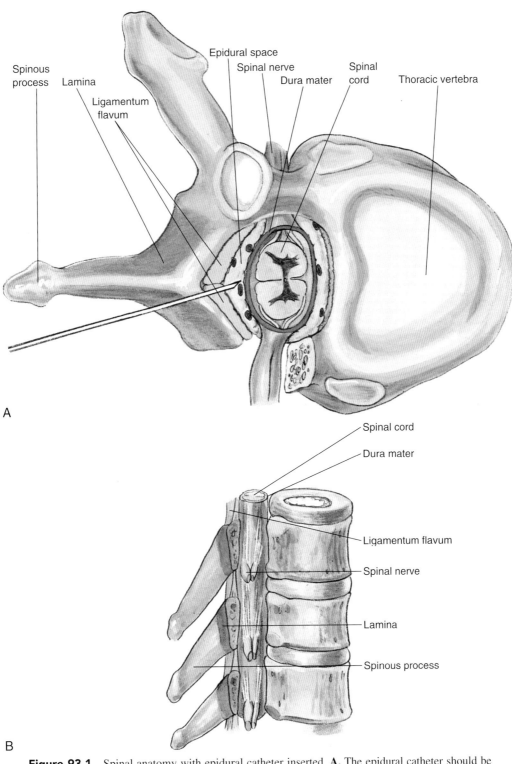

Figure 93.1   Spinal anatomy with epidural catheter inserted. **A,** The epidural catheter should be inserted into the epidural space. **B,** Epidural block. *(A, From Brown DL: XXXX, 2017. B, From Farag E, Mounir-Soliman L, Brown DL, editors:* Brown's atlas of regional anesthesia, *ed 5, Philadelphia, PA, Elsevier, 279–290.)*

- Sterile towels
- Sterile forceps
- Sterile gauze, 4 × 4 pads
- Face masks with eye shields
- Sterile gloves and gowns
- 20 mL 0.9% NaCl solution[14]

- 5 to 10 mL local anesthetic as prescribed (e.g., 1% lidocaine) for local infiltration[14,16]
- Test dose of local anesthetic (e.g., 3 mL 2% lidocaine with epinephrine, 1:200,000)[4,6,14,21]
- 5-mL local anesthetic bolus dose as prescribed to establish the block[21]

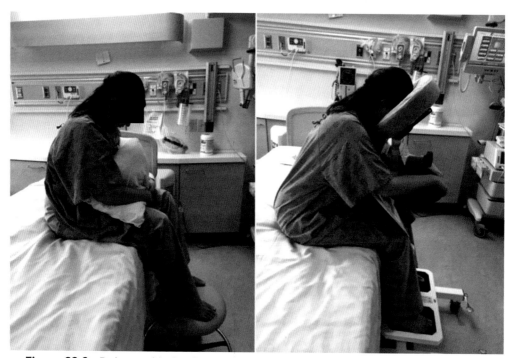

Figure 93.2   Patient positioning for insertion of an epidural catheter. This figure shows one of the positions patients can assume for the epidural catheter insertion procedure *(left)*, which may be facilitated by an epidural positioning device *(right)*. *(From Sebbag I, Qasem F, VedagiriSai R, et al: Efficacy of the Epidural Positioning Device© in optimizing the acoustic target window for neuraxial needle placement in term pregnancy.* Int J Obstet Anesth *41:47–52, 2020.)*

- Sterile gauze or transparent dressing to cover the epidural catheter entry site[2,10]
- Tape to secure the epidural catheter to the patient's back and over the patient's shoulder[4,10]
- "Epidural only" and "Not for intravenous (IV) injection" labels
- Pump for administering analgesia (e.g., volumetric or PCEA pump)
- Dedicated yellow-lined, portless epidural administration set
- Equipment for monitoring blood pressure, heart rate, and pulse oximetry

Additional equipment to have available as needed includes the following:
- Epidural positioning device (Fig. 93.2)[20]
- Ice or alcohol swabs for demonstrating level of block after catheter insertion[4,14]
- Emergency medications (e.g., naloxone for respiratory depression; IV colloids, vasopressors, and/or vasoconstrictors for hypotension; and Intralipid, a 20% fat emulsion, for local anesthetic toxicity)[4,9,14,15,16,21]
- Bag-valve-mask device and oxygen[16,21]
- Intubation equipment[16,21]

PATIENT AND FAMILY EDUCATION

- Review the principles and indications of epidural use with the patient and family. If the patient's needs are not met, an assessment of the therapy will be completed and the physician, advanced nurse practitioner, or other healthcare provider may change the dosage or therapy to meet those needs. If available, supply easy-to-read, written information in the patient's primary language. *Rationale:* This information prepares the patient and family for what to expect and may reduce anxiety and misconceptions about epidural use.[1] (Level C)*

- Explain to the patient and family that the insertion procedure will require a specific position and can be uncomfortable, but that a local anesthetic will be used at the insertion site to facilitate comfort.[16] *Rationale:* Explanation promotes patient cooperation and comfort, decreases anxiety and fear, and facilitates the insertion procedure.[4]

- During insertion and therapy, instruct the patient to immediately report adverse side effects that are indicative of local anesthetic toxicity (e.g., ringing in the ears, a metallic taste in the mouth, or numbness or tingling around the mouth), changes in pain management, numbness of extremities, loss of motor function of lower extremities, acute onset of back pain, loss of bladder and bowel function, itching, and nausea and vomiting. *Rationale:* Education regarding adverse side effects allows for more rapid assessment and management of potential complications.[4,14]

- Review an appropriate pain rating scale with the patient. The physician, advanced practice nurse, or other healthcare provider and the patient must establish a mutually agreeable pain level goal. *Rationale:* Review ensures that the patient understands the pain rating scale and enables the nurse to obtain a baseline assessment. Establishing a pain level goal allows the physician, advanced practice nurse, or other healthcare provider to know an acceptable goal for pain management.[1]

- When using PCEA, ensure that patient and family understand that only the patient is to activate the medication release (see Procedure 94, Patient-Controlled Analgesia).[1] *Rationale:* The patient should remain alert enough to administer his or her own dose.

---

*Level C: Qualitative studies, descriptive or correlational studies, integrative reviews, systematic reviews, or randomized controlled trials with inconsistent results.

PATIENT ASSESSMENT AND PREPARATION

Patient Assessment

- Review the patient's allergies. *Rationale:* This information may decrease the possibility of an allergic reaction.
- Review the patient's current anticoagulation and antiplatelet therapy. *Rationale:* Anticoagulant medications may increase the risk for epidural hematoma and spinal cord damage or paralysis, so it is recommended for these medications to be withheld before insertion and removal of the epidural catheter. The amount of time that a medication should be withheld depends on the specific medication.[4,11] (Level D)* Antiplatelet medications by themselves do not pose an increased risk for epidural hematoma if the patient's coagulation status is within normal limits.[4,11,21] Fibrinolytic and thrombolytic medications are contraindications for epidural therapy; if the patient receives epidural therapy at or near the time of fibrinolytic and/or thrombolytic medication administrations, monitoring should be done at least every 2 hours.[4] (Level D)*, (Level D)*
- Obtain the patient's vital signs. *Rationale:* Baseline data are provided.[14,16]
- Assess the patient's pain. *Rationale:* Baseline data are provided.[1]
- Assess the patient for local infection and/or generalized sepsis. Rationale: A contraindication for epidural catheter placement is active, untreated infection; the patient may need to be treated with preprocedure antibiotics.[2,4]

*Level D: Peer-reviewed professional and organizational standards with the support of clinical study recommendations.

Patient Preparation

- Verify the correct patient with two identifiers. *Rationale:* Before performing a procedure, the nurse should ensure the correct identification of the patient for the intended intervention.
- Verify that consent has been obtained. *Rationale:* Informed consent protects the rights of the patient and allows the patient to make a competent decision about the procedure.[4,21]
- Consider nothing by mouth (NPO), especially if sedation or general anesthesia is to be used. *Rationale:* NPO status decreases the risk for vomiting and aspiration.
- Establish IV access, or ensure the patency of IV catheters. Administer IV fluids as prescribed before epidural catheter insertion. *Rationale:* IV access ensures that medications can be given quickly if needed. However, there is some evidence that administration of preprocedure IV fluids fails to treat hypotension that may occur during epidural infusion, and it has been recommended that epidural-related hypotension is best treated with vasopressors or vasoconstrictors.[4] (Level D)*
- Open the gown in the back. Wash the patient's back with soap and water. *Rationale:* This action cleanses the skin and allows easy access to the patient's back.
- Perform a preprocedure verification and time out including all team members present for the epidural catheter insertion procedure. *Rationale:* This action ensures patient safety.[12]

*Level D: Peer-reviewed professional and organizational standards with the support of clinical study recommendations.

Procedure	for Pain Management: Epidural Catheters (Assisting With Insertion and Initiating Continuous Infusion)	
Steps	Rationale	Special Considerations
1. **HH**		
2. **PE**		Physicians, advanced practice nurses, and other healthcare providers present during epidural insertion should don **PE** (e.g., face mask, eye shield, hair covering). The individual performing the procedure should wear a face mask, eye shield, hair covering, and sterile gloves; there is inconsistent evidence that a sterile gown worn during insertion affects catheter infection risk.[2] **(Level B*)**[5,14,21]
3. Obtain and verify the prescribed epidural infusion medication.	Ensures that the correct medication is being administered and reduces the risk of medication errors.	The medication should be prepared with aseptic technique by the pharmacy with laminar flow or prepared commercially to decrease the risk for epidural infection. All epidural solutions are preservative-free to avoid neuronal injury.[4] **(Level D*)**
4. Connect the epidural tubing to the epidural infusion medication, and prime the tubing.	Removes air from the infusion system and tubing.	

*Level B: Well-designed, controlled studies with results that consistently support a specific action, intervention, or treatment.
*Level D: Peer-reviewed professional and organizational standards with the support of clinical study recommendations.

UNIT III

Procedure **for Pain Management: Epidural Catheters (Assisting With Insertion and Initiating Continuous Infusion)—*Continued***

Steps	Rationale	Special Considerations
5. Assist as needed in positioning the patient into the lateral decubitus knee-to-chest position; sitting and leaning over a bedside table; or sitting and leaning into an epidural positioning device (see Fig. 93.2).	Facilitates ease of insertion of the epidural catheter, as each position opens the interspinous spaces (see Fig. 93.1).[4,14,21]	Movement of the back may increase the risk of complications, such as misplacement of the catheter.[4] Use of an epidural positioning device or preprocedure analgesia/sedation may increase patient comfort and facilitate correct positioning throughout the procedure.[14,20] **(Level D*)**
6. Assist as needed with antiseptic preparation of the intended insertion site.	Reduces the transmission of microorganisms into the epidural space.	Povidone-iodine or chlorhexidine as an antiseptic agent is appropriate as long as the prepping agent dries completely[2,5,7,18,21] **(Level B*)**
7. Assist as needed with draping the patient with exposure only of the insertion site.	Aids in maintaining sterility.[4,14]	Patient privacy and normothermia should be considered as the patient's back is exposed.
8. Assist the provider as needed while the epidural catheter is placed.	Provides needed assistance.	
9. After the catheter is placed, monitor the patient as the physician or advanced practice nurse administers the test dose medication.	Assists in confirming proper placement of the epidural catheter.[4,6,14,21]	An immediate increase in heart rate indicates that the catheter has inadvertently penetrated an epidural vein.[4,14] If this occurs, the healthcare provider inserting the catheter should withdraw the catheter slightly or remove it and insert a new catheter.
10. After the epidural catheter placement is confirmed, assist as needed with application of a sterile, occlusive dressing.	Reduces insertion site contamination by microorganisms.[2]	Use of a transparent dressing allows for ongoing assessment of the insertion site for infection, leakage, or dislodgment.[2,10]
11. Secure the epidural tubing and filter to the patient with gauze padding and tape.	Avoids disconnection between the epidural catheter and filter.[2,4,10]	Gauze padding prevents discomfort and pressure on the skin from the filter.
12. Monitor the patient as the provider administers a bolus dose of medication.	Facilitates a therapeutic level of analgesia.[13,21]	If a local anesthetic is used for the bolus, monitor the blood pressure frequently, with assessment for possible hypotension.[8,16] Epidural medications may have a slower onset, so longer monitoring may be needed.[4,8,9]
13. Connect the prescribed medication infusion system.	Prepares the infusion system.	
14. Initiate therapy: A. Place the system in the epidural pump or PCEA pump, and set the rate and volume to be infused as ordered.	Prepares the epidural medication to be administered.	No other solution or medication (e.g., IV antibiotic, total parenteral nutrition) should be given through the epidural catheter.
B. Attach "Epidural only" and "Not for intravenous (IV) injection" labels to the epidural tubing.[6]	Reduces the risk of inadvertent medication administration via the epidural catheter or IV line.	Inadvertent IV administration of some epidural solutions can cause serious adverse reactions, including hypotension and cardiovascular collapse.[4,16] Use a portless system.
C. Lock the epidural or PCEA pump.	Prevents tampering with the pump settings and provides patient safety.	

*Level B: Well-designed, controlled studies with results that consistently support a specific action, intervention, or treatment.
*Level D: Peer-reviewed professional and organizational standards with the support of clinical study recommendations.

Procedure continues on following page

Procedure | **for Pain Management: Epidural Catheters (Assisting With Insertion and Initiating Continuous Infusion)—*Continued***

Steps	Rationale	Special Considerations
15. Assess the effectiveness of the therapy and medication: A. Assess the patient's pain score.	Identifies the need for additional medication and/or interventions.[1]	Tolerable pain scores should be reported at rest, and very little pain should be experienced with deep breathing, coughing, and movement.
B. Assess the level of the epidural block with ice or an alcohol swab.	Verifies the level placement of the epidural catheter.[4,14]	The preferred insertion level of an epidural block varies based on the indication for epidural catheter placement (e.g., surgical incision, trauma site, labor). The level and efficacy of therapy can be assessed by affected dermatomes (Fig. 93.3).[16]

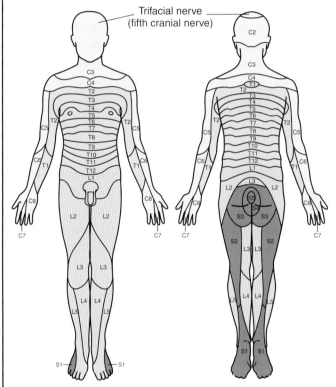

Figure 93.3 Dermatomes. Dermatomes are specific skin surface areas innervated by a single spinal nerve or group of spinal nerves. During epidural therapy, the dermatomes can be assessed to determine the level and efficacy of treatment.[4,14] *C,* Cervical segments; *T,* thoracic segments; *L,* lumbar segments; *S,* sacral segments. *(From Phillips N, Hornacky A. Anesthesia: techniques and agents. In Phillips N, Hornacky, editors:* Berry & Kohn's operating room technique, *ed 14, St. Louis, 2021, Elsevier, 421–454.)*

| 16. Remove **PE**, and discard used supplies in an appropriate receptacle. | Removes and safely discards used supplies. | |
| 17. **HH** | | |

Procedure	for Pain Management: Epidural Catheter (Bolus Dose Administration After Insertion)		
Steps		**Rationale**	**Special Considerations**
1. 🅷🅷			
2. 🅿🅴			Physicians, advanced practice nurses, and other healthcare providers administering a bolus dose should don 🅿🅴 (e.g., gloves).[2,5]
3. Label the epidural catheter used for intermittent bolus dosing (suggest color-coding).[6]		Reduces the risk of inadvertent medication administration via the epidural catheter or IV line.	Inadvertent IV administration of some epidural solutions can cause serious adverse reactions, including hypotension and cardiovascular collapse.[4,16]
4. Obtain, verify, and prepare (if necessary) the ordered epidural bolus medication.		Ensures that the correct medication is being administered and reduces the risk of medication errors.	Use only preservative-free solution to dilute, which decreases the risk of neuronal injury.[4] **(Level D)*** Do not use multidose solutions because they increase the risk for contamination and the risk for an epidural infection.[2]
5. Prepare and cleanse the epidural port with an antiseptic agent.		Maintains aseptic technique.	Povidone-iodine or chlorhexidine as an antiseptic agent is appropriate as long as the prepping agent dries completely.[2,5,7,18,21] **(Level B*)**
6. Aspirate the epidural catheter with an empty syringe using aseptic technique.[4,6,14,15,21] **(Level D*)**		Verifies that the catheter is in the epidural space.	Institutional policies may limit the amount of aspirated fluid allowed. If more than 3 mL of blood or 5 mL of clear fluid is aspirated, the catheter may have migrated into a vessel or the subarachnoid space.[4,6,21] Do not reinject the aspirated blood or clear fluid, and do not inject the epidural bolus. Notify the physician, advanced practice nurse, or healthcare provider.
7. Connect the syringe with the bolus medication to the epidural catheter port, and administer the medication slowly.		Facilitates a therapeutic level of analgesia while assessing for resistance of the bolus medication.[13,21]	Some resistance will be felt because the diameter of the epidural space is small, and the epidural filter is in place. If excessive resistance occurs, assess for kinks in the catheter, or reposition the patient.[10] Excessive resistance may be more pronounced if the epidural catheter is placed at the lumbar dermatomes as opposed to the thoracic dermatomes (see Fig. 93.3). If resistance continues to impair administration of a bolus dose, contact the physician or advanced practice nurse.
8. Assess the effectiveness of the therapy and medication.		Identifies the need for additional medication and/or interventions.[1]	Report ineffective therapy despite bolus administration or signs of impending complications to the physician or advanced practice nurse.
9. Remove 🅿🅴, and discard used supplies.		Removes and safely discards used supplies.	
10. 🅷🅷			

*Level B: Well-designed, controlled studies with results that consistently support a specific action, intervention, or treatment.
*Level D: Peer-reviewed professional and organizational standards with the support of clinical study recommendations.

Procedure for Assisting With Removal of the Epidural Catheter

Steps	Rationale	Special Considerations
1. **HH**		
2. **PE**		All healthcare providers present during epidural catheter removal should don **PE** (e.g., face mask, eye shield, gloves).[2,5]
3. Assist the provider as needed with removal of the catheter (e.g., patient positioning, infusion medication disposal)	Facilitates catheter removal.	If encountering resistance with removal, reposition the patient. If encountering excessive resistance or abnormal patient symptoms (e.g., pain, paresthesia), do not remove the catheter.[19] **(Level D*)** Epidural catheters may shear and remain retained in the patient.[6,19] Assess that the entire catheter has been removed; if the catheter breaks, evidence suggests leaving the broken pieces and observing the patient. Surgical intervention may be needed.[4,19] **(Level D*)**
4. Assist as needed with applying a sterile, occlusive dressing.	Reduces insertion site contamination by microorganisms.[2]	Use of a transparent dressing allows for ongoing assessment of the insertion site for infection or leakage.[2,10,19]
5. Remove **PE**, and discard used supplies in an appropriate receptacle.	Removes and safely discards used supplies.	
6. **HH**		

*Level D: Peer-reviewed professional and organizational standards with the support of clinical study recommendations.

Expected Outcomes

- The epidural catheter is inserted into the epidural space using sterile technique
- The epidural catheter, tubing, and filter are secured to the patient and properly labeled[4,6,10]
- Medications can be given with minimal resistance via epidural catheter
- The patient receives a bilateral, equal block at the indicated level[4]
- The patient's pain is decreased and maintained at a tolerable level[9,13]
- The patient experiences minimal physiological or adverse effects from the block or medications administered[4,13]
- The patient remains free from infection during epidural insertion, therapy, and after catheter removal
- The epidural catheter is removed with minimal complications or patient discomfort

Unexpected Outcomes

- Inability to insert the epidural catheter[6]
- Accidental dural puncture into the subarachnoid space, which may result in a dural puncture headache[4,6,14,16]
- Epidural catheter tip dislodgement or migration into a vessel or adjacent structure (e.g., subarachnoid space)[4,6,10]
- Cracked epidural filter
- Accidental connection of the epidural solution to the IV fluids or accidental connection of IV fluids to the epidural catheter[4]
- Occlusion/excessive resistance of medication administration via epidural catheter[19]
- Inadvertent block (e.g., patchy block, unilateral block, high or total spinal blockade)[4,6,14,16,21]
- Motor blockade of limbs or lower extremity weakness[2,19]
- Sensory loss in the limbs, which may result in redness or signs of skin breakdown at pressure area sites (e.g., sacrum, heels) from decreased sensation[2,19]
- Suboptimal pain relief
- Physiological or adverse effects from the block or medications administered, such as hypotension, respiratory depression, hypoxia, nausea, vomiting, pruritus, oversedation, drowsiness, urinary retention, local anesthetic systematic toxicity, anaphylaxis, or cardiopulmonary arrest[1,2,4,8,9,15,16,21]
- Leakage, local erythema, or drainage at the insertion site[19]
- Dressing disruption exposing the insertion site
- Catheter shearing or retention during insertion or removal[4,6,14,19]
- Epidural abscess or hematoma[3,4,11,14,19]

UNIT III

UNIT III

Patient Monitoring and Care

Steps	Rationale	Reportable Conditions
Unless stated, the frequency of patient assessment and monitoring should be determined by institutional standards. 1. Monitor vital signs:[14,16,19] A. Assess respiratory function (rate, oxygenation status, and end-tidal carbon dioxide if prescribed) the first 20 minutes after epidural medication administration and/or bolus, then every 1–2 hours and as needed.	These steps assist to monitor the patient before epidural catheter insertion, during catheter insertion, throughout therapy, and after catheter removal. Identifies the patient's baseline respiratory rate, oxygenation status, and any changes in respiratory function. A decrease in oxygen saturation is a late sign of opioid oversedation and should not be solely relied on to detect oversedation.	These conditions should be reported if they persist despite nursing interventions. • Increasing respiratory depression • Sudden change in respiratory rate • Oxygen saturation <93% • Decreasing trend in oxygenation
B. Assess heart rate every 2 hours, then every 4 hours when stable.	Identifies the patient's baseline heart rate and any changes in heart rate. Tachycardia may indicate a condition such as shock. Bradycardia may indicate opioid overmedication and sympathetic blockade by the local anesthetic.	• Change in heart rate • Abnormal heart rate or rhythm
C. Assess blood pressure at least once every 2 hours, then every 4 hours when stable.	Identifies the patient's baseline blood pressure and any changes in blood pressure. Epidural therapy containing a local anesthetic may cause hypotension from vasodilation.[4,8,9,16] This adverse effect is most common when the patient has underlying hypovolemia.[21] If the patient is hypotensive: turn off the epidural infusion, place the patient in the supine position, and administer IV fluids, vasopressors, and/or vasoconstrictors as prescribed.[4] **(Level D*)**	• Hypotension
D. Assess the patient's temperature every 4 hours, or more often if febrile.	Identifies the patient's baseline temperature and any changes in temperature.	• Temperature >38.5°C (101.3°F)
2. Label and monitor the medication infusion supplies and equipment: A. Label the epidural tubing and pump, and monitor that the labeling system remains clearly identifiable.[6]	Reduces the risk of inadvertent medication administration via the epidural catheter or IV. Cardiopulmonary arrest and seizures may occur if the epidural solution is infused intravenously.[4] Consider placing the epidural pump away from other equipment and using a specific colored label to differentiate it from other supplies and equipment.	• Infusion of IV fluid into the epidural space • Infusion of epidural solution into the IV
B. Monitor the medication infusion rate, and, if applicable, assess that the medication infusion pump is locked.[19]	Ensures that the correct medication is administered safely.	• Unlocked medication pump • Tampered or broken medication pump
3. Monitor the patient's motor and sensory function.[2,19] A. Assess the patient's motor function at least every 4 hours and as needed.	Identifies the patient's baseline motor function and any changes in function. Motor loss in the extremities (e.g., leg numbness or inability to bend knees) may be an early warning sign of an epidural abscess or hematoma or may indicate an excessive dose of a local anesthetic.[3,4,9,11,14,19]	• Change in motor function in extremities • Sudden onset of back pain with decreasing motor weakness • Loss in bladder and bowel function (e.g., incontinence)

*Level D: Peer-reviewed professional and organizational standards with the support of clinical study recommendations.

Procedure continues on following page

Patient Monitoring and Care —*Continued*

Steps	Rationale	Reportable Conditions
B. Monitor the patient's sensory function and skin integrity of pressure area sites every 2 hours and as needed.	Identifies the patient's baseline sensory function, skin integrity, and any changes. If a local anesthetic is used in the epidural solution, check for pressure injuries and decubitus ulceration.	• Changes in sensory function • Altered skin integrity • Increasing redness or blistering of the skin on pressure area sites
4. Assess the patient's level of pain using the agreed-upon pain rating scale.[19]	Identifies the efficacy of epidural therapy and the need for additional medication and/or interventions.[1]	• Moderate to severe pain scores
5. Monitor the patient for any physiological or adverse effects from the block or epidural medication administration:[19]		
A. Assess for nausea and vomiting	Identifies potential adverse effects of medication administration.[2,4,8,16,21] Nausea and vomiting may be a sign of severe hypotension and may be treated with antiemetics, epidural medication adjustment, or low-dose opioid antagonists, such as naloxone.[9] **(Level D*)**	• Unrelieved nausea and vomiting
B. Assess for pruritus.	Identifies potential adverse effects of medication administration.[2,4,8,16] Pruritus may be treated with low-dose opioid antagonists such as naloxone (e.g., 0.04 mg).[9] **(Level D*)** Treatment with antihistamines, such as diphenhydramine or hydroxyzine, may cause increased sedation and are ineffective for spinally mediated itching.	• Unrelieved itching • Redness • Rash
C. Assess the patient's level of sedation.	Identifies the patient's baseline sedation status and potential adverse effects of medication administration.[4,8,19] Sedation precedes opioid-related respiratory depression, or a sudden change in sedation may indicate that the epidural catheter has migrated into an epidural blood vessel or the intrathecal space.	• Increasing sedation and drowsiness • Sudden change in sedation
D. Assess the patient's ability to void and ability to completely empty the bladder.	Identifies the patient's baseline bladder habits and function and potential adverse effects of medication administration or hematoma.[4,9,16,19,21] If the urinary retention is opioid-related, it may be treated with low-dose opioid antagonists such as naloxone.[9] **(Level D*)** If the urinary retention is hematoma-related, immediately notify the physician, advanced practice nurse, or other healthcare provider, as this is a late sign.[19] **(Level D*)**	• Urinary retention • Change in bladder function • Lack of urination for >6–8 hours
E. Assess for local anesthetic systematic toxicity.	Identifies potential adverse effects of medication administration.[4,15,19]	• Ringing in the ears • Tingling around the lips • Metallic taste
6. Assess the epidural catheter insertion site every 4 hours.[19]	Identifies epidural insertion site complications, such as leakage, local erythema, drainage, infection, dressing disruption, epidural abscess, or epidural hematoma.[2,3,4,10,11,19]	• Redness, pain, tenderness, swelling, or paresthesia at the insertion site • Increasing diffuse back pain • Presence of exudate

*Level D: Peer-reviewed professional and organizational standards with the support of clinical study recommendations.

UNIT III

Patient Monitoring and Care —*Continued*

Steps	Rationale	Reportable Conditions
A. Assess the epidural catheter dressing, and change as ordered or if soiled, wet, or loose.	Identifies epidural catheter dressing integrity.[10]	• Exposed catheter insertion site • Repetitive soiled or wet dressings
7. Change the epidural solution, tubing, and filter at a defined interval.[4] **(Level D*)**	Reduces epidural tubing and contamination by microorganisms.	• Contaminated epidural solution

*Level D: Peer-reviewed professional and organizational standards with the support of clinical study recommendations.

Documentation

Documentation should include the following:
- Patient and family education
- Completion of informed consent[21]
- Preprocedure verification and time out[12]
- Patient assessments, such as the following[1,2]:
  - Vital signs (e.g., respiratory rate and oxygen saturation, heart rate, blood pressure, temperature)
  - Sedation status
  - Pain assessments and efficacy of epidural analgesia
  - Levels of motor and sensory blockade
  - Insertion site appearance
  - Dressing integrity
- Any complications associated with the insertion or removal procedures[19]
- Confirmation of epidural catheter placement (e.g., decrease in blood pressure, demonstrable block to ice/alcohol swab)
- Medications, such as the following:
  - Test dose medication during catheter placement
  - Continuous epidural medication concentration and infusion rate
  - Bolus dose medication administration
  - PCEA medication concentration, amount of medication administered in a specific period, and associated pump settings (e.g., lockout intervals)
- Occurrence of physiological or adverse effects of the block or medication administration
- Type of dressing used[10]

References and Additional Readings

For a complete list of references and additional readings for this procedure, scan this QR code with your smartphone, or visit https://www.elsevier.com/__data/assets/pdf_file/0009/1319868/Chapter0093.pdf.

CHAPTER

94 Patient-Controlled Analgesia

Misti Tuppeny

PURPOSE: Intravenous (IV) patient-controlled analgesia (PCA) empowers patients to manage their pain by allowing them to administer smaller analgesic doses more frequently. Nurses are responsible for ensuring appropriate patient selection, maintaining the IV delivery system, and ensuring that patients are able to safely meet their own needs for pain management through frequent assessment and patient education.

PREREQUISITE NURSING KNOWLEDGE

- Pain is defined as an "unpleasant sensory and emotional experience associated with, or resembling that associated with, actual or potential tissue damage" by the International Association for the Study of Pain.[15] An estimated 25.3 million adults (11.2% of total U.S. adult population) had pain every day for the preceding 3 months. Nearly 40 million adults (17.6%) experience severe levels of pain.[24]
- The management of acute pain remains inadequate across various treatment settings, with a substantial proportion of patients continuing to experience intense pain despite the availability of effective treatment.[26]
- Several perceived barriers to adequate pain management are clearly defined standards and pain protocols, patient reluctance to report pain and take analgesics, and physician reluctance to prescribe opioids.[1]
- Tables 94.1 and 94.2 list guidelines for dosing and considerations for selection of opioids.
- Poorly controlled acute postoperative pain is associated with increased morbidity, functional and quality-of-life impairment, delayed recovery time, prolonged duration of opioid use, and higher healthcare costs.[14] Negative clinical outcomes related to ineffective pain management for patients after surgery include deep vein thrombosis, pulmonary embolism, coronary ischemia, myocardial infarction, pneumonia, poor wound healing, impairment of the immune system, insomnia, readmissions, and negative emotions.[11] Unrelieved pain may delay recovery and prolong hospital stays.[14]
- Self-report of pain is the single most reliable indicator of pain intensity.[6]
- Although pain is prevalent, underdiagnosed and undertreated populations include racial and ethnic minorities, people with lower levels of education and income, women, older adults, military veterans, postsurgical and cancer patients, and patients nearing the end of life.[21]
- Studies and meta-analyses have shown that patients receiving PCA report an increased satisfaction level with pain management and an improvement in pain control.[4,18,20,30,33] IV PCA may be used for both acute and chronic pain,[26,32] although IV administration of opioids is most often used for acute pain.[26]

- IV PCA can be an effective method of pain relief for pediatric and adult patients.[9,14,27,31,33] Table 94.1 lists dosing guidelines. PCA is not recommended in situations in which oral opioids can readily manage pain (e.g., chronic and relatively stable cancer pain).[26]
- IV PCA can be administered as a continuous (basal) infusion along with patient-initiated boluses or as patient-initiated boluses exclusively. Use caution with continuous infusion because of accumulation of the medication.[2]
- Patient assessment at frequent, regular intervals[13] (at least every 4 hours) should include an evaluation of the patient's vital signs, sedation level with a valid and reliable scale, pain level with a valid and reliable scale, and common opioid side effects, such as pruritus, nausea,[5,9] constipation, and urinary retention.[20] Table 94.2 lists side effects associated with PCA opioids. Patients need more frequent assessments during the first 24 hours after initiation of IV PCA and during the night.[8,16]
- PCA pump settings should be confirmed at regular intervals.[8,16] See Box 94.1 for common terms used when administering PCA. Adverse events during IV PCA may include sedation, respiratory depression, and hypoxemia. Opioid antagonists should be readily available.
- Adjuvant medications such as nonsteroidal antiinflammatory drugs (NSAIDs)[2] and cyclooxygenase (COX-2) inhibitors[2,16,24,33] can be used to improve pain management[5] or to improve opioid side effects.[22,30,31]
- The Joint Commission does not support PCA by proxy (someone other than the patient pushing the PCA button) on the recommendation of the Institute of Safe Medication Practices (ISMP). According to the ISMP, patients have experienced oversedation, increased respiratory depression, and death from PCA by proxy.[8,31,33] A safety feature of PCA therapy is that an oversedated patient cannot press the button to obtain additional pain medication.
- PCA by an authorized user (typically nurse or designated family member of patient) is a potential alternative to PCA by proxy. Healthcare institutions that use PCA by an authorized user must have the following in place before this practice is initiated[8,9]
  - ❖ Policies that guide the practice, including the patient population
  - ❖ Definition of PCA by an authorized user

TABLE 94.1	Intravenous Patient-Controlled Analgesia Regimens		
Opioid	Demand Dose	Lockout Time (minutes)	Continuous Basal Infusion Rate
Fentanyl	20–50 mcg	5–15	0–60 mcg/kg/hr
Hydromorphone	0.1–0.6 mg	5–15	0–0.4 mg/b
Morphine	1–3 mg	5–15	0-2 mg/hr

Adopted from formulary at Virginia Commonwealth University Medical Center. Opioid-naive patients are typically set at a lower range for demand dose and higher range for lockout time. Basal infusion rates may be considered in opioid-tolerant patients.
From Sharma J, Tran B, Dhillon S: Acute postoperative pain: patient-controlled analgesia. In Banik RK, editors: *Anesthesiology in-training exam review,* Cham, 2022, Springer. https://doi.org/10.1007/978-3-030-87266-3_3.

TABLE 94.2	Patient-Controlled Analgesia: Considerations in Opioid Selection			
Opioid	Side Effects	Advantages	Disadvantages	Cautions/Contraindications
Morphine				
	Nausea	Vast clinical experience	Slow onset: 15 minutes	Allergy (use fentanyl)
	Sedation	Less expensive than other	Histamine release	Renal dysfunction
	Pruritus	opioids	Active metabolite (M6G) accumulates in	Hepatic dysfunction
	Reduced peristalsis		renal patients and causes excessive	Asthma (histamine release)
	Respiratory depression		sedation and other side effects	
Hydromorphone (Dilaudid)				
	Nausea	Faster onset than morphine	More expensive than morphine	Allergy
	Sedation	Less sedation	Less clinical experience than morphine	High doses can result in
	Pruritus	No active metabolites	Higher potential for abuse	excitation with impaired
	Reduced peristalsis			renal dysfunction
	Respiratory depression			
Fentanyl (Sublimaze)				
	Nausea	Rapid onset	More expensive than morphine	Allergy
	Sedation	No active metabolites	Less clinical experience than with	Rapid administration of drug
	Pruritus	Less constipation compared	morphine	can result in "stiff chest,"
	Reduced peristalsis	with morphine	Short duration of action	making ventilation difficult
	Respiratory depression			

From Mariano E: *Management of acute perioperative pain in adults.* UpToDate. Updated August 30, 2022. https://www.uptodate.com/contents/management-of-acute-perioperative-pain.

BOX 94.1	Key Terms for Patient-Controlled Analgesia

- *Basal rate:* The amount of analgesic administered continuously.
- *Breakthrough dose:* A bolus dose administered by the nurse, similar to a loading dose when pain is inadequately managed with the current PCA settings.
- *Cumulative dose limit:* The predetermined maximum drug amount that can be delivered over either 1 or more (usually 4) hours.
- *Demand or PCA dose:* The amount of drug administered each time the patient activates the pump.
- *Loading dose:* A bolus dose given before initiation of PCA therapy, usually higher than the dose administered when the patient activates the pump.
- *Lockout interval:* Predetermined period during which the patient cannot initiate doses.

Modified from Mariano E: *Management of acute perioperative pain in adults.* UpToDate. Updated August 30, 2022. https://www.uptodate.com/contents/managem ent-of-acute-perioperative-pain; Sharma S, Balireddy RK, Vorenkamp KE, Durieux ME: Beyond opioid patient-controlled analgesia: a systematic review of analgesia after major spine surgery. *Reg Anesth Pain Med* 37:79-98, 2012; Stewart D. Pearls and pitfalls of patient-controlled analgesia. *US Pharmacist* 42: HS24–HS27, 2017.

- ❖ Education plan for the authorized user
- ❖ Documentation of the authorized user and education given
- Serious adverse events from errors with opioids include "failure to control pain, oversedation, respiratory depression, seizures, and death[13,21]
- Risk factors for complications during IV PCA use include the following:
  - ❖ Age older than 61 years of age (greater incidence of desaturation)[16,30,32]
  - ❖ Morbid obesity (greater incidence of desaturation)[16,30]
  - ❖ Sleep apnea, sleep disorder or asthma, and snoring[8,16,30]
  - ❖ Concurrent medications that potentiate opiates (e.g., sedation)[8]
  - ❖ Impaired organ function[26]
  - ❖ No recent opioid use[16]
  - ❖ Postsurgery, especially if upper abdominal or thoracic, and longer times receiving anesthesia[16]
  - ❖ Increased opioid requirement[15]
  - ❖ Preexisting cardiac and pulmonary disease[16]
- Careful patient selection is imperative for effective pain management.[12,13,16]

- Patient assessment for management of pain helps prevent adverse events.[2]
    - Screen for those with increased risk of complications.[8]
    - Assess the patient's analgesic use and abuse potential.[8]
- Individualize pain treatment plans, and use multimodal strategies (pharmacology, nonpharmacology, psychosocial support, and complementary and behavioral approaches)[6,24,29]
- Extra precautions should be taken to prevent complications, such as a short-term trial to determine the patient's response and sufficient time for assessment of the patient and the pain.
- Patients who may be poor candidates for PCA include the following:
    - Anyone with cognitive abilities that prohibit understanding and following directions for IV PCA (e.g., patients with a decreased level of consciousness or developmental disabilities)[6,9,17,30]
    - Anyone without the physical ability to push the PCA button that controls the dose administration[11,12,22]
    - Anyone with a psychological reason that prohibits using the PCA button for pain management (e.g., psychological disability, refusal to operate the PCA administration button)[6,9]
- A number of medication errors have been reported with IV PCA. Factors associated with errors include improper patient selection, inadequate monitoring, inadequate patient education, medication product mix-ups, programming errors, PCA by proxy, inadequate medical and nursing staff education, prescription errors, and PCA pump design flaws.[8,14]
- PCA is available in various routes, including IV, epidural (patient-controlled epidural analgesia [PCEA]; see Procedure 93), subcutaneous, peripheral nerve catheter, oral, intranasal, and transdermal.[24] The focus of this procedure is IV PCA.
- An interprofessional team approach is beneficial for pain management.[22]

EQUIPMENT

- PCA pump
- PCA tubing with antisiphon valve (may also include a plunger for insertion into the PCA medication syringe barrel)
- IV pump
- IV tubing
- Prescribed medication (may be in a syringe, bag, or cassette)
- Antiseptic pad
- Nonsterile gloves
- Electrocardiogram (ECG) and blood pressure monitoring equipment
- Pulse oximetry equipment
- Normal saline solution or other compatible IV fluid
Additional equipment, to have as needed, includes the following:
- Emergency medications, including an opioid reversal agent to reverse oversedation or respiratory depression
- Bag-valve-mask device and oxygen
- End-tidal carbon dioxide ($Etco_2$) monitoring equipment

PATIENT AND FAMILY EDUCATION

- Review an appropriate pain rating scale with the patient. The physician, advanced practice nurse, nurse, or other healthcare professional and patient must establish a mutually agreeable pain level goal. *Rationale:* Review ensures that the patient understands the pain rating scale and enables the nurse to obtain a baseline assessment. Establishing a pain level goal allows the physician, advanced practice nurse, or other healthcare professional to know an acceptable goal for pain management.
- Review the principles of PCA use with the patient and family members.[2,13,26] If a basal rate has been prescribed, inform the patient that pain medication will be infusing at all times. Explain that if the pain is not relieved with the steady dose, extra medicine can be delivered by pressing the patient bolus button. Be sure the patient understands what the lockout interval is. If the patient's pain needs are not met, an assessment of the therapy will be completed, and the physicians, advanced practice nurses, or other healthcare professionals may change the dosage or therapy to meet those needs. *Rationale:* This review may reduce anxiety and preconceptions about PCA use.
- IV PCA is designed for the patient to administer the pain medication. The patient should be the only one to deliver the demand dose. The Institute for Safe Medication Practices (ISMP), the American Society for Pain Management Nursing (ASPMN), and The Joint Commission do not support PCA by proxy because of adverse events such as oversedation, respiratory depression, cardiopulmonary arrest, and death that have occurred with PCA by proxy.[7,11] *Rationale:* The patient should remain alert enough to administer his or her own dose. A safeguard to oversedation is that a patient cannot administer additional medication doses if sedated.
- Instruct the patient and family members to report common side effects such as oversedation, pruritus, nausea or vomiting, constipation, or urinary retention. *Rationale:* Side effects are identified by the patient and family.

PATIENT ASSESSMENT AND PREPARATION

Patient Assessment

- Assess the patient's ability to properly use IV PCA as a method for pain management. *Rationale:* The patient will not achieve adequate pain management if unable to use the PCA.
- Assess the patient's pain, and document the intensity, location, and characteristics.[25-27] *Rationale:* A baseline assessment permits an accurate evaluation of the efficacy of the PCA.
- Assess the patient's level of sedation with the use of a sedation scale.[6,16,24,26] *Rationale:* Sedation generally precedes respiratory depression; a patient who is less alert should be closely monitored if PCA is prescribed.
- Review the patient's medication allergies. *Rationale:* Review of medication allergies before administration of

a new medication decreases the chances of an allergic reaction.

Patient Preparation

- Verify the correct patient with two identifiers. *Rationale:* Before performing a procedure, the nurse should ensure the correct identification of the patient for the intended intervention.

- Ensure that the patient understands the teaching. Having the patient demonstrate the procedure helps evaluate patient education. Answer questions as they arise, and reinforce information as needed.[25] *Rationale:* Understanding of previously taught information is evaluated and reinforced.
- Obtain IV access, and ensure patency of the IV. *Rationale:* Analgesia is delivered intravenously.

Procedure	for Initiating Intravenous Patient-Controlled Analgesia	
Steps	Rationale	Special Considerations
1. HH		
2. PE		
3. Review the prescription for the PCA, including the medication, concentration, basal rate, loading dose, demand PCA dose, lockout interval, cumulative dose limit (over 1 or more hours), and basal rate as prescribed.[9]	Ensures that the correct PCA prescription is administered to the patient.	Ensure coverage for common side effects, such as pruritus, constipation, or nausea. Follow institutional standards. A medication such as naloxone may be prescribed. Naloxone is an opioid reversal agent that is used to reverse oversedation or respiratory depression. Ensure that the patient is physically, psychologically, and cognitively able to use the PCA for pain management. The use of a basal rate is controversial and may result in oversedation in patients who are opioid naive.[20]
4. Check for medication allergies or sensitivities. Check for medications that may potentiate the opioid and for adverse effects of the opioid.[9,14] **(Level E*)**	Prevents allergic or adverse reactions.	
5. Attach the antisiphon valve of the tubing to the medication syringe.	Prepares the equipment.	Many PCA pumps use syringe delivery of the medication. Other PCA pumps use bags and cassettes rather than syringe delivery.
6. Purge the PCA tubing of air.	Removes air from the system.	If the injector is the plunger of the syringe, attach the antisiphon valve on the tubing to the syringe, and manually purge. The PCA may offer the option of purging via the PCA pump before it is attached to the patient.
7. Insert the syringe into the PCA pump by first placing the bottom of the syringe in the lower flanges of the cradle and then positioning the top portion of the syringe in place. If using a cassette system, snap and lock the cassette in place on the infusion pump.	Prepares the PCA system.	Place the syringe barrel into the pump within the area provided by the upper and lower flanges of the cradle. If a cassette system is used, unlock the system, and place the new cassette into the bottom of the infusion pump, where it can be snapped into place and then locked.

*Level E: Multiple case reports, theory-based evidence from expert opinions, or peer-reviewed professional organizational standards without clinical studies to support recommendations.

Procedure for Initiating Intravenous Patient-Controlled Analgesia—*Continued*

Steps	Rationale	Special Considerations
8. Position the medication syringe or cassette so the name and concentration of the drug and the volume markings are visible.	Ensures ready identification of the medication.	
9. Secure the syringe in the cradle.	Ensures proper positioning of the syringe.	
10. Occlude the PCA tubing with the slide clamp.	Contains the medication until the infusion begins.	
11. Insert the IV tubing of the continuous IV solution into the IV pump.	Prepares the infusion pump.	
12. Connect the IV tubing of the continuous IV solution to the lowest Y-site on the PCA medication tubing, and ensure that the tubing from the Y-site to the end of the PCA medication tubing is purged with the IV fluid.	Prepares the system and prevents an air bolus.	
13. Program the PCA pump with the medication name and concentration, the loading dose (as prescribed), PCA dose, lockout interval, cumulative dose limit (over 1 or more hours), and basal rate (as prescribed).	Prepares the system.	
14. Independently verify the patient's identification, medication and medication concentration, PCA pump settings, and tubing[3,9,11,16] with another physician, advanced practice nurse, or other healthcare professional. **(Level E*)**	Adverse events can occur as a result of programming errors.	Independent verification of patient identification, medication and concentration, PCA pump settings, and the line attachment before use and before pump refill or programming change may lessen the risk of programming errors.[7,11,16]
15. Program the compatible IV solution at a rate to provide not less than the minimal acceptable rate for a continuous IV solution per institutional standards.	Ensures delivery of the prescribed medication. Highly concentrated medications such as hydromorphone may be administered in bolus doses of <1 mL, but do not reach the patient quickly through most IV tubing without a continuous IV infusion. Some PCA pumps do not use continuous IV solution; however, the PCA tubing is much smaller, increasing the likelihood that the medication will reach the patient, although the infused volume is small.	The medication's basal rate combined with any other IV fluids should total the prescribed hourly IV rate. If the PCA is programmed for bolus dosing only, set the IV solution on no less than the minimal rate for the maintenance IV.

*Level E: Multiple case reports, theory-based evidence from expert opinions, or peer-reviewed professional organizational standards without clinical studies to support recommendations.

Procedure continues on following page

UNIT III

Procedure for Initiating Intravenous Patient-Controlled Analgesia—*Continued*

Steps	Rationale	Special Considerations
16. Clean the IV catheter cap with an appropriate antiseptic cleanser, and connect the PCA tubing directly to the patient's IV line.[28] Release the slide clamp from the PCA tubing. Initiate continuous IV delivery and PCA therapy.	Connects the PCA to the IV access.	Verify patent IV access before connecting or infusing medication. Extension tubing may result in errors in the medication delivery and should not be used.
17. Label the PCA pump and the IV infusion pump.	Ensures quick and clear identification of IV fluids and medications.	
18. Label the IV tubing and the PCA tubing.	Ensures identification of IV fluids and PCA medications infusing via each IV tubing.	
19. Secure the PCA tubing at two points of tension.	Prevents accidental removal of the IV.	
20. Remove **PE**, and discard used supplies in an appropriate receptacle.	Removes and safely discards used supplies.	
21. **HH**		

Expected Outcomes

- Pain is minimized or relieved (at an acceptable level for the patient)
- No unmanaged side effects
- Continuous IV access

Unexpected Outcomes

- Extravasation
- Oversedation or respiratory depression
- Loss of IV access and interruption of medication delivery
- Pain not relieved

Patient Monitoring and Care

Steps	Rationale	Reportable Conditions
		These conditions should be reported if they persist despite nursing interventions.
1. Ensure that the medication is infusing properly through the IV.	New infusions may precipitate extravasation; an IV catheter may become dislodged through patient movement.	• Extravasation
2. Assess the patient's pain and level of sedation.[8] Follow institutional standards.	Monitors effectiveness of therapy; identifies the need for adjustment. Institutional assessment policies should take into account the expected.	• Pain is unrelieved • Altered level of sedation
3. Monitor the patient's vital signs, including heart rate, blood pressure, respirations, oxygen saturation (Sao_2), and $Etco_2$ according to institutional standards.[10,13,16,26]	Determines the presence of potential complications.	• Change in sedation level, respiratory status or other vital signs (e.g., respiratory rate, oxygenation via pulse oximetry, $Etco_2$)
4. Verify all PCA prescription changes and pump changes with another registered nurse (independent double-check verification).[10,13] (**Level E***)	Decreases the risk of a medication error or programming error.	• Medication dosage and/or programming errors

*Level E: Multiple case reports, theory-based evidence from expert opinions, or peer-reviewed professional organizational standards without clinical studies to support recommendations.

Patient Monitoring and Care —*Continued*

Steps	Rationale	Reportable Conditions
5. Ensure patient comprehension of PCA use and analgesic goal. Reinforce patient education.	Comprehension can be assessed with patient report, with review of the PCA history for frequency of attempts and through return patient demonstration.	• Patient unable to use PCA • Inability to achieve analgesia goal
6. Assess for the presence of side effects such as nausea, pruritus, urinary retention, or constipation.[7]	Many side effects from opioid use can be managed.[7]	• Nausea • Pruritus • Constipation • Urinary retention
7. Ensure prevention of constipation by encouraging mobilization and adequate fluid intake, adding fiber to the diet if applicable, and using stool softeners if indicated.	This is a significant complication of opioid use and can lead to other complications.	• Unresolved constipation despite prevention measures
8. Ensure that the patient continues to be an appropriate candidate for IV PCA.	Pain management may be ineffective, and the patient may be at higher risk for adverse events if not an appropriate candidate.	• Patient is cognitively, psychologically, or physically unable to manage IV PCA

Documentation

Documentation should include the following:
- Medication, concentration, basal rate, loading dose, any breakthrough dosing, demand dose, lockout interval, and cumulative dose (independent double check verification by another registered nurse after initiation of treatment and with all changes thereafter)[11,15,28]
- Pain assessment, interventions, and effectiveness of PCA and other adjunctive pain management[8]
- Patient's baseline and follow-up pain scores using a valid and reliable scale[8]
- Patient's baseline and follow-up sedation scores using a valid and reliable scale
- Total dose of medication administered, per institutional standards
- Time the PCA pump was cleared, per institutional policy
- Patient teaching and any reinforcement needed
- Side effects of opioids
- Unexpected outcomes
- Vital signs, oxygen saturation, and if used, $Etco_2$ level
- Appearance and patency of the IV site
- Additional interventions that were needed

References and Additional Readings

For a complete list of references and additional readings for this procedure, scan this QR code with your smartphone, or visit https://www.elsevier.com/__data/assets/pdf_file/0010/1319869/Chapter0094.pdf

UNIT III

PROCEDURE

95

Esophagogastric Tamponade Tube

Rosemary Lee

PURPOSE Esophagogastric tamponade therapy is used to provide temporary control of bleeding from gastric or esophageal varices.

PREREQUISITE NURSING KNOWLEDGE

- Tamponade therapy exerts direct pressure against the varices with the use of a gastric and/or esophageal balloon and may be used for patients who are unresponsive to medical therapy or are too hemodynamically unstable for endoscopy or sclerotherapy.[1-3]
- Esophagogastric tamponade tubes are used to control bleeding from either gastric and/or esophageal varices. The suction lumens allow the evacuation of accumulated blood from the stomach or esophagus. The suction lumens also allow for the intermittent instillation of saline solution to assist with evacuation of blood or clots and provide a means of irrigation if indicated.
- Three types of tubes are available for esophagogastric tamponade therapy. The two most common tubes are the Sengstaken-Blakemore tube (Bard, Inc., Covington, Georgia) (Fig. 95.1) and the Minnesota esophagogastric tamponade tube. The Sengstaken-Blakemore tube has a gastric and esophageal balloon and a gastric aspiration lumen. The four-lumen Minnesota tube (Fig. 95.2) has gastric and esophageal balloons and separate gastric and esophageal aspiration lumens. The third, the Linton or Linton-Nachlas tube[4] (Mallinckrodt Inc., Tyco Health Care Group, Hampshire, UK), has a gastric balloon and separate gastric and esophageal aspiration lumens and is used only for treatment of bleeding gastric varices. The Minnesota tube is considered the preferred tube for esophagogastric tamponade therapy because it allows for aspiration of drainage above the esophageal balloon and below the gastric balloon.
- Esophagogastric tamponade tubes may be introduced via either the nasogastric or the orogastric route by an expert provider.[5,6] The tubes are then advanced through the oropharynx and esophagus and into the stomach.
- Contraindications include latex allergy, esophageal strictures, and recent esophageal surgery. Relative contraindications are heart failure, respiratory failure, hiatal hernia, severe pulmonary hypertension, and cardiac dysrhythmias.[7,8]

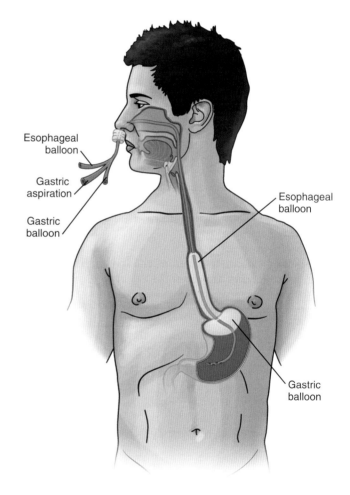

Figure 95.1 Sengstaken-Blakemore tube in place with both the esophageal and gastric balloons inflated. *(From Carlson KK, editor: AACN advanced critical care nursing, Philadelphia, 2009, Saunders.)*

- Because of the risk for aspiration, it is recommended that the patient be endotracheally intubated for airway protection before esophagogastric tamponade tube insertion.[3,9]
- Sedation should be considered, but dosing should be individualized on the assessment of each patient. Sedation

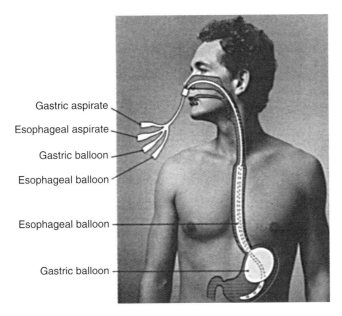

Figure 95.2 Minnesota four-lumen tube. *(From Swearingen PL: Photo atlas of nursing procedures, Reading, MA, 1991, Addison-Wesley.)*

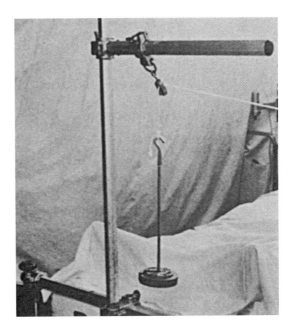

Figure 95.3 Balanced suspension traction securing tamponade tube and placement. *(From DeGroot KD, Damato M: Critical care skills, Norwalk, CT, 1987, Appleton & Lange.)*

should be used with caution in the setting of liver injury and/or failure due to these patients' impaired metabolism of sedating medications. The plan for sedation, if needed, is individualized with the goal to achieve patient comfort.

- The head of the bed should be at least 30 to 45 degrees at all times to reduce the risk of aspiration.[8,10]
- The use of esophageal tamponade can stop variceal bleeding in 80% of patients, yet 50% of patients rebleed after the balloons are deflated.[5,7,10] Its use is decreasing in clinical practice due to lack of provider expertise and major complications that may occur with the use of esophageal balloon tamponade therapy.[6,7,11] However, esophagogastric tubes are still used in areas where esophagogastric duodenoscopy is not readily available. The use of esophageal tamponade is designed to be a temporary intervention until more definitive therapy can be carried out. Balloon tamponade is recommended to be used for only 24 hours.[3,8,9]
- Potential complications include the following:
  - ❖ Aspiration
  - ❖ Medical device–associated pressure injury to the nares, tongue, or lips
  - ❖ Tube migration causing airway compromise/asphyxia
  - ❖ Esophageal/gastric necrosis and/or rupture
  - ❖ Arrhythmia (bradycardia)
  - ❖ Chest pain

EQUIPMENT

- Tamponade tube (Sengstaken-Blakemore, Minnesota, or Linton-Nachlas)
- Irrigation kit (or catheter-tip, 60-mL syringe and basin)
- Nasogastric (NG) tubes (one for Sengstaken-Blakemore tube)
- Normal saline (NS) solution for irrigation
- Water-soluble lubricant
- Topical anesthetic agent
- Sphygmomanometer or pressure gauge

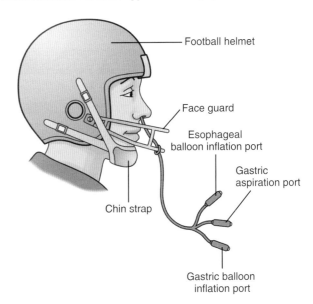

Figure 95.4 Tamponade tube secured in position with helmet.

- Four rubber-shod clamps or plastic plugs that may come with the balloon kit
- Adhesive tape
- Two to three suction setups and tubing for esophageal, gastric, and endotracheal suctioning
- Rigid pharyngeal suction-tip (Yankauer) catheter for oral secretions
- Cardiac monitor
- Scissors; must be kept at bedside

Additional equipment, to have available as needed, includes the following:

- Rubber cube sponge (used for nasal tamponade tube placement)—may be used for traction
- Balanced suspension traction apparatus with 1 pound of weights, 500-mL bag of IV fluid (Fig. 95.3), or football helmet with face mask (Fig. 95.4)

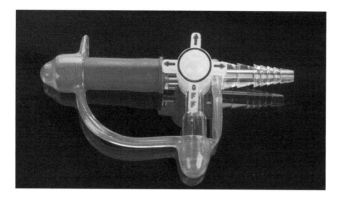

Figure 95.5 Lopez valve. *(Courtesy ICU Medical, Inc,. San Clemente, CA.)*

- Lopez enteral valve (Fig. 95.5) (ICU Medical, San Clemente, CA) or a three-way stopcock used to attach a 60-mL catheter-tip syringe and the handheld manometer to the tube
- Emergency medications and equipment, including transcutaneous pacemaker and intubation equipment (if not already intubated)
- Endotracheal suction equipment
- Marker
- Cervical collar

PATIENT AND FAMILY EDUCATION

- Explain the procedure and reason for the esophagogastric tube insertion. *Rationale:* This may decrease patient and family anxiety.
- Explain the patient's role (if applicable) in assisting with the passage of the tube and maintenance of tamponade traction. *Rationale:* Patient cooperation is elicited during the insertion and tamponade therapy.
- Explain to the patient that the procedure may be uncomfortable because the gag reflex may be stimulated, causing the patient to be nauseated or to vomit. *Rationale:* This explanation prepares the patient for what to expect during the procedure.

PATIENT ASSESSMENT AND PREPARATION

Patient Assessment

- Assess signs and symptoms of major blood loss. *Rationale:* Esophageal or gastric varices can cause significant blood loss:
  - Tachycardia
  - Tachypnea
  - Hypotension
  - Decreased urine output
  - Decreased filling pressures (pulmonary artery pressure, pulmonary artery wedge pressure, central venous pressure, stroke volume, stroke volume index)
  - Decreased platelet counts
  - Decreased hematocrit and hemoglobin values
  - Change in level of consciousness

- Assess the baseline cardiac rhythm. *Rationale:* Passage of a large-bore tube into the esophagus may cause vagal stimulation and bradycardia.
- Assess the baseline respiratory status (i.e., rate, depth, pattern, and characteristics of secretions). *Rationale:* Use of topical anesthetic agents in the nares or oropharynx may alter the gag or cough reflex, increasing the risk for aspiration. Passage of a large-bore tube may impair the airway. Large amounts of blood in the stomach predispose a patient to vomiting and potential aspiration.
- Assess the patient's ability to protect the airway. *Rationale:* Multiple factors can influence the patient's ability to protect the airway, including the presence of vomiting and depressed mental status. Inserting an endotracheal tube before inserting the esophageal balloon is recommended.[3,8,9]
- Assess the patient's level of consciousness. *Rationale:* If the patient has an altered level of consciousness, he or she may need to be intubated and mechanically ventilated prophylactically to prevent airway complications.
- If anticipating a nasal esophageal tube placement:
  - Assess for medical history of nasal deformity, surgery, trauma, epistaxis, or coagulopathy. *Rationale:* The risk for complications and bleeding with nasal insertion is increased.
  - Evaluate the patency of the nares. Occlude one naris at a time, and ask the patient to breathe through the nose. Select the naris with the best airflow. *Rationale:* Choosing the most patent naris eases insertion and may improve patient tolerance of the tube.
  - The nasal route is not recommended in patients with coagulopathy. *Rationale:* The risk for bleeding and complications is increased.
- Assess for allergy to latex. *Rationale:* Balloon tamponade tubes contain natural latex and may cause anaphylaxis in patients with a latex allergy.

Patient Preparation

- Ensure that the patient and family understand the preprocedural teaching. Answer questions as they arise, and reinforce information as needed. *Rationale:* Understanding of previously taught information is evaluated and reinforced. Typically this is an emergency procedure, and the patient and family will be under stress.
- Ensure that informed consent has been obtained for esophagogastric tamponade tube placement and endotracheal intubation. *Rationale:* Informed consent protects the rights of the patient. If the procedure is done emergently, obtain two-provider emergent consent.
- The provider measures the tube from the bridge of the nose to the earlobe to the tip of the xiphoid process. Mark the length of the tube to be inserted. *Rationale:* Estimating the length of the tube to be inserted helps place the distal tip in the stomach.
- If the patient is alert, elevate the head of the bed to 30 to 45 degrees. If the patient is unconscious or obtunded, place the patient's head down in the left lateral position.[8,10] *Rationale:* Positioning facilitates the passage of the tube into the stomach and reduces the risk for aspiration.

Procedure for Inserting an Esophagogastric Tamponade Tube		
Steps	Rationale	Special Considerations

1. 🔲
2. 🔲
   Exposure to blood and gastric fluids is likely.
3. Assist the provider with sedation as needed. The provider may anesthetize the oropharynx.[7] The provider may elect to perform endotracheal intubation to protect the airway.[7]

   Sedation may be needed for the patient to tolerate endotracheal tube and tamponade tube insertion.

   The provider performing the procedure may elect to omit this step in the case of a medical emergency.
4. Assist the provider with assessing gastric balloon integrity before insertion.

   The provider performing the procedure may elect to omit this step in the case of a medical emergency.

   A. Attach the gastric balloon port to the sphygmomanometer or pressure gauge (Fig. 95.6) before insertion.
   B. The provider inflates the gastric balloon with 100, 200, 300, 400, and 500 mL of air, noting the pressure reading at each stage of inflation.

   Knowing the pressure required at each stage of inflation before insertion may prevent inadvertent perforation of the esophagus after insertion.[1]

   C. If applicable, the provider inflates the esophageal balloon with the volume indicated in the package insert.

   Verifies the integrity of the esophageal balloon.[1]

   D. Hold the air-filled balloon under water to test for air leaks.

   Verifies the integrity of the balloon.[1]

   E. Actively and completely deflate the balloon and clamp. **(Level M*)**

   A deflated balloon eases insertion.[1]

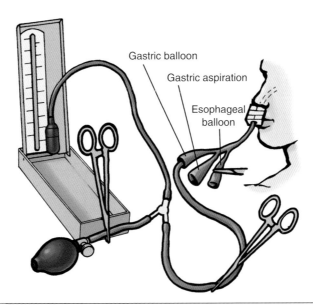

Figure 95.6 Inflation of esophageal balloon. *(Courtesy Davol, Inc., Warwick, RI)*

*Level M: Manufacturer's recommendations only.

Procedure continues on following page

UNIT IV

Procedure for Inserting an Esophagogastric Tamponade Tube—*Continued*

Steps	Rationale	Special Considerations
5. Insert a nasogastric tube (see Procedure 100) into the stomach, drain contents, and then remove the tube.	Emptying the stomach of blood/gastric contents decreases the risk for aspiration and minimizes occlusion of the tube with blood clots.	There is a risk of lacerating the varices with NG tube insertion.
6. Lubricate balloons and the distal 15 cm of the tube with water-soluble lubricant.	Minimizes mucosal injury and irritation during insertion; facilitates insertion.	Use only water-soluble lubricant. Oil-based lubricants, such as petroleum jelly, may cause respiratory complications if inadvertently aspirated. Oil-based lubricants may also damage the latex in the tube and may cause the balloon to rupture.[1]
7. Apply topical anesthetic agent to the posterior oropharynx as prescribed by the provider (apply to the nostril if nasally inserted).	Decreases discomfort caused by insertion.	*Caution:* Gag and cough reflexes may be compromised by topical anesthetic, increasing the risk for aspiration. Keep emergency intubation equipment easily available.
8. Position the patient in the supine position with the head of the bed elevated 45 degrees.	Facilitates tube placement and reduces the risk of aspiration.	If patient is sedated or unresponsive, place them in the left lateral decubitus position. This facilitates passage of the tube.
9. Assist the provider with insertion of the tamponade tube into the mouth or selected nostril. The tube is advanced into the stomach to at least the 50-cm mark on the tube or 10 cm beyond the estimated length needed to reach the stomach (Fig. 95.7).	Helps placement of the entire gastric balloon in the stomach.[1]	The patient's heart rate may decrease as a result of vagal stimulation. Should symptomatic bradycardia occur, atropine may be administered or transcutaneous pacing initiated as prescribed (or per institutional protocol).

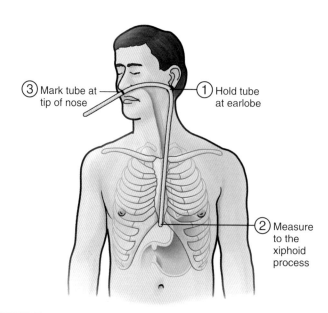

③ Mark tube at tip of nose
① Hold tube at earlobe
② Measure to the xiphoid process

Figure 95.7   Measuring the nasogastric tube. *(From Luckmann J: Saunders manual of nursing care, Philadelphia, 1997, Saunders.)*

Procedure	for Inserting an Esophagogastric Tamponade Tube—*Continued*	
Steps	Rationale	Special Considerations
10. Lavage the stomach via the gastric aspiration port with room temperature NS solution until clear of large blood clots. (**Level E***)	Ensures patency and prevents clots from blocking the tube.[7,12]	
11. Connect the gastric aspiration port to intermittent suction between 60–120 mm Hg as ordered. (**Level E***)	Provides for evacuation of gastric contents and for assessment of continued bleeding.[1,7,8]	
12. Connect the esophageal aspiration port to intermittent suction between 120 and 200 mm Hg as ordered (Minnesota tube only). (**Level E***)	Provides for evacuation of secretions and for assessment of continued bleeding.[1,7,8]	
13. Tube placement must be confirmed:		
A. Aspirate drainage from the gastric aspiration port. (**Level M***)	Prevents the gastric balloon from being inflated in the esophagus, causing rupture.[1]	The ability to simply aspirate fluid from the tube is often interpreted as confirmation of gastric intubation. Caution is needed because several reports have shown that fluid can also be aspirated after endotracheal intubation. The gold standard for confirming placement is an abdominal or chest radiograph to ensure proper placement of the tamponade tube. Before inflating the gastric balloon more than 50 mL, placement should be confirmed via radiography.[1,7-9,13]
B. The provider slowly inflates the gastric balloon with increments of 100 mL of air, up to a total 500 mL, observing the pressure on the sphygmomanometer or pressure gauge at each increment. (If the pressure exceeds preinflation pressure for a particular volume by more than 15 mm Hg, all of the air is withdrawn, and the tube is advanced an additional 10 cm.) (**Level E***)	A pressure difference of more than 15 mm Hg indicates that the gastric balloon is in the esophagus.[1,7-9]	pH testing of gastric secretions may also be used to assess placement. However, this may not be accurate because the patient is actively bleeding. Auscultation to confirm gastric tube placement by placing a stethoscope over the stomach and instilling 20–50 mL of air via syringe is no longer accepted practice.[13](www.aacn.org/clinical-resources/practice-alerts/initial-and-ongoing-verification-of-feeding-tube-placement-in"/>) Alternatively, the gastric balloon can be inflated with 100 mL of air and the position verified by a portable x-ray. Once verified the balloon may be completely inflated.

*Level E: Multiple case reports, theory-based evidence from expert opinions, or peer-reviewed professional organizational standards without clinical studies to support recommendations.
*Level M: Manufacturer's recommendations only.

Procedure continues on following page

UNIT IV

Procedure	for Inserting an Esophagogastric Tamponade Tube—*Continued*	
Steps	**Rationale**	**Special Considerations**
C. On full inflation of the gastric balloon, clamp the gastric balloon lumen with a rubber-shod clamp or plug with the white plastic plug. An abdominal radiograph is obtained.	The outline of the gastric balloon can be visualized on a radiograph. Verifies placement of the entire gastric balloon within the stomach.[7,8,10,14]	The gastric balloon inflation process may be simplified with the use of a Lopez enteral valve (see Fig. 95.5), which can be connected to one side of the gastric balloon. The catheter-tip syringe goes into the large port, the manometer goes into another, and the tapered end of the valve goes into the Minnesota tube. This alternative may eliminate the need to repeatedly clamp and unclamp the tubing while measuring the volume of air injected through the 60-mL catheter-tip syringe. Alternately a three-way stopcock may also be used.
14. After radiographic confirmation of placement, the tube is withdrawn until slight resistance is met. The provider double-clamps the gastric balloon lumen with the rubber-shod clamp or plugs it with the white plug. Disconnect the sphygmomanometer or pressure gauge from the gastric port. **(Level M*)**	Positions the gastric balloon at the gastroesophageal junction where the inflated balloon fills the stomach and creates the tamponade effect.[7,8] The clamp or plug prevents an air leak from the gastric balloon.[1,7]	Interval assessment of gastric balloon pressures is not indicated and may result in accidental deflation and loss of tamponade.
15. Use permanent marker or tape to mark the tamponade tube placement at the opening at either the mouth or nose. Place the tape marker around tube as it exits the mouth or nose.	Provides a reference point to assess placement of the tube.	Document the marking and assess the tube for possible migration.
16. Attach the sphygmomanometer or pressure gauge to the esophageal balloon port. **(Level M*)**	Allows for direct measurement of balloon pressures to prevent excess pressure on esophageal tissue.	The provider may opt to inflate only the gastric balloon if only gastric varices are present.
17. The provider inserting the tube should inflate the esophageal balloon if bleeding is not controlled with gastric tamponade.	Produces direct pressure on esophageal vessels.[1,11]	Maintain esophageal balloon pressures as prescribed or per institutional protocol.
A. The provider gradually inflates the esophageal balloon to 25–45 mm Hg. **(Level M*)**	Higher pressures may cause esophageal necrosis or rupture[1,8,9]	The patient may have chest pain or bradycardia with inflation. Monitor electrocardiographic (ECG) changes during placement, removal, or inflation of the balloon.
B. Double-clamp or plug the esophageal balloon port. **(Level M*)**	Prevents air leaks from the esophageal balloon.[1]	
18. Gentle traction is applied to the tube. **(Level E*)**	Positions the gastric balloon and exerts pressure on the varices.[1,7,8,10,14]	

*Level E: Multiple case reports, theory-based evidence from expert opinions, or peer-reviewed professional organizational standards without clinical studies to support recommendations.

*Level M: Manufacturer's recommendations only.

Procedure for Inserting an Esophagogastric Tamponade Tube—*Continued*		
Steps	Rationale	Special Considerations

A. Apply gentle traction.
  1. Use 1 pound of weight attached to the tube with balance suspension traction (see Fig. 95.3).
  2. For alternative traction, use a bag with 500 mL of IV fluid. Attach the bag to the tube with the balance system (see Fig. 95.3).

B. Tape the tube to the sponge cube at the naris if the tube is passed nasally.
  Or
C. Apply a semirigid cervical collar, and tape the tube to the collar.[12] (**Level E***)

   Rationale: Prevents excessive pressure on the nares.

19.
A. Maintain the head of the bed at 30–45 degrees.

   Rationale: Promotes comfort, minimizes aspiration, and may prevent ventilator-associated pneumonia (if the patient is intubated).[8]

B. Connect the gastric and esophageal ports to intermittent suction between 120 and 200 mm Hg as ordered. (**Level E***)

   Rationale: Reduces secretions and accumulated blood.[1,5,7,10,14]

   Special Considerations: Connect the gastric and esophageal ports to intermittent suction between 120 and 200 mm Hg as ordered. (**Level E***)

C. The position of the tube should be checked and documented every 3 hours.[2,7]

   Special Considerations: The position of the Sengstaken-Blakemore tube should be checked and documented every 3 hours.[2,7]

20. Sengstaken-Blakemore tube only:
A. Insert an NG tube to just above the esophageal balloon. (**Level E***)

   Rationale: Reduces secretions and accumulated blood in the esophagus that may result in aspiration into the lungs.[1,5,7,10,14]

B. Use permanent marker or tape to mark the tamponade tube placement at the opening of either the mouth or nose.

   Rationale: Creates a reference point to assess migration of the tube.

   Special Considerations: If the gastric tube migrates upward, it may result in complete blockage of the airway.

C. Connect the gastric and esophageal ports to intermittent suction between 120 and 200 mm Hg as ordered. (**Level E***)

   Rationale: Reduces secretions and accumulated blood.[1,5,7,10,14]

D. The position of the Sengstaken-Blakemore tube should be checked and documented every 3 hours.[2,7]

21. The provider inflates the gastric balloon:

*Level E: Multiple case reports, theory-based evidence from expert opinions, or peer-reviewed professional organizational standards without clinical studies to support recommendations.

Procedure continues on following page

UNIT IV

Procedure   for Inserting an Esophagogastric Tamponade Tube—*Continued*

Steps	Rationale	Special Considerations
A. The inflated esophageal balloon should be kept at the minimal pressure required to control bleeding (approximately 25 mm Hg for at least 24 hours) and deflated by the provider for 12–24 hours to assess for any new bleeding. (**Level M***)	Underinflation can lead to tube displacement into the esophagus. Overinflation can lead to mucosal and submucosal ischemia.[1]	Maximum pressure is 45 mm Hg.[2,7]
B. The Sengstaken-Blakemore tube should remain in place for a short period. (**Level E***)	Minimizes the opportunity for mucosal trauma.[3,9,11]	
22. Inflation or deflation of the tamponade tube should be performed or prescribed by a provider.		
A. Connect the sphygmomanometer to the esophageal balloon port.	The esophageal balloon is inflated if the bleeding continues after the inflation of the gastric balloon. Do not inflate the esophageal balloon first.	
B. With use of the second access port, the provider gradually inflates the esophageal balloon to 25–45 mm Hg.	High pressures can lead to mucosal and submucosal ischemia or esophageal rupture.	Higher pressures may cause pain with inflation. Monitor the ECG for changes during placement, inflation, or removal of the esophageal balloon.
C. Double-clamp the esophageal balloon port with rubber-shod clamps, or use the white plug. (**Level M***)	Prevent loss of balloon pressure.	
D. The provider must deflate the esophageal balloon to make any changes to the tube's position. (**Level E***)	Ensures adequate balloon inflation for tamponade. Prevents mucosal ischemia, necrosis, and injury.[1,7] Prevents air leaks from the esophageal balloon.[1]	

Discontinuing Tamponade Therapy

Steps	Rationale	Special Considerations
23. Discontinue tamponade therapy in stages. (**Level E***)	Provides for gradual reduction in tamponade to assess cessation of bleeding.[1,8,14]	
A. The provider must deflate the esophageal balloon (if inflation was needed to control bleeding) by unclamping the esophageal balloon port and aspirating to actively deflate the balloon.	Removes the tamponade effect exerted against the esophagus.	Never deflate the gastric balloon while the esophageal balloon remains inflated. A deflated gastric balloon may allow an inflated esophageal balloon to migrate in the airway. If the airway becomes obstructed, immediately cut both balloon ports to deflate the balloons, and remove the tube immediately. If a provider is not present, the registered nurse may be able to deflate the balloon and remove the tube to clear the airway; follow institutional protocols.

*Level E: Multiple case reports, theory-based evidence from expert opinions, or peer-reviewed professional organizational standards without clinical studies to support recommendations.
*Level M: Manufacturer's recommendations only.

Procedure for Inserting an Esophagogastric Tamponade Tube—*Continued*		
Steps	Rationale	Special Considerations
B. Observe for recurrence of bleeding over 24 hours. If bleeding recurs, notify the provider as the esophageal balloon may need to be inflated.	Bleeding may recur with the release of pressure on the esophageal varices.[1,8,14]	
C. If no further bleeding is noted, the provider deflates the gastric balloon by unclamping the gastric balloon port and aspirating with an irrigation syringe to actively deflate the balloon.		
D. Observe for recurrence of bleeding over 24 hours. If bleeding recurs, notify the provider as the gastric balloon may need to be reinflated.	Bleeding may recur with the release of pressure on esophageal varices.	
E. If bleeding has not recurred in 24 hours, assist with removal of the tube by cutting the balloon lumens with scissors and slowly withdrawing the tube. (**Level E***)	Ensures complete balloon deflation before removal.[1,8,14]	
24. Remove 🅿🅴, and discard used supplies in an appropriate receptacle.	Standard precautions.	
25. 🅷🅷		

Expected Outcomes

- Control of variceal bleeding
- Gastric decompression and evacuation

Unexpected Outcomes

- Rebleeding of varices
- Inappropriate placement of the tamponade tube
- Gastric or esophageal necrosis
- Esophageal rupture
- Airway obstruction
- Cardiac dysrhythmias (during insertion or removal)
- Aspiration of gastric or oropharyngeal contents
- Erosion of mucosa around the nares, lips, mouth, or tongue

UNIT IV

Patient Monitoring and Care

Steps	Rationale	Reportable Conditions
		These conditions should be reported to the provider if they persist despite nursing interventions.
1. Assess for pain and sedation using a validated tool per hospital protocol. Use end-tidal carbon dioxide ($EtCO_2$) continuous waveform capnography.	Both the tamponade tube and the endotracheal tube may cause pain and distress.	• Validated tools for pain are the Critical Care Pain Observation Tool (CPOT), Nonverbal Pain Scale (NVPS). Validated tools for sedation are the Aldrete, Ramsey, and Richmond Agitation/Sedation Scale (RASS). • Monitor the $EtCO_2$ waveform for indication of obstruction. Report values with an increase or decrease of more than 10% (see Procedure 12)
2. Maintain tamponade therapy as needed: maximum of 24 hours.	A longer inflation time may cause necrosis, ulceration, or esophageal rupture.[5,6]	• Continued bleeding
3. Assess and monitor for changes in position of the permanent marker mark or tape mark to ensure that the tamponade tube has not slipped out of place.	Allows for rapid identification of proper placement or dislodgement of the tamponade tube.	• Significant changes in tube position

4. Provide care to the nares every 2 hours when the tube is inserted nasally.[2,7]
   A. Remove dried blood or secretions from the nasal orifice and proximal nares.
   B. Apply lubricating ointment or lotion to keep the mucosa moist.
	Prevents drying and ulceration of the mucosa.	• Breakdown of tissue around the nares

5. Provide oral care every 4 hours.[13] (www.aacn.org/clinical-resources/practice-alerts/initial-and-ongoing-verification-of-feeding-tube-placement-in"/>)	Prevents drying and ulceration of the mucosa and is also a strategy to thwart the development of ventilator-associated pneumonia.	• Mouth, tongue, or lip ulcerations
6. Provide frequent oral suctioning as needed. (**Level E***)	The esophageal balloon prevents swallowing of secretions and saliva.[5,7]	• Bloody oral secretions
7. Monitor the esophageal balloon pressure as prescribed. Maintain esophageal balloon pressures at 25–45 mm Hg (pressures vary with respirations and may intermittently reach 70 mm Hg).[10] (**Level E***)	Prevents excessive pressure on esophageal tissues.[1,7,8] Sudden loss of pressure may indicate rupture of the balloon or esophagus.	• Continued esophageal bleeding • Sudden loss of balloon pressure
8. Decrease the esophageal balloon pressure by 5 mm Hg every 3 hours as prescribed until the pressure is 25 mm Hg, without evidence of bleeding. Follow institutional standards. (**Level E***)	Use of the lowest possible pressure to create a tamponade effect reduces the risk of necrosis.[1,7,8]	• Continued esophageal bleeding

*Level E: Multiple case reports, theory-based evidence from expert opinions, or peer-reviewed professional organizational standards without clinical studies to support recommendations.

Patient Monitoring and Care —*Continued*

Steps	Rationale	Reportable Conditions
9. Assist with complete deflation of the esophageal balloon for 30 minutes every 8 hours, or perform this step as prescribed; follow institutional standards. **(Level E*)**	Intermittent relief of the pressure may prevent necrosis of esophageal tissue.[1]	• Continued esophageal bleeding
10. Evaluate for the recurrence of variceal bleeding.	Bleeding may occur despite tamponade therapy.	• Continued bleeding
11. Monitor for airway patency and respiratory status.	Presence or movement of a large-bore tube may occlude the upper airway.	• Tachypnea • Stridor • Cough • High-pressure alarms on the mechanical ventilator
12. Keep scissors at the bedside to immediately deflate the balloons.	Emergency deflation of both balloons may be needed in case of life-threatening complications such as airway occlusion or esophageal rupture. Scissors are used to cut the balloon tubes, resulting in rapid deflation.	• Airway problems such as airway occlusion by a migrating balloon • Physiological instability related to displacement of the balloon (i.e., bleeding)
13. Obtain an abdominal radiograph as prescribed if there is any indication of displacement of the tamponade tube. **(Level E*)**	Inadvertent deflation of the gastric balloon may cause blockage of the airway by the esophageal balloon.[1,7,8,14]	• Balloon deflation • Airway problems (such as occlusion by migrating balloon) • Physiological instability related to displacement of the balloon (i.e., bleeding)
14. Monitor the gastric output. Irrigate the gastric aspiration port with 50 mL of NS solution every 30 minutes or as needed and prescribed to keep the lumen patent.[7]	Maintains patency of the gastric lumen.[1,7,8,14]	• Continued gastric bleeding • Change in characteristics of output (e.g., color, quantity)
15. Monitor the esophageal output. Irrigate the esophageal aspiration port (or NG with Sengstaken-Blakemore) with 5–10 mL of NS solution every 2–4 hours or as needed to maintain patency. **(Level M*)**	Blood clots may occlude the esophageal aspiration lumen (or NG tube).[1]	• Continued esophageal bleeding • Change in characteristics of drainage (e.g., color, quantity)
16. Follow institutional standards for assessing pain. Administer analgesia as prescribed.	Identifies the need for pain interventions.	• Continued pain despite pain interventions

*Level E: Multiple case reports, theory-based evidence from expert opinions, or peer-reviewed professional organizational standards without clinical studies to support recommendations.

*Level M: Manufacturer's recommendations only.

UNIT IV

UNIT IV

Documentation

Documentation should include the following:
- Patient and family education
- Date and time of the insertion
- Name of the physician, advanced practice nurse, or other healthcare professional inserting the tube
- Location of the tube placement marker (marker or tape)
- Tube type
- Any difficulties with the insertion
- Patient tolerance of the tube insertion, including pressures with specific balloon volumes
- Confirmation of placement with an abdominal radiograph
- Type and maintenance of the traction device
- Amount and type of suction applied to the various lumens
- Esophageal and gastric balloon pressures as applicable
- Periodic deflation of the esophageal balloon as prescribed
- Appearance and volume of gastric and esophageal drainage if present
- Nasal or oral care
- Tube site assessments (nasal or oral)
- Unexpected outcomes
- Deflation sequence of the esophageal and gastric balloons
- Medications administered during the tube insertion (if applicable)

References and Additional Readings

For a complete list of references and additional readings for this procedure, scan this QR code with your smartphone, or visit https://www.elsevier.com/__data/assets/pdf_file/0011/1319870/Chapter0095.pdf.

PROCEDURE

96 Focused Abdominal AP Assessment With Sonography

Cynthia Anne Blank-Reid, Zoë Maher, Thomas A. Santora, and Valeda L. Yong

PURPOSE The focused assessment with sonography for trauma (FAST) as we know it today is a tool for the rapid assessment of an injured patient that allows reliable bedside identification of internal hemorrhage.

PREREQUISITE NURSING KNOWLEDGE

- When first introduced in the United States,[2] the FAST examination was performed by properly trained individuals and afforded a sensitive bedside evaluation to detect the presence of hemoperitoneum and hemopericardium. As experience and expertise accrued, the FAST examination has now expanded to reliably detect significant hydrothorax and hemothorax and with advanced training, the presence of pneumothorax (PTX).[5,6] Thus ultrasound examination provides a rapid, noninvasive, accurate, and inexpensive means of diagnosing internal injury of the torso results in hemorrhage within the chest (pleural or pericardial) or the abdominopelvic region.
- The FAST is a "patient-centric" diagnostic intervention performed at the bedside in the resuscitation room while other diagnostic or therapeutic procedures are performed simultaneously. This noninvasive diagnostic intervention can be easily repeated to evaluate either equivocal initial results or clinical deterioration. A traditional or extended FAST may be obtained:
  - Traditional FAST
    - Pericardial sac (Fig. 96.1)
    - Hepatorenal fossa or the right upper quadrant (RUQ) view to include the diaphragm-liver interface and Morrison's pouch (liver–right kidney) interface (Fig. 96.2)
    - Splenorenal fossa or the left upper quadrant (LUQ) view to include the diaphragm-spleen interface and spleen–left kidney interface (Fig. 96.3)
    - Pelvic or suprapubic view (cul-de-sac of the peritoneum; also known as the *pouch of Douglas*) (Fig. 96.4)

  - Extended FAST (above views, plus the following):
    - Right supradiaphragmatic or the right lung–diaphragm interface (Fig. 96.5)
    - Left supradiaphragmatic or the left lung–diaphragm interface
    - Right pleural slide or the right lung–pleural interface (Fig. 96.6)
    - Left pleural slide or the left lung–pleural interface (see Fig. 96.6)
- Pertinent anatomy
  - Solid organs of the abdominal cavity are the spleen, liver, kidneys, and uterus.
  - Hollow organs of the abdominal cavity are the stomach, small and large intestines, and urinary bladder.
- Basic ultrasound physics[7]: Ultrasound (US) involves using several distinct sound frequencies above the 20,000-Hz range (above the human hearing range). The usual frequencies used clinically are between 2 and 10 MHz (1 MHz = 10,000 Hz). In general, the lower-frequency probes (3.5 MHz and 5 MHz) provide better penetration but less resolution, whereas higher-frequency probes (7.5 MHz and 10 MHz) provide better image detail resolution but less depth of penetration. Typically, a 3.5-MHz probe is typically used for abdominal evaluations, and a 7.5-MHz probe is used for detection of hemothorax or PTX and evaluations of superficial vascular structures.[2,3,6]
- US waves cannot travel through air, therefore the probe must be completely coated with acoustic gel to make for an air-free interface between the probe and the skin. Bone and calcium-containing objects have a very high acoustic impedance, making them impenetrable by US waves; any wave that reaches a bone interface will be reflected. Any structures on the other side of the bone will not receive any US wave and will not be seen (referred to as *acoustic shadowing*).
- The probe acts as both a transmitter of these waves (1%) and a receiver (99%) of waves reflected back from the tissues. As the US wave travels through tissues, it will lose power because of acoustic impedance imposed by the tissues. Different tissues have different acoustic impedance

919

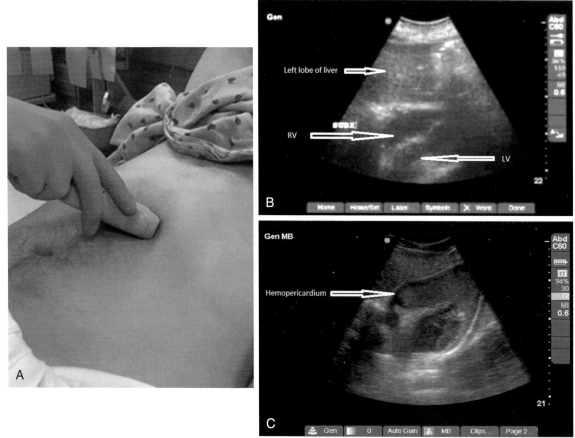

Figure 96.1   Pericardial view. **A,** The 3.5-MHz transducer is positioned below the operator's hand, so with gentle pressure, a satisfactory pericardial view can be obtained. The orientation indicator (on this particular probe) is directed to the patient's right. **B,** The resulting pericardial four-chamber view from the subxiphoid orientation. **C,** Subxiphoid pericardial view of a patient after a stab wound to the precordium with evidence of hemopericardium. On dynamic evaluation of this ultrasound, the anterior black stripe seen on this static image resulted in compression of the right ventricular free wall, suggestive of early tamponade physiology. *(From the Temple University Hospital Department of Emergency Medicine Teaching Files.)*

that results in a unique characteristic reflection (similar to an individual's reflection of light in a mirror) called an *echo.*

- Bone and gases are very dense. As such, US waves cannot permeate them, and they will be reflected. Therefore any structures that are below the bone or gas will not receive any US wave and therefore will not be seen. Fluids, soft tissues, and solid organs will transmit US waves and allow them to pass through.
- The reflected US waves are displayed on a screen as a two-dimensional image with varying echoic appearances. Bone and calcium-containing calculi appear as a white surface with an acoustic shadow beneath. Blood, urine, and water appear black, while solid organs appear in varying shades of gray.
- Tissues are described by their relative echo patterns.
  - *Anechoic* refers to the lack of an echo (e.g., simple fluid, blood). An anechoic finding appears black.
  - *Isoechoic* refers to adjacent tissues/organs with similar echo amplitudes (e.g., solid organs such as liver, spleen, and kidneys). Isoechoic structures appear gray.

  - *Hyperechoic* refers to higher-amplitude echoes than adjacent tissues (e.g., diaphragm and liver or spleen). Hyperechoic structures appear white.
  - *Hypoechoic* refers to echoes of lower amplitude than surrounding tissues.
- The US identification of tissues is dependent on the difference in acoustic impedance at the organ interface. The greater the difference in impedance between adjacent structures, the better the US delineation of the structures will be.
- The rate of US wave transmission through a given tissue is constant; therefore the waves returning from the depths of penetration (far field) take longer to return to the probe than those returning from the near field. This understanding is needed to appropriately set up the US machine for optimal visualization.
- A negative FAST does not exclude the possibility of a significant intraabdominal injury producing small volumes of fluid. Although it is difficult to say with certainty, the minimal amount of blood required for US detection has been shown to be 100 mL[4]; however, others have shown in a prospective study done on adults that the average volume

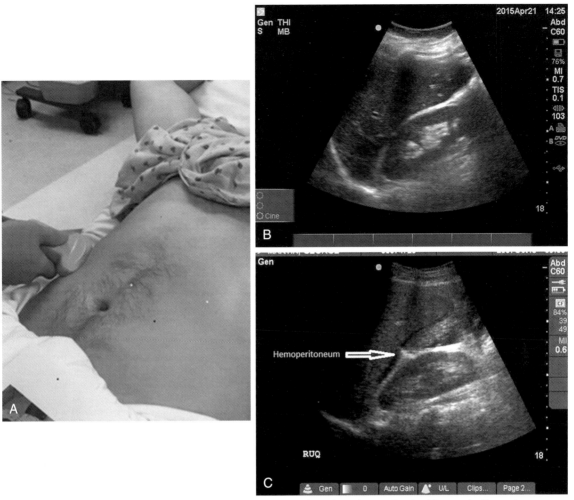

Figure 96.2   Right upper quadrant view. **A,** Note the orientation marker in this case is directed cephalad. If a vertical orientation of the transducer encounters rib artifact, the transducer can be angled diagonally to look between the rib spaces. This maneuver is particularly important to obtain the diaphragm-liver interface in individuals who have high-riding diaphragms. If the patient is able to cooperate, holding a deep breath can facilitate visualization of the diaphragm-liver interface. **B,** In this particular view, the bright interfaces between the diaphragm and liver as well as the liver and right kidney are well visualized. **C,** Hemoperitoneum is demonstrated in this image by the black stripe between the liver and kidney. Note that at the right side of the image is a complex fluid collection (just in front of the *arrowhead*) representing a clot in Morrison's pouch. *(From the Temple University Hospital Department of Emergency Medicine Teaching Files.)*

needed is 619 mL, with only 10% of the evaluators able to detect volumes less than 400 mL.[3]

- *US machines:* These machines vary from extremely portable devices about the size of a standard laptop computer to the large machines used in radiology departments. Regardless of the exact machine, there is a minimal amount of technological understanding of particular machines needed to obtain useful US images. The necessary terms to be familiar with are as follows:

  ❖ *Power:* Controls the strength of the US wave. Use the minimal power setting to obtain interpretable images. More power may create distortion and artifact.

  ❖ *Gain:* Amplifies the echo signal returning to the probe. Increasing gain will make the image appear whiter.

  ❖ *Time-gain compensation* (also called *near-field, far-field time compensation*): Used to compensate for the

time delay from echoes at the depth of penetration. Generally the gain is increased in the far field relative to the near field. Adjustments may be required to create a consistent echogenicity of the organ or structures of interest.

  ❖ *Depth of penetration:* Should be set to visualize the entire structure of interest.

- *Transducers:* There are a variety of probe configurations available for clinical use. Most US machines allow rapid exchange of these probes to allow for differing clinical imaging requirements. In general, the following are commonplace probes:

  ❖ *Annular array*: This probe has a semicircular contact surface and creates a pie-shaped image. This probe configuration is common in the lower-frequency probes used to perform the abdominal and pericardial portions of the FAST.

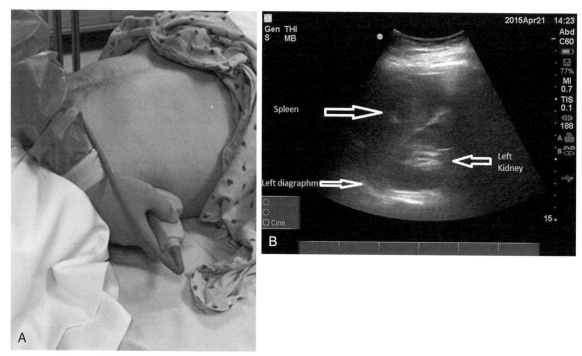

Figure 96.3   Left upper quadrant view. **A,** To obtain this view, the transducer is directed with the orientation marker cephalad *(not shown)*. Because of the posterior position of the spleen, the operator's knuckles frequently need to touch the examining table while directing the transducer slightly anteriorly to obtain the spleen–left kidney interface. As with the right upper quadrant view, a cooperating patient should be asked to take a deep breath and hold it to facilitate visualization of the diaphragm-spleen interface. In the event that rib shadowing occurs, the transducer can be positioned diagonally into the space between the ribs, directing the orientation marker cephalad and posterior. **B,** In this static image, only the most posterior aspect of the diaphragm-spleen interface is visualized. Dynamically, with a slight tilt of the transducer, the entirety of this interface can frequently be visualized. *(From the Temple University Hospital Department of Emergency Medicine Teaching Files.)*

❖ *Linear array:* The probe has a linear patient contact surface and produces a linear image. This arrangement is frequently found in the higher-frequency probes used for superficial vascular imaging and is the probe of choice to perform the extended portion of the FAST to evaluate potential PTX.

❖ *Phased array:* This probe has a small profile that allows placement between the ribs to obtain a high-quality cardiac image; it creates a pie-shaped image. It is used primarily for the parasternal cardiac view.

• Regardless of the probe utilized, it is imperative to orient the probe properly. All probes have an indicator for this orientation. This indicator is oriented to the patient's right side when doing the pericardial and pelvic transverse views or toward the head when doing the RUQ, LUQ, pelvic sagittal, and the pleural evaluation for PTX. When properly oriented, the indicator side of the view will be shown on the left side of the monitoring screen. A trick that many physicians, advanced practice nurses, and other healthcare professionals use if the indicator is no longer recognizable is to apply gel to the probe and gently scratch one edge of the probe; this will create a disturbance of one edge of the image on the screen. The probe should be oriented to have this disturbance on the left side of the monitoring screen.

• FAST is safe in pregnancy and children because it produces no ionizing radiation.

• Indications are as follows:

❖ *Blunt trauma:* FAST affords rapid bedside evaluation of potential torso cavitary hemorrhage and cardiac tamponade and assists in the clinical diagnosis of PTX.

❖ *Penetrating trauma:* Evaluation of the pericardial and upper abdominal views allows for identification of the appropriate body cavity before surgical exploration.

❖ *Unexplained hypotension regardless of injury mechanism:* The portability and noninvasive nature of the FAST allows repeated assessments that may detect changes that occasionally occur in the dynamic natural history of traumatic injury. It is helpful when the same operator does repeat FAST examinations because the operator can best evaluate (or assess) any changes. This is especially true if pictures were not taken during previous FAST examinations.

• The FAST is extremely operator dependent and should be performed only by physicians, advanced practice nurses, or other healthcare professionals who have been adequately trained. Training requires an understanding of basic US physics and an understanding of the general operations of the US machine used. Most courses offered include didactic and hands-on experience. Additionally,

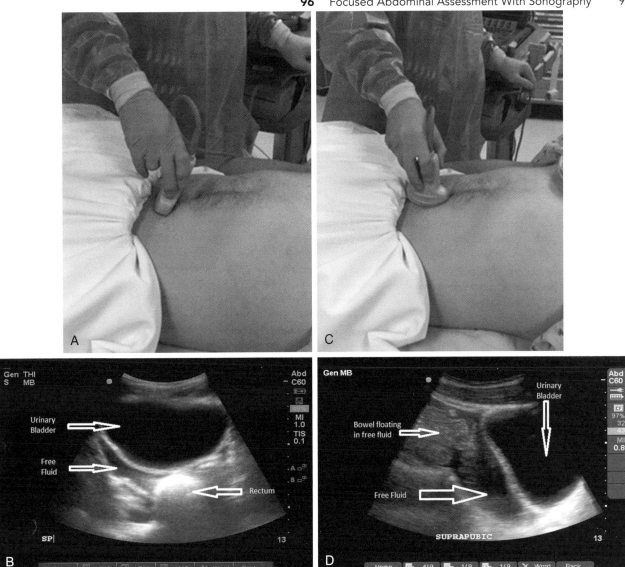

Figure 96.4 Pelvic view. **A,** This view can be obtained in a transverse orientation as depicted in this image; the orientation marker is directed to the patient's right. **B,** Free fluid in the transverse orientation is seen as having a "bowtie" appearance dorsal to (behind) the urinary bladder and anterior to the rectum. **C,** A sagittal image can be obtained by positioning the transducer vertically with the orientation marker directed cephalad. **D,** In this transverse image, free fluid is seen in the rectovesicular pouch of Douglas. The bowel is seen floating in free fluid, which is readily seen at the urinary bladder interface. *(From the Temple University Hospital Department of Emergency Medicine Teaching Files.)*

demonstration of clinical proficiency (usually requiring proctored scans that are correlated with computed tomography [CT] or operative findings) has been debated over the years. In a prospective study, Shackford demonstrated the learning curve for the nonradiologist to detect hemoperitoneum at an acceptable error rate of less than 5% varies based on the prevalence of hemoperitoneum in the study population; if hemoperitoneum occurs in less than 30% of the population, 50 scans are needed, whereas if hemoperitoneum occurs in more than 20% of the population, 30 scans are needed to reach the acceptable error rate of less than 5%.[8]

- Obesity may make it difficult to interpret images; adjusting the gain and frequency (either on the machine or by

changing the transducer) may improve the image quality. Lower-frequency transducers may be necessary for adequate penetration in patients who are obese.

- If there is an indication for a laparotomy or immediate surgery, there is no clinical indication for the FAST. However, a FAST may allow the surgeon to know which body cavity to explore initially (e.g., if there is minimal abdominal fluid but a hemopericardium, open the chest first to decompress the hemopericardium and fix the cardiac wound).[1]

- If emergency treatments and therapies are indicated, such as IV fluids, blood transfusions, intubation, pericardiocentesis, or needle decompression of the chest, they should not be delayed for the performance of a FAST. Ideally the

UNIT IV

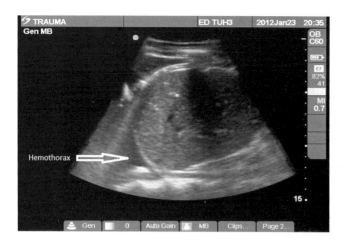

Figure 96.5 Supradiaphragmatic view of the right upper quadrant. This image clearly shows the bright reflectance from the right hemidiaphragm. Just above the diaphragm is a triangular-shaped black area, sometimes called a *sail sign,* indicative of free fluid in the pleural space. In this instance, a hemothorax was found. *(From the Temple University Hospital Department of Emergency Medicine Teaching Files.)*

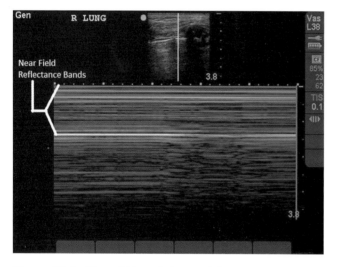

Figure 96.6 Normal M-mode image of the pleura. This evaluation requires a higher-resolution transducer, usually 7.5 to 10 MHz. This static image shows separation of the reflectance of the ultrasound beam off of the pleural surface over time, sometimes referred to as the *beach sign.* The separation of these bands in the near field *(top* of ultrasound image) results from movement of the pleura with normal respiration. This M-mode appearance is seen in patients who have no pneumothorax. Separation of these reflectance bands is much easier to see in real time and is known as a *pleural slide.* *(From the Temple University Hospital Department of Emergency Medicine Teaching Files.)*

FAST and interventions can be conducted simultaneously by multiple physicians, advanced practice nurses, or other healthcare professionals.[1]

- Factors that can compromise the utility of US and the accuracy of the FAST include the following:
  - Obesity (unable to penetrate for adequate imaging). This can sometimes be improved by either adjusting the gain or using a lower-frequency probe to allow deeper penetration.

- Presence of subcutaneous air (air blocks transmission of US waves, thus impeding evaluation of deeper structures)
  - Bowel gas (same rationale as described earlier)
  - Pelvic fractures (FAST detection of blood in the pelvic view cannot discriminate peritoneal from retroperitoneal sources of blood)
  - Previous abdominal surgeries (adhesions may not allow blood to pool in the usual dependent portions of the abdominal cavity)
- Clotted blood can generate various degrees of echogenicity and may be mistaken for normal surrounding soft tissue.
- Ascites, hydrothorax, or pericardial effusion from medical causes will be seen on FAST/eFAST, and these findings could confound a diagnosis of torso cavitary hemorrhage due to injury.
- The FAST is not as sensitive with smaller volumes of blood; serial examinations may be required. It will not identify retroperitoneal bleeding. The FAST will not allow for the grading of organ injuries but will show the provider only that fluid is present.

EQUIPMENT

- US machine
- Transducer
- Water-based gel
- Gown
- Gloves
- Goggles

PATIENT AND FAMILY EDUCATION

- Explain why the FAST is needed to acquire an accurate diagnosis and to decrease the time to diagnosis. ***Rationale:*** Explanation may allay anxiety and elicit cooperation to facilitate the procedure.
- Explain that the FAST is noninvasive, performed at the bedside, and can be repeated as needed. ***Rationale:*** Explanation may allay anxiety.
- Outline the steps of the procedure and the patient's role during the FAST (e.g., positioning). ***Rationale:*** Patient cooperation may facilitate completion of the procedure.
- Describe the typical sensations experienced during a FAST (the application of cool gel and minor pressure, especially for the subxiphoid view). ***Rationale:*** Explanation may alleviate anxiety and promote patient cooperation.

PATIENT ASSESSMENT AND PREPARATION

Patient Assessment

- Evaluate the patient for hemodynamic stability during the primary survey assessment.[1] ***Rationale:*** Hemodynamic instability may preclude the use of FAST and other

diagnostic testing because it may require immediate surgical intervention.
- Obtain a baseline pain assessment. ***Rationale:*** Changes in level of pain during or after the procedure may be an indicator of complications.

Patient Preparation

- Verify the correct patient with two identifiers. ***Rationale:*** Before performing a procedure, the nurse should ensure the correct identification of the patient for the intended intervention.
- Ensure that the patient and family understand the preprocedural teaching. Answer questions as they arise, and reinforce information as needed. ***Rationale:*** Understanding of previously taught information is evaluated and reinforced.

- Obtain informed consent in the nonemergent situation. ***Rationale:*** This protects the rights of the patient.
- Perform a preprocedure verification and time out, if nonemergent. ***Rationale:*** This ensures patient safety.
- The FAST should be performed before Foley catheter insertion to obtain a good pelvic view. ***Rationale:*** The urine in the bladder provides a way for the US waves to penetrate the depths of the peritoneal cavity surrounding the bladder.
- In cases in which a Foley catheter has already been placed, if time allows and the patient is not critical, it should be clamped, and sufficient time should be allowed for the bladder to fill. ***Rationale:*** The fuller the bladder, the more urine there is. A normal full bladder will be black in color and triangular in shape. This helps distinguish it from other abdominal structures.

Procedure FAST and Extended FAST		
Steps	Rationale	Special Considerations
1. HH		
2. PE		
3. Keep the patient as warm as possible using the following: A. Warming lights B. Warmed IV fluids C. Warm blankets	Preservation of body heat; minimizes conductive and convection losses.	The patient must be kept warm when exposed for FAST. Keep bare skin area exposure to a minimum.
4. Assist the patient to the supine position with the arms slightly away from the lower torso.	This arm position allows the operator to position the probe at the lower chest to obtain the RUQ and LUQ views.	
5. Evaluate the patient in the supine position, and then adjust the patient's position to the Trendelenburg or lateral decubitus position if there are no contraindications (i.e., spinal precautions).	The Trendelenburg position may be required to visualize free fluid during perihepatic and perisplenic examination.	Consider the reverse Trendelenburg position while evaluating for hemothorax or pelvic free fluid.
6. Place gel on the transducer.	A water-soluble gel between the transducer and the body is necessary to initiate transmission of the ultrasound waves into the body.	Gel is needed to eliminate any air between the surface of the probe and the body contact surface. Air between the probe and the contact surface will block transmission of the US wave, thus preventing visualization.

Procedure continues on following page

Procedure	FAST and Extended FAST—*Continued*	
Steps	**Rationale**	**Special Considerations**

7. Begin with the cardiac view.
  A. The heart can be imaged using the subxiphoid or parasternal view.
  B. The subxiphoid approach. The transducer probe (3.5 MHz) should be placed in the subxiphoid area and directed into the chest toward the left shoulder to view the diaphragm and heart. The view may be difficult to obtain if the patient has significant abdominal pain. It often requires pressing the probe into the abdomen and angling the probe so it is nearly parallel and deep into the level of the sternum.
  C. Parasternal approach: the transducer-probe should be placed in the subxiphoid area and directed into the chest toward the left shoulder to view the diaphragm and heart.
  D. The view may be difficult to obtain if the patient has significant abdominal pain.
  E. You may need to press the probe into the abdomen and angle the probe so it is nearly parallel to the sternum.
  F. You may need to place the palm of your hand over the top of the probe (the surface furthest away from the skin).
  G. The probe indicator is always to the patient's right side.
  H. This approach gives a long-axis four-chamber view of the heart (see Fig. 96.1).
	Pericardial anechoic or hypoechoic stripes that are circumferential usually represent pericardial fluid. A focal anterior hypoechoic region may be normal pericardial fat. Fluid within the heart should be black.
	The subxiphoid long-axis view is the best view to assess for pericardial effusions and allows the examiner to assess the size of the effusion and collapsibility of the free wall of the right ventricle.
		This is particularly important in the unstable patient, especially for those with thoracoabdominal penetrating wounds. It will allow the operator to determine which body cavity requires exploration initially.
		When using the parasternal approach, the curved array transducer or the phased array cardiac transducer can be used. The smaller footprint fits more easily between the ribs. Regardless of the probe used, the indicator is place to the patient's right in the third or fourth intercostal space between the ribs. A focal posterior effusion, seen on the parasternal long-axis view, may be a left pleural effusion rather than a pericardial effusion. The hypoechoic stripe of a pericardial effusion usually wraps around the apex of the heart. If the patient is experiencing significant abdominal pain or is obese, consider changing to a parasternal long-axis view.

8. The second view is the RUQ, which is a sagittal view in the midaxillary line at approximately the 10th or 11th intercostal space (see Fig. 96.2).
  A. The probe is held with the palm upward under the probe.
  B. To view Morrison's pouch, the transducer-probe should be placed in the RUQ or laterally along the thoracoabdominal junction.
	Structures to visualize include the diaphragm, liver, and right kidney.
	
	The entire hepatorenal fossa (Morrison's pouch) should be visualized.
		The RUQ is usually the easiest view to obtain because of the large acoustic windowing effect of the liver.
		
		Not all abdominal injuries produce free fluid.
		Bowel injury and solid organ injury without significant bleeding will not be detected by US.

Procedure · FAST and Extended FAST—*Continued*

Steps	Rationale	Special Considerations
C. The placement uses the liver as an acoustic window and avoids interference from air-filled bowel.		US will not allow the grading of organ injuries.
D. The probe should be moved toward the inferior margin of the liver to obtain improved images of the right kidney.	Scanning is frequently needed to fully visualize the diaphragm, liver, and right kidney completely.	CT imaging can detect things that US cannot and can grade organ injuries.
		Remember to assess the hepatodiaphragmatic space; blood often accumulates here. A common pitfall is to scan only through the hepatorenal spaces.
9. The third view is a sagittal view of the LUQ in the midaxillary line at approximately the 8th or 9th intercostal space.	Structures to visualize include the diaphragm, spleen, and kidney.	Air artifacts from the stomach and colon, in addition to the smaller acoustic window, make this the most difficult view to obtain.
A. The probe is held with the palm upward under the probe.	The entire splenorenal fossa should be visualized.	It may be necessary to move the transducer posteriorly.
B. To adequately visualize the diaphragm, spleen, and left kidney, the operator's knuckles should be on the patient bed and the probe tilted anteriorly (see Fig. 96.3).	This view allows the spleen to be used as an acoustic window and avoids interference from air-filled bowel.	Free fluid is not always blood; consider ascites, fluid related to a ruptured ovarian cyst, ruptured bladder, or peritoneal dialysis.
C. The probe should then be moved superiorly (toward the thoracoabdominal junction) and inferiorly to assess for the presence of free fluid above the spleen and along the spleen tip.	Scanning is frequently needed to fully visualize the diaphragm, spleen, and left kidney completely.	Remember to assess the splenodiaphragmatic space; blood often accumulates here. A common pitfall is to scan only through the splenorenal space.
10. The fourth view is a suprapubic view (see Fig. 96.4).	This view is easier to obtain with a full bladder.	Optimally this should be obtained before placement of a Foley catheter. A distended bladder is helpful in seeing free pelvic fluid.
A. Obtain both a transverse and sagittal view.	It is utilized to view the bladder, lower abdomen, uterus, and pelvic area.	
B. The probe should be placed just above the symphysis and directed inferiorly into the pelvis.	Artifact may be introduced as a result of posterior enhancement.	Do not look too low; the seminal vesicles are in the retroperitoneum.
C. If areas of fluid disappear with side-to-side movement of the transducer, they are likely artifact.		

Procedure continues on following page

UNIT IV

UNIT IV

Procedure FAST and Extended FAST—*Continued*

Steps	Rationale	Special Considerations
11. Extended FAST (see Fig. 96.6).	This technique is used to rule out PTX.	Lack of pleural sliding may indicate PTX, right mainstem intubation, or poor ventilation.
A. If an extended FAST examination is being performed, place a high-frequency linear probe (8–12 MHz) with the indicator toward the patient's head in a long-axis orientation.		Chest US can only detect a PTX that is directly under the probe; consider looking in several sites on the anterior chest.
B. Place the probe high on the patient's chest, just below the clavicles in the midclavicular line.		Comparing one side of the chest to the other is helpful but can be confusing if bilateral PTXs are present.
C. Look for the pleural line sitting at the back of the ribs.		Dimming the lights in the examination room may provide the examiner with an improved display of US findings.
D. The presence of sliding between the visceral and parietal pleura indicates the absence of a PTX in the area being scanned.		
E. The absence of sling implies the presence of a PTX.		
12. Clean the ultrasound gel off of the patient, and cover the patient.	Keeps the patient's skin clean.	
13. Reposition the patient.	Promotes comfort.	
14. Remove **PE**, and discard used supplies.		
15. **HH**		

Expected Outcomes

- If the patient is experiencing internal bleeding, the source of the bleeding will be determined.
- Rapid bedside detection of potentially life-threatening injuries.
- Consider CT as a complementary test, especially when a FAST detects intracavitary fluid in a stable patient. CT can help determine the nature of the fluid, assess the integrity of the solid organs, and assess the retroperitoneal structures.

Unexpected Outcomes

- Bowel injury and solid organ injury without significant bleeding will not be detected by FAST
- Patient will continue to deteriorate despite FAST being interpreted correctly

Patient Monitoring and Care

Steps	Rationale	Reportable Conditions
		These conditions should be reported to the provider if they persist despite nursing interventions.

Patient Monitoring and Care —*Continued*

Steps	Rationale	Reportable Conditions
1. Monitor vital signs and the patient's electrocardiogram during and after the procedure. Follow institutional standards.	FAST is commonly performed if there is unexplained hypotension, increased abdominal pain, or deterioration in the patient's condition.	• Worsening hypotension • Dysrhythmias • Abnormal heart rate
2. Perform serial abdominal examinations as prescribed.	Changes in a patient's abdominal status may be detected before other changes (i.e., alterations in vital signs).	• Guarding • Decreased bowel sounds • Increased girth • Nausea and/or vomiting
3. Monitor the patient's pain level.	If the patient continues to have pain or the pain is increasing, it could be a sign of increased internal bleeding. Follow institutional protocols for assessing pain. Identifies the need for pain interventions.	• Continued pain despite pain interventions, if performed

Documentation

Documentation should include the following:
- Patient and family education
- Date and time the examination is performed
- Documentation of the FAST written report and select photos
- Results of the FAST
- Adequacy of the technique to obtain interpretable images in all views
- Interpretation of the study as positive or negative for fluid (in the extended FAST, the presence or absence of PTX)
- Unexpected outcomes
- If the FAST is repeated, the above documentation should be undertaken for each procedure
- Pain assessment, interventions, and response to interventions

References and Additional Readings

For a complete list of references and additional readings for this procedure, scan this QR code with your smartphone, or visit https://www.elsevier.com/__data/assets/pdf_file/0003/1319871/Chapter0096.pdf.

UNIT IV

PROCEDURE

97 Gastric Lavage in Hemorrhage and Overdose

Melanie Roberts

PURPOSE When gastric hemorrhage is suspected, gastric lavage can be used for the initial assessment of upper gastrointestinal (GI) bleeding to potentially identify the severity of bleeding and clear the stomach of blood and clots. Gastric lavage may improve visualization of the gastric fundus in preparation for endoscopy or endoscopic treatments. In overdose, gastric lavage may be used to evacuate drugs or toxins within 1 hour of ingestion, potentially minimizing the consequences of systemic absorption of drugs or toxins.

PREREQUISITE NURSING KNOWLEDGE

- Gastric lavage is not recommended as a routine procedure in the management of hemorrhage and overdose. Current evidence shows no improvement in patient outcomes after lavage. The procedure may contribute to additional complications, including gastric or esophageal perforation, aspiration, laryngospasm, dysrhythmias, hypothermia, fluid and electrolyte abnormalities, pain, and hypoxia.[3,8,11] The risk-benefit ratio of gastric lavage should be considered before the procedure is performed.
- The use of gastric lavage may be of potential benefit in some cases of hemorrhage and overdose. Specific indications for the use of gastric lavage include the following:
  - ❖ GI hemorrhage: The patient who has had GI hemorrhage may present with signs and symptoms of volume loss and a decrease in oxygen-carrying capacity. These symptoms include tachypnea, tachycardia, hypotension, orthostatic changes, decreased hemodynamic filling pressures, decreased urine output, pallor, cold and clammy skin, confusion, anxiety, and somnolence. The patient may also show signs of hematemesis, maroon or tarry stools, or hematochezia. Gastric lavage in GI hemorrhage may help clear the stomach of blood and clots to facilitate the evaluation of the source of bleeding and improve visualization of the gastric fundus in preparation for endoscopic treatment.[12] The presence of bright red blood in the aspirate could indicate the need for urgent endoscopy.[12] Bloody aspirate might also be predictive of higher-risk gastric lesions when the patient is hemodynamically stable and has no hematemesis, while clear aspirate might indicate a lower-risk lesion.[12]
  - ❖ Current guidelines for the management of GI hemorrhage recommend early endoscopy, defined as less than 24 hours.[2,8] Very early endoscopy (less than 12 hours) is recommended for patients with high-risk clinical features: hemodynamic instability despite ongoing volume resuscitation, in-hospital bloody emesis

or nasogastric aspirate, and or contraindication to the interruption of anticoagulation.[2,8] Administration of IV erythromycin before endoscopy is recommended for patients with severe, ongoing upper GI hemorrhage to improve endoscopic visualization.[2,8] For patients with active bleeding and no access to endoscopy, gastric lavage with hemostasis powder may prove helpful.[2,10]

- ❖ Overdose: The American Academy of Clinical Toxicology and European Association of Poisons Centres and Clinical Toxicologists do not recommend using gastric lavage in the routine management of poisoned patients because of the limited evidence of improved patient outcomes and potential risks of the procedure.[3,5,9] Supportive care should be considered as the primary treatment before initiating the use of gastric lavage.[3,5,9] If gastric lavage is utilized for decontamination, it should be performed by individuals specifically trained and skilled in gastric lavage.[3] Lavage may be initiated in symptomatic patients within 1 hour (60 minutes) of ingestion of a potentially life-threatening amount of a highly toxic substance or when recommended by the poison control center.[3,5] Gastric lavage is contraindicated in the following circumstances: unprotected airway, ingestion of caustic agents or hydrocarbons, or the patient is at risk for GI hemorrhage (recent surgery, underlying anatomical abnormality, coagulopathy).[9] The administration of activated charcoal has been used in combination with gastric lavage for specific toxins; however, its use must be approached cautiously because the combination of therapies may result in an increased risk for aspiration. It should be noted that the endpoint of gastric lavage is not clearly defined if particulate cannot be clearly observed; however, the amount of lavage fluid instilled should approximate the amount of fluid returned. Gastric lavage after an overdose or toxin ingestion has variable efficacy. The amount of toxin or drug recovered depends on variables such as time from ingestion, whether liquid or pills were ingested, the specific agent ingested, and the size of lavage tube used. Even if lavage is performed close to the time of

930

ingestion, not all ingested toxins will be recovered, and treatment related to effects of the overdose will still be necessary.[3,5] For the most part, gastric lavage has been abandoned because of the efficacy of activated charcoal.[9]

- Nonintubated patients who need gastric lavage must be alert and have adequate pharyngeal and laryngeal reflexes. If the patient has a limited gag reflex or is unable to protect the airway, the he or she should be intubated before gastric lavage is performed.[3,8]
- A colorimetric carbon dioxide detector or capnography is a helpful tool to assist with gastric tube insertion to avoid the complication of inadvertent airway intubation.[1,4,6,7,11,13] Studies show that the colorimetric carbon dioxide detector and capnography have a sensitivity ranging from 0.88 to 1.00 and a specificity ranging from 0.95 to 1.00.[4,7] There is insufficient evidence for carbon dioxide detection to replace the radiograph to confirm the gastric tube.[1,4,6,7,11,13]
- Passage of the lavage tube may cause vagal stimulation and precipitate bradydysrhythmias.
- Patients with esophageal varices, coagulopathy, a recent history of upper GI tract surgery, craniofacial abnormalities, head trauma, or an underlying pathology should be carefully evaluated for the risk-benefit ratio before gastric lavage is performed.[3,12]

EQUIPMENT

- Nonsterile gloves
- Eye and face protection
- Barrier gowns and underpads
- Large-bore (36 to 40F for adults) nasogastric (NG) or orogastric (OG) tube
- 60-mL irrigating syringe
- Water-soluble lubricant
- Colorimetric carbon dioxide detector or capnography if available[1,4,6,7,11,13]
- Lavage fluid (warm normal saline solution or tap water)
- Measurable container for lavage fluid
- Disposable basin or suction canister for aspirate
- Suction source and connecting tubing
- Rigid pharyngeal suction-tip (Yankauer) catheter
- Endotracheal suction equipment
- Tape for securing the NG or OG tube
- Stethoscope
- Cardiac monitor
- Pulse oximeter
- Automatic blood pressure cuff

Additional equipment, to have available as needed, includes the following:

- Specimen container for aspirate (for overdose)
- Absorptive agent for instillation (for overdose, if prescribed)
- Emergency intubation and cardiac equipment
- Bite block or oral airway (if patient needs intubation for the procedure)
- Emergency medications (e.g., atropine)

PATIENT AND FAMILY EDUCATION

- ❖ Explain the indications and procedure for gastric lavage. *Rationale:* Patient and family anxiety may be decreased.
- ❖ Evaluate the patient's and family's understanding of the risks and benefits of gastric lavage. *Rationale:* The patient and family may be unaware of the risks and benefits of the procedure.
- ❖ Explain the patient's role in assisting with passage of the tube and lavage of the stomach. *Rationale:* The patient's cooperation during the procedure is elicited.
- ❖ Explain the purpose of the cardiac monitor, automatic blood pressure cuff, and pulse oximeter. *Rationale:* Patient and family anxiety may be decreased.
- Assess the need for family presence during the procedure. *Rationale:* Patient and family anxiety may be decreased and patient cooperation during the procedure could potentially be improved.
- Evaluate the patient's and family's need for information on prevention of accidental ingestion of drugs or toxic agents. *Rationale:* The patient and family may be unaware or uninformed that the agent or drug is potentially toxic.
- Evaluate the patient's and family's need for information on emergency treatment for accidental ingestion of drug or toxic agents. *Rationale:* Emergency first aid measures may be helpful with some ingestions to decrease potential toxicity or systemic absorption.
- Evaluate the patient's and family's need for information regarding postprocedure monitoring and restrictions, including dietary restrictions, and assessment for aspiration and other complications. *Rationale:* The patient and family may be unaware or uninformed about what to expect postprocedure.

PATIENT ASSESSMENT AND PREPARATION

Patient Assessment

- Perform baseline cardiovascular and neurological assessments, and assess hemodynamic status, cardiac rhythm, and vital signs. *Rationale:* Passage of the lavage tube may cause heart rate or blood pressure changes or vagal stimulation, which can precipitate bradydysrhythmias or other electrocardiographic (ECG) changes, including ST elevation. In the overdose case, toxic levels of certain classes of drugs can also cause ECG changes.
- Perform baseline respiratory assessment and pulse oximetry. *Rationale:* Gastric lavage has been shown to cause changes in oxygen saturation, leading to hypoxia. Patients who are unable to protect the airway should be intubated before gastric lavage.
- Signs and symptoms of major blood loss are as follows. *Rationale:* Esophageal or gastric varices can cause significant blood loss. The clinical presentation is dependent on amount of blood lost.

- ❖ Tachycardia (if the patient has not received beta blockers or calcium channel blockers)
- ❖ Tachypnea
- ❖ Decreased urine output
- ❖ Hypotension
- ❖ Decreased hemodynamic filling pressures
- ❖ Pallor, cold and clammy skin
- ❖ Changes in mental status or somnolence
- ❖ Hematemesis
- ❖ Maroon or tarry stools
- ❖ Hematochezia
- Evaluate the patient for a history of esophageal varices, recent GI surgery, coagulopathy, or underlying pathology. *Rationale:* Varices, recent surgery, coagulopathies, or other contraindications may predispose the patient to complications during lavage tube insertion.
- Obtain baseline coagulation studies as prescribed, and assess hematocrit and hemoglobin values, basic metabolic panel, renal and liver function tests, and blood type. *Rationale:* Baseline information is provided so treatment can be determined and progress can be more accurately monitored.
- Obtain and assess serum toxicology screen, urinalysis, urine toxicology screen, and anion gap (overdose case) as prescribed. *Rationale:* Baseline information for diagnosis is provided so interventions can be made appropriately and patient progress can be more accurately monitored.
- Obtain and assess arterial blood gas (ABG) values as prescribed. *Rationale:* Overdose victims with hypoventilation and patients with GI hemorrhage with significant blood loss or comorbid disease are at risk for hypoxia, hypercapnia, and acid-base disorders.
- Assess the adequacy of the patient's gag reflex. *Rationale:* Lack of an adequate gag reflex indicates the need for endotracheal intubation before lavage begins.
- Assess the type of drugs or toxic substances ingested, quantity ingested, and time since ingestion. Use of common toxidromes (classifications of the signs and symptoms that develop with poisoning) can help identify unknown ingested substances (for the overdose case). *Rationale:* Certain substances may require neutralization before tube evacuation is attempted. A poison control center should be contacted if the practitioner is unsure that lavage is

indicated. Side effects can be anticipated if the drugs or toxins that were swallowed and the quantity are known.
- Perform careful skin assessment (overdose case). *Rationale:* Assessment may give evidence regarding toxin ingested because various drugs can cause cutaneous changes. Changes to look for include diaphoresis, bullae, acneiform rash, flushed appearance, and cyanosis.
- Assess any odors present (overdose case). *Rationale:* Some toxins have a distinctive odor, which can aid in identification of the substance ingested.
- Perform and assess a 12-lead ECG and continuous cardiac monitoring. *Rationale:* In an overdose case, the drug or toxin ingested may be cardiotoxic. For the patient with a GI hemorrhage, comorbid disease states may increase the risk for tissue hypoxia and ischemia.

Patient Preparation

- Ensure that the patient understands the preprocedural teaching. Answer questions as they arise, and reinforce information as needed. *Rationale:* Understanding of previously taught information is evaluated and reinforced.
- Place the patient on a cardiac monitor, automatic blood pressure cuff, and pulse oximeter. *Rationale:* Allows for close cardiovascular and respiratory system monitoring during the procedure.
- Set up oropharyngeal suction. *Rationale:* Ensures that suction is available for the procedure.
- Establish and maintain intravenous (IV) access. For the patient with GI hemorrhage, place a minimum of two large-bore IVs, or provide central venous access. *Rationale:* IV access is necessary for emergency IV medication administration and volume resuscitation in the case of GI hemorrhage.[2,8]
- If not contraindicated, position the patient in the left lateral decubitus position. *Rationale:* This position facilitates passage of the tube into the stomach. The left lateral position is the position of choice to prevent aspiration if the patient should vomit.
- Apply oxygen via nasal prongs or mask as needed. Continue to evaluate the patient for possible need of airway intubation. *Rationale:* Supplemental oxygen may optimize the patient's oxygen saturation.

Procedure for Gastric Lavage in Hemorrhage and Overdose		
Steps	Rationale	Special Considerations
1. **HH**		
2. **PE**		
3. Coat the distal end of the lavage tube with water-soluble lubricant.	Minimizes mucosal injury and irritation during tube insertion.	

Procedure for Gastric Lavage in Hemorrhage and Overdose—*Continued*		
Steps	**Rationale**	**Special Considerations**

4. Position the patient (if not contraindicated):
  A. Assist the patient to the left lateral decubitus position.
  B. Elevate the head of the bed 10–20 degrees, or elevate the bed using a slight (10–20 degree) reverse Trendelenburg position.
	The left lateral decubitus position maximizes access to the stomach and minimizes pyloric emptying. The elevation of the head of the bed or the slight reverse Trendelenburg position also decreases movement of stomach contents into the duodenum and possibly helps minimize the risk of aspiration during the procedure.	Ensure adequate ventilation and oxygenation while the patient is positioned for gastric lavage.

5. Prepare suction, lavage fluids, tape, and emergency equipment.	Preprocedural setup facilitates smooth technique, minimizes complications, and prepares for emergency situations.	If the patient does not have an intact gag reflex, endotracheal intubation should be done before the procedure.[2,8,9]
6. Insert a large OG or NG tube (36–40F) for adults.	A large-bore OG or NG tube is preferred for the evacuation of blood, clots, undigested pills, or pill fragments. A smaller bore tube may become occluded with solid material.	For overdose situations, an OG or NG tube should be placed that is large enough to capture the pill particulate. A smaller-bore NG tube may be used if only known liquid poisons were ingested. Do not cut the end of the tube to create a larger opening because rough edges on the tube can injure the mucosal lining of the GI tract.
A. Measure the distance from the bridge of the patient's nose to the ear (see Fig. 9.2A) and then from the earlobe to the tip of the xiphoid process (Fig. 97.1). Mark this distance on the tube.		

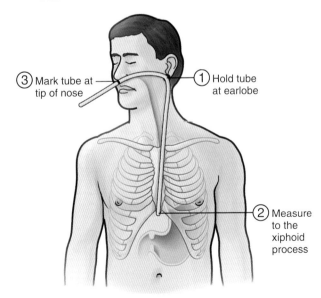

③ Mark tube at tip of nose

① Hold tube at earlobe

② Measure to the xiphoid process

Figure 97.1 Measuring the nasogastric tube. *(From Luckmann J: Saunders manual of nursing care, Philadelphia, 1997, Saunders.)*

B. Attach a colorimetric carbon dioxide detector or capnography to the gastric tube if available.[1,4,6,7,11,13]	Carbon dioxide detection has been shown to be an effective tool to avoid inadvertent tracheal intubation with the gastric tube[1,4,6,7,11,13]	

Procedure continues on following page

UNIT IV

Procedure for Gastric Lavage in Hemorrhage and Overdose—*Continued*

Steps	Rationale	Special Considerations
C. Insert an oral airway (see Procedure 9, Surgical Cricothyrotomy [Perform]) or bite block if necessary.		Remove patient dentures.
D. Position the tube toward the posterior pharynx over the tongue.	Prevents patient from biting on the lavage tube or harming the practitioner during insertion of the lavage tube.	
E. Pass the tube slowly into the stomach assessing for the presence of carbon dioxide (if available), and encourage the patient to attempt to swallow as the tube is advanced. Continue to advance the tube until the mark previously placed on the tube is reached. If carbon dioxide is detected, remove the gastric tube, and start the insertion procedure from the beginning.	Rapid passage of the tube may lead to perforation or stimulate vomiting, leading to an increased risk of aspiration. Detection of carbon dioxide indicates inadvertent airway intubation with the gastric tube.[1,4,6,7,11,13]	Asking the patient to flex the head forward may facilitate advancement of the tube. Heart rate may decrease as a result of vagal stimulation. Have emergency medication (e.g., atropine) ready for use as necessary. Have oropharyngeal suction available. Follow the manufacturer's instructions for the specific colorimetric carbon dioxide detector used.
7. Utilize a variety of bedside practices to assess tube location during the insertion procedure, including: A. Aspirating with a 60-mL syringe for return of stomach contents.[1,11] B. Obtaining radiographic confirmation of placement.[1,11] **(Level D*)**	The position of the lavage tube must be confirmed to be in the stomach because of the risk for endotracheal placement of the lavage tube and subsequent pulmonary complications. Radiographic confirmation of lavage tube placement is currently the only definitive way to confirm tube placement.[1,11]	If not contraindicated, ask the patient to phonate to ensure that the tube has not been placed improperly in the trachea. Be aware that auscultating an air bolus in the stomach is an unreliable method of placement confirmation.[1,11]
8. After placement is confirmed, secure the tube with tape, and aspirate gastric contents through the lavage tube with a 60-mL syringe.	Manual aspiration withdraws gastric contents and toxic agents or blood and clots out of the stomach.	In cases of overdose, save the aspirate in a specimen container, and send it to the laboratory for analysis as prescribed.
9. Perform intermittent lavage (with either room-temperature normal saline solution or tap water).	In overdose cases, lavage might aid in removing toxic substances from the stomach before absorption. In GI hemorrhage, lavage might aid in clearing the stomach of blood and clots to help identify the severity of bleeding and improve visualization of the gastric fundus in preparation for endoscopic evaluation or treatment.	
A. Slowly instill lavage fluid into the lavage tube with a 60-mL irrigating syringe.	Small amounts of lavage fluid are used to limit fluid from entering the duodenum during lavage.	Lavage fluid should be slightly warmed or at room temperature to prevent hypothermia, particularly in individuals receiving large amounts of lavage fluids.
B. Aspirate gastric contents through the lavage tube with an irrigating syringe.*or*	Evacuates stomach contents, blood, clots, or ingested toxic agents.	The amount of lavage fluid returned should approximate the amount instilled.
C. Connect the lavage tube to low intermittent suction.	Low levels of suction (<60 mm Hg) should be used to prevent suction-induced mucosal damage to the GI tract.	

Procedure for Gastric Lavage in Hemorrhage and Overdose—*Continued*

Steps	Rationale	Special Considerations
D. For patients with GI hemorrhage, continue intermittent lavage until the aspirate is clear of blood and clots.[12]	Gastric lavage may help identify the severity of bleeding and clear the stomach of blood and clots to improve visualization for endoscopic evaluation and treatment.[12] The presence of bright red blood can be an indicator of the need for urgent endoscopic treatment.[12]	The presence of coffee-ground aspirate may indicate a resolving or previous GI bleed. Note that the absence of blood or coffee-ground aspirate does not rule out the presence of current or past bleeding.[12]
E. For patients with overdose, continue intermittent lavage until the aspirate is clear of the toxic substance or particulate matter. Once lavage is complete, activated charcoal can be instilled through the tube if indicated.	Gastric lavage may help remove life-threatening levels of ingested toxic substances from symptomatic patients if performed within 1 hour of ingestion.[3,5,9,11] Activated charcoal is used for absorption of the residual substance ingested (unable to be removed with lavage). If the patient is alert and has an intact gag reflex, activated charcoal can be swallowed.	Note that the endpoint of gastric lavage is not clearly defined if particulate cannot be clearly observed and that the lack of lavage return does not rule out significant ingestion of the toxic substance.
10. Remove the OG or NG tube.	The OG or NG tube should be for single use only.	
Remove the tape holding the OG or NG tube in place.	Prepares for removal.	If the lavage tube does not remove easily, discontinue removal and evaluate for causes of obstruction.
Pull the OG or NG tube out slowly and steadily.	Minimizes the risk for vomiting or complications.	
11. Remove **PE**, and dispose of equipment in an appropriate receptacle.	Reduces transmission of microorganisms; standard precautions.	
12. **HH**		

*Level D: Peer-reviewed professional and organizational standards with the support of clinical study recommendations.

Expected Outcomes

- Evacuation of blood and clots from the stomach
- Prevention of blood aspiration
- Improved visualization of the gastric fundus for endoscopy
- Identification of the severity of GI hemorrhage
- Prevention or minimization of systemic complications from the absorption of drugs or toxic agents
- Minimization of mucosal damage by toxic agents

Unexpected Outcomes

- Endotracheal intubation rather than gastric intubation with lavage tube
- Esophageal or gastric perforation
- Trauma to the nose, throat, or esophagus
- Epistaxis if NG route is used for lavage
- Hypothermia in the elderly patient
- Bradydysrhythmias or ECG changes
- Vomiting
- Pulmonary aspiration of gastric contents, with risk for aspiration pneumonia
- Movement of gastric contents into the duodenum, potentially increasing the amount of toxin absorbed
- Fluid and electrolyte imbalance
- Laryngospasm
- Hypoxia or hypercapnia
- Intubation as a result of hypoxia, aspiration, or other respiratory compromise
- Prolonged absence of the gag reflex

UNIT IV

UNIT IV

Patient Monitoring and Care

Steps	Rationale	Reportable Conditions
		These conditions should be reported to the provider if they persist despite nursing interventions.
1. Monitor vital signs every 15 minutes throughout the procedure and every hour after lavage for at least 4 hours or longer, depending on patient condition.	Continued blood loss or side effects of drugs or toxins ingested may cause changes in vital signs. Cold lavage fluid may cause hypothermia. Complications from the procedure may not present during or immediately after the procedure.	• Increase in heart rate 10–20 beats or more above baseline • Decrease in systolic blood pressure 20–30 mm Hg or more below baseline • Respiratory rate <8 or >24 breaths/min or rate changes >20% of baseline normal • Temperature <97.5°F (36.5°C) or >101°F (38°C)
2. Monitor the neurological status continuously throughout the procedure and after lavage.	Side effects from toxic agents ingested or significant blood loss may lead to a decrease in level of consciousness.	• Decreasing level of consciousness • Loss of gag reflex
3. Monitor respiratory status continuously throughout the procedure and after lavage.	Determines pulmonary complications.	• Decrease in oximetry below baseline or 92% • Increase in respiratory rate above baseline • Shortness of breath • Increasing oxygen requirements
4. Monitor cardiac status continuously throughout the procedure and after lavage.	Bradydysrhythmias may be caused by passage of the lavage tube, or an increase in heart rate may indicate continued blood loss. Toxic effects of drugs ingested may also cause ECG changes, including prolongation of the PR, QRS, and QT intervals.	• Heart rate <60 beats/min or >100 beats/min with or without a decrease in blood pressure below baseline • Chest pain, diaphoresis, change in level of consciousness, and shortness of breath • Change in ECG rhythm or length of PR, QRS, and QT intervals from baseline • Prolonged absence of gag reflex
5. Assess for normal pharyngeal function and laryngospasm. After lavage, keep the patient in the left lateral position with slight head elevation until normal gag reflex returns.	The left lateral position is the position of choice to prevent aspiration should the patient not be able to control secretions or emesis.	
6. For the patient with GI hemorrhage:		• Bright red emesis or bleeding from the OG or NG tube • Decrease in hemoglobin or hematocrit below baseline • Decrease in systolic blood pressure 20–30 mm Hg or more below baseline • Increase in pulse 10–20 beats/min or more above baseline • Urine output <0.5–1 mL/kg/hour • Increasing confusion or decreasing level of consciousness • Continued bleeding • Changes in pulmonary status
A. Measure blood volume loss.	Aids in assessment of fluid balance and volume resuscitation requirements.	

Steps	Rationale	Reportable Conditions
B. Monitor for recurrence of bleeding, color, and consistency of gastric drainage, serial hemoglobin and hematocrit, postural vital signs, urine output, and change in level of consciousness.	Bleeding may recur despite interventions.	
C. Administer crystalloid IV fluids as prescribed for volume resuscitation. Switch to the administration of packed red blood cells and fresh-frozen plasma or platelets when available for volume replacement and reversal of coagulopathies.	Replaces volume, prevents hemorrhagic shock, and improves oxygen-carrying capacity. Goal hemoglobin level should be 7–9 g/dL.[8]	
D. Administer proton pump inhibitors (PPIs) as prescribed.	PPIs inhibit the proton pump in the parietal cells of the stomach, suppressing gastric acid secretion.	
E. Prepare for possible administration of intravenous erythromycin (250 mg) before endoscopy as prescribed when a diagnosis of GI hemorrhage is suspected.[2,8,14]	Administration of erythromycin may help accelerate gastric emptying and might decrease the need for repeat endoscopy.[2,8,14]	
F. Prepare the patient for possible endoscopy.	Endoscopic evaluation is the gold standard in the diagnosis and treatment of GI hemorrhage and should occur within 24 hours of initial presentation.[2,8]	
7. For the patient with drug overdose:		• Patient reporting intent to harm self • Patient reporting that ingestion was a suicide attempt • Deviation of test results outside normal limits
A. Evaluate the patient's need for follow-up psychiatric support for suicide ideation.	The drug or toxin ingestion may be a result of suicidal ideation.	
B. Institute suicide precautions until the patient has been cleared by psychiatric services. Precautions include removal of objects from the patient's room that could be used by the patient to inflict self-harm.		
C. In the hours and days after ingestion, repeat laboratory tests, including electrolytes, glucose, blood urea nitrogen and creatinine, liver function, and drug or toxin levels.	Laboratory tests ordered depend on the drug or toxin ingested. Lavage may cause electrolyte abnormalities. Liver function tests may be necessary if the drug is toxic to the liver. Drug or toxin level tests validate the clearance of the drug or toxin from the patient's system.	

Patient Monitoring and Care —*Continued*

UNIT IV

Documentation

Documentation should include the following:
- Patient and family education
- History of ingestion of drug or toxin or upper GI bleeding
- Date, time, and reason for lavage
- Type and size of lavage tube inserted
- Patient tolerance of tube placement and lavage procedure
- Verification of lavage tube placement (method used)
- Type and amount of lavage fluid used
- Unexpected outcomes
- Nursing interventions
- Amount and characteristics of aspirate
- Assessment of gastric drainage after lavage
- Name and dosage of medications given after lavage
- Aspirated specimen sent to the laboratory for analysis
- Referral to psychiatry if potential for suicide is suspected
- Occurrence of rebleed in the patient with GI hemorrhage
- Blood products given during volume resuscitation

References and Additional Readings

For a complete list of references and additional readings for this procedure, scan this QR code with your smartphone, or visit https://www.elsevier.com/__data/assets/pdf_file/0004/1319872/Chapter0097.pdf.

98   Endoscopic Therapy

Eleanor Fitzpatrick

PURPOSE Endoscopic therapy is performed to control or prevent bleeding from esophageal or gastric varices, gastric or duodenal ulcer sites, or other selected causes of upper gastrointestinal (GI) bleeding.

PREREQUISITE NURSING KNOWLEDGE

- Upper GI hemorrhage is a relatively common, potentially life-threatening emergency that requires rapid assessment and resuscitation.[1-5]
- Esophagogastroduodenoscopy is the diagnostic and therapeutic modality for nonvariceal and variceal upper GI bleeding.[1,3-5] Patients with hemodynamic instability and signs of upper GI bleeding should be offered urgent endoscopy, performed within 24 hours of presentation.[6] Endoscopic therapy reduces the occurrence of rebleeding, blood transfusion requirements, and the need for surgery.[2-4]
- Endoscopic therapies are often interventions of choice for upper and lower GI bleeding lesions. Upper endoscopic therapies include injection therapy, ablative therapy, such as heater probe, and mechanical therapy, such as endoclips or endoscopic banding.[2-4,7]
- Most recent technologies for upper GI bleeding include new rotatable clips, over-the-scope clip (OTSC) systems, and new hemostatic agents in the form of powders and gels.[4,8-10]
- For all upper endoscopic interventions, a fiberoptic endoscope is passed through the esophagus and into the stomach and duodenum to identify the source of bleeding. The nurse (or other clinician) assisting the endoscopist typically prepares all of the equipment potentially needed during the procedure. Once the site of bleeding is located, any of the endoscopic techniques identified previously may be used.
- Endoscopic variceal ligation (EVL) is a form of mechanical therapy and the preferred endoscopic method for control of acute esophageal bleeding and for prevention of rebleeding, unless excess bleeding prevents effective band placement and ligation.[11-14] Endoscopic sclerotherapy (EST), which involves injection of a sclerosant into or adjacent to a varix, may also be used; however, EST has largely been replaced by the use of EVL.[11-14]
- For gastric varices, a promising intervention is gastric variceal occlusion with tissue adhesives such as *N*-butyl-cyanoacrylate.[11-13] Varied new hemostatic agents, including powders, sprays, and gels, which can be delivered via the endoscope, have also been developed and promote clotting in the setting of GI hemorrhage.[11,13]
- Injection therapy with epinephrine or other sclerosant is used for hemostasis for bleeding from peptic ulcer disease, Mallory-Weiss tears, other lesions, and postprocedure bleeding.[3,4,13,15] Epinephrine is the injection agent of choice

for these conditions in the United States. Injection therapy alone is not recommended and therefore is often used with additional modalities such as thermal coagulation or endoscopic clipping to achieve or enhance thrombosis.[3,4,13,15]
- The several proposed mechanisms of action of the various sclerosing agents include vasoconstriction, esophageal or vascular smooth muscle spasm, compression of the bleeding vessel by submucosal edema or by the volume of sclerosing agent used (tamponade effect), and actual coagulation of the vessel. Ultimately, vessel thrombosis occurs.[3,4,13,15]
- A variety of sclerosing agents are available (Table 98.1). The physician who performs the endoscopy prescribes the agents to be used during the procedure.
- Ablative therapies, such as the use of a heater probe or bipolar electrocoagulation, are other endoscopic techniques for the management of bleeding from peptic ulcer disease and other nonvariceal causes of upper GI bleeding. These therapies are effective as they result in coagulation of a bleeding vessel.[3,4,15]
- Endoscopic therapy can combine several interventions to promote hemostasis, including esophageal band ligation, endoscopic clipping, injection therapy, laser therapy, and thermal coagulation.[3,4,13,15]
- The U.S. Food and Drug Administration (FDA) has approved a new device for endoscopic clipping. The over-the-scope clip is approved for achieving hemostasis in the upper and lower GI tract and for closure of some luminal perforations. This technique appears to be especially effective after failure of other hemostatic techniques for nonvariceal bleeding episodes.[3,4,15–17]
- Passage of the large-bore therapeutic endoscope may stimulate the vagal response in the patient and precipitate bradydysrhythmias.[18,19]
- As a result of sedation or the use of topical anesthetics, the patient's gag reflex may be diminished or absent, putting the patient at risk for aspiration.[18,19]
- Moderate sedation is recommended for use during endoscopic procedures. Sedation may increase the risk of respiratory depression; thus appropriate monitoring and emergency equipment should be readily available.

EQUIPMENT

- Safety goggles for each healthcare provider and the patient
- Nonsterile gloves
- Barrier gowns

TABLE 98.1   Sclerosing Agents

Sclerosants Used for Bleeding Varices	Sclerosants Used for Other Causes of Upper Gastrointestinal Bleeding
Sodium morrhuate (5%)	Epinephrine (1:10,000–1:20,000)
Ethanolamine oleate (5%)	Ethyl alcohol (volumes >1–2 mL can lead to tissue damage)
Sodium tetradecyl sulfate	Thrombin
Ethanolamine acetate	Polidocanol
Polidocanol (0.5–1%)	Sodium tetradecyl sulfate
Ethanol (can cause ulceration)	

From Mujtaba S, Chawla S, Massaad JF: Diagnosis and management of non-variceal gastrointestinal hemorrhage: a review of current guidelines and future perspectives. *J Clin Med* 9(2):402, 2020; Kovacs TO, Jensen DM: Varices: esophageal, gastric, and rectal. *Clin Liver Dis* 23(4):625–642, 2019.

- Two suction setups with connecting tubing: one for airway use and one for the procedure
- Rigid pharyngeal suction-tip (Yankauer) catheter
- Additional suction setup with connecting tubing for endoscopic procedure
- Oral airway or bite block
- Bag-valve-mask (BVM) device
- Cardiac monitor
- Pulse oximeter
- End-tidal carbon dioxide ($Etco_2$) monitor
- Automatic blood pressure cuff
- Emergency intubation and resuscitation equipment
- Premedications (as prescribed by the physician or advanced practitioner)
- Topical anesthesia
- Nonsterile 4-inch gauze or washcloth
- Water-soluble lubricant
- Two 30- to 60-mL syringes
- Normal saline solution or tap water for irrigation
- Therapeutic large-caliber endoscope (rigid or flexible; however, the flexible scope is the usual type used for upper endoscopy)
- Endoscopic injector needle (23- to 26-gauge, 2- to 5-mm needle; as ordered by the provider)
- Three 10-mL syringes filled with sclerosing agent, as prescribed by physician
- Additional therapeutic equipment should be available for management of nonvariceal upper GI bleeding (i.e., laser or thermal equipment, endoloops, or endoclips)
- Esophageal bands should be available for management of known or suspected variceal upper GI bleeding

Additional equipment to have available as needed includes the following:

- Nasogastric (NG) tube, Minnesota tube, or Sengstaken-Blakemore tube for esophagogastric tamponade (see Procedure 95)

PATIENT AND FAMILY EDUCATION

- Explain the procedure and indication for endoscopic therapy and the patient's role in the procedure. *Rationale:* Patient and family anxiety may be decreased.

- Explain that sedation will be provided for comfort and ease in passing the endoscope. *Rationale:* Patient and family anxiety may be decreased.
- Explain that the patient will be monitored closely during and after the procedure. *Rationale:* Patient and family anxiety may be decreased.

PATIENT ASSESSMENT AND PREPARATION

Patient Assessment

- Assess for a history of upper GI bleeding, the source of current bleeding, and baseline hematocrit and hemoglobin levels. *Rationale:* This information provides an assessment of risk for bleeding or continued bleeding after endoscopic therapy.
- Assess baseline cardiac rhythm. *Rationale:* Passage of a large-bore tube may cause vagal stimulation and bradydysrhythmias.
- Obtain baseline coagulation study results (i.e., prothrombin time, partial thromboplastin time, platelet count). *Rationale:* Abnormal coagulation values increase the potential for bleeding after endoscopic therapy.
- Review respiratory, hemodynamic, and neurological assessment before the administration of any sedative agents. *Rationale:* Baseline assessment data provide comparison information for further evaluation once medications have been administered.
- Obtain baseline vital signs, pulse oximetry, and $Etco_2$ level, if applicable. *Rationale:* Close monitoring of vital signs and pulse oximetry during the procedure and comparison with baseline values are essential to assess the patient's tolerance of the procedure.
- Assess sedation using a validated tool (i.e., Aldrete score, Ramsay scale, or the Richmond Agitation/Sedation score). *Rationale:* Use of a scoring system standardizes the assessment of the patient's tolerance of moderate sedation.

Patient Preparation

- Ensure that informed consent has been obtained. *Rationale:* Informed consent protects the rights of the patient.
- Check that all relevant documents and studies are available before beginning the procedure. *Rationale:* Provides information needed before performing the procedure.
- Ensure that the patient understands the preprocedural teaching. Answer questions as they arise, and reinforce information as needed. *Rationale:* Understanding of previously taught information is evaluated and reinforced.
- Verify the correct patient with two identifiers, and perform a procedural time out. *Rationale:* Before performing a procedure, the nurse should ensure the correct identification of the patient for the intended intervention.
- Place the patient on a cardiac monitor, and apply a pulse oximeter and automatic blood pressure cuff. *Rationale:* This allows for continuous cardiovascular and respiratory monitoring during the procedure.
- Place the patient on the $Etco_2$ monitor per institiution guidelines as applicable. *Rationale:* This allows for continuous $Etco_2$ monitoring during the procedure, which may identify oversedation.
- Ensure that venous access is in place. *Rationale:* Venous access is needed for procedural and emergency medications.

- Ensure that the patient has received nothing-by-mouth (NPO status) for at least 4 hours before the procedure. ***Rationale:*** Undigested material in the stomach increases the risk for aspiration and decreases visualization of the GI tract.
- Remove the patient's dentures. ***Rationale:*** Dentures interfere with safe passage of the endoscope.
- Have sedatives and analgesics (common sedatives include midazolam, diazepam, and fentanyl for analgesia) available (as prescribed), and administer when requested by the provider. Naloxone (for narcotic reversal) and flumazenil (for benzodiazepine reversal) should be available for analgesic or sedative reversal. ***Rationale:*** Sedation and analgesia provide for patient comfort during the procedure,

decrease patient anxiety, and help facilitate cooperation. Overdose of sedative or analgesic medications my lead to respiratory decompensation and clinical deterioration.
- Set up suction with connecting tubing, and attach the rigid pharyngeal suction tip. Ensure that suction is on and ready for use. ***Rationale:*** This setup is necessary for suctioning the patient's oral secretions during the procedure.
- Have atropine available at the bedside. ***Rationale:*** Atropine is necessary if a vagal reaction occurs with the insertion and passage of the endoscope.
- Protect the patient's eyes with goggles or a waterproof covering. ***Rationale:*** Protection is provided against accidental exposure to blood or the sclerosing agents. Sclerosing agents are eye irritants.

Procedure for Assisting With Endoscopic Therapy

Steps	Rationale	Special Considerations
1. **HH**		
2. **PE**		
3. Position the patient in the left-lateral position. **(Level E*)**	The left-lateral position allows predictable views of the stomach as the scope is advanced. This position allows secretions to collect in the dependent areas of the mouth for ease of suctioning and is the position of choice to prevent aspiration should the patient vomit.[13,18,19]	
4. Administer analgesic and sedative medications as prescribed. **(Level C*)**	Promotes patient cooperation during the endoscopy, promotes patient comfort, and facilitates passage of the endoscope.[18,19]	
5. Assist the physician or advanced practice provider if needed with insertion of the endoscope.	Provides assistance.	Gag and cough reflexes may be compromised by topical anesthetics; the patient may vomit as the endoscope is passed, increasing the risk for aspiration. Have emergency intubation equipment available. Monitor heart rate, rhythm, and respiratory status during the endoscopy.
A. Assist as needed in anesthetizing the posterior pharynx with a topical agent as prescribed. **(Level A*)**	Decreases the discomfort caused by passage of the endoscope.[18,19]	
B. Insert an oral airway (see Procedure 9, Surgical Cricothyrotomy [Perform]) or bite block.	Prevents the patient from biting the endoscope or the inserter's fingers.	
C. Lubricate 20–30 cm of the distal end of the endoscope with water-soluble lubricant. (Many physicians prefer to lubricate the scope themselves.)	Minimizes mucosal injury and irritation and facilitates ease of passage of the endoscope.	
D. Encourage the patient to simulate swallowing while the endoscope is passed.	The swallowing maneuver causes the epiglottis to close the trachea and directs the endoscope into the esophagus.	

*Level A: Meta-analysis of quantitative studies or metasynthesis of qualitative studies with results that consistently support a specific action, intervention, or treatment (including systematic review of randomized controlled trials).

*Level C: Qualitative studies, descriptive or correlational studies, integrative reviews, systematic reviews, or randomized controlled trials with inconsistent results.

*Level E: Multiple case reports, theory-based evidence from expert opinions, or peer-reviewed professional organizational standards without clinical studies to support recommendations.

Procedure continues on following page

Procedure | for Assisting With Endoscopic Therapy—*Continued*

Steps	Rationale	Special Considerations
E. Suction the oral pharynx as needed throughout the procedure.	Because of the diminished gag reflex and the presence of the endoscope in the patient's pharynx, oral secretions may not be able to be swallowed. Blood from the GI tract may be vomited and could be aspirated because of the diminished gag reflex.	
6. Perform or assist the physician or advanced practice provider with gastric lavage (see Procedure 109, Bone Marrow Biopsy and Aspiration).	Large amounts of blood or clots in the stomach or esophagus can impair visualization of varices and increase the risk for aspiration during the procedure.	
7. The physician or advanced practice provider performing the esophagogastroduodenoscopy may ask the nurse to assist with preparing equipment for thermal or laser coagulation of a bleeding site.	This technique is frequently used to control bleeding from many upper GI sites.	
8. Assist as needed with injecting an irrigant via the endoscope.	Cleanses the area to increase visualization of the tissue.	
9. If a bleeding site is to be sclerosed, manipulate the sclerosing needle as requested (Fig. 98.1). Inject sclerosant if requested.	Ensures that the sclerosing needle is in proper position for injection and does not injure tissue during movement of the endoscope.	The needle must be retracted before manipulation of the endoscope.
10. Endoscopic bands or endoclips may also be requested by the physician performing the intervention (Fig. 98.2).	In EVL, or banding, a rubber band is deployed from the endoscope and contracts around a lesion that has been raised with endoscopic suction into a specially fitted, transparent endoscopic cap (see Fig. 98.2).[18,19]	

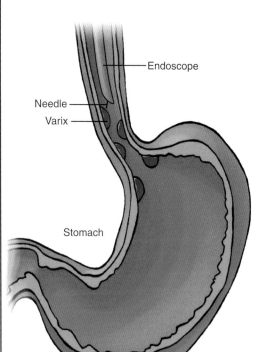

Endoscope

Needle

Varix

Stomach

Figure 98.1 Injection of a sclerosing agent into an engorged varix. *(From Pierce JD, Wilkerson E, Griffiths SA: Acute esophageal bleeding and endoscopic injection therapy.* Crit Care Nurse *10:67–72, 1990.)*

Procedure	for Assisting With Endoscopic Therapy—*Continued*	
Steps	Rationale	Special Considerations

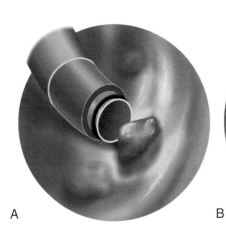

A

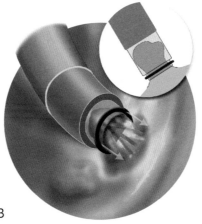

B

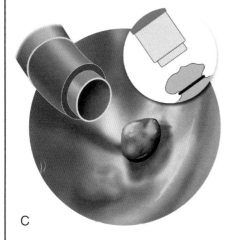

C

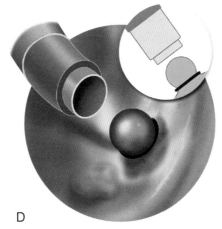

D

Figure 98.2 Endoscopic variceal ligation. **A,** Endoscope placement over the varix. **B,** The varix is drawn into the distal portion of the endoscope. **C,** A rubber band is dropped over the varix. **D,** The rubber band contracts around the varix, causing it to sclerose and eventually slough. *(Drawings courtesy Paul Schiffmacher, Medical Illustrator, Medical Media Services at Thomas Jefferson University Hospital, Philadelphia.)*

UNIT IV

Steps	Rationale	Special Considerations
11. Assist with insertion of an NG tube or esophagogastric tamponade tube (see Procedures 107 and 112, Donor Site Care, after removal of the endoscope if assistance is needed.	An NG tube provides assessment of continued or recurrent bleeding. An esophagogastric tamponade tube may be used to apply pressure to bleeding varices.	Suction applied to an NG tube can cause mucosal damage or disrupt fragile varices and initiate bleeding. A chest radiograph may be performed to rule out aspiration or esophageal perforation.
12. Remove **PE**, and discard used supplies in appropriate receptacles.	Removes and safely discards used supplies, reduces the transmission of microorganisms; standard precautions. Safely removes sharp objects.	The endoscope should be returned to the GI laboratory for proper disinfection. Follow institutional standards.
13. **HH**		

Procedure continues on following page

Expected Outcomes

- Visualization and identification of the bleeding source
- Hemostasis at the site of GI bleeding without recurrent bleeding or prevention of bleeding from esophageal varices
- Stabilization of hematocrit and hemoglobin values

Unexpected Outcomes

- Continued or recurrent bleeding from ligated (banded) or injected varices
- Continued or recurrent bleeding from the ulcer site treated with injection, ablative, or mechanical therapy
- Esophageal, gastric, or duodenal sloughing or ulceration
- Esophageal, gastric, or duodenal perforation
- Substernal chest pain
- Fever
- Temporary dysphagia
- Allergic response to sclerosing agent
- Aspiration pneumonia
- Pleural effusion
- Atelectasis
- Bacteremia/sepsis

Patient Monitoring and Care

Steps	Rationale	Reportable Conditions
		These conditions should be reported to the provider if they persist despite nursing interventions.
1. Monitor cardiovascular, respiratory, and neurological status continuously during and after the procedure. Document heart rate, cardiac rhythm, respiratory rate, pulse oximetry, $Etco_2$ (if used), and level of consciousness frequently during and after the procedure as per institutional protocols. A. Capnography may be used for moderate sedation but is recommended for patients undergoing endoscopic procedures with deep sedation.[18] **(Level B*)**	Changes in vital signs, heart rhythm, oximetry, and capnography may indicate complications related to the procedure.	• Altered level of consciousness from baseline • Oximetry reading below baseline • Abnormal or changed $Etco_2$ from baseline • Pulse rate above or below baseline • Fever >101°F • Decrease in blood pressure 20–30 mm Hg below baseline • Dysrhythmias
2. Follow institutional standards for assessing pain.	May indicate continued bleeding or reaction to sclerosant. Identifies the need for pain interventions.	• Same pain rating as before procedure • New onset of chest pain • Continued pain despite pain interventions
3. Monitor output from NG tube or any vomitus.	Signs of continued or recurrent bleeding.	• Sudden change in condition, bright red vomitus or NG drainage, or decreased patency of NG tube
4. Monitor serial hematocrit and hemoglobin results as prescribed.	Continued decrease in the hematocrit and hemoglobin value indicates continued or recurrent bleeding.	• Decreasing hematocrit and hemoglobin value below baseline
5. Monitor postural vital signs once the patient is able to be out of bed.	Postural changes may indicate volume loss.	• Decrease in blood pressure 20–30 mm Hg below baseline • Increase in pulse 10–20 beats per minute above baseline

*Level B: Well-designed, controlled studies with results that consistently support a specific action, intervention, or treatment.

Patient Monitoring and Care —*Continued*		
Steps	**Rationale**	**Reportable Conditions**
6. Assess for return of normal pharyngeal function. 　A. Keep the patient on the left side with slight head elevation until gag, swallow, and cough reflexes are intact. 　B. Remain with the patient until reflexes return. 7. Provide clear liquids when prescribed after return of pharyngeal function. Diet should be progressed slowly to solid food.	Some endoscopic therapies can cause transient dysphagia. Topical anesthesia decreases the gag reflex and increases the risk for aspiration. The left-lateral position is the position of choice to prevent aspiration should the patient not be able to control secretions or vomit. Food may act as an irritant to the sclerosed ulcer or variceal sites.	• Prolonged absence of gag, swallow, or cough reflex • Nausea • Vomiting of bright red blood
8. Administer antacids, histamine (H$_2$) blockers, sucralfate, proton pump inhibitors, somatostatin, or octreotide as prescribed.[3,15,20] **(Level A*)** For patients with bleeding ulcers with high-risk stigmata who have undergone successful endoscopic therapy, PPI therapy via an intravenous loading dose followed by continuous intravenous infusion is recommended over no treatment or H$_2$-receptor antagonists.[7,21] 9. Continue patient and family education. 　A. Explain signs and symptoms to report (fever, chest pain, difficulty swallowing, vomiting bright red blood, and difficulty breathing). 　B. Explain diet progression. 　C. Explain medication therapy.	Antacids neutralize gastric acid. Histamine blockers decrease gastric acid secretion. Sucralfate reacts with gastric acid, forming a paste that adheres to ulcer sites. Proton pump inhibitors inhibit the proton pump in the parietal cells of the stomach, suppressing gastric acid secretion. Somatostatin and octreotide (synthetic somatostatin) lower portal pressure with splanchnic vasoconstriction.[3,5,12,13,20,22] Unexpected outcomes can occur within hours or may be delayed days or weeks after endoscopic therapy. Decreases the risk for aspiration of liquid or food before the patient is ready for swallowing. Knowledge and understanding about the medication regimen promotes safe, effective medication use.	

*Level A: Meta-analysis of quantitative studies or metasynthesis of qualitative studies with results that consistently support a specific action, intervention, or treatment (including systematic review of randomized controlled trials).

Procedure continues on following page

Documentation

Documentation should include the following:
- Completion of informed consent
- Date and time of procedure
- Initial patient assessment
- Preprocedure verifications and time out
- Baseline vital signs
- Baseline pulse oximetry
- Baseline capnography
- Date and start time of the procedure including the time moderate sedation begins
- Premedications administered
- Vital signs, cardiac rhythm, pulse oximetry, capnography, level of consciousness every 5 minutes (or per institutional standards) during endoscopic therapy
- Gastric lavage with results (if performed) and patient's tolerance
- Type of intervention: injection, ablative, or mechanical; sclerosing agents administered and amount or dose; number of bands or clips placed; and location if applicable
- Time of insertion of NG or esophagogastric tamponade tube (if inserted), patient's tolerance, characteristics of any drainage from the NG tube, radiographic documentation of placement of the NG or tamponade tube, and initial pressure applied
- Postendoscopic therapy vital signs and pulse oximetry
- Date and end time of procedure
- Position of the patient after the procedure
- Vital signs, cardiac rhythm, pulse oximetry, capnography, level of consciousness every 15 minutes (or per institutional standards) after the procedure until the patient returns to preprocedure condition. Include the time the patient returns to baseline.
- Recovery from sedation
- Assessment of gag, swallow, and cough reflexes
- Postprocedure medications administered
- Unexpected outcomes
- Nursing interventions
- Sedation score
- Pain assessment, interventions, and effectiveness
- Preprocedure and postprocedure patient and family education

References and Additional Readings

For a complete list of references and additional readings for this procedure, scan this QR code with your smartphone, or visit https://www.elsevier.com/__data/assets/pdf_file/0005/1319873/Chapter0098.pdf.

99 Intraabdominal Pressure Monitoring

Rosemary Lee

PURPOSE The purpose of this procedure is to present the correct method of measuring intraabdominal pressure (IAP) via the urinary bladder. Intraabdominal hypertension (IAH) and abdominal compartment syndrome (ACS) occur when the abdominal contents expand in excess of the capacity of the abdominal cavity, compromising abdominal organ perfusion and resulting in organ dysfunction or failure and associated mortality. Research has identified that at least 50% to 80% of critically ill patients have some degree of IAH.[1-8]

PREREQUISITE NURSING KNOWLEDGE

- Understanding of the anatomy and physiology of the abdominal contents.
- Knowledge of aseptic technique.
- The abdominal cavity should be viewed as a "closed box" with the spine, costal arch, and pelvis as rigid margins and the diaphragm and abdominal wall as flexible margins.[4]
- IAH and ACS occur when the abdominal contents expand in excess of the capacity of the abdominal cavity, compromising abdominal organ perfusion and resulting in organ dysfunction or failure and associated mortality.[1-3,9,10]
- Five major categories of risk are associated with the development of IAH and ACS (Box 99.1). They include the following[1,4,11,12]:
  - Diminished abdominal wall compliance
  - Increased intestinal intraluminal contents
  - Increased peritoneal cavity contents
  - Capillary leakage into the bowel wall and mesentery/fluid resuscitation[20]
  - Miscellaneous/other
- IAH is defined as a sustained or repeated pathological elevation of IAP greater than or equal to 12 mm Hg.[1,3-5]
- IAH is graded by severity.[1,3-5]
  - Grade I: IAP 12 to 15 mm Hg
  - Grade II: IAP 16 to 20 mm Hg
  - Grade III: IAP 21 to 25 mm Hg
  - Grade IV: IAP greater than 25 mm Hg
- The abdominal perfusion pressure (APP) is proposed as a more accurate predictor of visceral perfusion and a potential endpoint for resuscitation. Both IAH and ACS may compromise perfusion to the visceral organs represented by this parameter, APP. APP is derived as follows[1,4,5,11,12]:
  - $APP = MAP - IAP$, where MAP is mean arterial pressure.
  - A target APP of at least 60 mm Hg has been demonstrated to correlate with improved survival.[4,5,11,12]

- ACS is defined as an IAP greater than or equal to 20 mm Hg that is associated with new organ dysfunction or failure with or without an APP <60 mm Hg.[1,4,5,11,12]
- ACS is categorized into three types. Primary ACS is a condition associated with injury or disease in the abdominopelvic region that frequently requires early surgical or interventional radiological intervention. Secondary ACS is a condition that does not originate from the abdominopelvic region. Recurrent ACS is a condition in which ACS redevelops following previous surgical or medical treatment of primary or secondary ACS. Primary ACS occurs more frequently, but secondary ACS has a higher mortality rate.
- Measurement of bladder pressure via an indwelling urinary bladder catheter is considered the reference standard for the measurement of IAP and may be performed with equipment readily available in the critical care environment (Fig. 99.1). Bladder pressure monitoring may be performed using a transducer method or manometer method. Another device that is FDA approved for measuring IAP is the Accuryn Monitoring System (Potrero). The Accuryn Monitoring System is designed to accurately measure IAP at the push of a button with a continuous-trend, high-resolution Urine Output (U/O) and Core Body Temperature. The Accuryn Monitoring System measures IAP directly from a special self-calibrating balloon on the tip of the Accuryn urinary catheter (Fig. 99.2), which transmits the pressure from inside the bladder to the Accuryn Monitoring System on-demand, regardless of Accuryn monitor position (Fig. 99.3).
- Commercially prepared kits designed for the measurement of IAP are also available and may provide advantages in efficiency, standardization of measurement technique, and data reproducibility.
- Instructions for specific setup and operation of commercially prepared devices are provided by the manufacturer.
- Regardless of the device used, a standardized procedure for measurement should be used to prevent measurement variability among physicians, advanced practice nurses, and other healthcare professionals.[4,5,13-16]

BOX 99.1 **Patients at Risk for Development of Intraabdominal Hypertension and Abdominal Compartment Syndrome**[1,4,11,12]

DIMINISHED ABDOMINAL WALL COMPLIANCE
- Abdominal surgery
- Major trauma
- Major burns
- Prone positioning

INCREASED INTESTINAL INTRALUMINAL CONTENTS
- Gastroparesis
- Gastric distention
- Ileus
- Colonic pseudo-obstruction
- Volvulus

INCREASED INTRAABDOMINAL CONTENTS
- Distended abdomen
- Peritoneal dialysis
- Laparoscopy with excessive insufflation pressures
- Acute pancreatitis
- Hemoperitoneum/pneumoperitoneum or intraperitoneal fluid collections
- Intraabdominal infection/abscess
- Intraabdominal or retroperitoneal tumors
- Liver dysfunction/cirrhosis with ascites

CAPILLARY LEAK/FLUID RESUSCITATION
- Metabolic acidosis, pH <7.20
- Hypothermia (core temperature <33°C or <91.4°F)
- Massive fluid resuscitation (>5 L/24 hours) or positive fluid balance
- Polytransfusion (>10 units of blood/24 hours)
- Damage-control laparotomy
- Increased severity of disease classification score such as Acute Physiology and Chronic Health Evaluation II (APACHE-II) or Sequential Organ Failure Assessment (SOFA) score

OTHERS/MISCELLANEOUS
- Age (>69 years)
- Coagulopathy (not on anticoagulation)
  - Platelets <55,000/mm³ **OR**
  - A partial thromboplastin time greater than twice normal **OR**
  - International normalized ratio >1.5
- Increased head of bed angle (>20 degrees)
- Large hernia repair
- Mechanical ventilation
- Positive end-expiratory pressure >10 cm H_2O
- Obesity or increased body mass index (BMI >30)
- Diagnosis of:
  - Intraabdominal infections/peritonitis
  - Pneumonia
  - Bacteremia
  - Sepsis
- Shock or hypotension

Bladder Pressure Monitoring Setup

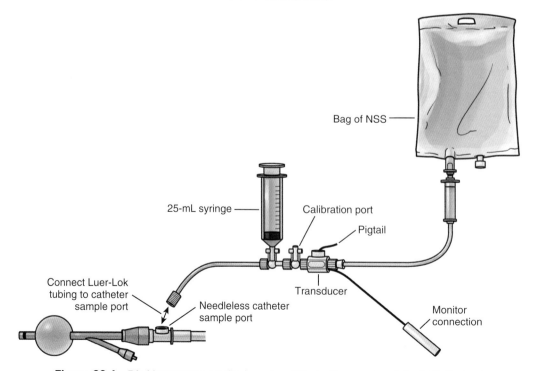

Figure 99.1   Bladder pressure monitoring setup. *(Illustration courtesy John J. Gallagher.)*

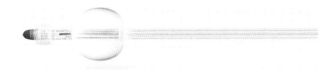

Figure 99.2   Accuryn catheter.

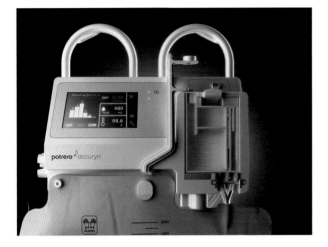

Figure 99.3   Accuryn monitoring system.

- The bladder acts as a passive reservoir and accurately reflects IAP when intravesicular volumes of 25 mL or less are used. Larger volumes previously suggested (50 to 100 mL) are not necessary and may in fact overdistend the bladder, falsely elevating measured bladder pressure (IAP).[4,5,14-16]
- Normal IAP is 0 to 5 mm Hg. The typical critically ill patient averages an IAP of 5 to 7 mm Hg.[1,3-5,11]
- Bladder pressure measurement may be contraindicated in certain conditions, such as bladder trauma or bladder surgery. IAP readings are inaccurate in patients with a neurogenic bladder. Risks and benefits of measurement should be discussed with the provider before the procedure is performed in these patients.
- In patients who do not have a urinary catheter in place, the risks and benefits of catheter placement for the purpose of bladder pressure measurement should be considered.

EQUIPMENT

- Nonsterile gloves
- Intravenous (IV) pole
- If using transducer technique:
  - Cardiac monitor and pressure cable for interface with the monitor
  - 250-mL or 500-mL IV bag of normal saline (NS) solution
  - Pressure transducer system, including pressure tubing with flush device, transducer, and two stopcocks
  - 25- to 30-mL Luer-lock syringe
  - Clamp
  - Chlorhexidine or alcohol swabs

- If using manometer technique:
  - 20 mL of sterile saline
  - 20-mL Luer-lock syringe
  - Urinary manometer kit

  Note: A commercial bladder pressure monitoring system may be substituted for the previous list.

PATIENT/FAMILY EDUCATION

- Explain the procedure of bladder pressure measurement and its purpose to the patient and family. *Rationale:* Patient and family anxiety may be decreased. Understanding of how the procedure is performed may promote the patient's ability to cooperate.
- Inform the patient that fullness may be felt in the bladder when the normal saline solution is injected into the bladder during the procedure. *Rationale:* Patient anxiety may be decreased. The patient is prepared for what to expect.

PATIENT ASSESSMENT AND PREPARATION

Patient Assessment

- Obtain the patient's health history to determine whether risk factors are present that may predispose the patient to IAH or ACS. These conditions are outlined in Table 99.1. *Rationale:* Patients with these conditions may experience an increase in abdominal cavity fluid collection or tissue edema, placing them at risk for IAH and ACS. It is recommended that patients with any one risk factor have IAPs measured.[6]
- Assess the patient for signs of progression of IAH to ACS. These findings include decreased cardiac output and blood pressure, oliguria and anuria, increased peak inspiratory pressures, hypercarbia and hypoxia, and increased intracranial pressure (ICP) (see Table 99.1). *Rationale:* These physical findings indicate pathophysiological organ system changes associated with the progression of IAH to ACS.

Patient Preparation

- Ensure that the patient and family understand the preprocedural teaching. Answer questions as they arise, and reinforce information as needed. *Rationale:* Understanding of previously taught information is evaluated and reinforced.
- Ensure the presence of a conventional (single-lumen) urinary catheter connected to a drainage system. *Rationale:* A urinary catheter with a drainage system is required to obtain bladder pressure measurements.
- Verify the correct patient with two identifiers. *Rationale:* Before performing a procedure, the nurse should ensure the correct identification of the patient for the intended intervention.
- Perform a preprocedural verification and time out if required by institutional policy, if the procedure is nonemergent. *Rationale:* This ensures patient safety.

UNIT IV

TABLE 99.1	Physiological Changes Associated With Intraabdominal Hypertension and Abdominal Compartment Syndrome[3,4,10-12,14,18,19,21]	
Organ System	**Rationale**	
Cardiovascular ↑ Central venous pressure (CVP), pulmonary artery pressure (PAP), pulmonary capillary wedge pressure (PCWP), systemic vascular resistance (SVR) ↓ Cardiac output (CO) (more pronounced with hypovolemia) ↓ Venous return from lower extremities (risk for deep vein thrombosis)	Up to 50% of the IAP is reflected into the thoracic cavity. This leads to compression of the heart and decreased venous return (preload reduction), and impedes arterial outflow (increase in afterload). Transmitted backpressure from the abdominal cavity can falsely elevate CVP, PAP, and PCWP. The World Society of the Abdominal Compartment Syndrome recommends using volumetric indices rather than pressure indices for assessment of fluid responsiveness. Indices recommended for use are stroke volume, stroke volume index, global ventricular end-diastolic volume, pulse pressure variation, and stroke volume variation in appropriate situations. Note: The passive leg-raise maneuver is not accurate in assessing fluid responsiveness when the IAP is greater than or equal to 12 mm Hg.	
Pulmonary ↑ Intrathoracic pressures ↑ Peak inspiratory pressures ↑ Plateau pressures ↓ Functional residual capacity ↑ Dead space shunt ↓ Tidal volume → ↑ hypercarbia + ↓ partial pressure of oxygen in arterial blood ↓ Compliance ↑ Compression atelectasis ↑ Pulmonary infection rate	Increased IAP causes an increase in intrathoracic pressure and limits diaphragm excursion, resulting in hypoventilation and hypoxia. IAH can cause prolonged ventilator time. Patients with primary IAH are at higher risk for developing acute lung injury/acute respiratory distress syndrome.	

Renal
↓ Renal blood flow → ↓ glomerular filtration rate (GFR) → ↓ urine output
	Increased IAP:
	    Reduces cardiac output to the kidney
	    Compresses the renal artery and vein, which reduces perfusion pressure to the glomerulus.
	    IAP simultaneously increases the pressure within the renal parenchyma, leading to a reduction in filtration. The combination leads to a marked reduction in GFR and urine production. The patient is at risk for acute kidney injury (AKI). AKI is known to occur with persistent IAPs of 10–12 mm Hg.	

Neurologic ↑ Intracranial pressure (ICP) ↓ Cerebral perfusion pressure (CPP)	Increased IAP impedes venous outflow from the brain, increasing cerebral venous congestion.	

Hepatic
↓ Hepatic artery and portal vein blood flow
↓ Liver function:
  • Lactate clearance
  • Glucose metabolism
  • Cytochrome P450 function
  • Clearance of toxic metabolites
	Increased IAP compresses the hepatic artery and portal vein, leading to decreased liver perfusion and decreased hepatic function.	

Gastrointestinal
↓ Blood flow to the celiac axis and the superior mesenteric artery
↓ Perfusion of the abdominal organs
↑ Compression of mesenteric veins leading to abdominal venous hypertension
↓ Successful enteral nutrition
↑ Ileus
↑ Intestinal edema and permeability
↑ Bacterial translocation
↑ Visceral swelling
↑ Bowel ischemia
↑ Abdominal wound complications:
  • Edema
  • Ischemia
  • Dehiscence
  • Infection
	Increased IAP compresses the major arteries feeding the abdominal organs. The compression of the veins leads to venous congestion. Poor perfusion leads to the gastrointestinal complications listed.	

Endocrine ↑ Antidiuretic hormone ↑ Renin, angiotensin, aldosterone	As a result of decreased cardiac output and blood pressure, the baroreceptors stimulate the sympathetic nervous system to maintain homeostasis.	

Procedure for Intraabdominal Pressure Monitoring

Steps	Rationale	Special Considerations
1. HH		
2. PE		
3. Assemble the entire pressure transducer system (see Fig. 99.1): A. Attach the two stopcocks between the transducer and the pressure tubing. B. Spike the normal saline bag with the pressure transducer system, and flush it.	Ensures that all air is out of the system.	If the pressure transducer already has a stopcock attached to the transducer, only one stopcock is needed. Note that a pressure bag is not required.
4. Attach the 25- or 30-mL syringe to the distal stopcock (see Fig. 99.1).	The syringe is used to fill the bladder with normal saline solution.	
5. Cleanse the sampling port on the urinary drainage system with an antiseptic solution, and aseptically attach the end of the pressure tubing to the sampling port.	Cleansing the sampling port reduces the incidence of catheter-associated urinary tract infection (CAUTI) from system contamination.	
6. Connect the system to the pressure module of the monitoring system with the transducer cable. Select a 30–mm Hg scale, and use an IAP label if available, or label as "P."	Connects the system for monitoring. The 30–mm Hg scale is sufficient to measure most IAP ranges. Monitors may not have an IAP label; it is best to use the "P" for pressure.	Using the label "CVP" or "ICP" can cause confusion.
7. Level the transducer: A. With the patient in the supine position and the head of the bed flat, level the transducer (zeroing stopcock) to the iliac crest at the level of the midaxillary line (Fig. 99.4).[1,4,5,14-17] **(Level D*)** B. If the patient must remain with the head of the bed elevated, the transducer must be placed at the level of the bladder (iliac crest; see Fig. 99.4).	The supine position limits the effect of the abdominal cavity contents on the bladder that may falsely elevate bladder pressure measurements. Approximates the level of the bladder and should be used as the reference point.	Marking the position ensures consistent use of the same reference point. The transducer system may be secured to an IV pole beside the patient, or it can be secured to the patient. If the patient is unable to be placed in the supine position, note the degree of elevation of the head of the bed on the medical record along with the bladder pressure to allow future measurements to be performed in the same position and compared accurately. Note that the phlebostatic axis should not be used to level the transducer for bladder pressure measurement.

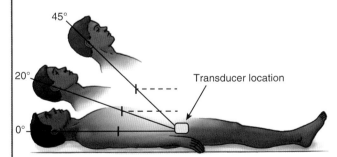

The correct transducer position at the iliac crest in the mid-axillary line in the supine position and with head of bed elevation

Figure 99.4   Correct position of the transducer for bladder pressure measurement. *(Illustration by John J. Gallagher.)*

*Level D: Peer-reviewed professional and organizational standards with the support of clinical study recommendations.

Procedure continues on following page

UNIT IV

Procedure | **for Intraabdominal Pressure Monitoring—*Continued***

Steps	Rationale	Special Considerations
8. Zero the IAP monitoring system.	Negates the effect of atmospheric pressure. Ensures accuracy of the system with the established reference point.	
9. Clamp the bladder drainage system just distal to the catheter and drainage bag connection on the drainage bag tubing.	Prevents drainage of the normal saline solution out of the bladder during bladder filling. Provides a closed loop from the bladder to the transducer for an accurate reading.	
10. Turn the stopcock attached to the syringe off to the patient and open to the fluid bag and syringe. Activate the fast-flush mechanism while pulling back on the syringe plunger to fill the syringe to 25 mL.[1,4,5,14-16] **(Level D*)**		
11. Turn off the stopcock to the fluid bag and open to the syringe and patient. Inject 25 mL of saline solution into the bladder.[1,4,5,14-16] **(Level D*)**	The fluid-filled bladder accurately reflects IAP. Use of a volume of 25 mL prevents overdistention of the bladder and false elevation of the bladder pressure.	
12. Expel any air seen between the clamp and the urinary catheter by opening the clamp and allowing the saline solution to flow back past the clamp; then reclamp it.	Air in the system may dampen the pressure reading.	
13. Measure the IAP at end expiration with the graphic scale on the monitor display and numeric display of the mean pressure (Fig. 99.5). IAP should be measured with the patient in the supine position. Ensure that the patient is relaxed and not coughing or moving.	Measurement at end expiration is most accurate when the effects of pulmonary pressures are minimized. Patient movement and coughing can elevate the IAP.	The numeric mean IAP pressure displayed on the monitor may be used in most circumstances. The numeric reading is a mean pressure value reflecting the average of both inspiratory and expiratory IAP. Consider reading the IAP from the monitor graphic scale or a printed strip if noticeable excursions or variations are found in the waveform with ventilation.

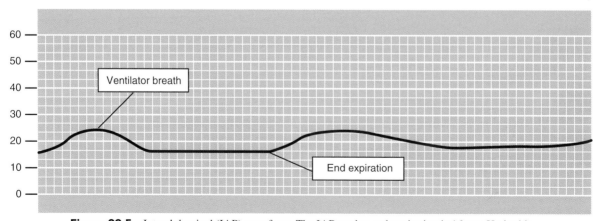

Figure 99.5   Intraabdominal (IAP) waveform. The IAP read at end expiration is 16 mm Hg in this patient on mechanical ventilation.

*Level D: Peer-reviewed professional and organizational standards with the support of clinical study recommendations.

Procedure for Intraabdominal Pressure Monitoring—*Continued*		
Steps	**Rationale**	**Special Considerations**
14. Once a reading has been obtained, unclamp the urinary drainage system. The pressure monitoring system may be left connected or disconnected and capped to maintain the sterility of the system. Note: The urinary drainage system should be left unclamped between readings.	Unclamping the drainage system discontinues pressure measurement and resumes the normal urinary drainage function of the catheter system. If the monitoring system is maintained connected to the urinary catheter, repeated reentry into the catheter tubing is avoided.	Monitoring requires clamping the drainage system and filling the bladder to obtain a reading. Minimizing entry into the urinary drainage system may reduce the chance of CAUTI. Specific data to support this practice in IAP measurement do not exist.
15. Record the bladder pressure in the patient's record, and remember to subtract the 25 mL of instilled saline solution from the hourly urine output.	The volume of instilled normal saline solution falsely elevates the calculation of hourly urine output if it is not subtracted.	
16. Discard used supplies and gloves in the appropriate receptacles.		
17. 🄷🄷		

Procedure for Intraabdominal Pressure Monitoring With the Foley Manometer LV System		
Steps	**Rationale**	**Special Considerations**
Note: Intended for patients who are at least 10 kg.		
1. 🄷🄷		
2. 🄿🄴		
3. Open the Foley Manometer LV pouch, and close the tube clamp.	The clamp is left open for effective device sterilization. During urine drainage, the filter must be clamped; the clamp is open only when IAP is measured.	
4. Place the urine collection device below the patient's bladder, and tape the drainage tube to the bedsheet (Fig. 99.6). **(Level M*)**	Prevents dependent loops in the drainage tubing.	
5. Carefully cleanse the catheter connection with an antiseptic before disconnecting the urinary catheter system.	Maintains sterility and prevents a CAUTI.	
6. Using aseptic technique, insert the Foley Manometer LV between the catheter and the drainage device.	Maintains sterility and prevents a CAUTI.	This step is key in preventing contamination of the urinary drainage system.
7. Prime the Foley Manometer LV with 20 mL of sterile saline solution through its needle-free injection/sampling port. **(Level M*)**	Removes air from the system.	Prime only once, at initial setup or subsequently, to remove any air from the manometer tube. The manometer tube should always be fluid filled. Note: In patients who are anuric, repriming at each pressure determination is not necessary. The fluid returned to the bladder from the manometer tube provides an adequate volume for a reliable pressure determination. Carefully disinfect the needle-free port before urine sampling.

*Level M: Manufacturer's recommendations only.

Procedure continues on following page

Procedure for Intraabdominal Pressure Monitoring With the Foley Manometer LV System—*Continued*

Steps	Rationale	Special Considerations

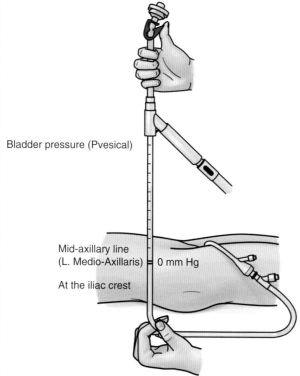

Bladder pressure (Pvesical)

Mid-axillary line
(L. Medio-Axillaris) = 0 mm Hg

At the iliac crest

Figure 99.6 Commercially prepared Foley Monitor LV pressure monitoring system. *(Redrawn with permission from Holtech Medical, Charlottenlund, Denmark.)*

8. Place the "0 mm Hg" mark of the manometer tube at the midaxillary line at the iliac crest, and elevate the filter vertically above the patient (Fig. 99.7). Place the patient in the supine position, and ensure that the patient is relaxed and not coughing or moving.	Approximates the level of the bladder and should be used as the reference point. Limits the effect of the abdominal cavity contents on the bladder that may falsely elevate bladder pressure measurements. Patient movement or coughing can elevate the IAP.	Note that the phlebostatic axis should not be used to level the transducer for bladder pressure measurement.
9. Open the clamp and read the bladder pressure (end-expiration value) when the fluid meniscus has stabilized (see Fig. 99.7).	Allows for equilibration of the fluid column to accurately represent bladder pressure.	Slow descent (>20–30 seconds) of the meniscus during a bladder pressure determination suggests a blocked or kinked urinary catheter.
10. Close the clamp, and place the Foley Manometer LV in its drainage position (see Fig. 99.6).	Allows normal flow through the urinary drainage system.	Avoid a U-bend of the large urimeter drainage tube (which will impede urine drainage). Never empty the manometer tube into the urine drainage device during use. The Foley Manometer LV tube should be fluid filled during drainage. Only reprime with sterile normal saline solution to remove any air or bladder debris in the manometer tube. Note: Never use the Foley Manometer LV for more than 7 days. **(Level M*)**
11. Discard used supplies gloves in the appropriate receptacles.		
12. **HH**		

*Level M: Manufacturer's recommendations only.

Procedure	**for Intraabdominal Pressure Monitoring With the Foley Manometer LV System—*Continued***	
Steps	Rationale	Special Considerations

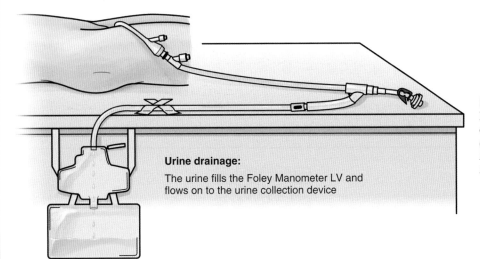

Urine drainage:
The urine fills the Foley Manometer LV and
flows on to the urine collection device

Figure 99.7 The urine fills the Foley Manometer LV and flows on to the urine collection device. *(Redrawn with permission from Holtech Medical, Charlottenlund, Denmark.)*

Expected Outcomes

- IAP is monitored in at-risk patients.
- IAP is within normal limits.
- Elevated IAP is detected and therapeutic interventions are initiated.

Unexpected Outcomes

- Inability to monitor IAP
- Inaccurate pressure readings obtained
- Development of a CAUTI from urinary drainage system manipulation
- Patient discomfort
- Abdominal compartment syndrome

Patient Monitoring and Care

Steps	Rationale	Reportable Conditions
		These conditions should be reported to the provider if they persist despite nursing interventions.
1. Monitor IAP every 4 hours or more frequently, as prescribed and depending on clinical need.[4,11,17] **(Level E*)**	Serial measurements detect a trended increase in IAPs, reflecting development of IAH or ACS.	• IAP ≥12 mm Hg
2. Assess the patient for signs of increasing IAP.[3,4,12,18-21]	Patients may have symptoms develop slowly over time. The symptoms may mimic other clinical conditions, such as acute respiratory distress syndrome, acute renal failure, congestive heart failure, and intracranial hypertension.	• Decrease in blood pressure and cardiac output • Oliguria or anuria • Increase in peak inspiratory pressures • Hypoxia and hypercarbia • Elevated ICP
3. Monitor for signs and symptoms of CAUTI.[13,16] **(Level E*)**	Frequent breaks in the integrity of the urinary drainage system may contribute to the development of CAUTI.	• Temperature elevation • Elevated white blood cell count • Increased urine sediment or cloudiness of urine
4. Follow institutional standards for assessing pain.	Increasing abdominal pain may indicate an increase in IAP or impending ACS.	• Same pain rating as before interventions • Continued pain despite pain interventions

*Level E: Multiple case reports, theory-based evidence from expert opinions, or peer-reviewed professional organizational standards without clinical studies to support recommendations.

Documentation

Documentation should include the following:
- Patient and family education
- Assessment findings before obtaining IAPs
- IAP value
- Degree of elevation of the head of the bed if measurements are not obtained in the supine position[1,4,5,11,14,15]
- Postprocedure assessment
- Changes in the patient's assessment that indicate onset of IAH or ACS
- The amount of fluid instilled into the bladder to be subtracted from the hourly urine output
- Unexpected outcomes
- Additional interventions
- Pain assessment, interventions, and effectiveness
- Reportable conditions

References and Additional Readings

For a complete list of references and additional readings for this procedure, scan this QR code with any freely available smartphone code reader app, or visit https://www.elsevier.com/__data/assets/pdf_file/0006/1319874/Chapter0099.pdf

100 Nasogastric and Orogastric Tube Insertion, Nursing Care, and Removal

Carol Marie McGinnis

PURPOSE Nasogastric (NG) and orogastric (OG) tubes are inserted to facilitate gastric decompression and drainage. This may involve removal of air, retained food materials, secretions, blood, or ingested drugs or toxins. These tubes are also used to deliver fluid and medication. Enteral tube feeding via the gastric route is sometimes implemented on a short-term basis until a smaller feeding tube or percutaneous tube can be inserted. OG tubes might be inserted when nasal tubes are contraindicated or unable to be placed (e.g., basilar skull fracture or nasal fracture) or sometimes preferentially, as in critical care settings. Consider that the OG tube position may be more difficult to maintain in a conscious, nonintubated patient who might be at risk for tube displacement secondary to tongue movement or difficulty securing the tube.

PREREQUISITE NURSING KNOWLEDGE

- Knowledge of the anatomy and physiology of the gastro-intestinal (GI) tract.
- Knowledge about use and care of the variety of tubes that may be used in clinical practice can help guide practice. Knowing the intended use and anticipated duration for the NG tube may help determine the best type and size of tube to be used.
- Knowledge of means to guide and comfort the patient during a potentially uncomfortable procedure.[10,15]
- Critical thinking skills are important, especially in terms of determining and monitoring appropriate tube position and assessing that the tube is functioning properly for its intended purpose.
- Knowledge of evidence-based measures to verify appropriate tube position.
- Knowledge of means to prevent or monitor for adverse effects that could be related to an NG tube, including sinus infection, tube misplacement and displacement, tube clogging, pressure injuries related to tube securement, and patient discomfort.

EQUIPMENT

- NG tube, preferably with numeric marks to identify depth of insertion and to determine whether the external tube amount has changed. The smallest size that can achieve the intended purpose will typically be more tolerable for the patient.
- Water-soluble lubricant
- A 50- or 60-mL syringe with a tip that is appropriate for the tube being inserted that also meets the standards to prevent administration into an inappropriate port.[8]
- Small towel
- Clean gloves
- Personal protective equipment (PPE) as indicated as exposure to body fluids with this procedure is possible
- Stethoscope
- pH strips or paper; follow institutional protocol for quality control and bedside testing
- Capnometry device if this is to be used in the procedure
- Emesis bag or basin (keep discretely out of sight) and tissues for eye watering, and so on
- Tape and securement device of choice, which may include transparent dressing or nasal securement device
- Skin prep agent or other agent to promote adherence to skin, such as tincture of benzoin; optional (e.g., if skin is oily)
- Indelible marker
- Tape measure
  Additional equipment to have available as needed includes the following:
- Local anesthetic agent (e.g., lidocaine gel) per provider order or institutional protocol, such as per nurse-driven protocol. If using lidocaine gel administered via syringe, use a tip that meets standards to prevent administration into an inappropriate port.[8,9]
- Clean cup and supplies if specimens are to be obtained.
- Provide ice chips or a cup of water with a straw if the patient is able to safely swallow fluid.

PATIENT AND FAMILY EDUCATION

- Explain the purpose of the NG or OG tube, and reassure the patient that efforts will be made to minimize discomfort and provide support. Some patients may appreciate that having an NG tube is less unpleasant than abdominal distention and vomiting. *Rationale:* Patient and family anxiety may be decreased.
- Explain what the patient might expect as well as the patient's role in assisting with the passage of the tube. *Rationale:* This information may decrease patient anxiety and help during the procedure.

PATIENT ASSESSMENT AND PREPARATION

Patient Assessment

- Assess history for factors that might be relevant to this procedure, including recent facial or head injury with basilar skull fracture or transsphenoidal surgery. Determine whether the patient has had prior nasal or upper GI surgery, esophageal stent, or anatomical anomalies (e.g., deviated nasal septum, esophageal diverticulae or varices, known hiatal hernia). *Rationale:* Contraindications to placing an NG tube include basilar skull fracture and may include nasal or pharyngeal, esophageal, or gastric injury or surgery. Other conditions may require special care or complicate placement.
- If the patient is susceptible to epistaxis or sinusitis, determine which naris is more susceptible. Inquire whether the patient has a preference for which naris should be used for NG intubation. *Rationale:* Preliminary assessment provides an alert to contraindications or potential issues that can be avoided or minimized related to tube placement.

- Assess the nares to determine patency by assessing air exchange and by visual inspection. *Rationale:* The naris with the best airflow may be easiest to access.
- Assess physical status before tube insertion, including assessing for abdominal distention, firmness, tenderness, tympany, and presence or absence, as well as quality of bowel sounds. *Rationale:* This provides preliminary information that will be useful in monitoring patient status.

Patient Preparation

- Verify the correct patient with two identifiers. *Rationale:* Before performing a procedure, the nurse should ensure the correct identification of the patient for the intended intervention.
- Perform a preprocedure verification of patient need for the procedure and a time out, if nonemergent. *Rationale:* This promotes patient safety.
- Ensure that the patient understands what the procedure entails and how the tube will be helpful. *Rationale:* Patient understanding can reduce anxiety and increase cooperation.
- Assess what helps the patient deal with stressful procedures, and offer suggestions for dealing with temporary discomfort (e.g., related to tube insertion, such as distraction, using a focal point, providing a washcloth or other item to squeeze, breathing techniques). If the patient is restless, having a support person present may be helpful. *Rationale:* This maintains the patient's sense of self-control.
- If the patient may safely sip on water, he or she may find this to be helpful during the NG insertion, or it may be overwhelming; assess patient preference. *Rationale:* Following the swallow mechanism may facilitate tube insertion if it is not distracting.

Procedure for Nasogastric or Orogastric Tube Insertion		
Steps	Rationale	Special Considerations
1. **HH**		
2. Don **PE** as indicated.	Exposure to body fluids can occur with this procedure.	
3. Position the patient in the Fowler's or semi-Fowler's position, as possible, providing for patient comfort as well as easy access. If water is to be sipped during the procedure, the head of the bed must be appropriately elevated.	Patient and staff comfort are important for any procedure. Provide for safety of patient swallowing if there is to be sipping of water.	The lateral decubitus position may be helpful for the unconscious patient who is at risk for backward tongue displacement.[19]
4. Discuss and provide comfort measures, including administration of lidocaine gel[10] or other agent per provider order via the appropriate naris for NG insertion. If used, follow proper medication administration procedure.	Reduces patient discomfort.	A calming nurse presence also provides comfort and a sense of security. An order set via the electronic medical record with supplies readily available (as via a medication supply station) can reduce time to provide for patient comfort.[16]

Procedure for Nasogastric or Orogastric Tube Insertion—*Continued*

Steps	Rationale	Special Considerations
5. Place a clean towel over the patient's upper chest area.	Provides a clean work surface and keeps supplies as clean as possible.	Although this is not a sterile procedure, optimal cleanliness is important.
6. Prepare supplies for easy access (e.g., on a clean overbed table).	Aids in organization and avoids unnecessary delays in the procedure.	
7. Perform **HH** again, and don clean gloves.	Aids in cleanliness of procedure.	Repeat if interrupted for non–procedure-related reasons.
8. Estimate the length of tube to be inserted: A. The traditional method of measuring insertion distance (from the tip of the nose to the ear or earlobe to the xiphoid process) may underestimate the amount of tube needed to access the gastric fluid pool.[4,5,14,17,18] Adding 10 cm to this measurement may help ensure that the tube tip opening(s) reach the gastric pool.[7,17] **(Level C*)** The term *NEMU* (or nose to ear to mid umbilicus) has been used to refer to this concept.[5] B. Identify the corresponding number on the tube to be inserted or, if without numbers, mark the tube or note identifier at the intended exit point.	Helps determine the appropriate amount of tube insertion length. For gastric decompression, appropriate placement will help ensure that all NG openings are within or as close to the gastric pool as possible for optimal decompression.	Anatomy differs from patient to patient. There is no exact method to determine the best tube insertion length; therefore the clinician must correlate with placement verification, clinical condition, aspirated returns, and so on.
9. Lubricate the end of the tube with water-soluble lubricant.	Facilitates easier tube passage across potentially dry tissue and help decrease patient discomfort.	
10. For NG tube insertion: Insert the tube gently through the naris at an angle parallel to the floor of the nasal canal and then with a gentle downward motion as the tube advances through the nasal passage toward the distal pharynx. If resistance is felt, try gentle rotation of the tube tip until it advances beyond the nasal passage. If resistance continues, withdraw the tube, and allow the patient to rest; relubricate the tube; and retry or insert the tube via the other naris. **Do not force the tube past resistance.**	Helps guide the tube through the opening in the naris toward the nasopharynx.	This may be the most uncomfortable portion of the procedure for the patient. One naris may be more patent than the other.

*Level C: Qualitative studies, descriptive or correlational studies, integrative reviews, systematic reviews, or randomized controlled trials with inconsistent results.

Procedure continues on following page

UNIT IV

Procedure for Nasogastric or Orogastric Tube Insertion—*Continued*

Steps	Rationale	Special Considerations
11. Position the head forward in a chin-tuck position, if not contraindicated.	May aid in accessing the GI tract versus the trachea.	The chin-tuck position has been shown to be more successful in accessing the GI tract than the neutral head position (opposite of CPR position).[2,11] A slight chin-tuck position might be possible if a cervical collar is being used.
12. For NG tube insertion: If the patient agrees and is able to swallow safely, sipping on water may enhance NG insertion after the tube is in the oropharynx. If swallowing is not safe, the patient could try dry swallowing to facilitate tube insertion, if desired.	The tube may follow the swallow mechanism and aid insertion. However, this may be distracting to a patient who prefers to have the tube inserted quickly.	Swallowing is not necessary for successful NG insertion.
13. For OG tube insertion: Insert the tube via the oral cavity, guiding it downward toward the esophagus. If resistance is met, rotate the tube end to guide it toward the esophagus. **Do not force the tube.** If continued resistance is met, stop the procedure and investigate barriers to tube advancement.	Guides the tube into the esophagus and then the stomach.	The tongue might provide a barrier to tube insertion. Gentle guidance over the tongue using a tongue depressor to slightly depress the tongue may facilitate tube insertion.
14. Watch for patient cues (e.g., cough, discomfort) as the tube is advanced.	Patient coughing or other signs of discomfort could signal potential tube advancement via the respiratory tract. It could also signal that the tube is kinked or curled in the nasopharyngeal or oral cavity.	Sense of gagging may not be unexpected, but do not advance the tube if the patient is coughing, because the tube is more likely to enter the respiratory tract during a cough. If coughing is noted, pull back to the nasopharyngeal area, and readvance. Patient cues can be very helpful, although respiratory intubation can occur with no overt signs such as coughing.
15. If capnometry is to be used to help detect inadvertent tracheal placement, attach the colorimetric capnometry device, and assess for color at about the 30-cm mark. If the color on the device is purple, the tube may be further advanced. If it is yellow or brown, withdraw the tube, and repeat the process.	Purple color reflects the absence of CO_2, whereas brown or yellow reflects placement other than gastric.	This method may be more reliable than auscultation for reflecting placement in the GI tract versus the respiratory tract,[3,6] but it has not been found to be accurate for determining gastric versus duodenal placement (**Level C***); therefore radiographic verification for tube confirmation is still indicated.

*Level C: Qualitative studies, descriptive or correlational studies, integrative reviews, systematic reviews, or randomized controlled trials with inconsistent results.

Procedure	for Nasogastric or Orogastric Tube Insertion—*Continued*	
Steps	Rationale	Special Considerations
16. Continue to advance the tube to the intended distance as previously determined. If there is any resistance, **do not force the tube past resistance.** If the tube is difficult to advance, pull it back to the nasopharyngeal or oropharyngeal area, and gently advance again. Insertion of a small amount of air via syringe can help assess for tube kinking. Gentle resistance may be felt when the tube has been inserted to the distal stomach.	Advance tube to the stomach with sliding motion through the esophagus. Forcing the tube can cause kinking or trauma.	Anatomical anomalies such as hiatal hernias may present challenges to NG insertion. It is important to guide, **but never force** tube insertion. For typical adults, gastric placement might be noted in the range of ~50–65 cm for tubes with these markings.
17. Instill 20–30 mL of air into the tube with a large syringe while listening for the air bolus over the epigastric region.	*Although this is unreliable in assessing tube placement alone,* it can provide valuable information to add to other information regarding tube placement.	Consider that if air is difficult to hear, the tube may not be in the stomach. If the injected air is audible in the mouth area, the tube tip may have curled in the upper GI tract. If unable to instill air, the tube may be kinked.
18. Once the tube has been inserted to the predetermined length, aspirate using a 50- to 60-mL syringe to assess for gastric content. The tube may need to be advanced or withdrawn slightly to best obtain gastric contents, which may help determine the best placement.	Gastric returns can indicate that the openings or hole(s) of the tube are in a pool of gastric fluid.	To facilitate aspiration of gastric returns, it may be necessary to insert a small volume of air to clear the tube of thick secretions.
19. Observe the quantity, color, and quality of the aspirated returns, and store in the syringe or a clean container to assess pH when the tube has been secured.	Can help differentiate between gastric fluid and returns from the upper small bowel. Also provides valuable clinical information (e.g., evidence of recent gastric bleeding or a large volume of dark fluid, which might predispose to reflux or emesis).	Returns from the small bowel might be gold in color and perhaps thick and oily as opposed to typical gastric returns. Gastric decompression may not be effective if the tube terminates in the upper small bowel.

Procedure continues on following page

Procedure for Nasogastric or Orogastric Tube Insertion—*Continued*		
Steps	Rationale	Special Considerations
20. Cleanse the area for tube securement. Use a skin prep agent if indicated. If using the split-tape method to secure the tube to the nasal area: A. Split the tape lengthwise, leaving 1–2 inches unsplit. B. Cleanse the top of the nose with alcohol or a skin prep agent, and apply an adhesive or tacifier agent (e.g., tincture of benzoin) for adhesiveness as indicated. C. Secure the unsplit tape to the nose, and wrap the split ends around the tube in opposite directions, leaving a gap at the tip of the nose to avoid pressure on nasal tissue. Pull up on the tip of the naris during taping to prevent the tube from pressing against the external aspect of the nares *or* Secure the tube using a nasal securement device, also avoiding pressure on nasal tissue as possible *or* If the tube is relatively small and soft, it may be secured across the cheek using transparent dressing up to the naris, overlapping two dressings as needed. Secure to the neck area to reduce pressure on the cheek dressings; pinch the tape around the tube and then to the neck for additional security.	Reduces potential for inadvertent tube misplacement. **Avoid pressure from the tube against the nasal mucosa with tube securement.** Ensure that there is space between the tube and internal or external aspects of the naris or skin; serious pressure injury can develop related to NG securement. Using a skin prep agent may aid the adhesiveness of the tape or other dressing material. Taping to the neck area reduces pressure on the securement to the cheek (or nose).	If it is possible to adequately secure the tube to the cheek and neck area, the patient may prefer this as opposed to having it hang from the nose. On occasion, an NG tube might be bridled for situations where there is increased risk of displacement. When taping to the neck, pinch the tape around the tube and then to the neck to provide additional security. This taping method may be likened to the Greek symbol omega (Ω).
21. For OG tube securement, the tube might be secured to the endotracheal tube that is often present when this method is used. If the endotracheal tube is not present, secure the tube to the corresponding cheek and neck area, monitoring frequently for potential tube displacement.	The risk of displacement for an orally placed tube is increased when there is difficulty securing it.	Ongoing need for oral gastric access is reassessed when endotracheal extubation is planned.
22. Measure the amount of tube that is external (from the naris to the distal tube end), and/or note the numeric mark on the tube at the exit point; mark the tube where it exits the naris with an indelible marker.	Provides an objective measure to determine placement; marking aids in quickly determining tube misplacement.	Document this information in a place that is visible for ongoing monitoring.
23. Assess the pH of aspirated returns.	Gastric returns are typically acidic, with a pH of 1–5.5,[1,13] unless affected by medication or feeding. **(Level C*)**	Assess the pH before administering proton pump inhibitors (PPIs) or histamine (H_2) antagonists when possible to avoid the alkalinizing effect of these agents.

*Level C: Qualitative studies, descriptive or correlational studies, integrative reviews, systematic reviews, or randomized controlled trials with inconsistent results.

Procedure | for Nasogastric or Orogastric Tube Insertion—*Continued*

Steps	Rationale	Special Considerations
24. Remove gloves, and wash hands.	As per any procedure involving patient contact.	
25. Utilize a variety of bedside practices to assess tube location during the insertion procedure, including: A. Obtaining an abdominal x-ray before instillation of fluid or medication into a blindly placed tube (either small or large bore) in the absence of other reliable confirmatory methods of placement verification[1,13] (**Level D***) B. Aspirating with a 60-mL syringe for gastric returns, assessing quantity, quality, color, as well as pH for acidity.	Confirms tube placement. NG tubes can be misplaced into the esophagus, small intestine, or even lung, and placement must be ascertained before use. Radiographic confirmation of tube placement is currently the only definitive way to confirm placement.[1,13] (**Level D***)	Auscultation of air bolus may be heard in the gastric region, even if the tube terminates in the esophagus, and this should not be relied on for verification of placement.

*Level D: Peer-reviewed professional and organizational standards with the support of clinical study recommendations.

Procedure | for NG or OG Tube Removal

Steps	Rationale	Special Considerations
1. **HH**		
2. **PE**	Splash and exposure to body fluids can occur with this procedure.	
3. Place a clean hand towel on the patient's upper chest area.	Keeps the patient's clothing and linens clean.	
4. Verify the order to remove the tube, and verify the correct patient with two identifiers.	Prevents the wrong patient or wrong procedure.	Sometimes clamping of the tube is done before discontinuing the tube to ascertain patient tolerance before removal.
5. Explain the procedure to the patient and what to expect; reassure the patient that tube removal is less uncomfortable than insertion.	Prevents undue patient anxiety.	
6. Ensure that the patient is comfortably positioned.	For the patient's comfort as well as ability to cooperate with the procedure.	
7. Disconnect from suction if indicated.	Avoids suction and potential trauma to tissues as the tube exits the GI tract.	
8. Have available, or offer the patient, a facial tissue.	If indicated for dripping nose or eye watering.	
9. Remove the tube securement.	Aids in tube removal.	
10. Instill a small air bolus into the tube to clear secretions from it.	Reduces potential aspiration of gastric fluid with tube removal.	If air is difficult to insert, the tube may have a kink; withdrawing slightly may reduce the kink.

Procedure continues on following page

UNIT IV

Procedure for NG or OG Tube Removal—*Continued*

Steps	Rationale	Special Considerations
11. Kink or clamp the tubing, ask the patient to hold his or her breath, and then pull out steadily and smoothly into the towel.	Reduces potential aspiration of any fluid and provides a focal point for the patient.	
12. Inspect the tube to ensure that it is intact, and discard it into the appropriate container.	It is unlikely that the tube would be damaged, but evidence of tube damage warrants further investigation.	Use caution as one would with any equipment that has been a carrier of body fluids.
13. Cleanse or assist the patient in cleaning the naris, and assist with oral care.	Nasal secretions are likely after tube removal; oral care may be very welcome.	Ascertain that damage resulting from the tube or tube securement has not occurred on related body tissue.

Expected Outcomes

- The NG tube is inserted safely with no adverse effects or unintended consequences.
- The NG tube remains appropriately positioned for as long as it is needed, with no adverse effects, including displacement or pressure injury related to the tube and its securement.
- The tube helps accomplish its intended purpose (e.g., the patient will experience relief from gastric distention and emesis, and potential aspiration will be avoided).
- The patient will experience as little discomfort as possible related to the NG tube.

Unexpected Outcomes

- Difficulty is experienced in inserting the tube: If two attempts are unsuccessful, consider obtaining assistance.
- The tube inadvertently intubates the respiratory tract. Immediate recognition of this will reduce other potential adverse events.
- The tube becomes displaced. Monitoring the external amount can help in recognizing this, and tube securement may prevent displacement.[1] To determine the amount of tube that is internal, subtract the length of the external tube from the total length of the tube (see manufacturer package insert). Compare with typical measurement assessment, but also consider that the tube could have become coiled in the back of the pharynx or esophagus, and monitor for this possibility as well.
- Inability to aspirate gastric content manually or with suction. Reassess tube placement; the tube tip may not be deep enough, or the tube may have intubated the upper small intestine. Ensure that the tube is not clogged.
- The patient will develop a pressure injury from pressure of the tube against nasal or other tissue. Secure the tube without pressure on surrounding tissue, and monitor for pressure frequently.

Patient Monitoring and Care

Steps	Rationale	Reportable Conditions
		These conditions should be reported to the provider if they persist despite nursing interventions.
1. Monitor tube securement and amount externally before use and every 4 hours or per institutional protocol.	Ensures that the NG or OG tube is secure.	- Report deviations to the provider.

Patient Monitoring and Care —*Continued*

Steps	Rationale	Reportable Conditions
2. Monitor for signs of pressure on surrounding tissue before use and every 4 hours or per institutional protocol. The tube should be secured in a different manner if there are signs of pressure on surrounding tissue. Report signs of tissue damage to the physician, advanced practice nurse, or other healthcare professional.	Reduces the potential for tissue injury.	• Report signs of tissue damage to the provider. • Report to and enlist assistance from wound/skin specialists as available.
3. Ensure that the tube is connected to low suction, as prescribed. Consider manual aspiration of gastric contents if suction is not being used and the patient exhibits nausea, the potential for emesis, or other signs of potential for aspiration.	Avoids a high level of continuous suction. Maintains the sump feature of the tube, if used, to reduce potential tissue damage.	• Nausea, increasing abdominal firmness, discomfort or distention, change in bowel sounds or status; emesis despite NG to suction • Signs of aspiration
4. Assess and measure output (volume, color, quality) every 4 hours and as indicted. Document output and intake via the tube. Compare intake to output daily as well as the trending pattern.	Helps quantify and characterize output for ongoing clinical correlation. Detects potential fluid imbalance. Patients with large NG output are at risk for fluid, electrolyte, and possibly acid-base imbalance. Correlate with laboratory values that might reflect a trend toward dehydration and/or electrolyte imbalance.	• Sudden cessation of output, especially if coupled with increased patient discomfort, may signal tube misplacement or clogging, problem with suction, and so on. • Report a pattern of output greater than intake.
5. Assess and monitor patient status including abdominal assessment every 4 hours and as indicated.	Provides information about clinical condition as well as effectiveness of NG suction.	• Increased abdominal distress
6. Irrigate the NG or OG tube as needed.	Maintains tube patency. Clean warm water, if used, may be better tolerated than cold fluid.	• Lack of patency despite interventions
7. Unless contraindicated, keep the head of the bed elevated 30 degrees or more.	A patient with an NG tube may not be able to clear secretions well; reduces risk for aspiration.[12] (**Level C***)	
8. Follow institutional standards for assessing pain. Provide comfort measures, and administer analgesia as prescribed.	Identifies the need for pain interventions. NG use can be associated with patient discomfort.	• Continued pain despite pain interventions
9. Keep equipment used for the NG tube (e.g., syringes) as clean and dry as possible, and change per institutional standards.	Moisture provides media for microbial growth.	

*Level C: Qualitative studies, descriptive or correlational studies, integrative reviews, systematic reviews, or randomized controlled trials with inconsistent results.

Procedure continues on following page

Documentation

Documentation in the medical record should include the following:

- Type and size of tube
- Naris of insertion
- Numeric mark at the tube exit and/or external length in an area where it can be monitored on an ongoing basis
- Description and volume of aspirated returns
- How placement was verified
- Use of anesthetic agent if used (including in medication record as indicated)
- Assessment of changes in patient condition (e.g., increased abdominal distention, firmness or discomfort, nausea or emesis)
- Any adverse events related to insertion or the indwelling tube
- NG tube removal date and time and any adverse events related to tube removal

References and Additional Readings

For a complete list of references and additional readings for this procedure, scan this QR code with your smartphone, or visit https://www.elsevier.com/__data/assets/pdf_file/0007/1319875/Chapter0100.pdf

101

Fecal Microbiota Transplant AP (Perform)

Anna Alder, Katherine Dickerman, and Michael Schnake

PURPOSE Fecal microbiota transplant (FMT) is the infusion of stool from a healthy individual to a patient with gut dysfunction.[7] FMT may be used for treatment of recurrent *Clostridium difficile* infection (CDI) and other disorders after treatment with antimicrobial therapy alone has been trialed. CDI, also known as *Clostridioides difficile* or *C. difficile,* can invade the colonic mucosa and result in colitis, generally caused by exposure to antibiotic therapy. The initial treatment of this condition is to withdraw the offending antibiotic, treat the sequelae, such as severe diarrhea, and begin the first-line agent, which is oral vancomycin. CDI can recur, requiring extended courses of vancomycin or the use of alternative antibiotics. FMT may be employed for cases that are refractive to the usual therapy.

PREREQUISITE NURSING KNOWLEDGE

- Anatomy and physiology of the gastrointestinal (GI) tract.
- Pathophysiology of CDI and consequences of this untreated infection with the understanding that CDI must be confirmed before FMT.[6,8,12]
- The mechanism of action of this intervention is the establishment of new gut microbiota and restoration of normal gut function.[4,6,7]
- Universal precautions, contact isolation precautions, donning, and doffing PPE.[8]
- Various approaches for FMT including upper endoscopy, colonoscopy, and enema. Capsule delivery is the newest method of FMT. This can be used for patients with contraindications to other delivery methods or other risks[7,10]
- Donor selection is a rigorous process including patient-selected donor and stool banks that screen for particular infections.[7,12] This process is necessary to minimize the risk of infection and disease transmission.[7]
- The safety profile and costs of FMT as an option for treatment of CDI.[5,8,12]
- The indications of or against bowel preparation on an individual patient basis, considering that bowel preparation may be contraindicated in severely ill patients.[10] Providers will determine the need for bowel preparation.
- FMT for CDI is still considered investigational by the U.S. Food and Drug Administration (FDA). There are potential significant risks (e.g., allergic or immune reaction, fever,

diarrhea, abdominal pain, infection, or other disease transmissions), but significant risks from the transplant itself are believed to be rare.[2,5,6]

EQUIPMENT

- Personal protective equipment (PPE): Contact isolation precautions including gloves, fluid-resistant gown, face shield, surgical mask, and eye protection
- 60-mL slip-tip syringe: Six syringes for administration via colonoscope (during colonoscopy); two syringes for administration via endoscope (via upper endoscopy)
- Graduated cylinder
- One large towel
- Sterile water
- Fecal microbiota donor sample: 30-mL sample for upper GI tract administration via endoscope; 250-mL sample for lower GI tract administration via colonoscopy[10]
- Delivery device: Endoscope, nasojejunal tube, nasogastric tube, enema bottle or colonoscope
- Lubrication for scope or tube if indicated

PATIENT AND FAMILY EDUCATION

- Explain the purpose and anticipated outcomes of FMT to the patient and family. Explain to them the risks and benefits of the procedure, including bleeding, perforation, or treatment failure.[2,9] ***Rationale:*** It is important for patients and families to understand the purpose and anticipated outcomes of FMT. This may decrease patient and family anxiety. In patients who are clinically stable, providers will discontinue antibiotics being used for *C. difficile* 24 to 48 hours before the procedure. The patient will need to retain the donor sample. If delivery is via colonoscopy, this will require the patient to perform rectal tension to retain stool for as long as possible following

---

AP This procedure should be performed only by clinicians who have demonstrated competence and are credentialed to perform it. In addition, the procedure must be within the scope of practice defined by their professional licensure, and in accordance with professional practice acts. Physicians, advanced practice nurses, and physician assistants may be credentialed to perform this procedure.

the procedure.[10] Administration of an antidiarrheal agent before and/or after the procedure may be appropriate, depending on institutional standards and provider orders.[1] If delivery is via endoscopy or enteral tube, antiemetics may be administered.[1]

- The patient may experience bloating and diarrhea following the procedure. This does not indicate that the transplant was ineffective.[8] Most patients generally have formed stool by 1 to 2 weeks. Persistent watery, loose stools with abdominal cramping should be reported to the provider.[4,7]
- Symptoms of postprocedure complications should be thoroughly explained. These include nausea, vomiting, persistent diarrhea, risk of bowel perforation, and bleeding.[9]

PATIENT ASSESSMENT AND PREPARATION

Patient Assessment

- Assess vital signs before the procedure. *Rationale:* This is used as baseline for monitoring after the procedure and to determine if interventions are needed because of volume and electrolyte losses from frequent diarrhea stools.
- Assess the patient's ability to tolerate bowel preparation (if ordered by the provider). *Rationale:* Bowel preparation is contraindicated in those who are acutely ill because they may not be able to tolerate oral/enteral bowel preparation medications. If a patient's colon is significantly inflamed, there is risk of worsening the inflammation or of causing a bowel perforation.
- Assess for clinical signs of severe infection including sepsis. *Rationale:* This is performed to assess for improvement in response to FMT.

- If administering via a nasogastric tube or other enteral tube, placement should be verified by radiographic confirmation. *Rationale:* This will ensure safe delivery of the material into the GI system.

Patient Preparation

- Verify the correct patient with two identifiers. *Rationale:* Before performing a procedure, the nurse should ensure the correct identification of the patient for the intended intervention.
- Explain the steps of the procedure, including sedation if applicable. Answer questions that arise, and reinforce information as needed. *Rationale:* Understanding of previously communicated information is evaluated and reinforced.
- Ensure that a written informed consent form has been obtained by the provider. *Rationale:* Esophagogastroduodenoscopy (EGD) and colonoscopy are both invasive procedures that require signed informed consent.
- Check that all relevant documents and studies are available before the procedure is started. *Rationale:* This measure ensures that the correct patient receives the correct procedure.
- Place the patient in the appropriate position for either an EGD or colonoscopy, depending on delivery method. Positioning for an EGD involves placing the patient in the left lateral position with the head of the bed elevated to approximately 30 degrees. Positioning for a colonoscopy involves placing the patient in the left side-lying position with the head of the bed flat and the knees drawn up toward the chest. *Rationale:* Appropriate positioning allows the provider to more easily maneuver the scope to the appropriate delivery location. Left lateral positioning for EGD reduces the risk of aspiration.[11]

Procedure	Fecal Microbiota Transplant	
Steps	Rationale	Special considerations
1. **HH**	Prevents infection.	
2. **PE**	Prevents infection.	
3. If the specimen is frozen, thaw the specimen by placing in a designated sink filled with warm water. This process takes about 30 minutes and can be performed while the patient is preparing for the procedure. If the specimen is not frozen, the stool will need to be diluted, typically with saline, strained. Position the patient according to procedure (i.e., EGD or colonoscopy)	Donor specimen will need to be at room temperature for administration. Mixing the nonfrozen stool with saline improves viscosity and allows the sample to be administered with ease.	Protocols among institutions are not standardized. Mixing of stool varies from stirring with a spoon to blending in a standard blender. Samples should never be refrozen. If thawed and not used within 8 hours, the material should be disposed of. Repeating the freeze-thaw cycle can compromise the viability of the stool.

Procedure   Fecal Microbiota Transplant—*Continued*

Steps	Rationale	Special considerations
4. Perform a time-out according to universal protocol requirements.	Provides patient safety. Reduces the risk of "wrong patient, wrong site, wrong procedure" errors	Protocols vary among institutions.
5. For colonoscopic or endoscopic delivery: Once the patient is comfortably sedated, the scope is inserted, and the provider will begin with assessment and biopsies if needed.	Evaluation before administering FMT.	
6. Prepare equipment. Using the 60-mL slip-tip syringes, draw up contents of the sample until the container is empty. Place full syringes in a clean graduated cylinder (tip down). Use the final syringe to draw up 60 mL of sterile water, and place it in the cylinder with the other syringes. For enema administration, place the full sample into the enema bottle and lubricate the tip.	Proper use of equipment to prepare the sample for administration.	Protocols vary among institutions.
7. Before discarding the sample packaging and bottle, ensure that the lot number and expiration date has been captured and that the information card that will be given to the patient following the procedure has been set aside. Discard the remaining packaging, and empty the bottle.	Safety and documentation.	If stool is provided by the patient rather than a stool bank, the lot number would not be applicable.
8. For administration via endoscope, colonoscope: Once the provider has reached the designated delivery location and has requested the sample, start by handing the first full syringe to the provider. The provider will open the cap to the biopsy channel cover, insert the tip of the syringe into the biopsy channel cylinder, and then inject the contents of the syringe into the biopsy channel by depressing the plunger on the syringe. Continue this process until the entire sample has been administered, and then follow with a 60-mL syringe of normal saline administered through the same channel. Discard empty syringes into a biohazard container. The provider will immediately withdraw the scope to conclude the procedure.	Proper use of equipment to optimize delivery of the sample. Provides patient safety.	Protocols may vary among institutions for enema administration and placement of nasogastric and nasojejunal tubes

UNIT IV

Procedure continues on following page

UNIT IV

Procedure   Fecal Microbiota Transplant—*Continued*

Steps	Rationale	Special considerations
For administration via enema: Lubricate the tip of the enema, and assist (if needed) with insertion of the enema bottle into the anus. Instruct the patient (or assist the patient) to squeeze the bottle until the entire sample has been administered. Then remove the enema bottle while the patient attempts to retain the sample. Discard the enema bottle into a biohazard container. For administration via a nasojejunal or nasogastric tube: Lubricate the tip of the tube, and place the tube via the nare per nursing protocol. Once positioning has been confirmed, administer the full sample from the syringe into the tube. Then flush the tube with 200-mL of normal saline. Remove the tube, and discard the syringe and tube into a biohazard container.		
9. 🔲	Prevents infection	
10. Document the implant in the electronic health record (EHR), including the date/time, delivery method, lot number, volume of sample, volume of normal saline flush, and expiration date of the sample.	Allows for documentation. Provides patient safety.	
11. Upon arrival to the postanesthesia care unit (PACU) or other recovery area: After administration via colonoscopy or enema, the provider may order the antimotility agent loperamide immediately before and following the procedure, and again 2 hours after the procedure to maximize the retention of transplanted fecal microbiota.[4] Instruct the patient to attempt to avoid having a bowel movement for as long as possible following the procedure.[1,4] For administration via endoscopy or gastrostomy tube, give antiemetics as needed. **(Level E*)**	Provides symptom management. Optimizes the time the sample remains in the GI tract.	The role of loperamide is inconclusive, but it is deemed safe and possibly effective in helping with retention of FMT administered via colonoscopy.

*Level E: Multiple case reports, theory-based evidence from expert opinions, or peer-reviewed professional organizational standards without clinical studies to support recommendations.

Procedure *Fecal Microbiota Transplant—Continued*

Expected Outcomes

- Donor stool is administered successfully.
- Patient is able to retain the donor stool without difficulty.
- CDI will be eradicated.

Unexpected Outcomes

- Patient is unable to tolerate the procedure.
- Patient sustains procedural complications.
- Patient is unable to eradicate the infection.

Patient Monitoring and Care

Steps	Rationale	Reportable Conditions
• Monitor temperature, blood pressure, heart rate, respiratory rate, oxygen saturation ($Spco_2$), end-tidal capnography ($Etco_2$) (intra- and postprocedure if sedation is used), cognition according to institutional standards, and patient illness severity. • Monitor for retention of stool if transplant is administered via enema or colonoscopy. • Monitor for nausea, vomiting, and GI bleeding.	• Patient safety • Monitoring after administration of sedation and after procedure • Longer retention may be associated with improved outcomes.[3]	• Abnormal vital signs or vital signs that are greater 10% from baseline levels: fever, tachycardia, tachypnea, hypotension or hypertension, changes in $Etco_2$ • Abdominal pain • Rectal pain • Blood from rectum • Nausea and vomiting • Adverse reaction to the sedatives (if used)

Documentation

Documentation should include the following:
- Patient and family education
- Date and time of procedure
- Patient verification
- Performing provider and others present during the procedure
- Description of the procedure including specific steps taken
- Stool volume, lot number, and route of administration
- Any medications administered (e.g., antiemetics, antidiarrheals)
- All equipment used
- Patient tolerance of the procedure
- Postprocedure vital signs and patient assessment
- Any unexpected outcomes
- Nursing interventions

References and Additional Readings

For a complete list of references and additional readings for this procedure, scan this QR code with your smartphone, or visit https://www.elsevier.com/__data/assets/pdf_file/0008/1319876/Chapter0101.pdf

UNIT IV

102 Molecular Adsorbent Recirculating System (MARS)

Lynelle N.B. Pierce and Claire Sutherlin

PURPOSE Molecular adsorbent recirculating system (MARS), or liver dialysis, is an extracorporeal detoxification method, used in conjunction with continuous renal replacement therapy (CRRT), in which an albumin dialysis is used to clear protein-bound toxins. The MARS system supports rapid removal of toxic substances that accumulate due to acute liver injury.

PREREQUISITE NURSING KNOWLEDGE

- The liver is a remarkable organ responsible for a myriad of functions including synthesis of clotting factors, detoxification, breakdown of hormones and medications, metabolism of essential nutrients, and biotransformation. When the liver fails, the loss of these functions leads to the accumulation of lethal toxins with life-threatening complications.
- Acute liver failure (ALF) is a highly specific, rare syndrome characterized by an acute abnormality of liver blood tests in an individual without underlying chronic liver disease, development of a coagulopathy of liver etiology, and altered level of consciousness (LOC) due to hepatic encephalopathy.[4,5,15] It may progress to multisystem organ failure.
- In the United States and United Kingdom, the most common cause of ALF is paracetamol (acetaminophen) toxicity and idiosyncratic drug reactions (i.e., antibiotics, antiseizure medications, and antidepressants).[4] Herbal supplements, mushroom poisoning (most commonly by the *Amanita* species), and postoperative or traumatic events are also implicated in ALF. Viral infections are the most common cause in developing countries.[4,5,15] The overall outcome for these patients is dependent on early recognition and intervention to address the cause of the disease.[15]
- Over the past 10 years, new technology, collaborative medical management, and liver transplantation have improved the outcome for these patients. However, despite advances in critical care therapies, ALF is a life-threatening disease with a high mortality rate.[4,5,14,15]
- MARS is an albumin liver-dialysis system designed to filter toxins from the blood, thus supporting the lost detoxification functions of the liver.[1,7,8] MARS has been shown to reduce bilirubin and to improve hepatic encephalopathy, coagulopathy, and systemic hemodynamics.[8,10] Supporting the injured liver with MARS provides time for recovery of liver function or liver transplantation.[4]
- MARS technology is approved for use in ALF from drug overdoses and poisonings by the U.S. Food and Drug Administration (FDA). The only requirement is that the drug or chemical be dialyzable (in unbound form) and bound by charcoal and/or ion exchange resins.[3] MARS therapy generally consists of 8-hour treatment sessions for 3 consecutive days. Patient selection and early initiation are critical to the success of this treatment.
- Substances removed by the MARS therapeutic system include but are not limited to albumin-bound and water-soluble substances (Table 102.1).[10]
- The MARS therapy system consists of two systems working in tandem: the MARS and the Prismaflex CRRT machines (Fig. 102.1). CRRT is an integral part of the MARS system. The CRRT machine blood pump drives the blood through an extracorporeal circuit into the MARS dialyzer (MARSFLUX), where large protein-bound toxins are removed from the blood using albumin as the dialysate. The MARS machine albumin pump drives the albumin bound with toxins to the CRRT machine into the CRRT dialysis filter (diaFLUX), where it is dialyzed using a standard bicarbonate dialysate, removing water-soluble substances. It is in the CRRT dialyzer where diffusion and hemofiltration (predilution and/or postdilution) of water-soluble toxins and controlled fluid removal (ultrafiltration) occurs.[8,14]
- The key to MARS is that it is an albumin recirculating system, meaning that the albumin solution returns to the MARS machine where it is reprocessed, making it ready to bind toxins again. This is achieved by means of adsorbents in a two-stage filtering procedure. The first stage uses an activated carbon adsorber (diaMARS AC250) to bind nonionic toxins. During the second stage, toxic ionic molecules bound to the albumin such as bilirubin are removed from recirculating albumin by the ion exchange resin filter (diaMARS IE250).[3,14] This process regenerates the albumin, making it ready for recirculation through the circuit to remove more toxins for the entire duration of the therapy.
- CRRT may be used between therapy sessions to support impaired renal function and continue the filtration of smaller particles such as ammonia. CRRT is a critical adjunct in the management of ALF because it removes ammonia, a substrate believed to play a large role in

hepatic encephalopathy and subsequent cerebral edema and potential herniation.[8] Even in the absence of impaired renal function, CRRT may be needed between MARS treatments to remove ammonia and manage volume overload to prevent neurological deterioration between MARS treatments.

- MARS is associated with the same risk as other extracorporeal devices, including air embolus, bleeding, thrombocytopenia, infection, and hypothermia.[8] Careful patient monitoring and knowledgeable response to circuit alarms is required to mitigate risk and prevent adverse patient events.

TABLE 102.1	Substances Removed During Albumin Dialysis[10]

Albumin-Bound Substances	Water-Soluble Substances
Benzodiazepines*	Ammonia
Bilirubin (conjugated)	Aromatic amino acids
Bilirubin (unconjugated)	Creatinine
Bile acids	Urea
Copper	Tryptophan
Fatty acids (medium and short chain)	Interleukin 6
Nitric oxide	
Indoles	
Mercaptans, phenols, prostacyclins	

*Endogenous and exogenous

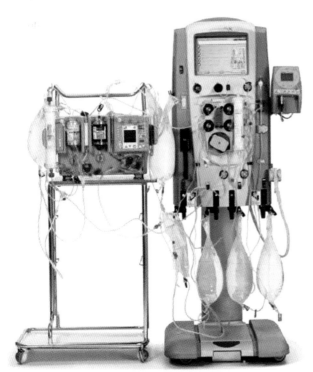

Figure 102.1 The MARS system setup consists of a combination of the MARS Monitor and the Prismaflex System *(From Gambro. Operating Instructions, MARS Monitor 1TC and MARS Treatment Kit. Illinois, 2015, Baxter Healthcare Corporation.)*

- Frequent laboratory testing is performed to aid in identification of adverse effects of MARS therapy. This includes coagulation studies, including thromboelastography (TEG) or rotational thromboelastometry (ROTEM), which are noninvasive studies that measure the ability of whole blood to form a clot.
- Setting up the MARS requires the concentrated attention of one to two competent RNs for approximately 2 hours. The kit requires detailed assembly, and the system requires careful priming. The cumulative cost of the MARS treatment kit and the albumin is considerable.

EQUIPMENT

- Prismaflex CRRT machine with MARS software enabled
- MARS machine
- MARS kit containing three filters (MARSFLUX, dia-MARS AC250 activated carbon adsorber, ion exchange resin diaMARS IE250); Prismaflex filter (diaFLUX), units 1 to 4 and accessory kit to set up the MARS dialysis system
- Priming solutions:
  - ❖ Two to three 1-L bags of heparinized priming solution (per manufacturer's recommendations) or solution per institutional policy for priming the blood circuit (Prismaflex system). One 5-L bag of heparin-free priming solution for priming the albumin circuit (MARS)
- Prescribed replacement solutions
- Albumin dialysate: 16 g of albumin in a 600-mL solution resulting in a 16.6% concentration. For example: 400 mL (100 g) 25% human serum albumin in 200 mL of 0.9% normal saline = total volume 600 mL
- Anticoagulant (heparin or citrate) if prescribed
- Nonsterile gloves
- Antiseptic solution

PATIENT AND FAMILY EDUCATION

- Explain the purpose and anticipated outcome of MARS therapy to the patient (if possible) and family. ***Rationale:*** It is important for patients and families to understand that in the absence of a healthy liver, MARS therapy supports liver function. The MARS system removes the toxic substances that are injuring the liver and substances in the body normally removed by a healthy liver, allowing the liver to rest and recover.
- Explain in general terms the MARS procedure to the patient (if possible) and family before initiating treatment. Explain that typically in the United States the patient is given three treatments lasting 8 hours or longer for 3 sequential days; however, the number of treatments and duration may vary based on patient response and overall goals of care and is evaluated daily. Review what to expect during and after the treatments. Answer any questions that develop during the process of preparing the system and delivering therapy. For example, you may explain that as the blood is cleaned by the albumin, the white resin filter will turn dark, reflecting the removal of toxic particles. ***Rationale:*** This information may decrease patient and family anxiety.

• Explain the need for careful monitoring of the patient throughout the procedure for expected outcomes as well as for complications. Introduce yourself as a specialty trained critical care nurse who will provide care and be in close communication with other members of the healthcare team throughout the treatment. *Rationale:* Both the underlying disease process and the MARS therapy can result in complications. Explanation provides information and reassurance and may decrease patient and family anxiety.

PATIENT ASSESSMENT AND PREPARATION

Patient Assessment

• Perform baseline cardiovascular, neurological, respiratory, and integumentary assessments before initiating therapy. *Rationale: Cardiovascular:* Attention should be paid to fluid management and hemodynamic monitoring. Monitor for dysrhythmias related to electrolyte imbalance and fluid shifts. Hypotension may also occur as a result of decreased plasma proteins in the blood. *Respiratory:* Assess for the ability to protect the airway. Change in mental status may alter this, and intubation may be required to protect the airway. *Neurological:* Neurological changes can range from simple personality changes to coma. The onset of encephalopathy can also occur quickly with the development of asterixis, delirium, hyperreflexia, seizures, and coma. The pathophysiology of this is not fully understood but may be related to circulating toxins such as ammonia and other substances that cross the blood-brain barrier and affect neurological status, LOC, and level of activity.[4,15] Signs of increased intracranial pressure should also be monitored such as changes in LOC, pupillary response and ability to follow commands. Hepatic encephalopathy, arterial ammonia greater than 150 mmol/L, hyponatremia, seizures, and pupil changes may indicate a poor prognosis.[13] *Integumentary:* Special attention should also be given to the patient's skin integrity, not only because of the disease process, but also because of limited mobility. Minimize pressure, and maintain function with active and passive range of motion.

• If computed tomography (CT) or magnetic resonance imaging (MRI) is required, these and any other diagnostic tests should be performed before initiation of MARS therapy. Once the therapy is operational, transport of the patient for testing should be avoided to limit discontinuation of the therapy. *Rationale:* CT or MRI of the head provides baseline evidence of cerebral edema. Manufacturer guidelines for MARS, unlike the CRRT system, do not support recirculation via the albumin circuit. The MARS circuit is bathed with albumin, presenting a greater risk

of clogging. No studies have been completed to date that validate recirculation, which would allow for temporary disconnection of the patient from the system for transport.

• Obtain laboratory specimens as prescribed, including toxicology screens, ammonia, phosphorus, coagulation studies including TEG or ROTEM, hematocrit and hemoglobin values, basic metabolic panel, renal and liver function tests, and blood type. *Rationale:* Baseline information is necessary so appropriate interventions can be implemented before initiation of CRRT MARS. This will also allow the effect of therapy to be more accurately monitored.

Patient Preparation

• Verify the correct patient with two identifiers. *Rationale:* Before performing a procedure, the nurse should ensure the correct identification of the patient before the intervention is initiated.

• Ensure that informed consent has been obtained. *Rationale:* Informed consent protects the rights of the patient.

• Assist the licensed independent provider (LIP) with insertion of a dialysis catheter, 13F or greater in size. *Rationale:* Dialysis catheter access must be at least 13F because of required flow rates and increased resistance due to the expanded circuit.[12]

MARS is unable to be used with other high-flow circuits such as extracorporeal membrane oxygenation (ECMO) or temporary left ventricular assist devices (LVADs). *Rationale:* The excess positive pressure on the return limb of the MARS circuit can cause the transmembrane pressure to be outside the operational limits.

• The recommended site for line placement of vascular access of the appropriate length for MARS is the right internal jugular vein.[12] *Rationale:* Tip placement of the catheter at the junction of the superior vena cava and the right atrium ensures optimal blood flow.

• Ensure that there is adequate blood flow in the dialysis catheter, and instill appropriate anticoagulation per institutional guidelines and/or manufacturer recommendations. *Rationale:* this prevents clotting or occlusion of the lumens.

• Prophylactic fresh-frozen plasma transfusion to improve coagulopathy in patients with ALF is not recommended.[14,15] *Rationale:* This action does not reduce the risk of significant bleeding or transfusion requirements, and it can mask the trend of international normalized ratio (INR) as a prognostic marker as well as increase the risk of volume overload and occlusion of the circuit.

• Ensure that the patient and/or family understands the pre-procedural teaching. Answer questions as they arise, and reinforce information as needed. *Rationale:* Understanding of previously taught information is evaluated and reinforced.

Procedure	for Molecular Adsorbent Recirculating System (MARS)	
Steps	**Rationale**	**Special Considerations**
1. **HH**		
2. **PE**		
3. Secure MARS and CRRT machines to the bedside. Gather the MARS machine, Prismaflex dialysis/replacement, solutions, ordered priming solutions, anticoagulation if ordered, MARS Treatment kit, and supplies for accessing the HD catheter.	Ensures efficient set up	
4. Verify that MARS/CRRT orders, including anticoagulation, if necessary, are completed by the appropriate provider.	Anticoagulation may be used to prevent clotting of the blood circuit. Heparin may be prescribed for patients with a lower risk of bleeding and trisodium or ACD-A citrate may be prescribed for patients with a higher risk of bleeding[12] Regional citrate anticoagulation in patients with liver failure is feasible. Citrate anticoagulation was identified as providing superior patency of the extracorporeal circuit[2,9], Avoidance of anticoagulation during MARS can result in significant loss of treatment time, due to downtime[9]	If citrate is used, calcium replacement must be initiated. Titration of a continuous infusion is based on the level of ionized calcium.[12]
5. Confirm accurate placement and size (13F or greater) of the hemodialysis catheter, and verify blood flow of the dialysis catheter to ensure patency.	This size is necessary to provide adequate blood flow to the CRRT and MARS circuits.	
6. Place the MARS machine and the Prismaflex machine side by side with the Prismaflex to the right of the MARS machine close enough to ensure that the Prismaflex/MARS circuit will reach hemodialysis catheter access (Fig. 102.2).	The MARS is dependent on the Prismaflex blood pump to circulate blood through both machines.	The machines will ideally be located on the patient's right side due to required order of the machines and circuit length

Procedure continues on following page

Procedure for Molecular Adsorbent Recirculating System (MARS)—*Continued*

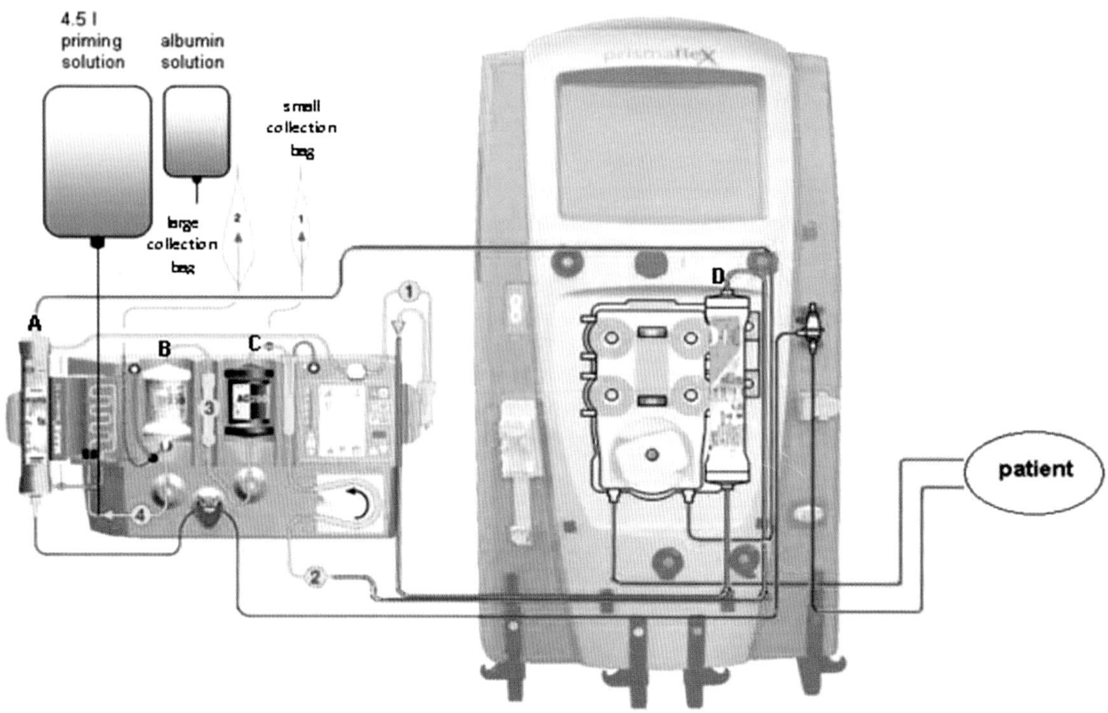

Figure 102.2 Combined MARS and Prismaflex machine therapeutic system. MARS units 1-4 assembled to create the albumin circuit. **A,** MARSFLUX filter. **B,** diaMARS ion exchanger adsorber. **C,** diaMARS activated carbon adsorber. **D,** diaFLUX filter. The small and large collection bags are removed after prime is complete, before beginning therapy. *(Modified from Gambro. Operating Instructions, MARS Monitor 1TC and MARS Treatment Kit. Illinois, 2015, Baxter Healthcare Corporation.)*

Steps	Rationale	Special Considerations
7. Level the holder for the MARS Flux dialyzer on the MARS machine and the holder for the diaFLUX filter on the Prismaflex machine with one another.	The blood lines connecting the blood flow between the machines require that the filters be aligned to eliminate flow resistance.	
8. Plug machines into emergency power outlets, and turn on both machines.	Emergency outlets are necessary to prevent interruption of blood pump and continuation of treatment.	There are two power buttons on the MARS machine. One is located on the back and the other on the front of the machine. The Prismaflex machine power button is located on the right side of the machine.

UNIT IV

Procedure	for Molecular Adsorbent Recirculating System (MARS)—*Continued*

Steps	Rationale	Special Considerations
9. Open the MARS treatment kit and supplies in preparation of assembling on the MARS machine (Fig. 102.3). Follow directions on the Prismaflex screen to set up the system: A. Follow initial setup screens for entering patient information and select CRRT MARS therapy mode. Then select CVVHDF mode. B. Select each instruction line on the Prismaflex screen, complete the step, and then select the next step to proceed. C. If use of the MARS heater is prescribed: Complete the heater installation following the steps on the Prismaflex. D. Install the MARSFLUX dialyzer and two adsorbers, (resin and charcoal) on the MARS machine. Install units 1–4 as directed. E. Install the Prismaflex filter system as directed. F. Connect the Prismaflex filter set to the MARS set as directed by the Prismaflex screen. G. Install the syringe containing heparin anticoagulation if ordered or normal saline if heparin not ordered. H. Hang the prescribed CRRT solutions as prompted. **(Level M*)**	Step-by-step instructions are displayed on the Prismaflex screen and should be used for set up. Verify that each step on each screen has been completed before moving to the next screen. Syringe must be installed and primed during set up to ensure its availability should heparin anticoagulation be ordered at any time during therapy.	Follow manufacturer's recommendations when initiating set up of the MARS/Prismaflex system. Any deviation from the directions can result in delays in patient care and the MARS/CRRT system not working properly. Syringe use for heparin is not universal. Follow institutional guidelines. If citrate regional anticoagulation is used hang the citrate (trisodium citrate or citrate ACD-A) on the preblood pump white scale. If citrate is used, systemic calcium replacement must be initiated.

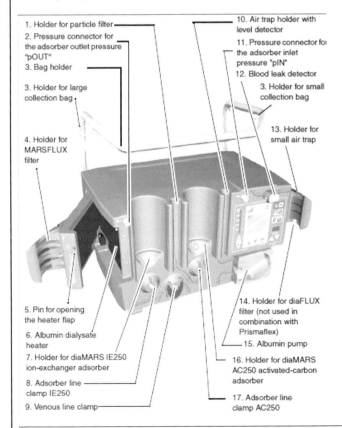

1. Holder for particle filter
2. Pressure connector for the adsorber outlet pressure "pOUT"
3. Bag holder
3. Holder for large collection bag
4. Holder for MARSFLUX filter
5. Pin for opening the heater flap
6. Albumin dialysate heater
7. Holder for diaMARS IE250 ion-exchanger adsorber
8. Adsorber line clamp IE250
9. Venous line clamp
10. Air trap holder with level detector
11. Pressure connector for the adsorber inlet pressure "pIN"
12. Blood leak detector
3. Holder for small collection bag
13. Holder for small air trap
14. Holder for diaFLUX filter (not used in combination with Prismaflex)
15. Albumin pump
16. Holder for diaMARS AC250 activated-carbon adsorber
17. Adsorber line clamp AC250

Figure 102.3 MARS Monitor. *(From Gambro. Operating Instructions, MARS Monitor 1TC and MARS Treatment Kit. Illinois, 2015, Baxter Healthcare Corporation.)*

*Level M: Manufacturer's recommendations only.

Procedure continues on following page

UNIT IV

Procedure   for **Molecular Adsorbent Recirculating System (MARS)**—*Continued*

Steps	Rationale	Special Considerations
10. Step 1. Prime the Prismaflex system according to the instructions on the screen. *Prismaflex Prime:* Two 1-L normal saline bags are used for the Prismaflex prime.		Prismaflex system does not provide a prompt to hang the second bag. Monitor closely to prevent air from entering the system. Consider use of a Y-site connector between the two 1-L bags.
11. Step 2: Prime the MARS. One 5-L bag dialysate solution is used for the MARS prime. *Prime Cycle 1:*First prime of small collection bag *Prime Cycle 2*: Second prime of small collection bag *Prime Cycle 3*: Prime of large collection bag *Albumin filling:* 600 mL albumin solution is used for the albumin prime. **(Level M*)** *Albumin circulation* Set the circulation time (range from 15 minutes to 1 hour and 15 minutes) according to amount of time needed before connecting to patient.		Screen prompts user to Luer-Lok tubing to the priming solution. It is acceptable to use the spike from the accessory kit. This spike will remain in place and be used to connect to the albumin solution. Carefully monitor solution level in container and stop prime to prevent air from entering the system. Albumin solution:16 Grams of albumin in a 600 mL solution resulting in a 16.6% concentration. For example: 400 mL (100 g) 25% human serum albumin in 200 mL of 0.9% normal saline = total volume 600 mL[3]

12. Initiating therapy
Step 1: Set the Prismaflex rates as prescribed:
   A. Blood flow rate (BFR): Set the initial rate at 100 mL/min. When therapy is initiated, the rate will gradually be increased to the prescribed rate as described below.
   B. Replacement solution(s)
   C. Anticoagulant if prescribed
     • Heparin
     • Citrate via the preblood pump (PBP) white scale and calcium replacement in a central line
   D. Dialysis solution
   E. Fluid removal rate
Step 2: Prepare hemodialysis catheter for connection to the patient circuit using aseptic technique (see Procedure 105).
Step 3: Connect to the patient using aseptic technique following prompts on the Prismaflex.
Step 4: Start therapy on the Prismaflex.
Step 5: Start the albumin pump on the MARS; Prismaflex will alert when to start Albumin pump.
    a. Initiate at 100 mL/min
    b. Gradually (within ~15 minutes) increase both the albumin and blood flow rates simultaneously to ordered rates.
    c. Monitor Pressure In (pIN) with each incremental increase in albumin pump rate. If pIN rises too high (maximum 500), then temporarily decrease the albumin rate to allow the pIN to drift back down.
    d. When at full ordered rates, set the lower alarm limit 100 mm Hg below the pIN pressure.
	Flow rates for the blood pump and albumin pump must match and be titrated to keep the albumin "in" pressure (pIN) limit below 450 mm Hg. The albumin pump max rate is 250 mL/min.
	At beginning of the run, flow rates are started low and gradually increased to prevent sudden rise in pIN. Rise in pIN triggers an alarm that stops the albumin pump and may result in backflow of fluid in the pressure line.
	Maximum pIN is 500. If 500mmHg is reached, albumin pump will stop, and the MARS will alarm.
		If citrate is prescribed, initiate calcium infusion.
		Allow time for Prismaflex pressures and patient to equilibrate prior to starting the albumin pump (MARS).
		Due to filter capacity, preblood pump (PBP) solution, post filter replacement, and ultrafiltration rate (UFR) cannot exceed 1500 mL/hr.
		The blood and albumin pump rates should be equal during therapy.[3]
		If unable to reach ordered flow on albumin pump due to high pIN, then notify provider to modify ordered albumin pump rate and BFR.

*Level M: Manufacturer's recommendations only.

Procedure for Molecular Adsorbent Recirculating System (MARS)—*Continued*

Steps	Rationale	Special Considerations
13. Document start time and initial pressures.	Allows trending of pressures with awareness of the baseline.	
14. During therapy, monitor the system pressures and alarms and troubleshoot.[3] A. Start the pump. • Start the albumin pump by using the START/STOP button. B. pIN too high • Try to find increase in pressure (clamp closed or line kinked, wet hydrophobic pIN transducer protector, fluid level too high in unit 2 air trap (see "Level" below), or kinked heater bag tubing). C. pIN too low • Try to find the cause of the pressure drop, such as leaks caused by loose connections in the albumin circuit. • If no leaks or loose connections are identified, shift the pressure window, or increase the flow rate of the albumin pump. D. pOUT too high • Try to find the cause of increase in pressure (clamp closed or line kinked) E. Blood leak detected • Albumin pump will stop, and blood return line clamp will close. • Ensure that the albumin line is correctly installed in the blood leak detector. • Inspect the albumin line for gross blood. If no blood is visible, send the albumin sample from the MARS unit 1 line port for a red blood cell check. If no red blood cells are detected, re-initialize the MARS monitor BLD.	The albumin pump has stopped for more than two minutes. pIN and Pressure out (pOUT) alarms are most often related to a line being clamped or kinked. The circuit is not intact or the albumin flow rate is too low pOUT exceeds pIN by 35 mm Hg If blood enters the albumin circuit, this results in a change in light intensity received at the blood leak detector (BLD). The blood compartment of the filter is not intact, and treatment will need to be discontinued. Microscopic blood could be present, indicating the filter is not intact and treatment will need to be discontinued This resets the BLD to a new normal to prevent future misleading alarms	If increased albumin pump rate required, obtain order for new flow rate TMP value in the MARSFLUX filter is not considered for filter is clotting alarm during CRRT MARS therapy. Due to this, the filter pressure drop is the only value used to provide notification about clotting in the MARSFLUX filter. Additional troubleshooting instructions can be found in the MARS operating instructions manual.[3]
F. Level • Maintain the level of the albumin dialysate in the large air trap of unit 2 between the two red LED lights. • Manual adjustment is performed using a 20-mL syringe attached to the tubing with clamp on the top of the large air trap. • To raise the level, cautiously open the clamp to allow the albumin level to rise until it is between the two LED lights • To lower the level, cautiously open the clamp, and insert air from the 20-mL syringe until the albumin level is between the LED lights. • Clamp the tubing. • Resume therapy by pressing the start button.	An advisory alarm will occur if the pressure rises to a level where manual adjustment is needed. This chamber reflects pressure in the albumin circuit. As pressure increases, this level will rise and the pIN pressure alarm will sound.	

Procedure continues on following page

UNIT IV

Procedure for Molecular Adsorbent Recirculating System (MARS)—*Continued*

G. Transmembrane pressure (TMP) too high
- Assess if volume being pulled across the filter, the UFR, exceeds the 1500-mL limit (UFR equals patient fluid removal rate plus replacement solution rate plus preblood pump rate).
- Decrease replacement and/or patient fluid removal and/or PBP rate.

TMP: MARS Flux filter and diaFLUX filter combined transmembrane pressure exceeds membrane pressure limit.

H. Filter is clotting
- Increase blood flow rate and/or adjust anticoagulation prescription and/or increase prefilter fluids

Clotting can occur in the blood compartment of the filter causing the filter pressure drop to increase.

15. Remove **PE**, and discard used supplies.
16. **HH**

Expected Outcomes

- Effective removal of dialyzable toxic drugs or chemicals.
- Reduction in ammonia levels and potential improvement in severe hepatic encephalopathy[7,13,14]
- Improvement in hemodynamic impairment due to decompensating liver disease.[14]
- Improvement in acid-base and electrolyte disturbances, BUN, and creatinine in patients with renal insufficiency due to the therapeutic effect of CRRT.[12]

Unexpected Outcomes

- Decreased protein-bound drug levels
- Hypothermia
- Bleeding secondary to use of anticoagulant[2,6,9]
- Clotting and clogging of the system or catheter
- Problems related to the extracorporeal circuit: decreased hemoglobin level or platelet count
- Progressive cerebral edema, brainstem herniation[13]

Patient Monitoring and Care

Steps	Rationale	Reportable Conditions
		These conditions should be reported to the provider if they persist despite nursing interventions.
1. Patients may be maintained on bed rest during the entire therapy to prevent alarms and ensure circuit patency. In addition, the patient's LOC and overall stability will determine how interactive and mobile the patient can be. A. The patient should be turned every 2 hours during treatment if hemodynamically stable. B. Passive range-of-motion exercises may be needed to decrease issues related to limited mobility and prevent the complications of immobility.	ALF results in altered mental status ranging from simple confusion to coma.[4] Interventions can reduce the risk of complications of immobility.	• Complications of immobility, such as pressure injury formation
2. Monitor the neurological status every hour. Avoid conditions and interventions that might increase intracranial pressure (ICP) when possible. These include high positive end-expiratory pressure, frequent movements (agitation), neck vein compression, fever, arterial hypertension, hypoxemia, coughing, seizures, head-low position, and respiratory suctioning.	Neurological changes may indicate increasing intracranial pressure and the need for intervention. Elevated ICP is a dangerous sequela of ALF and is worsened by these conditions and interventions.[4]	• Abnormal pupil size and/or reactions • Changes in LOC

Patient Monitoring and Care —*Continued*

Steps	Rationale	Reportable Conditions
3. Monitor heparin anticoagulation if ordered with aPtt, and adjust per provider orders to achieve a therapeutic goal.	Anticoagulation improves patency of the circuit and therefore improves therapy time.	
4. Monitor citrate anticoagulation using postfilter and systemic ionized calcium levels.[6] • Titrate citrate solution to *postfilter* ionized calcium level levels. • Titrate calcium replacement infusion to *systemic* ionized calcium levels. • Adjust citrate and calcium per provider orders to achieve target lab range(s). • Monitor postfilter and systemic ionized levels at frequency outlined in institutional citrate protocol. • Administer calcium supplementation as needed based on systemic ionized calcium. • Monitor for alkalosis. • Assess for citrate lock, a condition that occurs when the total serum calcium level rises with a serious decreasing level of ionized calcium, and acidosis.	Calcium is needed for clotting. Citrate added to the blood prefilter binds free calcium (ionized) in the blood, rendering it unavailable to assist in the clotting cascade, thus inhibiting clotting in the filter. To restore normal patient blood calcium levels, calcium is administered post filter.[6] Patients may require additional supplements of calcium during treatment beyond what a continuous infusion can provide. Citrate is converted into bicarbonate by a functional liver. The goal is to clear the citrate/calcium complex from the patient's blood by the dialysate and replacement solution into the effluent, however some citrate may reach the patient. Therefore metabolic alkalosis may develop if the liver is able to metabolize citrate that is spilling over into the patient.[2,6] Citrate lock occurs when the citrate/calcium complex is not sufficiently dialyzed off in the CRRT filter enters the patient and then exceeds the capacity of the failing liver to metabolize the citrate.[2,6] Therefore patients with liver failure are at greater risk of developing citrate toxicity, resulting in metabolic complications. However, citrate toxicity is prevented in protocols that prescribe a higher hemofiltration rate and UFR and thereby provide greater citrate/calcium complex clearance. Monitor the total to ionized calcium ratio.[2,6,9]	• Hypocalcemia: Report ionized calcium level less than 1.0 for replacement • Alkalosis • Citrate lock: Ratio of total to systemic ionized calcium level greater than 2.5 and acidosis[6]
5. Obtain laboratory specimens as prescribed or per institutional standards. Results to monitor include: A. Complete blood count (CBC) B. Albumin C. Coagulation panel including INR; factors VII, V, and VIII; antithrombin, TEG or ROTEM D. AST, ALT, total bilirubin, alkaline phosphatase E. Arterial ammonia level F. Sodium G. Phosphorus H. Electrolyte and acid/base I. Glucose	CBC: Address for evidence of bleeding. This may occur as a result of liver failure Albumin: Protein is broken down by the liver. Albumin will be decreased in liver failure. resulting in decreased oncotic pressure within the vasculature. Monitor changes in clotting. TEG and ROTEM both measure the functional abilities of the overall coagulation pathways rather than specific pathways.[4,11] Ammonia is an important factor related to cerebral edema and encephalopathy.[4,5] For patients with ALI/ALF, hyponatremia should be strictly avoided as it may exacerbate cerebral edema.[5] Phosphorus replacement is critical in the liver recovery process; hypophosphatemia should be monitored for and treated aggressively.[5,15]	• Report hemoglobin less than 7.5g/dL • Report INR greater than 2.0 • Report elevated ammonia level • Abnormal sodium levels less than 145 mEq/L or greater than 155 mEq/L • Hypophosphatemia with levels less than 0.8–1.5 mmol/L • Blood glucose less than 80 mg/dL • Abnormal TEG or ROTEM measurement

Procedure continues on following page

Patient Monitoring and Care —*Continued*

Steps	Rationale	Reportable Conditions
	Other electrolyte and acid/base concentrations including potassium, magnesium, pH, and bicarbonate should be kept within the normal range by the CRRT.[12] Glycogen stores are depleted in ALF, and gluconeogenesis is impaired resulting in hypoglycemia.[4,11] Hypoglycemia is associated with increased mortality and should be corrected with a target serum blood glucose of 110–180.[4,11,15]	
6. Monitor the dialysis access site and lines for kinks, clots, leaking, redness, swelling, or drainage (see Procedure 106).	Access pressure alarms are built into the system of the CRRT machine and will alert staff to any significant risk issues. The greatest risks associated with the catheter are kinking of the line, dislodgement, and infection.	• Accidental catheter dislodgement, clots, leaking • Signs of central-line–associated bloodstream infection
7. Monitor vital signs every hour for the duration of therapy and more frequently if needed. Titrate vasoactive medications to a MAP of 65–70 mm Hg.[4]	Hemodynamic instability is often associated with acute liver insufficiency as a consequence of cytokines and circulating endotoxins causing proinflammatory effects.[4] This results in systemic vasodilatation, a decrease of systemic vascular resistance, arterial hypotension, and an increase of cardiac output that gives rise to a hyperdynamic circulation. If cerebral edema is identified on CT, mean arterial pressure (MAP) may be required to be greater than or equal to 70 mm Hg to maintain cerebral perfusion pressure, the pressure necessary to effectively perfuse the brain.[4]	• MAP less than 70 mm Hg or below the prescribed level • Increase in heart rate 20% or more above baseline • Decrease in systolic blood pressure 20–30 mm Hg or more below baseline
8. Closely monitor respirations, oxygen saturation, and lung sounds.	Respiratory stability may be affected by decreased neurological status and impaired airway protection, fluid overload related to renal failure, decreased compliance caused by intrapleural effusions, and acute lung injury due to inflammation.[4]	• Respiratory rate less than 10 breaths/min or greater than 20 breaths/min • SpO_2 less than 92% • Respiratory decompensation
9. Monitor renal function with BUN, creatinine, urine output, and fluid balance	Renal failure is present in about 50% of patients with ALI/ALF.[4] Positive fluid balance is associated with higher mortality in ALF.[15]	• Urine output 0.5–1 mL/kg/hour
10. Follow institutional standards for assessing pain. Administer analgesia as prescribed.	Identifies the need for pain interventions.	• Continued pain despite pain interventions

Documentation

Documentation should include the following:
- Patient and family education
- Patient tolerance of therapy
- Date and time therapy initiated
- Mode of CRRT (CVVHD, CVVHDF, or CVVH), CRRT system data per institutional policy (blood flow rate, patient fluid removal rate, access, return pressure, effluent and filter pressure, TMP, and filter pressure drop)
- Anticoagulation rate, monitoring laboratory tests and titrations
- Dialysis fluid and rate (green scale)
- Replacement fluid and rate (purple scale)
- From the MARS system: pIN and pOUT (optional), albumin flow rate, and alarm limits
- Location and condition of insertion site and any signs or symptoms of infection
- Vital signs throughout the treatment
- Unexpected outcomes
- Nursing interventions
- Laboratory assessment data

References and Additional Readings

For a complete list of references and additional readings for this procedure, scan this QR code with your smartphone, or visit https://www.elsevier.com/__data/assets/pdf_file/0009/1319877/Chapter0102.pdf.

103 Paracentesis (Perform)

Eleanor Fitzpatrick

PURPOSE Abdominal paracentesis is performed to remove fluid from the peritoneal cavity for diagnostic or therapeutic purposes.

PREREQUISITE NURSING KNOWLEDGE

- Knowledge of anatomy and physiology of the abdomen is important to avoid unexpected outcomes.
- The intestines and bladder lie immediately beneath the abdominal surface.
- Large volumes of ascitic fluid tend to float in the air-filled bowel toward the midline, where the bowel may be perforated during the procedure.
- The cecum is relatively fixed and is much less mobile than the sigmoid colon; therefore bowel perforations are more frequent in the right lower quadrant than in the left.
- Peritoneal fluid is normally straw-colored serous fluid secreted by the cells of the peritoneum. Grossly bloody fluid in the abdomen is abnormal.
- The peritoneal fluid collected is used in evaluation and diagnosis of ascites, acute abdominal conditions such as peritonitis or pancreatitis, and blunt or penetrating trauma to the abdomen.
- Therapeutic paracentesis is used to reduce intraabdominal and diaphragmatic pressures, to relieve dyspnea and respiratory compromise, and to prevent hernia formation and diaphragmatic rupture.[1,9,12,16,17,20] These complications are seen in patients with tense, refractory ascites and failed medical interventions such as sodium restriction and diuresis.[1,9,10,16,17]
- Cirrhosis is the most common cause of ascites formation. However, ascitic fluid is produced as a result of a variety of other conditions.[1,9,10,12,16] These conditions may include interference in venous return because of heart failure, constrictive pericarditis, or tricuspid valve insufficiency; obstruction of flow in the vena cava or portal vein; disturbance in electrolyte balance, such as sodium retention; depletion of plasma proteins because of nephrotic syndrome or starvation; lymphoma, leukemia, or neoplasms that involve the liver or mediastinum; ovarian malignant disease; and chronic pancreatitis.
- Analysis of the ascitic fluid can determine the cause of ascites. A serum-to-ascites albumin gradient should be calculated by subtracting the ascitic fluid albumin level from the serum albumin value. This calculation differentiates portal hypertensive from nonportal hypertensive ascites.[1,8-10,16,17]
- Paracentesis is contraindicated in patients with an acute abdomen who need immediate surgery. Coagulopathy should preclude paracentesis only in the case of clinically evident fibrinolysis or clinically evident disseminated intravascular coagulation.[1,9,10] Absolute contraindications include an acute abdomen, an uncooperative patient, and disseminated intravascular coagulopathy. Relative contraindications include coagulopathy, abdominal adhesions, an infected abdominal wall at the entry site, a distended bowel or bladder, and pregnancy.[1,8,9,10,15]
- Caution should be used when paracentesis is performed in patients with severe bowel distention, previous abdominal surgery (especially pelvic surgery), pregnancy (use open technique after the first trimester), a distended bladder that cannot be emptied with a Foley catheter, or obvious infection at the intended site of insertion (cellulitis or abscess).
- The insertion site should be midline one-third the distance from the umbilicus to the symphysis or 2 to 3 cm below the umbilicus (Fig. 103.1). An alternate position is a point one-third the distance from the umbilicus to the anterior iliac crest (left side is preferred, especially in obese patients or in those requiring removal of large volumes of fluid).[6,9,15,17]
- Ultrasound scan can be used before paracentesis to locate fluid and during the procedure to guide insertion of the catheter.[3]
- If ascitic fluid is difficult to localize with physical examination because of obesity or other conditions, ultrasound is effective in identifying the fluid and critical structures that must be avoided during the procedure.[9,15] Endoscopic transgastric ultrasound scan has also been used in the diagnosis of malignant ascites.[15,16]
- A semipermanent catheter or a shunt may be an option for patients with rapidly reaccumulating ascites.[1,10,16]
- For patients with refractory ascites, a battery-operated pump that removes ascitic fluid and continuously moves it to the bladder may be considered.[5,13]
- When large-volume paracentesis (>5 L) is performed in patients with cirrhosis and other disorders, the infusion of albumin (6 to 8 g/L) may prevent the onset of circulatory compromise associated with massive fluid shifting.[1,2,4,16-18] Albumin administration may be effective in preventing paracentesis-induced circulatory dysfunction, the most common complication after the procedure.[1,2,4,16] Albumin infusion is recommended with large-volume paracentesis.[1,2,4,16]

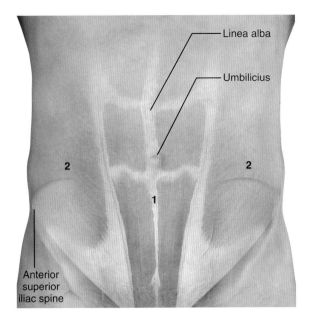

Figure 103.1   Preferred sites for paracentesis: *1,* The primary site is infraumbilical in midline through the linea alba. *2,* The preferred alternate (lateral rectus) site is in either lower quadrant, approximately 4 to 5 cm cephalad and medial to the anterior superior iliac spine. *(From Roberts JR:* Roberts and Hedges' clinical procedures in emergency medicine, *ed 7, Philadelphia, 2019, Saunders.)*

EQUIPMENT

- Commercially prepared paracentesis kit if available
- Nonsterile gloves, sterile gloves, mask, gown
- Antiseptic solution (e.g., 2% chlorhexidine-based preparation)
- Sterile marking pen
- Sterile towels or sterile drape
- Local anesthetic for injection: 1% or 2% lidocaine with epinephrine
- 5- or 10-mL syringe with 21- or 25-gauge needle for anesthetic
- Trocar with stylet, needle (16-, 18- or 20-gauge), or angiocatheter, depending on abdominal wall thickness
- 25- or 27-gauge 1½-inch needle
- 20- or 22-gauge spinal needles
- 20-mL syringe for diagnostic tap
- 50-mL syringe if using stopcock technique
- Four sterile tubes for specimens
- Scalpel and No. 11 knife blade
- Three-way stopcock
- Sterile 1-L collection bottles with connecting tubing
- Nylon skin suture material on cutting needle (4-0 or 5-0) and needle holder
- Mayo scissors and straight scissors
- Four to six sterile 4 × 4 gauze pads
- Sterile gauze dressing with tape or adhesive strip
  Additional equipment, to have available as needed, includes the following:
- Soft wrist restraints
- Stoma bag
- Ultrasound equipment

PATIENT AND FAMILY EDUCATION

- Explain the indications, procedure, and risks to the patient and family. *Rationale:* Explanation may decrease patient anxiety and encourages patient and family cooperation and understanding of the procedure.
- Explain the patient's role in assisting with the procedure and postprocedure care. *Rationale:* Patient cooperation during and after the procedure is elicited.
- Explain the signs and symptoms to report, such as fever, abdominal pain, decreased urine output, bleeding, and leakage of fluid from the surgical wound site. *Rationale:* Unexpected outcomes may not manifest themselves for a period after the procedure.

PATIENT ASSESSMENT AND PREPARATION

Patient Assessment

- Obtain the medical history, and perform a review of systems for abdominal injury, major gastrointestinal pathology, liver disease, and portal hypertension. *Rationale:* Certain conditions of the gastrointestinal tract may be diagnosed and treated with paracentesis. Contraindications to paracentesis may be identified.
- Identify the presence of any allergies to medications or other substances. *Rationale:* Patients may have allergies to skin preparations or anesthetics used before the invasive procedure is performed. Identification assists the practitioner in choosing the most appropriate skin preparation and anesthetic.
- Assess respiratory status (i.e., rate, depth, excursion, gas exchange, use of accessory muscles, pulse oximetry). *Rationale:* Paracentesis may be indicated to decrease the work of breathing.
- Obtain baseline vital signs. *Rationale:* Hypotension and dysrhythmias may occur with rapid changes in intraabdominal pressure.
- Obtain baseline pain assessment. *Rationale:* Changes in level of pain during or after the procedure may be an indicator of complications.
- Obtain baseline fluid and electrolyte status. *Rationale:* Removal of peritoneal fluid may cause compartment shifting of intravascular volume, electrolytes, and proteins, leading to decreased circulating volume.
- Assess bowel or bladder distention. *Rationale:* Distension increases the risk for bowel or bladder perforation during the procedure.
- Examine the abdomen, including assessment of abdominal girth, fluid wave, and shifting dullness; mark landmarks as needed. *Rationale:* Knowledge of abdominal landmarks and an understanding of the amount of fluid present are helpful in determining the amount to drain as well as where to best insert the catheter.
- Obtain coagulation study results (i.e., prothrombin time, partial thromboplastin time, and platelets). *Rationale:* Abnormal clotting may increase the risk for bleeding during and after the procedure, although this complication

is rare.[9,15] Therapy may be necessary to correct clotting abnormalities before the procedure, though this would be rare as bleeding risks are quoted as approximately 0.5% when patients are consented for the procedure.[1,15]

Patient Preparation

- Verify the correct patient with two identifiers. ***Rationale:*** Before performing a procedure, the nurse should ensure the correct identification of the patient for the intended intervention.
- Ensure that the patient understands preprocedural teaching. Answer questions as they arise, and reinforce information as needed. ***Rationale:*** Understanding of previously taught information is evaluated and reinforced.
- Obtain a written informed consent form. ***Rationale:*** Paracentesis is an invasive procedure that requires signed informed consent.
- Decompress the bladder either by having the patient void or by inserting a Foley catheter. ***Rationale:*** A distended bladder increases the risk for bladder perforation during the procedure.
- Obtain plain and upright radiographs of the abdomen before the procedure is performed. ***Rationale:*** Air is introduced during the procedure and may confuse the diagnosis later.
- Perform a preprocedure verification and time out, if nonemergent. ***Rationale:*** This ensures patient safety.
- Check that all relevant documents and studies are available before the procedure is started. ***Rationale:*** This measure ensures that the correct patient receives the correct procedure.
- Place the patient in the supine position (may tilt to side of collection slightly for improved fluid positioning). ***Rationale:*** Fluid accumulates in the dependent areas.
- If the patient has altered mental status, soft wrist restraints may be needed. ***Rationale:*** The patient must not move his or her hands into the sterile field once it has been established.

Procedure for Performing Paracentesis

Steps	Rationale	Special Considerations
1. HH		
2. PE		
3. Prepare the equipment and sterile field. Label all medications, medication containers (e.g., syringes, medicine cups, basins), and other solutions that are to be used during the procedure.	Provides a sterile field to decrease risk for infection	Maintain aseptic technique.
4. With the patient in the supine position, determine the site for trocar insertion. The site should be midline one-third the distance from the umbilicus to the symphysis (2–3 cm below the umbilicus; see Fig. 103.1).	Determines correct site for trocar placement. An alternate position, frequently chosen in obese patients or when large volumes of fluid are to be removed, is a point one third the distance from the umbilicus to the anterior iliac crest (left side preferred).	Avoid the rectus muscle because of increased risk for hemorrhage from epigastric vessels; surgical scars because of increased risk for perforation caused by adhesion of bowel to the wall of the peritoneum; and upper quadrants because of the possibility of undetected hepatomegaly[9,15]
5. Cleanse the insertion site with antiseptic solution (e.g., 2% chlorhexidine-based preparation.[9,15] **(Level C*)**	Reduces risk for infection.	Allergies should be identified before a skin preparation product is chosen. Use sterile technique.
6. Wash hands, and apply sterile gloves and a sterile gown.	Reduces transmission of microorganisms and body secretions.	
7. Apply sterile drapes to outline the area to be accessed.	Provide sterile field to decrease risk for infection.	

*Level C: Qualitative studies, descriptive or correlational studies, integrative reviews, systematic reviews, or randomized controlled trials with inconsistent results.

Procedure continues on following page

Procedure	for Performing Paracentesis—*Continued*	
Steps	**Rationale**	**Special Considerations**
8. Inject the area with local anesthetic (lidocaine with epinephrine preferred). Initially infiltrate the skin and subcutaneous tissues in a circumferential wheel; then direct the needle perpendicular to the skin, and infiltrate the peritoneum.	Local anesthesia minimizes pain and discomfort. Epinephrine helps eliminate unwanted abdominal wall bleeding and false-positive results.	Usually 1% lidocaine is used, but 0.5% lidocaine with 1:200,000 epinephrine has been shown to provide equivalent anesthetic effect as 1% lidocaine with 1:100,000 epinephrine. The maximum dosage is generally accepted to be 5 mg/kg of 1% plain lidocaine and 7 mg/kg of 1% lidocaine with epinephrine.[8,9] Assess for anesthesia of the area. Resistance is felt as the needle perforates the peritoneum.
9. With the No. 11 blade and scalpel holder, create a skin incision large enough to allow threading a 3- to 5-mm catheter.	Promotes easier insertion of the catheter.	If lavage is necessary, the opening is large enough to thread the lavage catheter.
10. Insert an 18-gauge needle attached to a 20- or 50-mL syringe through the anesthetized tract into the peritoneum. The needle is inserted through the small stab wound created as noted in **Step 9.** The stab wound should be made at the midline below the umbilicus. Apply slight suction to the syringe as it is advanced. Grasp the needle close to the skin as it is advanced.	Provides access to peritoneal fluid for evacuation. Slight suction is applied to indicate when the peritoneum is entered and if a blood vessel is entered. Grasping the needle as it is advanced prevents accidental thrusting into the abdomen and possible viscus perforation.	A small pop is felt as the needle advances through the anterior and posterior muscle fascia and enters the peritoneum.
11. Once in the cavity, direct the needle at a 60-degree angle toward the center of the pelvic hollow. When fluid returns, fill the syringe (Fig. 103.2). A flexible catheter/drain can be threaded into the abdominal cavity over the needle and left in place if needed.	Removes fluid for laboratory analysis.	Usually, diagnostic tests are ordered dependent on the patient's status and reason for paracentesis.[7,9,15] Tests may include the following: tube 1: lactate dehydrogenase, glucose, albumin; tube 2: total protein, specific gravity; tube 3: cell count and differential; tube 4: additional tests as needed. If there is suspicion of infection: gram stain, acid-fast bacillus stain, bacterial and fungal cultures, amylase, and triglyceride tests may be performed.[7,9,14,15,16] Also, send a specimen for cytology if malignancy is suspected.[7,14,15]
12. Attach syringes or stopcock and tubing, and gently aspirate or siphon fluid via gravity or vacuum into the collection device. Drains may be left in and allowed to drain for 6–12 hours.[9,15] **(Level E*)**	Initiates therapy.	Monitor the amount of fluid removed. Removal of large amounts of ascitic fluid (>5L) is associated with a reduction of circulating blood volume, a condition known as postparacentesis circulatory dysfunction (PPCD). This condition is seen in up to 70% of patients undergoing LVP.[11] The clinical manifestations of PPCD are hypotension, renal dysfunction, hepatic encephalopathy and lowered survival.[2,7,9,11,14,15,16] If large volume paracentesis is performed (>5–6L) an albumin infusion of 6–8 g/L of fluid removed improves survival and is recommended to prevent circulatory dysfunction.[2,7,11,14-16] **(Level A*)**

*Level A: Meta-analysis of quantitative studies or metasynthesis of qualitative studies with results that consistently support a specific action, intervention, or treatment (including systematic review of randomized controlled trials).

*Level E: Multiple case reports, theory-based evidence from expert opinions, or peer-reviewed professional organizational standards without clinical studies to support recommendations.

UNIT IV

Procedure	for Performing Paracentesis—*Continued*	
Steps	Rationale	Special Considerations

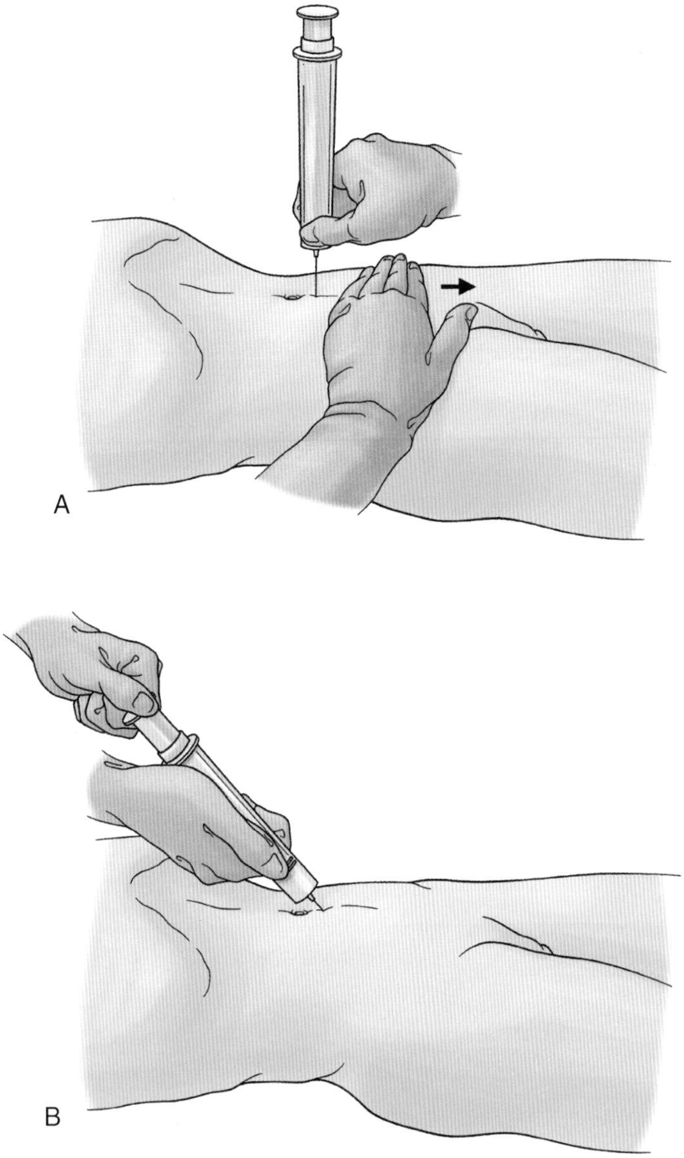

A

B

Figure 103.2 **A,** Z-track method of paracentesis. The skin is pulled approximately 2 cm caudal in relation to the deep abdominal wall by the non–needle-bearing hand while the paracentesis needle is slowly being inserted directly perpendicular to the skin. **B,** After the peritoneum is penetrated and fluid return is obtained, the skin is released. Note that the needle is angulated caudally. *(From Roberts JR: Roberts and Hedges' clinical procedures in emergency medicine, ed 7, Philadelphia, 2019, Saunders.)*

13. After the fluid is removed, gently remove the catheter, and apply pressure to the wound. If the wound is still leaking fluid after 5 minutes of direct pressure, suture the puncture site with a mattress suture.	Keeps insertion site clean and dry. Reduces risk for infection.	Inspect catheter to ensure if it intact. If significant leakage is found, apply a stoma bag over the site until drainage becomes minimal.
14. Apply a sterile dressing to the wound site.	Provides a barrier to infection and collects fluid that may leak from wound site.	
15. Remove **PE** and sterile equipment and equipment used during the procedure, and dispose in appropriate receptacles.	Standard Precautions.	
16. **HH**		

Expected Outcomes

- Evacuation of peritoneal fluid for laboratory analysis
- Decompression of the peritoneal cavity
- Relief of respiratory compromise
- Relief of abdominal discomfort

Unexpected Outcomes

- Perforation of the bowel, bladder, or stomach
- Lacerations of major vessels (mesenteric, iliac, aorta)
- Abdominal wall hematomas
- Laceration of the catheter and loss in the peritoneal cavity
- Incisional hernias
- Local or systemic infection
- Hypovolemia, hypotension, shock
- Bleeding from the insertion site
- Ascitic fluid leak from the insertion site
- Peritonitis

Patient Monitoring and Care

Steps	Rationale	Reportable Conditions
		These conditions should be reported to the provider if they persist despite nursing interventions.
1. Evaluate changes in abdominal girth.	Provides evidence of fluid accumulation.	• Increasing abdominal girth
2. Monitor for changes in respiratory status.	Removal of ascitic fluid should relieve pressure on the diaphragm and the resulting respiratory distress.	• Respiratory rate >24 breaths per minute or significant increase from baseline • Increased depth of breathing • Irregular breathing pattern • Pulse oximetry less than 92%, or significant decrease from baseline
3. Monitor for potential complications, including bowel or bladder perforation, bleeding, and intravascular volume loss.	Paracentesis interrupts the integrity of the skin and underlying peritoneum.	• Hematuria • Hypotension • Tachycardia
4. Monitor vital signs, temperature, and insertion site for drainage or evidence of infection.	Rapid changes in intraabdominal pressure may affect heart rate and blood pressure. Infection is a complication of paracentesis.	• Hypotension • Dysrhythmias • Increased temperature • Purulent drainage from the insertion site • Redness, swelling at the insertion site • Abnormal laboratory results (e.g., increased white blood cell count)
5. Monitor intake and output.	Provides data for evaluation of fluid balance status.	• Inappropriate fluid balance or changes from baseline fluid status
6. Monitor abdominal pain and level of weakness.	Patients often feel weak and have abdominal discomfort for a few hours after the procedure. Follow institutional standards for assessing pain. Identifies the need for pain interventions.	• Continued pain despite pain interventions, if performed
7. Evaluate laboratory data when returned.	Provides for evaluation of the patient's condition and aids in diagnosis.	• Red blood cell count >100,000/ mm^3 • Amylase value >2.5 times normal • Alkaline phosphatase value >5.5 mg/dL • White blood cell count >100/mm^3 • Positive culture results[19]

UNIT IV

Documentation

Documentation should include the following:
- Patient and family education
- Date and time of procedure
- Step-by-step description of the procedure
- Patient tolerance of the procedure
- Assessment of the insertion site after the procedure
- Amount and characteristics of fluid removed
- Specimens sent for laboratory analysis
- Postprocedure vital signs, respiratory status
- Postprocedure comfort/pain level
- Abdominal girth
- Unexpected outcomes
- Nursing interventions

References and Additional Readings

For a complete list of references and additional readings for this procedure, scan this QR code with your smartphone, or visit https://www.elsevier.com/__data/assets/pdf_file/0010/1319878/Chapter0103.pdf.

104 Paracentesis (Assist)

Eleanor Fitzpatrick

PURPOSE Abdominal paracentesis is performed to remove fluid from the peritoneal cavity for diagnostic or therapeutic purposes.

PREREQUISITE NURSING KNOWLEDGE

- Knowledge of anatomy and physiology of the abdomen is important to avoid unexpected outcomes.
- Intestines and bladder lie immediately beneath the abdominal surface.
- Large volumes of ascitic fluid tend to float the air-filled bowel toward the midline, where it may be easily perforated during the procedure.
- The cecum is relatively fixed and is much less mobile than the sigmoid colon; therefore bowel perforations are more frequent in the right lower quadrant than in the left.
- Peritoneal fluid is normally straw-colored, serous fluid secreted by the cells of the peritoneum. Grossly bloody fluid in the abdomen is abnormal.
- The peritoneal fluid collected is used to evaluate and diagnose the cause of ascites, acute abdominal conditions such as peritonitis or pancreatitis, and blunt or penetrating trauma to the abdomen.
- Therapeutic paracentesis is used to reduce intraabdominal and diaphragmatic pressures to relieve dyspnea and respiratory compromise and to prevent hernia formation and diaphragmatic rupture.[1,7,9,10,16,17,20] These complications are seen in patients with tense, refractory ascites with failed medical interventions, such as sodium restriction and diuresis.[1,7,9,10,16,17,20]
- Cirrhosis is the most common cause of ascites formation. However, ascitic fluid is produced as a result of a variety of other conditions.[1,9,10,12,16] These conditions may include interference in venous return because of heart failure, constrictive pericarditis, or tricuspid valve insufficiency; obstruction of flow in the vena cava or portal vein; disturbance in electrolyte balance, such as sodium retention; depletion of plasma proteins because of nephrotic syndrome or starvation; lymphoma, leukemia, or neoplasms that involve the liver or mediastinum; ovarian malignant disease; and chronic pancreatitis.
- Analysis of the ascitic fluid can determine the cause of ascites. A serum-to-ascites albumin gradient should be calculated by subtracting the ascitic fluid albumin level from the serum albumin. This calculation differentiates portal hypertensive from nonportal hypertensive ascites.[1,8,9,10,16,17]
- Paracentesis is contraindicated in patients with an acute abdomen who need immediate surgery. Coagulopathies

and thrombocytopenia are considered relative contraindications. Coagulopathy should preclude paracentesis only in the case of clinically evident fibrinolysis or clinically evident disseminated intravascular coagulation.[1,9,10] Absolute contraindications include an acute abdomen, an uncooperative patient, and disseminated intravascular coagulopathy. Relative contraindications include coagulopathy, abdominal adhesions, an infected abdominal wall at the entry site, a distended bowel or bladder, and pregnancy.[1,8,9,10,15]

- Caution should be used when paracentesis is performed in patients with severe bowel distention, previous abdominal surgery (especially pelvic surgery), pregnancy (use open technique after the first trimester), a distended bladder that cannot be emptied with a Foley catheter, or obvious infection at the intended insertion site (cellulitis or abscess).
- The insertion site should be midline one-third the distance from the umbilicus to the symphysis (2 to 3 cm below the umbilicus; see Fig. 103.1). An alternate position is a point one-third the distance from the umbilicus to the anterior iliac crest (the left side is preferred, especially in obese patients or in those requiring removal of large volumes of fluid).[6,9,15,17]
- Ultrasound scan can be used before paracentesis to locate fluid and during the procedure to guide catheter insertion.[3]
- If ascitic fluid is difficult to localize with a physical examination due to obesity or other conditions, ultrasound is effective in identifying the fluid and critical structures that must be avoided during the procedure.[9,15]
- Endoscopic transgastric ultrasound scan has also been used in the diagnosis of malignant ascites.[15,16]
- A semipermanent catheter or a shunt may be an option for patients with rapidly reaccumulating ascites.[1,10,16]
- For patients with refractory ascites, a battery-operated pump that removes ascitic fluid and continuously moves it to the bladder may be considered.[5,13]
- When large-volume paracentesis (>5 L) is performed in patients with cirrhosis and other disorders, the infusion of albumin (6 to 8 g/L) may prevent the onset of circulatory compromise associated with massive fluid shifting.[1,2,4,16,17,18] Albumin administration may be effective in preventing paracentesis-induced circulatory dysfunction, the most common complication after the procedure.[1,2,4,16] Albumin infusion is recommended with large-volume paracentesis as its use has shown improved survival.[1,2,4,16]

EQUIPMENT

- Commercially prepared paracentesis kit if available
- Nonsterile gloves, sterile gloves, mask, goggles, and gown
- Antiseptic solution (e.g., 2% chlorhexidine-based preparation)
- Sterile marking pen
- Sterile towels or sterile drape
- Local anesthetic for injection: 1% or 2% lidocaine with epinephrine
- 5- or 10-mL syringe with 21- or 25-gauge needle for anesthetic
- Trocar with stylet, needle (16-, 18-, or 20-gauge), or angiocatheter, depending on abdominal wall thickness
- 25- or 27-gauge 1½-inch needle
- 20- or 22-gauge spinal needles
- 20-mL syringe for diagnostic tap
- 50-mL syringe if using the stopcock technique
- Four sterile tubes for specimens
- Scalpel and No. 11 knife blade
- Three-way stopcock
- Sterile 1-L collection bottles with connecting tubing
- Nylon skin suture material on cutting needle (4-0 or 5-0) and needle holder
- Mayo scissors and straight scissors
- Four to six sterile 4 × 4 gauze pads
- Sterile gauze dressing with tape or adhesive strip
  Additional equipment to have available as needed includes the following:
- Soft wrist restraints
- Stoma bag
- Ultrasound equipment

PATIENT AND FAMILY EDUCATION

- Explain the indications, procedure, and risks to the patient and family. *Rationale:* Explanation may decrease patient anxiety and encourages patient and family cooperation and understanding of the procedure.
- Explain the patient's role in assisting with the procedure and postprocedure care. *Rationale:* This elicits patient cooperation during and after the procedure.
- Explain the signs and symptoms to report, such as fever, abdominal pain, decreased urine output, bleeding, and leakage of fluid from the surgical wound site. *Rationale:* Unexpected outcomes may not manifest themselves for a period after the procedure.

PATIENT ASSESSMENT AND PREPARATION

Patient Assessment

- Obtain the medical history and a review of systems for abdominal injury, major gastrointestinal pathology, liver disease, and portal hypertension. *Rationale:* Certain conditions of the gastrointestinal tract may be diagnosed and treated with paracentesis. Contraindications to paracentesis may be identified.

- Identify the presence of any allergies to medication or other substances. *Rationale:* Patients may have allergies to skin preparations or anesthetics used before the invasive procedure is performed. Identification assists the practitioner in choosing the most appropriate skin preparation and anesthetic.
- Assess respiratory status (i.e., rate, depth, excursion, gas exchange, use of accessory muscles, and pulse oximetry). *Rationale:* Paracentesis may be indicated to decrease the work of breathing.
- Obtain baseline vital signs. *Rationale:* Hypotension and dysrhythmias may occur with rapid changes in intraabdominal pressure.
- Obtain a baseline pain assessment. *Rationale:* Changes in the level of pain during or after the procedure may be an indicator of complications.
- Obtain baseline fluid and electrolyte status. *Rationale:* Removal of peritoneal fluid may cause compartment shifting of intravascular volume, electrolytes, and proteins, leading to a decreased circulating volume.
- Assess for bowel or bladder distention. *Rationale:* Distension increases the risk for bowel or bladder perforation during the procedure.
- Assess abdominal girth. *Rationale:* Information on changes in fluid accumulation within the peritoneal cavity is provided.
- Obtain coagulation study results (i.e., prothrombin time, partial thromboplastin time, and platelets). *Rationale:* Abnormal clotting may increase the risk for bleeding during and after the procedure, although this complication is rare.[9,15] Therapy may be necessary to correct clotting abnormalities before the procedure, though this would be rare as bleeding risks are quoted as approximately 0.5% when patients are consented for the procedure.[1,15]

Patient Preparation

- Verify the correct patient with two identifiers. *Rationale:* Before performing a procedure, the nurse should ensure the correct identification of the patient for the intended intervention.
- Ensure that the patient understands the preprocedural information. Answer questions as they arise, and reinforce information as needed. *Rationale:* Understanding of previously taught information is evaluated and reinforced.
- Ensure that a written informed consent form has been obtained by the practitioner performing the procedure. The assisting practitioner may be a witness to the signing of the consent if needed. *Rationale:* Paracentesis is an invasive procedure and requires a signed informed consent form.
- Decompress the bladder either by having the patient void or by inserting a Foley catheter. *Rationale:* A distended bladder increases the risk for bladder perforation during the procedure.
- The physician, or advanced practice provider (nurse practitioner, physician assistant and in some areas, clinical nurse specialist) orders plain and upright radiographs of the abdomen before the procedure is performed. *Rationale:* Air is introduced during the procedure and may confuse the diagnosis later.

- Perform a preprocedure verification and time out with the provider if nonemergent. *Rationale:* Ensures patient safety.
- Check that all relevant documents and studies are available before the procedure is started. *Rationale:* This measure ensures that the correct patient receives the correct procedure.
- Place the patient in the supine position (may tilt to the side of the collection slightly for improved fluid positioning). *Rationale:* Fluid accumulates in the dependent areas.

- The provider will examine the abdomen for areas of shifting dullness, find landmarks, and mark appropriately. *Rationale:* Shifting dullness indicates fluid.
- If the patient has altered mental status, soft wrist restraints may be prescribed. *Rationale:* The patient must not move his or her hands into the sterile field once it has been established.

Procedure	for Assisting With Paracentesis	
Steps	**Rationale**	**Special Considerations**
1. HH		
2. PE		
3. Assist in preparing the equipment and sterile field. Label all medications, medication containers (e.g., syringes, medicine cups, basins), and other solutions that will be used during the procedure.	Provides a sterile field to decrease the risk for infection.	Maintain aseptic technique.
4. As needed, assist the physician or advanced practice provider to cleanse the insertion site with antiseptic solution (e.g., 2% chlorhexidine-based preparation).[9,15] (**Level C***)	Reduces the risk for infection.	Allergies should be identified before a skin preparation product is chosen.
5. As needed, assist the provider with the application of sterile gloves, gown, and mask as well as sterile drapes to outline the area to be tapped.	Provides a sterile field to decrease the risk for infection.	
6. As needed, assist the provider to draw up local anesthetic (lidocaine with epinephrine preferred).	Local anesthesia minimizes pain and discomfort. Epinephrine helps eliminate unwanted abdominal wall bleeding and false-positive results.	Usually 1% lidocaine is used, but 0.5% lidocaine with 1:200,000 epinephrine has been shown to provide an equivalent anesthetic effect as 1% lidocaine with 1:100,000 epinephrine. The maximum dosage is generally accepted to be 5 mg/kg of 1% plain lidocaine and 7 mg/kg of 1% lidocaine with epinephrine.[8] Assess for anesthesia of the area.
7. Assist in collection and labeling of peritoneal fluid for laboratory analysis.	Assists in collecting and labeling fluid for laboratory analysis.	Usually diagnostic tests are ordered depending on patient status and reason for paracentesis.[7,9,15] Tests may include the following: tube 1: lactate dehydrogenase, glucose, albumin; tube 2: total protein, specific gravity; tube 3: cell count and differential; tube 4: additional tests as needed. If there is suspicion of infection: Gram stain, acid-fast bacillus stain, bacterial and fungal cultures, amylase, and triglyceride tests may be ordered.[7,9,14,15,16] Also, collect a specimen for cytology if malignancy is suspected.[7,14,15]

*Level C: Qualitative studies, descriptive or correlational studies, integrative reviews, systematic reviews, or randomized controlled trials with inconsistent results.

Procedure continues on following page

UNIT IV

Procedure for Assisting With Paracentesis—*Continued*

Steps	Rationale	Special Considerations
8. Assist the provider in attaching syringes or the stopcock and tubing and aspirating or siphoning fluid via gravity or vacuum into the collection device. A flexible catheter/drain can be threaded into the abdominal cavity over the needle and left in place if needed. Drains may be left in and allowed to drain for 6–12 hours.[9,15] **(Level E*)**	Initiates therapy.	Monitor the amount of fluid removed. Removal of large amounts of ascitic fluid (>5 L) is associated with a reduction of circulating blood volume, a condition known as postparacentesis circulatory dysfunction (PPCD). This condition is seen in up to 70% of patients undergoing large-volume paracentesis.[11] The clinical manifestations of PPCD are hypotension, renal dysfunction, hepatic encephalopathy and lowered survival.[2,7,9,11,14,15,16] If large-volume paracentesis is performed (>5–6 L), an albumin infusion of 6–8 g/L of fluid removed improves survival and is recommended to prevent circulatory dysfunction.[2,7,11,14,15,16] **(Level A*)**
9. After the fluid and catheter are removed, apply pressure to the wound. If the wound is still leaking fluid after 5 minutes of direct pressure, the provider may suture the puncture site and apply a pressure dressing.	Keeps the insertion site clean. Reduces the risk for infection.	Inspect the catheter to ensure that it is intact. If significant leakage is found, apply a stoma bag over the site until drainage becomes minimal.
10. Assist with applying a sterile dressing to the wound site.	Provides a barrier to infection and collects fluid that may leak from the wound site.	
11. Remove **PE** and sterile equipment used during the procedure and place in appropriate receptacles.	Standard precautions.	
12. **HH**		

---

*Level A: Meta-analysis of quantitative studies or metasynthesis of qualitative studies with results that consistently support a specific action, intervention, or treatment (including systematic review of randomized controlled trials).

*Level E: Multiple case reports, theory-based evidence from expert opinions, or peer-reviewed professional organizational standards without clinical studies to support recommendations.

Expected Outcomes

- Evacuation of peritoneal fluid for laboratory analysis
- Decompression of peritoneal cavity
- Relief of respiratory compromise
- Relief of abdominal discomfort

Unexpected Outcomes

- Perforation of the bowel, bladder, or stomach
- Lacerations of major vessels (mesenteric, iliac, aorta)
- Abdominal wall hematoma
- Laceration of the catheter and loss in the peritoneal cavity
- Incisional hernias
- Local or systemic infection
- Hypovolemia, hypotension, shock
- Bleeding from the insertion site
- Ascitic fluid leak from the insertion site
- Peritonitis

Patient Monitoring and Care

Steps	Rationale	Reportable Conditions
		These conditions should be reported to the provider if they persist despite nursing interventions.
1. Evaluate changes in abdominal girth.	Provides evidence of fluid reaccumulation.	• Increasing abdominal girth
2. Monitor for changes in respiratory status.	Removal of ascitic fluid should relieve pressure on the diaphragm and the resulting respiratory distress.[7]	• Respiratory rate >24 breaths/min or significant increase from baseline • Increased depth of breathing • Irregular breathing pattern • Pulse oximetry <92%, or significant decrease from baseline
3. Monitor for potential complications, including bowel or bladder perforation, bleeding, and intravascular volume loss.	Paracentesis interrupts the integrity of the skin and underlying peritoneum.	• Hematuria • Hypotension • Tachycardia
4. Monitor vital signs, temperature, and the insertion site for drainage or evidence of infection.	Rapid changes in intraabdominal pressure may affect heart rate and blood pressure. Infection is a complication of paracentesis.	• Hypotension • Dysrhythmias • Increased temperature • Purulent drainage from the insertion site • Redness, swelling at the insertion site • Abnormal laboratory results (increased white blood cell [WBC] count)
5. Monitor intake and output.	Provides data for evaluation of the fluid balance status.	• Altered fluid balance or changes from baseline fluid status
6. Monitor abdominal pain and level of weakness. Follow institutional standards for assessing pain.	Patients often feel weak and have abdominal discomfort for a few hours after the procedure. Identifies the need for pain interventions.	• Continued pain despite pain interventions, if performed
7. Evaluate the laboratory data when results are obtained.	Provides for evaluation of the condition and aids in diagnosis.	• Red blood cell count >100,000/mm³ • Amylase value >2.5 times normal • Alkaline phosphatase value >5.5 mg/dL • WBC count >100/mm³ • Positive culture results[19]

Documentation

Documentation should include the following:
- Patient and family education
- Date and time of the procedure
- Patient tolerance of the procedure
- Assessment of the insertion site after the procedure
- Amount and characteristics of fluid removed
- Specimens sent for laboratory analysis
- Postprocedure vital signs and respiratory status
- Postprocedure comfort/pain level
- Abdominal girth
- Unexpected outcomes
- Nursing interventions

References and Additional Readings

For a complete list of references and additional readings for this procedure, scan this QR code with your smartphone, or visit https://www.elsevier.com/__data/assets/pdf_file/0011/1319879/Chapter0104.pdf

UNIT IV

PROCEDURE

105 Continuous Renal Replacement Therapies

Heather L. Przybyl and Amanda J. Golino

PURPOSE Continuous renal replacement therapies are used in the critical care unit setting for volume regulation, acid-base control, electrolyte regulation, drug intoxications, management of azotemia, and immune modulation. These methods are most often used in critically ill patients whose hemodynamic status does not tolerate the rapid fluid and electrolyte shifts associated with intermittent hemodialysis or who need continuous removal or regulation of solutes and intravascular volume.[11,20]

PREREQUISITE NURSING KNOWLEDGE

- Continuous renal replacement therapy (CRRT) is an extracorporeal blood-purification therapy intended to substitute for impaired renal function over an extended period for, or attempted for, 24 hours per day.[11,22,37]
- The Risk, Injury, Failure, Loss, End-Stage (RIFLE) or the Acute Kidney Injury Network (AKIN) scales are commonly used by nephrologists to determine the level of kidney impairment. The scales assess variations in serum creatinine levels, glomerular filtration rate, and urine output to determine the level of impairment. These values assist the provider in determining the best modality to treat the patient based on the stage of acute renal injury.[20,22,37,39]
- Basic knowledge is required to understand the principles of diffusion, convection, ultrafiltration (UF), osmosis, oncotic pressure, and hydrostatic pressure and how they pertain to fluid and solute management during dialysis.[27,31]
  - ❖ *Diffusion:* The passive movement of solutes through a semipermeable membrane from an area of higher concentration to an area of lower concentration until equilibrium is reached.
  - ❖ *Convective transport:* The rapid movement of fluid across a semipermeable membrane from an area of high pressure to an area of low pressure with transport of solutes. When water moves across a membrane along a pressure gradient, some solutes are carried along with the water and do not require a solute concentration gradient (also called *solute drag*). Convective transport is most effective for removal of middle-molecular-weight and large-molecular-weight solutes.
  - ❖ *UF:* The bulk movement of solute and solvent through a semipermeable membrane in response to a pressure

difference across the membrane. This movement is usually achieved with positive pressure in the blood compartment in the hemofilter and negative pressure in the dialysate compartment. Blood and dialysate run countercurrent. The size of the solute molecules compared with the size of molecules that can move through the semipermeable membrane determines the degree of UF.
  - ❖ *Osmosis:* The passive movement of solvent through a semipermeable membrane from an area of higher concentration to an area of lower concentration.
  - ❖ *Oncotic pressure:* The pressure exerted by plasma proteins that favor intravascular fluid retention and movement of fluid from the extravascular space to the intravascular space.
  - ❖ *Hydrostatic pressure:* The force exerted by arterial blood pressure that favors the movement of fluid from the intravascular space to the extravascular space.
  - ❖ *Absorption:* The process by which drug molecules pass through membranes and fluid barriers and into body fluids.
  - ❖ *Adsorption:* The adhesion of molecules (solutes) to the surface of the hemofilter, charcoal, or resin.

VARIATIONS IN CONTINUOUS RENAL REPLACEMENT THERAPY MODALITIES

- These therapies are used to remove both plasma water and solutes.[5,11,13,]
- The following methods of CRRT are included as listed (details are outlined in Table 105.1):
  - ❖ Slow, continuous ultrafiltration (SCUF)[5,27,28,32]
    - ○ SCUF (Fig. 105.1) is used primarily to remove plasma water. A hemofilter with a large surface area,

TABLE 105.1	Continuous Renal Replacement Therapies				
Mode of Therapy	Principle Involved	Fluids Used	Indications	Advantage	Considerations
SCUF (slow, continuous ultrafiltration)[27,28]	Ultrafiltration, convection • Movement of plasma water through a semipermeable membrane that is driven by a pressure gradient[5,31] • Volume controlled by the effluent pump[4,15]	• None	• Achieve volume control with patients who are volume overloaded and are diuretic-resistant[27] • Adjunct therapy for heart failure patients[27] • Refractory fluid volume overload with or without renal dysfunction[32]	• Smaller-bore catheter may be used	• Filtration fraction may need to be examined once the volume of plasma water is removed. This phenomenon may give the appearance of an elevated filtration fraction because of the constant hematocrit and decreasing volume.
CVVH (continuous venovenous hemo-filtration)[5,27,31,32]	Ultrafiltration, convection • Movement of plasma water through a semipermeable membrane that is driven by a pressure gradient[5,31] • Unwanted solutes are removed while plasma volume is replaced by repla-cement solutions infused either pre- or postfilter • "Solute drag" across a semipermeable membrane • Typically removes large- to medium-sized molecules[31]	• Replacement fluids	• Solute clearance • Volume control	• Blood flow is typically 200-400 mL/min, therefore it can be initiated in a patient who is hemodynamically unstable	• Complications associated with anticoagulation, therapy, and access
CVVHD (continuous venovenous hemodialys is)[5,27,31,32]	Ultrafiltration, diffusion • Unwanted solutes are moved from an area of higher concentration to an area of lower concentration • Fluids move countercurrent to the patient's blood flow • Small to medium molecules[31]	• Dialysate	• Solute clearance • Volume control	• Blood flow is typically 200–400 mL/min; therefore it can be initiated in a patient who is hemodynamically unstable	• Complications associated with anticoagulation, therapy, and access
CVVHDF (continuous venovenous hemodiafiltra-tion)[5,27,31,32]	Ultrafiltration, convection, diffusion • All sized molecules removed (dependent on filter specifications)[31]	• Replacement fluids • Dialysate	• Solute clearance of all size molecules • Volume control	• Blood flow is typically 200–400 mL/min; therefore it can be initiated in a patient who is hemodynamically unstable	• Complications associated with anticoagulation, therapy, and access

high sieving coefficient (potential for solutes to pass across a membrane), and low resistance is used to facilitate slow continuous fluid removal.[19]
- ○ SCUF can be achieved via a pumped or nonpumped system and can be used even if acute kidney injury has resolved.
- ❖ Continuous venovenous hemofiltration (CVVH)[5,19,27,32,42]
  - ○ CVVH (Fig. 105.2) removes fluids and solutes via convective clearance. Replacement solution is part of the setup; the replacement solution creates a sol-ute drag effect and is effective for large-molecule removal.
  - ○ CVVH is a pump-driven modality.
- ❖ Continuous venovenous hemodialysis (CVVHD)[5,19,27,32,42]

- ○ CVVHD (Fig. 105.3) is used to remove solutes pri-marily via diffusion.
- ○ Dialysate solution is part of the setup; flow of the dialysate is countercurrent to the blood flow.
- ○ CVVHD is a pump-driven modality.
- ❖ Continuous venovenous hemodiafiltration (CVV HDF)[5,19,27,32,42]
  - ○ CVVHDF (Fig. 105.4) removes fluids and solutes via diffusion and convection.
  - ○ Dialysate runs countercurrent to the blood flow and clears toxins by diffusion.
  - ○ Replacement fluid is infused at a prescribed rate and clears by convection.
  - ○ CVVHDF is a pump-driven modality.

UNIT V

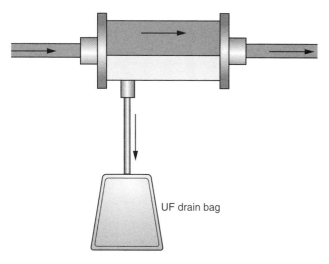

Figure 105.1 Slow continuous ultrafiltration (SCUF). Fluid removal and no fluid replacement. *(Copyright Rhonda K. Martin.)*

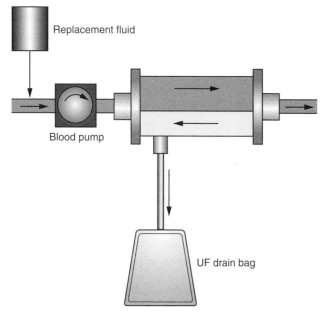

Figure 105.2 Continuous venovenous hemofiltration (CVVH). Fluid removal and fluid replacement. *(Copyright Rhonda K. Martin.)*

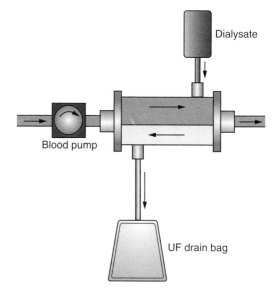

Figure 105.3 Continuous venovenous hemodialysis (CVVHD). Fluid and solute removal with dialysate. *(Copyright Rhonda K. Martin.)*

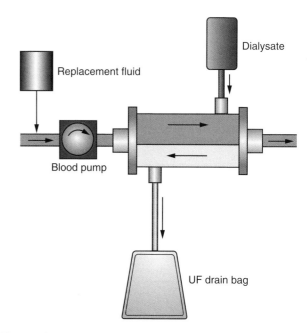

Figure 105.4 Continuous venovenous hemodiafiltration (CVVHDF). Fluid replacement with dialysate. *(Copyright Rhonda K. Martin.)*

Other extended renal replacement therapy techniques or "hybrid" techniques (sustained low-efficiency dialysis, extended daily dialysis) generally use standard hemodialysis equipment with reduced blood flow and dialysate rates to gradually remove plasma water and solutes. They are typically used from 6 to 12 hours a day.[32,33,42,40] These therapies can also have modified run times depending on patient presentation and hemodynamic stability. Preliminary studies show that new modes of CRRT such as cascade filtration may benefit patients by reducing the loss of micronutrients. More research is needed to determine clinical benefits.[44]

THE CRRT PUMP

- A blood pump provides the pressure that drives the extracorporeal system; the blood circuit consists of blood lines, a blood pump, and various monitoring devices. The blood lines are connected to the vascular access and carry the blood to and from the patient. The blood pump controls the speed of the blood through the circuit. The monitoring devices include pressure monitors and an air detection monitor to prevent air that may have entered the circuit from being infused to the patient. Anticoagulant, dialysate, and replacement fluids can also be added to the system.[30,32]

- Integrated pump systems have separate pumps for blood, dialysate, ultrafiltrate/effluent, and replacement fluids (Fig. 105.5). The pumps are controlled by a computerized control module. Blood flow rate, dialysate flow rate, replacement fluid rate, anticoagulation rate, and fluid-removal rates are entered by the nurse as prescribed. Dialysate, ultrafiltrate/effluent, and replacement fluids are measured by weight or volumetric scales on the machine. The module calculates and adjusts pump speeds to achieve the selected fluid goal. The module also records and displays treatment data.[30,32]

CENTRAL VENOUS CATHETER HEMODIALYSIS ACCESS

- Most commonly, CRRT can be accomplished through venovenous (VV) access.[22,28]
- The VV access is used almost exclusively because of its less invasive nature. There are many variations of the hemodialysis central venous catheter on the market, all with pros and cons for use.[3,6,28,30]
- Without the use of a dual-lumen catheter and blood pump for CRRT, dialysis access required both arterial and venous cannulation (AV access). With AV access, the patient's systemic blood pressure is required for blood to flow into the extracorporeal circuit, making it unreliable for hypotensive patients. The newer-generation CRRT machines have an added extracorporeal blood pump that pulls the patient's blood into the circuit, so it is better suited to treat hemodynamically unstable patients.[22,28,41] Common sites for the vascular access catheter (VAC) are the internal jugular, subclavian, and femoral veins. The internal jugular approach is the preferred access (particularly for those with a higher body mass index (BMI). Cannulation of the subclavian vein may cause stenosis and prevent placement of upper extremity grafts or fistulas if long-term dialysis is necessary. Femoral cannulation is associated with increased infection.[3,6,18,21,22,34,37,41]
  ❖ Hemodialysis shunts or surgically created hemodialysis anastomoses have been used in the past for CRRT; however, because of increased incidence rates of vascular injury, bleeding, and infection, they are *not* recommended for CRRT access.[22,28,41]

EXTRACORPOREAL FILTER/DIALYZER

- CRRT uses an artificial kidney (i.e., hemofilter, dialyzer) with a semipermeable membrane to create two separate compartments: the blood compartment and the dialysis solution or dialysate compartment. The semipermeable membrane allows the movement of small molecules (e.g., electrolytes) and middle-sized molecules (e.g., creatinine, vasoactive substances) from the patient's blood into the dialysis solution but is impermeable to larger molecules (e.g., red blood cells, plasma proteins).[14,21,33]
- Each dialyzer has four ports: two end ports for blood (blood flows in one end and out the other) and two side ports for dialysis solution ultrafiltrate (dialysate solution flows in one end and out the other). In most cases, the

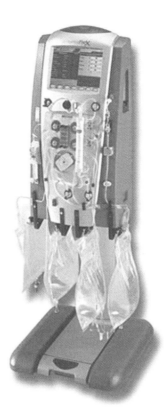

Figure 105.5 Gambro Prismaflex Continuous renal replacement therapy machine. *(Courtesy Gambro USA, Lakewood, CO.)*

blood and dialysate run through the dialyzer in opposite or countercurrent directions.[28,32]
- Hollow-fiber dialyzers are used almost exclusively for CRRT. The blood flows through the center of hollow fibers, and the dialysis solution (dialysate) flows around the outside of the hollow fibers. The advantages of hollow-fiber filters include a low priming volume, low resistance to flow, and a high amount of surface area. The major disadvantage is the potential for clotting as a result of the small fiber size.
- All dialyzers have a UF coefficient; thus the dialyzer selected varies in different clinical situations. The higher the UF coefficient, the more rapid the fluid removal. UF coefficients are determined with in vivo measurements done by each dialyzer manufacturer.[14,33]

Clearance refers to the ability of the dialyzer to remove metabolic waste products or drugs from the patient's blood. The blood flow rate, the dialysate flow rate, and the solute concentration affect clearance. Clearance occurs by the processes of diffusion, convection, and UF.

FLUIDS USED IN CRRT

- The dialysate (when used during CRRT) is composed of water, a buffer (i.e., lactate or bicarbonate), and various electrolytes. Most solutions also contain glucose. The buffer helps neutralize acids that are generated as a result of normal cellular metabolism. The concentration of electrolytes is usually the normal plasma concentration, which helps create a concentration gradient for removal of excess electrolytes. The glucose aids in increasing the oncotic pressure in the dialysate (thus aiding in fluid removal) and in caloric replacement. Although glucose comes in various concentrations, it is mostly used in normal plasma concentrations to prevent hyperglycemia.[32]

- Replacement fluids can be either the same formula as the dialysate or a combination of saline fluids. There is a wide range of fluid types that can be utilized as replacement fluids. Providers will base these choices on the patient's laboratory values (e.g., electrolytes) to formulate their decision.[28]

The patient's volume status and serum electrolyte levels are changed gradually so patients have fewer problems maintaining hemodynamic stability than with hemodialysis. Specifics of these therapies are outlined in Table 105.1.[10,12,43,45]

ANTICOAGULATION

- Citrate or heparin is often used during CRRT to prevent clotting of the extracorporeal circuit during treatment. Saline solution flushes can be used alone or with other anticoagulants to maintain circuit patency.[1,2,23-25,36,38]
  - ❖ Anticoagulation choice is dependent on patient status and laboratory values. The provider may choose citrate, heparin, no anticoagulation, or any other variation of anticoagulation.[1,2,18,22-25,28,36-38]
- Citrate will anticoagulate the CRRT filter and is considered regional anticoagulation, whereas heparin is used systemically and is considered systemic anticoagulation.[22,36]
- Citrate anticoagulation must be used in conjunction with a calcium infusion to replace the amount of ionized calcium in the patient's blood.[36]

An anticoagulant may be used to maintain vascular access patency when CRRT is not in use.

EQUIPMENT

- Dedicated vascular access catheter (VAC)
- CRRT machine
- Dialyzer/filter
- Fluid warmer (or alternative method to warm the patient)
- Heparin or citrate (for priming if indicated, as prescribed)
- Drainage bag
- Dialysate fluid as prescribed
- Replacement fluid as prescribed
- Sterile normal saline (NS) solution (1 to 2 L) for priming the dialyzer/filter
- Fluid shield, face mask, or goggles
- Two sets of clean or sterile gloves; follow institutional standards[36,37]
- Two empty 5- or 10-mL (dependent on VAC fill volume) syringes to aspirate VAC contents before flushing and connecting the line
- Two 10-mL prefilled syringes with NS solution
- Dressing supplies (alcohol wipes, sterile barrier, gauze pads, transparent dressing, tape)
- Antiseptic solution (e.g., 2% chlorhexidine–based preparation)

- Intravenous (IV) accessory spike to connect NS bag if additional priming is needed
- Two dialysis luer caps for the VAC
- Two alcohol-impregnated caps for the VAC for use when the line is not in use

Additional equipment to have available as needed includes the following:

- Two 5- or 10-mL syringes and blunt-tip needles (if needed to draw up NS for injection)
- NS for injection (if prefilled NS syringes are not used)
- Plastic hemodialysis clamps

PATIENT AND FAMILY EDUCATION

- Explain the purpose of CRRT—specifically why the treatment is performed and the expected clinical outcomes.[16] *Rationale:* The patient and family should understand that CRRT is necessary to perform the physiological functions of the kidneys if the patient is hemodynamically unstable.
- Explain the procedure, including risks, anticipated length of treatment, and patient positioning, and review any questions the patient may have.[16] *Rationale:* Explanation provides information and may decrease patient anxiety.
- Explain the need for careful sterile technique for the duration of treatment. *Rationale:* The patient and family must know the importance of sterile technique to decrease the likelihood of systemic infection.
- Explain the need for careful monitoring of the patient during the treatment, particularly for fluid and electrolyte imbalance. *Rationale:* The patient and family should understand that careful monitoring is a routine part of CRRT.
- Explain the signs and symptoms of possible complications during CRRT.[42] *Rationale:* The patient and family should be fully prepared if complications occur (e.g., hypotension, hemorrhage, manifestations of fluid/electrolyte/acid-base imbalance).
- Explain the CRRT circuit setup to the patient and family. *Rationale:* It is important that the patient and family know that blood will be removed from the patient's body and will be visible during the CRRT treatment.

PATIENT ASSESSMENT AND PREPARATION

Patient Assessment

- Assess baseline vital signs, including hemodynamic parameters, weight, current medications, laboratory values (blood urea nitrogen, creatinine, electrolytes, hemoglobin, and hematocrit), neurological status, and nutritional needs.[11,16,17,20,22,28,42] *Rationale:* Patients in renal failure often have altered baseline assessment results, both in physical assessment and in laboratory values. Knowledge of this information before treatments are started is helpful so interventions, including net fluid balance and dialysate fluid, can be individualized. Alterations during treatment are common because of the rapid removal of fluid and solutes.

- Assess the VAC insertion site for signs and symptoms of infection.[3] *Rationale:* Insertion sites provide a portal of entry for organisms, which may result in septicemia if unrecognized or untreated. If the insertion site appears to be infected, further interventions (e.g., site change, culture, antibiotic treatment) may be necessary.
- Assess the patency of the VAC and the ability to easily aspirate blood from both ports.[3] *Rationale:* Adequate blood flow is necessary during treatment to facilitate optimal fluid and solute removal. Patent catheter ports are necessary for adequate blood flow.
- Assess adequate circulation to the distal parts of the access limb. *Rationale:* The placement of vascular access may compromise circulation.

Patient Preparation

- Verify the correct patient with two identifiers. *Rationale:* Before performing a procedure, the nurse should ensure the correct identification of the patient for the intended intervention.
- Before CRRT initiation, ensure that informed consent has been obtained. *Rationale:* Informed consent protects the rights of the patient.
- Ensure the patient understands the preprocedural teaching. Answer questions as they arise, and reinforce information as needed. *Rationale:* Understanding of previously taught information is evaluated and reinforced.
- Position the patient in a comfortable position (that also facilitates optimal blood flow through the vascular access). *Rationale:* The patient and family must understand that movement may affect blood flow through the system and that a comfortable position is important.
- Following initiation of treatment, continue to reposition the patient at regular intervals. *Rationale:* Critically ill patients are at a high risk for pressure points and skin breakdown.

Procedure for Initiation and Termination of Continuous Renal Replacement Therapy		
Steps	Rationale	Special Considerations
Systems (SCUF, CVVH, CVVHD, CVVHDF)		
1. **HH**		
2. **PE**		
3. Verify orders, which should include the following: A. Modality B. Vascular access C. Type of hemofilter/dialyzer D. Anticoagulant type, concentration, infusion rate, monitoring parameters, and calcium replacement if indicated E. Replacement fluid and rate (CVVH or CVVHDF) F. Hourly net fluid goal G. Calculate hourly UF rate H. Dialysate solution and rate (CVVHD or CVVHDF) I. Blood pressure/vital sign parameters J. Laboratory testing	Familiarizes the nurse with the individualized patient treatment and reduces the possibility of error.[3,5,6,13,14,16-18,21,27,28,30-34,39,40,42]	Ensure that patient weight and laboratory values are assessed and recorded before initiation of therapy. Communicate with the nephrologist/intensivist ordering therapy if questions arise.[10,42,43]

UNIT V

UNIT V

Procedure for Initiation and Termination of Continuous Renal Replacement Therapy—*Continued*

Steps	Rationale	Special Considerations

4. Prepare the system:
   A. Turn the machine on.
   B. Load the circuit according to the manufacturer's instructions.
   C. Follow the manufacturer's instructions and prompts from the control screen for solution setup, connections, and so on.
   D. Attach solutions as prescribed.
   E. Prepare the anticoagulant infusion as prescribed.
   F. Prepare the replacement fluid, dialysate, and flush infusion as prescribed.
   G. Automated setup instructions include the following:
     1. Selecting therapy/modality
     2. Calibrating (if indicated)
     3. Loading the set
     4. Priming
     5. Anticoagulant
     6. Dialysate and replacement fluid rates
     7. Blood flow rate
     8. Fluid removal rate
   H. After priming per manufacturer's instructions, **go to Step 5.**
	Correct system setup is imperative for safety and optimal functioning. The use of anticoagulants prolongs the function of the hemofilter.[32]	Each CRRT machine will have specific instructions for setup; follow as directed, and troubleshoot if needed.[4,15,35]

5. Leave the priming bag, collection bag, and protective caps in place until the blood lines are attached to the VAC.	Preserves the sterility of the system.	Some systems have a collection bag for the priming solution, which stays attached to the venous blood line until it is attached to the VAC.
6. Remove gloves, and discard **PE** in the appropriate receptacles.	Reduces transmission of microorganisms; standard precautions.	
7. Wash hands.	Reduces transmission of microorganisms on the hands after removal of gloves and before performing a sterile procedure.	
8. Everyone in the room should have a face mask in place before opening a sterile field or accessing the VAC. Limit the number of visitors while the procedure is taking place.	Reduces transmission of microorganisms; standard precautions.	Prevents the chance of airborne contamination.[3,8,9,26]
9. Prepare a "No Touch"/ sterile field with a barrier under the VAC.[8,9,26]	Prepares material and maintains aseptic technique.	Always handle the catheter using aseptic technique.[9]
10. Open sterile antiseptic wipes (chlorhexidine gluconate, alcohol, or any other combination per facility guidelines), empty 5- or 10-mL syringes, prefilled NS syringes, or blunt-tip needles and NS to fill additional empty 5- or 10-mL syringes, and place on the sterile field.	Prepares material and maintains aseptic technique.	Should at minimum have two NS flushes and two empty syringes. Empty syringes will be used with withdraw contents from the VAC.

Procedure continues on following page

Procedure	**for Initiation and Termination of Continuous Renal Replacement Therapy—*Continued***	
Steps	Rationale	Special Considerations
11. If prefilled antiseptic wands or wipes are not available, add 4 × 4 gauze sponges to the sterile field. Then add an antiseptic solution (e.g., 2% chlorhexidine–based preparation) to the sterile container.	Prepares solution used to cleanse VAC ports; 10% povidone-iodine, 70% alcohol, or greater than 0.5% chlorhexidine with alcohol solutions are acceptable bactericidal agents.[8,9,26]	There is not enough evidence to recommend one solution over the other for cleaning the catheter hubs.[8,9,26]
12. Wash hands, and apply new clean or sterile gloves.[8,9,26]	Maintains aseptic technique.	Follow facility-based guidelines for recommendations on clean versus sterile gloves.
13. If prefilled syringes are not available, attach the blunt-tip needles to two 10-mL syringes; with help of an assistant, fill with NS, or use prefilled syringes per institutional standards.	Prepares syringe for VAC flushing.	Follow the manufacturer's guidelines for flushing and accessing the VAC. Many of the catheters have varying fill volumes.
14. Use the prepackaged antiseptic wipes/wands to scrub the hub on the VAC.[9] Follow institutional guidelines regarding the length of the scrub. At minimum, perform for 15–30 seconds[7,29] with friction scrub of the access and return ports of the VAC.	Prevents introduction of pathogens.	Be sure to remove any residual, old blood or drainage at the catheter insertion site. Use a new antiseptic pad for each lumen. Scrub the sides (threads) and the end of each hub.
15. Using an antiseptic pad, apply antiseptic with friction to the VAC, moving from the hub to at least several centimeters toward the body. Hold the catheter while allowing the antiseptic to dry.[9]	Prevents introduction of pathogens.	
16. Ensure that clamps are closed on the access and return ports of the VAC, then remove the cap from the access port of the VAC and discard. Alternatively, many facilities are using dialysis-specific luer caps and an antiseptic soaking cap[4] that lock into the VAC. If using the dialysis-specific luer cap, replace the cap with every new filter tubing change.	The VAC is not opened to air unless caps require changing, reducing the chance of contamination and infection.	Always handle the catheter hubs aseptically. Once disinfected, do not allow the catheter hubs to touch nonsterile surfaces.[9] Ensure that the VAC clamp is closed before removing the access and return port caps. Minimize the time that the ports are exposed.[3] The soaking cap has an antiseptic-impregnated sponge designed to be placed on the top of the catheter hub to provide a level of protection from pathogens. There are inconclusive recommendations about whether an additional scrub is necessary, but it is recommended at this time until further evidence is brought forward.[9]
17. Attach an empty 5- or 10-mL syringe to the access port, open the clamp, and gently aspirate fill volume of the catheter (listed on the lumen) of blood and anticoagulant. Close the clamp, remove the syringe, and discard it in an appropriate receptacle.	Verifies the patency of the access port. Note any resistance, which may indicate a clotted or kinked port. Prevents bolus of anticoagulant to the patient (if used) and decreases transmission of microorganisms.	Always handle the catheter hubs aseptically. Once disinfected, do not allow the catheter hubs to touch nonsterile surfaces.[9] Do not forward-flush an indwelling port before aspirating. This prevents dislodgment/embolism of clots and prevents a bolus of anticoagulant to the patient. Observe for clots. A clotted or kinked port decreases blood flow and reduces efficacy of the treatment.

UNIT V

Procedure	for Initiation and Termination of Continuous Renal Replacement Therapy—*Continued*

Steps	Rationale	Special Considerations
18. Attach a 10-mL syringe with NS flush solution to the access port. Open the clamp and flush; then close the clamp.	Prevents clotting of blood until dialysis is initiated.	Always handle the catheter hubs aseptically. Once disinfected, do not allow the catheter hubs to touch nonsterile surfaces.[9] Note any resistance on flushing.
19. **Follow steps 16–18** for the VAC return port.		Limit the time that the port is open to air.[9]
20. Follow the filter manufacturer's guidelines regarding the amount of time between priming the filter and connecting the circuit to the patient.	Prevents reactions to sterilization products used during manufacturing process of the filter.	These reactions occur due to AN69 and have a bradykinin response.
21. Disconnect the access line from the primed circuit, and attach it to the access port of the VAC; secure the connection. Ensure a tight connection from the filter to the VAC.	Loose connections introduce air into the circuit.	
22. Disconnect the return line from the primed circuit, and attach it to the return port of the VAC; secure the connection. Ensure a tight connection from the filter to the VAC.	Loose connections introduce air into the circuit.	
23. Open the clamps on the VAC ports and the access and return blood lines.	Opens the circuit in preparation for starting the blood pump.	Perform a final check for air in the circuit.
24. Ensure that all connections are secure on the filter and lines that are connected to the VAC.		
25. Ensure that all clamps on the filter tubing are unclamped.		
26. Check that all alarms are on and parameters are set.	Ensures safe delivery of therapy.	
27. Watch the machine pressures and patient hemodynamics. Gradually increase the blood flow to the prescribed rate.	Prevents hypotension from rapid blood and fluid shifts.	Observe for blood leaks, air in the system, and pressure alarms. Assess the patient's vital signs, which should remain within 20% of baseline parameters.
28. Note the blood pump flow rate, access and return monitor pressures, transmembrane (TMP) filter pressure, pressure drop, filtration fraction, the amount and color of UF, and vital signs on initiation and hourly or per institutional standards.	Ensures safe delivery of therapy.	Document per protocol.
29. Remove **PE**, and discard supplies in the appropriate receptacles.	Safely discards used supplies.	
30. **HH**		
31. Prepare a fluid balance flow sheet, and calculate the net fluid gain/loss prescribed each hour, or document in the electronic health record.	Accurate calculations of hourly fluid balance prevent hypervolemia and hypovolemia and ensure that clinical goals are being met.	Hourly fluid balance is usually calculated by subtracting the total output (including UF removed) from the total intake.

Termination

1. **HH**		
2. **PE**		
3. Turn off all infusions into the circuit.	Prepares for termination of therapy.	

Procedure continues on following page

Procedure	for Initiation and Termination of Continuous Renal Replacement Therapy—*Continued*	
Steps	**Rationale**	**Special Considerations**
4. With the IV accessory spike, attach the NS flush solution to the access infusion line of the circuit.	Prepares for flushing blood from the tubing.	The machine may require 1–2 L of NS fluid for blood return; follow the manufacturer's guidelines.
5. Follow onscreen directions for blood return.		
6. Return the blood in the circuit to the patient. Follow the manufacturer's guidelines for the recommended volume of fluid to return to the patient (may be the volume kept in the circuit).	Follow instructions on the pump for termination. The blood should be flushed from the circuit back to the patient to prevent unnecessary blood loss.	If clots are identified beyond the venous bubble trap, stop the pump; do not return blood to the patient.
7. Continue terminating the procedure according to the manufacturer's guidelines.		
8. If the VAC is to be discontinued, remove it per institutional standards.	CRRT therapy may no longer be needed.	Frequently, patients are transitioned from CRRT to intermittent hemodialysis (HD).
9. Record the volume of NS infused.	Ensures accurate fluid balance.	The flush solution infused to the patient must be recorded as intake.
10. If the VAC will not be removed, prepare supplies for the catheter lock and dressing change per institutional standards.	Maintains aseptic technique.	
11. Prepare a "No Touch"/sterile field with a barrier under the VAC.[8,9,26]	Prepares material and maintains aseptic technique.	Always handle the catheter using aseptic technique.[8,9,26]
12. Open the sterile antiseptic wipes (chlorhexidine gluconate, alcohol, or any other combination per facility guidelines), empty 5- or 10-mL syringes, prefilled NS syringes, or blunt-tip needles and NS to fill additional empty 5- or 10-mL syringes, and place it on the sterile field.	Prepares material and maintains aseptic technique.	There should be a minimum of two NS flushes and two empty syringes. Empty syringes will be used with withdraw contents from the VAC.
13. If prefilled antiseptic wands or wipes are not available, add 4 × 4 gauze sponges to the sterile field. Then add an antiseptic solution (e.g., 2% chlorhexidine–based preparation) to sterile container.	Prepares solution used to cleanse VAC ports; 10% povidone-iodine, 70% alcohol, or greater than 0.5% chlorhexidine with alcohol solutions are acceptable bactericidal agents.[8,9,26]	
14. Wash hands, and apply new clean gloves.[4]	Maintains aseptic technique.	
15. If prefilled syringes are not available, attach blunt-tip needles to two 10-mL syringes; with help of an assistant, fill with NS, or use prefilled syringes per institutional standards.	Prepares the syringe for VAC flushing.	Follow manufacturer guidelines for flushing and accessing the VAC. Many of the catheters have varying fill volumes.
16. Ensure that all lines are clamped. Disconnect the lines from the filter that attach to the access.		

UNIT V

Procedure	for Initiation and Termination of Continuous Renal Replacement Therapy—*Continued*		
Steps	**Rationale**	**Special Considerations**	
17. Use the prepackaged antiseptic wipes/wands to scrub the hub on the VAC.[9] Follow institutional guidelines regarding the length of the scrub. At minimum, perform a 15- to 30-second[7,29] with friction scrub of the access and return ports of the VAC.	Prevents introduction of pathogens.	Be sure to remove any residual, old blood or drainage at the catheter insertion site. Use a new antiseptic pad for each lumen. Scrub the sides (threads) and the end of each hub.	
18. Using an antiseptic pad, apply antiseptic with friction to the VAC, moving from the hub to at least several centimeters toward the body. Hold the catheter while allowing the antiseptic to dry.[9]	Prevents introduction of pathogens.		
19. Follow facility specific guidelines related to the flushing and locking the VAC. Instill the prescribed anticoagulant into each access port according to institutional standards. Use only the "fill" amount listed on the VAC ports to avoid instilling anticoagulant into the patient. (Many facilities are now using NS instead of heparin or citrate.)	Maintains patency of the accesses.	Label each port with the date, time, anticoagulant used, and your initials.	
20. Apply new sterile needleless dialysis-specific luer caps and antiseptic soaking cap[9] per institutional policy.	Maintains sterility of the VAC.		
21. **Follow steps 16–20** for the VAC return port.		Limit the time that the port is open to air.[9]	
22. Change the vascular access dressings according to institutional guidelines.	Prevents infection.		
23. Remove **PE**, and discard used equipment in the appropriate receptacle.	Safely discards used supplies.		
24. **HH**			

Expected Outcomes

- VAC accessed without complications
- Blood easily aspirated from the access site
- Accumulated fluid and waste products removed
- Acid-base balance restored
- Blood urea nitrogen and creatinine values restored to baseline levels
- Electrolyte levels within baseline values
- Hemodynamic stability and maintenance of optimal intravascular volume
- Nutritional status maintained[42]

Unexpected Outcomes

- Clotting/decreased patency of access sites
- Crack in the VAC or end caps leading to air embolus
- Bleeding from the VAC insertion site or access/return lines
- Signs and symptoms of infection at the insertion or access site
- Dislodgment or migration of the VAC
- Decreased circulation in the extremity with the vascular access
- Hematoma formation at the VAC insertion site
- Physiological complications (dysrhythmias, chest pain, fluid or electrolyte imbalance, complications related to anticoagulation, air embolism, hypotension, seizures, nausea and vomiting, headache, muscle cramping, dyspnea, exsanguination, hemorrhage)
- Introduction of pathogens or air into the circuit
- Technical problems with the equipment (blood leak, air leak, clotting, disconnection of circuit, hemolysis, hemofilter rupture)
- Hypothermia[42]
- Electrolyte disturbances[42]
- Medication errors[42]
- Malnutrition

Patient Monitoring and Care

Steps	Rationale	Reportable Conditions
		These conditions should be reported to the provider if they persist despite interventions.
1. Obtain and record predialysis and daily weight.	Predialysis weight is an important factor in deciding how much UF is needed and helps guide ongoing treatment.[11,16,17,20,22,28,42]	• Increase or decrease in weight
2. Perform ongoing assessments, including the following: A. Vital signs B. Jugular vein distention C. Presence of edema D. Intake and output E. Neurological assessment F. Pulmonary assessment G. Cardiac monitoring	Provides information in response to treatment.[16,17,28] Monitors for complications.	• Hypotension • Hypertension • Tachycardia/bradycardia • Tachypnea • Fever • Hypothermia[42] • Jugular vein distention • Crackles in lung fields • Edema • Change in level of consciousness, dizziness • Change in cardiac rhythm • Diminished capillary refill
3. Monitor the circulation to the extremity where the VAC is located.	Assesses for any decrease in perfusion distal to the VAC site.[3,6,28,30]	• Diminished or absent peripheral pulses, numbness, tingling, or pain in the extremity • Pale, mottled, or cyanotic color • Cool to touch • Diminished or absent movement or sensation

UNIT V

Patient Monitoring and Care —*Continued*

Steps	Rationale	Reportable Conditions

4. Monitor electrolytes, glucose, and albumin during treatment as prescribed or per institutional standards.	Must be monitored because of continued fluid and electrolyte shifts during treatment. Amino acids are also lost through the hemofilter.	• Electrolyte disturbances (either hypo or hyper)[42]
		  • Potassium
		  • Sodium
		  • Calcium
		  • Magnesium
		  • Phosphate
		• Hyperglycemia or hypoglycemia
		• Hypoalbuminemia

5. Administer medications to correct electrolyte abnormalities as needed during treatment. **(Level D*)**	Patients with renal failure are predisposed to many electrolyte abnormalities. During CRRT, medications or electrolyte replacements may be given as prescribed for individual patients.[11,20,42] The patient is required to have a renal diet with adjusted protein, potassium, phosphorous, carbohydrate, and fluid intake that accounts for the patient's current catabolic state, renal function, adequacy of dialysis, and removal of amino acids via dialysis.[28,42]	• Electrolyte disturbances (either hypo or hyper)[42]
		  • Potassium
		  • Sodium
		  • Calcium
		  • Magnesium
		  • Phosphate
		• Hyperglycemia or hypoglycemia
		• Hypoalbuminemia
		• Unexpected change in weight (loss or gain)

6. Monitor the CRRT circuit (e.g., occlusions; kinks in UF, blood, or vascular access lines; hemofilter).	Disconnections or introduction of air into the circuit are always possible during treatment. Bleeding or exsanguination can also occur.[2,6,23-25,28,34,36,38,42] Clotting of the circuit is a potential complication.[2,23-25,36,38] If the hemofilter needs replacing, the extracorporeal blood volume should be returned to the patient if possible. Blood leaks from the filter into the dialysate may occur and necessitate termination of treatment. In the event of a filter leak, do *not* return circuit blood to the patient. Access or return pressures that are out of range may indicate filter or access malfunction.	• Disconnections, cracks, or leaks • Excessive clotting • Blood leaks/hemofilter rupture • Malfunction of dialyzer or access
7. Monitor UF for rate, clarity, and air bubbles.	A decrease in UF production can occur from clotting of the dialyzer.[2,23-25,28,36,38] Pink or blood-tinged UF is indicative of a filter leak or rupture. In the event of a filter leak, do *not* return circuit blood to the patient.	• Decreases in UF production • Change in color or characteristics of UF • Air in UF
8. Administer anticoagulant as prescribed.	Heparin or citrate is often used to prevent clotting of the circuit.[2,22-25,28,36,38] The heparin/citrate dose varies according to patient condition and laboratory values.	• Suspicion of clotting in the circuit
9. Monitor anticoagulation per institutional standards.	Because heparin or citrate is commonly used to prevent system clotting, coagulation studies should be routinely monitored.	• Abnormal coagulation study results
10. Monitor the vascular access.	Bleeding and/or infection can occur from the access site. Clotting of the access can occur.[2,6,23-25,28,34,36,38,42]	• Decrease in access function or patency • Bleeding • Site redness or edema • Warmth • Purulent drainage • Pain or tenderness • Fever

*Level D: Peer-reviewed professional and organizational standards with the support of clinical study recommendations.

Procedure continues on following page

Patient Monitoring and Care —*Continued*

Steps	Rationale	Reportable Conditions
11. Monitor the patient for complications associated with CRRT treatment.	Complications are possible with CRRT.[28,42]	• Muscle cramps • Air embolism • Dialyzer reaction (hypotension, pruritus, back pain, angioedema, anaphylaxis) • Hypoxemia • Hypothermia[28,42] • Dialysis disequilibrium syndrome (headache, nausea and vomiting, hypertension, decreased sensorium, seizures, coma)
12. Monitor the equipment for proper functioning.	Alerts the nurse to problems with the procedure.	• Problems with the equipment
13. Follow institutional guidelines for assessing pain. Administer analgesia as prescribed.	Identifies the need for pain interventions.	• Continued pain despite pain interventions

Documentation

Documentation should include the following:
- Patient and family education
- Completion of informed consent
- Date and time of treatment initiation, mode of therapy, filter change
- Condition of vascular access regarding patency, quality of blood flow, ease of access procedure
- Date and time of VAC insertion and dressing change
- Condition of insertion site and any signs or symptoms of infection
- Blood flow rate and access and return monitoring pressures
- Other machine pressures as required by facility standards (e.g., transmembrane pressure drop)
- Prescribed dose and delivered dose[31]
- Type and content of dialysate and replacement fluids
- Anticoagulation type and dose
- Vital signs/hemodynamic parameters
- Status of pulse distal to the vascular access site
- Hourly fluid balance calculation
- Patient's response to CRRT and daily progress toward treatment goals
- Unexpected outcomes
- Nursing interventions
- Daily weight
- Laboratory assessment data
- Pain assessment, interventions, and effectiveness

For a complete list of references and additional readings for this procedure, scan this QR code with your smartphone, or visit https://www.elsevier.com/__data/assets/pdf_file/0003/1319880/Chapter0105.pdf.

UNIT V

106 Hemodialysis

Heather L. Przybyl and Amanda J. Golino

PURPOSE Hemodialysis is performed for volume regulation, acid-base control, electrolyte regulation, management of azotemia, and the treatment of drug intoxication.

DEFINITIONS

- Disease process[34,35,59]
  - Acute kidney diseases and disorders (AKD): Signs of alterations in kidney function and/or kidney damage occurring within 1 week or up to 3 months.[35]
  - Chronic kidney disease (CKD): Kidney abnormalities that have been present over 3 months, including either alterations in kidney function or kidney damage.
  - Acute kidney injury (AKI): Clinical syndrome of kidney injury with multiple etiologies. Can be a subset of either AKD or CKD and is characterized by an increase in serum creatinine: 1.5 times the baseline that evolves over 48 hours.
- Therapy[29,60]
  - Kidney replacement therapy (KRT), previously known as *renal replacement therapy* (RRT), is a therapy that compensates kidney function in patients with renal failure. KRT encompasses the following therapies:
    - Intermittent hemodialysis (IHD) (Fig. 106.1) is used in hemodynamically stable patients. IHD may be needed for the onset of AKI, maintenance therapy for patients with chronic kidney failure, or for patients with acute drug intoxication or medication toxicity (e.g., Lithium, Tylenol). IHD can be prescribed as daily or every other day. IHD typically runs for 3 to 4 hours.[26,57]
    - Continuous renal replacement therapy (CRRT) used in hemodynamically unstable patients that runs continuously for 24 hours (see Procedure 105, Continuous Renal Replacement Therapies, for more information on CRRT).
    - Sustained low-efficiency dialysis (SLED) and sustained low-efficiency daily dialysis (SLEDD) are used in hemodynamically unstable patients. The therapy does not run continuously as the therapies run typically for 6 to 12 hours.[26]
    - Peritoneal dialysis (PD) uses the lining in the abdominal cavity and dialysate fluid to remove waste products not accomplished by the patient's native kidney (see Procedure 107, Peritoneal Dialysis for more information on PD).
- Access[2,4,5,7,41,55]
  - Arteriovenous fistula (AVF) is surgically created by anastomosis between an artery and vein. The increased blood flow from the artery to the vein results in engorgement, dilation, and thickening of the vein wall. AVF is the gold standard for vascular access.[4,5,21,41,55]

- Arteriovenous graft (AVG) a surgical connection between the artery and vein using a synthetic tube.[4,55] AVG is considered when patient's vessels are too small to create a successful AVF.
- Hemodialysis vascular access catheter (VAC): A dual-lumen catheter that can be tunneled (cuffed) or not tunneled (uncuffed). Right internal jugular (RIJ) is the preferred location of the VAC.

PREREQUISITE NURSING KNOWLEDGE

- Knowledge of the principles of diffusion, ultrafiltration (UF), osmosis, oncotic pressure, and hydrostatic pressure as they pertain to fluid and solute management during dialysis.[3,47]
  - *Diffusion:* Passive movement of solutes through a semipermeable membrane from an area of higher to lower concentration until equilibrium is reached. Diffusion primarily effects small-molecule solutes.[3,25] Diffusion is the primary principle that drives hemodialysis.[3]
  - *Convective* transport: Rapid movement of fluid across a semipermeable membrane from an area of high pressure to an area of low pressure with transport of solutes. When water moves across a membrane along a pressure gradient, some solutes are carried along with the water and do not require a solute concentration gradient (also called *solute drag*). Convective transport is most effective for removal of medium-molecular-weight and large-molecular-weight solutes.[3]
  - *UF:* Bulk movement of solute and solvent through a semipermeable membrane with a pressure movement. This movement is usually achieved with positive pressure in the blood compartment of the hemodialyzer and negative pressure in the dialysate compartment. Blood and dialysate flow countercurrent to each other. The size of the solute molecules compared with the size of molecules that can move through the semipermeable membrane determines the degree of UF.[3]
  - *Osmosis:* Passive movement of solvent through a semipermeable membrane from an area of higher to lower concentration.[3]
  - *Oncotic pressure:* Pressure exerted by plasma proteins that favors intravascular fluid retention and movement of fluid from the extravascular to the intravascular space.[3]

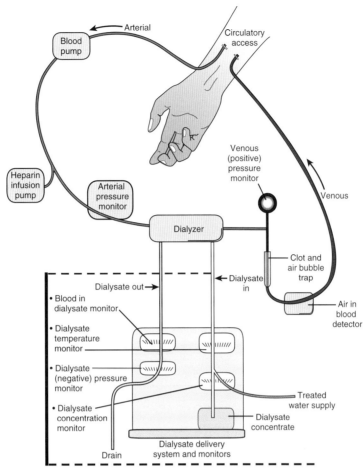

Figure 106.1 Components of a typical hemodialysis system. *(From Thompson JM, et al, editors: Mosby's manual of clinical nursing, St. Louis, 1989, Mosby.)*

❖ *Hydrostatic pressure:* Force exerted by arterial blood pressure that favors the movement of fluid from the intravascular to the extravascular space.[3]

❖ *Absorption:* Process by which drug molecules pass through membranes and fluid barriers and into body fluids.[3]

❖ *Adsorption*: Adhesion of molecules (solutes) to the surface to the hemodialyzer, charcoal, or resin.[3]

❖ *Azotemia:* Abnormally elevated levels of nitrogen-containing compounds (i.e., urea, creatinine, other waste products created in the body) in the blood.[20,57]

INDICATIONS, RIFLE/AKIN CRITERIA FOR HD INITIATION

- Indications for IHD[29,57]
  - ❖ Renal indications include the following:
    - ○ Azotemia
    - ○ Volume overload or oliguria
    - ○ Electrolyte disturbances, commonly hyperkalemia[42,57]
    - ○ Metabolic acidosis[26]
  - ❖ Nonrenal indications[29]
    - ○ Sepsis
    - ○ Thermoregulation

- ○ Drug overdose, intoxication
- ○ Rhabdomyolysis
- ○ Radiocontrast-induced AKI
- The RIFLE (Risk, Injury, Failure, Loss, End-Stage) or the AKIN (Acute Kidney Injury Network) scales are commonly used by nephrologists to determine the level of kidney impairment. The scales assess variations in serum creatinine levels, glomerular filtration rate, and urine output to determine the level of impairment. These values assist the provider in determining the best modality to treat the patient based on the stage of renal failure.[20,29,49]

Vascular Access[2,4]

- Vascular access is needed to perform hemodialysis and can be provided with a double-lumen vascular access catheter (VAC) or a surgically created arteriovenous (AV) anastomosis (e.g., fistula or graft).[2,4,5,12,21] The AV fistula or graft is used for long-term dialysis management.[2,4,39]
- Advantages and disadvantages of the AVF/AVG/VAC (Table 106.1)
- Decision tree for location of vascular access of a temporary VAC[30,38]
  1. Right jugular vein

TABLE 106.1   **Advantages and Disadvantages of the AVF/AVG/VAC**

	AVF	AVG	VAC

Advantages	• Patency of AVF is typically 3 years[4]
	• Lower rates of
	  • Infection[4,5,7,21]
	  • Thrombosis[4,5,7,21]
	  • Morbidity[4,5]
	• Less chance of allergic response to foreign material[4]
	• Cardiac complications
	  • High-output heart failure[7,15]
	• Can use buttonhole technique for cannulation[4]
		• Surface area is larger than AVF, providing needle insertion with less chance of complications[4]
		• Shorter healing time[4]
		• Able to be placed in more shapes and locations than the AVF[4]
		• Easier to repair than the AVF if needed[4]
			• No limitations on patient selection for VAC[4]
			• No time needed for line to mature; can be utilized immediately
			• Can be in place for months depending on location and type (tunneled versus nontunneled)[4]

Disadvantages	• Vein may fail to enlarge or increase thickness[4]
	• Vein may take weeks to months to mature[4]
	• Difficult to cannulate vein[4]
	• Body image may be distorted due to enlarged vein[4]
	• Specialized training is required to access AVF; technique is different to access compared with AVG[4,29]
		• Higher rates of
		  • Stenosis[4,7]
		  • Infections[4,7]
		• May have a reaction to the foreign material that makes the graft[7]
		• Higher mortality rate[4]
		• Shorter length of patency compared with AVF. Typically, 1–2 years[4]
		• Specialized training is required to access AVG; technique is different compared with AVF[4,29]
			• Highest infection rates compared with AVF/AVG[4,7]
			• Risk of permanent stenosis or occlusion[4]
			• Specialized training required to access VAC[4]

AVF, Arteriovenous fistula; *AVG,* arteriovenous graft; *VAC,* vascular access catheter.

2. Right external jugular vein[38]
3. Femoral vein
4. Left jugular vein
5. Subclavian vein with preference for the dominant side
6. Tunneled transhepatic, typically the final option
• Common locations for AVF[38]
1. Forearm radial or ulnar basilic
2. Antecubital vessel
3. Brachiocephalic
4. Brachiobasilic
5. Other combination of brachial or basilic
• Common locations for AVG[38]
1. Forearm loop
2. Upper arm straight
3. Upper arm loop
4. Thigh loop
• The subclavian vein is not recommended for temporary access because of the increased incidence of vascular stenosis, which makes the vein of the ipsilateral arm unsuitable for chronic dialysis if needed.[30]
• When discussing long-term access goals of IHD, there was a focus ensuring that optimal access was available to patients in a timely manner. These initiatives were "Fistula First" in 2003 and then "Fistula First, Catheter Last" in 2007. The initiatives encouraged patients to move to getting an AVF as soon as possible. Now the focus has a patient-centered approach, additionally taking into consideration the patient's preferences. This is called *Life-Plan* or *Patient Life-plan Access Needs* (PLAN).[7,38,58]

Hemodialysis Dialyzer/Filter[3]

• Hemodialysis uses an artificial kidney (hemodialyzer, dialyzer, filter) with a semipermeable membrane to create two separate compartments: the blood compartment and the dialysis solution (dialysate) compartment.[3]
  ❖ The semipermeable membrane allows the movement of small molecules (e.g., electrolytes, urea, drugs) and medium-weight molecules (e.g., creatinine) from the patient's blood into the dialysate but is impermeable to larger molecules (e.g., blood cells, plasma proteins).
• Each dialyzer has four ports: two end ports for blood (in one end and out the other) and two side ports for dialysis solution (also in one end and out the other). In most cases, the blood and dialysate are run through the dialyzer in opposite or countercurrent directions.
• The hollow-fiber dialyzer is the most commonly used dialyzer. With this dialyzer, the blood flows through the center of hollow fibers, and the dialysate flows around the outside of the hollow fibers.
  ❖ The advantages of hollow-fiber filters include a low priming volume, low resistance to flow, and high amount of surface area.
  ❖ The major disadvantage is the potential for clotting because of the small fiber size.[46]
• All dialyzers have UF coefficients; thus the dialyzer selected varies in different clinical situations. The higher the UF coefficient, the more rapid the fluid removal. UF coefficients are determined with in vivo measurements performed by each dialyzer manufacturer.[36,46]

- *Clearance* refers to the ability of the dialyzer to remove metabolic waste products from the patient's blood. The blood flow rate, the dialysate flow rate, and the solute concentration affect clearance. Clearance occurs by the processes of diffusion, convection, and UF.[25,46]
- The blood circuit consists of blood lines, a blood pump, and various monitoring devices. The blood lines carry the blood to and from the patient. The blood pump controls the speed of the blood through the circuit. The monitoring devices include arterial and venous pressure monitors, an air detection monitor to prevent air entering the circuit from being returned to the patient, and conductivity detectors to measure dialysate chemistry.
- Transmembrane filter pressures (TMP) measures pressures across the filter and are closely associated with clotting or clogging of the filter. Analysis of these pressures in addition to the blood filter prevents clots from going to the patient.

Dialysate and Other Fluids

- The dialysate is composed of water, a buffer (e.g., bicarbonate), and various electrolytes.[18]
  - The buffer helps neutralize acids that are generated as a result of normal cellular metabolism and usually are excreted by the kidney.
  - The composition of electrolytes reflects normal plasma levels, which help create a concentration gradient for removal of excess electrolytes.
  - A fundamental goal of IHD is to maintain serum potassium levels within normal range during both intradialytic (during) and interdialytic (period between) treatment sessions.[52]
  - Most solutions also contain glucose, which promotes the removal of plasma water.[44]
- Because large volumes of water are used during treatments to generate the dialysate, the water must be purified before patient use to prevent patient exposure to potentially harmful substances present in the water supply (e.g., calcium carbonate, sodium chloride, iron).[18,26,31,56]

Anticoagulation

- Use of anticoagulants during dialysis is aimed at preventing the inflammatory response and thereby inhibiting the clotting cascade during therapy due to bio-incompatibility between the patient's blood and the synthetic materials it comes into contact with during therapy.[16,23,26,31]
- Unfractionated heparin (UFH) or low-molecular-weight heparin (LMWH) is recommended during dialysis to prevent clotting of the circuit.[16]
- In patients with coagulopathies, normal saline (NS) solution flushes can be used to keep the blood circuit patent.[30,31] Other options for anticoagulation therapies can be considered (e.g., regional citrate anticoagulation, citrate dialysate, argatroban, lepirudin or Flolan), but these are not as common as UFH or LMWH.[31]

- Heparin should be avoided in patients with a history of heparin-induced thrombocytopenia (HIT).[16,30,31]
- One advantage of IHD compared with CRRT is the amount of anticoagulation needed to perform the therapy, with IHD needing much less than CRRT.[23]

Outcome Measures[32,33,40,54]

- The adequacy of dialysis and assessment of the patient's residual renal function should be evaluated on a periodic basis.
  - Adequacy of dialysis can be measured with urea kinetic modeling (Kt/V) or urea clearance.[25,40,54]
  - Measurement of fluid status and volume overload.[9,10,19,36]
  - Residual renal functioning can be monitored with urine creatinine clearance.[32,40]
- Collaboration with the nephrology team is necessary to ensure efficacy of these parameters.[40]
- In addition to the efficacy of IHD outcome measures, focus also must be on the long-term effects that IHD has on the patient and family. Long-term indicators for patients on IHD include quality of life, mental health, family impact, fatigue, and employment.[54,61]

The Future of Hemodialysis

- Future innovations in hemodialysis include portable options for patients that will decrease limitations and pose promise to improve quality of life. These innovations include options such as the artificial and wearable kidney. Further research is anticipated as these products evolve and have the potential to play a significant role in the future of renal care.[28,31]

REQUIRED EQUIPMENT FOR INITIATION OF IHD

- Dedicated vascular access, either AVF, AVG, or VAC
- Dialysis machine, tubing, dialyzer, and dialysate solution/water treatment setup
- Dialysate fluid as prescribed
- PPE as defined by institutional standards
- Clean or sterile gloves[13,14,38] (follow facility-specific guidelines)
- Gowns, fluid shield, face masks or goggles
- Two empty 5- or 10-mL syringes with (dependent on VAC fill volume) syringes to aspirate VAC contents before flushing and connecting the line
- Two 10-mL prefilled syringes with NS solution
- Dressing supplies per facility policy (alcohol wipes, sterile barrier, gauze pads, transparent dressing, tape)
- Antiseptic solution (e.g., 2% chlorhexidine-based preparation)
- Anticoagulant as prescribed (Heparin 1000 units/mL for both priming and infusion)
- Alcohol wipes
- Two dialysis luer caps for VAC (as per institution standards)

UNIT V

- Two alcohol-impregnated caps for the VAC, used when the line is not in use (as per institutional protocols)
- For patients with AVF or AVG, additional equipment may include two plastic hemodialysis clamps (if used by the institution)

REQUIRED EQUIPMENT FOR TERMINATION OF INTERMITTENT HEMODIALYSIS

- PPE as defined by the facility
- Gown, fluid shield, face mask or goggles
- Four hemostats
- 2 × 2 gauze pads
- Bandages and tape
- Nonsterile gloves
- Catheter locking solution (VAC) as prescribed

PATIENT AND FAMILY EDUCATION

- Explain the procedure, and review any questions the patient may have. *Rationale:* Explanation provides information and may decrease patient anxiety.
- Explain the purpose of hemodialysis. *Rationale:* This explanation ensures that the patient and family know that hemodialysis is necessary to perform the physiological functions of the kidneys when kidney failure is present.
- Explain the need for careful monitoring of the patient during the treatment for fluid and electrolyte imbalance. *Rationale:* This explanation prepares the patient for what to expect.
- Explain the importance of input from the patient about how they are feeling during the treatment. *Rationale:* Hypotension is a common occurrence during treatment; the patient may experience lightheadedness or dizziness if hypotension is present. Patient knowledge of this possibility should help decrease anxiety.
- Explain the hemodialysis circuit setup to the patient. *Rationale:* The patient and family must be aware that blood will be removed from the patient's body and will be visible during the hemodialysis treatment.

PATIENT ASSESSMENT AND PREPARATION

Patient Assessment

- Assess baseline vital signs, weight, and neurological status, and perform a physical assessment of all body

systems and fluid and electrolyte status.[27] *Rationale:* Patients in kidney failure often have altered baseline assessments, both in the physical assessment and laboratory values. Having this information before treatments are started is helpful so interventions, including the dialysate, can be individualized. Alterations during treatment are common because of the rapid removal of fluid and solutes.
- Assess the graft, fistula, or VAC site for signs or symptoms of infection.[27] *Rationale:* Because dialysis access sites are used frequently, infection is always a potential risk. Dialysis access sites should only be used for dialysis, and not for other intravenous (IV) access needs, except in an emergency. Insertion sites provide a portal of entry for infection, which may result in septicemia if unrecognized or untreated. If the insertion site appears to be infected, further interventions (e.g., site change, culture, and antibiotic treatment) may be necessary.
- Assess VAC patency and the ability to easily aspirate blood from both ports. *Rationale:* Adequate blood flow is necessary during treatment to facilitate optimal fluid and solute removal. Patent VAC ports are necessary for adequate blood flow.
- With AVF or AVG use, assess the site for the presence of bruit, thrill, erythema, swelling, aneurysms, pseudoaneurysms, and quality of blood flow. *Rationale:* Physical assessment of the fistula can indicate patency of the graft and the possible presence of infection.
- Assess the circulation to the distal parts of the access limb. *Rationale:* Placement of vascular access may cause ischemic steal syndrome (ISS).

Patient Preparation

- Verify the correct patient with two identifiers. *Rationale:* Before performing a procedure, the nurse should ensure the correct identification of the patient for the intended intervention.
- Ensure that the patient understands the preprocedural instructions. Answer questions as they arise, and reinforce information as needed. *Rationale:* Understanding of previously taught information is evaluated and reinforced.
- Position the patient in a comfortable position (that also facilitates optimal blood flow through the access site and allows for setup of the field). *Rationale:* Facilitation of patient comfort helps minimize the amount of patient movement during treatment, which can change the amount of blood flow through the access site. Different access sites may require different patient positions to facilitate optimal blood flow. Patient comfort is promoted, and anxiety may be reduced.

Procedure for Hemodialysis

Steps	Rationale	Special Considerations
Cannulation of the AV Fistula or Graft		
1. 🅷🅷		
2. 🅿🅴	Everyone in the room is required to wear a face mask in place before opening the sterile field.	
3. Locate, inspect, and palpate needle cannulation sites before skin preparation.[4,12,38] Prepare supplies needed to cleanse the access site using an antimicrobial product. Follow the manufacturer's guidelines and facility protocols.[4]	Reduces transmission of microorganisms.	Inspect the whole arm, and compare it against the other extremity. Assess for swelling, circulation, and signs of infection.[4] The first access on a new fistula must be performed with a team member with specialized training.[4,55]
4. Place the patient's arm on a clean barrier.	Maintains aseptic technique.	
5. Wearing clean gloves, starting at the site of insertion and moving out in concentric circles for 2–3 inches, or alternatively a back-and-forth friction scrub to site for 30 seconds minimum.[11,13,37,38] Allow the area to dry completely before proceeding to the next step. **(Level D*)**	Povidone-iodine, 70% isopropyl alcohol, or chlorhexidine bactericidal solution reduces the transmission of microorganisms. • Chlorhexidine has a rapid and prolonged antimicrobial effect; apply solution with back-and-forth friction scrub for 30 seconds.[38] • Isopropyl alcohol is applied using a circular friction motion for 1 minute.[38] • Povidone-iodine solution requires a 2- to 3-minute scrub for bacteriostatic effect.[38]	This is one of the most important steps in the cannulation process. Skin asepsis is crucial to prevent infection. Repeat all steps if the area is touched by the patient or there was a break in aseptic technique.
6. Prepare two 10-mL NS flush syringes: A. Obtain prefilled syringes. *Or* B. Prepare the syringes.	The flush syringes can be used to assess the placement and patency of the fistula/graft.	
7. Attach the flush to the fistula needle tubing, and prime through the fistula needle.	Prevents clotting of blood in the fistula needles.	Do not prime the needle until ready to be used immediately.[4] This creates a "wet needle," which is recommended for cannulation.[4,45]
8. Clamp the tubing.	Prevents loss of solution and backflow of blood.	
9. Apply a tourniquet to the upper portion of the access limb (AVF cannulation).	Facilitates site determination for cannulation.	
10. Determine the technique to access AVF • The rope ladder technique in which the site is rotated between each dialysis session to allow for healing of the vessel is the most commonly used technique. • The buttonhole technique in which a constant site is used at the same angle and same depth each time the vessel is accessed can also be used.	Decreases recirculation of dialyzed blood. The rope ladder technique uses the entire length of the anastomosis. Needles are kept 1.5 to 2 inches apart. Uses a sharp needle to access the vessel. The buttonhole technique uses a sharp needle until a matured opening is formed (usually around 10 cannulations), which is covered by a scab and then switched to a blunt needle.[4]	The venous needle must be in the direction of venous blood flow.[4] The arterial needle can be placed either in the same direction of blood flow (antegrade) or in the opposite direction of blood flow in the vessel (retrograde).[4,12]

*Level D: Peer-reviewed professional and organizational standards with the support of clinical study recommendations.

UNIT V

Procedure	for Hemodialysis—*Continued*	
Steps	**Rationale**	**Special Considerations**
11. Grasp the butterfly wings or the hub of the fistula needle between the thumb and index finger of the dominant hand with the needle tip bevel up.	Provides a secure grasp of the needle on cannulation.	Always insert the needle with the bevel facing up.
12. Remove the needle guard.	Exposes the fistula needle.	
13. Hold the skin taut with the nondominant hand.	Prevents rolling of the vessel.	
14. With the dominant hand: • AVF: Insert the needle at a 25-degree angle to the skin.[4,38] • AVG: Insert the needle at a 45-degree angle to the skin.[4,38]		An angle that is too shallow increases the risk of dragging the needle's cutting edge on the vessel's surface.[4,45] An angle that is too steep increases the risk of perforating the back wall of the vessel.[4,45]
• Slowly advance the bevel up to the hub of the needle.	Accesses the arterial vascular system.	Do not flip or rotate the needle as it may cause trauma to the vessel.[4]
15. AVF: Remove the tourniquet before infusing NS or the prescribed heparin solution.	Prevents clotting or infiltration.	
16. Unclamp the tubing, and aspirate blood.	Verifies the correct placement and patency of the access.	
17. Infuse the flush solution, and then reclamp the tubing.	Prevents clotting and backflow of blood.	
18. Secure the needle with adhesive tape over the insertion site.	Maintains the angle of the needle so it floats freely in the vessel/graft. Assists with prevention of migration of bacteria into the bloodstream.[4]	Three pieces of tape are required:[4] 1. Place the first piece over the wings of the needle. 2. Place the second piece under the needle tubing with the sticky side up, and then cross over in a chevron V shape. 3. The last piece is placed over the chevron tape and applied with a 2 × 2 gauze. This dressing should completely cover the needle puncture site.
19. Repeat **Steps 10–18** for insertion of the second needle.	Cannulation of the venous site. Vascular access and needles must be visible during the duration of therapy, to intervene promptly if dislodgement occurs.	Hemodialysis can now be initiated.
20. Remove **PE**, and discard used equipment in the appropriate receptacle.		
21. **HH**		

Decannulation of the AV Fistula or Graft
1. **HH**
2. **PE**

| 3. Remove both cannulas from the patient's access site, one at a time. With a sterile 2 × 2 gauze pad, apply moderate pressure using two fingers per access site once the needle has been removed until bleeding has stopped. Repeat this for each access site. Hold pressure for a minimum of 10 minutes.[4] | Discontinues vascular access. Promotes hemostasis at access sites. Remember that two holes were created when the needle was inserted: one to the skin and one to the vessel wall. Compression to both sites is crucial to prevent complications such as bleeding or hematoma at the access site.[4] | Removing the needles one at a time prevents unnecessary loss of blood due to the force of pressure in the access. |

Procedure continues on following page

Procedure for Hemodialysis—*Continued*

Steps	Rationale	Special Considerations
4. Apply a sterile dressing to the site.	Provides a protective barrier.	
5. Remove **PE**, and discard used equipment in the appropriate receptacle.		
6. **HH**		
Accessing a VAC		
1. **HH**		
2. **PE**	Everyone in the room is required to wear a face mask in place before opening the "No Touch" field or accessing the VAC.	
3. Prepare a "No Touch"/sterile field with barrier under the VAC.[13,37,38]	Prepares supplies and maintains aseptic technique.	Always handle the catheter using aseptic technique.
4. Open sterile antiseptic wipes (CHG, alcohol, or any other combination per facility guidelines), empty 5- or 10-mL syringes, prefilled NS syringes or blunt-tip needles and NS to fill additional empty 5- or 10-mL syringes, and place on the sterile field.	Prepares material and maintains aseptic technique.	Should at minimum have two NS flushes and two empty syringes. Empty syringes will be used with withdraw contents from the VAC.
5. If prefilled antiseptic wands or wipes are not available, add 4 × 4 gauze sponges to the sterile field. Then add an antiseptic solution (e.g., 2% chlorhexidine-based preparation) to the sterile container.	Prepares solution used to cleanse VAC ports; 10% povidone-iodine, 70% alcohol, or greater than 0.5% chlorhexidine with alcohol solutions are acceptable bactericidal agents.[11,13,37,38]	There is not enough evidence to recommend one solution over the other for cleaning the catheter hubs.[11,13,37,38]
6. Wash hands, and apply new clean or sterile gloves.[11,13,37,38]	Maintains aseptic technique.	Follow institutional protocols for recommendations on clean versus sterile gloves.
7. If prefilled syringes are not available, attach blunt-tip needles to two 10-mL syringes; with help of an assistant, fill with NS, or use prefilled syringes per institutional standards.	Prepares the syringe for VAC flushing.	Follow the manufacturer's guidelines for flushing and accessing the VAC. Many catheters have varying fill volumes.
8. Use the prepackaged antiseptic wipes/wands to "Scrub the Hub" on the VAC.[11,13,37,38] Follow institution guidelines regarding the length of the scrub. At minimum, perform a 15- to 30-second with friction scrub of the access and return ports of the VAC.[4,11,13]	Prevents introduction of pathogens.	Be sure to remove any residual, old blood or drainage at the catheter insertion site. Use a new antiseptic pad for each lumen. Scrub the sides (threads) and the end of each hub.
9. Using an antiseptic pad, apply antiseptic with friction to the VAC, moving from the hub to at least several centimeters toward the body. Hold the catheter while allowing the antiseptic to dry.[13,14]	Prevents introduction of pathogens.	

UNIT V

Procedure for Hemodialysis—*Continued*

Steps	Rationale	Special Considerations
10. Ensure that clamps are closed on the access and return ports of the VAC; then remove the cap from the access port of the VAC and discard. Alternatively, many facilities are using dialysis-specific luer caps and an antiseptic soaking cap[13,14] that lock into the VAC. If using the dialysis-specific luer cap, replace the cap with every new filter tubing change.	The VAC is not opened to air unless caps require changing, reducing the chance of contamination and infection.	Always handle the catheter hubs aseptically. Once disinfected, do not allow the catheter hubs to touch nonsterile surfaces.[11,13,37,38] Be sure the VAC clamp is closed before removing access and return port caps. Minimize the time that the ports are exposed.[4] The soaking cap has a sponge that is impregnated with antiseptic and designed to be placed on the top of the catheter hub to provide some protection from pathogens. There are inconclusive recommendations regarding whether an additional scrub is necessary, but it is recommended at this time until further evidence is brought forward.[13,14]
11. Attach an empty 5- or 10-mL syringe to the access port, open the clamp, and gently aspirate fill volume of the catheter of blood and anticoagulant. Close the clamp, remove the syringe, and discard it in an appropriate receptacle.	Verifies the patency of the access port. Note any resistance, which may indicate a clotted or kinked port. Prevents bolus of anticoagulant to the patient (if used) and decreases transmission of microorganisms.	Always handle the catheter hubs aseptically. Once disinfected, do not allow the catheter hubs to touch nonsterile surfaces.[13,14] Do not forward flush an indwelling port before aspirating. This prevents dislodgment/embolism of clots and prevents a bolus of anticoagulant to the patient. Observe for clots. A clotted or kinked port decreases blood flow and reduces efficacy of the treatment.
12. Attach a 10-mL syringe with NS flush solution to the access port. Open the clamp and flush; then close the clamp.	Prevents clotting of blood until dialysis is initiated.	Always handle the catheter hubs aseptically. Once disinfected, do not allow the catheter hubs to touch nonsterile surfaces.[13,14] Note any resistance on flushing. Limit the time that the port is open to air.[13,14]
13. Follow **Steps 7–12** for the VAC return port.		
14. Follow the filter manufacturer's guidelines regarding the amount of time between priming the filter and connecting the circuit to the patient.	Prevents reactions to sterilization products used during manufacturing process of the filter.	These reactions occur due to AN69 and have a bradykinin response.
15. Disconnect the access line from the primed circuit, and attach it to the access port of the VAC; secure the connection. Ensure a tight connection from the filter to the VAC.	Loose connections introduce air into the circuit.	
16. Disconnect the return line from the primed circuit, and attach it to the return port of the VAC; secure the connection. Ensure a tight connection from the filter to the VAC.	Loose connections introduce air into the circuit.	

Procedure continues on following page

Procedure for Hemodialysis—*Continued*

Steps	Rationale	Special Considerations
17. Open the clamps on the VAC ports and the access and return blood lines.	Opens the circuit in preparation for starting the blood pump.	Perform a final check for air in the circuit.
18. Ensure that all connections are secure on the filter and lines that are connected to the VAC.		
19. Ensure that all clamps on the filter tubing are unclamped.		
Disconnecting from the VAC		
1. 🅷🅷		
2. 🅿🅴	Everyone in the room is required to wear a face mask in place before opening the "No Touch" field or accessing the VAC.	
3. Prepare a "No Touch"/sterile field with barrier under the VAC.[11,13,37,38]	Prepares materials and maintains aseptic technique.	Always handle the catheter using aseptic technique.[11,13,37,38]
4. Open sterile antiseptic wipes (CHG, alcohol, or any other combination per facility guidelines), empty 5- or 10-mL syringes, prefilled NS syringes, or blunt-tip needles and NS to fill additional empty 5- or 10-mL syringes, and place on the sterile field.	Prepares materials and maintains aseptic technique.	Should at minimum have two NS flushes.
5. If prefilled antiseptic wands or wipes are not available, add 4 × 4 gauze sponges to the sterile field. Then add an antiseptic solution (e.g., 2% chlorhexidine-based preparation) to the sterile container.	Prepares solution used to cleanse VAC ports; 10% povidone-iodine, 70% alcohol, or greater than 0.5% chlorhexidine with alcohol solutions are acceptable bactericidal agents.[11,13,37,38]	
6. Wash hands, and apply new clean gloves.[13,14]	Maintains aseptic technique.	
7. If prefilled syringes are not available, attach blunt-tip needles to two 10-mL syringes; with help of an assistant, fill with NS, or use prefilled syringes per institutional standards.	Prepares the syringe for VAC flushing.	Follow the manufacturer's guidelines for flushing and accessing the VAC. Many of the catheters have varying fill volumes.
8. Ensure that all lines are clamped. Disconnect the lines from the dialyzer that attach to the access.		
9. Use the prepackaged antiseptic wipes/wands to scrub the hub on the VAC.[13,14] Follow institutional guidelines regarding the length of the scrub. At minimum, perform a 15- to 30-second[4,11] with friction scrub of the access and return ports of the VAC.	Prevents introduction of pathogens.	Be sure to remove any residual, old blood or drainage at the catheter insertion site. Use a new antiseptic pad for each lumen. Scrub the sides (threads) and the end of each hub.

UNIT V

UNIT V

Procedure for Hemodialysis—*Continued*		
Steps	**Rationale**	**Special Considerations**
10. Using an antiseptic pad, apply antiseptic with friction to the VAC, moving from the hub to at least several centimeters toward the body. Hold the catheter while allowing the antiseptic to dry[13,14]	Prevents introduction of pathogens.	
11. Follow facility-specific guidelines related to the flushing and locking of the VAC. Instill the prescribed anticoagulant into each access port according to institutional standards. Use only the "fill" amount listed on the VAC ports to avoid instilling anticoagulant into the patient. (Many facilities are now using NS instead of heparin or citrate).	Maintains patency of the accesses.	Label each port with the date, time, anticoagulant used, and your initials.
12. Apply new sterile needless dialysis-specific luer caps and an antiseptic soaking cap if applicable.[13,14]	Maintains sterility of the VAC.	
13. Follow **Steps 8–12** for the VAC return port.		Limit the time that the port is open to air.[13,14]
14. Change the vascular access dressings according to institutional guidelines.	Prevents infection.	
15. Remove **PE**, and discard used equipment in the appropriate receptacle.	Safely discards used supplies.	
16. **HH**		

Initiation and Termination of Hemodialysis

1. Verify orders, which should include:[3] A. Vascular access B. Hours of treatment C. Type of hemodialyzer/ dialyzer D. Blood flow rate E. Anticoagulant type, concentration, infusion rate, monitoring parameters F. UF goal G. Dialysate solution and rate H. Blood pressure and vital sign parameters I. Laboratory testing	Familiarizes the nurse with the individualized patient treatment and reduces the possibility of error.[3]	Ensure that the patient's weight and laboratory values are recorded before initiation of therapy.
2. Set up the dialysis machine according to the manufacturer's instructions.	Ensures safe and proper assembly and allows for testing of all patient alarms and the proper functioning of the machine before the VAC/ graft/fistula is accessed.	
3. **HH**		
4. **PE**		

Procedure continues on following page

Procedure for Hemodialysis—*Continued*

Steps	Rationale	Special Considerations
5. Access the VAC, graft, or fistula.	Allows access to the site.	
6. Connect the arterial access to the arterial blood line with a Luer-Lok connector. Repeat the steps with the venous blood line.	Provides a circuit between the patient and dialyzer.	
7. Remove the clamps from the arterial and venous blood lines.	Permits the flow of blood.	
8. Adjust the blood pump to 50–100 mL/min until blood reaches the venous drip chamber.[3]	The slow rate prevents symptoms of rapid blood loss and allows for assessment of blood flow from the arterial line.	If a heparin loading dose is prescribed, it can be given via bolus in the arterial line.
9. Adjust the blood level in the arterial and venous drip chambers to three-fourths full per the manufacturer's specifications.[3]	Prevents accumulation of air in the tubing and dialyzer.	
10. Turn the dialyzer over so the arterial (red) port is at the bottom. Follow the manufacturer's specifications as some machines vary related to this practice.	Establishes the countercurrent flow.	
11. If the patient is receiving systemic heparinization, set the parameters on the heparin infusion pump as prescribed.[3,16]	Provides anticoagulation.	
12. Secure the cannula connections.	Additional precaution against accidental disconnection.	
13. Slowly increase the blood pump speed to the prescribed rate while continuing to assess the patient (level of consciousness, symptoms of chest pain, dysrhythmias, and changes in hemodynamic variables).[3,19]	Prevents complications of rapid removal of blood.	If any question exists as to how well the patient will tolerate hemodialysis, the pump speed should be started at 100 mL/min and gradually increased to goal.
14. Set the arterial and venous alarm parameters.[3]	Sets the safety alarm system.	
15. Observe the patient's transmembrane pressure (TMP) display.[3]	Removes the desired UF.	Most dialysis machines automatically calculate the TMP.
16. Set the TMP alarms.	Allows for UF.	Most machines automatically adjust based on the treatment time and volume removal goal. TMP may indicate clotting or clogging of the dialyzer. It is important to know the maximum TMP for the dialyzer; levels approaching or above the maximum TMP can result in dialyzer membrane rupture or blood leak.
17. Remove PE, and discard used equipment in an appropriate receptacle.	Safely discards used supplies.	
18. HH		

Procedure for Hemodialysis—*Continued*

Steps	Rationale	Special Considerations
19. Continuously monitor the patient's status and machine function throughout treatment.[3]	Prevents complications and minimizes the effects of fluid and electrolyte shifts.	Patient assessment should include vital signs and symptoms related to fluid and electrolyte shifts (e.g., cramping, hypotension, nausea, vomiting). Monitor the machine for blood flow rate, arterial and venous pressure readings, dialysate pressure, TMP, and blood circuit for clotting or air.

Termination

Steps	Rationale	Special Considerations
1. **HH**		
2. **PE**		
3. Set the arterial, venous, and dialysate pressure alarms to the maximum low/high limits.	Prevents the machine from alarming when terminating dialysis as pressures drop.	
4. Turn off the TMP or negative pressure.	Removes the negative pressure, thereby stopping UF.	
5. Turn off the heparin infusion pump.	Discontinues heparinization before the end of dialysis, thus allowing clotting times to return to normal shortly after treatment.	May be performed 30 minutes to 1 hour before termination of treatment; follow institutional standards.
6. Decrease the blood pump flow rate.	Reduces blood flow.	
7. Check the amount of NS solution left in the circuit for adequate blood return; hang a new NS solution bag if necessary.	Minimizes the danger of air embolism on return of blood to the patient.	NS solution (100–300 mL) is used to return blood to the patient.
8. Maintain the blood level in the arterial and venous drip chambers at three-fourths full per the manufacturer's guidelines.	Prevents air in the tubing and dialyzer.	
9. Turn off the blood pump.	Stops the blood flow.	
10. Clamp the arterial line: A. Disconnect the line from the patient, and connect it to the NS flush port on the circuit. B. Unclamp the arterial arm of the catheter.	Prevents the loss of blood.	
11. Unclamp the NS: A. Turn the pump on at a low speed, and return the blood to the patient. B. Allow the NS flush to infuse until the lines are pink-tinged.	Promotes the slow return of blood in the tubing back to the patient.	
12. Turn off the blood pump.	Terminates the flow of blood.	
13. Place a sterile 4 × 4 gauze pad under the vascular access, and disconnect the dialysis tubing from the vascular access.	Prevents contamination.	
14. Flush the fistula/graft/VAC according to institutional standards.	Prevents clotting.	
15. Sanitize the single-patient machine according to institutional standards.	Reduces transmission of microorganisms and readies it for future use.	

Procedure continues on following page

Procedure	**for Hemodialysis—*Continued***	
Steps	**Rationale**	**Special Considerations**
16. Remove **PE**, and discard used equipment in an appropriate receptacle.	Safely discards used supplies.	
17. **HH**		

Expected Outcomes

- Catheter/fistula/graft accessed without complications
- Blood is easily aspirated from the access site
- Pulsating blood flow occurs in the dialysis tubing set (does not occur with a wet stick technique which involves connecting a NS-filled syringe to the needle before insertion/cannulation)
- Accumulated waste products are removed
- Blood urea nitrogen (BUN) and creatinine values are restored to baseline levels
- Acid-base balance is restored
- Electrolyte values are restored to baseline levels
- Accumulated fluid is removed; dry weight is achieved[9,10,19]

Unexpected Outcomes

- Dislodgment of the catheter
- Decreased circulation in the vascular access limb
- Hematoma formation at the access site[1]
- Prolonged bleeding from the insertion site or access site
- Clotting or decreased patency of the AV fistula or catheter lumens
- Poor blood flow
- Signs or symptoms of infection at the insertion or access site or systemically.[1] Physiological complications (dysrhythmias, chest pain, fluid-electrolyte imbalance, hypotension, seizures, nausea and vomiting, headaches, muscle cramping, dyspnea)
- Technical problems with the dialysis machine

Patient Monitoring and Care

Steps	**Rationale**	**Reportable Conditions**
		These conditions should be reported to the provider if they persist despite nursing interventions.
1. Perform and record a predialysis weight.[3,9] **(Level D*)**	Predialysis weight is an important factor in deciding how much UF is needed during treatment. It also helps guide ongoing treatment.[3,9,10,19,29]	- Abnormal increase or decrease in weight
2. Perform ongoing assessments, including the following: A. Vital signs B. Jugular vein distention C. Presence of edema D. Intake and output E. Neurological assessment F. Pulmonary assessment	Provides information in response to treatment.[3,27,29] Monitors for complications.	- Hypotension - Hypertension - Tachycardia/bradycardia - Tachypnea - Fever - Hypothermia - Jugular vein distention - Crackles - Edema - Change in level of consciousness, dizziness - Change in cardiac rhythm[15,22]
3. Monitor the circulation to the extremity where the graft/fistula is located for the following: A. Capillary refill B. Pulses distal to access C. Color/temperature of extremity D. Sensation **(Level D*)**	Assesses for decrease in perfusion distal to the graft site.[4]	- Diminished capillary refill - Diminished or absent peripheral pulses - Pale, mottled, or cyanotic extremity - Cool to touch - Diminished or absent movement - Pain[8,17]

*Level D: Peer-reviewed professional and organizational standards with the support of clinical study recommendations.

UNIT V

Patient Monitoring and Care —*Continued*

Steps	Rationale	Reportable Conditions

4. Monitor electrolytes and glucose pretreatment or posttreatment as prescribed or per institutional standards.[18]	Must be monitored because of continued fluid and electrolyte shifts during treatment.	• Electrolyte disturbances (either hypo or hyper)[18,43,52]
		  • Potassium
		  • Sodium
		  • Calcium
		  • Phosphate
		  • Magnesium
		  • Hyperglycemia or hypoglycemia

5. Adjust the dialysis bath to correct electrolyte abnormalities as prescribed during treatment.[18]	Patients with renal failure are predisposed to many electrolyte abnormalities. During dialysis, several medications/electrolyte replacements may be given as prescribed for individual patients.[18]	• Electrolyte disturbances (either hypo or hyper)[18,43,52]
		  • Potassium
		  • Sodium
		  • Calcium
		  • Phosphate
		  • Magnesium
		  • Hyperglycemia or hypoglycemia

6. Monitor the dialysis circuit (e.g., occlusions, kinks, or leaks; blood or clots in vascular access lines). **(Level E*)**	Disconnections or introduction of air into the circuit are always possible during treatment. Bleeding or exsanguination can occur.[3] Clotting of the circuit is a potential complication. If the hemodialyzer becomes excessively clotted, the extracorporeal blood volume should be returned to the patient quickly. Blood leaks from the dialyzer into the dialysate may occur and necessitate termination of treatment without returning of blood. Venous or arterial pressures, which are out of range, may indicate dialyzer or access malfunction.	• Disconnections, cracks, or leaks • Bleeding • Excessive clotting • Blood leaks, hemodialyzer rupture • Malfunction of the dialyzer or access
7. Monitor UF for rate, clarity, and air bubbles.	A decrease in UF production can occur from clotting of the dialyzer.[3] Pink- or blood-tinged UF could be indicative of a filter leak or rupture. Some medications, such as vitamin K, rifampin, and methylene blue, cause discoloration of the UF; therefore a test for RBC is required to ensure that there is no rupture of the membranes if discoloration is noted.	• Decrease in UF production • Change in color or characteristic of UF • Air in UF
8. Administer heparin as prescribed.	Heparin is often used to prevent clotting of the circuit.[55] The heparin dose varies according to patient condition, laboratory values, and type of vascular access.	• Suspicion of clotting in the circuit
9. Monitor anticoagulation per institutional standards.	Because heparin is commonly used to prevent system clotting, coagulation studies should be routinely monitored.	• Abnormal coagulation studies

*Level E: Multiple case reports, theory-based evidence from expert opinions, or peer-reviewed professional organizational standards without clinical studies to support recommendations.

Procedure continues on following page

Steps	Rationale	Reportable Conditions

Patient Monitoring and Care —*Continued*

10. Monitor the patency of vascular access.
    A. Gently palpate along the entire length of the graft or over the access for a thrill (feeling of vibration or purring under the fingers).

Bleeding can occur from either the venous or arterial catheter or AV fistula. Clotting of the access can occur.[4]

    B. Auscultate for the presence of a bruit (sounds like rushing water).

Absence of a bruit does not confirm occlusion. Use a Doppler scan if unable to hear a bruit with a stethoscope.

- Decrease in access function or patency
- Absence of bruit or thrill

11. Monitor the patient for complications associated with dialysis treatment.

Complications are possible with dialysis treatments.[3,15,19,51]

- Muscle cramps[51]
- Dialysis disequilibrium (headache, nausea/vomiting, hypertension, decreased sensorium, convulsions, coma)—rare
- Air embolism[51]
- Dialyzer reaction (hypotension, pruritus, back pain, angioedema, anaphylaxis)[51]
- Hypoxemia[51]
- Cardiac abnormalities[15,22]
- Abnormal laboratory values

12. Administer medications to correct metabolic abnormalities as prescribed.

Patients with renal failure are predisposed to many metabolic abnormalities. Common medications administered to patients with renal failure include the following[1,5,6,12]:
    A. Vitamin D and calcium carbonate to increase the serum calcium level and prevent or treat bone disease
    B. Erythropoietin and iron to treat anemia[24]
    C. Phosphate binders to treat hyperphosphatemia
    D. Deferoxamine mesylate to remove excessive iron

13. Reinforce the prescribed renal diet.[6,42,48,50]

Encourage a BMI between 18.5 and 25 kg/m^2 to avoid patient obesity.[6,42] Collaboration with a dietitian/nutritionist at the facility should be considered.[27]

14. Place a sign above the patient's bed and arm band when available to indicate which limb has the vascular access (AV graft or fistula).

Blood pressures and blood draws should not be performed on the access arm.

UNIT V

Patient Monitoring and Care —*Continued*

Steps	Rationale	Reportable Conditions
15. Follow institutional standards for assessing pain. Administer analgesia as prescribed.	Identifies the need for pain interventions.[8,17] Many patients report pain and will have a rating of moderate to severe. The etiology can be multifactorial. Pain is commonly caused by peripheral vascular disease, osteoarthritis, or complications from kidney disease, or it can be related to the dialysis procedure.[8]	• Continued pain despite pain interventions

Documentation

Documentation should include the following:
- Patient and family education
- Date and time of treatment initiation
- Condition of catheter or AVF/AVG regarding patency, quality of blood flow, and ease of access procedure
- Condition of insertion site and any signs or symptoms of infection
- Presence of thrill or bruit if an AVF/AVG is used
- Needle gauge size used for cannulation
- Type of machine used for dialysis
- Pain assessment, interventions, and effectiveness
- Arterial and venous pressures, TMP during treatment
- Pump speed
- Length of dialysis treatment
- Vital signs throughout the treatments
- Unexpected outcomes
- Medications/IV fluids given during treatment
- Nursing interventions
- Predialysis and postdialysis weight
- Laboratory assessment data

References and Additional Readings

For a complete list of references and additional readings for this procedure, scan this QR code with your smartphone, or visit https://www.elsevier.com/__data/assets/pdf_file/0004/1319881/Chapter0106.pdf.

107 Peritoneal Dialysis

Heather L. Przybyl and Amanda J. Golino

PURPOSE Peritoneal dialysis (PD) is used for the removal of fluid and toxins, the regulation of electrolytes, and the management of azotemia.

DEFINITIONS

- Disease process[12,25,30,31]
  - ❖ Acute kidney diseases and disorders (AKD): Signs of alterations in kidney function and/or kidney damage occurring within 1 week or up to 3 months.
  - ❖ Chronic kidney disease (CKD): Kidney abnormalities that have been present over 3 months, including either alterations in kidney function or kidney damage.
  - ❖ Acute kidney injury (AKI): Clinical syndrome of kidney injury with multiple etiologies. Can be a subset of either AKD or CKD. Characterized by an increase in serum creatinine that is 1.5 times the baseline and evolves over 48 hours.
- Therapy
  - ❖ Kidney replacement therapy (KRT): A therapy that compensates nonendocrine kidney function in patients with renal failure. Encompasses the following therapies:
    - ○ Intermittent hemodialysis (IHD) used in hemodynamically stable patients. IHD may be needed for the onset of AKI, maintenance therapy for patients with chronic renal failure, or for patients with acute drug intoxication. Can be prescribed as daily or every other day, or any variation of the two. Therapy typically runs for 3 to 4 hours. See Procedure 106, Hemodialysis, for more information.
    - ○ Continuous renal replacement therapy (CRRT) used in hemodynamically unstable patients that runs continuously for 24 hours per day. (see Procedure 106, Hemodialysis, for more information on CRRT).
    - ○ Peritoneal dialysis (PD) uses the lining in the abdominal cavity and dialysate fluid to remove waste products not accomplished by the patient's native kidney. Table 107.1 reviews the variety of modalities used in PD.
- Access[1,9]
  - ❖ Flexible catheter: The Tenckhoff catheter is regarded as the gold standard catheter for PD.[9] Improved flow of dialysate is achieved with the flexible catheters because of a large diameter with multiple holes located on the side of the catheter. Commonly the catheters are made of a silicone material, however there are other materials that are being marketed.[1] PD catheters can be straight (Tenckhoff) with one or two cuffs, coiled, or Swan neck.[1,41]

  - ○ Dacron cuffs allows the tissue to adhere to the cuff and stabilize the catheter.[1] Catheters come with varying number of cuffs depending on the manufacturer.
  - ○ Rigid catheter: Rigid catheters use a stiff trochanter inserted into the abdomen and toward the iliac fossae. These catheters are temporary and usually in place for maximum of 3 days. Higher infection rates are associated with prolonged duration of use. They have decreased efficacy compared with flexible catheters.[9] These catheters are no longer used in North America because of their limitations and high infection rates.
- Principles: PD works on the principles of diffusion and osmosis; thus a basic knowledge of these concepts is necessary. Lymphatic uptake of fluids and solutes is influenced by convection.[4]
  - ❖ *Diffusion:* Passive movement of solutes through a semipermeable membrane from an area of higher concentration to one of lower concentration. When this concept is applied to PD, diffusion occurs because the patient's blood contains waste products (solute), which gives it a higher osmolarity (concentration) than the dialysate. Therefore waste products in the blood diffuse across the semipermeable membrane into the dialysate solution.
  - ❖ *Osmosis:* Passive movement of solvent through a semipermeable membrane from an area of lower concentration to one of higher concentration. The dextrose added to the dialysate gives it a higher osmotic gradient than that of the patient's blood. Therefore excess water in the blood is pulled into the dialysate via osmosis.
  - ❖ *Convective transport:* Rapid movement of fluid across a semipermeable membrane from an area of high pressure to an area of low pressure with transport of solutes. When water moves across a membrane along a pressure gradient, some solutes are carried along with the water and do not require a solute concentration gradient (also called *solute drag*). Convective transport is most effective for the removal of middle-molecular-weight and large-molecular-weight solutes.
  - ❖ *Ultrafiltration (UF):* Bulk movement of solute and solvent through a semipermeable membrane with a pressure movement. This movement is usually achieved with positive pressure in the blood compartment of the hemodialyzer and negative pressure in the dialysate compartment. Blood and dialysate flow is countercurrent to each other. The size of the solute molecules compared with the size of molecules that can move

TABLE 107.1	Comparison of PD Techniques

Modality	Number of Exchanges	Dwell Time	Advantages	Disadvantages	Key Aspects of the Modality
Continuous ambulatory peritoneal dialysis (CAPD)	• 3–5 manual or manual assisted[1,27]	• Day: dwell 4–6 hours • Night: dwell 8–10 hours[1,27] • Many exchanges take place during meal schedules	• Mobility flexibility • Most commonly used PD in the United States		• Preferred modality for anuric patients[51] • *Level D Evidence*
Continuous-flow peritoneal dialysis (CFPD)[3,5,17,27,42]	• Day: 1 exchange • Night: 3–5 exchanges using a cycler	• Day: dwell 12–16 hours • Night: dwell 1.5–2 hours	• Improved small solute clearance[20] • Effective in treating volume overload[5]	• Effective CFPD must achieve a dialysis rate of 100–300 mL/min[5,17,27] • High rate of complications • Costly[20]	• Uses a catheter for inflow and another for outflow (total of 2 catheters)[17] or a double Y-lumen catheter[1,42] • Preferred modality for anuric patients[51] • Considered to be opposite of CAPD modality and most closely mimics hemodialysis[27]
Intermittent peritoneal dialysis (IPD)[17]	20–30 manual or manual-assisted exchanges[1]	30 minutes		Poor efficiency due to low small solute clearance	
Chronic equilibrated peritoneal dialysis (CEPD)[17]	4–6 manual exchanges	4–6 hours	Low cost	Poor clearance of small molecules	
High-Volume peritoneal dialysis (HVPD)[17]	18–22 mechanical (cycler)	30–60 minutes			
Tidal peritoneal dialysis (TPD)[17]			• Shorter inflow and outflow time • Improved UF compared with CEPD[20]	• Requires higher flow rates, up to 20 L per session, to achieve enhanced small solute clearance • Higher solute clearance than CEPD • Not typically used in the United States[1]	• Chronic PD • PD dialysate is drained from patient at scheduled intervals Drained volume is replaced with fresh dialysate (tidal volume), and a variable amount of dialysate is left in the peritoneal cavity (residual volume) after each PD session.

Exchange, process of draining waste, filling new dialysate and dwell;[1] *F,* Ultrafiltration.

through the semipermeable membrane determines the degree of UF.[29]

PREREQUISITE NURSING KNOWLEDGE

• PD has been an intervention to manage complications related to kidney injury since the 1920s and can be utilized in both CKD and AKI. Improvements made in the 1940s to solutions and PD catheters increased positive outcomes in this patient population.[9] However, advances in technology, equipment, and central venous catheters led to a decline in prescribing PD for patients in technologically

advanced countries, while the therapy is still prevalent in low- to middle-income countries.[9,15,17,34,38,44,49] The COVID-19 pandemic brought a resurgence of the use of PD for the treatment of AKI because of a lack of dialysis resources and the increased AKI population.[34]

• The RIFLE (Risk, Injury, Failure, Loss, End-Stage) or the AKIN (Acute Kidney Injury Network) scales are commonly used by nephrologists to determine the level of kidney impairment in AKI. The scales assess variations in serum creatinine levels, glomerular filtration rate (GFR), and urine output within a 48-hour period. These values assist the provider in determining the best modality to treat the patient based on the stage of AKI.[12,25]

- ❖ Determination of the time frame in which to initiate therapy based on one value alone, such as GFR, has not resulted in improved mortality rates.[22,40]
- PD can be utilized in the critical care setting for both acute kidney injury and can be classified as acute-on-chronic (AoC) kidney disease.[11,40,50]
- Indications for PD[15,28]
  - ❖ Fluid removal
  - ❖ Electrolyte abnormalities
  - ❖ Acid-base derangements
- Solutes are transported via two routes: membrane layers and the lymphatic system.[1,42]
  - ❖ Transport of solutes is achieved using three membrane layers.
  1. Mesothelium: Touches the dialysate with no resistance to solute transport
  2. Interstitium: Normally thin but can thicken over time. Builds fibrin after repeated exposure.
  3. Endothelium "Capillary wall": Site where fluid and solute transport takes place
     - ○ Three-pore model[1,29,41,42]
     - ○ Transcellular (ultra-small) pore: Smallest pore that only allows free water to pass via specialized protein "aquaporin." The opening is approximately 8A (angstroms) (<0.5 nm).
     - ○ Small extracellular pore: Allows small solutes (urea, creatinine, potassium, sodium) approximately 40 to 50A (4 to 5 nm)
     - ○ Large extracellular pore: Allows passage of medium (B_{12}, microglobulin) and large (protein-bound solutes) macromolecules approximately 150A (>15 to 25 nm)
  - ❖ Primary role of the lymphatic system in PD is to absorb fluids, electrolytes, proteins, colloid materials, cells, and inert particles that are present in the peritoneal cavity.[14,24]
- Catheter insertion, PD prescription, and technique
  - ❖ The provider may insert the PD catheter using surgical dissection, laparoscopic technique, or percutaneous insertion.[1,6,8,36]
    - ○ Catheters can be placed at various locations on the abdomen, with the exit site positioned in an area with the least risk for infection, either above or below the belt line based on body habitus and best option for the catheter to sit in the pelvis.[8,53]
    - ○ Successful functioning of a PD catheter depends more on the technique used during placement (e.g., laparoscopic, open) than the catheter design (e.g., straight, coiled).[6]
    - ○ Some common causes of catheter dysfunction include migration, fibrin clots, and omental wrapping.[36,53]
  - ❖ Bowel prep before insertion
    - ○ 2 L polyethylene glycol solution
    - ○ Stimulant suppository
    - ○ Enema
    - ○ Avoid phosphate- and magnesium-containing agents[1]
  - ❖ Antibiotic prophylaxis before insertion[41,51]

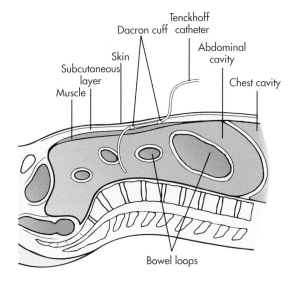

Figure 107.1 Tenckhoff catheter used in peritoneal dialysis. *(From Lewis SM, et al: Medical-surgical nursing: assessment and management of clinical problems, ed 7, St. Louis, 2007, Mosby.)*

- ❖ Recommendations from the International Society for Peritoneal Dialysis (ISPD) include daily topical application of antibiotic at the exit site.[1,51]
- ❖ Postinsertion catheter healing time is typically 2 weeks; however, there may be times when an emergent start is initiated by the provider. An urgent start would be classified as starting therapy between 72 hours and 2 weeks postinsertion.[1,8]
  - ○ Patient should be placed in the supine position with small fill volumes with urgent starts.[1]
- ❖ Sterile dialysis fluid (dialysate) is infused into the peritoneal cavity of the abdomen through a flexible catheter (Fig. 107.1).
- ❖ PD requires an infusion of 1.5 to 3 L of dialysate into the abdominal cavity. The volume is dependent on the prescription and patient condition.[41]
- ❖ When dialysate is infused into the abdominal cavity, intraperitoneal hydrostatic pressure (IPP) is created. Absorption typically occurs with an IPP above 3 to 4 mm Hg.[14] The larger the volume infused, the larger the IPP. IPP is dependent on the size of the patient, volume, patient positioning (e.g., sitting, standing).[14,41]
- ❖ The prescription should be adjusted on goals of therapy and the patient's condition.[28]
  - ○ Modality choice: Intermittent or continuous
  - ○ PD can be performed either manually with a dialysis administration set (continuous ambulatory PD) or with a cycler machine (automated PD [APD], also known as *continuous cycling peritoneal dialysis* [CCPD]) (Fig. 107.2).
  - ○ With a cycler machine, multiple exchanges are programmed into the machine and run automatically.[27]
  - ○ Causality of AKI and the goal of fluid and solute removal determine the duration of therapy.
  - ○ Number of exchanges and volume of dialysate: This is dependent on the patient's size and medical issues, such as hernias or respiratory status. The volume can range from 1.5 L to 3.5 L. An average-sized

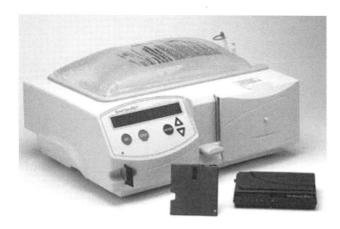

Figure 107.2 Baxter HomeChoice Pro PD Cycler. *(Courtesy Baxter International, Inc, Deerfield, IL.)*

patient with no respiratory dysfunction or hernia could tolerate a 2-L volume of dialysate, whereas a large-framed adult may tolerate over 3 L of dialysate. Additionally, a small-framed adult patient with respiratory failure and a hernia may only be able to tolerate 1.5 L.[28,41]

- ○ The most limiting factor for the volume of dialysate is that it may cause direct pressure on the diaphragm and cause respiratory compromise.[28]
- ○ Inflow, dwell, and outflow time[28]
- ○ **Inflow:** The time it takes to infuse the volume of dialysate into the peritoneal cavity (typically between 10 and 15 minutes)
- ○ **Outflow:** The time it takes to completely drain the dialysate (typically between 20 and 30 minutes)
- ○ **Dwell time:** Time between the inflow and outflow time. The highest exchange of solutes is achieved during the first hour rather than in the subsequent hours.[27]
- ○ Formula of dialysate and potential additives[28,48]
- ❖ Osmotic agent: The glucose concentration determines the osmotic strength and UF
  - ○ 1.5% dextrose (75 mmol/L): May be used in patients who are hemodynamically unstable with slight volume overload, cannot tolerate shifts of volume
  - ○ 2.5% (125 mmol/L)
  - ○ 4.25% (214 mmol/L): May be used in patients who are severely volume overloaded and hemodynamically stable
  - ○ The PD dialysate contains higher concentrations of glucose than normal serum levels.
  - ○ These higher concentrations aid in the removal of water via osmosis and small- to medium-weight molecules (urea, creatinine) via diffusion.
  - ○ The higher the concentration of glucose in the dialysate, the greater the amount of fluid removal.
  - ○ 7.5% Icodextrin may also be used as the osmotic agent for PD requiring long dwell times (greater than 8 hours).[48]
  - ○ Use of icodextrin has been shown to enhance UF and clearance.[28,48]

- ○ This glucose polymer is metabolized to maltose and is not readily absorbed.
- ○ Metabolites may cause erroneously high glucose levels; check the manufacturer's recommendations to ensure that icodextrin metabolites will not interfere with the glucose analyzer being used for patient testing.
- ○ Icodextrin may affect blood glucose readings up to 14 days after the last icodextrin use. There is a black box warning about use of icodextrin and type of glucose meters as a result of untreated severe hypoglycemia leading to coma and death.
- ○ Buffer agent: Most widely used is lactate because of stability in the presence of calcium and magnesium. Bicarbonate buffered solutions can be prescribed in patients with hepatic failure, septic shock, or lactic acidosis.[28]
- ○ Electrolytes including sodium, chloride, magnesium, and calcium standard concentrations include:
- ○ Calcium ranging from 1.25 to 1.75 mmol/L (2.5 to 3.5 mEq/L)[28,48]
- ○ Sodium 131 to 134 mEq/L/mmol/L[28,48]
- ○ Magnesium 0.25 to 0.75 mmol/L (0.5 to 1.5 mEq/L)[28,48]
- ○ No potassium in commercially prepared solutions
- ○ Additional agents added to the dialysate prescription may include heparin, insulin, antibiotics, and potassium[28]
- ❖ Efficiency of PD
  - ○ Urea kinetic modeling Kt/V_{urea} (Kt/V)[41] target >2 to 2.2 weekly[1,9,43]
  - ○ K = rate of passage blood through the dialyzer expressed in mL/min
  - ○ t = duration of therapy, time
  - ○ V = volume of water in body: 0.5 female or 0.6 male multiplied by body weight[9]
  - ○ Multiply above value by 7 to get a weekly Kt/V_{urea}[9]
  - ○ Normalized creatinine clearances[49,51] target >60 L/week/1.73 m²
  - ○ Solute reduction[49]

- PD involves repeated fluid exchanges or cycles. Each cycle has three phases: drain, instill, and dwell. If this is the patient's first dialysis cycle, the instillation phase will be first; however, if the patient has been on routine peritoneal dialysis at home, for example, the drain phase will be done first, followed by instillation and dwell.
  - ❖ During the drain phase, the dialysate and excess extracellular fluid, wastes, and electrolytes are drained via gravity from the peritoneal cavity via a peritoneal catheter.
  - ❖ During the instillation phase, the dialysate is infused via gravity into the patient's peritoneal cavity through a peritoneal catheter.[1]
  - ❖ During the dwell phase, the dialysate remains in the patient's peritoneal cavity, allowing osmosis and diffusion to occur. Dwell time varies based on the patient's clinical need and the delivery method of PD.[1]
- PD dialysate should be warmed using a commercial warmer or other warming techniques as determined by your institution to normal body temperature. Never warm

the solution in a standard microwave oven, which heats unevenly and does not regulate the fluid temperature.[1,28]

- Complications of PD[37,49]
  - ❖ Prevention of peritonitis is at the cornerstone for management of patients receiving PD; must be a primary consideration with PD.[10,19,39]
  - ❖ Peritonitis frequently occurs within the first 48 hours of treatment
    - ○ Exit-site infections are often related to the following organisms
    - ○ Gram-positive
    - ○ *Staphylococcus aureus*[37,39,49,51] most common and accounts for approximately one-half of exit-site infections.[49]
    - ○ *Staphylococcus epidermidis* accounts for approximately 20% of exit-site infections.[49]
    - ○ Coagulase-negative *Staphylococcus*[45,47]
    - ○ Concern for peritonitis caused by the following species, which are slow to respond to antibiotic treatment. An ultrasound evaluation should be ordered by the provider.[8]
    - ○ Gram-positive: *Staphylococcus aureus*[8,37,39,45]
    - ○ Gram-negative: *Pseudomonas aeruginosa*[8,39]
    - ○ Rare but emerging pathogens common with peritonitis
    - ○ Gram-positive organisms
  - ❖ *Corynebacterium striatum*[26]
  - ❖ *Mycobacterium abscessus*[23]
  - ❖ *Streptococcus vestibularis*[52]
    - ○ Cases of severe inflammation of the viscera or perforation could be considered to be an abdominal catastrophe.[34]
  - ❖ Also called secondary peritonitis, intrinsic peritonitis, or peritonitis due to bowel perforation.[34]
  - ❖ Mortality rate is extremely high in this population.[34]
  - ❖ Bleeding[49]
  - ❖ Inflow and outflow malfunctions[10,29,49]
    - ○ Inflow difficulty[49] 2-L bag should typically take 15 minutes to infuse into the peritoneal cavity[10]
    - ○ Check for mechanical issues such as kinked tubing or clamped rollers[10]
    - ○ PD catheters can become clogged with the buildup of fibrin. Heparin or other anticoagulant medications are sometimes added to thedialysate or used as a separate flush to prevent occlusion.[10]
    - ○ Outflow issues
    - ○ Constipation accounts for the majority of outflow issues.[10,49]
    - ○ Impaired UF caused by impaired solute transport, reduced membrane efficiency, or fibrosis.[29]
  - ❖ Dialysate leaks
    - ○ Leaks that occur within the first 4 weeks of initiation of PD are considered "early," and those occurring after 4 weeks are considered "late."[16]
    - ○ Early leaks typically manifest as the fluids are moving across the catheter track[16]
    - ○ Late leaks typically manifest as leaking of fluids that accumulate in the adjacent anatomic spaces outside the peritoneum[16]
      - ○ Both categories of leaks could lead to an increase in IPP[16]
    - ❖ Hemoperitoneum[34]
- Elevated IPP puts the patient at risk for the following[1,49]:
  - ❖ Peri-catheter or subcutaneous dialysate leaks[16]
  - ❖ Inguinal or umbilical herniation with potential for bowel incarceration[53]
  - ❖ Hemorrhoids
  - ❖ Altered respiratory system
  - ❖ Potential for vagal stimulation leading to bradycardia[1]
  - ❖ Hydrothorax[2,10]

EQUIPMENT

- Masks (for everyone in the room)
- Signage outside the room stating that sterile procedure is taking place
- Goggles or fluid shield face masks
- Sterile gloves are required for connecting the tubing to the PD catheter (the inner lumen of catheter and peritoneal cavity are sterile; therefore aseptic technique is paramount)[1]
- Nonsterile gloves required for all other preparation or discarding of equipment
- Two to four packs of sterile 4 × 4 gauze pads
- Antiseptic solution (follow institutional standards)
- Tape
- Sterile barriers (towels or pads)
- Plastic hemostats (or clamps)
- PD administration set (most facilities use closed-delivery systems with an attached drainage bag)
- Intravenous (IV) pole
- Warmed dialysate solution (use a commercial warmer or other warming techniques as determined by your institution)
- Sterile catheter caps (may be impregnated with antiseptic solution per facility standards)
- Labels for catheter
- Scale

Additional equipment to have available as needed includes the following:
- Sterile container
- Three plastic clamps (if not included in the PD administration set)
- Cycler with tubing
- Equipment for gram stain, culture, and/or cell count with differential/hematocrit[35]

PATIENT AND FAMILY EDUCATION

- Explain the purpose of PD. *Rationale:* PD is necessary to perform the physiological functions of the kidneys when renal failure is present. PD uses the lining inside the abdomen, called the *peritoneal cavity* as a filter to clean the blood and remove excess fluid.
- Explain the procedure, and review any questions. *Rationale:* Explanation provides information and may decrease patient anxiety.

- Explain the need for careful sterile technique when the abdominal catheter is accessed in the inpatient setting. This may be different from techniques performed in their home because of infection risks while hospitalized. ***Rationale:*** Sterile technique is used to decrease the chance of peritoneal infection because pathogens can be introduced into the abdominal cavity via the catheter.[1]
- Explain the three phases of PD. ***Rationale:*** Because each phase is different, the patient must be informed of all three phases and the purposes, interventions, and possible complications of each.
- Explain the potential for feelings of fullness and possibly shortness of breath during the dwell phase. ***Rationale:*** The pressure of the dialysate fluid on the diaphragm may cause the patient to have these feelings, which are normal for the dwell phase.

PATIENT ASSESSMENT AND PREPARATION

Patient Assessment

- Obtain baseline vital signs, respiratory status, abdominal assessment, blood glucose level with compatible glucose meter, and pertinent laboratory results (potassium, sodium, calcium, phosphorus, magnesium, renal function tests, complete blood count). ***Rationale:*** Patients in renal failure often have altered baseline assessments, according to both physical assessment and laboratory values. The availability of this information before treatments are started is helpful so interventions, including the type and amount of dialysate fluid, can be individualized.[18]
- Assess volume status, as indicated by the following: skin turgor, mucous membranes, edema, lung sounds, weight, intake, and output. ***Rationale:*** PD is often initiated for the control of hypervolemia. Knowledge of a patient's pretreatment volume status is essential to allow for individualization of treatment goals and interventions.[18]

- Assess the PD catheter and abdominal exit site for signs and symptoms of infection, leakage or drainage, or peritonitis. ***Rationale:*** The catheter insertion site provides a portal of entry for pathogens that can result in septicemia or peritonitis. If the insertion site or effluent appears to be infected, further interventions (e.g., site change, culture, antibiotics) may be necessary.[1,7,10,47]
  - ❖ Cloudy or bloody dialysate solution
  - ❖ Leakage at the catheter site
  - ❖ Subcutaneous fluid in the abdomen, groin, or upper thighs
  - ❖ Abdominal pain
  - ❖ Fever
  - ❖ Chills
  - ❖ Rebound tenderness
- Check the peritoneal catheter and tubing for kinks, puncture sites, and loose connections. ***Rationale:*** Adequate flow is essential for optimal treatment. A dysfunctional catheter can alter outcomes.

Patient Preparation

- Verify the correct patient with two identifiers. ***Rationale:*** Before performing a procedure, the nurse should ensure the correct identification of the patient for the intended intervention.
- Ensure that the patient understands the preprocedural education. Answer questions as they arise, and reinforce information as needed. ***Rationale:*** Understanding of previously taught information is evaluated and reinforced.
- Assist the patient and everyone present in the room with applying a mask. ***Rationale:*** This decreases the risk for pathogen transmission.
- Reposition the patient to a comfortable position. ***Rationale:*** Proper positioning is important to ensure patient comfort, optimize respiratory status, and facilitate optimal flow through the abdominal catheter.

Procedure	for Peritoneal Dialysis	
Steps	Rationale	Special Considerations
Sterile Administration Set Change		
1. Verify PD orders, which should include: A. Manual or automated delivery system B. Dialysis solution type, volume, dextrose/icodextrin and calcium concentrations, and additional medications C. Fill volume/time, dwell time, drain volume/time D. Vital sign parameters E. Laboratory testing	Familiarizes the nurse with the individualized patient treatment and reduces the possibility of error.	Ensure that patient weight and laboratory values are recorded before initiation of therapy and that the patient is wearing a mask and properly positioned.
2. 🅷🅷		
3. 🅿🅴		

Procedure for Peritoneal Dialysis—*Continued*

Steps	Rationale	Special Considerations
4. Assemble equipment in a clean, draft-free area.	Maintains aseptic technique.	A bathroom is not an appropriate place to prepare supplies or perform PD.
5. Remove the warmed dialysate bag from the protective pouch; check the concentration of solutions; check for an expiration date, clarity, and leaks.[1]	Assesses for contamination of dialysate.	
6. Hang the PD administration set on the IV pole, and clamp the tubing between the dialysate bag and the patient.	Fills tubing with dialysate; decreases the chance of introducing air into the abdominal cavity.	The dialysate solution may have a frangible pin that must be broken to allow the solution to flow into the administration tubing. APD/CCPD do not utilize an IV pole. For this procedure, the cycler and specialized tubing set is used. Priming of the tubing does not occur until the operator is prompted by the cycler.
7. Ensure that the twist clamp on the catheter adaptor or extension set is in the locked position and the cap is secured.	Prevents inadvertent disconnection.	
8. Don a mask, and assist the patient in applying a mask. Everyone in the room must wear a mask.	Reduces transmission of pathogens.	Place a sign outside the door stating that a sterile process is taking place.
9. Prepare a sterile field. Open a sterile container package or sterile 4 × 4 gauze packs.	Maintains aseptic technique.	
10. Pour antiseptic solution into a sterile container or onto sterile 4 × 4 gauze pads.	Maintains aseptic technique.	
11. Scrub the catheter cap, and allow the cap to soak in a disinfectant-soaked gauze pad for the recommended period (follow the manufacturer's guidelines regarding soak times). Dry the catheter cap connection.[1,13]	The effectiveness of the antiseptic is dependent on the scrub and soak time.[1,13] • Povidone-iodine • Sodium hypochlorite. Although there are no recommendations on specific solutions to use, the recommendation for a 1-minute scrub followed by a 5-minute soak showed a clear elimination of bacteria on the catheter external and internal surfaces.[13]	Allow to air-dry. Follow the manufacturer's recommendations as soak times may vary. Chlorhexidine cannot be used for some catheters.
12. Remove the cap, and soak the open catheter adapter in disinfectant (follow the manufacturer's guidelines regarding soak times).	The effectiveness of the antiseptic is dependent on the scrub and soak time.[1,13] • Povidone-iodine • Sodium hypochlorite. Although there are no recommendations on specific solutions to use, the recommendation for a 1-minute scrub followed by a 5-minute soak showed a clear elimination of bacteria on the catheter external and internal surfaces.[13]	Allow to air dry. Follow the manufacturer's recommendations. Chlorhexidine cannot be used for some catheters. In addition, some caps may have a disinfectant imbedded into the cap, so follow the manufacturer's guidelines or institutional policies.

Procedure continues on following page

Procedure for Peritoneal Dialysis—*Continued*

Steps	Rationale	Special Considerations
13. Connect the catheter to the administration set or to the cycler line.	Ensures a tight connection.	If a cycler is used, follow the manufacturer's instructions for system setup.
14. Remove PE, and discard used supplies.		
15. HH		
Drain Cycle		
1. HH		
2. PE		
3. Place the drainage bag below the midabdominal area on a clean surface.	Enhances flow by gravity.	
4. Assure that the drainage tubing to the empty drainage bag is open.	Allows flow into the drainage bag.	
5. Unclamp the twist clamp on the catheter adaptor or extension set of the catheter.	Allows flow from the peritoneal cavity to the drainage bag.	Allow 20–30 minutes for outflow; observe and record characteristics (e.g., cloudy, bloody, clear, yellow) and amount of outflow. Reposition the patient if flow stops or is sluggish. Notify the physician or advanced practice nurse if drainage is cloudy or bloody.
6. Monitor vital signs as prescribed during outflow.	Assesses for hypotension, tachycardia related to hypovolemia, and sudden release of IPP.	Notify the physician or advanced practice nurse if the patient becomes hypotensive, has tachycardia, or has abdominal pain.
7. Observe the outflow of the PD cycle.	Turning the patient from side to side ensures that the patient's abdomen is empty of dialysate.	
8. Clamp the catheter when the effluent is completely drained.	Decreases leakage and contamination.	
9. Remove PE, and discard used supplies.	Safely discards used supplies.	
10. HH		
Instillation Cycle		
1. HH		
2. PE		
3. Ensure that the tubing to the catheter is clamped, and unclamp the tubing between the dialysate and the drainage bag.	Allows flow between the dialysate bag and the drainage bag.	
4. Flush the tubing between the dialysate bag and the drainage bag with approximately 100 mL of dialysate or for approximately 5 seconds.	The "flush before fill" assures the effluent drainage left in the tubing to the drainage bag does not backflow into the peritoneal cavity.[1,41,51]	This technique is a key factor in potentially lowering the risk of peritonitis from contamination.
5. Clamp the tubing to the drainage bag.	Allows flow from the dialysate bag to the peritoneal cavity.	
6. Open the clamp on the catheter.	Allows flow from the dialysate bag to the peritoneal cavity.	
7. Open the clamp from the dialysate bag to the catheter.	Provides open access between the catheter and the PD tubing, allowing inflow of dialysate to the peritoneal cavity.	

Procedure for Peritoneal Dialysis—*Continued*

Steps	Rationale	Special Considerations
8. Set the flow rate as prescribed.	Time for inflow depends on the height of the dialysate bag, the position of the patient, and the patency of the catheter.	Monitor for signs of increased peritoneal volume.
9. Remove **PE**, and discard used supplies.	Safely discards used supplies.	
10. **HH**		

Discontinuation of PD

Steps	Rationale	Special Considerations
1. **HH**		
2. **PE**		
3. When inflow is complete, clamp the dialysate tubing and the patient's catheter.	Prepares the catheter for disconnection.	
4. Don a mask, and assist the patient in applying a mask.	Maintains aseptic technique.	
5. Open a sterile cap.	Maintains aseptic technique.	Follow institutional standards regarding the use of a betadine-impregnated cap.
6. Disconnect the PD administration set from the patient's catheter.	Prepares to end the current dialysis cycle.	
7. With the transfer/extension set tubing pointing in a downward position, apply the sterile cap.	Maintains aseptic technique.	
8. Securely tape the catheter to the patient's abdomen.	Prevents accidental dislodgment.	
9. Obtain and record drainage bag weight.	Accurately assesses intake and output values.	
10. Remove **PE**, and discard used supplies.	Safely discards used supplies.	
11. **HH**		

Catheter Exit Site Care

Steps	Rationale	Special Considerations
1. **HH**		
2. **PE**		
3. Don a mask, and assist the patient in applying a mask.		
4. Prepare a sterile field. Open sterile 4 × 4 gauze pads and a sterile container.	Maintains aseptic technique.	
5. Pour antiseptic solution into a sterile container.	Reduces transmission of microorganisms.	
6. Remove the old dressing.	Allows for visualization of the catheter site.	Be careful not to tug or dislodge the catheter. Note any odor or drainage on the old dressing.
7. Inspect the catheter exit site and surrounding area for leakage, infection, or trauma.	Provides assessment for complications.	Note any pain, warmth, crusting, bleeding, tenderness, redness, or swelling that may indicate infection.
8. Gently palpate the subcutaneous catheter segments and cuff.	Assesses for pain, erythema, edema, or accumulated drainage.	Obtain a culture if drainage is present, and notify the provider if the listed signs or symptoms are present.
9. Remove nonsterile gloves, and perform meticulous hand hygiene.[46]		

Procedure continues on following page

UNIT V

Procedure for Peritoneal Dialysis—*Continued*

Steps	Rationale	Special Considerations
10. Apply sterile gloves.	Maintains aseptic technique.	Sterile gloves are used for newly placed PD catheters until the site is healed (2–4 weeks). Once healed, aseptic procedure with clean gloves is used.
11. Use a sterile 4 × 4 gauze pad to hold the catheter off the skin.	Helps prevent contamination of the catheter by skin flora.	
12. Cleanse the catheter and exit site with antiseptic solution.	Several cleansing strategies are available, although there are no studies that definitively show one solution or method to be superior to another: • Antibacterial soap and water • 10% Povidone-iodine • Chlorhexidine • 0.55% Sodium hypochlorite[1,37,46]	Allow to dry. Recommended to cleanse the exit site at minimum twice per week and every time after showering.[46]
13. Apply a new catheter site dressing with sterile gauze, or leave it open to the air.[37,46] Application of antibiotic cream to the exit site may be ordered.[39,45,51] Follow institutional standards.	Gauze wicks drainage away from the site. At this point, the patient may choose to immobilize the catheter, either with tape or a commercial securement device, although there have been no clinical trials showing efficacy of this practice.[46]	Some patients prefer to leave their well-healed catheter sites open to air. Some patients apply prophylactic antibiotic cream to their exit site for maintenance.[1,37,46]
14. Remove **PE**, and discard used supplies in appropriate receptacles.	Safely discards used supplies.	
15. **HH**		

Expected Outcomes

- Respiratory status not compromised during treatment
- Catheter and exit site maintained without complications
- Instillation and drainage of dialysate without complications
- BUN and creatinine values restored to baseline levels
- Electrolyte values restored to baseline levels
- Glucose control maintained
- Accumulated fluid removed
- Peritoneum and abdomen intact

Unexpected Outcomes

- Signs and symptoms of peritonitis
- Signs or symptoms of infection at the insertion or access site
- Introduction of pathogens into the abdominal catheter
- Diaphragmatic impingement
- Drainage/leakage from the exit site
- Poor dialysate flow during instillation or drainage.
- Inability to drain the total amount of instilled dialysate.
- Dislodgment of the abdominal catheter
- Viscus perforation by the PD catheter
- Protein or blood loss from peritonitis
- Increased IPP
- Physiological complications during treatment
- Tubing disconnection

UNIT V

Patient Monitoring and Care

Steps	Rationale	Reportable Conditions
		These conditions should be reported to the provider if they persist despite nursing interventions.
1. Perform and record predialysis and postdialysis weights.[1,18,33,51] **(Level D*)**	Predialysis weight is an important factor in deciding how much PD is needed during treatment. It also helps guide ongoing treatment and nutritional status. Postdialysis weight measures the effectiveness of the dialysis treatment.[1,18,33] Weight gain is associated with PD as a result of increased carbohydrate intake of approximately 50 to 150 g per day due to glucose added to PD solutions.[33]	• Abnormal increase or decrease in weight.
2. Perform baseline and ongoing assessments, including the following: A. Vital signs B. Jugular vein distention C. Presence or absence of edema D. Skin turgor E. Mucus membranes F. Intake and output G. Pulmonary assessment, including expiratory tidal volume and peak inspiratory pressures on the mechanically ventilated patient H. Abdominal assessment	Important to establish a baseline before initiation of treatment.[1,18] Monitors for complications.	• Hypotension • Hypertension • Fever • Hypothermia • Jugular vein distention • Dry mucous membranes • Shortness of breath • Crackles • Edema • Abdominal distention or tenderness • Rebound tenderness • Decreased tidal volume • Increased peak inspiratory pressures
3. Monitor BUN, creatinine, and electrolyte levels during treatment at a frequency determined by institutional standards.[21]	Fluids and electrolyte levels shift during treatment.[1,18]	• Hyperglycemia • BUN or creatinine levels abnormal for the patient • Hyperkalemia or hypokalemia • Hypernatremia or hyponatremia • Hypercalcemia or hypocalcemia
4. Administer medications to correct metabolic abnormalities as prescribed.[9,33]	Patients with renal failure are predisposed to many metabolic abnormalities. Common medications administered to patients with renal failure include the following:[1,18,21] • Vitamin D and calcium carbonate to increase the serum calcium level and prevent or treat bone disease • Erythropoietin and iron to treat anemia • Deferoxamine mesylate to remove excessive iron • Stool softeners because constipation can impair drainage of PD fluid • Phosphate binders to treat hyperphosphatemia	• Abnormal hemoglobin or hematocrit values • Hypercalcemia or hypocalcemia • Hyperphosphatemia or hypophosphatemia • Decreased albumin or prealbumin levels

Procedure continues on following page

UNIT V

Patient Monitoring and Care —*Continued*

Steps	Rationale	Reportable Conditions
5. Monitor serum glucose at the beginning of the treatment and throughout the treatment according to institutional standards. Administer insulin as prescribed to maintain glucose control.[51]	The glucose in the dialysate solution predisposes patients to hyperglycemia, especially patients with diabetes.[33,51]	• Hyperglycemia or hypoglycemia[9,33,51]
6. Monitor the integrity of the PD setup.[51]	Disconnections in the setup provide a portal of entry for pathogens that can lead to peritonitis.[1,46]	• Fever
7. Monitor for signs and symptoms of infection/cracking or damage to the catheter or catheter exit site.	Identifies the need for intervention.	• Tachycardia • Cloudy or bloody dialysate • Site redness or edema • Warmth • Bleeding • Purulent drainage • Pain or tenderness • Fever • Crack/leaking/damage to the catheter[1,46]
8. Monitor the ease with which the dialysate is both instilled and drained through the abdominal catheter.	Patients may need repositioning to facilitate flow through the abdominal catheter. Mixing of new solution/retained fluid reduces potency and effectiveness. Catheters may also become kinked or occluded. Fibrin clots can obstruct outflow; heparin may be added to the dialysate solution if prescribed. Rapid infusion can cause abdominal pain.[51]	• Inability to instill or drain fluid through the abdominal catheter
9. Follow institutional standards for assessing pain. Administer analgesia as prescribed.[51]	Identifies the need for pain interventions.	• Continued pain despite pain interventions
10. Monitor for signs and symptoms related to quality of life.[32,50]	A primary goal is to enable patients and families to be empowered while developing the plan of care, flexibility, and freedom while the patient is undergoing treatment.[32] Patient may require further treatment management. A renal diet may also be prescribed, with adjusted protein, phosphorus, carbohydrate, and fluid intake that takes into account the patient's current catabolic state, residual renal function, adequacy of dialysis, and removal of amino acids by dialysis.[21]	• Fatigue[32] • Depression • Headache • Poor appetite • Pruritus • Constipation

*Level D: Peer-reviewed professional and organizational standards with the support of clinical study recommendations.

Documentation

Documentation should include the following:
- Patient and family education
- Vital signs/hemodynamic parameters throughout the treatment
- Pain assessment, interventions, and effectiveness
- Date and time of treatment initiation
- Treatment/exchange number
- Dialysate solution used
- Length and parameters of treatment
- Condition of the abdominal catheter and exit site at the time of treatment
- Intake and output
- Total UF output
- Patient weight before and after treatment
- Date and time of dressing application
- Unexpected outcomes with associated nursing interventions
- Laboratory assessment data

References and Additional Readings

For a complete list of references and additional readings for this procedure, scan this QR code with your smartphone, or visit https://www.elsevier.com/__data/assets/pdf_file/0005/1319882/Chapter0107.pdf.

UNIT V

PROCEDURE

108 Apheresis and Therapeutic Plasma Exchange (Assist)

Erin Reynolds

PURPOSE Apheresis techniques are used to remove cells, plasma, and other substances from blood. Apheresis is an extracorporeal therapy in which components of the blood are removed from the patient to reduce or manage a life-threatening or significant symptom caused by the blood component.[2] These procedures are used as adjunctive treatments in many diseases, especially in antibody-mediated conditions that produce autoantibodies.

PREREQUISITE NURSING KNOWLEDGE

Therapeutic apheresis is a technique for selective removal of cells, plasma, and substances from the patient's circulation to promote clinical improvement. The different apheresis techniques vary according to the component of the blood removed or replaced or the substance removed.[7]

Procedure/Term	Definition
Adsorptive cytapheresis	A therapeutic procedure in which blood from the patient is passed through a medical device containing a column or filter that selectively adsorbs activated monocytes and granulocytes, allowing the remaining leukocytes and other blood components to be returned to the patient.
β_2-microglobulin column	A therapeutic apheresis procedure that uses a column containing porous cellulose beads specifically designed to bind to β_2-microglobulin as the patient's blood passes over the beads.
Double-filtration plasmapheresis (DFPP)	A filter-based therapeutic procedure that removes pathogenic substances from separated plasma based on their size, which is mainly determined by molecular weight and three-dimensional configuration (e.g., autoantibodies, immune complexes, lipoproteins) using plasma filters with different pore sizes.
Erythrocytapheresis	A procedure in which blood from the patient or donor is passed through a medical device that separates red blood cells (RBCs) from other components of blood. The RBCs are removed and replaced with crystalloid or colloid solution, when necessary.
Extracorporeal photopheresis (ECP)	A therapeutic procedure in which the buffy coat is separated from the patient's blood, treated extracorporeally with a photoactive compound (e.g., psoralens), exposed to ultraviolet A light, and subsequently reinfused to the patient during the same procedure.
Immunoadsorption (IA)	A therapeutic procedure in which plasma of the patient, after membrane-based or centrifugal separation from the blood, is passed through a medical device (adsorber column) with the capacity to remove immunoglobulins by binding them to select ligands on the backing matrix surface (membranes or beads) of the adsorber column.
Leukocytapheresis	A procedure in which blood of the patient is passed through a medical device that separates out white blood cells (e.g., leukemic blasts or granulocytes), collects the selected cells, and returns the remainder of the patient's blood with or without the addition of replacement fluid such as colloid and/or crystalloid solution.
Lipoprotein apheresis (LA)	The selective removal of lipoprotein particles from the patient's blood with the return of the remaining components. A variety of methodologies are available and include DFPP, HELP-apheresis, polyclonal-sheep-anti-apoB-immunoadsorption, dextran-sulfate plasma adsorption, dextran-sulfate whole-blood adsorption, and polyacrylate whole-blood adsorption.

Procedure/Term	Definition
RBC exchange	A therapeutic procedure in which blood of the patient is passed through a medical device that separates RBCs from other components of blood. The patient's RBCs are removed and replaced with donor RBCs and colloid solution.
Rheopheresis	A therapeutic procedure in which blood of the patient is passed through a medical device that separates out high-molecular-weight plasma components such as fibrinogen, α_2-macroglobulin, low-density lipoprotein cholesterol, and IgM to reduce plasma viscosity and RBC aggregation. This is done to improve blood flow and tissue oxygenation. LA devices and selective filtration devices utilizing two filters, one to separate plasma from cells and a second to separate the high-molecular-weight components, are used for these procedures.
Therapeutic plasma exchange (TPE)	A therapeutic procedure in which blood of the patient is passed through a medical device that separates out plasma from other components of blood. The plasma is removed and replaced with a replacement solution such as colloid solution (e.g., albumin and/or plasma) or a combination of crystalloid/colloid solution.
Thrombocytapheresis	A therapeutic procedure in which blood of the patient is passed through a medical device that separates out platelets, removes the platelets, and returns the remainder of the patient's blood with or without the addition of replacement fluid such as colloid and/or crystalloid solution.

- During plasma exchange procedures, the plasma volume removed must be replaced; the most common replacement fluids are 5% albumin, fresh frozen plasma (FFP), thawed plasma (derived from thawed FFP and maintained at low temperatures for use within 1 to 5 days), and normal saline.[3] Because clotting factors are transiently reduced by plasma exchange, FFP can also be used as a fluid replacement in patients when bleeding is an issue as it contains all of the coagulation factors and other proteins of blood.
- Plasma volume is an estimate of the patient's total volume based on gender, height, weight, and hematocrit value. Exchange volume is the ratio of the patient's plasma volume to be removed and replaced; this is usually 1:1 or 1.5:1 of the patient's estimated plasma volume.[3]
- In plasma exchange, an average of 3 to 5 L of plasma is removed and replaced.[3]
- Treatments can be done with two different systems: centrifugal and filtration.[3]
  - *Centrifugal:* Separates plasma and other blood components with use of a centrifuge in which substances are separated and various layers can be obtained based on specific gravity[3] (Fig. 108.1).
  - *Filtration:* A hollow-fiber cell separator, permeable to plasma proteins, is used to remove the patient's plasma via an apheresis machine or continuous renal replacement machines adapted for apheresis (Fig. 108.2).
    - *Cascade filtration:* A second filter is used following centrifugal or filtration techniques to further filter so only larger components are removed and smaller components of plasma can be recirculated[3]
    - *Immune absorption:* An additional filter with biologic or physiochemical components that allow for absorption of a specific component[3]
- Treatment urgency can depend on several factors:
  - Emergent: For critically ill patients when treatment must be administered within 4 to 6 hours as treatment can quickly remove or delay the pathogenesis of the disease or supplement a vital component. It can be used

as both a definitive treatment or as a bridging therapy to mitigate patient decline while further evaluation and treatment is administered.[5] These procedures are generally performed in the critical care setting where advanced monitoring can be ensured.
  - Urgent: For acutely but not critically ill patients. Although indications can be the same as the emergent patient indications, the symptomatology associated with the disease process is not as severe or life threatening. In general, the patient should receive treatment within 24 hours.[5]
  - Routine: For stable or scheduled treatments. Clinical indications per the disease process necessitating treatment.
- Treatment length and frequency vary according to the disease being treated, rate of production of the substance being removed, and the patient's response to treatment. Acute conditions, such as thrombotic thrombocytopenia purpura or graft-versus-host disease, usually require daily treatments for 5 to 7 days, depending on the response to treatment.[6,7] Other conditions usually require plasma exchanges two or three times weekly for up to 6 weeks.[3] The total amount of plasma to be exchanged is used as a guide for treatment. A single treatment, referred to as a *plasma exchange,* usually takes 2 to 3 hours with a centrifugal machine and 2 to 6 hours with filtration methods.[2]
- Apheresis procedures are performed by healthcare professionals, such as registered nurses or blood bank personnel, with special knowledge and skills in apheresis. These procedures are commonly performed both in critical care units and on an outpatient basis, depending on the type of disease being treated and on the patient's condition.
- The most commonly used apheresis access systems use either two large-bore peripheral venous catheters, double-lumen vascular access catheters (VAC), vortex ports, or a dialysis graft/fistula. Peripherally inserted central venous catheters do not provide adequate blood flow and are not acceptable for use.[5]

UNIT VI

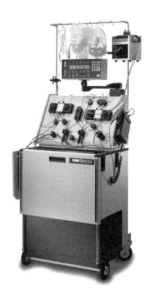

Figure 108.1   COBE Spectra Apheresis System. *(Photo courtesy CaridianBCT, Inc.)*

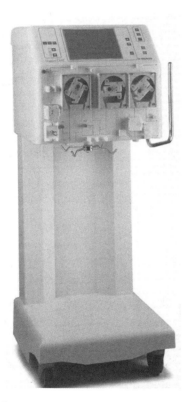

Figure 108.2   The B. Braun Diapact CRRT system can also be used for therapeutic plasma exchange and plasma adsorption/perfusion. *(Photo courtesy B. Braun Medical, Inc.)*

- ❖ A discontinuous or single-needle system can be used with peripheral venous access when component removal and reinfusion to the patient occur sequentially.[1,8]
- ❖ A continuous or dual-needle system can be used when component removal and reinfusion occur concurrently.[1,8]
- The system should be primed with an anticoagulant (e.g., heparin or citrate) to prevent clotting. If citrate is used, the patient must be monitored closely for hypocalcemia.

Citrate works as an anticoagulant by binding calcium (Ca^{++}), therefore decreasing the amount of Ca^{++} available for normal clotting.[3]

- ❖ If citrate is used, clinicians should be vigilant to monitor calcium levels and signs and symptoms of hypocalcemia during and following treatment.
- Plasma exchange is used to treat antibody-mediated disorders because the pathogenic antibodies are contained in the plasma. Removal of these antibodies through plasma exchange reduces the number of circulating antibodies, temporarily decreasing the patient's symptoms.
- Conditions treated by plasma exchange may include the following[7]:
  - ❖ Myasthenia gravis
  - ❖ Guillain-Barré syndrome
  - ❖ Various hematological disorders
  - ❖ Nephrological disorders
  - ❖ Rheumatological disorders
  - ❖ Poisoning
  - ❖ Drug overdose/drug toxicity
  - ❖ Acute liver failure
  - ❖ Solid organ transplantation for ABO incompatibility and rejection
  - ❖ Cytokine-mediated injury, such as sepsis, burns, and multisystem organ dysfunction syndrome (MODS)
- Current indication categories for therapeutic apheresis, as endorsed by the American Association of Blood Banks (AABB) and the American Society for Apheresis (ASFA), are listed in Table 108.1.
- If the patient is taking angiotensin-converting enzyme (ACE) inhibitors, contact with certain filters or membranes in the apheresis system can cause an anaphylactic reaction and severe hypotension as a result of increased levels of bradykinin, a potent vasodilator. The provider may withhold ACE inhibitors for 48 to 72 hours before treatment.
- Because of an anticoagulated state, invasive procedures should be delayed until the treatment is completed unless FFP is used as a replacement fluid.
- Potential complications of apheresis techniques include the following:
  - ❖ Bleeding
  - ❖ Thrombocytopenia
  - ❖ RBC lysis/hemolysis
  - ❖ Air embolism
  - ❖ Blood leak
  - ❖ Circuit clotting
  - ❖ Hypovolemia
  - ❖ Hypotension
  - ❖ Hypothermia
  - ❖ Vascular access complications
  - ❖ Fever/chills
  - ❖ Shock
  - ❖ Anaphylaxis
  - ❖ Allergic reactions
  - ❖ Transfusion reactions
  - ❖ Electrolyte imbalances
  - ❖ Dysrhythmias
  - ❖ Citrate toxicity
  - ❖ Infection

TABLE 108.1 American Society for Apheresis (ASFA) 2019 Indication Categories for Therapeutic Apheresis

Disease	TA modality	Indication	Category	Grade
Acute disseminated encephalomyelitis (ADEM)	TPE	Steroid refractory	II	2C
Acute inflammatory demyelinating polyradiculoneuropathy (Guillain-Barré syndrome)	TPE/IA	Primary treatment	II	1A, 1B
Acute liver failure	TPE-HV		I	1A
	TPE		III	2B
Age-related macular degeneration, dry	Rheopheresis	High-risk	II	2B
Amyloidosis, systemic	β₂-microglobulin column	Dialysis-related amyloidosis	II	2B
	TPE	Other causes	IV	2C
Anti-glomerular basement membrane disease (Goodpasture syndrome)	TPE	Diffuse alveolar hemorrhage (DAH)	I	1C
	TPE	Dialysis independence	I	1B
	TPE	Dialysis independence, no DAH	III	2B
Atopic (neuro-) dermatitis (atopic eczema), recalcitrant	ECP		III	2A
	IA		III	2C
	TPE/DFPP		III	2C
Autoimmune hemolytic anemia, severe	TPE	Severe cold agglutinin disease	II	2C
	TPE	Severe warm autoimmune	III	2C
Babesiosis	RBC exchange	Severe	II	2C
Burn shock resuscitation	TPE		III	2B
Cardiac neonatal lupus	TPE		III	2C
Catastrophic antiphospholipid syndrome (CAPS)	TPE		I	2C
Chronic focal encephalitis (Rasmussen encephalitis)	TPE		III	2C
Chronic inflammatory demyelinating polyradiculoneuropathy (CIDP)	TPE/IA		I	1B
Coagulation factor inhibitors	TPE		III	2C
	IA		III	2B
Complex regional pain syndrome	TPE	Chronic	III	2C
Cryoglobulinemia	TPE	Severe/symptomatic	II	2A
	IA	Severe/symptomatic	II	2B
Cutaneous T-cell lymphoma (CTCL); Mycosis fungoides; Sézary syndrome	ECP	Erythrodermic	I	1B
	ECP	Non-erythrodermic	III	2C
Dilated cardiomyopathy, idiopathic	IA	NYHA II-IV	II	1B
	TPF	NYHA II-IV	III	2C
Erythropoietic protoporphyria, liver disease	TPE		III	2C
	RBC exchange		III	2C
Familial hypercholesterolemia	LA	Homozygotes	I	1A
	LA	Heterozygotes	II	1A
	TPE	Homozygotes/heterozygotes	II	1B
Focal segmental glomerulosclerosis (FSGS)	TPE/IA	Recurrent in kidney transplant	I	1B
	LA	Recurrent in kidney transplant/steroid resistant in native kidney	II	2C
	TPE	Steroid resistant in native kidney	III	2C
Graft-versus–host disease (GVHD)	ECP	Acute	II	1C
	ECP	Chronic	II	1B
Hemolysis, elevated liver enzymes, and low platelets (HELLP) syndrome	TPE	Postpartum	III	2C
	TPE	Antepartum	IV	2C
Hemophagocytic lymphohistiocytosis (HLH); hemophagocytic syndrome; macrophage-activating syndrome	TPE		III	2C

TABLE 108.1	American Society for Apheresis (ASFA) 2019 Indication Categories for Therapeutic Apheresis—cont'd			
Disease	**TA modality**	**Indication**	**Category**	**Grade**
Heparin-induced thrombocytopenia and thrombosis (HIT/HITT)	TPE	Precardiopulmonary bypass	III	2C
	TPE	Thrombosis	III	2C
Hereditary hemochromatosis	Erythrocytapheresis		I	1B
Hyperleukocytosis	Leukocytapheresis	Symptomatic	II	2B
	Leukocytapheresis	Prophylactic or secondary	III	2C
Hypertriglyceridemic pancreatitis	TPE/LA	Severe	III	1C
	TPE/LA	Prevention of relapse	III	2C
Hyperviscosity in hypergammaglobulinemia	TPE	Symptomatic	I	1B
	TPE	Prophylaxis for rituximab	I	1C
IgA nephropathy (Berger disease)	TPE	Crescentic	III	2B
	TPE	Chronic progressive	III	2C
Immune thrombocytopenia (ITP)	TPE/IA	Refractory	III	2C
Inflammatory bowel disease	Adsorptive cytapheresis	Ulcerative colitis/Crohn's disease	III	1B
	ECP	Crohn's disease	III	2C
Lambert-Eaton myasthenic syndrome	TPE		II	2C
Lipoprotein(a) hyperlipoproteinemia	LA	Progressive atherosclerotic cardiovascular disease	II	1B
Malaria	RBC exchange	Severe	III	2B
Multiple sclerosis	TPE	Acute attack/relapse	II	1A
	IA	Acute attack/relapse	II	1B
	TPE	Chronic	III	2B
	IA	Chronic	III	2B
Myasthenia gravis	TPE/IA	Acute, short-term treatment	I	1B
	TPE/IA	Long-term treatment	II	2B
Myeloma cast nephropathy	TPE		II	2B
Nephrogenic systemic fibrosis	ECP/TPE		III	2C
Neuromyelitis optica spectrum disorders (NMOSDs)	TPE	Acute attack/relapse	II	1B
	IA	Acute attack/relapse	II	1C
	TPE	Maintenance	III	2C
N-methyl-ᴅ-aspartate receptor antibody encephalitis	TPE/IA		I	1C
Overdose, envenomation, and poisoning	TPE	Mushroom poisoning	II	2C
	TPE	Envenomation	III	2C
	TPE	Drug overdose/poisoning	III	2C
Paraneoplastic neurological syndromes	TPE/IA		III	2C
Paraproteinemic demyelinating neuropathies; Chronic acquired demyelinating polyneuropathies	TPE	IgG/IgA/IgM	I	1B
	TPE	Anti-MAG neuropathy	III	1C
	TPE	Multiple myeloma	III	2C
	TPE	Multifocal motor neuropathy	IV	1C
Pediatric autoimmune neuropsychiatric disorders associated with streptococcal infections (PANDAS); Sydenham chorea	TPE	PANDAS, exacerbation	II	1B
	TPE	Sydenham chorea, severe	III	2B
Pemphigus vulgaris	TPE	Severe	III	2B
	ECP/IA	Severe	III	2C
Peripheral vascular diseases	LA		II	1B
Phytanic acid storage disease (Refsum disease)	TPE/LA		II	2C
Polycythemia vera; erythrocytosis	Erythrocytapheresis	Polycythemia vera	I	1B
	Erythrocytapheresis	Secondary erythrocytosis	III	1C

Continued

TABLE 108.1	American Society for Apheresis (ASFA) 2019 Indication Categories for Therapeutic Apheresis—cont'd			
Disease	TA modality	Indication	Category	Grade
Posttransfusion purpura (PTP)	TPE		III	2C
Progressive multifocal leukoencephalopathy (PML) associated with natalizumab	TPE		III	1C
Pruritus due to hepatobiliary diseases; psoriasis	TPE	Treatment resistant	III	1C
	ECP	Disseminated pustular	III	2B
	Adsorptive cytapheresis	Disseminated pustular	III	2C
	TPE	Disseminated pustular	IV	2C
Red cell alloimmunization, prevention, and treatment	RBC exchange	Exposure to RhD + RBCs	III	2C
	TPE	Pregnancy, GA <20 weeks	III	2C
Scleroderma (systemic sclerosis)	TPE		III	2C
ECP	ECP		III	2A
Sepsis with multiorgan failure	TPE		III	2B
Sickle cell disease, acute	RBC exchange	Acute stroke	I	1C
	RBC exchange	Acute chest syndrome, severe	II	1C
	RBC exchange	Other complications	III	2C
Sickle cell disease, non–acute	RBC exchange	Stroke prophylaxis	I	1A
	RBC exchange	Pregnancy	II	2B
	RBC exchange	Recurrent vaso-occlusive pain crisis	II	2B
	RBC exchange	Preoperative management	III	2A
Steroid-responsive encephalopathy associated with autoimmune thyroiditis (Hashimoto encephalopathy)	TPE		II	2C
Stiff-person syndrome	TPE		III	2C
Sudden sensorineural hearing loss	LA/rheopheresis/TPE		III	2A
Systemic lupus erythematosus (SLE)	TPE	Severe complications	II	2C
Thrombocytosis	Thrombocytapheresis	Symptomatic	II	2C
	Thrombocytapheresis	Prophylactic or secondary	III	2C
Thrombotic microangiopathy, coagulation mediated	TPE	THBD, DGKE, and PLG mutations	III	2C
Thrombotic microangiopathy, complement mediated	TPE	Factor H autoantibody	I	2C
	TPE	Complement factor gene mutations	III	2C
Thrombotic microangiopathy, drug associated	TPE	Ticlopidine	I	2B
	TPE	Clopidogrel	III	2B
	TPE	Gemcitabine/quinine	IV	2C
Thrombotic microangiopathy, infection associated	TPE/IA	STEC-HUS, severe	III	2C
	TPE	pHUS	III	2C
Thrombotic microangiopathy, thrombotic thrombocytopenic purpura (TTP)	TPE		I	1A
Thrombotic microangiopathy, transplantation associated	TPE		III	2C
Thyroid storm	TPE		II	2C
Toxic epidermal necrolysis (TEN)	TPE	Refractory	III	2B
Transplantation, cardiac	ECP	Cellular/recurrent rejection	II	1B
	ECP	Rejection prophylaxis	II	2A
	TPE	Desensitization	II	1C
	TPE	Antibody mediated rejection	III	2C

UNIT VI

TABLE 108.1	American Society for Apheresis (ASFA) 2019 Indication Categories for Therapeutic Apheresis—cont'd			
Disease	**TA modality**	**Indication**	**Category**	**Grade**
Transplantation, hematopoietic stem cell, ABO incompatible (ABOi)	TPE	Major ABOi HPC(M)	II	1B
	TPE	Major ABOi HPC(A)	II	2B
	RBC exchange	Minor ABOi HPC(A)	III	2C
	TPE	Major/Minor ABOi with pure RBC aplasia	III	2C
Transplantation, hematopoietic stem cell, HLA desensitization	TPE		III	2C
Transplantation, liver	TPE	Desensitization, ABOi living donor	I	1C
	TPE	Desensitization, ABOi deceased donor/ antibody-mediated rejection	III	2C
	ECP	Desensitization, ABOi	III	2C
	ECP	Acute rejection/immune suppression withdrawal	III	2B
Transplantation, lung	ECP	Bronchiolitis obliterans syndrome	II	1C
	TPE	Antibody-mediated rejection/ desensitization	III	2C
Transplantation, renal, ABO compatible	TPE/IA	Antibody-mediated rejection	I	1B
	TPE/IA	Desensitization, living donor	I	1B
	TPE/IA	Desensitization, deceased donor	III	2C
Transplantation, renal, ABO incompatible	TPE/IA	Desensitization, living donor	I	1B
	TPE/IA	Antibody-mediated rejection	II	1B
Vasculitis, ANCA-associated (AAV)	TPE	MPA/GPA/RLV: RPGN, Cr ≥5.7	I	1A
	TPE	MPA/GPA/RLV: RPGN, Cr <5.7	III	2C
	TPE	MPA/GPA/RLV: DAH	I	1C
	TPE	EGPA	III	2C
Vasculitis, IgA (Henoch-Schönlein purpura)	TPE	Crescentic RPGN	III	2C
	TPE	Severe extrarenal manifestations	III	2C
Vasculitis, other	TPE	Hepatitis B polyarteritis nodosa	II	2C
	TPE	Idiopathic polyarteritis nodosa	IV	1B
	Adsorptive cytapheresis	Behçet disease	II	1C
	TPE	Behçet disease	III	2C
Voltage-gated potassium channel (VGKC) antibody– related diseases	TPE/IA		II	1B
Wilson disease, fulminant	TPE		I	1C

Categories: *I,* Disorders for which apheresis is accepted as first-line therapy, either as a primary standalone treatment or in conjunction with other modes of treatment; *II,* Disorders for which apheresis is accepted as second-line therapy, either as a standalone treatment or in conjunction with other modes of treatment; *III,* Optimum role of apheresis therapy is not established. Decision making should be individualized; *IV,* Disorders in which published evidence demonstrates or suggests apheresis to be ineffective or harmful. IRB approval is desirable if apheresis treatment is undertaken in these circumstances.

Grades: *1A,* Strong recommendation, high-quality evidence; *1B,* Strong recommendation, moderate quality evidence; *1C,* Strong recommendation, low-quality or very-low-quality evidence; *2A,* weak recommendation, high-quality evidence; *2B,* weak recommendation, moderate-quality evidence; *2C,* weak recommendation, low-quality or very-low-quality evidence

ANCA, Antineutrophil cytoplasmic antibody; *CNS,* central nervous system; *ECP,* extracorporeal photopheresis; *DAH,* diffuse alveolar hemorrhage; *HLA,* human leukocyte antigen; *HSCT,* hematopoietic stem cell transplant; *IA,* immunoadsorption; *IgG,* immunoglobulin G; *IgM,* Immunoglobulin M; *IUT,* intrauterine transfusion; *IVIG,* intravenous immunoglobulin; *MCP,* membrane cofactor protein; *NYHA,* New York Heart Association; *PANDAS,* pediatric autoimmune neuropsychiatric disorders associated with streptococcal infections; *PEOMS,* polyneuropathy, organomegaly, endocrinopathy, M protein and Skin changes; *PML,* progressive multifocal leukoencephalopathy; *RBC,* red blood cell; *TPE,* therapeutic plasma exchange; *WAHA,* warm autoimmune hemolytic anemia.

From Padmanabhan A, Connelly-Smith L, Aqui N, et al: Guidelines on the use of therapeutic apheresis in clinical practice. Evidence-based approach from the writing committee of the American Society for Apheresis: the eighth special issue. *J Clin Apher* 34:171– 354, 2019.

EQUIPMENT

- Blood cell separator or filter machine
- Blood cell separator or filter tubing set
- Replacement intravenous (IV) fluids
- Hemostats
- Vascular access dressings and flushes
- Nonsterile gloves
- Fluid shield face masks or goggles
- End caps for IV lines

Additional equipment, to have available as needed, includes the following:

- Laboratory specimen tubes
- Sterile gloves if accessing central lines such as VAC or vortex port

PATIENT AND FAMILY EDUCATION

- Explain the procedure, including risks, length of treatment, and patient positioning, and answer any questions the patient may have. *Rationale:* Explanation provides information and may decrease patient anxiety.
- Explain the purpose of the apheresis procedure, why this treatment is being performed, and the expected clinical outcomes. *Rationale:* Knowledge about the procedure helps the patient understand the treatment plan and will decrease anxiety.
- Explain the need for careful sterile technique for the duration of treatment. *Rationale:* Sterile technique is important to decrease the chance of systemic infection because pathogens can be transported throughout the entire body via the circulation.
- Explain the need for careful monitoring of the patient for complications. *Rationale:* Hypocalcemia, hypotension, bleeding, and hypothermia are all potential complications of apheresis.
- Explain the importance of the patient informing the nurse any symptoms felt during the treatment. *Rationale:* Patient symptoms can be important signs of complications related to the procedure. Examples include lightheadedness as a sign of hypotension and numbness and tingling as a sign of hypocalcemia.
- Explain the importance of preventing bleeding complications: pressure dressings at vascular sites, avoiding shaving, and care of the access catheter. *Rationale:* Alterations in blood composition and anticoagulation can put the patient at risk for bleeding.
- Explain the apheresis circuit setup to the patient and family. *Rationale:* Blood will be removed from the patient's body and will be visible during apheresis treatment.

PATIENT ASSESSMENT AND PREPARATION

Patient Assessment

- Obtain baseline vital signs, body system assessment, hemodynamic parameters (if appropriate), weight, and pretreatment fluid balance. *Rationale:* Total body assessment should be based specifically on the patient's diagnosis and reason for treatment. Pretreatment assessment provides a baseline for comparison once the treatment is started, allowing for appropriate modification of the intervention as needed. Changes in weight during and after treatment are an indicator of fluid balance.
- Review prescribed medications, and ensure that the patient has not taken an ACE inhibitor within the previous 48 hours. *Rationale:* Contact with certain fibers or membranes in the apheresis system can cause an anaphylactic reaction and severe hypotension.
- Assess pretreatment laboratory values. *Rationale:* Baseline values of the complete blood count (CBC) with differential, platelet count, and electrolytes are needed before these are altered by treatment. Coagulation parameters are particularly important: fibrinogen, prothrombin time (PT), activated clotting time (ACT), and partial thromboplastin time (PTT) if heparin is used, and ACT and ionized Ca^{++} if citrate is used. Serum sodium and serum bicarbonate levels/pH also should be evaluated in patients when citrate is used as the anticoagulant. Disease-specific tests should also be obtained pretreatment as needed.
- Obtain vascular access. *Rationale:* A properly functioning vascular access is necessary to perform plasmapheresis.

Patient Preparation

- Verify the correct patient with two identifiers. *Rationale:* Before performing a procedure, the nurse should ensure the correct identification of the patient for the intended intervention.
- Ensure that informed consent has been obtained. *Rationale:* Informed consent protects the rights of the patient and makes a competent decision possible for the patient.
- Ensure that the patient understands the preprocedural instructions. Answer questions as they arise, and reinforce information as needed. *Rationale:* Understanding of previously taught information is evaluated and reinforced.
- Assist the patient to a position of comfort that also facilitates optimal blood flow through the vascular access. *Rationale:* Facilitating patient comfort helps minimize the amount of patient movement during treatment. Movement can change the blood flow through the access site. Different access sites may require different patient positions to facilitate optimal blood flow.

Procedure for Assisting With Apheresis/Plasmapheresis

Steps	Rationale	Special Considerations
1. Verify apheresis orders.	Familiarizes the nurse with the individualized patient treatment and reduces the possibility of error.	
2. 🅗🅗		
3. 🅟🅔		
4. Confirm access placement.	Validates that the line is in correct placement.	

5. Review the following with the apheresis nurse:
A. Exchange volume
B. Anticoagulant
C. Replacement fluids
D. Baseline patient assessment, including
   i. Vital signs
   ii. Jugular vein distention
   iii. Presence of edema
   iv. Intake and output
   v. Neurological assessment
   vi. Pulmonary assessment
   vii. Renal assessment
   viii. Parameters/treatment for heart rate and blood pressure
   ix. Laboratory monitoring
   x. Procedure for emergency resuscitation
	Sets joint goals and actions to provide for patient safety and optimize the patient's outcome.[6]	

6. Gather supplies for vascular access.	Prepares for the procedure.	The process of vascular access depends on whether the site is central or peripheral.
7. Assist in gathering supplies for the apheresis procedure.	Prepares for the procedure.	Obtaining and sending laboratory specimens may be part of the apheresis setup as the vascular system is accessed.
8. Ensure that appropriate replacement fluid is available. Warm replacement fluids as prescribed.	Maintains the correct electrolyte balance; avoids hypothermia.[6]	Replacement fluids should be slightly warmed before infusion unless contraindicated (e.g., blood products should be maintained at a specific temperature before infusion to maintain viability of the product). Never use a microwave to warm fluids. Some patients also may need an increase in the ambient room temperature or ventilator heating system and warming blankets to avoid hypothermia. Most apheresis systems have inline blood warmers.
9. Infuse fluid boluses as needed before initiation.	Maintains hemodynamic stability.	Ensure the ability to continuously assess and monitor volume status and the available equipment to continue to assess throughout treatment.
10. Assist with setup and priming of the apheresis circuit as needed.	Ensures safe and proper assembly and complete removal of air from the circuit.	
11. Secure all connections.	Prevents inadvertent disconnection of the system.	
12. Remove gloves, and discard used supplies.		
13. 🅗🅗		

Procedure continues on following page

Expected Outcomes

- Therapeutic goals are achieved
- Optimal fluid balance is maintained
- Laboratory values are maintained within the expected range
- Properly functioning access site
- Patient remains pain free or has pain controlled to an acceptable goal
- Therapeutic medication levels will be maintained
- Patient/family will verbalize understanding of the procedure

Unexpected Outcomes

- Complications related to the treatment (e.g., hypotension, hypocalcemia, hypothermia, hypokalemia, hypernatremia, metabolic alkalosis, air embolism, blood leak, bleeding, infection)
- Poor blood flow through the vascular access
- Bleeding from the access site
- Dislodgment of the access catheter
- Hematoma formation at the access site
- Technical problems with apheresis circuit
- Hemolysis

Patient Monitoring and Care

Steps	Rationale	Reportable Conditions
		These conditions should be reported to the provider if they persist despite nursing interventions.
1. Monitor the patient during and after the apheresis treatment: A. Vital signs B. Hemodynamic parameters C. Jugular vein distention D. Presence of edema E. Intake and output F. Neurological assessment G. Pulmonary assessment H. Renal assessment I. Apheresis circuit J. Laboratory values as prescribed (if plasma is removed, include PT/international normalized ratio [INR], fibrinogen, and platelet count)	Patients can experience complications, such as hypotension, hypothermia, blood leak, air embolism, transfusion reactions, hypocalcemia, RBC hemolysis, thrombocytopenia, citrate toxicity, and bleeding, that may need intervention.[3,4]	• Hypotension • Hypertension • Tachycardia/bradycardia • Tachypnea/bradypnea • Fever • Hypothermia • Jugular vein distention • Crackles/rales • Edema • Change in level of consciousness • Dizziness • Change in cardiac rhythm • Blood leak • Hemolysis • Thrombocytopenia • Dysrhythmias • Coagulopathies • Allergic reaction • Transfusion reaction
2. Monitor serum ionized Ca^{++}, magnesium, serum sodium, and serum bicarbonate levels/pH (if citrate is used as an anticoagulant).	Citrate binds with Ca^{++} and can cause hypocalcemia. It also metabolizes to sodium and bicarbonate, which may cause hypernatremia, metabolic alkalosis, and citrate toxicity.[4]	• Hypocalcemia • Hypernatremia • Metabolic alkalosis • Increased anion gap
3. Monitor ACT/PTT (if heparin is used as an anticoagulant).	These values primarily reflect the activity of the intrinsic clotting pathway.	• Prolonged ACT/PTT
4. Administer replacement fluid as prescribed and needed.	Replacement fluids are important during the treatment to maintain adequate intravascular volume.	• Hypotension • Tachycardia • Decreased central venous and pulmonary artery pressures • Decreased urine output
5. Hold medications as prescribed during the procedure.	Many medications are withheld during treatment, including vasopressors and pain medications, especially those that are protein-bound.[6] Some medications, such as antihypertensive agents, anticholinergic agents, and Ca^{++} supplements, may be withheld during treatment.[6] Analgesics and antipyretics may be indicated during treatment, although these medications may mask the symptoms of a transfusion reaction.[6]	• Medications needed (e.g., analgesics, antipyretics) • Transfusion reaction

UNIT VI

Patient Monitoring and Care —*Continued*

Steps	Rationale	Reportable Conditions
6. Monitor the access and dressing sites after termination of the apheresis procedure.	Bleeding or signs or symptoms of infection can be complications of the vascular access.[3]	• Bleeding • Redness, tenderness, pain, or warmth at the access insertion site • Generalized bleeding or fever
7. Appropriately label VACs that contain indwelling anticoagulant.	Prevents infusion of anticoagulant into the patient.	• Bleeding • Bruising • Oozing
8. Review the following with the apheresis nurse, including:	Provides proper patient evaluation and documentation.	
A. Amount and type of fluids removed		• Unexpected volume
B. Amount and type of fluids given		• Unexpected volume
C. Exchange volume and fluid balance		• Unexpected volume
D. Patient reactions during treatment		• Flushing • Dysrhythmias • Tachypnea
E. Medications given during treatment	Identify possible side effects of administered medications, and anticipate patient change if this occurs.	• Unexpected side effects
1. Follow institutional standards for assessing pain. Administer analgesia as prescribed.	Identifies the need for pain interventions.	• Continued pain despite pain interventions
2. Resume or administer medications held during the procedure as prescribed.	Medications held for apheresis may need to be resumed per the patient treatment plan.	• Side effects or consequences of medication being delayed

Documentation

Documentation should include the following:
- Patient and family education
- Completion of informed consent
- Date and time of treatment initiation
- Condition of vascular access
- Intake/output/fluid balance
- Vital signs throughout the apheresis treatment
- Daily weight
- Patient's response to apheresis and daily progress toward treatment goals
- Unexpected outcomes
- Nursing interventions
- Laboratory assessment data
- Pain assessment, interventions, and effectiveness.

References and Additional Readings

For a complete list of references and additional readings for this procedure, scan this QR code with your smartphone, or visit https://www.elsevier.com/__data/assets/pdf_file/0006/1319883/Chapter0108.pdf

UNIT VI

109 Bone Marrow Biopsy and Aspiration

Sandra Kurtin

PURPOSE The bone marrow aspiration and biopsy is performed to obtain information on initial diagnosis, staging, or treatment response for patients with suspected or established hematological or oncological malignancies or blood abnormalities.

PREREQUISITE NURSING KNOWLEDGE

- **Physiology:** The majority of bone marrow is produced in the pelvis.[7]
- Multiple tests are required depending on the diagnosis. Common diagnostic tests include morphology, flow cytometry, cytogenetics, fluorescence in situ hybridization (FISH), and molecular studies. Much less commonly, infectious disease testing may be requested, including culture and Gram stain, fungal culture, viral culture, polymerase chain reaction (PCR), acid-fast bacillus (AFB), or Gomori methenamine silver (GMS) stain.[10]
- A thorough understanding is needed of the anatomy and physiology of the posterior and anterior iliac crest and the sternum. The preferred site for a bone marrow aspirate and biopsy is the posterior iliac crest.[7] The sternum may be used to aspirate marrow; however, a core biopsy cannot be obtained from the sternum because of risk of damage to underlying organs, most significantly the heart.
- **Indications:** The bone marrow biopsy and aspirate provide two distinct samples, the bone marrow aspirate, and the trephine core biopsy. They are most often performed as one procedure.
  - ❖ The procedure is essential for diagnostic and prognostic classification and evaluation of response to treatment for hematological malignancies. It may also be performed to evaluate metastatic disease in the setting of solid tumors or isolate potential infectious or genetic etiologies.
  - ❖ The aspirate is essential to differential diagnosis and is sent for hematopathology review including morphology and immunohistochemistry, flow cytometry, cytogenetics, FISH, PCR, next-generation sequencing (NGS), and chimerism analysis.

- ❖ The trephine biopsy is used to describe the architecture of the bone marrow including cellularity, organization, fibrosis, iron stores, and the presence of abnormal morphological inclusions.
- ❖ Collectively, these samples are used to answer specific questions including morphology, immunohistochemistry, cellularity, flow cytometry, FISH, cytogenetic and molecular profiling, chimerisms, and in some cases cultures.

PROCEDURE

- Clinicians including physicians, advanced practitioners, and, in some settings, advanced practice nurses with special training and experience may perform the procedure.[4] In the majority of cases, the procedure can be performed with a local anesthetic, allowing for bedside procedures. In some patients, moderate sedation is necessary and requires the safety procedures necessary for this approach.
- Approximately 70% of bone marrow is produced in the pelvis. Therefore the superior posterior iliac crest provides the most accessible location for sampling. The patient may be positioned prone or in the lateral (side-lying) position. Sternal aspirates (no trephine biopsy possible) may be obtained in patients who cannot be placed in the prone position, patients for whom direct access to the iliac crest is limited (morbidly obese patients or those who cannot assume the prone position), or patients who have received pelvic radiation exposure that may limit the sample accuracy.[9]
- The bone marrow biopsy is generally a safe procedure; however, infection, bleeding, and nerve damage (usually due to nerve compressive hematoma or improper location) may occur. Care should be taken to prevent such complications by proper site selection, maintaining strict sterile technique, and ensuring that coagulation laboratory parameters are met, anticoagulation therapy is managed appropriately, and local hemostasis is maintained.
- Clinical and technical competence in performing a bone marrow aspirate and biopsy is necessary.
- An underlying understanding of the physiology of the pelvis and sternum is necessary for proper site selection and a reduction in the potential for adverse procedural events.

AP This procedure should be performed only by clinicians who have demonstrated competence and are credentialed to perform it. In addition, the procedure must be within the scope of practice defined by their professional licensure, and in accordance with professional practice acts. Physicians, advanced practice nurses, and physician assistants may be credentialed to perform this procedure.

- The procedure is performed using sterile technique. Thus essential knowledge of sterile technique is necessary.
- Pain during a bone marrow biopsy and aspirate is generally due to the sensory nerves in the periosteum and the negative pressure induced during the bone marrow aspirate. Adequate local anesthesia and technique during the aspirate is essential to minimize procedural pain.[5]
- The majority of bone marrow biopsy and aspirate procedures may be performed using local anesthesia (lidocaine in most cases; procaine may be used in cases of lidocaine allergy). This is applied both to the skin at the designated site using a wheal, and to the underlying periosteum.
- For patients requiring moderate sedation, review and adhere to institutional policies and procedures for administration of intravenous (IV) pharmacological agents and the monitoring required. In many cases, procedures requiring moderate sedation require locations designated for these procedures (interventional radiology or inpatient). Procedural care of the patient receiving IV moderate sedation, oral or intravenous anxiolytics, or pain medication should be reviewed before performing the procedure.
- Before performing a bone marrow biopsy and aspirate, the clinician must review the indications for the procedure and confirm the requirements for sampling to ensure that all required testing can be performed.[2-3,6,8]
- Indications for bone marrow aspiration and biopsy include the following:
  - Diagnose a hematological abnormality or malignancy
  - Monitor a hematological disease state after initial diagnosis or therapy
  - Diagnose bone marrow involvement before stem cell collection and for staging of various malignant states
  - Assess the status of disease after autologous bone marrow or hematopoietic stem cell transplant
  - Assess chimerism disease status and immune reconstitution after an allogeneic bone marrow or hematopoietic stem cell transplant
  - Evaluate immunodeficiency syndromes or to confirm an infectious disease process in the marrow
- Contraindications to bone marrow biopsy and aspirate are generally related to the risk of bleeding. Patients with hemophilia, severe disseminated intravascular coagulopathy, or other related severe bleeding disorders will require special considerations before performing the procedure. Thrombocytopenia alone is not a contraindication to bone marrow examination, although a platelet transfusion may be indicated if the patient is severely thrombocytopenic or if bleeding develops or persists after the procedure.[10] The use of anticoagulant medications may pose a serious bleeding risk; therefore coagulation studies may be required in these patients. The decision on whether anticoagulation can be safely withheld before and restarted after the procedure is patient dependent and may require specialty consultation.

EQUIPMENT

- Bone marrow aspiration and biopsy kit, which includes the following:
  - Antiseptic solution (e.g., 2% chlorhexidine-based preparation)

- Two sterile fenestrated drapes
- One to two vial(s) of lidocaine (1% or 2%; 5 to 10 mL, as per institutional standards); administration should not exceed 4.5 mg/kg or 300 mg.
- 5- or 10-mL syringe for drawing up lidocaine
- Filter needle (if lidocaine drawn from glass vial)
- Needles of appropriate lengths to anesthetize both skin and periosteum
- 3½- to 6-inch spinal needle (may be required for anesthetizing periosteum in the obese patient)
- Sterile 4 × 4 and 2 × 2 gauze pads
- Small scalpel blade
- Bacitracin or Bactroban ointment (optional; for incision site postprocedure)
- Pressure tape or pressure dressing
- Biopsy needle options:
  - Illinois needle (16 gauge for bone marrow aspirate only)
  - Jamshidi bone biopsy needle (for aspirate and core biopsy, 8 or 11 gauge, 4 inches or longer)
  - TrapLok bone marrow biopsy needle (for aspirate and core biopsy, 8 or 11 gauge, 4 inches or longer)
  - SNARECOIL bone marrow biopsy needle (for aspirate and core biopsy, 8 or 11 gauge, 4 inches or longer)
  - Powered bone marrow biopsy system (for aspirate and core biopsy, 8 or 11 gauge, 4 inches or longer)
  - Extra-long bone marrow biopsy needle may be required for obese patients
- 10–20 mL syringes for bone marrow aspirate
- Blunt-tip needles for drawing up ethylenediaminetetraacetic acid (EDTA), heparin
- Sterile gloves
- Sterile gowns
- Fluid shield, face mask, or goggles
- Specimen bags and labels
- Required tubes for specimen processing (variable based on required tests; follow institutional standards) including edetate disodium (liquid EDTA and/or EDTA lavender top) and sodium heparin (green top) tubes.
- Eight glass slides and cover plate
- Container for bone core biopsy specimen, including appropriate fixative (10% formalin)

Additional equipment to have available as needed includes the following:
- Power drill (institution-specific)
- One vial of 100 units/mL heparin (follow institutional standards)
- One vial of buffered lidocaine (optional: The addition of sodium bicarbonate may minimize pain during lidocaine administration)
- Equipment for patients receiving moderate sedation:
  - Pulse oximeter with telemetry
  - Automated blood pressure monitor
  - Oxygen
  - Suction
  - Bag-valve-mask device
  - IV pharmacological agents for sedation (e.g., midazolam, 1 to 4 mg; lorazepam, 1 to 2 mg; fentanyl, 25 to 100 µg; morphine 2 to 4 mg; hydromorphone 0.5 to 2 mg)
  - IV opiate and benzodiazepine antagonist agents (i.e., naloxone and flumazenil)
  - Emergency equipment

PATIENT AND FAMILY EDUCATION

- Assess patient and family understanding of the bone marrow aspiration and biopsy procedure and the reason for it. *Rationale:* Clarification of the procedure and reinforcement of information may reduce patient and family anxiety and stress.
- Inform the patient and family (if permitted by patient) that the results will be shared with them as soon as they are available. *Rationale:* The patient and family are usually anxious about the results.
- Explain the actual procedure to the patient and family. *Rationale:* The patient and family are prepared for what to expect, and anxiety may be decreased.
- Review safety requirements for patients who will receive pharmacological agents for sedation (i.e., must have transportation and escort home and may not drive until the next day). *Rationale:* Review ensures patient safety and accountability of the physician, advanced practice nurse, or other healthcare professional for patients receiving sedation.
- Encourage the patient to verbalize any pain experienced during the procedure. *Rationale:* Additional lidocaine, pain medication, or sedation medication can be administered. The patient becomes a participant in care. Poor relaxation can cause the large gluteal muscles to spasm, making the procedure more difficult for all involved.

PATIENT ASSESSMENT AND PREPARATION

Patient Assessment

- Assess the patient's allergies and home medications, including over-the-counter medications that can increase the risk of bleeding. Anticoagulant medications may need to be held. Specialty consultation may be required to clarify risks and benefits related to anticoagulation. *Rationale:* Assessment can decrease the risk of bleeding, hematoma, and allergic reaction.
- Assess the need for antianxiety or analgesic medication or moderate sedation. *Rationale:* If the patient is very anxious before the procedure or has had severe pain with previous bone marrow procedures, small doses of analgesia or sedation promote patient comfort. Tense muscles can create a technically difficult procedure and add to pain and anxiety.
- Assess coagulation studies (PT/INR, PTT) in patients who are taking anticoagulant medications. No recommendations exist regarding minimal requirements for coagulation studies before bone marrow biopsy; however, based on clinical guidelines for similar procedures and expert opinion, a PTT goal of less than 1.5 times the control and INR less than 2 (≤1.5 if platelet count <20,000/mL) are recommended. *Rationale:* Patients at risk for bleeding complications are identified, and anticoagulant medications may need to be held.
- Assess current complete blood count (CBC) for severe thrombocytopenia requiring pre- or postprocedure transfusion. No recommendations exist regarding minimal requirements for platelet counts before bone marrow biopsy; however, based on clinical guidelines for similar procedures

and expert opinion, a platelet count ≥20,000 mL is recommended. If the procedure must be performed emergently and the platelet count is ≥10,000/mL but not ≥20,000/mL, platelet transfusion during and possibly after the procedure is recommended. Additionally, patients with platelets counts <50,000/mL who are on antiplatelet medications may require a hold on those mediations and/or platelet transfusion to reduce the risk of bleeding. *Rationale:* Patients at risk for bleeding complications are identified, and interventions for bleeding prevention are completed.
- Assess the ability of the patient to lie in the prone or lateral position, with the head of the bed at no greater than a 25-degree elevation. *Rationale:* Access to and control of the posterior iliac crest are best obtained with the patient lying flat or with the head of the bed only slightly raised with the patient in the side-lying or prone position.
- Assess vital signs and oxygenation status. *Rationale:* Baseline data are provided. Assessment ensures that the blood pressure and oxygenation status can be maintained if the patient is placed on his or her side or prone.
- Assess the posterior iliac crest with palpation. In select cases, the anterior iliac crest may be used as a result of positioning limitations or excessive tissue surrounding the posterior iliac crest. However, an increased risk of injury to the surrounding nerves and blood vessels makes this procedure more complicated. The sternum is used for aspiration only in very select cases because of potentially fatal complications with this procedure. It should only be performed in the absence of lower-risk techniques and with special equipment and close cardiac monitoring by an experienced physician. *Rationale:* Assessment identifies the most suitable area for obtaining optimal samples with a minimum of risk of discomfort and danger to the patient.
- Assess for recent bone marrow aspiration and biopsy sites. *Rationale:* The patient may have a painful experience if an additional biopsy is performed at a site that has not yet healed from a previous procedure. Penetration of scar tissue from previous bone marrow biopsy sites may also be difficult and yield inadequate results.

Patient Preparation

- Ensure that the patient and family understand the information taught. Answer questions as they arise, and reinforce information as needed. *Rationale:* Understanding of previously taught information is evaluated and reinforced.
- Verify the correct patient with two identifiers. *Rationale:* Before performing a procedure, the nurse should ensure the correct identification of the patient for the intended intervention.
- Obtain informed consent for bone marrow aspiration and biopsy and, if indicated, for moderate sedation. *Rationale:* Informed consent protects the rights of the patient and makes a competent decision possible for the patient.
- Perform a preprocedural verification and time out. *Rationale:* This ensures patient safety.
- Obtain a CBC and differential on the day of the procedure. *Rationale:* Review of the peripheral smear on the same day of the bone marrow sampling provides the hematopathologist with a view of the bone marrow capacity and resulting peripheral counts.[1]

- Assist the patient to an appropriate position depending on the patient's comfort and the preference of the physician, advanced practice nurse, or other healthcare professional. *Rationale:* Positioning ensures good visualization and control of the posterior iliac crest.
- Ensure that site markings have been made where appropriate. *Rationale:* This identifies the procedure site.
- For patients requiring moderate sedation:
  - ❖ Prescribe analgesia or sedation, if needed. *Rationale:* The patient may need analgesia or sedation to ensure adequate cooperation and minimize discomfort during the procedure.
  - ❖ Follow institutional standards for a patient receiving moderate sedation. *Rationale:* Preparation ensures that appropriate emergency equipment and medical staff are available.
  - ❖ Obtain IV access for patients receiving sedation. *Rationale:* A secure patent IV line is necessary for administration of IV pharmacological agents and, if necessary, emergency antagonist agents.
  - ❖ Place the patient on a cardiac monitor. *Rationale:* This allows for assessment of patient status during the procedure.

Procedure for Performing Bone Marrow Aspiration and Biopsy

Steps	Rationale	Special Considerations
Bone Marrow Aspiration and Biopsy		
1. Provide preprocedural patient education, obtain consent for the procedure, and perform a time-out.	Informed consent, including risks and benefits as well as patient safety.	• Rationale • Risks • Alternatives • Procedure description • After care
2. Confirm availability of personnel who will assist with the procedure.	Slide preparation, specimen processing, and additional supplies require an appropriately trained assistant for the procedure if available.	If the procedure is to be performed without assistance, prepare all equipment, and walk through the procedure for concise and accurate specimen acquisition.
3. Open the bone marrow procedure tray; add any additional supplies in a manner that preserves sterility. Ensure that you have adequate syringes and any other procedural equipment needed for the procedure before donning sterile gloves.	Maintains sterility of the procedure.	An extra overbed table works well as a procedure table. Clean before and after each use.
4. Don sterile gloves (gown if indicated)	Maintains sterility of the procedure.	Refer to institutional procedure.
5. Prepare all necessary syringes, including lidocaine syringe and those requiring anticoagulant.	Ensures adequate preparation for the procedure and reduces distraction once the procedure is started.	
6. Site selection A. Review the anatomy of the pelvis. B. Establish landmarks by placing your index finger on the anterior iliac crest and your thumb on the posterior iliac crest, approximately 3 fingerbreadths from the spine. This is the posterior iliac crest, the most common site for biopsy. C. The anterior superior iliac spine may be used in selected patients (e.g., those with extensive radiation to the pelvis for prostate or rectal cancers). D. In patients who are unable to be placed in a position for access to the posterior iliac crest, the sternal site may be used for aspirates only using a special needle and only by physicians with specialized training.		

Procedure	**for Performing Bone Marrow Aspiration and Biopsy—*Continued***	
Steps	**Rationale**	**Special Considerations**
7. Prepare the intended site with the antiseptic swabs (e.g., chlorhexidine-based preparation), and place a sterile drape.	Minimizes the risk for infection.	
8. With a 25-gauge needle, inject the skin with lidocaine, creating a wheal.	A small-gauge needle lessens the discomfort associated with administration of local anesthesia.	The use of buffered lidocaine may minimize the pain associated with administration compared with lidocaine alone.
9. With a 21-gauge 1½ inch needle (or spinal needle if necessary), infiltrate the periosteum with lidocaine in a "peppering" fashion with 5–15 mL of lidocaine (1%–2%) with 1–2 mL bicarbonate buffer solution, if available. Downward pressure on the tissue and stabilization of the needle with the thumb and forefinger of the opposite hand are helpful.	This allows the clinician to establish the geography of the site and to anesthetize an area large enough for the aspirate and the biopsy at two sites. While allowing the anesthesia to work, prepare the remaining syringes for aspirate, check the bone marrow needle (remove cap and inner sheath and replace). If the periosteum is not anesthetized, the patient may have extreme discomfort. Also, assessing the area of the posterior iliac crest in an obese patient is often difficult. Use of the spinal needle helps the provider locate an appropriate site. Buffered lidocaine reduces pain.[3]	If additional lidocaine is needed, ask the critical care nurse or person assisting to invert the extra vial. If the 1½-inch needle does not reach the bone, use the 3½-inch spinal needle to reach it. The spinal needle can also be used to assess the geography of the posterior iliac crest and allows the provider to assess the depth of the bone. It is helpful to anesthetize an area of about a quarter to half dollar size so that adjustments can be made in needle placement.
10. Make an incision over the biopsy site with a small scalpel.	Assess adequate anesthesia on skin with scalpel using the pin-prick test; if adequate, make a small incision horizontal to the vertebral column at the landmark site. Prevents tearing of the tissue that may occur with needle-only access.	Provider preference for needle-only access is allowed based on experience.
11. Advance the bone marrow needle or power device through the incision (with stabilization of the needle with the thumb and forefinger of the opposite hand) to the periosteum with firm pressure and slight rotation. Confirm with the patient that the site is numb by gently tapping on the periosteum. Either reposition or administer additional lidocaine if any sensation of sharpness is reported. Penetrate the outer cortex using a rotating motion. If a power drill device is used, DO NOT hold the needle. A slight sensation of "giving" is often noticed as the marrow cavity or medulla is reached.	Slight rotation of the needle allows for smooth entry into the marrow cavity. Attempting to stabilize the drill needle by holding will tear sterile gloves.	If the patient experiences pain, it is recommended that the needle be placed in another section of bone or additional lidocaine be applied to the outer surface of the bone. Repositioning the needle even 2–3 mm from the site of pain may reduce or eliminate the pain sensation. Follow institutional guidelines for use of the power drill device.

Procedure continues on following page

UNIT VI

Procedure for Performing Bone Marrow Aspiration and Biopsy—*Continued*

Steps	Rationale	Special Considerations
12. Remove the stylet, and attach the 10- to 20-mL syringe without heparin to obtain 1 cc of aspirate. Immediately hand this syringe to the critical care nurse or person assisting. If performing the procedure alone, place a small portion of aspirate onto a glass slide or petri dish to verify the presence of spicules (small pieces of bone) in the sample.	The first aspirate sample is used to make the slides and to form the clot section. Confirm that spicules (appear as grains of tapioca) are present. If there is no technician available, this sample will be placed into a lavender-top EDTA tube.	Follow institutional guidelines for sample requirements.
13. Draw subsequent samples in the appropriate syringes (heparinized, nonheparinized as per institutional policy). In the event that the patient is slow to aspirate, multiple syringes may be required to prevent clotting in the syringe.	Each sample requires specific sampling techniques to ensure that the sample can be processed for the requested study. Heparinized aspirate is used for chromosome analysis and FISH. Invert the syringe to mix the heparin and marrow. Nonheparinized tubes are used for molecular studies, flow cytometry, and measurable residual disease (MRD) studies. Follow institutional standards for use of heparinized and nonheparinized tubes.	The number of viable cells is reduced with each subsequent sample. Sampling for MRD requires the first pull. Preparation of slides for hematopathology review requires spicules. Refer to institutional guidelines for sampling requirements.
14. If aspirate is not obtained or is aparticulate, replace the stylet, reposition the needle, and attempt to aspirate again. With each pull, rotate the needle slightly.[5] **(Level C*)**	If marrow cannot be obtained after several attempts, another needle may be needed because of blunting.	At times, it is difficult to obtain a bone marrow aspirate. Difficulty can occur if a patient is aplastic, fibrosed, or if the marrow space is packed by disease. This is known as a *dry tap.* In these cases, the provider should try to obtain an additional core biopsy specimen for pathology analysis that may include flow cytometry and cytogenetics/ FISH analysis. The specimen should be placed in RPMI tissue transport medium. The touch preparation in this case also becomes a crucial step in providing the pathologist with suitable material for morphological examination.[5]
15. Have the assisting personnel help by inverting all of the tubes several times.	Aspirate samples can clot quickly if not thoroughly mixed with anticoagulant.	
16. Remove the aspiration needle from the site with a gentle twisting and pulling motion.	Ensures adequate hemostasis and reduces the chance of hemorrhage, hematoma, and infection.	Replacing the stylet decreases discomfort with removal of the aspirate needle.

*Level C: Qualitative studies, descriptive or correlational studies, integrative reviews, systematic reviews, or randomized controlled trials with inconsistent results.

UNIT VI

Procedure for Performing Bone Marrow Aspiration and Biopsy—*Continued*

Steps	Rationale	Special Considerations
17. If a bone marrow biopsy is not being obtained: A. Hold very firm pressure for 5 minutes or until bleeding has stopped. B. Cleanse the site with antiseptic swab (e.g., chlorhexidine-based preparation). C. Apply bacitracin or Bactroban ointment, an adhesive bandage, and a 4 × 4 pressure dressing with paper or Medipore tape (follow institutional standards). D. Reposition patient into the supine position for 10–15 minutes to maintain pressure at the biopsy site.	Ensures adequate hemostasis and reduces the chance of hemorrhage, hematoma, and infection.	Very firm pressure is key. If the patient is at high risk for bleeding (e.g., severely thrombocytopenic, other coagulopathy, anticoagulation therapy), have the patient lie on a firm surface (e.g., book, sandbag, firmly rolled towel), or a large ice pack may be helpful.
18. Label samples in the presence of the patient and send them for laboratory analysis.	Ensures accuracy of results and timeliness of laboratory analyses.	Ensure that paperwork for specimens is correctly completed to avoid delays in processing.
19. If a biopsy is not being obtained, remove and discard used supplies in an appropriate receptacle.	Safely discards used supplies.	Never allow another individual to clear the biopsy tray of sharps. The provider should clear the tray.

Bone Marrow Biopsy

Steps	Rationale	Special Considerations
1. It is rare that a bone marrow biopsy is performed without first attempting an aspirate. Therefore the procedure continues with obtaining a trephine biopsy after the aspirate.		
2. Once the aspirate is obtained, there are two options to obtain the core: (1) advance the needle further in the same site to obtain the biopsy, or (2) move to a second site to obtain the core.	Some sections of bone are extremely hard or sloped, making placement of the needle difficult. If hard bone is encountered, another section of bone should be used. If a section of bone is extremely soft, it is often difficult to obtain an adequate biopsy, and another section of bone should be chosen. Be sure all of the periosteum is anesthetized. Follow institutional guidelines for use of the power drill device if indicated.	Obtaining the core from the same site as the aspirate may be complicated by crush artifact. Moving to an adjacent site requires verification of anesthesia.
3. If using the same site, advance the needle using steady pressure, monitoring patient tolerance. Use the inner sheath to measure the core. The core should be 1.5–2 cm in length.	Requires constant smooth pressure.	
4. If using a second site, bring the needle just out of the bone, but not out of the skin. Reposition to an adjacent site. Secure the needle into the periosteum. Remove the stylet, replace the cap on the needle, and advance the needle approximately 2 cm with a firm and slightly rotating motion.	Removing the stylet allows the core section of bone to fill the needle. Replacing the cap provides suction to keep the specimen in the needle and protects the hand.	

UNIT VI

Procedure continues on following page

Procedure for Performing Bone Marrow Aspiration and Biopsy—*Continued*

Steps	Rationale	Special Considerations
5. Verify the length of the biopsy sample using the stylet as a guide.	Gently insert the stylet so as not to push the core back or damage it.	The optimal length of biopsy sample should be between 1.5 and 2.0 cm.
6. Before removal, the manual biopsy needle should be rotated 360 degrees in each direction three to five times. Place the cap back on the hub, and gently rotate the needle back out of the bone, skin, and muscle while applying firm gentle pressure.	Giving the manual needle a few 360-degree turns and creating a vacuum by placing the cap over the top of the needle during removal increases the likelihood that the bone core will be retained within the needle.	If no cap is available for the needle, place the thumb over the needle to create a vacuum.
7. Specialty needles include core severing devices. See the instructions for the individual needles for proper use.		
8. Apply firm pressure to the site for 5 minutes or until bleeding has stopped. A. Cleanse the site with an antiseptic swab (chlorhexidine-based preparation). B. Apply bacitracin or Bactroban ointment, an adhesive bandage, and a 4 × 4 pressure dressing with paper or Medipore tape (follow institutional standards). C. Reposition the patient into the supine position for 10–15 minutes to maintain pressure at the biopsy site.	Reduces the chance of bleeding at the site. Prevents hemorrhage, hematoma, and infection.	Very firm pressure is key. If the patient is at high risk for bleeding (e.g., severely thrombocytopenic, other coagulopathy, anticoagulation therapy), have the patient lie on a firm surface (e.g., book, sandbag, firmly rolled towel), or a large ice pack may be helpful.
9. Slide preparation requires specialized training and generally includes laboratory trained staff. Refer to institutional guidelines for securing samples for bone marrow biopsy and aspirate.		
10. Label samples in the presence of the patient, and send then for laboratory analysis.	Specimens require staining and decalcification for studies.	
11. Remove and discard used supplies in an appropriate receptacle.	Safely discards used supplies.	Never allow another individual to clear the biopsy tray of sharps. The provider should clear the tray.

Expected Outcomes

- Adequate bone marrow aspirate and core biopsy specimens obtained
- Spicules in the aspirate (unless the patient is aplastic, fibrosed, or packed); aspirate not clotted
- Minimal bleeding and discomfort (patient may feel a dull ache for a few days after the procedure)
- Absence of additional complications

Unexpected Outcomes

- Difficulty obtaining a bone marrow aspirate or core biopsy
- Excessive pain
- Inability to perform the procedure because of patient fear or intolerance
- Hematoma
- Retroperitoneal bleed
- Local infection
- Nerve damage

Patient Monitoring and Care

Steps	Rationale	Reportable Conditions
		These conditions should be reported to the provider if they persist despite nursing interventions.
1. Follow institutional standards for assessing pain. Administer analgesia as prescribed. **(Level B*)**	Identifies the need for pain interventions. Promotes patient comfort.	• Continued pain despite pain interventions
2. Assess vital signs, oxygenation, level of consciousness, and cardiac rhythm during the procedure and until the patient is completely recovered from sedation medications.	Monitors patient response to positioning, the procedure, and medications.	• Changes in vital signs • Decreases in oxygen saturation (SpO_2) • Changes in cardiac rhythm • Changes in level of consciousness
3. Assess the site at regular intervals with consideration of patient-specific risk factors for bleeding.	Monitors for signs and symptoms of complications.	• Bleeding • Hematoma • Pain • Nerve damage • Infection
4. Instruct the patient and family to keep the pressure dressing clean, dry, and in place for 24 hours after the procedure. Ask the patient or family to assess for bruising or hematoma.	Proper dressing care reduces the chance of bleeding and minimizes the chance of infection at the site.	
5. Advise the patient and family to apply a wrapped ice bag to the site over clothing if experiencing discomfort. This will also reduce the risk of bleeding. The ice should never be applied directly to the skin.	Ice reduces swelling, decreases the chance of hematoma, and adds comfort.	
6. Instruct the patient and family to notify the physician, advanced practice nurse, or other healthcare professional immediately if the patient develops fever, increasing pain, erythema, excessive warmth, bruising, and/or bleeding at the biopsy site. Also report numbness, tingling, and/or loss of strength in the extremity of the corresponding biopsy site.	Increasing pain (especially radiating down the leg), numbness, tingling, and/or loss of strength may be signs of a compressive hematoma. Fever, pain, excessive warmth, and erythema may be signs of infection requiring immediate intervention.	
7. Avoid applying heat to the procedure site.	Heat may exacerbate bleeding.	
8. Advise against nonsteroidal antiinflammatory drugs or aspirin for 24 hours after the biopsy.	This measure reduces the chance of bleeding or hematoma at the site.	
9. Advise the use of acetaminophen for pain relief, if not contraindicated.	Acetaminophen relieves pain and does not promote bleeding.	
10. If the patient has been on prophylactic or treatment-dose anticoagulation, instruct the patient and family on the appropriate time frame to restart anticoagulation if being held.	Clear instruction is required to prevent bleeding complications related to anticoagulation and/or thromboembolism related to a lapse in anticoagulation.	

*Level B: Well-designed, controlled studies with results that consistently support a specific action, intervention, or treatment.

UNIT VI

Documentation

Documentation should include the following:
- Patient and family education
- Completion of informed consent
- Procedure verification and time out
- Date and time of the procedure
- Indication for the procedure
- Preparation for the procedure
- Any complications that occurred
- Any medications used
- Specimens obtained
- Additional interventions
- For patients receiving moderate sedation, documentation that institution-approved discharge criteria have been met
- Pain assessment, interventions, and effectiveness

References and Additional Readings

For a complete list of references and additional readings for this procedure, scan this QR code with your smartphone, or visit https://www.elsevier.com/__data/assets/pdf_file/0007/1319884/Chapter0109.pdf

PROCEDURE

110 Bone Marrow Biopsy and Aspiration (Assist)

Sandra Kurtin

PURPOSE The bone marrow aspiration and biopsy are performed to obtain information on initial diagnosis, staging, or treatment response for patients with suspected or established hematological or oncological malignancies or blood abnormalities.

PREREQUISITE NURSING KNOWLEDGE

- **Physiology:** The majority of bone marrow is produced in the pelvis.
- Multiple tests are required depending on the diagnosis. Common diagnostic tests include morphology, flow cytometry, cytogenetics, fluorescence in situ hybridization (FISH), and molecular studies.[1] Much less commonly, infectious disease testing may be requested, including culture and Gram stain, fungal culture, viral culture, polymerase chain reaction (PCR), acid-fast bacillus (AFB), or Gomori methenamine silver (GMS) stain.
- A thorough understanding is needed of the anatomy and physiology of the posterior and anterior iliac crest and the sternum. The preferred site for a bone marrow aspirate and biopsy is the posterior iliac crest. The sternum may be used to aspirate marrow; however, a core biopsy cannot be obtained from the sternum because of the risk of damage to underlying organs, most significantly the heart.
- **Indications:** The bone marrow biopsy and aspirate provide two distinct samples: the bone marrow aspirate and the trephine core biopsy.[1-3,6,9-10] They are most often performed as one procedure.
  ❖ The procedure is essential for diagnostic and prognostic classification and evaluation of response to treatment for hematological malignancies. It may also be performed to evaluate metastatic disease in the setting of solid tumors or to isolate potential infectious or genetic etiologies.
  ❖ The aspirate is essential to the differential diagnosis and is sent for hematopathology review including morphology and immunohistochemistry, flow cytometry, cytogenetics, FISH, PCR, next-generation sequencing (NGS), and chimerism analysis.
  ❖ The trephine biopsy is used to describe the architecture of the bone marrow including cellularity, organization, fibrosis, iron stores, and the presence of abnormal morphological inclusions.
  ❖ Collectively, these samples are used to answer specific questions including morphology, immunohistochemistry, cellularity, flow cytometry, FISH, cytogenetic and molecular profiling, chimerisms, and in some cases cultures.

PROCEDURE

- Clinicians, including physicians, advanced practitioners, and, in some settings, advanced practice nurses with special training and experience may perform the procedure. In the majority of cases, the procedure can be performed with a local anesthetic, allowing for bedside procedures. In some patients, moderate sedation is necessary and requires the safety procedures necessary for this approach.
- Approximately 70% of bone marrow is produced in the pelvis. Therefore the superior posterior iliac crest provides the most accessible location for sampling. The patient may be positioned in the prone or lateral (side-lying) position. Sternal aspirates (no trephine biopsy possible) may be obtained in patients who cannot be placed in the prone position, patients for whom direct access to the iliac crest is limited (morbidly obese patients or those who cannot assume the prone position), or patients who have received pelvic radiation exposure that may limit the sample accuracy.[8]
- The bone marrow biopsy is generally a safe procedure; however, infection, bleeding, and nerve damage (usually due to nerve compressive hematoma or improper location) may occur. Care should be taken to prevent such complications by proper site selection, maintaining strict sterile technique, and ensuring that coagulation laboratory parameters are met, anticoagulation therapy is managed appropriately, and local hemostasis is maintained.
- Clinical and technical competence in performing a bone marrow aspirate and biopsy is necessary.
- An underlying understanding of the physiology of the pelvis and sternum is necessary for proper site selection and a reduction in the potential for adverse procedural events.
- The procedure is performed using sterile technique. Thus essential knowledge of sterile technique is necessary.
- Pain during a bone marrow biopsy and aspirate is generally due to the sensory nerves in the periosteum and the negative pressure induced during the bone marrow aspirate. Adequate local anesthesia and technique during the aspirate is essential to minimize procedural pain.[5]
- The majority of bone marrow biopsy and aspirate procedures may be performed using local anesthesia (lidocaine in most cases; procaine may be used in cases of lidocaine allergy). This is applied both to the skin at the designated site using a wheal, and to the underlying periosteum.

- For patients requiring conscious sedation, review and adherence to institutional policies and procedures for administration of intravenous (IV) pharmacological agents, including moderate sedation (if indicated) is required. In many cases, procedures requiring conscious sedation require locations designated for these procedures (interventional radiology or inpatient). Procedural care of the patient receiving IV moderate sedation, oral anxiolytics, or pain medication should be reviewed before performing the procedure.
- Before performing a bone marrow biopsy and aspirate, the clinician must review the indications for the procedure and confirm the requirements for sampling to ensure that all required testing can be performed.[3,8-10]
- Indications for bone marrow aspiration and biopsy include the following:
  - Diagnose a hematological abnormality or malignancy
  - Monitor a hematological disease state after initial diagnosis or therapy
  - Diagnose bone marrow involvement before stem cell collection and for staging of various malignant states
  - Assess the status of disease after autologous bone marrow or hematopoietic stem cell transplantation
  - Assess chimerism disease status and immune reconstitution after an allogeneic bone marrow or hematopoietic stem cell transplant
  - Evaluate immunodeficiency syndromes or confirm an infectious disease process in the marrow
- Contraindications to bone marrow biopsy and aspirate are generally related to the risk of bleeding. Patients with hemophilia, severe disseminated intravascular coagulopathy, or other related severe bleeding disorders require special considerations before performing the procedure. Thrombocytopenia alone is not a contraindication to bone marrow examination, although a platelet transfusion may be indicated if the patient is severely thrombocytopenic or if bleeding develops or persists after the procedure. The use of anticoagulant medications may pose a serious bleeding risk; therefore coagulation studies may be required in these patients. The decision on whether anticoagulation can be safely withheld before and restarted after the procedure is patient dependent and may require specialty consultation.

EQUIPMENT

- Bone marrow aspiration and biopsy kit, which includes the following:
  - Antiseptic solution (e.g., 2% chlorhexidine-based preparation)
  - Two sterile fenestrated drapes
  - One to two vial(s) of lidocaine (1% or 2%; 5 to 10 mL, should not exceed 4.5 mg/kg or 300 mg)
  - 5- or 10-mL syringe for drawing up lidocaine
  - Filter needle (if lidocaine drawn from a glass vial)
  - Needles of appropriate lengths to anesthetize both the skin and periosteum
  - 3½- to 6-inch spinal needle (may be required for anesthetizing the periosteum in obese patients)
  - Sterile 4 × 4 and 2 × 2 gauze pads
  - Small scalpel blade
  - Bacitracin or Bactroban ointment (optional; for incision site postprocedure)
  - Pressure tape or pressure dressing

- Biopsy needle options:
  - Illinois needle (16 gauge for bone marrow aspirate only)
  - Jamshidi bone biopsy needle (for aspirate and core biopsy, 8 or 11 gauge, 4 inches or longer)
  - TrapLok bone marrow biopsy needle (for aspirate and core biopsy, 8 or 11 gauge, 4 inches or longer)
  - SNARECOIL bone marrow biopsy needle (for aspirate and core biopsy, 8 or 11 gauge, 4 inches or longer)
  - Powered bone marrow biopsy system (for aspirate and core biopsy, 8 or 11 gauge, 4 inches or longer)
  - Extra-long bone marrow biopsy needle may be required for obese patients
- 10- to 20-mL syringes for bone marrow aspirate
- Blunt-tip needles for drawing up ethylenediaminetetraacetic acid (EDTA), heparin
- Sterile gloves
- Sterile gowns
- Fluid shield, face mask, or goggles
- Specimen bags and labels
- Required tubes for specimen processing (variable based on required tests; follow institutional standards) including edetate disodium (liquid EDTA and/or EDTA lavender top) and sodium heparin (green top) tubes
- Eight glass slides and cover plate
- Container for bone core biopsy specimen, including appropriate fixative (10% formalin)

Additional equipment, to have available as needed, includes the following:
- Power drill (institution-specific)
- One vial of 100 units/mL heparin (follow institutional standards)
- One vial of buffered lidocaine (optional: The addition of sodium bicarbonate may minimize pain during lidocaine administration.)
- Equipment for patients receiving moderate sedation:
  - Pulse oximeter with telemetry
  - Automated blood pressure monitor
  - Oxygen
  - Suction
  - Bag-valve-mask device
  - IV pharmacological agents for sedation (e.g., midazolam, 1 to 4 mg; lorazepam, 1 to 2 mg; fentanyl, 25 to 100 µg; morphine, 2 to 4 mg; hydromorphone, 0.5 to 2 mg)
  - IV opiate and benzodiazepine antagonist agents (i.e., naloxone and flumazenil)
  - Emergency equipment (e.g., cardiac monitor/defibrillator, code cart)

PATIENT AND FAMILY EDUCATION

- Assess patient and family understanding of the bone marrow aspiration and biopsy procedure and the reason for it. **Rationale:** Clarification of the procedure and reinforcement of information may reduce patient and family anxiety and stress.
- Inform the patient and family (if permitted by patient) that the results will be shared with them as soon as they are available. **Rationale:** The patient and family are usually anxious about the results.

- Explain the actual procedure to the patient and family, or participate in the informed consent process if the rationale and description is explained by the clinician performing the procedure. *Rationale:* The patient and family are prepared for what to expect, and anxiety may be decreased.
- Review safety requirements for patients who will receive pharmacological agents for sedation (e.g., must have transportation and escort home and may not drive until the next day). *Rationale:* Review ensures patient safety and accountability of the physician, advanced practice nurse, or other healthcare professional for patients receiving sedation.
- Encourage the patient to verbalize any pain experienced during the procedure. *Rationale:* Assist with administration of additional lidocaine, pain medication, or sedation medication if ordered. The patient becomes a participant in care. Poor relaxation can cause the large gluteal muscles to spasm, making the procedure more difficult for all involved.

PATIENT ASSESSMENT AND PREPARATION

Patient Assessment

- Assess the patient's allergies and home medications, including over-the-counter medications that can increase the risk of bleeding. Anticoagulant medications may need to be held. Specialty consultation may be required to clarify risks and benefits related to anticoagulation. *Rationale:* Assessment can decrease the risk of bleeding, hematoma, and allergic reaction.
- Assess the need for antianxiety or analgesic medication or moderate sedation. Assist with administration as ordered by the physician or advanced practitioner. *Rationale:* If the patient is very anxious before the procedure or has had severe pain with previous bone marrow procedures, small doses of analgesia or sedation will promote patient comfort. Tense muscles can create a technically difficult procedure and add to pain and anxiety.
- Assist in obtaining and review relevant laboratory measures including:
  - ❖ Coagulation studies (PT/INR, PTT) in patients who are taking anticoagulant medications. No recommendations exist regarding minimal requirements for coagulation studies before bone marrow biopsy; however, based on clinical guidelines for similar procedures and expert opinion, a PTT goal of less than 1.5 times the control and INR less than 2 (≤1.5 if platelet count <20,000/mL) are recommended. *Rationale:* Patients at risk for bleeding complications are identified, and anticoagulant medications may need to be held.
  - ❖ Complete blood count (CBC) for severe thrombocytopenia requiring pre- or postprocedure transfusion. No recommendations exist regarding minimal requirements for platelet counts before the bone marrow biopsy; however, based on clinical guidelines for similar procedures and expert opinion, a platelet count ≥20,000/mL is recommended. If the procedure must be performed emergently and the platelet count is >10,000/mL but not >20,000/mL, platelet transfusion during and possibly after the procedure is recommended.

Additionally, patients with platelets counts <50,000/mL who are on anti-platelet medications may require a hold on those medications and/or platelet transfusion to reduce the risk of bleeding. Assist with obtaining blood products, and administer as per institutional guidelines. *Rationale:* Patients at risk for bleeding complications are identified, and interventions for bleeding prevention are completed.
- Assess the ability of the patient to lie in the prone or lateral position, with the head of the bed at no greater than a 25-degree elevation. Assist with positioning to ensure maximal comfort during the procedure. *Rationale:* Access to and control of the posterior iliac crest are best obtained with the patient lying flat or with the head of the bed only slightly raised with the patient in the side-lying or prone position.
- Assess vital signs and oxygenation status. *Rationale:* Baseline data are provided. Assessment ensures that the blood pressure and oxygenation status can be maintained if the patient is placed on the side or prone.

Patient Preparation

- Ensure that the patient and family understand the information taught. Answer questions as they arise, and reinforce information as needed. *Rationale:* Understanding of previously taught information is evaluated and reinforced.
- Assist with obtaining informed consent for bone marrow aspiration and biopsy and, if indicated, for moderate sedation. *Rationale:* Informed consent protects the rights of the patient and makes a competent decision possible for the patient.
- Assist with a preprocedural verification and time out. Verify the correct patient with two identifiers. *Rationale:* Before performing a procedure, the nurse should ensure the correct identification of the patient for the intended intervention.
- Facilitate obtaining a CBC and differential on the day of the procedure. *Rationale:* Review of the peripheral smear on the same day of the bone marrow sampling provides the hematopathologist with a view of the bone marrow capacity and resulting peripheral counts.
- Assist the patient to an appropriate position depending on the patient's comfort and the preference of the physician, advanced practice nurse, or other healthcare professional. *Rationale:* Positioning ensures good visualization and control of the posterior iliac crest.
- For patients requiring sedation:
  - ❖ Assist with administration of prescribed analgesia or sedation, if needed. *Rationale:* The patient may need analgesia or sedation to ensure adequate cooperation and minimize discomfort during the procedure.
  - ❖ Follow institutional standards for a patient receiving moderate sedation. *Rationale:* Preparation ensures that appropriate emergency equipment and medical staff are available.
  - ❖ Obtain IV access for patients receiving sedation. *Rationale:* A secure patent IV line is necessary for administration of IV pharmacological agents and, if necessary, emergency antagonist agents.
  - ❖ Place the patient on a cardiac monitor. *Rationale:* This allows for assessment of patient status during the procedure.

Procedure for Assisting With Bone Marrow Aspiration and Biopsy[4,7]

Steps	Rationale	Special Considerations
1. Assist the physician, advanced practice nurse, or other clinician in obtaining informed consent.	Informed consent, including risks and benefits as well as patient safety.	• Rationale • Risks • Alternatives • Procedure description • After care
2. Assist the physician, advanced practice nurse, or other healthcare professional performing the procedure with patient positioning as needed.	Prepares for the procedure.	
3. Assist the physician, advanced practice nurse, or other healthcare professional performing the procedure if needed with opening and assembling necessary supplies.	Prepares supplies. Maintains sterile technique.	
4. Assist the physician, advanced practice nurse, or other healthcare professional performing the procedure with applying personal protective and sterile equipment (sterile gown, sterile gloves, mask, goggles).	Maintains sterile technique.	Gowns may be required in some settings, such as the blood and marrow transplant unit. Follow institutional standards.
5. Assist with or draw up 2 mL of EDTA into one of the sterile syringes (10–20 mL) depending on the number of specimens needed.	Ensures adequate slide preparation because EDTA is used to preserve spicules (small pieces of bone).	EDTA tubes usually have a lavender top. Follow institutional guidelines for using EDTA in syringes and tubes.
6. Assist with drawing up heparin into one of the syringes (10-mL or 20-mL) depending on the number if specimens needed.	Heparinized aspirate is used for flow cytometry, chromosome analysis, FISH, and chimerism studies (chimerism may also be performed on EDTA tubes).	Heparinized tubes usually have a green top. Follow institutional standards for use of heparinized and nonheparinized tubes for obtaining samples.
7. Follow institutional standards for administration of prescribed IV pharmacological agents, including moderate sedation. (**Level B***)	Promotes patient comfort and reduces anxiety.	Ensure that emergency equipment is available and functional.
8. Assist with processing the aspirate obtained in the nonheparinized (EDTA) syringe first. A. The aspirate in the 20-mL nonheparinized (EDTA) syringe should be placed in lavender-top tubes. B. The aspirate in the heparinized syringes should be placed into green-top sodium heparin tubes.	Nonheparinized (EDTA) bone marrow aspirate can clot if it is not placed in the appropriate tubes soon after it is obtained. These will be used for slide preparation, clot analysis, and PCR studies.	If no spicules are visible in the aspirate syringe, there will be no hematopoietic elements for morphological analysis. It may be necessary to attempt aspiration after repositioning the aspirate needle to an alternate site, or the patient may have an "empty marrow." If no blood can be aspirated at all, the procedure may be documented as a "dry tap."
9. Assist as needed with performing the touch preparation with the bone biopsy core sample, and place the sample in 10% formalin fixative or sterile saline solution–soaked sterile gauze in a container.	A touch preparation can be useful for a complete pathology analysis, especially if the aspirate is a particulate or a "dry tap."	

*Level B: Well-designed, controlled studies with results that consistently support a specific action, intervention, or treatment.

Procedure | for Assisting With Bone Marrow Aspiration and Biopsy—*Continued*

Steps	Rationale	Special Considerations
10. Assist with holding pressure for 5 minutes or until bleeding has stopped (use sterile technique). Once bleeding stops, assist as needed with applying a sterile pressure dressing.	Ensures adequate hemostasis and reduces hemorrhage, hematoma, and infection.	Very firm pressure is key. If the patient is at high risk for bleeding (e.g., severely thrombocytopenic, other coagulopathy, anticoagulation therapy), it may be helpful to have the patient lie on a firm surface (e.g., book, sandbag, firmly rolled towel) or use a large ice pack.
11. Follow institutional standards for recovering a patient who has received IV moderate sedation.	Ensures that recovery parameters have been met.	
12. Label samples in the presence of the patient, and send for laboratory analysis.	Ensures accuracy of results and timeliness of laboratory analyses.	Ensure that the paperwork for specimens is correctly completed to avoid delays in processing.
13. Remove PE, and discard used supplies in an appropriate receptacle.	Safely discards used supplies.	Never clear the tray of sharps. This will be done by the practitioner.

Expected Outcomes

- Adequate bone marrow aspirate and core biopsy specimens obtained
- Spicules in the aspirate (unless the patient is aplastic, fibrosed, or packed); aspirate not clotted
- Minimal bleeding and discomfort (patient may feel a dull ache for a few days after the procedure)
- Absence of additional complications

Unexpected Outcomes

- Difficulty obtaining a bone marrow aspirate or core biopsy
- Excessive pain
- Inability to perform the procedure because of patient fear or intolerance
- Hematoma
- Retroperitoneal bleed
- Local infection
- Nerve damage

Patient Monitoring and Care

Steps	Rationale	Reportable Conditions
		These conditions should be reported to the provider if they persist despite nursing interventions.
1. Follow institutional standards for assessing pain. Administer analgesia as prescribed. **(Level B*)**	Identifies the need for pain interventions. Promotes patient comfort.	• Continued pain despite pain interventions
2. Monitor vital signs, level of consciousness, oxygenation, and cardiac rhythm during the procedure and until the patient is completely recovered from sedation medications.	Determines the patient response to positioning and the procedure.	• Changes in vital signs or level of consciousness • Decreased oxygen saturation (SpO_2) • Cardiac dysrhythmias
3. Assess the site at regular intervals with consideration of patient-specific risk factors for bleeding.	Monitors for signs and symptoms of complications.	• Bleeding • Hematoma • Infection
4. Instruct the patient and family to keep pressure dressing clean, dry, and in place for 24 hours after the procedure. Ask the patient or family to assess for bruising or hematoma.	Proper dressing care reduces the chance of bleeding and minimizes the chance of infection at the site.	

*Level B: Well-designed, controlled studies with results that consistently support a specific action, intervention, or treatment.

UNIT VI

Procedure continues on following page

Patient Monitoring and Care —*Continued*

Steps	Rationale	Reportable Conditions
5. Advise the patient and family to apply a wrapped ice bag to the site over clothing if experiencing discomfort. This will also reduce the risk of bleeding. The ice should never be applied directly to the skin.	Ice reduces swelling, decreases the chance of hematoma, and adds comfort.	
6. Instruct the patient and family to notify the physician, advanced practice nurse, or other healthcare professional immediately if the patient develops fever, increasing pain, erythema, excessive warmth, bruising, and/or bleeding at the biopsy site. Also report numbness, tingling, and/or loss of strength in the extremity of the corresponding biopsy site.	Increasing pain (especially radiating down the leg), numbness, tingling, and/or loss of strength may be signs of a compressive hematoma. Fever, pain, excessive warmth, and erythema may be signs of infection requiring immediate intervention.	
7. Do not apply heat to the procedure site.	Heat may exacerbate bleeding.	
8. Advise against nonsteroidal anti-inflammatory drugs or aspirin for 24 hours after the biopsy.	This measure reduces the chance of bleeding or hematoma at the site.	
9. Advise the use of acetaminophen for pain relief, if not contraindicated.	Acetaminophen relieves pain and does not promote bleeding.	
10. If the patient has been on prophylactic or treatment-dose anticoagulation, instruct the patient and family on the appropriate time frame to restart anticoagulation if being held.	Clear instruction is required to prevent bleeding complications related to anticoagulation and/or thromboembolism related to a lapse in anticoagulation.	

Documentation

Documentation should include the following:
- Patient and family education
- Completion of informed consent
- Procedure verification and time out
- Indication for the procedure
- Date and time of the procedure
- Practitioner performing the procedure
- Person assisting with procedure
- Any complications that occurred
- Any medications used
- Specimens obtained
- Additional interventions
- Pain assessment, interventions, and effectiveness

References and Additional Readings

For a complete list of references and additional readings for this procedure, scan this QR code with your smartphone, or visit https://www.elsevier.com/__data/assets/pdf_file/0008/1319885/Chapter0110.pdf.

PROCEDURE

111   Burn Wound Care

Susan Ziegfeld

PURPOSE Burn wound care is performed to promote healing, to maintain function, and to prevent infection and burn wound sepsis. A major focus during burn wound care also incorporates strategies to effectively manage pain.

PREREQUISITE NURSING KNOWLEDGE

- Burns destroy the structural integrity of the skin, disrupting its normal functions of regulating temperature, maintaining fluid status, protecting against infection, and covering nerve endings. The skin is composed of three layers, the epidermis, dermis, and subcutaneous fat, which is rich in blood vessels (Fig. 111.1).
  - ❖ The *epidermis* is the outermost layer. It is capable of rapid regeneration through division of cells closest to the dermis; older epidermal cells are pushed outward as the epidermis is regenerated. The epidermis provides a barrier to the environment, containing melanocytes (protection from the sun) and Langerhans cells (protection against foreign organisms).
  - ❖ The *dermis* contains blood vessels, sensory fibers (for pain, touch, pressure, and temperature), collagen, sebaceous glands, and sweat glands.
  - ❖ Epidermal cells line deep dermal structures (hair follicles and sweat glands); these epidermal elements provide the ability for the skin to regenerate (the more epidermal cells remaining in the wound bed, the faster the healing).
- Burn depth has historically been classified as first, second, third, or fourth degree. A more meaningful way to classify burn injury is in terms of the anatomy. *Superficial* injury is restricted to the outer layer (epidermis); *superficial partial thickness* injury crosses the epidermis and reaches the dermis; *deep partial-thickness* injury crosses into the deeper dermis; *full-thickness* injury crosses into the entire epidermis, dermis, and hypodermis; and *deep full-thickness* injury crosses into all layers of the skin and underlying tissue and can include the nerves, muscle, and bone (Table 111.1).[1,14]
- Superficial (first-degree) burns extend only partially through the epidermis, thereby maintaining the barrier function of the skin. Burns involving only the epidermis are very painful but do not form blisters. The epidermis is usually regenerated in 3 to 4 days.[9] These burns are not included when estimating the percentage of total body surface area burned (%TBSA) because they do not result in an open wound.
- Superficial partial-thickness (second-degree) burns involve loss of the epidermis and part of the dermis.

- Deep partial thickness (second degree) burns destroy most of the dermis (Fig. 111.2). These wounds heal by epithelialization from epidermal cells remaining in the dermis. Deep partial-thickness burns may result in slow healing (more than 21 days) and are fragile wounds prone to hypertrophic scarring. For this reason, surgical excision of partial-thickness wounds that affect functional and cosmetic areas and application of skin grafts may be considered.
- A full-thickness (third-degree) burn involves complete destruction of the dermis and extends into the subcutaneous tissue. Because the skin is unable to regenerate, the dead tissue is removed and the wound is grafted with skin from another part of the patient's own body (autograft).[6,7,15] The grafted wound loses epidermal appendages and is unable to sweat, maintain lubrication, or protect from sun exposure after healing (Fig. 111.3).
- Fourth-degree burns extend through the entire layer of skin into the underlying fat, muscle, and bone. The goal of treatment is to provide adequate soft tissue coverage of the burn and restore function. Negative pressure wound therapy, skin grafts, and skin flaps are potential treatment strategies.[14,16]
- The depth of a burn wound is directly related to the temperature and the duration of contact with the burning agent. The burning agent can be thermal (i.e., flame, contact, or scald), chemical, electrical, or radiation. An inhalation injury should always be suspected if the patient was in an enclosed space with a fire; the mortality rate is significantly increased when burns are compounded by smoke inhalation.[10,21]
- The burn injury produces three zones of injury: the zone of coagulation (cellular death), the zone of stasis (vascular impairment, potentially reversible tissue injury), and the zone of hyperemia (increased blood flow and inflammatory response). Decreased perfusion or poor fluid resuscitation of the burn wound can cause the burn to convert to the next severe zone deepening the initial wound. This progressive destruction can be minimized by providing adequate oxygenation and fluid resuscitation, alleviating pressure on the injured tissue, maintaining local and systemic warmth, and decreasing edema by elevating the burned area.[1,2,8]
- Assess areas where full-thickness eschar is circumferential. Because of the inelastic nature of eschar, it acts like a tourniquet as edema develops. Surgical release

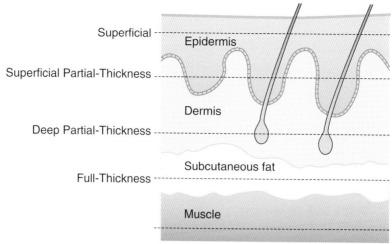

Figure 111.1 Depth of burn wound injury. *(From Townsend CM et al., editors: Sabiston textbook of surgery, ed 19, Philadelphia, 2012, Saunders.)*

TABLE 111.1	**Depth Characteristics of Burn Wounds**	
Type	Physical Characteristics	Healing
Superficial burn (first degree): destruction of epidermis, usually caused by overexposure to sun or brief exposure to hot liquid. This type of injury is not included in calculations of burn size.	Red; hypersensitive; no blisters.	Injured layers peel away from totally healed skin at 5–7 days without residual scarring.
Superficial partial-thickness burn (superficial second degree): destruction of epidermis and upper dermis. Usually results from scalding or brief contact with hot objects.	Blistered; very moist; red or pink in color; exquisitely painful; capillary refill intact.	Reepithelializes from epidermal appendages in 7–14 days. Usually has minimal scarring but variable repigmentation.
Deep partial-thickness burn (deep second degree): destruction of epidermis through to lower dermis. May result from grease or longer contact with hot objects.	Mottled pink to white; drier than superficial burns; less sensitive to pinprick; does not blanch to pressure; hair follicles and sweat glands intact. Can be dark red with a "starry night" appearance.	Slower regeneration from epidermal elements: 14–21+ days in absence of grafting. Prone to hypertrophic scars and contracture formation. May require grafting to reduce healing time and complications.
Full-thickness burn (third degree): destruction of epidermis and all of the dermis. Results from exposure to flames, chemicals that are not immediately washed, electrical injury, or prolonged contact with a heat source.	Dry; leathery and firm to touch; pearly white, brown, or charred in appearance; no blanching to pressure; no pain; may see thrombosed vessels.	Incapable of self-regeneration. Preferred treatment is early excision and autografting.
Full-thickness burn (fourth degree). Extends through the entire skin and into underlying fat, muscle, and bone.	Black; charred with eschar, dry; no pain.	Incapable of self-regeneration. Preferred treatment is early excision and autografting. Potential for tissue engineering and regenerative medicine.[16]

(escharotomy) is imperative to prevent respiratory compromise or circulatory impairment, which could lead to limb loss (Fig. 111.4).[4,6,7]

- Monitor pulses, capillary refill, and sensation distal to circumferential eschar, especially after fluid resuscitation. Signs and symptoms that indicate a need for escharotomy include cyanosis of distal unburned skin, unrelenting deep tissue pain, progressive paresthesia, and progressive decrease or absence of pulse.[1,4]
- Circumferential eschar of the trunk can lead to decreased tidal volume and agitation (Fig. 111.5)[1]; therefore adequacy of respiratory excursion must be assessed.

- Escharotomy is performed at the bedside by a physician, with a scalpel or electrocautery used to cut the eschar longitudinally. Bleeding should be minimal because only dead tissue is cut; any bleeding can be controlled with sutures, silver nitrate sticks, collagen packing, or electrocautery.[1,2] Pain is usually managed with small intravenous doses of opiates and benzodiazepines.
- Burn size may be determined with several methods.[5,14,19]
  - ❖ The *rule of nines* may be used to quickly calculate burn size. In an adult, the head and neck and each upper extremity represent 9% of the patient's body surface area. The anterior trunk, posterior trunk, and each leg

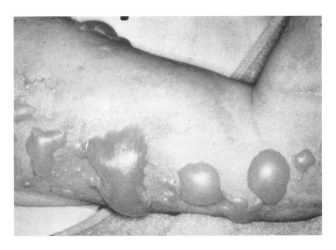

Figure 111.2 Blisters of a partial-thickness burn wound on the arm.

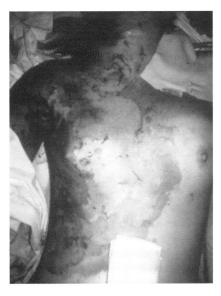

Figure 111.3 A fresh partial-thickness burn toward the patient's left side progressed to a full-thickness burn on the patient's right side.

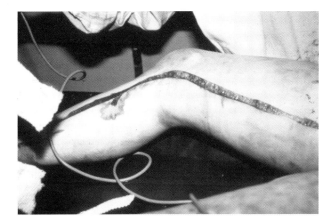

Figure 111.4 Escharotomy of the leg to improve circulation.

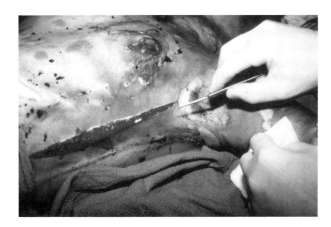

Figure 111.5 Full-thickness burn with chest escharotomy to improve chest expansion.

represent 18% of the patient's body surface area. This rule only applies to adults; infants and young children have much larger heads and smaller legs in proportion to body size.[1,19]

❖ The *Lund and Browder chart,* best used for pediatric patients (Fig. 111.6), breaks the body into smaller areas and takes into consideration the proportional differences of persons of different ages.[14]

❖ The *rule of the palm (Palmar method)* notes that the patient's entire hand, including the fingers, may be used as a template to represent roughly 1% of the TBSA.[1,14]

• Burn inflammatory response occurs during the first 24 hours and causes a massive fluid shift to the interstitial space. It is imperative not to over-resuscitate during this time; urine output should be the driving factor in resuscitation. Mobilization of fluid starts after 72 hours. Fluid resuscitation with a balanced salt solution is based on the patient's weight and burn size (partial-thickness and full-thickness wounds).[5,8] Large wounds are prone to huge

evaporative water losses that require close monitoring of volume status.[8,11]

• Effective resuscitation results in adequate urinary output (0.5 mL/kg/hour) as a surrogate marker of end-organ perfusion.[1,11]

• Burns of specific anatomical areas need special consideration. Assess the eyes for injury, and treat chemical exposure with copious normal saline solution irrigation; treat burned ears with a topical antimicrobial cream that can penetrate the cartilage and protect from pressure by eliminating the use of pillows or dressings about the head; elevate burned extremities; cautiously consider the need for an indwelling urinary catheter in the patient with perineal burns, paying particular attention to reevaluating the need to reduce the risk of a catheter-associated urinary tract infection (CAUTI); and clip hair growing through the burn wounds. Two burned surfaces that contact each other need dressings between them to prevent fusing as they heal (e.g., between toes, skin folds).

• Criteria for transferring patients to a specialized burn-care facility have been adopted by the American Burn Association and the American College of Surgeons. These criteria are listed in Box 111.1 and are available at the American Burn Association website at www.ameriburn.org.

• Emergency treatment of thermal injuries includes initially cooling the burned skin with tepid water (never ice) and

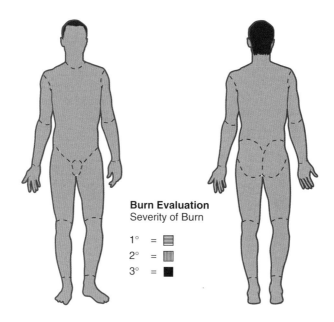

Burn Evaluation
Severity of Burn

1° = ▤
2° = ▦
3° = ■

Lund and Browder chart								
AREA	**AGE–YEARS**					% 2º	% 3º	% TOTAL
	0–1	1–4	5–9	10–15	ADULT			
Head	19	17	13	10	7			
Neck	2	2	2	2	2			
Ant. Trunk	13	17	13	13	13			
Post. Trunk	13	13	13	13	13			
R. Buttock	2½	2½	2½	2½	2½			
L. Buttock	2½	2½	2½	2½	2½			
Genitalia	1	1	1	1	1			
R.U. Arm	4	4	4	4	4			
L.U. Arm	4	4	4	4	4			
R.L. Arm	3	3	3	3	3			
L.L. Arm	3	3	3	3	3			
R. Hand	2½	2½	2½	2½	2½			
L. Hand	2½	2½	2½	2½	2½			
R. Thigh	5½	6½	8½	8½	9½			
L. Thigh	5½	6½	8½	8½	9½			
R. Leg	5	5	5½	6	7			
L. Leg	5	5	5½	6	7			
R. Foot	3½	3½	3½	3½	3½			
L. Foot	3½	3½	3½	3½	3½			
					Total			

Figure 111.6   The Lund and Browder chart is used to assess and graphically document size and depth of the burn wound is *(From Carlson, K.K. (2009). AACN advanced critical care nursing, St. Louis, Elsevier).*

recognizing the importance of preventing hypothermia.[1] In preparation for transfer, the airway should be assessed and 100% oxygen administered; large-bore intravenous (IV) access should be established and fluid resuscitation started. Pediatric patients should be started on maintenance fluid until further instructed by the burn team to avoid fluid overload; patients should initially have nothing by mouth status; wounds should be wrapped with a clean, dry sheet and a warm blanket; pain medication should be given in small IV doses, with recognition that coexisting injuries or medical conditions exacerbate the effects of opiates; tetanus prophylaxis should be administered; and all initial treatment should be documented.[1,5]

- Initial treatment of chemical burns includes removing saturated clothing, brushing off any powdered chemical, and continuously irrigating involved skin with copious amounts of water for 20 to 30 minutes. If at all possible, determine whether the chemical is acidic or alkaline. Neutralizing chemical burns with another chemical is contraindicated because the procedure generates heat. Burned eyes must be irrigated with large volumes of normal saline solution followed by an eye examination.[1] Some chemicals

- Partial-thickness burns on more than 10% total body surface area
- Burns that involve the face, hands, feet, genitalia, perineum, or major joints
- Third-degree burns in any age group
- Electrical burns, including lightning injury
- Chemical burns
- Inhalation injury
- Burn injury in patients with preexisting medical disorders that could complicate management, prolong recovery, or affect mortality
- Any patient with burns and concomitant trauma (such as fractures) in which the burn injury poses the greatest risk for morbidity or mortality
- Burned children in hospitals without qualified personnel or equipment to care for children
- Burn injury in patients who will need special social, emotional, or long-term rehabilitative intervention

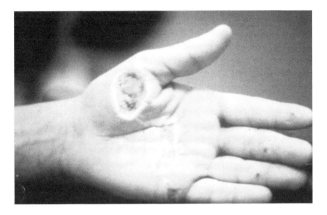

Figure 111.7 Entry site of an electrical burn.

are absorbed systemically through burn wounds; contact the local poison control center to determine whether further treatment is indicated.[1,2] Ensure that all physicians, advanced practice nurses, and other healthcare professionals wear appropriate personal protective equipment to prevent unintentional chemical exposure.

- Initial treatment of tar burn consists of cooling the tar with cold water until the product is completely cooled.
    - ❖ After cooling, adherent tar should be covered with a petrolatum-based ointment (such as white petroleum jelly) and dressed to promote emulsification of the tar.[1] Electrical injuries (Fig. 111.7) result when the body becomes part of the pathway for the electrical current. Deep burns may occur from tissue resistance where the patient contacted the electrical source and where the patient was grounded. Initially of greater concern than the burns is the high incidence of cardiac dysrhythmias, myoglobinuria resulting in acute tubular necrosis, and neurological sequelae. Monitoring electrocardiographic (ECG) results, increasing urine output to 1 to 1.5 mL/kg/hour in the presence of dark port-colored urine, assessing for associated trauma, and establishing baseline neurological status are vital in the treatment of the electrical injury patient.[1,7,19]

- Inhalation of smoke may cause localized airway inflammation and edema that can lead to airway obstruction. Signs and symptoms that increase suspicion for inhalational injury include but are not limited to fire in a closed compartment, prolonged entrapment, singed nares, cough, carbonaceous sputum, stridor, and hoarseness. Bronchoscopy on admission should be used for evaluation when these are present to assess for airway edema and mucosal injury. Significant findings may necessitate endotracheal intubation as a precautionary measure. Inhalational injury/burns are not included in the calculation for estimating the percentage of total body surface area burned.[21]
- Care of the burn wound and associated healing are determined by the extent and depth of the injury and the overall condition of the patient.
- Most burn centers use clean technique for dressing removal and wound cleansing, with sterile technique for sterile dressing application only.[7]
- Wound care should be performed in a warm area. Many burn units have replaced traditional hydrotherapy tanks with shower tables for large wound care procedures to allow water runoff, thus decreasing leaching of electrolytes and minimizing wound exposure to perineal-contaminated water. Emergency equipment must always be immediately available during hydrotherapy procedures. As wounds decrease in size and patients approach discharge, bathtubs and showers offer reasonable options for wound cleansing.
- Initial wound cleansing requires thorough debridement of all devitalized tissue. Blisters >2 cm are generally unroofed.[6] Use of a moistened washcloth is effective to gently remove burned tissue, with use of a slow and deliberate wiping motion. Wash the wounds with gentle pH-neutral liquid soap solution or wound cleanser, and pat dry with clean towels.[4,19]
- Topical antimicrobial agents limit bacterial proliferation and fungal colonization in burn wounds. There are numerous dressings used to limit bacterial burden in the wound, including antimicrobial ointments and creams and silver-based long-wear dressings.[14] Systemic antibiotics are not routinely administered to burn patients because of the high risk for development of antibiotic resistance (Table 111.2).[7]
- Burn wounds should be assessed daily for infection, cellulitis, burn progression, and the wound care plan tailored to the needs of the patient. Moist healing may speed the time of burn wound healing.
- An *autograft* (skin graft taken from the patient) typically is required to heal a full-thickness burn wound.[6] A debrided full-thickness wound may be protected from infection and drying through the use of biologic or biosynthetic dressings when donor sites are not available for autografting. An *allograft*, or *homograft*, refers to the use of "nonself" human skin grafts; typically cadaver skin, these grafts become vascularized by the patient and risk rejection if they stay in place too long. A *xenograft*, or *heterograft*, is nonhuman skin obtained from commercial pigskin (porcine)-processing companies; it forms a collagen bond with the wound and protects it for a period until donor sites are available for autografting. Porcine xenografts may be placed over clean partial-thickness wounds to protect the wound while it heals beneath the

TABLE 111.2   Topical Antimicrobial Agents[14]

Agent	Activity	Advantages	Disadvantages
Silver sulfadiazine 1% cream (Silvadine)	Bactericidal effect on cell membrane and wall; excellent against *Pseudomonas aeruginosa*, *Staphylococcus aureus*, other burn flora, and yeast	Broad-spectrum antimicrobial coverage; low toxicity; no discomfort on application; easy to remove; rare hypersensitivity to sulfa component; may increase neovascularization	Poor eschar penetration; infrequent hypersensitivity; macerates surrounding tissues; contraindicated in pregnant women and newborns (risk for kernicterus); early transient neutropenia when applied to large burns. Pseudo-eschar masks the appearance of the burn making assessment difficult
Mafenide acetate 10% cream (Sulfamylon)	Broad-spectrum against gram-positive and gram-negative organisms; not effective against yeast; diffuses through devascularized areas; is absorbed, metabolized, and excreted by kidneys	Highly soluble and penetrates eschar well; persistent activity against *Pseudomonas*	Pain on application of cream; systemically absorbed; may cause metabolic acidosis (through carbonic anhydrase inhibition – monitor ABGs); cutaneous hypersensitivity reactions occur; may see yeast overgrowth
Mafenide acetate (Sulfamylon) 5% solution	Broad-spectrum against gram-positive and gram-negative organisms; not effective against yeast	Moist dressings may be used over wounds, such as a new graft, when a liquid soak antibiotic is desired	Expensive; the wet dressings are often uncomfortable and may result in hypothermia
Silver nitrate, 0.5% in water (if dressing is allowed to dry, concentration of silver nitrate increases and becomes caustic at 2%)	Bacteriostatic against many organisms; does not penetrate drainage or debris	Painless application; few organisms are resistant to silver	Must be kept wet; poor penetration of eschar; stains unburned tissue and environment brown-black; hypotonicity of dressing may lead to hyponatremia and hypochloremia. Monitor serum sodium and potassium); requires thick dressings and resoaking every 4 hours to prevent drying
Silver nylon (a nonadherent nanocrystalline silver-coated dressing with sustained silver release for several days)	Lower minimal inhibitory concentration; a lower minimal bactericidal concentration; faster bacterial killing than other topicals	Decreases dressing changes by being left in place for 3 days	Decreases ability to visualize the wound
Acticoat delivers a uniform antimicrobial concentration of silver to the wound bed for up to 5 days	Broad-spectrum against gram-positive and gram-negative organisms and some yeasts and molds	Decreases dressing changes	May produce a pseudo eschar from silver after application; requires remoistening with sterile water every 3 hours; costly

xenograft.[6,7] Skin regeneration with autologous stem cells is currently being investigated.[18]

- Negative-pressure wound therapy may be used to maintain fresh-graft placement, improve wound bed vascularization, and reduce microbial activity.[4,14]
- The burn patient's condition is hypermetabolic until burn wounds are closed and healing is complete, and it can last up to 12 months after the injury.[4,6] Dietary consultation is recommended, and adjunctive supplemental therapies may be ordered to optimize wound healing.[4,7,15] Increased caloric and protein requirements for wound healing are usually met through nasogastric or nasoduodenal tube feeding to maintain mucosal integrity in large burns. Supplementation with high-calorie nutritional drinks can facilitate energy needs, and vitamins can promote wound healing. Large quantities of free water should be discouraged because the risk for hyponatremia is high after a large burn.
- An individualized plan for pain control should be in place for both background pain (pain that is continuously present), breakthrough pain (associated with activities of daily living), and procedural pain (intermittent pain related to procedures).[4,5,12,20] Unrelieved pain can lead to stress-related immunosuppression, increased potential for infection, delayed wound healing, decreased quality of life, and depression.[12] Subcutaneous and intramuscular injections should be avoided because absorption is poor and unreliable as a result of edema.[1] As the wound heals, the patient may experience more discomfort from itchiness and less discomfort from pain.[12,] A moisturizing lotion prevents drying and reduces pruritus. Nonpharmacological techniques can be learned to assist with the management of pain and itch.[4]
- Burn wounds contract during the healing phase. Self-care and range-of-motion exercises are encouraged. Stretching exercises and proper positioning are vital to prevent contractures and loss of function.[7] Static splinting is sometimes added to maintain sustained stretch.[7] Hypertrophic scar formation is countered through the use of topical silicone gel sheeting and pressure garments worn 24 hours a day until the scars mature and soften (6 to 18 months).[13] Keloids as well as hypertrophic scars may

require surgery, laser therapy, steroid injections, and pressure treatment.[6,7,22]

- Grafts and donor sites on the lower extremities require support during healing when the patient is out of bed. Application of elastic bandages to extremities may prevent pooling of venous blood, permanent discoloration, or skin breakdown.
- The burn wound should not be exposed to the sun for 1 year because new scars sunburn easily.
- Patients should be instructed to select clothing that blocks sun and to use sunscreen on exposed grafts, generally for life.

EQUIPMENT

- Personal protective equipment as needed (e.g., gown, mask, goggles)
- Nonsterile gloves
- Sterile gloves
- Warm water
- Mild pH-neutral liquid cleansing agent
- Normal saline solution
- Washcloths
- Towels
- Scissors and forceps (clean and sterile)
- Topical agents, as ordered
- Tongue depressors
- Sterile dressings as needed (e.g., gauze)
- Rolled dressing, gentle tape, or netting to secure dressings
- Pillows to elevate extremities
- Pain and sedation medication (as prescribed)

Additional equipment, to have available as needed, includes the following:

- Emergent intubation and advance airway equipment
- Nasolaryngoscope

PATIENT AND FAMILY EDUCATION

- Involve the patient and family in wound care during their hospital stay, and encourage them to ask questions. Demonstrate wound care, and have the patient and family return the demonstration before the planned discharge. Provide detailed wound care instructions electronically or in writing. Arrange for home care or clinic visits to follow up on wound care. ***Rationale:*** Education validates patient and family understanding and ability to perform wound care, and it allows time for them to develop a level of comfort. The opportunity to reinforce important points is provided.
- Explore resources the patient will have for wound care at home (e.g., availability of running water, shower versus tub, burn supplies, insurance coverage. ***Rationale:*** This measure ensures that the patient is knowledgeable about care based on what adjustments need to be made at home.
- Simplify wound care, and assess the family's ability to provide care at home. ***Rationale:*** Continued care of the wound may be necessary after discharge.
- Teach the patient and family about the signs and symptoms of infection and the importance of reporting these in a timely manner. ***Rationale:*** The patient and family can recognize problems early so appropriate measures can be instituted by the physician, advanced practice nurse, and other healthcare professionals.
- Teach the patient and family about pain control; assess the patient's personal acceptable level of pain. ***Rationale:*** Education and assessment decrease concerns about pain, facilitate an individualized pain-relief plan, and foster cooperation with care.
- Teach the patient and family about pain management, including types of medications prescribed, timing of medications in relation to wound care, and nonpharmacological pain strategies.[4] ***Rationale:*** Comfort at home is supported.
- Provide instructions to the patient and family about the normal changes seen in the wound, including epithelial islands, healing margins, dryness on epithelialization, epidermal fragility on shearing, hypervascularization of the healed wound, and venous congestion in the dependent wound. ***Rationale:*** Anxiety about appearance is reduced.
- Teach the patient and family about care of healed burns, including medications to reduce itching,[4,20] use of nonscented moisturizers, protection from shear, and protection from sun exposure for a minimum of 1 year. ***Rationale:*** Education reduces complications and promotes patient satisfaction.
- Explain the rationale to the patient and family for the wearing and care of pressure garments. Also explain that the duration of treatment can be up to 18 months; children will have to get remeasured as they grow. ***Rationale:*** Pressure garments must fit properly to reduce scar formation, and they can be difficult to apply.[2]
- Discuss the importance of mobility and proper positioning (e.g., splinting) on function. Self-care (activities of daily living) and range-of-motion exercises should be encouraged during the healing phase. ***Rationale:*** Contractures associated with healing skin, improper positioning, and immobility are prevented.
- Identify caloric needs for healing, and suggest appropriate nutritional supplements. ***Rationale:*** Metabolic needs are increased for months after discharge, and a balanced diet facilitates gain of muscle mass versus adipose tissue.
- Inform the patient and family that many burn patients experience nightmares, alterations in body image, and psychological disturbances.[2,17] Provide resources, including consultation to a psychologist or burn survivor group, if desired. ***Rationale:*** Information increases awareness of these problems and reassures the patient and family that these experiences, although unpleasant, are not abnormal.
- Provide the patient and family with follow-up appointments and contact information of the burn provider in case of a question. ***Rationale:*** Necessary information for further care and follow-up is provided.

PATIENT ASSESSMENT AND PREPARATION

Patient Assessment

- Assess vital signs, including temperature. ***Rationale:*** Baseline vital signs allow for comparison during and after the procedure to evaluate patient tolerance, normothermia, and adequacy of pain medication.

- Evaluate for signs of healing, including the following. **Rationale:** Healing should occur within a predictable time frame determined by the depth of burns, unless complications occur.
  - ❖ Decreased pain
  - ❖ Reepithelialization from epithelial islands within the wound
  - ❖ Decreasing wound size
  - ❖ Decreased edema
  - ❖ Compare the patient's level of healing with the expected level of healing for the number of days after the burn.
- Evaluate for the following signs and symptoms of infection.[4,10] **Rationale:** Infection can result in delayed wound healing, prolonged hospitalization, and death.
  - ❖ Foul odor
  - ❖ Purulent drainage
  - ❖ Increased pain
  - ❖ Increasing edema
  - ❖ Cellulitis
  - ❖ Fever
  - ❖ Development of eschar or early eschar separation
  - ❖ Wound discoloration
  - ❖ Increase in burn size or depth
- Monitor for distal circulation (pulses, pain, color, sensation, movement, and capillary refill) to areas with circumferential burns and increased edema. **Rationale:** Edema and circumferential burns impede distal circulation and cause worsening tissue perfusion and cell death.
- Determine the patient's understanding of pain management strategies. Assess the patient's pain level on a standardized pain scale (such as the 0 to 10 scale) before, during, and after the procedure. Explore discrepancies between the patient's level of pain and desired level of pain. **Rationale:** An individualized plan for pain control should be in place for background, breakthrough, and procedural pain.[4,5,12] In addition to the traditional use of pain and anxiety medications, alternative therapies should be included (e.g., relaxation techniques, distraction, massage

therapy, music therapy). The patient's needs change based on changes in the wound (e.g., healing, debridement, conversion to a deeper wound).

- Evaluate the patient's general level of function, particularly in burned areas. **Rationale:** An individualized plan for range-of-motion exercises, positioning, and splinting should be made to optimize the patient's level of function. Burns contract during the healing phase, and immobility enhances loss of function.

Patient Preparation

- Ensure that the patient understands the preprocedural teaching. Answer questions as they arise, and reinforce information as needed. **Rationale:** Understanding of previously taught information is evaluated and reinforced.
- Verify the correct patient with two identifiers. **Rationale:** Before performing a procedure, the nurse should ensure the correct identification of the patient for the intended intervention.
- Notify other appropriate healthcare providers who need to assess the burn wound or perform a task (e.g., quantitative wound biopsies, range-of-motion exercises by physical therapist) at the time of dressing changes. **Rationale:** Organization of care allows important assessment and intervention to take place without causing extra pain and stress to the patient.
- After checking previous requirements for patient comfort during the dressing change, premedicate the patient with pain medication and any sedative as prescribed, allowing an appropriate amount of time before starting wound care. **Rationale:** Premedication allows time for medication to take effect and promotes optimal comfort for the patient.
- Consider the synergistic effects of opioids, sedatives, and drugs that affect the central nervous system. Closely monitor the patient for 30 to 60 minutes after the wound care procedure is completed or until there is a return to baseline. **Rationale:** Stimulatory effects that counteract central nervous system depression are reduced after wounds are covered; decreased noxious stimuli and respiratory depression may occur.

Procedure for Care of Burn Wounds

Steps	Rationale	Special Considerations
1. Prepare all necessary equipment and supplies. The treatment area should be warmed.	Preparation facilitates efficient wound care and prevents needless delays. Warming the room decreases the risk for hypothermia.	Providers who need to observe the wound should be notified ahead of time so they can be present while the wound is uncovered.
2. 🔲		
3. 🔲		For larger dressing changes, all physicians, advanced practice nurses, and other healthcare professionals participating in the wound care should apply caps, masks, and gowns. Smaller graft changes may require less personal protective equipment.

Procedure for Care of Burn Wounds—*Continued*

Steps	Rationale	Special Considerations
4. Remove old dressings, and discard them in infectious waste containers. Place a towel or pad under the exposed extremity.	Old dressings can contain large amounts of body secretions and blood. A clean field under the extremity helps prevent the wound from getting soiled once clean and helps prevent infection.	Remove dressings only from areas that can be redressed within 20–30 minutes at one time. Finish wound care to these areas before moving to new areas (decreases heat loss and pain related to nerve endings being exposed to air).
5. Remove and discard gloves, and apply a pair of clean gloves.	Used gloves are contaminated by handling of the burn dressing. Aseptic technique is necessary for wound care.	
6. Wash the wound with mild soap solution or wound cleanser, rinse with warm water or saline, and pat dry.	Cleanses the wound of debris with mechanical débridement and reduces microorganisms.	Cleanse beyond the wound to reduce the microbial count on surrounding tissue. Patient tolerance may improve if allowed to cleanse one's own wounds.
7. Use scissors and forceps or gauze to remove loose necrotic tissue and any broken blister tissue.	Bacteria proliferate in necrotic tissue.	Typically, physicians perform this function in hospitals that do not specialize in burn wound care.
8. Assess the burn wound for color, size, odor, depth, drainage, bleeding, edema, cellulitis, epithelial budding, eschar separation, sensation, movement, peripheral pulses, and any signs of pressure areas from splints. For wet dressings, proceed to **Step 9.**	Validates the healing process and identifies complications.	
9. *Creams:* Use a sterile tongue depressor to remove the required amount of topical agent from the container. *Ointments:* Apply a thin layer to the wound as prescribed; apply a dressing as needed.	Use of a sterile tongue depressor and removal of only what is needed from the container prevent contamination of the topical agent.	If the area to be covered has folds and crevices or if the wound consists of scattered areas, topical agents should be placed directly on the wound rather than on the burn dressing (ensures good coverage without applying unnecessary amounts of an absorbable topical agent to uninjured areas).
10. *Soaks:* Pour the prescribed solution onto sterile gauze pads. Squeeze out excess fluid, and apply to the wound.	Ideal moisture is when the dressing is similar to a damp sponge. Excess fluid may macerate tissue.	
11. Loosely wrap extremities with gauze rolls. Secure dressings with elastic net. Wrap extremities from distal to proximal. Wrap fingers and toes separately to allow for movement and therapy.	Holds the dressings in place.	Wrapping distally to proximally assists with circulation and prevents pooling of blood. Check pulses and capillary refill after wrapping to ensure that circulation is not compromised.

Procedure continues on following page

UNIT VII

Procedure for Care of Burn Wounds—*Continued*

Steps	Rationale	Special Considerations
12. Assess the need for additional pain medication before continuing.	Patients have a right to good pain control. The success or failure of pain control for the current dressing change affects the way the patient responds to future dressing changes.	The first dressing change is very important to set up future dressing change successes.
13. Repeat steps starting at **Step 4** until all burn wounds have been cared for.	Isolating areas for dressing changes prevents unnecessary temperature loss, pain from increased nerve ending exposure to air movement, and cross-contamination of wounds.	The size of the team doing the dressing and the amount of débridement time required determine how much of the wound should reasonably be exposed at any given time.
14. Work closely with PT and OT. Apply splints as ordered, and elevate burned extremities with pillows, elastic net sling, or both; elevate the head of the bed.	Maintains position of function, prevents contractures and pressure ulcers, and reduces edema. Elevation of donor sites facilitates healing.	Do not bend the knees if the popliteal space is burned. Do not put pillows under the patient's head if the neck or ears are burned. Do not inhibit movement with splints if the patient is awake and able to use the involved extremity.
15. Remove gloves, and discard used supplies.		
16. ▢▢		

Expected Outcomes

- Wounds heal as expected without infectious complications
- Patient maintains a self-identified acceptable level of pain relief
- Patient attains comfort from measures taken for anxiety and itching
- Patient and family verbalize knowledge of patient condition and plan of care
- An optimal level of function is maintained or attained
- Patient and family response and interactions demonstrate adaptation to injury
- Patient and family collaborate in management of care
- At the time of discharge, patient and family verbalize and demonstrate an understanding of post-hospital care

Unexpected Outcomes

- Wound converts to deeper injury
- Wound infection or systemic sepsis occurs
- Wound heals with unnecessary loss of function

Patient Monitoring and Care

Steps	Rationale	Reportable Conditions
		These conditions should be reported to the provider if they persist despite nursing interventions.
1. Follow institutional standards for assessing pain. Administer analgesia as prescribed. Evaluate and treat the patient for pain, consider using the FACES scale for children. Ask the patient to rate the pain on a scale of 0–10; check the orders for pain and sedation for dressing changes; check the patient's medication requirements with previous dressing changes, and have that amount of medication available in the room before starting the procedure; assess the need for more medication throughout the dressing change. Incorporate alternative pain relief techniques (e.g., relaxation techniques, massage therapy, distraction, music, visual imaging).	Identifies the need for pain interventions. The burn patient has baseline pain that requires analgesia, increased pain medication requirements, and possibly sedation requirements for the pain involved in dressing changes. Attention to the patient's pain fosters the patient's trust in healthcare personnel to control pain and promotes cooperation with future burn wound care. The goal of pain management is an alert patient who is able to cooperate, follow commands, and respond to verbal stimuli. Use child life therapy if they are available.	• Continued pain despite pain interventions • Nonverbal indications of pain (restlessness, grimacing, teeth clenching) • Increased respiratory rate • Verbalization of pain • Inability to cooperate with dressing change • Increased heart rate • Increased or decreased blood pressure • Oversedation, decreased respiratory rate, not being arousable
2. Obtain baseline vital signs before the procedure, monitor throughout the procedure, and continue to check regularly until back to baseline.	Changes in vital signs can be an indication that the patient is experiencing pain or anxiety. Decreasing blood pressure, heart rate, and respiratory rate can be complications of pain medication (especially after the dressing change is complete and stimulation has stopped).	• Increased or decreased heart rate • Increased or decreased blood pressure • Increased or decreased respiratory rate; increased need for higher oxygen supplementation • High peak pressures on ventilator
3. Check the patient's temperature before large dressing changes. Ensure that the patient's environment is warm; cover the portions of the patient's body that are not involved in dressing changes. Check the patient's temperature at the end of dressing changes.	Heat is lost through burn wounds. Hypermetabolism and shivering increase caloric demand.	• Hypothermia • Shivering
4. Monitor peripheral pulses and circulation in the burned extremity during the dressing change, within 1 hour after applying the dressing, and every 2 hours thereafter. Keep extremities elevated and assess for increased edema.	Circumferential burns can decrease or prevent blood flow to the involved extremity. The dressing can be too tight, especially if edema increases.	• Increased peripheral edema • Pain or numbness in the extremity • Prolonged or absent capillary refill in the extremity • Decreased or absent pulses • Conversion to a deeper burn wound

Procedure continues on following page

UNIT VII

Patient Monitoring and Care —*Continued*

Steps	Rationale	Reportable Conditions
5. Assess the burn wound for color, size, odor, depth, drainage, bleeding, pain, early eschar separation, healing, and cellulitis in the surrounding tissue.	Observes for usual progression of wound healing versus complications of infection, progression of burn to a deeper wound, and bleeding. Wound colonization is common. Histological determination of the level of organism invasion in the presence of systemic symptoms is diagnostic for burn wound infection.	• Foul odor • Purulent or increased amounts of drainage • Elevated body temperatures • Cellulitis • Healthy granulation tissue vs. developing eschar • Increasing necrosis, loss of graft • Discoloration of the wound or the presence of fungal elements • Early eschar separation • Bleeding • Contractures • Loss of function
6. Encourage exercise and activities of daily living; perform range-of-motion exercises during dressing changes; place the patient in a position of optimal function, with splints used as needed, to maintain maximal function.[4,7,15] Use pain medication as needed to facilitate mobility.[4,12,14] (**Level C***)	Burns and grafts contract during the healing phase if not correctly splinted and exercised; loss of function is a complication of immobility. Pain inhibits patients from moving.	
7. Monitor the patient's tolerance of tube feedings or ingestion of a high-calorie and high-protein diet with supplements; encourage a nutritious diet, and discourage empty calories.[14,15] Limit free water intake. (**Level D***)	Nutrition is necessary for wound healing; patients with larger burns can become hypermetabolic. Protein-rich fluids promote healing; free water decreases intake of nutritional supplements and can lead to hyponatremia.	• Refusal to eat or inability to ingest adequate amounts of nutrition • Poor wound healing

*Level C: Qualitative studies, descriptive or correlational studies, integrative reviews, systematic reviews, or randomized controlled trials with inconsistent results.
*Level D: Peer-reviewed professional and organizational standards with the support of clinical study recommendations.

Documentation

Documentation should include the following:
- Patient and family education
- Date, time, and duration of wound care
- Areas of burn, other wounds, and pressure ulcers; weekly diagrams (or digital photographs) of unhealed wounds to monitor healing and wound changes
- Appearance of the wound (color, size, odor, depth, drainage, bleeding)
- Assessment of wound areas for level of pain (appropriate for depth and level of healing)
- Progression toward healing (e.g., presence of epithelial budding)
- Evidence of cellulitis around the wound (red, warm, tender)
- Assessment of peripheral pulses; color, movement, sensation, and capillary refill distal to a circumferential wound or an extremity wrapped in dressings
- Pain assessment, interventions, and effectiveness
- Medications given for pain, anxiety, and sedation
- Other comfort measures used
- Dressings and topical agents applied
- Patient's tolerance of the procedure
- Unexpected outcomes
- Nursing interventions

References and Additional Readings

For a complete list of references and additional readings for this procedure, scan this QR code with your smartphone, or visit https://www.elsevier.com/__data/assets/pdf_file/0009/1319886/Chapter0111.pdf.

UNIT VII

PROCEDURE

112 Donor-Site Care

Susan Ziegfeld

PURPOSE Care of the donor site is performed to promote wound healing and maintain function. A major focus during donor-site care incorporates strategies to effectively manage pain.

PREREQUISITE NURSING KNOWLEDGE

- Across the United States, diversity is found among burn units concerning policy, practice, and procedure in the care of thermal injuries and donor-site care. This procedure does not reproduce this diversity in practice but strives to provide common tenets that may be used for donor-site care.
- A partial-thickness wound is surgically created when a donor site (Fig. 112.1) is harvested to obtain skin for a full-thickness defect.[2] The more dermis moved with the skin graft, the less the graft shrinks with healing; therefore deeper donor sites may be created to obtain skin for cosmetically significant areas such as the face or hands.[12] Creation of donor sites adds new wounds that can create significant pain. Depending on the percentage of dermis moved for the graft, donor sites created may be superficial, partial-thickness, or deep partial-thickness wounds that heal in 10 to 20 days (typically 10 to 14 days; Fig. 112.2).[12]
- Factors that can disrupt or prolong healing include infection, desiccation, edema, adherent dressing changes, poor nutrition, hemodynamic instability, dependent donor sites, and a variety of preexisting medical conditions.[4,7]
- The longer a partial-thickness wound takes to heal, the more significant the scarring; therefore donor sites can produce minimal or hypertrophic scars.[2,4,7] Donor sites retain deep epidermal appendages, so they are generally capable of sweating and bearing hair after they heal. The site may be procured again once healing is complete, but skin from the first procurement of a donor site is always of higher quality than that of repeat procurements.
- Because the dermis is richly supplied with capillaries and nerve endings, donor sites are at risk for bleeding in the first 24 hours and are exquisitely tender to touch. They produce large volumes of serous exudate.[2,10]
- Donor-site treatment goals include minimizing bleeding, supporting reepithelialization, managing exudate, preventing infection, controlling pain, and minimizing scarring.[5,6,10] Epinephrine-soaked dressings, thrombin spray, or compression dressings may be applied in the operating room to attain hemostasis.[10] A compression dressing is usually used for the first 12 to 24 hours to ensure hemostasis.[10] After this initial period, compression may be applied for comfort.
- Wounds epithelialize most rapidly in a moist environment.[4,12] If donor sites are small enough, use of a thin-film

polyurethane or hydrocolloid dressing has been shown to promote rapid healing while providing comfort through dressing flexibility and occlusive coverage of nerve endings. Occlusive dressings (sealed on all sides) can be difficult to maintain on larger donor sites because of the substantial volume of exudate.[10] Calcium alginates can be used under occlusive dressings to manage exudate.[10]
- One of the oldest and most cost-effective methods for treatment of donor sites is to apply Xeroform wrap with an outer wrap for 12 to 24 hours and then remove the outer wrap to expose the inner dressing (Xeroform) and allow it to dry until the wound heals beneath.[4] The technique is only effective if the dressing dries well and becomes impermeable to bacteria, essentially acting as a scab. Positioning the patient for maximal exposure of the donor sites, preventing prolonged donor-site contact with sheets and clothing, and increasing airflow across the wound are important for this technique to work. If the donor site is large, this procedure creates a rather stiff and uncomfortable protective layer.
- Dressing selection should focus on patient comfort, symptom management, fewer dressing changes, and ease of application and removal while optimizing the healing environment.[3,9,10,12]
- Antimicrobial creams or ointments have also been used on donor sites, essentially treating the wounds in the same way as partial-thickness burns are treated. The disadvantage to this approach is that it requires daily washing of the wound and reapplication of cream and dressings, which is frequently a painful procedure.[2,6]
- Slow-release silver dressings are popular for donor-site use.[7] These dressings release silver for up to 7 days; ideally, they are placed on the donor site in the operating room, and the wound is allowed to heal beneath with infrequent or no dressing changes.
  - ❖ Donor sites must be assessed daily for signs of infection, including peri-wound warmth and erythema, increased pain, and purulent drainage.[1] The secondary dressing should be removed for this assessment while leaving the primary contact layer adherent to the donor site. Bacteria can delay healing and increase scarring or convert a partial-thickness donor site to a full-thickness wound.[2,10,13] Erythema should be outlined to monitor progression, with consideration of either removing the donor-site dressing or applying a topical antimicrobial to penetrate the donor-site dressing.[6] Reopening or

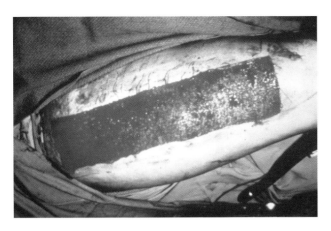

Figure 112.1 Fresh donor site.

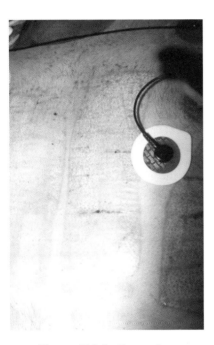

Figure 112.2 Donor sites.

"melting" of epithelium in previously healed donor sites is often the result of colonization with gram-positive organisms and may require antibacterial intervention.

⁕ Heavy hair-bearing donor sites such as the scalp provide special challenges. Heavy hair growth can lead to matting of hair in the exudate, which can lead to accumulation of protein, proliferation of bacteria, and ingrowth of hair, a condition referred to as *chronic folliculitis.*[11] This problem can lead to chronic, nonhealing, inflamed wounds or conversion of partial-thickness donor sites to full-thickness wounds. Dressings that prevent drying and wick away the exudate work well.

• Donor sites are often very painful, with the amount of pain variable depending on the dressing technique used. Patients with donor sites usually need scheduled, around-the-clock pain medication.[8]

• The donor site should not be exposed to the sun for 1 year after the burn. Apply full-spectrum sunblock to donor sites any time exposure to the sun is anticipated.[10]

• Protect fresh donor sites from dependent edema by wrapping with elastic bandages before sitting or ambulating.

Elastic wraps should be applied distal to proximal on a limb; therefore begin wrapping at the toes.

EQUIPMENT

• Personal protective equipment (gown, mask, goggles as needed)
• Nonsterile gloves
• Scissors
• Replacement dressing as needed
• Pain and sedation medication (as prescribed)

Additional equipment, to have available as needed, includes the following:

• Staple remover
• Marking pen

PATIENT AND FAMILY EDUCATION

• Teach the patient and family that donor sites generally heal in 10 to 12 days with variable scarring. ***Rationale:*** This provides realistic expectations about healing and scarring.

• Provide donor-site care instructions, and review them with the patient and family. Demonstrate how to assess and manage the donor-site dressing, and have the patient and family return the demonstration. Encourage the patient and family to ask questions. Provide positive feedback. Arrange for home care or clinic visits to follow up on dressings and wound care. ***Rationale:*** Return demonstration validates understanding and the ability to perform wound care. Once dressings are no longer needed, burns should be treated with moisturizing cream and massage. ***Rationale***: Moisturizing cream and scar massage assists with breaking down scar tissue.

• Patients should be encouraged to avoid smoking. ***Rationale:*** Smoking causes vasoconstriction, inhibits epithelialization, and decreases tissue oxygenation, all of which delay healing.[2]

• Explain to the patient about the pain and itching sensations associated with donor-site healing.[7,8] ***Rationale:*** Patients must know that donor-site pain and itching, although unpleasant, are normal and do not cause concern from a healing standpoint.

• Teach the patient and family about appropriate use of medications and nonpharmacological interventions to manage pain and itching.[8] Encourage application of a topical moisturizer after healing.[6] ***Rationale:*** This enhances patient comfort.

• Teach the patient and family about signs and symptoms of infection and the importance of reporting these in a timely manner.[1,4] ***Rationale:*** The patient and family can recognize infection early so appropriate measures can be instituted by the healthcare team.

• Provide the patient and family with follow-up appointments and a contact number to call with any problems. ***Rationale:*** This information is necessary for follow-up care.

• Assess the family's ability to provide care at home at each follow-up visit. ***Rationale:*** Continued care is necessary after discharge to ensure wound healing.

UNIT VII

- Stress the importance of wearing pressure garments if they are indicated. ***Rationale:*** Pressure garments reduce scarring.[3]
- Inform the patient and family that the donor site should not be exposed to the sun for 1 year after the burn. Patients should wear clothing that covers wounds or a sunscreen with sun protection factor (SPF) higher than 15.[6,10] ***Rationale:*** The patient and family understand that exposure to sunlight can damage the donor site.

PATIENT ASSESSMENT AND PREPARATION

Patient Assessment

- Evaluate for the following signs of healing. ***Rationale:*** Healing should occur within 10 to 12 days unless complications occur.
  - ❖ Decreased pain
  - ❖ Decreased edema
- Presence of epithelialized islands or skin buds
  - ❖ If using an adherent dressing: The dressing will separate at the wound edges when reepithelialization begins.
  - ❖ Compare the degree of healing with the expected rate of healing based on number of days post-procedure.
- Evaluate for signs and symptoms of infection. ***Rationale:*** Donor site infection may necessitate antimicrobial intervention.[6]
  - ❖ Foul odor
  - ❖ Purulent drainage
  - ❖ Discoloration
  - ❖ Increased pain
  - ❖ Increasing edema
  - ❖ Cellulitis
  - ❖ Delayed healing or wound reopening after previous epithelialization
  - ❖ Fever or increasing white blood cell (WBC) count[4]
- Evaluate the adequacy of the pain control by asking the patient to rate the pain on a scale of 0 to 10, both before and during wound care. ***Rationale:*** An individualized plan for pain control should be in place for background and procedural pain.[8]
- Evaluate the patient's range of motion in the vicinity of the donor site. Consultation with physical and occupational therapists may assist the patient with maintaining range of motion. ***Rationale:*** Wounds contract during healing; pain and tightness can decrease range of motion. The patient should be encouraged to continue normal movement and range-of-motion exercises.

Patient Preparation

- Ensure that the patient understands the preprocedural teaching. Answer questions, and reinforce information as needed. ***Rationale:*** Understanding of previously taught information is evaluated and reinforced.
- Verify the correct patient with two identifiers. ***Rationale:*** Before performing a procedure, the nurse should ensure the correct identification of the patient for the intended intervention.
- Premedicate the patient for pain and anxiety, as prescribed. Wait to perform the procedure until the medication has taken effect. ***Rationale:*** Waiting allows time for the medication to take effect and promotes optimal patient comfort. Medication reduces pain and anxiety and encourages patient trust and compliance with the procedure.

Procedure for Care of Donor Sites

Steps	Rationale	Special Considerations
1. Prepare all necessary equipment and supplies. The treatment area should be warmed.	Preparation facilitates efficient wound care and prevents needless delays. Warming the room decreases the risk for hypothermia.	Notify providers who must observe the wound ahead of time so they can be present while the wound is uncovered.
2. 🄷🄷		
3. 🄿🄴		For larger graft dressing changes, all healthcare professionals participating in the wound care should wear caps, masks, and gowns. Smaller graft changes may require less personal protective equipment.
4. Remove gauze roll and any padding covering the inner dressing.	The inner dressing is left in place until the wound heals, unless a problem with infection occurs or per provider orders.	Gauze roll or outer dressing is usually removed after 24 hours if the goal is for the inner dressing layer to be exposed to air and dry. Outer secondary dressings are changed daily as needed for drainage.

Procedure continues on following page

Procedure for Care of Donor Sites—*Continued*

Steps	Rationale	Special Considerations
5. Assess the donor site for signs of healing and complications; assess whether the inner dressing needs to be changed. If the inner donor dressing needs to be changed, refer to the procedure outlined ahead.	Validates the healing process and identifies complications. Avoid changing the inner dressing to facilitate healing.	If the inner dressing was stapled in place, staples must be removed when the inner dressing is fully adherent (generally between postoperative days 4 and 7).
6. Remove and discard gloves; perform **HH**, and apply a pair of clean gloves.	Handling the burn dressing contaminates the examination gloves, and clean gloves are needed for wound care.	
7. Gently wash exudate from wound edges with warm sterile water, and pat dry.	Clears exudate that can harbor microorganisms from the area of the donor site. Keep the covered donor site dry to improve healing.	
8. Use scissors to trim loose edges of the donor site dressing. If the inner dressing does not need to be changed, assess if a secondary dressing is needed, and apply if needed.	Because the dry inner dressing is not covered, loose edges of the dressing can snag and displace the inner dressing.	Assess the need for an outer dressing, and apply as needed.

Inner Dressing Change

1. Remove the inner dressing and discard it.		If the dressing is adherent, soak it with warm tap water to loosen it. Do not attempt to remove adherent dressings.
2. Remove and discard gloves; perform **HH**, and apply a pair of clean gloves.	Handling the burn dressing contaminates the examination gloves, and clean gloves are needed for wound care.	
3. Gently wash the wound with mild soap; rinse with warm, sterile water; and pat dry.	Cleanses the donor site.	Cleanse beyond the donor site to reduce the microbial count on surrounding tissue. Patients may do better if allowed to cleanse their own wounds.
4. Assess the donor site for progression of healing and complications; outline any inflammation with a marking pen.	Validates the healing process and identifies complications.	
5. Remove and discard gloves; perform **HH**, and apply a pair of sterile or clean gloves.	Clean gloves are applied after washing a wound.	Sterile gloves may be used when applying dressings to large burn wounds.
6. Cut the dressing to the size of the donor site with sterile scissors, apply, and secure it in place. Reapply the bulky outer dressing if indicated.	Ensures correct fit and adherence. Donor sites may be covered with bulky dressing to maintain a moisture barrier, maintain a moist wound surface, or apply a topical antimicrobial soak.	Dressing may be secured with tubular netting or cloth tape applied to the dressing margins.
7. Remove and discard gloves and used supplies.	Reduces the transmission of microorganisms.	
8. **HH**		

UNIT VII

Expected Outcomes

- Donor site heals within 2 weeks without complications.
- Patient maintains a self-identified, functional level of pain relief.
- Patient maintains comfort from measures taken for anxiety and itching.
- Patient and family verbalize knowledge of patient condition and plan of care.
- An optimal level of function is maintained or attained.
- Patient and family response and interactions demonstrate adaptation to the injury.
- Patient and family collaborate in management of care.
- At the time of discharge, patient and family verbalize and demonstrate an understanding of post-hospital care.

Unexpected Outcomes

- Bleeding
- Infection
- Conversion of donor site to deep partial-thickness or full-thickness wound

Patient Monitoring and Care

Steps	Rationale	Reportable Conditions
		These conditions should be reported to the provider if they persist despite nursing interventions.
1. Follow institutional standards for assessing pain. Administer analgesia as prescribed. Have the patient rate pain on a validated pain scale. Check pain medication orders, review the patient's previous response to pain medication, and assess the need to increase the dose. Incorporate nonpharmacological pain-relief techniques (e.g., relaxation techniques, massage therapy, music, visual imaging, child life therapist), and encourage patient participation in wound care.	Identifies the need for pain interventions. Minimizes donor site pain with an intact dressing that does not require a dressing change; the patient will have increased pain medication requirements if the dressing must be changed. Attention to the patient's pain fosters the patient's trust in the healthcare team.	• Continued pain despite pain interventions • Nonverbal indications of pain (e.g., restlessness, grimacing, teeth clenching) • Inability to cooperate with wound care • Increased respiratory rate • Increased heart rate • Increased or decreased blood pressure
2. Obtain baseline vital signs before the procedure, throughout the procedure, and for 30 minutes postprocedure.	Changes in vital signs can be a sign that the patient is experiencing pain or anxiety. Decreasing blood pressure, heart rate, and respiratory rate can be complications of pain medication (especially after the dressing change is complete and stimulation has stopped).	• Oversedation • Increased or decreased heart rate • Increased or decreased blood pressure • Increased or decreased respiratory rate
3. Assess the donor site for appearance (e.g., dressing wet or dry, dressing adherent, presence of drainage or bleeding, redness at edges) and progression toward healing (e.g., reepithelialization at wound edges).	Observe for the usual progression of wound healing versus complications of infection, progression of the donor site to a deeper wound, and bleeding.	• Foul odor • Purulent or increased amounts of drainage • Cellulitis or edema • Healing tissue developing eschar • Discoloration of wound • Bleeding

Procedure continues on following page

Patient Monitoring and Care —*Continued*

Steps	Rationale	Reportable Conditions
4. Encourage exercise and activities of daily living; place the patienst in a position of optimal function, and assess the need for pain medication to facilitate movement. Physical therapy and/or occupational therapy may be necessary to maintain range of motion.[2,10] (**Level D***)	Donor-site wounds contract during the healing phase. Pain also inhibits movement.	

*Level D: Peer-reviewed professional and organizational standards with the support of clinical study recommendations.

Documentation

Documentation should include the following:
- Patient and family education
- Date and time of wound care
- Appearance (e.g., dressing wet or dry, dressing adherence, presence of drainage or bleeding, redness at edges)
- Progression toward healing (e.g., reepithelialization at wound edges)
- Application of topical agents
- Type of dressing applied
- Pain assessment, interventions, and effectiveness
- Medications given for pain and sedation
- Patient's response to analgesic and sedatives
- Effective holistic comfort measures
- Emotional support
- Patient's tolerance of the procedure
- Unexpected outcomes
- Nursing interventions

References and Additional Readings

For a complete list of references and additional readings for this procedure, scan this QR code with your smartphone, or visit https://www.elsevier.com/__data/assets/pdf_file/0010/1319887/Chapter0112.pdf

UNIT VII

113 Skin-Graft Care

Susan Ziegfeld

PURPOSE Skin-graft care is performed to promote perfusion adherence of the graft and to prevent infection. Successful graft transplant and care result in maximal function and cosmetic outcomes.

PREREQUISITE NURSING KNOWLEDGE

- Skin grafts are used to replace skin on a patient's body that is unable to heal because of the size or thickness of the wound. The original wounds may be from a variety of causes (e.g., burns, infections, traumatic injury). An autograft is the only permanent treatment that can heal a large, full-thickness wound, and it may also be used to heal partial-thickness wounds with faster closure of the wound. An autograft is a type of skin graft that is created by taking a graft from one site of a patient's body (the donor site) and transplanting it to a different site of the same patient's body (the recipient site). The graft is applied over a clean, surgically excised wound that has been débrided of all nonviable tissue.[2]

- Autografts can be split-thickness skin grafts (STSG), containing the epidermis and part of the dermis, or full-thickness skin grafts (FTSG), containing the epidermis and all of the dermis. The donor site of an STSG is a new exposed wound area that will heal by reepithelization. The FTSG donor site is a full-thickness wound that heals by secondary intention due to harvest of the entire dermis, which may leave a scar.[2,13] The FTSG offers more functionality and a better cosmetic appearance but is limited by size due to the full-thickness donor site.[6] Therefore use of the STSG is more common.

- The STSG is procured from an appropriate donor site on the patient's body with a dermatome, a surgical instrument that shaves layers of skin at different depths to be grafted over the wound bed. The STSG is commonly meshed (Fig. 113.1) so it can be stretched to cover approximately 1.5 to 9 times more surface area than the original donor site.[2] The ability to stretch the donor graft is important when there is limited availability of suitable donor sites or when the wound area that requires grafting is extensive. Meshing the donor skin creates spaces, or interstices, that allow for fluid to escape, which can assist with graft adherence.[9]

- Nonmeshed grafts, called *sheet grafts* are used on the face, hands, and some joints because of cosmetic and functional concerns related to appearance and increased shrinkage.[13] Because sheet grafts are not meshed, a seroma or hematoma may form under the graft, causing it to lift and separate from the wound bed, therefore preventing graft to adherence or "take." For this reason, the sheet graft often has small pin holes made to allow for expected

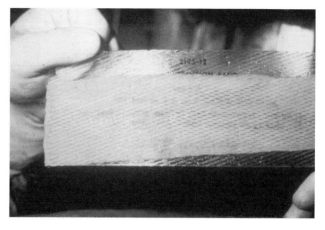

Figure 113.1 Meshed split-thickness skin graft.

fluid to leak through, not disturbing the graft. A sheet graft covers the same amount of surface area as the donor site. If fluid does form, evacuation of this fluid is imperative.[8] If the sheet graft has been in place for less than 48 hours and the fluid is near the edge of the sheet graft, the fluid can be rolled to the edge and out (Fig. 113.2).[2]

- Caution should be used when evacuating fluid after vascularization of the graft begins to avoid disruption of the graft attachment endangering graft take. Another option for fluid removal is to create a small nick in the sheet graft directly over the area of fluid accumulation and gently express the fluid through the hole. In either case, the fluid should be gently wicked away with gauze dampened with sterile normal saline solution or sterile water.[8] Seromas and hematomas tend to redevelop in the same areas, so careful documentation should reflect location of any fluid pockets (blebs). Close monitoring of these areas should occur at least every 8 hours until bleb formation is no longer noted.

- Cultured epidermal autografts (CEA) are grown from a sample of the patient's own epidermal cells in a laboratory. CEAs, most frequently used with burn injuries, are an option when the patient does not have enough unburned tissue for donor sites to cover the burn in a reasonable period.[3] The use of CEAs has been found to be a successful adjunct to the use of STSG. However, CEA use is very limited because of cost. In addition, the grafts are fragile, and successful take of the graft is dependent on experience of the burn team with this treatment.[3]

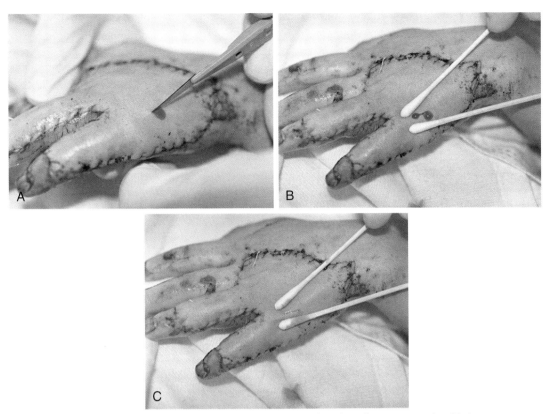

Figure 113.2   **A,** A No. 11 surgical blade and cotton-tipped applicator are used to blade a new sheet graft. Note that the blade is held so the tip of the cutting surface comes into contact with only the graft. **B,** Cotton-tipped applicators are rolled gently over the graft toward the slit to express fluid that has collected between the graft and the wound bed surface. When deblebbing thick grafts, adequate-size slits are important to avoid recurring buildup of fluid, which may jeopardize graft survivability and result in scarring. **C,** Blebs tend to recur in the same place. Vigilance about deblebbing at least once every 8 hours until bleb formation ceases is advisable. Documentation of bleb formation and location ensures that the next caregiver is aware of graft sites in need of close monitoring. *(From Carrougher GJ: Burn care and therapy, St Louis, 1998, Mosby.)*

- The use of artificial skin and other options for wound coverage has expanded in recent years. Currently, the use of these wound coverings is limited to providing temporary wound coverage or allowing for dermal regeneration while waiting for suitable donor sites for definitive wound closure with autografting.[10]
- Allografts, also called *homografts,* are fresh or cryopreserved grafts from human donors. Allografts are considered the gold standard for temporary coverage of wounds. Allograft benefits include prevention of wound desiccation, promotion of granulation tissue, and decreased water and heat loss.[1,5,7,14] Allografts can be used to cover widely meshed autografts to protect the fragile autograft and promote neovascularization of the interstices. Allografts and temporary skin substitutes can also assist in pain relief by covering raw nerve endings.
- The care for temporary grafts is different from care for permanent skin grafts and is generally unique to the type and manufacturer.
- In the operating room, all nonviable tissue is surgically excised to create a wound bed that is able to support a skin graft (Fig. 113.3); therefore the grafted area should be observed for bleeding for the first 24 hours.

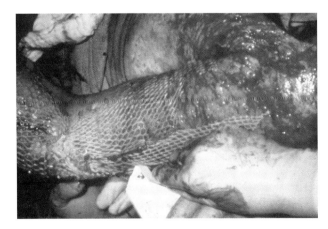

Figure 113.3   Meshed split-thickness skin graft covering the arm, with the remainder of the wound bed ready to be grafted.

- The goals after a graft placement are to protect the wound bed from infection and desiccation and to ensure that no movement (shearing) of the graft occurs while it is becoming vascularized. Neovascularization begins within the first 24 hours of surgery as capillaries grow

UNIT VII

up into the graft, securing the graft permanently to its new site. The newly grafted tissue must be well protected from shearing forces for 5 to 7 days to allow for graft adherence to the wound bed. With meshed skin grafts, the interstices of the autograft fill with granulation tissue, and the epidermis of the autograft migrates over the granulation tissues. Successful grafting is often expressed as a percentage of graft take or adherence and vascularization of the graft to the new site.[8] A barrier dressing may be used to protect the wound (with or without a bulky dressing added), or a minimal nonadherent dressing may be used with a bulky dressing over the grafted tissue to act as the barrier to infection and to prevent drying and shearing. The first dressing change is usually performed after 3 to 5 days. Most centers use clean technique for dressing removal, donor site cleansing, and dressing application and reserve sterile technique for unique dressing applications.[10]

- Negative-pressure wound therapy (NPWT) may also be used as a dressing on the STSG to enhance the take of the graft by providing fluid removal, bolstering, and protection of the graft. NPWT is a mechanical wound-care treatment that uses controlled negative pressure (via a machine, tubing, foam, and sealed dressing) to accelerate wound healing.[12,15] A nonadherent dressing is placed on the graft before the NPWT dressing during surgery. The NPWT dressing is usually changed every 3 to 7 days (see Procedure 118, Negative-Pressure Wound Therapy for more information on NPWT).
- The graft is usually stapled or sutured in place before covering with the dressings or NPWT. Fibrin sealants, a surgical hemostatic agent derived from human plasma, may also be used in place of staples for adherence of sheet grafts.[10]
- Initial healing of the grafted area should occur in 7 to 10 days. The graft area is immobilized for 4 to 5 days to prevent shearing. Splints and immobilizers may be used during this time to prevent disruption of grafts and to provide therapeutic positioning of the extremities.[8] If a patient is allowed to mobilize after surgery, leg grafts must be supported with elastic wraps or other compressive dressings when the patient's legs are dependent for the first 3 to 5 days after surgery. This prevents capillary engorgement and hematoma formation beneath the graft.[4] Grafted extremities should be elevated when the patient is supine.
- Signs of successful graft take include vascularization of the graft, reepithelialization of the interstices, decreased pain, and adherence of the graft. Signs of complications include bleeding, graft necrosis, graft loss, cellulitis, purulent drainage, and fever.
- Skin grafts contract during the healing and remodeling phases. Continuing mobility and proper positioning are vital to prevent contractures and loss of function. Self-care and range-of-motion exercises should be encouraged as soon as the graft is adherent. Once the wounds heal, pressure garments may be ordered to be worn at all times, except during bathing, to reduce hypertrophic scar formation.[4]
- Pain related to care of wounds is complicated by several components: background pain (pain that is continuously present), procedural pain (intermittent pain related to procedures

and routine care), and anxiety. Unrelieved pain can lead to stress-related immunosuppression, increased potential for infection, delayed wound healing, and depression. The management of pain should use a multidimensional approach, including pharmacological and nonpharmacological methods, tailored to individual patient needs.[11]

- Wound healing is dependent on energy production from nutrition. Nutrition that includes protein, carbohydrates, fat, amino acids, and micronutrients is paramount for energy production.[10]
- Exposure of the healed skin graft to the sun should be avoided.[8] The newly healed area is extremely sensitive to sunlight, and permanent discoloration can occur. To prevent discoloration, the patient should protect grafted areas with clothing or sunscreen. During the first year, as the patient's graft matures, the risk for skin discoloration slowly decreases.
- Smoking should be discouraged or reduced. Nicotine causes vasoconstriction, and the goal of care is to perfuse wounds and skin grafts to facilitate healing.

EQUIPMENT

- Personal protective equipment (i.e., gowns, mask, goggles)
- Nonsterile gloves
- Sterile gloves
- Scissors and forceps
- Sterile water or sterile normal saline solution for the first dressing change or per institutional protocol
- Clean washcloths
- Nonadherent dressing/gauze
- Secondary dressings, as needed
- Analgesic and anxiolytic medication (as prescribed)

Additional equipment, to have available as needed, includes the following:

- Splints (to be secured with gauze roll, elastic bandage wraps, or self-adherent wrap)
- Towels or waterproof pads
- Staple remover

PATIENT AND FAMILY EDUCATION

- Explain the procedure for skin-graft care to the patient and family. *Rationale:* Explanation diminishes fear of the unknown and ensures that the patient and family are knowledgeable about graft care.
- Inform the patient and family that the grafted area must be protected for 5 to 7 days to encourage graft take and reduce the risk of mechanical trauma to the graft site. *Rationale:* Patient and family assistance in protecting the graft site is increased.
- Inform the patient and family that the skin graft should not be exposed to the sun for approximately 1 year. Sunscreen and protective clothing should be used thereafter. Some scarring and discoloration will occur but will improve over the first year. Third-degree burns and skin grafts will result in permanent scars, which can involve color change, texture change, or both. Use of compression garments, continued exercises, and adjunct modalities such as scar

massage will help soften and smooth scar tissue. Explain that the grafted area will not grow hair or be able to sweat because of permanent loss of these dermal append-ages. *Rationale:* The patient and family are prepared for changes that will be present after hospital discharge, and anxieties about body image are addressed.

- Discuss the importance of proper positioning. Explain the need for continuing mobility through self-care and range-of-motion exercises as soon as the graft is adherent and throughout the healing phase. *Rationale:* Education prevents contractures and loss of function associated with healing skin grafts.
- Assess the family's ability to provide care at home. *Rationale:* Continued care of the wound is necessary after discharge. The patient and family may benefit from home health services or more frequent outpatient follow-up to ensure success in outpatient care.
- As appropriate, provide detailed wound care instructions in writing, and review them with the patient and family. Demonstrate exactly what to do and have the patient and family return demonstrations before the planned discharge. Continue to involve the patient and family in wound care for the remainder of the admission, and encourage them to ask questions. Provide positive feedback. Arrange for home care or clinic visits to follow up on dressings and wound care. *Rationale:* Education validates patient and family understanding and ability to perform wound care independently and allows time for them to develop a level of comfort. This provides the opportunity to reinforce important points.
- Teach the patient and family about pain and pruritus medications as prescribed. Pain medications should be given 30 minutes before wound care so the medications can be effective during the wound care process. Itching is a normal sign of healing. It can be managed with moisturizer application, compression wraps or garments, and scar massage. Over-the-counter antihistamines can help with pruritus. Nerve-targeting medications can also help with pruritus. Provide the name of a water-based lotion to apply to healed areas. *Rationale:* This supports patient comfort at home.
- Teach the patient and family about signs and symptoms of infection and the importance of reporting these in a timely manner. *Rationale:* The patient and family can recognize problems early so appropriate measures can be instituted by the healthcare team.
- Emphasize the importance of wearing pressure garments and splints. *Rationale:* This reduces scar formation and contractures.
- Schedule follow-up appointments, and provide the name of a healthcare provider to call with any problems. *Rationale:* This information is necessary for further care and follow-up.
- Work with a vocational rehabilitation counselor to formulate plan for the patient's return to work or school. *Rationale:* Depending on the severity of the patient's injuries, the patient may be physically unable to return to former employment or may need assistance with job modifications and accommodations. Developing a back-to-work plan based on any new limitations increases the patient's chance of successfully returning to work.

PATIENT ASSESSMENT AND PREPARATION

Patient Assessment

- Assess vital signs, including temperature. *Rationale:* Baseline vital signs allow for comparison during and after the procedure to evaluate patient tolerance and need for pain medication.
- Evaluate the success of graft take: vascularization of the graft; reepithelialization of the interstices; decreased pain; and adherence of the graft. *Rationale:* Graft success or adherence to the wound is assessed with each episode of care to evaluate healing.
- Monitor for signs of complications: fever, elevated white blood cell count, cellulitis, increased purulent drainage, or saturation of the secondary dressing. *Rationale:* Baseline and ongoing assessment for signs of graft failure to include possible infection are important for early identification of complications to minimize graft loss.
- Compare the patient's rate of healing with the expected rate of wound healing for the number of days after the skin graft. *Rationale:* Initial healing of the grafted area should occur in 7 to 10 days.
- Determine the adequacy of the pain-control regimen by asking the patient to rate the pain on a scale of 0 to 10 (or other scale as appropriate), both before wound care (background pain) and during the dressing change. *Rationale:* An individualized plan for pain control should be in place for background and procedural pain. In addition to the traditional use of pain and anxiety medications, alternative therapies should be included (e.g., relaxation techniques, distraction, massage therapy, music therapy). The patient's medication requirements should decrease as the grafted area heals.
- Assess the patient's level of function in the grafted area. *Rationale:* Skin grafts contract during the healing phase, and immobility enhances loss of function. The patient should be encouraged to continue normal movement and range-of-motion exercises after the graft take has been established.[1]
- Assess for graft loss. The graft does not adhere to the wound bed. *Rationale:* Skin-graft loss is usually caused by infection, an improperly prepared wound bed, seroma/hematoma formation, or shearing forces. Assure the patient that the wound bed may still be able to heal by secondary intention without the need to regraft the site.[8]

Patient Preparation

- Ensure that the patient understands the preprocedural teaching. Answer questions as they arise, and reinforce information as needed. *Rationale:* Understanding of previously taught information is evaluated and reinforced.
- Verify the correct patient with two identifiers. *Rationale:* Before performing a procedure, the nurse should ensure the correct identification of the patient for the intended intervention.
- Notify other appropriate physicians, advanced practice providers, and other healthcare professionals who need to assess the graft (e.g., a physician) or perform a task (e.g., range-of-motion exercises by a physical therapist)

UNIT VII

at the time of dressing change. ***Rationale:*** Organization of care allows important assessment and interventions to take place without causing extra pain and stress to the patient.

- Premedicate the patient with pain medication and any sedation and anxiolytic medications as prescribed. Allow

an appropriate amount of time for medications to begin to take effect before starting wound care. ***Rationale:*** Premedication reduces pain and anxiety and allows time for medication to take effect and promote optimal comfort for the patient. This encourages patient trust and compliance with the procedure.

Procedure for Care of Skin Grafts

Steps	Rationale	Special Considerations
1. Prepare all necessary equipment and supplies.	Preparation facilitates efficient wound care and prevents needless delays.	
2. **HH**		
3. **PE**		For large-graft dressing changes, all healthcare professionals participating in the wound care should apply a cap, mask, and gown. Small-graft changes may require less personal protective equipment. If the family will be performing dressing changes at home, a mask, cap, and gown are not used.
4. Remove bulky outer dressings, and discard them in an appropriate receptacle. Place a towel or pad under exposed extremity.	Old dressings can contain large amounts of body secretions and blood. A towel allows a place for the patient to rest an extremity during care.	The initial dressing is commonly left in place for 3–5 days, while the bulky outer dressings are changed and the nonadherent gauze is left in place. Follow provider orders and institutional standards.
5. Remove and discard gloves; perform **HH**, and apply clean gloves.	Examination gloves are contaminated by handling the burn dressing; clean gloves are needed for wound care.	
6. If prescribed, gently lift nonadherent gauze from the grafted site, anchoring the graft in place as needed. *Note:* The surgeon may have stapled on a dressing that must remain in place until the skin graft heals. Follow institutional standards.	Some grafts are not firmly attached to the wound bed and can be pulled loose for up to 5 days after grafting.	Normal saline solution or warm tap water may be used to loosen dressings stuck to the graft area.
7. Gently rinse the graft site and surrounding tissue with normal saline solution or warm tap water with gauze or washcloths.	Cleanses the wound of exudate and reduces microorganisms. Use pH-neutral cleansing agents.	Special care is necessary not to displace the skin graft during the cleansing process.
8. Use scissors and forceps to remove loose necrotic tissue. If the graft is a sheet graft, assess for and remove any pockets of fluid under the graft.	Clears debris that can harbor microorganisms. Pockets of fluid separate the graft from the wound bed, which is vital for blood supply, causing graft loss in that area of fluid collection.	If the sheet graft has been in place for <48 hours and the fluid is near the edge of the sheet graft, roll the fluid to the edge and out; otherwise, make a small nick in the sheet graft directly over the area of fluid accumulation, and gently express the fluid through the hole. Gently remove exudate with gauze dampened with sterile normal saline solution or sterile water. Follow institutional standards.

Procedure continues on following page

Procedure | for Care of Skin Grafts—*Continued*

Steps	Rationale	Special Considerations
9. Remove staples as prescribed that are no longer needed to hold graft or dressing in place.	Prevents embedding of staples, local irritation, infection, and scarring.	Staples can be removed starting 5–7 days after grafting. Removing a large number of staples may be very painful and may necessitate an anesthesia-assisted procedure. Follow institutional standards.
10. Assess the graft for progression of healing and for complications.	Validates the healing process and identifies complications.	
11. Apply a nonadherent dressing (if interstices are open), cover with secondary dressings, and secure; or apply moisturizer to healed adherent graft areas where interstices are closed, and cover with thin secondary dressings to promote mobility.	Protects the graft while healing.	A water-based lotion is used to moisturize the burn and reduce itching when interstices are closed.
12. Remove and discard gloves; perform **HH**, and apply clean gloves.	Reduces transmission of microorganisms.	
13. Apply splints to the appropriate limb, and elevate the involved extremity. The patient's hands and arms may be elevated with pillows or elastic net sling. Elevate the head of the bed.	Maintains the position of function, prevents contractures, and reduces edema and pain.	If possible, prevent the patient from lying on grafted areas. Consider the use of pressure-reduction mattress for grafts or donor sites on posterior surfaces. After the initial period of immobilization, splints are used only when the patient is unable to participate in range-of-motion exercises or self-care.
14. Remove and discard **PE**.		
15. **HH**		

Expected Outcomes

- Graft take of >90% is attained
- Patient maintains a self-identified acceptable level of pain relief
- Patient attains comfort from measures provided for anxiety and itching
- Patient and family verbalize knowledge of patient condition and plan of care
- An optimal level of function is maintained
- Patient and family response and interactions demonstrate adaptation to the injury
- Patient and family collaborate in management of care
- At the time of discharge, the patient and family verbalize and demonstrate an understanding of posthospital care

Unexpected Outcomes

- Bleeding
- Infection
- Graft failure

Patient Monitoring and Care

Steps	Rationale	Reportable Conditions
		These conditions should be reported to the provider if they persist despite nursing interventions.

UNIT VII

Patient Monitoring and Care —*Continued*

Steps	Rationale	Reportable Conditions
1. Follow institutional standards for assessing pain. Administer analgesia as prescribed. Ask the patient to rate pain on a scale of 0–10 (or other appropriate scale); check the orders for analgesic, sedative, and anxiolytic agents before dressing changes; evaluate the patient's medication requirements with previous dressing changes; and assess the need for more medication throughout the dressing change. Incorporate alternative pain-relief techniques (e.g., relaxation techniques, distraction, massage therapy, music therapy, visual imaging).[11]	Identifies the need for pain interventions. The patient with new skin grafts will have some baseline pain that requires pain medication; pain medication requirements may be increased, and sedation or anxiolytic agents may also be necessary for the procedural pain involved in graft care.[11] Attention to the patient's pain fosters the patient's trust in healthcare personnel to control pain and promotes cooperation with future graft care.	• Continued pain despite pain interventions • Increased heart rate • Increased or decreased blood pressure • Increased respiratory rate • Verbalization of pain • Nonverbal indications of pain (restlessness, grimacing, teeth clenching) • Inability to cooperate with the dressing change
2. Monitor vital signs throughout the procedure, and continue to assess for 30 minutes after the procedure is complete.	Changes in vital signs can be an indication that the patient is experiencing pain or anxiety. Decreasing blood pressure, heart rate, and respiratory rate can be complications of pain medication (especially after dressing change is complete and stimulation has stopped).	• Decreased level of consciousness • Increased or decreased heart rate • Increased or decreased blood pressure • Increased or decreased respiratory rate and depth of respirations • High peak pressures on a ventilator
3. Assess the graft site for appearance (e.g., color, drainage, bleeding, graft necrosis, graft loss, cellulitis) and progression toward healing (e.g., vascularization of the graft, reepithelialization of the interstices, decreased pain, adherence of the graft).	Observe for usual progression of wound healing versus complications.	• Foul odor • Purulent or increased amounts of drainage • Increased pain • Cellulitis • Hematoma or fluid collection under sheet grafts • Graft necrosis • Sloughing • Bleeding
4. Place the patient in a position of optimal function during the initial period of immobilization of newly grafted areas, with splints used to maintain position. After the first 5 days, encourage exercise, activities of daily living, and range-of-motion exercises during dressing changes. Use pain medication as needed to facilitate mobility.[11] **(Level E*)**	Grafted skin contracts during the healing phase if not correctly splinted and exercised. Loss of function is a complication of immobility. Pain inhibits patients from moving.	• Contractures • Loss of function
5. Monitor the patient's tolerance of tube feedings or ingestion of a high-calorie, high-protein diet with supplements; encourage a nutritious diet, and discourage empty calories. Limit free water.[10] **(Level D*)**	Nutrition is necessary for wound healing. Burn patients are hypermetabolic.[10]	• Poor wound healing • Graft failure

*Level D: Peer-reviewed professional and organizational standards with the support of clinical study recommendations.

*Level E: Multiple case reports, theory-based evidence from expert opinions, or peer-reviewed professional organizational standards without clinical studies to support recommendations.

Procedure continues on following page

UNIT VII

Patient Monitoring and Care —*Continued*

Steps	Rationale	Reportable Conditions
1. Continue to follow institutional standards for assessing pain. Administer analgesia as prescribed.	Identifies the need for pain interventions.	• Continued pain despite pain interventions

Documentation

Documentation should include the following:
- Patient and family education
- Date and time of graft care
- Appearance of graft site (e.g., color, drainage, bleeding, graft necrosis, sloughing, cellulitis)
- Progression toward healing (e.g., adherence and vascularization of the graft, reepithelialization of the interstices, decreased pain)
- Dressings and topicals applied (number and type of supplies used; this will help the next clinician prepare for future dressing change)
- Pain assessment, interventions, and effectiveness
- Medications given for pain and sedation
- Patient's response to analgesics and sedatives
- Other comfort measures used
- Patient's tolerance of the procedure
- Unexpected outcomes
- Nursing interventions

References and Additional Readings

For a complete list of references and additional readings for this procedure, scan this QR code with your smartphone, or visit https://www.elsevier.com/__data/assets/pdf_file/0011/1319888/Chapter0113.pdf.

UNIT VII

PROCEDURE

114 Intracompartmental Pressure Monitoring

Erin Reynolds

PURPOSE: Compartment syndrome can occur within any confined anatomical region when elevations in tissue pressure are sufficient to cause neurovascular compromise of the tissues in that region or compartment. Typically, diagnosis of this syndrome is made with serial clinical examinations of the involved extremity. However, in patients with inconclusive physical findings or with an altered level of consciousness, direct measurement of the intracompartmental pressure is a useful diagnostic adjunct.

PREREQUISITE NURSING KNOWLEDGE

- Nurses performing intracompartmental pressure monitoring (IPM) must have detailed knowledge of the anatomy of the involved limb compartments (Fig. 114.1), including external landmarks associated with each compartment. Compartment syndrome may also develop in the abdomen (abdominal compartment syndrome). See Procedure 99, Intraabdominal Pressure Monitoring, for information on intraabdominal pressure monitoring.
- All clinicians involved with performing and assisting with the procedure should have knowledge of aseptic technique.
- Providers and other healthcare professionals should be trained and approved by their facilities to perform IPM. This should include supervised training in the techniques used for IPM and opportunities to maintain clinical competence in IPM.
- Clinicians should have a high index of suspicion that the patient is at risk for developing compartment syndrome.
  - ❖ Etiologies can be divided into internal and external sources.
    - ○ Examples of internal causes include fractures, contusions, postoperative edema, and edema formation associated with crush injuries or reperfusion injuries.[1,2,6,7]
    - ○ External sources are generally related to compression of the limb and include such things as eschar from burn injuries, splints, casts, dressings, extravasation of intravenous (IV) medications and fluids, and immobility.[10,12,13]

- Definitive treatment may be as simple as releasing a splint, cast, or dressing. More advanced treatment may require release of the compartment with an escharotomy or fasciotomy.[3,4,9,11]
- The pathophysiology of compartment syndrome is related to compromised perfusion. Blood flow to any tissue or organ requires a sufficient perfusion pressure, which is generally calculated as the mean arterial pressure minus the intracompartmental pressure and should be 70 to 80 mm Hg.[13] Therefore, as the mean arterial pressure decreases or the intracompartmental pressure increases, the perfusion to the tissue is decreased.
- Compartment syndrome occurs when the pressure within the muscle compartment rises above the capillary perfusion pressure gradient, causing cellular anoxia, muscle ischemia, and tissue death.[13]
- Normal compartment pressure within an unaffected compartment is considered less than 10 mm Hg.[13] Clinically significant pressure changes are generally defined in one of two ways:
  - ❖ An absolute value of more than 30 mm Hg in the presence of other signs and symptoms of compartment syndrome. Injury of the area may lead to elevations of the intracompartmental pressure in the absence of actual compartment syndrome.[13] Positioning of the extremity may also cause elevations in intracompartmental pressure, particularly when assessing dependent compartments.
  - ❖ A delta compartment pressure (Δp) of less than 30 mm Hg: the diastolic blood pressure minus the intracompartmental pressure. This measurement may be a more reliable indicator of the risk for development of compartment syndrome because it takes into account blood pressure.[6]
- The diagnosis of compartment syndrome based solely on a single intracompartmental pressure measurement has a high false-positive rate and therefore should be used only to confirm clinical suspicion.[6]
- Acute compartment syndrome is a true orthopedic emergency. Signs and symptoms can develop in as little as 2 hours after injury. Ischemic damage to muscles and nerves

Compartments of the Calf

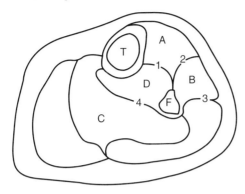

A Anterior compartment

B Lateral (peroneal) compartment

C Superficial posterior compartment

D Deep posterior compartment

T Tibia

F Fibula

1 Interosseous membrane

2 Anterior intermuscular septum

3 Posterior intermuscular septum

4 Intermuscular septum

Compartments of the Forearm

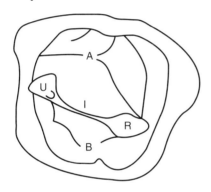

A Volar (anterior) compartment

B Dorsal (posterior) compartment

I Interosseous membrane

R Radius

U Ulna

Compartments of the Thigh

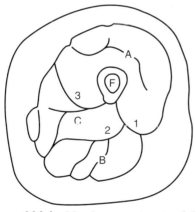

A Anterior compartment

B Posterior compartment

C Medial compartment

F Femur

1 Lateral intermuscular septum

2 Posterior intermuscular septum

3 Medial intermuscular septum

Figure 114.1 Muscle compartments of the calf, forearm, and thigh. *(From Tiwari A, Haq AI, Myint F, Hamilton G: Acute compartment syndromes,* Br J Surg *8:397–412, 2002.)*

can start in 4 to 6 hours, with permanent damage occurring in 12 to 24 hours.[2]

- Pressure measurements should be performed in all compartments within proximity to the suspected area of increased pressure to ensure complete assessment and avoid missing an evolving acute compartment syndrome beyond the suspected area.[13]
- Pressure monitoring devices/techniques:
  - ❖ Manometer: a device that uses resistance present against saline solution injected in the compartment. This is most commonly used.[5]

- ❖ Slit catheter and wick catheter: Allows for continuous monitoring of pressure. Data supporting the use are limited in current literature.

EQUIPMENT

- Electronic pressure monitoring device (bedside pressure monitor or a handheld monitoring device)
- Prefilled sterile saline solution syringes
- Dedicated disposable tubing with needle

- Chlorhexidine gluconate
- 1% lidocaine
- Sterile gloves
- Sterile dressing
- One roll of hypoallergenic tape

PATIENT AND FAMILY EDUCATION

- Explain the indications and rationale for performing this procedure to the patient and family (if applicable). **Rationale:** Explanation of the procedure may decrease patient and family anxiety and assist in patient cooperation.
- Explain the steps of the procedure to the patient and family. Answer any questions as they arise, and reinforce information as needed. **Rationale:** Explanation reinforces understanding of previously presented information and may assist in allaying anxiety.
- Inform the patient that pain medication will be given before the procedure is initiated. **Rationale:** This promotes patient comfort.

PATIENT ASSESSMENT AND PREPARATION

Patient Assessment

- Review the patient's history for conditions associated with the development of compartment syndrome. **Rationale:** This review raises the index of suspicion for diagnosis of compartment syndrome, leading to early detection and treatment.
- Clinical presentation of compartment syndrome is traditionally listed with a series of "Ps."[2,3] **Rationale:** Presence of these symptoms may be sufficient to diagnose acute compartment syndrome in neurologically intact patients. In patients with an impaired level of consciousness, these symptoms signal the need for IPM. Pain assessment in the setting of compartment syndrome is most useful in the conscious patient because of the patient's ability to identify the quality and location of pain.
  - *Pain:* In addition to being the most sensitive identifier, pain is the most commonly reported and earliest symptom of compartment syndrome.[7] Pain from compartment syndrome is often difficult to differentiate from that which is caused by the primary injury and

is described as out of proportion to the injury or minimally responsive to analgesic interventions (e.g., IV narcotics). It is also exacerbated by active or passive stretching of the muscle groups involved.
  - *Paresthesia:* This sign precedes loss of motor function and occurs as pressure increases on the affected nerve. Paresthesia and tingling are early *symptoms.* Loss of two-point discrimination may be an early *sign.*
  - *Paresis* or *paralysis:* This sign is a *late* finding that occurs as a result of pressure on the nerve or necrosis of the affected muscles.
- *Pulselessness:* Pulselessness is another late finding, from occlusion of the arterioles by the increasing intracompartmental pressure. This sign also results in pallor or coolness of the affected extremity.
- *Pressure:* Tense edema and firmness in the affected extremity are the earliest and only noninvasive objective findings in early compartment syndrome. It is important to remember that this may be the only initial sign of compartment syndrome in the sedated, unresponsive, or obtunded patient.[2,13] Pallor may be seen in the affected limb, which could also be mottled or cyanotic. Elevations in intracompartmental pressure are also considered part of the confirmatory diagnosis.

Patient Preparation

- Verify the correct patient with two identifiers. **Rationale:** Before performing a procedure, the nurse should ensure the correct identification of the patient for the intended intervention.
- Obtain a consent, if the procedure is not emergent. **Rationale:** Informed consent documents that the patient or family understands the explanation and need for the procedure.
- Remove constricting dressings and bandages. Assist with the modification of splints, casts, and other devices on the affected extremity. **Rationale:** Removal reduces external pressure on the tissue of the affected extremity.
- Place the patient in the supine position with the extremity at the level of the heart. **Rationale:** Provides access to the affected compartment and maintains the extremity in a neutral position. Positioning the extremity above the heart may impede circulation, and positioning it in a dependent position may worsen edema.
- Consider administration of a short-acting analgesic and/or anxiolytic. **Rationale:** An analgesic and/or anxiolytic can decrease patient discomfort during the procedure.

Procedure for Intracompartmental Pressure Monitoring Using a Handheld Pressure Monitoring System

Steps	Rationale	Special Considerations

Many one-time and continuous intracompartmental pressure-monitoring devices are available in healthcare settings (Fig. 114.2).

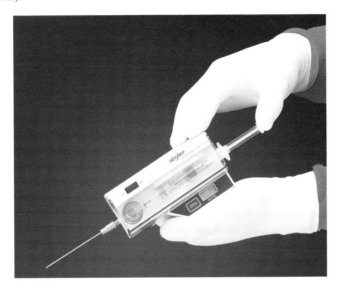

Figure 114.2 Stryker intracompartmental pressure monitor. *(Courtesy Stryker Instruments.)*

1. **HH**
2. **PE**
3. Cleanse the insertion site with antiseptic solution. | Reduces bacterial flora on the skin. | Allow the antiseptic solution to dry for maximal effectiveness.
4. Remove gloves and wash hands. | |
5. Assemble the disposable needle, prefilled sterile saline solution syringe, and pressure transducer using aseptic technique.
   A. Verify needle is the correct side port needle
   B. Maintain sterility of the needle | Prevention of infection by maintaining sterility during preparation of the monitoring system. | A. The needle cannot be exchanged for another same-gauge needle if dropped or damaged. A new setup will be needed.
6. Place the assembled disposable system into the pressure-monitoring device.
   A. Ensure that the system is securely inserted and that the wings of the syringe are flat against the device.
   B. Close the cover until an audible click is heard. (**Level M***) | Prepares the monitoring system. |
7. Tilt the device so the needle is at least 45 degrees upward, and purge the system with sterile saline solution. (**Level M***) | Removes air bubbles and ensures an accurate reading.[11] Avoids fluid flowing toward the sensor while performing the purge. |
8. Apply nonsterile gloves. | |
9. Inject the local anesthetic agent at the insertion site. | Increases patient comfort. | Consider concomitant use of IV analgesics or anxiolytics if appropriate for the patient's condition.
10. Determine landmarks for insertion. | Place the patient in the supine position to identify landmarks for anterior, deep posterior, superficial posterior, and lateral compartments of the calf.[5] | Differences in needle-insertion location can affect the measured value.

UNIT VII

Procedure	for Intracompartmental Pressure Monitoring Using a Handheld Pressure Monitoring System—*Continued*		
Steps	**Rationale**	**Special Considerations**	
11. A. Estimate the angle of insertion with the pressure-monitoring device. B. Turn the device on, and press the "zero" button. C. Wait until the display shows that the device is zeroed. **(Level M*)**	Eliminates atmospheric pressure.	Ensure that the device is zeroed at the angle of intended insertion to ensure accurate pressure measurement.	
12. Remove the needle cover, and insert 1–3 cm depending on which compartment is being measured.	Depth of needle insertion is dependent on the compartment being assessed.	Two areas of resistance will be felt on insertion as the needle passes through the skin/dermis and facia. To ensure that the side port is clear, the needle can be withdrawn by 1 mm.	
13. Inject 0.1–0.3 mL of saline solution into the compartment. **(Level M*)**	Equilibrates the device to allow for pressure measurement.		
14. Observe the pressure reading displayed on the device.	Allows the device to equilibrate to a constant reading.		
15. Verify placement by manually pressing on the tissue near the insertion site or by flexing and extending the extremity distal to the insertion site (e.g., ankle, wrist, or knee).	Fluctuations in pressure readings verify correct placement of the needle.	Patients with normal compartment physiology have a rapid increase in pressure during palpation or contraction of the muscle, with a rapid return to baseline pressure. Patients with compartment syndrome have a slow return to baseline pressure after relaxation of the muscle.	
16. Remove and discard the needle and syringe in appropriate receptacles. Apply an occlusive sterile dressing to the puncture site.	Reduces the risk of contamination.		
17. Discard used supplies.			
18. 🅷🅷			

*Level M: Manufacturer's recommendations only.

Expected Outcomes

- Procedure completed without complications in a timely manner
- Minimal patient discomfort
- Pressure readings consistent with clinical presentation of the patient's extremity
- If compartment syndrome is present, a rapid fasciotomy of the involved compartment is required; obtain immediate surgical consultation as necessary

Unexpected Outcomes

- Failure to recognize compartment syndrome, resulting in long-term morbidity for the patient
- Inaccurate pressure readings obtained
- Excessive bleeding from the catheter-insertion site
- Increased patient discomfort or pain
- Incorrect insertion of the needle resulting in tissue injury
- Signs and symptoms of procedure-related infection

Patient Monitoring and Care

Steps	Rationale	Reportable Conditions
		These conditions should be reported to the provider if they persist despite nursing interventions.

Procedure continues on following page

UNIT VII

Patient Monitoring and Care —*Continued*

Steps	Rationale	Reportable Conditions
1. Complete a neurovascular assessment of the affected extremity hourly and as necessary.	Documentation and review of serial trends in assessment detect the onset and development of compartment syndrome.	• Onset of pain or worsening of pain despite administration of analgesic agents • Paresthesia or hypoesthesia of the affected extremity • Changes in extremity skin color (mottling, cyanosis, pallor) and skin temperature • Decrease or loss of peripheral pulses • Paralysis of the affected extremity • Increase in circumference and tenseness of the extremity
2. Assess the insertion site for signs and symptoms of infection.	The needle insertion site may be a source of infection.	• Erythema, swelling, or drainage around the insertion site • Increase in skin warmth surrounding the insertion site • Increased pain and tenderness at the insertion site • Increase in white blood cell count on complete blood count • Fever
1. Follow institutional standards for assessing pain. Administer analgesia as prescribed.	Identifies the need for pain interventions.	• Continued pain despite pain interventions

Documentation

Documentation should include the following:
- Informed consent, fully explaining the procedure and associated risks
- Clinical findings and related assessment before and after compartment pressure measurement
- Description of the compartment(s) assessed
- Medications administered during the procedure
- Results of the compartment pressure measurement
- The condition of the puncture site and dressing after the needle was removed
- Description of how the patient tolerated the procedure
- Development of unexpected outcomes
- Additional interventions
- Pain assessment and response to interventions

References and Additional Readings

For a complete list of references and additional readings for this procedure, scan this QR code with your smartphone, or visit https://www.elsevier.com/__data/assets/pdf_file/0012/1319889/Chapter0114.pdf

UNIT VII

115 Wound Closure (Perform)

Gregory Simpson Marler

PURPOSE Proper and adequate wound closure is important to achieve hemostasis, reduce scarring and infection risk, and maintain secure placement of surgical tubes and drains. Appropriate healing of body structures can be mechanically supported by wound closure techniques.

PREREQUISITE NURSING KNOWLEDGE

- The skin is the largest organ of the body and has multiple functions (e.g., temperature regulation, fluid balance, and soft tissue protection). It consists of two major tissue layers: the outer epidermis and the inner dermis.
  - The epidermis consists of stratified, squamous cells with keratin and melanin. This layer provides thermoregulation, immunological activity, fluid balance, and pigmentation.
  - The dermis consists of fibro-elastic connective tissue with capillaries, lymphatics, and nerve endings. This layer provides energy, nourishment, and strength.
- A wound is any alteration to tissue that causes a disruption in the tissue's integrity, regardless of etiology. In some situations, formal wound closure is necessary to promote healing.
- Wound healing occurs at the cellular level in three overlapping phases: inflammation, proliferation, and maturation.
  - *Inflammation:* When an injury occurs, immediate local vasoconstriction decreases blood loss while the release of platelets and thromboplastin work to form a clot, leading to hemostasis. Bacterial growth and infection are suppressed by granulocytes and lymphocytes.[44,45] Cellular debris and foreign substances are phagocytized by macrophages that play a key role in wound healing.[41] Kinins and prostaglandins are subsequently released to enhance vasodilation and vascular permeability, leading to the production of inflammatory exudate to further promote wound repair. Wound scabs occur later in the healing process through fibrin formation. Wounds left open for up to 3 hours show a dramatic increase in vascular permeability, which results in thick inflammatory exudate and may limit the therapeutic value of antibiotics.[44,48] Early definitive closure may be essential in preventing infection, however, considerations should be given to the type of inciting injury (e.g., clean wound versus a bite).
  - *Proliferation and epithelialization:* Epithelialization occurs when epithelial cells migrate across the new tissue to form a barrier between the wound and the environment. The process of epithelialization is dependent on the type, location, and structure of the injury (e.g., depth, size, microbial contamination, partial thickness vs. full thickness).[41] Additionally, factors that affect the health of the patient plays a significant role in the healing process (e.g., genetics and epigenetics).[41] Fundamentally, neovascularization (the new flow of blood to the wound) plays a significant role in wound healing throughout the process, independent of the stages of healing.[10,11,41] The proliferation and epithelialization phase of wound healing usually occurs 2 to 3 days after the initial insult but can last up to 2 to 3 weeks. This stage is characterized by regeneration of new tissue, collagen, and blood vessels. Fibroblasts are released to rebuild collagen, fill in the wound defects, and aid in producing new capillaries. The wound defect decreases and epithelialization occurs as the wound edges contract. Multiple growth factors (e.g., hepatocyte, fibroblast, and epidermal) play key roles in epithelialization.[30] In general, epithelialization timing can vary, contingent on wound type and if any mechanical method of closure is utilized. Epithelialization in wounds that are formally closed with sutures or staples can occur within 18 to 48 hours, whereas wounds that are left open to heal by secondary intention may take longer. Adequate communication to the patient should include information on the multiple factors involved in wound closure, healing, and expectations.
  - *Maturation and Remodeling:* This is the final phase in wound healing. New collagen is formed and reorganized to increase the strength of the new tissue. This process can take from weeks to years to complete. Densely bundled tissues (e.g., scars) that contain collagen fibers can further develop during the healing process and can lead to aesthetic and functional limitations.[30]

AP This procedure should be performed only by clinicians who have demonstrated competence and are credentialed to perform it. In addition, the procedure must be within the scope of practice defined by their professional licensure, and in accordance with professional practice acts. Physicians, advanced practice nurses, and physician assistants may be credentialed to perform this procedure.

- Potential complications include infection and/or tetanus, wound dehiscence, loss of function or structure, scarring, and impaired cosmetic appearance.[30,33]
- Wound closure should focus on decreasing wound healing time and risk of infection, minimizing potential loss of function of the affected area, reducing scarring by minimizing dead space, and decreasing vulnerable open surfaces in a timely manner using aseptic technique.
- Wound closure occurs via primary or secondary intention or via delayed primary closure.
  - ❖ Closure via primary intention occurs when a wound is formally closed using sutures, staples, or adhesive strips. Success is dependent on contamination-free wounds, minimal tissue loss, and clean edges that are amenable to re-approximation and closure. The goals of primary wound closure are to stop bleeding, prevent infection, preserve function, and restore appearance.
  - ❖ Wound closure via secondary intention occurs when contributing factors (e.g., gross wound contamination and/or infection, traumatic wound with significant tissue loss, or jagged wound edges) prevent effective re-approximation, and wounds can require significant time to close.[8,45,48] In situations such as this, the wound often remains open to allow granulation tissue to develop for an extended period, thus allowing for close monitoring of the wound bed. Multiple wound-care techniques may be employed at this time to cleanse the wound and promote wound healing, and this is usually a planned healing process.[8] It is important to note that secondary intention wound healing has been linked with negative patient responses (e.g., physical and psychosocial stress); thus ramifications of this type of wound closure should be carefully considered and communicated to the patient.[31]
  - ❖ Delayed primary closure allows a grossly contaminated wound the time to be aggressively cleansed and potentially prepared for a formal wound closure, possibly in a delayed fashion. These wounds remain open with scheduled dressing changes and debridement over a 3- to 5-day period. The wound will be irrigated and closed after 3 to 5 days if it remains clean, has developed good granulation tissue, and signs of infection are not present. If an infection is present, the wound will remain open and be allowed to heal by secondary intention. If wounds have been open in excess of 8 hours or have been contaminated by saliva, feces, or purulent exudate, delaying the wound closure to decrease the risk for infection is beneficial.[28]
- Wounds with damage to the blood supply, nerves, or joints; wounds on the face; and wounds that have extensive tissue damage or infection may necessitate referral to an appropriate specialist (e.g., vascular, orthopedic, plastic, or general surgeon) depending on available resources. Wounds that require closure on the forehead and scalp should be closed with primary intention techniques if at all possible as opposed to secondary intention along with adjuvants (e.g., tissue expanders, dermal alternatives) as needed.[4]
- Adequate wound preparation is key for successful closure and healing. Irrigation of the wound is the first step in wound closure and is essential in minimizing the risk of infection.[38] Though not necessary, if hair can potentially interfere with wound closure, removal may be necessary using an electric clipper. Razors can cause abrasions and microscopic skin nicks that may increase the risk of infection and therefore should not be used.[14,23,27,29,34,45]
- Wound closure is performed traditionally by employing several methods including the use of sutures, staples, tissue adhesives, and adhesive skin strips (e.g., Steri-Strips). However, before would closure, an accurate wound assessment is key to determine the most effective closure techniques.[16]
  - ❖ Sutures and staples are secure, commonly used methods for wound closure. Staples have a distinct advantage over sutures in that they can be quickly and easily placed with minimal difficulty and are less reactive than sutures; therefore they may cause less scarring and infection. They are frequently used for lacerations on the scalp, trunk, and extremities.[28] Alternatively, sutures can be used on the hands and feet (overlying joints) and for deeper facial and neck lacerations. Skin adhesive or tape should be considered for straight and superficial lacerations and wounds of the hands, feet, neck, and face, avoiding any surfaces overlying joints, any surface tension, mucosa, or lips.[13] Cosmetically, the use of staples or sutures produces minimal scarring (unless the patient is predisposed to developing scar tissue or keloid) but can be slightly uncomfortable on removal.
  - ❖ Adhesive skin-closure strips are ideal in straight superficial lacerations that have good skin approximation without significant tension. They are most commonly used on the face, areas of flaps, and on any friable skin not amenable to sutures or stapling (e.g., skin in older adults or immunosuppressed patients).[7,39]
  - ❖ The use of tissue adhesives is newer than its counterparts in wound closure, having only been approved for use by the U.S. Food and Drug Administration (FDA) in the late 1990s.[45] The most common tissue adhesives in use today are cyanoacrylate polymers (e.g., n-butyl-2-cyanoacrylate [HistoAcryl or PeriAcryl] or 2-octyl-cyanoacrylate [Dermabond or SurgiSeal]).[21,22,36,45] Short, clean, dry wounds with easily approximated wound edges in areas with minimal to no tension are appropriate for tissue adhesives, in addition to any friable skin not amenable to sutures or stapling (e.g., older adults, immunosuppressed patients, or occasionally patients with oral wounds).[3,35] These adhesives will generally sluff off as the wound heals, typically over 5 days.[22] Adhesives should not be used over joints of the hands and feet, lips, or mucosa; on infected, puncture, or stellate wounds; or in patients with poor circulation or a propensity to form keloids.[14,28] They are best suited for short lacerations (<6 to 8 cm) with low-tension, clean-edge, straight to curvilinear wounds that do not cross joints or creases.[2,15,28,38] Though the tensile strength is not equivalent to sutures or staples at the time of application, the healing strength of the wound at the 1-week mark is about equivalent.[36] Overall, tissue adhesives have been found to be comparable in terms of cosmetic appearance and acceptability.[20,21,24,32] However,

UNIT VII

studies that compared sutures to adhesives found less dehiscence with the use of sutures.[12,16] Additionally, some studies support the use of adhesives in high-tension areas when combined with deeper tissue sutures.[49]

- Suture needles are curved and come either tapered or cutting. Tapered needles are used in soft tissues (intestine, blood vessels, muscle, and fascia) and produce minimal tissue damage. Cutting needles are typically used in tissue that is tougher (e.g., skin). Reverse cutting needles have a cutting edge on the outside of the curve. Most needles are swaged, or molded, around the suture, providing convenience, safety, and speed during suture placement. Needle drivers are necessary to prevent damage to surrounding tissue and injury to the user.
- Sutures come in varying sizes and materials, and they are classified as absorbable or nonabsorbable. Appropriate suture selection is subject to anatomical location and healing potential. Tissue reactivity, flexibility, knot-holding ability, wick action, and tensile strength are all important considerations when selecting sutures (Table 115.1).[5] Additionally, blood supply and the healing process are significantly affected by suture selection and the techniques used for closure.[42]
  - Suture size is indicated by a zero (0). The higher the number that precedes the zero, the smaller the suture (e.g., 4-0 is smaller than 3-0).
  - Absorbable sutures (i.e., natural gut, synthetic polymers) are used for layered closures. Gut sutures are broken down via phagocytosis and induce a moderate inflammatory reaction. Chromic gut sutures have increased strength and last longer in tissue. Severe tissue reaction prohibits this suture type from being used in skin. Synthetic absorbable sutures are favored over gut sutures because of decreased infection rates and increased strength and longevity.[3] Recent randomized controlled trials found few differences in overall types of sutures, although in abdominal wounds, nylon sutures reduced rates of incisional hernias when compared with absorbable sutures.[50] Synthetic braided absorbable sutures provide the best closure for interrupted dermal sutures and ligation of bleeding vessels.
  - Nonabsorbable sutures are either natural fibers (i.e., silk, cotton, linen) or synthetic fibers (i.e., nylon, Dacron, polyethylene) and are best for superficial lacerations because of their ease of handling and knot construction.
  - Although braided sutures provide more strength than monofilament, they also have small spaces between the braids that may harbor bacteria for infection. Monofilament is best suited for skin closure because it produces less inflammatory response; however, the knots are less dependable.
- Suture and knotting technique
  - The preferred knotting technique involves a square knot or double loop followed by a square-knot tie. The number of sutures required is dependent on the size of the wound, with the goal to only use as many needed to hold the wound edges together without crimping. Tension should be minimized but not eliminated on the wound edges. The more tension on a wound, the closer the sutures should be placed.
  - When performing a suture repair, the practitioner must remember not to tie the sutures too tightly during placement as injured tissue will become edematous and automatically tighten around the suture within 12 to 24 hours. If sutures are tied too tightly, there is a risk of developing tissue necrosis.

TABLE 115.1　Suggested Guidelines for Suture Material and Size for Body Region

Body Region	Percutaneous (Skin)	Deep (Dermal)
Scalp	5-0/4-0 monofilament*	4-0 absorbable†
Ear	6-0 monofilament	–
Eyelid	7-0/6-0 monofilament	–
Eyebrow	6-0/5-0 monofilament	5-0 absorbable
Nose	6-0 monofilament	5-0 absorbable
Lip	6-0 monofilament	5-0 absorbable
Oral mucosa	–	5-0 absorbable†
Other parts of face/forehead	6-0 monofilament	5-0 absorbable
Trunk	5-0/4-0 monofilament	3-0 absorbable
Extremities	5-0/4-0 monofilament	4-0 absorbable
Hand	5-0 monofilament	5-0 absorbable
Extensor tendon	4-0 monofilament	–
Foot/sole	4-0/3-0 monofilament	4-0 absorbable
Vagina	–	4-0 absorbable
Scrotum	–	5-0 absorbable†
Penis	5-0 monofilament	–

*Nonabsorbable monofilaments include nylon (Ethilon, Dermalon), polypropylene (Prolene), and polybutester (Novafil).
†Absorbable materials for dermal and fascial closures include polyglycolic acid (Dexon, Dexon Plus), polyglactin 910 (Vicryl), polydioxanone (PDS [monofilament absorbable]), and polyglyconate (Maxon [monofilament absorbable]).
From Newell K: Wound closure. In Dehn, RW, Aspry DP, editors. *Essential clinical procedures*, ed 3, St. Louis, MO, 2012, Saunders, Fig 23-3.

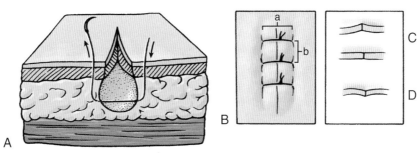

Figure 115.1 Interrupted dermal suture. **A,** Proper depth. **B,** Proper spacing (*a* = *b*). **C,** Proper final appearance. **D,** Improper final appearance. *(From Pfenninger JL, Fowler GC, editors:* Pfenninger and Fowler's procedures for primary care, *ed 3, St. Louis, 2011, Mosby.)*

- Lacerations are approximated using a variety of suturing techniques.[17]
  - Simple interrupted dermal sutures (Fig. 115.1) can be used when the skin margins are level or slightly everted. The needle should enter and exit the skin surface at a right angle. The stitch should be as wide as the suture is deep and no closer than 2 mm apart. The knot should be tied with an instrument tie and repeated four or five times. The first suture is placed in the midportion of the wound. Additional sutures are placed in bisected portions of the wound until it is appropriately closed.
  - Subcutaneous sutures with an inverted knot or buried stitch (Fig. 115.2) are used for deeper wounds or wounds under tension. Absorbable sutures are used in this setting, with the knot inverted below the skin margin. Begin at the bottom of the wound, come up and go straight across the incision to the base again, and tie. Deep, buried subcutaneous sutures are used to reduce the tension on skin sutures, close dead space beneath a wound, and allow for early suture removal.[18,19,26]
  - Vertical mattress sutures (Fig. 115.3) promote eversion of the skin, which promotes less prominent scarring.[26] Mattress sutures are used when skin tension is present or where the skin is very thick (palms and soles of feet). This suture is identical to a simple suture, but an additional suture is taken very close to the edge of each side of the wound.
  - Three-point or half-buried mattress sutures (Fig. 115.4) are used to close an acute corner of a laceration without impairing blood flow to the tip. The needle is inserted into the skin on the nonflap portion of the wound, passed transversely through the tip, and returned on the opposite side of the wound, paralleling the point of entrance. The suture is then tied, drawing the tip snugly in place.[19,26]
  - Subcuticular running sutures (Fig. 115.5) are used for linear wounds under little or no tension and allow for edema formation. Wound approximation may not be as meticulous as with an interrupted dermal suture. An anchor suture is placed at one end of the wound, and then continuous sutures are placed at right angles to the wound less than 3 mm apart. The wound is pulled together, and the other end secured with either another square knot or tape under slight tension.
- Sutures must be completely removed in a timely fashion to avoid further tissue inflammation and possible infection.

Sutures on extremities and the trunk should be removed in 7 to 14 days; those on the face should be removed in 3 to 5 days; and those on the palms, soles, back, and skin over mobile joints should be removed in 10 to 14 days. A thorough assessment of individual healing is performed before all suture removal (see Table 115.1).[37,42]

EQUIPMENT

- Local anesthetic
- Antimicrobial skin prep solution and sterile normal saline solution
- 8 to 10 4 × 4 gauze sponges
- Sterile metal prep basin
- 30- or 60-mL syringe and 18-gauge needle
- Sterile drape
- Fenestrated drape
- Sterile gloves, mask, eye protection
- For suturing
  - 6-inch needle holder
  - Suture material and needle
  - Curved dissecting scissors
  - Two mosquito hemostats: one curved, one straight
  - Suture scissors
  - Tissue forceps
  - Scalpel handle and No. 15 knife blade
  - Skin retractors (for atraumatic tissue handling)
- For other wound closures
  - Staple gun
  - Skin-closure strips
  - Skin adhesive
- *Note:* Frequently, hospitals use prepackaged suture kits; thus it may be not be necessary to assemble all of the items listed here if such a kit is available.

Appropriate dressing to cover the wound.

Additional equipment, to have available as needed, includes the following:
- Electric clippers (only if hair removal is necessary)
- 27- to 30-gauge needles

PATIENT AND FAMILY EDUCATION

- Explanation of the procedure, risks involved, potential benefits and alternatives, and expectations during and after the procedure should be included during patient education.

UNIT VII

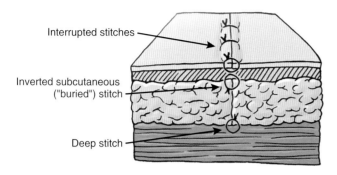

Figure 115.2   Inverted subcutaneous suture. Also shown is a layered closure. *(From Pfenninger JL, Fowler GC, editors:* Pfenninger and Fowler's procedures for primary care, *ed 2, St. Louis, 2006, Mosby.)*

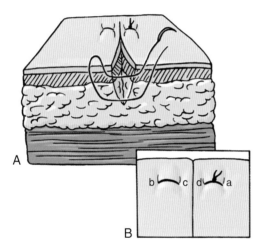

Figure 115.3   Vertical mattress suture. **A,** Cross-section. **B,** Overhead view. Begin at *a,* and go under skin to *b.* Come out, go in at *c,* and exit at *d. (From Pfenninger JL, Fowler GC, editors:* Pfenninger and Fowler's procedures for primary care, *ed 3, St. Louis, 2011, Mosby.)*

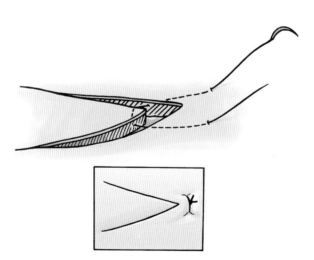

Figure 115.4   Three-point or half-buried mattress suture. *(From Pfenninger JL, Fowler GC, editors:* Pfenninger and Fowler's procedures for primary care, *ed 2, St. Louis, 2006, Mosby.)*

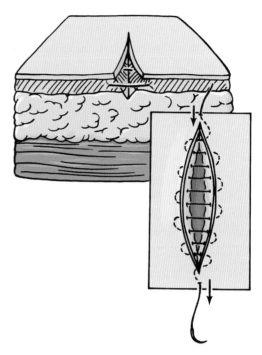

Figure 115.5   Subcuticular running suture. *(From Pfenninger JL, Fowler GC, editors:* Pfenninger and Fowler's procedures for primary care, *ed 3, St. Louis, 2011, Mosby.)*

Barriers to communication should be addressed appropriately before explaining the procedure (e.g., cultural, language, age, and level of understanding). ***Rationale:*** Explanation decreases patient anxiety, encourages patient and family cooperation, and improves understanding of the procedure.

- Once the explanation is complete and all patient/family questions have been answered, consent can be obtained. ***Rationale:*** Suturing is an invasive procedure that can have complications, so consent should be obtained before beginning the procedure. Having the patient/family describe the planned procedure in their own words demonstrates understanding.
- As appropriate, also provide instructions to the patient and family on the aftercare (i.e., pain medication, anticipated wound care, signs and symptoms of infection, and any follow-up appointments for removal of wound-closure material). ***Rationale:*** Instruction facilitates patient comfort, decreases the risk of infection, and encourages prompt intervention to treat possible infection.

PATIENT ASSESSMENT AND PREPARATION

Patient Assessment

- Assess the patient's current medical history, medications (prescribed and over the counter), and any pertinent information about the wound. Important factors in assessing the wound are how, when, and where the wound occurred. Additionally, assess comorbid conditions, medication history, vaccination status, and hand domination (if relevant). ***Rationale:*** This information allows a better understanding of the nature of the injury and any factors that could complicate wound healing.

- Wound assessment should always include type of wound, anatomical location, exact measurements, degree of severity and contamination, and any potential injuries to the peripheral nerves, vessels, or underlying structures. A full motor and sensory examination should be performed before any wound exploration or administration of anesthetic. Further imaging studies or specialist referrals may be indicated based on wound assessment. Consideration for tetanus vaccination should be made if the patient's status is unknown or expired. Administer the vaccination if criteria are met (visit http://www.cdc.gov/tetanus/index.html). ***Rationale:*** Provides baseline data. The

possibility of tetanus from an unclean wound is a preventable complication.

Patient Preparation

- Verify the correct patient with two identifiers. ***Rationale:*** Before performing a procedure, correct identification of the patient for the intended intervention is essential.
- Administer pain medication as necessary. Consider moderate procedural sedation for deep wounds and lacerations requiring repair.[32,39] Consider use of LET (lidocaine, 4%; epinephrine, 0.1%; and tetracaine, 0.5%) topically for local pain relief.[32,39] ***Rationale:*** Adequate pain control is essential to gain cooperation during the procedure and will provide the best opportunity for successful wound closure.

Procedure for Wound Closure

Steps	Rationale	Special Considerations
1. Prepare all necessary equipment and supplies.	Prepares for the procedure.	
2. **HH**		
3. **PE**		
4. Anesthetize the wound. Infiltrate the area with local anesthetic. May proceed with LET applied topically. Use local anesthetic with or without epinephrine and a 27- to 30-gauge needle to infiltrate the area.[1,40,46] **(Level C*)**	Provides for maximal patient comfort and cooperation during suturing.	Immobilization of the site also aids in decreasing pain.
5. Examine the wound thoroughly for foreign bodies, deep tissue layer damage, joint involvement, and injury to nerve, vessel, or tendon.	Prevents further damage. Assesses the need for referral.	Use aseptic technique to decrease contamination of wound. Radiographic imaging may be necessary to rule out a retained foreign body before wound closure.
6. Cleanse the wound.	Removes foreign substances and bacteria, and reduces the risk for infection.	
A. Mechanical: wiping, brushing, and irrigating with copious amounts of saline solution; use a 30- or 60-mL syringe with 18-gauge needle to generate pressure to remove debris as needed.	Mechanical cleansing is important for prevention of infection. The wound must be properly cleansed and irrigated before wound closure.	Too-aggressive cleansing of the wound can cause further trauma. A pressure of 8–12 psi is considered effective for cleansing and avoiding damage to tissues.
B. Chemical: antiseptic solution. Apply in concentric circles, moving toward the periphery.[25] **(Level A*)**	Reduces bacterial colony counts.[6,47]	Use a cleansing solution that is nontoxic to tissues.
C. Only if necessary, remove any hair in the area with an electric clipper.[23,27,29,43] **(Level A*)**	Do not remove hair at or around the suture site unless it interferes with the procedure.[9,14] Electric clippers (rather than razors) have been associated with significantly fewer infections.[9,14]	Consider use of hair-apposition techniques with longer hair to avoid shaving and promote wound closure without suturing.[21]

*Level A: Meta-analysis of quantitative studies or metasynthesis of qualitative studies with results that consistently support a specific action, intervention, or treatment (including systematic review of randomized controlled trials).

*Level C: Qualitative studies, descriptive or correlational studies, integrative reviews, systematic reviews, or randomized controlled trials with inconsistent results.

Procedure for Wound Closure—*Continued*

Steps	Rationale	Special Considerations
7. Remove nonsterile gloves, wash hands, and apply sterile gloves.		
8. Apply sterile drapes over and under the area as necessary.	Creates a sterile field. Reduces the risk for infection. Débridement reduces contamination and optimizes wound-healing potential.	Débridement should be conservative and limited to removal of devitalized tissue that could act as a medium promoting bacterial growth.
9. Examine the wound again for devitalized tissue that needs removal or débridement (see Procedure 132). Use a scalpel or sharp tissue scissors if necessary.		
10. If needed, loosen the wound from the subcutaneous tissue beneath the dermis with the scissors or scalpel. Note: For wound-closure methods other than suturing, skip to **Step 22.**	Promotes approximation of skin edges.	
11. Select the appropriate needle and suture material according to the type of wound.	Provides maximal support with the least amount of tissue trauma and encourages the best cosmetic outcome.	
12. Arm the needle between the jaws of the needle holder (Fig. 115.6).	Prevents needle bending and provides for guided insertion.	The needle holder should be perpendicular to the needle and should grasp the needle 3 mm beyond the wound opening. The handle of the needle holder should be closed to the first or second ratchet.
13. Grasp the needle holder (Fig. 115.7).	Correct grasp ensures smooth entry of the needle and proper stitch placement with minimal manipulation.	

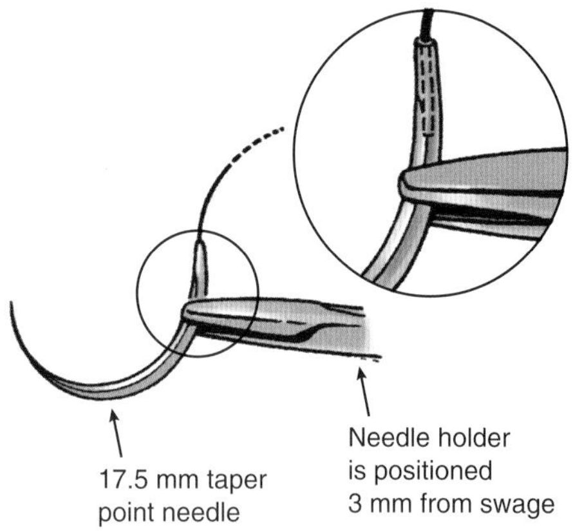

17.5 mm taper point needle

Needle holder is positioned 3 mm from swage

Figure 115.6   Because the laser-drilled hole is 15 mm long, this needle can be grasped by the needle holder 3 mm from the swage *(inset)*. The needle holder grasps the needle 3 mm from its swage. *(Copyright 1996, 2010. Courtesy Covidien.)*

Procedure continues on following page

Procedure for Wound Closure—*Continued*		
Steps	Rationale	Special Considerations

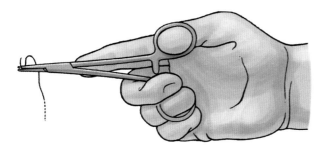

Figure 115.7 Thumb-ring finger grip of needle holder. *(Copyright 1996, 2010. Courtesy Covidien.)*

Steps	Rationale	Special Considerations
14. Position the free end of the suture away from the operator.	Allows optimal visualization of the free end of the suture and ensures that it does not become entangled during knot construction.	
15. Pass the needle through the tissue until the needle point is visualized.	Allows visualization of the needle.	The hand should start prone; supination of the wrist passes the needle in a direction toward the person suturing and in the direction of the curvature of the needle.
16. Using tissue forceps to grasp the needle point, unclamp the needle holder jaws.	Stabilizes the needle to maintain its position in the tissue.	
17. Regrasp the needle between the needle holder jaws, and pull the desired length of suture through the wound.	Prepares for tying a knot.	Keep the wrist in the prone position.
18. Tie the suture knot. Edges should be slightly everted.		Secure the precise approximation of the wound edges without strangulating the tissue. The suture should be tied snugly, but gently.
A. Form a suture loop: wrap the fixed suture end over and around the needle holder twice.	Double wrap provides increased strength.	Keep the length of free suture end less than 2 cm.
B. Pass the free end of the suture through the loop to create a throw.		Has a figure-of-eight shape.
C. Advance the throw to the wound surface by applying tension perpendicular to the wound.		
D. Repeat four or five times.		With each throw, your hands must reverse positions and apply equal and opposing tension to the suture ends in the same plane.
19. Cut the suture by holding the scissor blades perpendicular to the suture and keeping the knot in view between the blades, allowing 3-mm tails to remain.	Tails allow for easy identification of sutures on removal. The perpendicular positioning is helpful in preventing accidental cutting of the knot.	
20. Reposition the knot away from the wound edges.	Facilitates suture line care.	
21. Repeat **Steps 11–20** until the wound is closed. Dress the wound as indicated. Go to **Step 24.**		

UNIT VII

Procedure   for Wound Closure—*Continued*

Steps	Rationale	Special Considerations
22. Other wound-closure techniques: select the wound-closure technique to be used.		
A. Staples: Use fingers or forceps to approximate the edges. Apply firm pressure with the stapler, and dispense staples as directed. Place staples 0.5–1 cm apart. An assistant can help evert the wound edges while the primary operator uses the stapler.	Keep constant pressure and wound approximation to assist with even staple placement for wound closure.	
B. Adhesive skin strips: Ensure that the skin is not oily or hairy and that the wound has minimal drainage. The strips should overlap the wound about 2–3 cm on each side of the wound. Begin at the midpoint of the wound to approximate the sides, and work out to the ends of the wound. Strips should be placed about 2–3 cm apart. Additional strips can be placed over the cross tapes to prevent the ends from coming loose.[1]	Clean, smooth skin surfaces are optimal for the best adherence of skin-closure strips.	Should not be used for large wounds or on patients who may remove them (confused, uncooperative, or very young patients). Skin adherent (i.e., tincture of benzoin or Mastisol liquid adhesive) may be applied to the area to increase adhesion of skin strips. Although these adherents are widely used, their application should be limited only to intact skin, avoiding contact with the wound bed.
C. Skin adhesive: Apply to dry, well-approximated wound edges. Open the product, saturate the porous applicator tip, and paint the edges of the wound with short brush strokes in a multilayering process. Allow 15 seconds between layers. Usually four layers are applied. Hold edges together for 30–60 seconds.[13]	Precise application is important to avoid contaminating the wound with adhesive.	Avoid skin adhesive getting into the wound. If skin adhesive gets into the wound, it is ineffective, impairs healing, and increases the potential for foreign-body reaction.
23. After applying staples and adhesive skin strips, cover the wound with nonadherent dressing for the first 24–48 hours. Depending on institutional standards, a topical antimicrobial ointment may be added before dressing application. Skin adhesive: Dressing is unnecessary, but a dry gauze pad may be used. Do not use ointments, creams, or tape strips. Do not soak, scrub, or expose the wound to prolonged wetness. The patient may shower or gently bathe.[1]	Protects the wound from further injury; discourages microbial invsion[2]; minimizes bleeding, edema, and potential dead space; provides a physiological environment that is conducive to epithelial migration and scab formation; takes tension off the wound edges; cushions the wound from extraneous trauma; and restricts motion, which decreases lymphatic flow and minimizes the spread of wound microflora.[13,33]	For continued oozing, consider applying a pressure dressing. First assess for local perfusion to avoid dressing-related ischemia.

Procedure continues on following page

Steps	Rationale	Special Considerations
24. Dispose of equipment in appropriate receptacles. 25. 🄷🄷	Standard precautions.	

Expected Outcomes

- Bleeding ceases or is controlled
- Wound remains infection free
- Function is preserved
- Appearance is restored

Unexpected Outcomes

- Continued bleeding from the wound site or hematoma
- Wound infection and possible sepsis
- Skin necrosis
- Loss of function
- Abnormal appearance
- Wound dehiscence

Patient Monitoring and Care

Steps	Rationale	Reportable Conditions
		These conditions should be reported to the provider if they persist despite nursing interventions.
1. Serial examination of the wound.	Allows for early treatment and prevents systemic infection. Frequency of serial examination will depend on patient and wound history.	• Wound that is red, swollen, tender, or warm • Suppurative wound • Red streaks surrounding the wound • Tender lumps in the groin or under the arm • Chills or new fever
2. Administer prophylactic antibiotics as ordered if: A. Contamination of trauma site is suspected. B. Animal or human bite wounds exist. C. Preexisting medical conditions subject the patient to increased risk for infection (e.g., valvular heart disease, diabetes).	Prevents wound infection.	
3. Follow institutional standards for assessing pain. Administer analgesia as prescribed (agent and dose are determined by the extent of the trauma, the pain perception and threshold of the patient, age, and concerns of the patient).	Identifies need for pain interventions.	• Continued pain despite pain management interventions
4. Provide appropriate support to wounds under considerable tension (i.e., rigid splints, adhesive strips, or retention sutures, as clinically indicated).	Decreases lymphatic flow, thereby decreasing the spread of wound bacteria. Provides support and limitation of movement to allow for proper wound healing and patient comfort.	
5. Keep the wound and dressing clean and dry. If the dressing becomes wet, use sterile techniques to remove it, blot dry with a gauze pad, and reapply a clean, dry dressing.[24]	Decreases the opportunity for infection from wicking action of a wet dressing.	

UNIT VII

Patient Monitoring and Care —*Continued*

Steps	Rationale	Reportable Conditions
6. Keep dressed for 24–48 hours. If needed, cleanse with nontoxic cleansing solution, blot dry, apply triple antibiotic ointment (unless contraindicated), and reapply a sterile, nonadherent dressing.[13,33] Avoid the use of triple antibiotic ointments or topicals if the patient has a drug sensitivity or develops symptoms consistent with sensitivity.	Decreases the risk for wound contamination and infection. Beyond 48 hours, it is unclear whether an incision must be covered by a dressing or if showering or bathing is detrimental to healing.[12]	
7. Remove sutures or staples.[37] A. Facial wounds in 3–5 days. B. Scalp and extremity wounds in 7–14 days. C. Palms, soles, back, and skin over mobile joints in 10–14 days.	Prevents infection, enhances proper healing, and decreases the risk for undesirable scar formation.	
8. Provide detailed patient and family education, including wound care, medications, signs and symptoms of infection, and follow-up appointments.	Facilitates patient and family cooperation.	

Documentation

Documentation should include the following:
- Informed consent
- Patient and family education
- Location and appearance of the wound
- Time since injury
- The procedure used to clean wound
- The procedure and technique used to close wound
- How the patient tolerated the procedure
- Care of the wound after closure
- Instructions given to the patient and family
- Pain assessment and medication given
- Antibiotics given before wound closure and the need for continued antibiotics
- Tetanus status, if given
- Unexpected outcomes
- Nursing interventions

References and Additional Readings

For a complete list of references and additional readings for this procedure, scan this QR code with your smartphone, or visit https://www.elsevier.com/__data/assets/pdf_file/0004/1319890/Chapter0115.pdf

PROCEDURE

116 Cleansing, Irrigating, Culturing, and Dressing an Open Wound

Erin Reynolds

PURPOSE Cleansing, irrigating, and dressing open wounds are performed to optimize healing. Wound culturing may be necessary to isolate and allow for treatment of organisms and guide further management.

PREREQUISITE NURSING KNOWLEDGE

- Skin assessment and wound assessment techniques.[12]
- Goals of wound care must be clearly outlined so proper wound care products are used.
- Wound care products should be matched to the patient and wound conditions. Although no specific dressing is considered superior to others,[1] properties of dressing products are different and should be assessed relative to wound treatment goals and evaluated based on wound progress.[12]
  - ❖ Dressings may be categorized as semiocclusive or occlusive. Semiocclusive dressings are semipermeable to gases (O_2, CO_2, moisture) and are impermeable to liquids; they provide the moist wound healing environment that optimizes wound healing. Occlusive dressings lack permeability to gases and liquids.
  - ❖ Coarse gauze, used in a wet-to-dry dressing, nonselectively débrides the wound bed mechanically and absorbs wound fluid.
  - ❖ Dressings such as calcium alginates, foams, and hydrofibers enhance wound exudate absorption; hydrogels, hydrocolloids, and transparent films provide moisture to nondraining wounds with minimal absorption.
  - ❖ Wounds with excessive wound drainage also require protection of periwound skin (i.e., skin barrier wipes, skin barrier creams).
- Wounds heal by primary, secondary, or tertiary intention (Fig. 116.1).
  - ❖ Normal wound healing is often described as a progressive process that involves four overlapping phases: hemostasis, inflammation, proliferation, and maturation.
    - ○ The hemostasis phase is the initial phase marked by the cessation of bleeding at the wound site via the clotting cascade. This occurs immediately following tissue injury.
    - ○ The inflammatory phase, which may last for days, is marked for hemostasis, increased local vasodilation,

and migration of neutrophils and macrophages to the area.
    - ○ The proliferation phase begins 2 to 4 days after injury, may last for weeks, and is the healing phase of the wound process in which epithelialization, angiogenesis, and collagen synthesis predominate.[5]
    - ○ The maturation phase involves the body remodeling collagen fiber and increasing tissue tensile strength. Tissue maturation will occur after 2 weeks or longer and continue for 1 year or longer.
  - ❖ Most clean wounds heal by primary intention. Suturing each layer of tissue approximates the wound edges. These wounds typically heal quickly and require minimal wound care.
  - ❖ Open wounds heal by secondary intention by granulating from the base of the wound to the skin surfaces and contracting and epithelializing from the wound edges; care must be taken to allow for uniform granulation and prevention of open pockets or tunneling. Wounds should be assessed for signs of pocketing or tunneling as these will complicate and prolong the healing process and require additional intervention.
  - ❖ Tertiary intention involves a period of secondary healing to achieve edema reduction and decreased exudate production, followed by surgical closure for primary healing.
- Clean, moist wound beds allow for effective wound healing under the support of a dressing.
  - ❖ Open, granulating wounds heal slower, may result in drying of granulating tissue and tissue death, and may be more painful for the patient.
- The presence of exudate is not synonymous with infection but is the natural result of the inflammatory response to maintain moisture and allow movement and replication of epithelial cells necessary for healing. A change in volume, color, odor, or consistency of exudate may indicate impending infection.[2,4,11] Wound cleansing should be accomplished with minimal chemical or mechanical trauma.

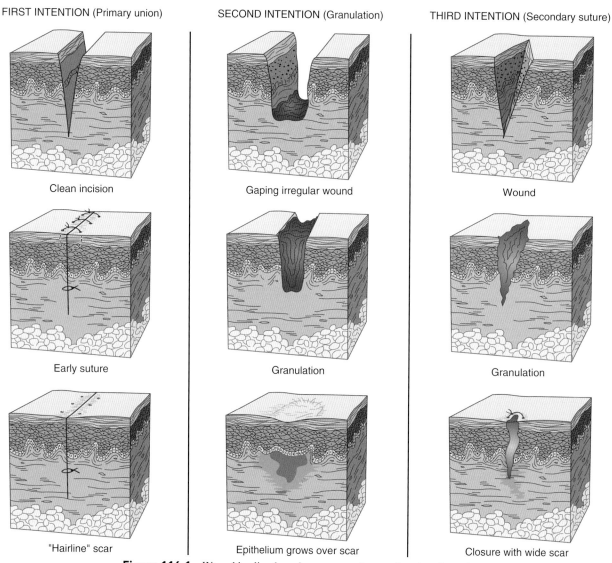

FIRST INTENTION (Primary union) SECOND INTENTION (Granulation) THIRD INTENTION (Secondary suture)

Clean incision   Gaping irregular wound   Wound

Early suture   Granulation   Granulation

"Hairline" scar   Epithelium grows over scar   Closure with wide scar

Figure 116.1 Wound healing by primary, secondary, and tertiary intention.

- ❖ Cytotoxic cleansing agents (i.e., chlorhexidine, iodine, hydrogen peroxide) should be limited because they can delay healing.[2,3,9,10]
- ❖ Wound cleansing solutions should be pH neutral to promote homeostatic conditions at the wound site.
- ❖ Normal saline (NS) solution or sterile water are the cleansing agents of choice; however, tap water is safe and effective for cleansing of most acute and chronic wounds if the water is potable and from a known safe source including water system contaminants such as *Listeria* and amoeboid populations.[6,8] The practice of using tap water is mostly used in remote and resource-limited and community situations.
- • All wounds should be cleansed to remove adherent and infectious material from the wound surface. Infected and deeper wounds typically require irrigation.
  - ❖ The irrigating solution must be delivered with enough force to physically loosen foreign materials and bacteria without injuring the tissue. Effective wound irrigation is best achieved when solution is delivered at 8 to 13 psi (Fig. 116.2). A 35-mL syringe attached to an 18-gauge angiocatheter tip only delivers fluid at 8 psi.

A 12-mL syringe with a 22-gauge angiocatheter tip provides 13 psi. A 20-mL syringe with an 18-gauge angiocatheter tip provides 10 psi. (Increasing syringe size decreases the pressure of the stream, and increasing the bore of the catheter tip increases the pressure.) Pressures greater than 15 psi may actually force bacteria and debris deeper into the wound bed.[5] The exception is first cleansing of heavily contaminated or debris-filled wounds in an emergent or operative setting in which the benefits are deemed to outweigh the risks.[9]

- ❖ The volume of isotonic irrigation fluid required is 50 to 100 mL per centimeter of wound size.
- • Wound infections delay wound healing. Wound cultures (obtained before antibiotic or antifungal therapy) may isolate organisms and differentiate between colonization and active infection. Proper collection of wound cultures is essential to therapeutic guidance of antimicrobial treatment; therefore care should be taken to minimize contamination of the specimen.
  - ❖ Wound contamination is the presence of bacteria on the wound surface that are not actively multiplying.

UNIT VII

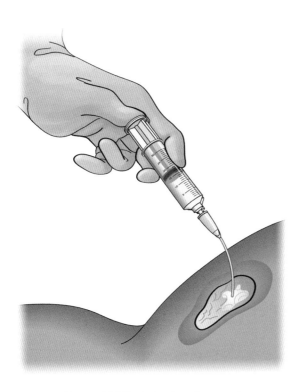

Figure 116.2 Irrigation of a wound.

❖ Colonization is the presence of bacteria in the wound that are actively multiplying or forming colonies. Colonization can delay healing but may not elicit signs of infection.

❖ Wound infection is present if organisms are present and have attached at $>10^5$ colony-forming units per milliliter in conjunction with clinical findings such as erythema, edema, pain, purulence, fever, and leukocytosis.

❖ With the proliferation of organisms like methicillin-resistant *Staphylococcus aureus* and aggressive bacteria that cause necrotizing soft tissue infections (e.g., group A *Streptococci* and *Streptococcus pyogenes*), knowledge of whether resistant strains of bacteria are present at the onset of treatment is critical to provide the optimal situation for healing and rapid intervention.[6,9,11]

❖ Bacterial invasion of wounds is managed with cleansing, débridement, and antibiotic therapy (local or systemic). Soaking can macerate the wound and periwound tissues and may not improve bacterial counts.[9]

❖ Biofilm, a polymicrobial structure that includes microorganisms (fungi protozoa as well as bacteria), proteins, polysaccharides, and lipids, prevent wound healing by forming a physical barrier that prevents access to topical treatments and proper granulation. They form within 24 hours of wound development and must be removed frequently through wound cleansing techniques to promote healing.[7,8]

❖ Critically ill patients commonly encounter factors that impair adequate wound healing, compounding the risks for poor patient outcomes. Nursing care should focus on early recognition and correction of underlying systemic disorders and patient-specific comorbidities that can impede wound healing goals.[4,5,9]

• Frequent comorbidities that can compromise optimal healing trajectories are diabetes mellitus, cardiovascular disease, chronic obstructive pulmonary disease, peripheral vascular disease, cancer, endocrine imbalances, renal failure, cerebral vascular accident, nicotine addiction, alcohol abuse, neurovascular deficit, obesity, and ascites. Of note, in the critically ill patient, hypotension and poor perfusion will compound the risk for delayed wound healing.

• Trauma-associated wound considerations include penetrating injuries that create anaerobic pockets and deep tissue injury; reperfusion of previously ischemic injuries that can trigger paradoxical injury extension; and possible contamination with organic and inorganic bodies that can inhibit effective wound healing, including feces, saliva, soils, and environmental vectors such as metal, rock, and glass.

• Sometimes medications and treatment interventions may jeopardize wound healing goals. Medications that impair tissue perfusion (e.g., vasoconstrictors) or the immune response (e.g., steroids, immunomodulators, antirejection drugs, antineoplastics) and treatments that impair tissue hydration (e.g., diuretics and fluid restrictions) may adversely affect wound healing.

• Poor nutritional status includes low serum protein, vitamin C, zinc, copper, and magnesium, and uncontrolled glucose.[5] Critically ill patients are also at risk for nutritional compromise, thus ensuring collaboration with the multidisciplinary team to address nutritional goals with the presence of wounds is necessary.

• Other factors that compound effective wound healing include hypothermia or hyperthermia, extended surgical procedures, intraoperative hypotension, immobility, hypoxemia, anemia, poor tissue oxygenation, sepsis, extremes of age, inadequate sleep or rest, uncontrolled pain,[10] clotting abnormalities, mechanical friction on the wound, and the development of adhesions or hypertrophic or keloid scars.

• Clean technique is used for most chronic wounds. Sterile technique is used for acute wounds and compromised host patients.[6]

• No evidence is found to support the use of sterile technique when changing dressings on chronic wounds.[6]

• Ultrasound and MRI can play a role in the diagnostic accuracy of the development of necrotizing fasciitis and abscess.

EQUIPMENT

• Nonsterile and/or sterile gloves (two pairs); sterile field (depending on type and age of wound)
• Two or three sterile cotton-tipped applicators
• NS solution or ordered commercial irrigation solution per institutional protocol
• Sterile basins
• Waterproof barriers
• Sterile gauze (4 × 4); large absorbent/ABD dressings (if the wound has excessive drainage, an absorptive dressing may be necessary; if the wound has minimal drainage, a moisture-enhancing dressing may be needed)
• Sterile 35-mL slip-tip syringe and 18-gauge angiocatheter sheath for irrigation (if necessary; other syringe selection to keep within the 8–13-psi recommendations may be used in place of the 35-mL syringe)

- Liquid skin barrier, cream, or wafer; apply around the wound edge to protect periwound tissue
- Hypoallergenic tape
  Additional equipment, to have available as needed, includes the following:
- Swab culture: two sterile serum-tipped swabs and culturettes
- Tissue biopsy: sterile field, scalpel, forceps, gauze for hemostasis, and container
- Needle aspiration: 10-mL syringe, 22-gauge needle, and syringe cap
- Montgomery straps, tubular mesh bandage, other closure/support supplies

PATIENT AND FAMILY EDUCATION

- Explain the procedure and rationale that supports wound cleansing, irrigating, and dressing management. ***Rationale:*** Patient anxiety and discomfort are decreased.[7]
- Discuss the patient's role in the procedure. ***Rationale:*** This elicits patient cooperation and prepares the patient for wound management on discharge (as appropriate).
- Explain the reason for obtaining a wound culture (if planning on obtaining one). ***Rationale:*** Patient anxiety is decreased.[10]
- Discuss signs and symptoms of local and systemic wound infection (erythema, pain, increased wound drainage, odor, fever), and inform the patient when to consult a physician, advanced practice nurse, or other healthcare professional. ***Rationale:*** The patient is prepared for wound management on discharge.

PATIENT ASSESSMENT AND PREPARATION

Patient Assessment

- Assess the following. ***Rationale:*** Assessment provides information about the healing process and assists in early identification of wound infection. True wound bed assessment cannot be completed until after the wound bed has been cleansed
- Wound drainage (amount, consistency, color, and possible odor)
- Size, shape, length, width, and depth of wound bed, including pockets (Fig. 116.3)
- Appearance of wound bed (color, presence of debris, i.e., necrotic or darkened areas on tissue bed are black, slough is green or cream yellow, and healthy tissue is red)
- Condition of wound margins and periwound skin (intact vs. maceration or xerosis; abnormal textures/undermining)
- Pain or tenderness at the wound site
- Elevated temperature or localized warmth at wound site

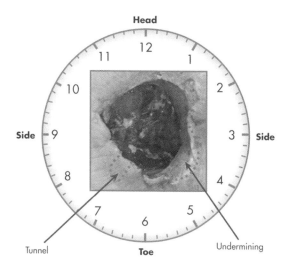

Figure 116.3   Measurement and assessment of a wound. (*From Lewis SL, Heitkemper MM, Dirksen SR, et al:* Medical-surgical nursing: Assessment and management of clinical problems, *ed 9, St. Louis, 2014, Mosby.*)

- Presence of erythema (blanches with pressure) or ecchymosis (does not blanch with pressure)
- White blood cell count; may be elevated or show a change from baseline
- Altered blood chemistries, especially hypokalemia and hyperglycemia (>200 mg/dL) and acid-base disturbances. Inadequate long-term glycemic control and major swings in glucose levels in diabetics are linked with three times the number of wound complications.[5]
- With advance age, subtle changes in activity and cognition may be the only indications of infection[10]
- Nutrition assessment including long-term glycemic control[7]

Patient Preparation

- Verify the correct patient with two identifiers. ***Rationale:*** Before performing a procedure, the nurse should ensure the correct identification of the patient for the intended intervention.
- Ensure that the patient understands the preprocedural teaching. Answer questions as they arise, and reinforce information as needed. ***Rationale:*** Understanding of previously taught information is evaluated and reinforced.
- Administer premedication with prescribed analgesic, if indicated, prior to procedure with enough time for medication to reach time to onset. ***Rationale:*** Medication decreases patient anxiety and increases comfort. Pain and stress are recognized deterrents for healing.
- Optimize lighting in the room, and provide privacy for the patient. ***Rationale:*** Lighting facilitates visualization.
- Place the patient in a position of optimal comfort and visualization for wound care procedures. ***Rationale:*** Proper positioning provides for effective wound visualization and enhances patient tolerance of the procedure.

Procedure	**for Cleansing, Irrigating, Culturing, and Dressing an Open Wound**	
Steps	Rationale	Special Considerations

Cleansing and Irrigating Wounds

1. **HH**
2. **PE**
3. Place a waterproof barrier under the wound area to collect drainage.

4. Position the wound-cleansing materials and soiled contamination container within reach of the provider; conform to the principles of aseptic technique.

5. **HH**
6. **PE**

7. Remove soiled dressing, noting any change in drainage and frequency of needed change. Discard in appropriate containers.

8. Assess the condition of the periwound skin and wound bed for shape and size, odor, and amount and consistency of drainage. Gently probe with a cotton swab to note the depth of tunnels and undermining. Remove soiled gloves.

9. For wounds requiring sterile technique:
   A. **HH**
   B. Don sterile gloves.
   C. Establish a sterile field.
   D. Open the sterile drape gauze.
   E. Place sterile water or NS cleansing solution in a sterile container. For clean technique, set up supplies per protocol to prevent cross-contamination. Use clean gloves.

10. If irrigation (see Fig. 116.2) is necessary, attach an angiocatheter sleeve to the syringe for irrigation.
   A. **HH**
   B. Apply gloves.
   C. Draw solution up into the syringe.
   D. Maintain a 1- to 3-cm distance from wound surface.
   E. Direct solution onto the wound bed from the area of least contamination to the greatest.
   F. Continue with irrigation until the return solution is clear.

Rationale column:

3. Controls the flow of cleansing solution and minimizes solution contact with intact skin.

4. Decreases cross-contamination during the wound-cleansing process; enhances body mechanics for the provider.

7. Increasing drainage and frequency of change may indicate impending infection.[7]

8. Assesses for indications of healing or deterioration (see Fig. 116.3).

9. Decreases cross-contamination during the wound-cleansing process. Cleansing solution should not be cytotoxic.[1,2]

10. Irrigation reduces the bacterial population and removes excess debris to enhance healing.

Special Considerations column:

6. Face and eye barriers are strongly suggested with irrigation of wounds to protect the provider against splash contaminant.

8. True wound bed assessment cannot be completed until after the wound bed has been cleansed. Measurements or photographs (per institutional protocol) should be taken intermittently to document progression.

9. No evidence is found to support the use of sterile techniques when changing dressings on chronic wounds.[5] The evidence for use of sterile water irrigation has generally been limited to acute wounds and open fractures (specifically excluding patients with a history of diabetes).[3]

10. Research does not support scrubbing or swabbing wounds.[9] Bulb syringes do not create enough psi to be effective.[12] A 35-mL syringe with an 18-gauge needle provides approximately 8 psi, which is sufficient force to remove debris without creating wound bed damage. The smaller the syringe, the greater the psi. Too great a force during irrigation can create tissue damage, drive bacteria deeper into the tissues, re-initiate the inflammatory process, and delay wound healing.[8,11] Not all open wound beds need irrigation.

Procedure continues on following page

UNIT VII

Procedure | for Cleansing, Irrigating, Culturing, and Dressing an Open Wound—*Continued*

Steps	Rationale	Special Considerations
11. Cleansing a closed wound: A. **HH** B. Apply nonsterile gloves. C. With moistened gauze, cleanse from the top of the wound to the base (or the center of the wound to the edges). D. Discard gauze. E. Cleanse from the area of least contamination to the greatest (Fig. 116.4).	Prevents wound contamination during the cleansing process.	If cleansing around a drain, cleanse from the drain site outward in a circular motion; discard gauze with each circle.

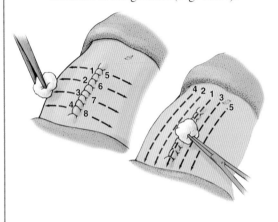

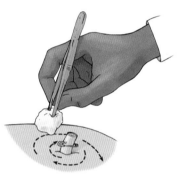

Figure 116.4   Cleansing of a wound. *(From Potter PA, Perry AG, Stockert PA, Hall A:* Fundamentals of nursing, *ed 9, St. Louis, 2017, Mosby.)*

Steps	Rationale	Special Considerations
12. Dry intact skin surrounding the wound with gauze.	Limits maceration of healthy skin surrounding the wound.	
13. Apply ointments/gauze/dressing prescribed.	Protects the wound.	
14. Discard uses supplies.		
15. **HH**		

Culturing Wounds

Swab Culture

Steps	Rationale	Special Considerations
1. **HH**		
2. Apply new gloves after cleansing, and remove the swab from the culturette tube; maintain sterile technique.	Must cleanse the wound before obtaining a culture to ensure that debris contamination and biofilm are not cultured.[5]	Sterile gloves may decrease inadvertent contamination to a statistically significant degree, but typically not a clinically significant rate.[6]
3. Swab firmly across the central surface of the wound in a zigzag manner, simultaneously rotating the swab between the finger and thumb with gentle pressure to extract any tissue fluid. **(Level D*)**	Tissue fluid, not superficial exudate, is desired for proper results. Swabbing the center of the wound and not the wound edges ensures collection of an adequate specimen.[10]	Culturing of wound edges may result in contamination from skin flora and wound debris.[10]

*Level D: Peer-reviewed professional and organizational standards with the support of clinical study recommendations.

Procedure	for Cleansing, Irrigating, Culturing, and Dressing an Open Wound—*Continued*	
Steps	Rationale	Special Cownsiderations
4. Carefully place the saturated swab into the culturette tube without touching the swab or inside of the container.	Enables adequate sample collection and prevents contamination.	
5. Crush the ampule of the medium in the culturette, and close securely; observe that the culture medium surrounds the swab.	Keeps the specimen from drying and provides a growth-supporting medium for culture.	With collection of an anaerobic culture, ensure that the tube is maintained upright to prevent carbon dioxide from escaping.
6. Apply a dressing as prescribed.	Protects the wound.	
7. Discard used supplies.		
8. **HH**		
9. Label the specimen with the patient's name, date, and wound site; transport the specimen to the laboratory as soon as possible.	Delays in culture transport increase the risk of invalid testing from exposure to temperature changes.	Bacterial overgrowth occurs with delays in plating and analysis.[10] Follow institutional guidelines on irretrievable specimen handling if the wound culture cannot be replicated should the specimen be lost.

Tissue Biopsy

1. **HH**		
2. Set a sterile field. Apply sterile gloves; with a sterile scalpel and forceps, curette, or punch biopsy, obtain a tissue sample approximately 1–2 mm in size (width and depth); apply pressure with sterile gauze to the tissue sampling site. (**Level D***)	Ensures that site markings have been made where appropriate. Ensures good tissue sample size free from necrotic tissue; provides for homeostasis of the tissue bed. A curette can obtain full biofilm organisms that can be missed by swabs.[9]	Caution must be exercised in obtaining a tissue biopsy; consider a local anesthetic to the site before the procedure; assess for excessive bleeding and damage to underlying and surrounding structures. Advanced training is required for nurses who perform this skill.
3. Place the tissue sample in a sterile container, and close it tightly; the sample may be placed on an agar plate, if indicated.	Prevents contamination of the sample.	
4. Apply a dressing as prescribed.	Protects the wound.	
5. Discard used supplies.		
6. **HH**		
7. Label the specimen with the patient name, date, and wound site; transport the specimen to the laboratory as soon as possible. Proceed to **"Dressing Open Wounds."**		Follow institutional guidelines on irretrievable specimen handling if the wound biopsy cannot be replicated should the specimen be lost.

Needle Aspiration

1. **HH**		
2. A. Cleanse the skin. B. Apply sterile gloves. C. Insert a sterile needle on the 10-mL syringe filled with 0.5 mL air into intact periwound tissue. D. Aspirate fluid from several vectors with a fan technique approach, and pull the plunger rapidly to draw tissue fluid into the syringe.	Ensures good specimen collection if two to four angles of aspiration are used.	The goal is to obtain tissue fluid, not wound exudate. Caution is required not to re-inject fluid back into tissues.
3. Express excess air out of the syringe.		
4. With sterile technique, remove the needle, and replace it with a blunt-end cap.	Maintains standard precautions; prevents contamination.	
5. Apply a dressing as prescribed.	Protects the wound.	
6. Discard used supplies.		
7. **HH**		

*Level D: Peer-reviewed professional and organizational standards with the support of clinical study recommendations.

UNIT VII

Procedure continues on following page

Procedure for Cleansing, Irrigating, Culturing, and Dressing an Open Wound—*Continued*

Steps	Rationale	Special Considerations
8. Label the specimen with the patient's name, date, and wound site; transport the specimen to the laboratory as soon as possible.		
Dressing Open Wounds	Apply a dressing that is appropriate to wound type and patient condition. Moisture-retentive dressings facilitate wound healing.	
1. HH		
2. PE		

3. Apply a wet dressing:
  A. Open 4 × 4 sterile gauze pads.
  B. Place it in a bowl, and saturate it with NS solution.
  C. Wring out excessive moisture.
  D. Apply 4 × 4 pads loosely over the wound bed.
  E. Gently pack the gauze to the wound edge, but do not exceed the wound edge.
	Saturating gauze on the packet greatly increases the risk of contamination unless the wrapping is coated to prevent bleed through of fluids. Open, moist gauze protects the wound bed and allows for placement of the dressing without creating open areas or pockets; the dressing must be moist but not wet to allow for absorption.[1]	Moist dressings must stay within the parameters of the wound bed to prevent surrounding skin maceration. Dressings packed too firmly into the wound compromise perfusion and wound healing. Wound care dressing products that absorb drainage or provide moisture may also be used. Gauze dressing may not control excessive wound exudate; alternative dressings to control exudate should be considered.

4. Place dry 4 × 4 gauze pads and ABDs over the moist dressing.	Provides protection and absorption.	
5. Secure the dressing. A. Tubular mesh dressings: sized to secure loose dressings underneath.	Conforming mesh dressings reduces the skin friction associated with tape removal and adhesive irritation. They allow airflow and increase security of coverage without added bulk.	
B. Tape: apply tape across the wound dressing, extending approximately 2 inches beyond the dressing onto the skin.	Hypoallergenic tape is less traumatic to noninjured skin and secures the dressing in place.	

C. Montgomery straps (Fig. 116.5):
    i. Apply a liquid or hydrocolloid barrier to surround the skin where straps will be applied.
    ii. Peel the paper backing off the straps, and apply to the skin surface with gentle, even pressure.
    iii. Lace the disposable ties (twill/trach tape; large rubber bands) through the holes in the straps in a crisscross fashion.
	Alternative if nonlatex mesh is unavailable for sensitive patients.
	1. Assists with providing a protective skin barrier and more effective anchoring of Montgomery straps.
	2. Secures Montgomery straps to the skin.
	3. Secures the dressing in place beneath the Montgomery strap.
		The straps, tapes, or twill used must be replaced if they become soiled or moist because they become a reservoir for contamination.

6. Discard uses supplies.		
7. HH		

Procedure for Cleansing, Irrigating, Culturing, and Dressing an Open Wound—*Continued*

Steps	Rationale	Special Considerations

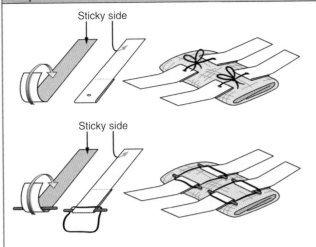

Figure 116.5   Montgomery straps.

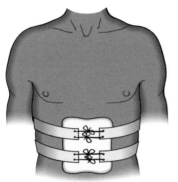

Expected Outcomes

- Healed wound
- Wound bed is free from devitalized tissue
- Wound culture specimen obtained confirms and identifies the causative organism of infection
- Wound heals uniformly without tunneling, abscess formation, or tracking
- Surrounding skin is free from maceration and erosion
- Wound is free from signs of infection or compromised perfusion

Unexpected Outcomes

- Cross-contamination of the wound
- Damage to the wound bed (hemorrhage, dehiscence) from excessive force during irrigation
- Maceration or inflammation of surrounding skin
- Hemorrhage from tissue biopsy culture technique
- Signs of infection; changes in amount and character of wound drainage
- Wound healing (granulation and contraction) not noticeably progressing on a weekly basis
- Development of wound tunneling, abscess, or tracking

Patient Monitoring and Care

Steps	Rationale	Reportable Conditions
		These conditions should be reported to the provider if they persist despite nursing interventions.
1. Follow institutional standards for assessing pain. Administer analgesia as prescribed.	Identifies the need for pain interventions and premedication to a noxious stimulus.	• Continued pain despite pain interventions

Procedure continues on following page

UNIT VII

Patient Monitoring and Care —*Continued*

Steps	Rationale	Reportable Conditions
2. Assess the patient, wound bed, and skin surrounding the wound.	Continued assessment is essential; wounds must be free from infection to heal. Healthy granulation tissue is pink or red. Discoloration may indicate infection, necrotic tissue, or poor perfusion or hypoxemia at the wound bed site.	• Foul drainage or odor • Darkened or pale areas on the tissue bed; red, green, or yellow tissue bed • Erythema; new ecchymosis • Pain • Change in wound drainage (amount, color, odor) • Elevated temperature • Elevated white blood cell count • Hyperglycemia in a patient with diabetes
3. Monitor the wound dressing site for bleeding.	The capillary bed of a healing wound is fragile. Excessive stimulation during cleansing, culturing, or biopsy may disrupt the capillary integrity, creating excessive bleeding.	• Bleeding that does not stop with mild pressure to the wound bed • Excessive bleeding
4. Assess the wound bed and edges for undermining, pockets, or tunnels.	Healing by secondary intention increases the risk for pockets or tunnels.	• Presence and depth of undermining, pocket, or tunnel

Documentation

Documentation should include the following:
- Patient and family education
- Pain assessment, premedication given, patient tolerance of the procedure, and response to pain medication
- Wound cleansing and irrigation procedure completed; date; time including whether clean or sterile technique was used
- Description of the wound bed before and after cleansing or irritation; drainage and odors if appropriate; presence of necrotic and granulation tissue
- Description of surrounding skin (color, moisture, integrity)
- Weekly measurements of wound size (measure or trace the wound area and depth when appropriate)
- Progression of difficult-to-heal or complex wounds (consider use of digital photography to document)
- Wound culture completed, date, time; type of culture obtained (swab, aerobic, anaerobic, needle aspiration, tissue biopsy)
- Description of approximate site where wound culture was obtained
- Description of wound drains, surrounding skin, and characteristics of wound drainage
- Type of dressing applied after wound care
- Unexpected outcomes
- Communication with provider/consulting service
- Nursing interventions

References and Additional Readings

For a complete list of references and additional readings for this procedure, scan this QR code with your smartphone, or visit https://www.elsevier.com/__data/assets/pdf_file/0005/1319891/Chapter0116.pdf.

117 Débridement: Pressure AP Ulcers, Burns, and Wounds

Gregory Simpson Marler

PURPOSE Wound débridement is the removal of necrotic, nonviable tissue to promote wound healing.

PREREQUISITE NURSING KNOWLEDGE

- The patient and wound aspects should be assessed for underlying causes or contributing factors (i.e., patient's physical condition, nutritional status, current healthcare treatment plan, and relevant medications before wound débridement is undertaken).[6,7]
- Normal wound healing progresses through an orderly sequence of four overlapping phases: hemostasis, inflammation, proliferation, and maturation.
- The presence of necrotic tissue or debris interrupts the normal sequence of wound healing, hinders healing processes, and provides a medium that promotes bacterial growth.[8]
- Acute wounds may be classified as either partial-thickness or full-thickness wounds.
  - Partial-thickness wounds penetrate the epidermis and part of the dermis and can further be delineated as superficial or deep partial-thickness wounds.
  - Full-thickness wounds extend to all skin layers, the epidermis and dermis, and may penetrate subcutaneous tissues.[21]
- *Pressure injury* is defined as localized injury to the skin or underlying tissue, usually over a bony prominence as a result of pressure.[21] The National Pressure Ulcer Advisory Panel staging system is used to describe pressure injuries.[14,21]
  - Stage I: Intact skin with nonblanchable erythema of a localized area usually over a bony prominence. Darkly pigmented skin may not have visible blanching, but the area may differ in color from surrounding tissues.[21] Visual changes may be preceded by alterations in sensation, temperature, or firmness.
  - Stage II: Presents as partial-thickness loss of the dermis and is seen as a shallow, open, nonsloughing injury that has a red-pink wound bed. It may also present as an intact or open/ruptured serum-filled blister.[20,21]

- Stage III: Presents as full-thickness tissue loss. Subcutaneous fat may be visible, however bone, tendon, and muscle are not exposed. Undermining, tunneling, and sloughing may be present.[21]
  - Stage IV: Presents as a full-thickness tissue injury that includes exposed bone, tendon, or muscle. Slough or eschar may be visible on some parts of the wound bed.
  - Unstageable: Tissue injury that cannot be adequately visualized and assessed because of the slough or eschar covering the wound base. Wound débridement should occur before staging the tissue injury.[21]
  - Deep tissue injury is suspected when a purple or maroon localized area of discolored intact skin or blood-filled blister is present. The area may be more painful, boggy, warmer, or cooler when compared with adjacent tissue.[1,21]
- Necrotic tissue is nonviable and presents in color from whitish gray to tan, yellow, or black. Enhanced bacterial growth and a delayed inflammatory phase of healing results from necrotic tissue.[24] Deeper penetration of bacteria into tissues results in cellulitis, osteomyelitis, and possible limb loss.
- Débridement provides a mechanism for removal of necrotic tissue and converts chronic wounds into acute wounds, thereby promoting epithelialization.[27] Biofilm is the adherence of microorganism cells on a surface. This can lead to a prolonged inflammatory state of the wound and possible chronic infection.[28] Débridement allows removal of biofilm from the wound surface and frequently leads to a positive outcome in healing.[18] Frequent débridements help suppress biofilm and accelerate healing.[18,28] Additionally, some literature advocates for débridement of acute wounds to adequately achieve primary closure for some wounds that historically have required secondary wound healing (e.g., animal bites).[19]
- Vascular evaluation is essential before non–burn wound débridement. Inadequate perfusion may result in the wound extending into a deeper dermal or full-thickness wound after débridement.[4] Pressure ulcers, burns, and chronic wounds may develop necrotic tissue that requires débridement for wound healing to progress.[23]

- Newer evidence suggests that biologic therapy using sterile maggots is effective in achieving débridement in chronic wounds.[1,27]
- Débridement may be achieved with several methods.[3]
    - Surgical débridement is an effective means of removal of devitalized tissue. It requires sedation, use of sterile instruments, and conditions and availability of a qualified clinician.[3] Large amounts of necrotic tissue may be removed. This may be considered in burn patients with large amounts of eschar or with necrotizing soft tissue infections (i.e., necrotizing fasciitis).[11,15] Surgical débridement requires a trained surgeon, anesthesia, and hospital admission, therefore making it more costly.[27]
    - Sharp débridement is similar to surgical débridement, but local anesthesia may or may not be administered. Sharp débridement procedures should be performed only by qualified physicians, advanced practice providers, and other healthcare professionals (including critical care nurses) with additional knowledge, skills, and demonstrated competence per professional licensure or institutional standards.[3] This kind of débridement may be performed at the hospital bedside, clinic, or office. Scalpels, scissors, and forceps may be used.[27] Sharp débridement is best for adherent dry eschar with or without infection present. When sharp débridement is used, the bacterial count can be rapidly reduced.[8] Sharp débridement may be difficult on hard, dry wounds in which enzymatic débridement may be a more appropriate option.[5] Sharp débridement should be discontinued in the presence of pain, excessive bleeding, or exposure of underlying structures. A key to successful safe sharp débridement is assessment and knowledge of anatomy.[15]
    - Chemical (enzymatic) débridement is a highly selective method of removal of necrotic tissue. It relies on naturally occurring enzymes that are exogenously applied to the wound surface to degrade tissue. This is a slower process that requires a moist wound bed with an adequate secondary dressing to absorb wound exudate. Enzymatic debriding agents may be selective or nonselective to viable tissues. Nonselective agents may be best for thick, leathery, adherent eschar. Selective agents may be best when excess protein buildup is present.[16] Patients who may benefit from chemical débridement include those with partial-thickness burn wounds or unstageable pressure ulcers and those who are not surgical candidates. Fortunately, patients typically do not require invasive management during enzymatic débridement (i.e., mechanical ventilation and deep sedation).[10]
    - Débridement alongside topical negative pressure therapy is used to enhance wound healing, not only in difficult-to-manage wounds and burns but also in prophylaxis format to prevent surgical wound infections, decreasing the need for future débridement.[2,9,11-13,22]
    - Mechanical débridement is a method of physical removal of debris from the wound. These methods include wet-to-dry gauze dressings, irrigation, pulsatile lavage, low-frequency ultrasonography (LFUS), negative pressure therapy, and hydrotherapy. Débridement is nonselective, meaning that healthy tissue, necrotic tissue, and any debris may be removed in the process, leading to bleeding and pain.
    - Autolytic débridement uses the properties of moisture-interactive dressings to facilitate digestion of devitalized tissue by the body's own enzymes. Typically, if tissue autolysis does not begin to appear in the wound in 24 to 72 hours, another method of débridement should be considered.[3]
- Wound care procedures should adhere to the principles of aseptic technique.
- Clinical judgment should be used in determining whether clean or sterile technique is indicated in the wound dressing procedure. Generally speaking, acute wounds may be cared for using sterile technique, and chronic wounds may be cared for using clean technique. When deciding which technique should be used in wound care, the clinician must assess the patient, type, and stage of the wound as well as the type of procedure.

EQUIPMENT

- Sharp débridement
    - Personal protective equipment (gown, goggles, mask)
    - Sterile gloves and field
    - Normal saline (NS) solution
    - 4 × 4 gauze pads
    - Sterile instrument set (scissors, forceps, No. 10 scalpel)
    - Wound dressing
    - Tape
- Chemical débridement
    - NS solution or water to cleanse the wound
    - Clean gloves or sterile gloves (depending on type and age of wound)
    - Enzymatic preparation or solution (prescribed)
    - Tongue blade
    - Filler dressing if needed; secondary absorptive dressing
    - Tape
- Mechanical débridement (wet-to-dry gauze dressing)
    - Clean or sterile gloves (depending on type and age of wound)
    - NS solution
    - Gauze (rolled or 4 × 4 pads)
    - Secondary absorptive dressing
    - Tape
- Autolytic débridement
    - Clean gloves
    - NS solution or water to cleanse wound
    - Moisture-retentive dressing (transparent film, hydrocolloid dressing, hydrogels)
    - Secondary absorptive dressing as indicated
    - Tape

PATIENT AND FAMILY EDUCATION

- Explain the procedure and the reason for wound débridement; educate the patient and family regarding potential complications such as bleeding if sharp débridement is the prescribed procedure. Barriers to communication should be addressed appropriately before explaining the procedure (e.g., cultural, language, age, level of understanding) *Rationale:* Explanation decreases patient anxiety and comfort and informs the patient.

- Discuss the patient's role during the procedure. *Rationale:* Patient cooperation is elicited.

PATIENT ASSESSMENT AND PREPARATION

Patient Assessment

- Vascular assessment should be completed before débridement. *Rationale:* Poor perfusion may result in extension of the wound after débridement.
- Assess tissues or underlying structures before sharp débridement. *Rationale:* Sharp débridement is contraindicated if underlying structures such as muscle, bone, tendon, and blood vessels may be exposed.
- Assess for signs and symptoms of local and systemic infection. *Rationale:* Débridement may seed bacteria into the systemic circulation; appropriate antibiotics should be considered before débridement in at-risk patient populations.[24] Surgical débridement, the most aggressive type of débridement, is the method of choice when signs of severe cellulitis or sepsis are present.
- Ensure that coagulation parameters are within normal limits. *Rationale:* Coagulation abnormalities may result in unwanted bleeding complications from the débridement process.
- Assess the patient for pain or anxiety, and consider premedication. *Rationale:* Medication decreases patient discomfort. Patients with neuropathy may still experience significant preprocedural anxiety.
- Assess and document wound length × width × depth in centimeters (cm). *Rationale:* This provides objective data to evaluate the wound healing trajectory.

Patient Preparation

- Ensure that the patient understands the preprocedural teaching. Answer questions as they arise, and reinforce information as needed. Fully review known risks, benefits, and alternatives. *Rationale:* Understanding of previously taught information is evaluated and reinforced.
- Verify the correct patient with two identifiers. *Rationale:* Before performing a procedure, ensure the correct identification of the patient for the intended intervention.
- Obtain informed consent for surgical and sharp débridement.[3,25] *Rationale:* Informed consent ensures patient knowledge of the procedure.
- Before the procedure, comply with universal protocol requirements.[25] Ensure that all relevant studies and documents, including informed consent, are available. Ensure that site markings have been made where appropriate. Before surgical or sharp débridement, perform a preprocedure verification and time out, if nonemergent. *Rationale:* This ensures patient safety.
- Premedicate the patient with the prescribed analgesia and/or sedation, if needed. Assess the patient's response to the analgesic before beginning the procedure. Reassess the patient's need for additional analgesic agents throughout the débridement procedure. Consider topical lidocaine. This will not be effective in the face of infection and should not be used on burns. *Rationale:* Patient anxiety and discomfort are decreased. Pain results in vasoconstriction of the cutaneous tissues from the increase in adrenergic activity. Adequate pain control improves tissue perfusion and results in improved healing.[7]
- Place the patient in a position of optimal comfort and visualization for dressing the wound. Keep the patient warm while the wound is exposed. *Rationale:* Positioning provides for effective wound visualization and enhances patient tolerance of the procedure. Keeping the patient warm prevents vasoconstriction that impairs wound healing.[23]
- Optimize lighting in the room, and provide privacy for the patient. *Rationale:* This facilitates visualization.

UNIT VII

Procedure	for Débridement: Pressure Ulcers, Burns, and Wounds	
Steps	Rationale	Special Considerations
Sharp débridement	Provides a fast and effective means of selective removal of devitalized tissue; should be performed by a qualified healthcare professional.	
1. Premedicate the patient for pain.	Systemic analgesic may be administered before and throughout the procedure as needed for patient tolerance and compliance.	Assess patient response to analgesia.
2. 🄷🄷		
3. 🄿🄴	Reduces transmission of microorganisms; standard precautions.	

Procedure continues on following page

Procedure for Débridement: Pressure Ulcers, Burns, and Wounds—*Continued*

Steps	Rationale	Special Considerations
4. Prepare the sterile drape and field of instruments, NS solution, gauze, and secondary dressing.	Maintains aseptic technique.	Gauze may be needed to provide hemostasis during the procedure.
5. Discard nonsterile gloves, **HH** and apply sterile gloves.		
6. With forceps, lift eschar and gently cut with a sterile scalpel or scissors. Débride tissue to the line of demarcation of healthy tissue.	The goal of sharp débridement is removal of devitalized tissue without damage to the healthy wound bed.	Pain and bleeding are signs of healthy tissue. Discontinue the procedure if pain or bleeding is excessive or if there is impending bone, tendon, or proximity to the fascial plane.[15]
7. Lavage the wound bed with NS solution.	Allows for removal of loose devitalized tissue and debris and reassessment of the wound bed.	
8. Apply a moist wound dressing of choice.	Promotes wound healing.	Assess for hemostasis before application of the dressing.
9. Discard used supplies in appropriate receptacles.		
10. **HH**		
Chemical débridement	Selective débridement technique.	Requires a prescription for the desired enzyme preparation.
1. Premedicate the patient for pain.	Systemic analgesic may be administered before and throughout the procedure as needed for patient tolerance and compliance.	Assess patient response to analgesia.
2. Perform hand hygiene, apply nonsterile gloves, and cleanse the wound.	Maintains aseptic technique.	
3. Discard gloves, perform hand hygiene, and apply a new pair of nonsterile gloves.	Maintains clean technique.	
4. If wound eschar is hard and dry, a No. 10 scalpel may be used to cross-hatch necrotic tissue. **(Level C*)**	A cross-hatching technique may allow better penetration of the enzymatic agent and enhance enzyme activity.[15]	
5. Discard gloves, perform hand hygiene, and apply nonsterile gloves.	Maintains aseptic technique.	
6. Establish a sterile field with an enzymatic agent, NS solution, and a secondary moist healing dressing.	Maintains aseptic technique.	
7. Apply the enzymatic agent with a tongue blade to the eschar in the wound bed, concentrating the enzymatic agent over the nonviable tissue.	Assists with even application of the enzymatic agent over the necrotic wound tissue.	
8. Place a moisture-retentive dressing (typically, gauze moistened with NS solution) over the wound.	Most enzymatic agents require a moist dressing to be applied over the agent for effective action.	Other dressings that promote moist wound healing may be used.
9. Secure a secondary dressing in place.	A secondary dressing is needed to absorb wound exudates.[17]	Assess the perimeter of the wound for irritation and breakdown from moisture. Consider application of a liquid skin barrier to the perimeter edge.

*Level C: Qualitative studies, descriptive or correlational studies, integrative reviews, systematic reviews, or randomized controlled trials with inconsistent results.

Procedure	for Débridement: Pressure Ulcers, Burns, and Wounds—*Continued*		
Steps	**Rationale**	**Special Considerations**

Steps	Rationale	Special Considerations
10. Discard used supplies in appropriate receptacles.		
11. **HH**		
Mechanical débridement: wet-to-dry gauze dressing	Nonselective débridement technique.	Nonviable and viable tissue may be lost with this method of débridement.
1. Assess patient response to analgesia.		
2. Perform hand hygiene, and apply clean gloves.	Maintains clean technique.	
3. Establish a sterile field: gauze dressing moistened with NS solution.	Maintains aseptic technique.	
4. Cleanse the wound.	Wound cleansing is a means of mechanical débridement; also removes nonadherent bacteria.	Remove any gauze particles left in the wound bed with gentle irrigation.
5. Wash hands, and apply nonsterile gloves.	Maintains aseptic technique.	
6. Place moistened gauze loosely into the wound bed.	Excessive packing of gauze into the wound bed may compromise perfusion.[21]	If more than one gauze dressing is used, place the ends of two dressings close to each other for easy removal, or consider using rolled gauze.
7. Cover the wound with a secondary absorptive dressing, and secure it.	Protects the wound from external contamination and absorbs exudates.	Consider changing the dressing if ≥75% area of the secondary dressing is saturated with wound drainage. Assess the wound perimeter for maceration; consider using a liquid skin barrier or hydrocolloid to protect the skin. A zinc oxide cream is useful to protect the wound perimeter. Apply a thin layer with each dressing change.
8. Discard gloves, and perform hand hygiene.		
9. After the prescribed time interval, wash hands, apply nonsterile gloves, and remove the dressing to create the mechanical débridement action.	The drying action of the gauze adheres it to the necrotic tissue, which is detached with the dressing removal.	If the dressing is dry and adherent to viable tissue, lightly moisten the gauze to prevent excessive débridement of viable tissue and to minimize pain.[3,23]
10. Apply the wound dressing as prescribed.	Protects the wound.	
11. Discard used supplies in appropriate receptacles.		
12. **HH**		
Autolytic débridement	Autolytic dressings should be used with caution if the wound bed has bacterial colonization and/or extensive necrotic tissue. This may lead to cellulitis and/or a systemic infectious process.	May not be effective for large wound surfaces. Can take several weeks to complete. Often used in conjunction with other methods of débridement.
1. Perform hand hygiene, and apply nonsterile gloves.		

Procedure continues on following page

UNIT VII

Procedure for Débridement: Pressure Ulcers, Burns, and Wounds—*Continued*

Steps	Rationale	Special Considerations
2. Cleanse the wound bed with NS solution or water.	Wound cleansing is a means of mechanical débridement; it also removes nonadherent bacteria.	
3. Apply a moisture-retentive dressing.	Provides a moist wound healing environment that enhances the autolytic débridement process.	Assess the dressing for absorptive properties. Consider changing the dressing if the area of the secondary dressing is ≥75% saturated with wound drainage.
4. Apply a secondary dressing as indicated.	Autolytic débridement results in production of wound exudates. Apply a secondary dressing to absorb exudate away from the wound bed.	
5. Discard used supplies in appropriate receptacles.		
6. **HH**		

*Level C: Qualitative studies, descriptive or correlational studies, integrative reviews, systematic reviews, or randomized controlled trials with inconsistent results.

Expected Outcomes

- Wound bed is free from necrotic tissue and debris
- Inflammatory progressing to proliferation stage of wound healing is reestablished, and wound healing progresses along a normal trajectory
- Wound is free from infection or signs of compromised perfusion
- Wound hemostasis is established after sharp débridement

Unexpected Outcomes

- Depth and width of wound extends, and necrotic tissue recurs
- Normal wound healing process is not reestablished by removal of devitalized tissue, and wound healing fails to progress[3,7]
- Bacterial infection is present; signs of local or systemic infection are present
- Excessive bleeding from lack of wound hemostasis

Patient Monitoring and Care

Steps	Rationale	Reportable Conditions
		These conditions should be reported to the provider if they persist despite nursing interventions.
1. Assess the patient, wound bed, and surrounding skin for signs of infection. (**Level D***)	Wound débridement may not effectively remove all bacteria; continued assessment for wound infection is essential for healing.[21,26]	• Erythema and warmth at the wound site • Pain and tenderness • Edema • Change in wound drainage amount, color, odor, or consistency • New fever • Elevated white blood cell count
2. Monitor the dressing for signs of bleeding.	Wound débridement may disturb newly formed, fragile blood vessels and established blood vessels and cause bleeding.	• Bleeding that does not stop with mild pressure to the wound bed • Excessive bleeding
3. Assess the wound for signs of healing after débridement. (**Level D***)	The goal of necrotic tissue débridement is to establish wound healing in the form of granulation tissue and wound contracture.[3,21,26]	• Discoloration of the wound bed noted (i.e., ecchymosis, ischemia) • Development of necrotic tissue in the wound bed • Changed, diminished, or absent pulses distal to the wound bed
4. Follow institutional standards for assessing pain. Administer analgesia as prescribed.	Identifies the need for pain interventions.	• Continued pain despite pain interventions

*Level D: Peer-reviewed professional and organizational standards with the support of clinical study recommendations.

Documentation

Documentation should include the following:

- Patient and family education
- Description of the wound bed before and after débridement
- Description of the wound perimeter skin assessment (e.g., color, maceration, integrity, evidence of infection)
- Size of the wound after the wound débridement procedure (document the length × width × depth in centimeters)
- Description of the dressing applied to the wound bed (primary and secondary dressings as appropriate) and count of gauze dressings left in the wound bed to prevent retained foreign bodies
- Pain assessment, interventions, and effectiveness
- Premedication given, patient tolerance of the procedure, and response to pain medication
- Description of the wound débridement process and any unexpected complications
- Vascular assessment
- Description of established wound hemostasis obtained at completion of the procedure
- Digital photography as approved by the institution is recommended to document the progression of wound healing
- Obtain patient consent per institutional standards

References and Additional Readings

For a complete list of references and additional readings for this procedure, scan this QR code with your smartphone, or visit https://www.elsevier.com/__data/assets/pdf_file/0006/1319892/Chapter0117.pdf.

UNIT VII

118 Negative-Pressure Wound Therapy

Sonia Astle

PURPOSE The purpose of negative-pressure wound therapy (NPWT) is to apply controlled subatmospheric (negative) pressure to the wound bed for stimulation of granulation tissue and edema reduction in order to enhance wound healing. Negative-pressure wound therapy has been available for over 20 years; there are many choices and possibilities for the use of NPWT for different indications.[3,4,8,10,12,14,19,29]

PREREQUISITE NURSING KNOWLEDGE

Negative-pressure wound therapy (NPWT) is an advanced wound care therapy that uses a wound filler dressing, a transparent device-specific semiocclusive or occlusive dressing, tubing, and a powered vacuum unit with a collection canister.[13] There is a growing body of evidence using NPWT with instillation and dwell time (NPWTi-d) to help with cleansing and removal of exudate to lessen the bacterial load in the wound.[9,11,13,16] During NPWTi-d, a topical solution such as normal saline or an antiseptic solution is instilled into the wound.[13] Solution dwell times range anywhere from less than 1 minute to 30 minutes.[13] Guidelines for application settings, wound characteristics, and various dressing types have recently been updated by an international multidisciplinary expert panel of clinicians.[13]

Additionally, the use of closed incision NPWT (ciN-PWT) has been extended to include closed surgical incisions to prevent surgical site infections, particularly for colorectal, cardiothoracic, and orthopedic surgery. Commercially available ciNPWT management systems include the VAC (KCI), PREVENTA (KCI), and PICO (Smith and Nephew).[17,23,28] Advantages of ciNPWT include protecting the incision from external contamination and its ability to decrease tension on the wound bed while increasing cutaneous blood perfusion to the site.[17] However, there is controversy with using prophylactic ciNPWT versus standard wound dressings.[2,27]

Other terms found in the literature for NPWT include topical negative pressure, vacuum-assisted closure (VAC), and subatmospheric pressure therapy.

- Many different U.S. Food and Drug Administration (FDA)–approved vacuum units are on the market for NPWT.[5,15,18,21] Common devices seen in the acute-care practice setting are the ActiV.A.C. and InfoV.A.C. Therapy Systems (KCI; Fig. 118.1). ActiV.A.C. and Info V.A.C.[24] use a patented open-cell foam wound contact dressing, and other units on the market use either an open-cell foam or the vacuum-pack method with an antimicrobial gauze packing dressing. The use of a moistened gauze

wound interface has also been reported in the literature as an effective dressing for NPWT.[1,6]

- Most randomized controlled studies and case studies on NPWT have been conducted with the VAC therapy. A few small, randomized controlled trials have compared alternate NPWT systems to the VAC therapy and found them to be comparable.[26] Further clinical research to evaluate wound closure outcomes with the different NPWT units is needed.[20]

- NPWT assists with wound closure by applying a controlled subatmospheric pressure evenly over the wound bed. This mechanical stress creates a noncompressive force on the wound bed that dilates the arterioles, increasing the effectiveness of local circulation and enhancing the proliferation of granulation tissue.[13,14,17] NPWT enhances lymphatic flow and removal of excessive fluid, decreasing wound edema and bacterial load at the wound site, further aiding wound healing (Fig. 118.2).[8,13,14,17]

- Wound healing is best achieved through adequate cleansing, irrigation, débridement, and dressing of the wound bed on the basis of patient and wound characteristics.[9,12,13]

- Wounds heal by either primary or secondary intention. Most clean surgical wounds heal by primary intention. Suturing each layer of tissue approximates the wound edges. These wounds typically heal quickly and require minimal wound care. Contaminated surgical or traumatic wounds (open wounds) heal by secondary intention. Wounds that heal by secondary intention granulate from the base of the wound to the skin surfaces; care must be taken to allow for uniform granulation and prevention of open pockets or tunneling.

- Openly granulating wounds heal more slowly and must remain moist to enhance tissue granulation. Wound care for these wounds focuses on maintaining a moist environment free from necrotic tissue.

- Open wounds may have excessive wound drainage that necessitates application of absorptive dressings, protection of periwound skin, and more frequent dressing changes to facilitate healing. NPWT provides wound drainage management and decreases the frequency of dressing changes with improved pain management.

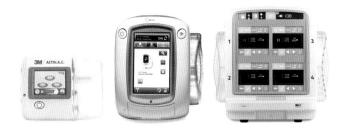

Figure 118.1 Components of the 3M NPWT Systems: 3M™ ActiV.A.C.™ Therapy System, 3M™ V.A.C.® Ulta Therapy System, 3M™ V.A.C.® Rx4 Therapy System, 3M™ V.A.C. Dermatac™ Drape and 3M™ V.A.C. ® Granufoam Dressing, V.A.C.® Granufoam™ Dressing Kit, and 3M™ V.A.C. Whitefoam™ Dressing. *(Courtesy of 3M. © 2022, 3M. All rights reserved.)*

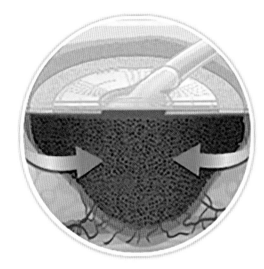

Figure 118.2 V.A.C.® Therapy System illustration. *(Courtesy of 3M. © 2022, 3M. All rights reserved.)*

- Goals of NPWT in wound management may include wound bed preparation for skin grafts, full wound closure, decrease in wound size, removal of wound edema for delayed primary closure, and increased perfusion to marginally viable flaps.[9,13] The effectiveness of NPWT should be evaluated with each dressing change to include a comprehensive wound assessment and weekly wound measurements. If wound measurements have not improved at least 15% after 2 weeks of therapy, reevaluate the continuation of NPWT with reassessment of wound healing variables.[24]
- Wounds with infections should undergo systemic antibiotic treatment before initiation of NPWT. If continued deterioration of the wound or infection persists, consider discontinuation of NPWT with possible evaluation for surgical drainage of the wound per the physician, advanced practice nurse, or other healthcare professional.
- Wounds treated with NPWT develop a characteristic, beefy red granulation bed. A pale wound bed or friable granulation

tissue is a secondary sign of infection and may be more reliable than the traditional indicators of infection.[25]
- Dehisced infected sternal wounds with use of NPWT require effective débridement of infected bone and a specific nonadherent wound contact layer before a NPWT dressing is placed.[7]
- Successful management of enteric fistulae with NPWT with use of special application techniques has been reported in case studies, but there are no clinical trials at this time. See NPWT device manuals for specific techniques in the management of fistulae.
- Rapid formation of granulation tissue with NPWT can lead to the development of abscesses. The surgically dehisced wound with NPWT should be monitored closely for abscess formation, particularly in patients with large irregular wounds with undermining present.
- The provider may perform a transcutaneous oxygen pressure ($TcpO_2$) evaluation before initiation of NPWT to lower extremity or toe wounds because of vascular flow requirements that are needed for optimal wound healing with NPWT.
- Contraindications to the use of NPWT include malignancy disease in the wound, untreated osteomyelitis, non-enteric and unexplored fistulae, and necrotic tissue with eschar present.[7,24] See the manufacturer's recommendations in the NPWT manual for special precautions required with exposed blood vessels, organs, tendons, and nerves.[14] Precautions should be used for wounds with active bleeding, for difficult wound hemostasis, and for patients undergoing anticoagulation therapy.[8,14] For significant bleeding, NPWT should be discontinued immediately, and direct pressure should be applied to the bleeding site. Consult the treating provider or emergency services.
- For optimal NPWT with the VAC device, at least 22 hours of daily uninterrupted therapy should be delivered.[24] With the newer vacuum units, there is limited evidence for the required time duration of uninterrupted therapy for wound healing. NPWT dressings are usually changed every 48 to 120 hours (2 to 5 days) depending on the clinical situation.[8,24] However, infected wound beds may require more frequent dressing changes (every 12 hours), and dressings over grafts may be changed less frequently (every 3 to 7 days).[1,8,24] The wound bed should be free from necrotic tissue and debris before application of the NPWT dressing.[14]
- In highly exudative wounds, drainage from the wound bed may be significant in the first 24 to 48 hours of therapy. Additional fluids may need to be provided for individuals with heavily draining wounds.
- Nutritional requirements for wound healing are great. These needs must be assessed, met, and monitored frequently because poor nutrition can impede successful NPWT wound healing.
- NPWT units offer home machines with increased portability. Smaller size and increased battery life allow for continuation of therapy outside of the acute hospital setting.

UNIT VII

EQUIPMENT

The following is generic equipment used for most NPWT units. Device- and wound-specific variations may need to be considered by the physician, advanced practice nurse, or other healthcare professional.

- Sterile and nonsterile gloves, gown (per institutional policy)
- Normal saline or wound cleanser with appropriate psi delivery device (see Procedure 116)
- Protective barrier film/wipe for periwound protection
- NPWT dressing with tubing/transparent drape kit (device specific)
- NPWT vacuum unit/collection chamber (device specific)
- Sterile scissors

PATIENT AND FAMILY EDUCATION

- Assess patient and family readiness to learn and any factors that may affect learning. Identification of the patient's preferred learning strategies (auditory, visualization, return demonstration) is also important. **Rationale:** The nurse can develop the most appropriate teaching strategy for each patient.
- Provide information about NPWT, the procedure, anticipated duration of therapy, and the equipment. **Rationale:** Information may decrease or alleviate anxiety by assisting patient and family to understand the procedure, why it is needed, and the preferred outcomes.
- Explain the procedure and the reason for changing the wound dressing. **Rationale:** This may decrease patient anxiety.
- Discuss the patient's role during the dressing change procedure and in maintaining the NPWT system. **Rationale:** Patient cooperation is elicited; the patient is prepared for wound management on discharge.

PATIENT ASSESSMENT AND PREPARATION

Patient Assessment

- Fully assess the wound with documentation of wound measurements, characteristics, and appropriateness for the procedure. **Rationale:** Assessment ensures that use of NPWT is not contraindicated. Data are provided for comparison at successive dressing changes.
- Assess for signs and symptoms of wound infection, including the following.[14] **Rationale:** Although NPWT assists

with removal of excessive fluid, thus reducing the potential of bacteria in the wound bed, assessment for signs and symptoms of wound infection is necessary, especially in patients with compromised conditions.
- Periwound erythema
- Increased periwound warmth
- Wound edema
- Increased pain associated with the wound
- Increased odor and amount of wound exudate
- Elevated temperature, white blood cell count, or chills
- Determine baseline pain assessment. **Rationale:** Data are provided for comparison with post-procedure assessment data. The nurse can plan for preprocedure and intraprocedure analgesia.
- Determine baseline nutritional and fluid volume status. **Rationale:** Adequate fluids and protein are necessary for optimal wound healing with NPWT.
- Assess medical history, especially related to bleeding problems, fistula formation, malignant disease, or vascular status. **Rationale:** NPWT may be contraindicated in these conditions.
- Assess current medications specifically related to anticoagulant use. **Rationale:** Possible areas of caution that should be monitored with NPWT use are identified.
- Assess current laboratory values, especially coagulation studies. **Rationale:** Abnormalities possibly associated with risks related to NPWT use are identified.

Patient Preparation

- Verify the correct patient with two identifiers. **Rationale:** Before performing a procedure, the nurse should ensure the correct identification of the patient for the intended intervention.
- Ensure patient and family understanding of the procedure. Reinforce teaching points as needed. **Rationale:** Understanding of previously taught information is evaluated, and a conduit for questions is provided.
- Validate the presence of patent intravenous access. **Rationale:** Access may be needed for administration of intravenous analgesic medications and fluid administration.
- Position the patient in a manner that will ensure patient comfort and privacy and facilitate dressing application. **Rationale:** This prepares the patient to undergo the procedure.
- Administer prescribed analgesics if needed. **Rationale:** Analgesics improve comfort level and tolerance of the procedure and decrease patient anxiety and discomfort.

Procedure for Negative-Pressure Wound Therapy

Steps	Rationale	Special Considerations
Procedure for KCI VAC Therapy for Wounds; VAC Application		
1. Obtain and prepare equipment.	Prepares for the procedure.	General principles of NPWT are consistent across devices; however, wound-specific and device-specific guidelines must be reviewed before NPWT. **Steps 1–8** are generic to all NPWT applications. This procedure uses clean technique; however, sterile technique may be desired per wound characteristics or clinician preference.[24]
2. HH		
3. PE		
4. Prepare a clean field for the dressing change, and remove gloves. Repeat HH and PE.	Prevents contamination of supplies and materials.	
5. Position the patient to facilitate wound cleansing with dressing application.	Provides for patient comfort and allows for visualization and access to the wound.	
6. Assess and measure the wound, and assemble supplies as indicated.[6,8,10] **(Level D*)**	Select the NPWT dressing type with appropriate size approximating the wound size. Multiple types of VAC-specialty size dressings are available (refer to the manufacturer's manual). VAC-specific dressings: A. Black polyurethane foam (GranuFoam) has larger pores and is considered to be more effective in stimulating granulation tissue formation and wound contraction. It is the most frequently used. B. White polyvinyl chloride foam (WhiteFoam) is denser, is premoistened, and has increased tensile strength. Because of its higher density, it requires higher pressure to obtain the same granulation rate as black foam. C. Black polyurethane foam, GranuFoam Silver, has antimicrobial silver and may reduce wound infections.[7,24]	The black VAC dressing does not hold moisture but allows exudates to pass through the dressing and be removed. Its design results in rapid growth of new granulation. The white VAC dressing holds moisture but also allows exudate to be removed through it. It is nonadherent and can be used in tunnels and shallow undermining because of its higher tensile strength. Additional precautions must be taken when using GranuFoam Silver. Refer to the specific product instructions when using GranuFoam Silver. It should not be used as a replacement for systemic therapy for infection.[6]
7. Cleanse the wound according to orders (see Procedure 116, Cleansing, Irrigating, Culturing, and Dressing an Open Wound) or institutional protocol.[25]	Wound bed cleansing and irrigation prepare the wound bed for application of the dressing.[12]	
8. The physician, advanced practice nurse, or other healthcare professional may débride (see Procedure 117, Debridement: Pressure Ulcers, Burns, and Wounds) necrotic tissue or eschar if applicable.	NPWT assists with autolytic and mechanical débridement of surface slough; it should not be used as a primary means of débridement. Sharp débridement of necrotic tissue should be performed before initiation of therapy for optimal healing with NPWT.[12]	If extensive débridement is needed, surgical débridement in the operative suite may be necessary.

*Level D: Peer-reviewed professional and organizational standards with the support of clinical study recommendations.

UNIT VII

Procedure continues on following page

Procedure   for Negative-Pressure Wound Therapy—*Continued*

Steps	Rationale	Special Considerations
9. Prepare the periwound by cleansing with warm solution. Clip the hair around the wound. Dry the skin, and prepare the periwound tissue with a barrier protective film.[24] **(Level D*)**	Moisture from perspiration, oil, or body fluids may interfere with the drape's adherence. Barrier films act as a protectant against periwound maceration.	Multiple removals of transparent drape may irritate hair follicles and result in folliculitis.
10. Remove gloves.		
11. 🄷🄷		
12. Apply nonsterile gloves.		
13. Open an intact package, and cut the VAC foam with sterile scissors; do not cut the foam directly over the wound.[24] **(Level E*)**	Prevents small particles of dressing from falling into the wound. The dressing should be cut to fit the size and shape of the wound, including tunnels and undermined areas. Tunneling can result in a cyst or abscess when vacuum pressure or granulation closes the entrance to the tunnel. Bacterial invasion and impaired healing result from unfilled dead space.[24]	Any exposed sutures, tendons, ligaments, or nerves should be protected with placement of a layer of nonadherent dressing over them.[14] Foam dressings should not be placed in direct contact with exposed blood vessels, anastomotic sites, organs, or nerves.[14] Any exposed vessels or organs in or near the wound must be fully protected before NPWT is applied.[24] See the manufacturer's recommendations in the NPWT manual for special precautions required.
14. Gently place the foam into the wound, ensuring contact with all wound surfaces. Do not allow the foam to overlap onto intact skin. Do not force the foam dressing into any area of the wound. Always note the total number of foam pieces used with notation on the transparent drape and in the patient's chart.[14] **(Level E*)**	Capillaries can be compressed if dressings are packed too tightly, and pressure on newly formed granulation tissue may prevent or delay healing.[14] Foam that is placed directly on intact skin may cause skin breakdown.	More than one dressing may be used to fill the wound bed. Foam pieces should be in contact with, but not overlapping each other to allow equalization of negative pressure applied to the wound bed by the suction device.[2,24] For small wounds, a larger piece of foam may need to be placed on top of the wound filler foam to provide an adequate surface for the Therapeutic Regulated Accurate Care T.R.A.C. Pad. Protect intact periwound skin with skin prep and drape under the foam.[24]
15. Trim and place the VAC transparent drape to cover the foam dressing and an additional 3–5 cm of intact periwound skin. Avoid stretching the drape over the wound.[24] **(Level M*)**	Avoids tension and shearing forces on the surrounding tissue.	Bridging of wounds can be done for more than one wound of similar pathology in close proximity with one vacuum pump. See manufacturer-specific instructions.

*Level D: Peer-reviewed professional and organizational standards with the support of clinical study recommendations.

*Level E: Multiple case reports, theory-based evidence from expert opinions, or peer-reviewed professional organizational standards without clinical studies to support recommendations.

*Level M: Manufacturer's recommendations only.

Procedure for Negative-Pressure Wound Therapy—*Continued*

Steps	Rationale	Special Considerations
16. Cut a 2.5-cm hole in the transparent drape for fluid to pass through. Cut a hole rather than a slit because a slit may self-seal during therapy. Apply the T.R.A.C. pad with tubing directly over the hole in the transparent drape. Apply gentle pressure around the pad to ensure complete adhesion.[24] **(Level M*)**	The vacuum does not function without an occlusive seal. The drape may also help maintain a moist wound environment. The drape is vapor-permeable and allows for gas exchange. It also protects the wound from external contamination.	The foam contracts into the wound bed if seal is obtained. If foam does not contract, reassess the outer dressing for possible leaks in the system or dressing seal.[2,10]
17. Ensure that the position of the T.R.A.C. tubing is not over bony prominences.[10,24] **(Level E*)**	Minimizes the risk of pressure related to tubing placement.	Extra foams with drape can be used under the tubing to reduce pressure and stabilize the tubing.
18. Remove the VAC canister from the packaging, and insert it into the vacuum unit. Connect the T.R.A.C. pad tubing to the canister tubing, and ensure that the clamps are open.	Closed clamps prevent activation of the negative therapy.	
19. Turn the power on to the vacuum unit, and select the prescribed therapy setting. Assess the dressing to ensure seal integrity. The dressing should collapse with a wrinkled appearance and no hissing sounds.[24] **(Level M*)**	Setting options include continuous or intermittent negative-pressure therapy. The settings are determined by type of wound, exudate, and goals as ordered by the provider (Table 118.1).	If the dressing does not collapse, check the tubing and transparent drape for leaks. Use an additional drape to seal leaks as necessary.
20. Discard used supplies; remove gloves.		
21. 🅷🅷		
VAC Dressing Removal Procedure		
1. Provide analgesia as appropriate for the patient's condition before the procedure.	Patients may experience discomfort during dressing changes or removal.[24]	

*Level M: Manufacturer's recommendations only.
*Level E: Multiple case reports, theory-based evidence from expert opinions, or peer-reviewed professional organizational standards without clinical studies to support recommendations.

TABLE 118.1   Recommended Therapy Setting for KCI VAC Therapy

Wound Characteristics	Continuous Therapy	Intermittent Therapy
Difficult dressing application	X	
Flap	X	
Highly exuding	X	
Grafts	X	
Painful wounds	X	
Tunnels or undermining	X	
Unstable structures	X	
Minimally exuding	X	X
Large wounds	X	X
Small wounds	X	X
Stalled wound-healing progress	X	X
VAC white foam dressing	X	X

A responsible provider should be consulted for individual patient conditions. Consult the device user manual and manufacturer's recommended guidelines before use.
Adapted from 2014 V.A.C. Therapy Clinical Guidelines, page 20, Table 1-1: Recommended Therapy Settings. Used with permission. Courtesy KCI, an Acelity Company.

UNIT VII

Procedure for Negative-Pressure Wound Therapy—*Continued*

Steps	Rationale	Special Considerations
2. **HH**		
3. **PE**		
4. To remove the dressing, raise the tubing connector above the level of the vacuum unit, and tighten the clamps on the dressing tubing. Disconnect the two tubings at the connection point.	Removes any remaining fluid from the tubing for purposes of infection control, thus preventing leakage.	
5. Allow the vacuum unit to pull the exudate through the canister tubing into the canister, and then tighten the clamp on the canister tube. Turn off the vacuum unit. Remove the canister from the vacuum unit, and discard.	Allows exudate to be contained; the canister should be discarded per institutional policy.	
6. Allow foam to decompress. Gently stretch the transparent drape horizontally to release adhesive from the skin. Do not peel vertically. Gently remove the foam dressing from the wound.[24] **(Level M*)**	Decreases patient discomfort and potential for skin and wound trauma.	
7. Discard used supplies; remove gloves.		
8. **HH**		

*Level M: Manufacturer's recommendations only.

Expected Outcomes

- Wound healing or granulation is enhanced by consistent negative-pressure therapy; early signs of contraction of wound margins
- Decreased volume of wound exudate (over time) and absence of foul odor or color
- Enhanced wound healing because of effective wound fluid or edema removal
- Decrease in the size of the wound with ability for surgical closure with flap/graft or skin graft; complete healing of the wound
- Decreased time to satisfactory healing (may decrease hospital length of stay and cost)

Unexpected Outcomes

- Infection
- Bleeding
- Fistula formation
- Disruption of underlying tissue or structures
- Pain
- Misplacement over exposed vessel, ligaments, other structures
- Lack of improvement in wound after 1 to 2 weeks of therapy
- Tissue loss
- Ischemia and necrosis
- Periwound maceration

Patient Monitoring and Care

Steps	Rationale	Reportable Conditions
		These conditions should be reported to the provider if they persist despite nursing interventions.
1. Assess the location of the VAC T.R.A.C. tubing to avoid excessive pressure on surrounding tissue or structures.	Excessive pressure may result in tissue breakdown from tubing over bony prominences.	- Tissue breakdown

Patient Monitoring and Care *—Continued*		
Steps	**Rationale**	**Reportable Conditions**
2. Assess the patency of the VAC system: drape has an occlusive seal, tubing is patent, and foam is compressed.	The VAC dressing should be collapsed when the seal is maintained and negative pressure is being delivered in a consistent manner. Alarms on the device indicate loss of seal; raised foam dressing indicates loss of negative-pressure therapy. See the manufacturer's clinical guidelines for troubleshooting difficulties with NPWT dressings.	• Loss of seal • Raised foam dressing • Wound drainage suddenly decreasing in amount or stopping • If therapy is interrupted for more than 2 hours, the entire VAC dressing should be removed and a wet-to-dry dressing applied (notify the provider before removing a VAC dressing).
3. Assess the amount and type of drainage.	Color of drainage can suggest bleeding, and the rate of canister filling can alert the caregiver to wound problems.	• Bright red blood or rapid filling of the canister
4. Monitor condition of the wound bed and periwound skin with dressing changes; observe for signs of wound infection.	Identifies any evidence of wound healing or any changes or abnormalities indicative of complications.	• Periwound erythema • Heat, edema, pain • Elevated temperature and white blood cell count • Cloudy or foul-smelling wound drainage • Increased wound drainage • Excess bleeding • Changes in tissue color within the wound bed • Macerated, broken, or discolored periwound skin • New tunneling or undermining • Stool in the wound bed • Signs or symptoms of infection
5. Change the dressing every 24-72 hours or as prescribed. If the wound is infected, the frequency of dressing changes should be increased per order.[22] **(Level D*)**	Removes exudate from the wound bed. If the dressing adheres to the wound base, consider interfacing a single layer of nonadherent porous material (e.g., meshed silicone, meshed petroleum-impregnated dressings, and meshed oil-emulsion–impregnated dressings),[24] also known as a *contact layer,* between the dressing and the wound when reapplying the dressing. If previous dressings were difficult to remove and painful, consider instillation of a topical anesthetic agent such as 1% lidocaine without epinephrine into the tubing or dressing ordered by the provider.[6]	
6. Monitor the mode (continuous or intermittent) and level of suction.[5] **(Level E*)**	Removal of edema and debris alleviates compressive forces, thus improving perfusion. Suctioning fluid from within the wound may remove wound fluid factors that inhibit healing.[7] Application and release of negative pressure on the wound bed stimulates cell proliferation and protein synthesis.[7] Mechanical stretch on the tissue by negative pressure draws the wound toward the center, closing the defect.[24]	• Patient discomfort • Excess granulation tissue overgrowth into the dressing with removal • Continued edema within the wound bed

*Level D: Peer-reviewed professional and organizational standards with the support of clinical study recommendations.

*Level E: Multiple case reports, theory-based evidence from expert opinions, or peer-reviewed professional organizational standards without clinical studies to support recommendations.

UNIT VII

Procedure continues on following page

Patient Monitoring and Care —*Continued*

Steps	Rationale	Reportable Conditions
7. Maintain an airtight seal[24] **(Level E*)**	Loss of an airtight seal can result in a decreased amount of drainage removal and desiccation of the wound.[24] Refer to the manufacturer's clinical guidelines for troubleshooting difficulties with maintaining a seal.	• Problems maintaining an airtight seal
8. Label the dressing with the date and time of application and amount of foam pieces placed in the wound.	VAC foam dressings are not bioabsorbable. Ensure that all pieces of foam are removed from the wound with each dressing change.	• Foam left in the wound for greater than the recommended period may foster ingrowth of tissue into the foam and create difficulty in removal of foam pieces from the wound or lead to infection.[12,14,24]
9. Change the canister when full, or at least weekly. Keep the canister position level.	Controls odor.	• Increased drainage amounts
10. Monitor the amount of wound drainage.[14] **(Level D*)**	If a wound produces excessive fluid, the patient may experience fluid imbalance, which will require oral or intravenous replacement. Excess drainage may also result in increased protein loss. A nutritional consultation to replace protein loss from wound exudates may be indicated.	• Increased drainage amounts • Wound drainage that is foul-smelling and cloudy
11. Follow institutional standards for assessing pain. Administer analgesia as prescribed. Pain can be associated with application of the dressing, initiation of initial therapy, intermittent cycling, or removal of the dressing.	Identifies the need for pain interventions. Use of analgesics at dressing changes can reduce the pain. The use of a wound contact layer may also decrease pain with dressing changes.[6,7] Additionally, lowering the initial amount of negative pressure or maintaining the pressure at continual versus intermittent levels can assist in pain control.[6,24] Some evidence has shown decreased pain with dressing changes when using gauze as a wound filler.[6,7] Pain during treatment may be alleviated through the use of the white foam rather than black foam.[24] See manufacturer-specific instructions.	• Continued pain despite pain interventions
1. See the manufacturer's guidelines for discharge considerations for patients with NPWT, and consult with the provider for assistance when discharging patients with NPWT.	Obtaining NPWT for home use can be complex, and there are important safety concerns.	

*Level D: Peer-reviewed professional and organizational standards with the support of clinical study recommendations.
*Level E: Multiple case reports, theory-based evidence from expert opinions, or peer-reviewed professional organizational standards without clinical studies to support recommendations.

UNIT VII

Documentation

Documentation should include the following:
- Patient and family education
- Patient tolerance of the procedure
- Condition of the wound bed and periwound skin description
- Characteristics of wound drainage
- Mode (continuous or intermittent) and degree (mm Hg) of suction
- Nursing interventions
- Pain medication given and patient's response to the pain medication
- Wound débridement procedure (if applicable); wound cleansing procedure completed, dated, and timed
- Size of the wound measured by length, width, and depth (consider obtaining a photograph of the wound, depending on institutional policy)
- Size and type of foam dressing applied, and total number of foam pieces placed in the wound
- Unexpected outcomes and reportable conditions

References and Additional Readings

For a complete list of references and additional readings for this procedure, scan this QR code with your smartphone, or visit https://www.elsevier.com/__data/assets/pdf_file/0007/1319893/Chapter0118.pdf

119 Wound Management With Excessive Drainage

Sonia Astle

PURPOSE Management of wound exudate is an essential step in wound healing. Pouching may be used to divert and contain excessive drainage. Suction may be used to remove drainage or used in conjunction with pouching. Drains may be placed in the wound for management of drainage.

PREREQUISITE NURSING KNOWLEDGE

- Wound exudate is produced in response to the inflammatory phase of the healing process. As wounds heal, the amount of exudate should diminish. Chronic, nonhealing wounds may produce exudate for prolonged periods, necessitating effective management of the fluid.[2,3,12,14,16,22,23]
- Goals of wound care must be clearly identified so proper wound care products are used.[1,3,16,19-24,26] Wound healing is best achieved through adequate cleansing, débridement, and dressing of the wound bed on the basis of wound characteristics.
- Excessive wound fluid may create pressure in the wound bed and compromise perfusion. Excessive moisture may cause periwound tissue damage and extend the wound or skin injury.[2,7,9,12,13,26]
- Assessment of wound exudate should include the quantity, color, consistency, and odor of drainage. When changes in wound exudate occur, the cause should be explored. These changes along with other clinical signs and symptoms (e.g., fever) may indicate a possible increase in bacterial burden or infection.
- Drains are placed in wounds to facilitate healing by providing a route for excessive fluid accumulating in or near the wound bed to escape. Most wound drains are surgically placed; drains may or may not be secured with sutures.[9]
- Excessive wound fluid may provide a source for proliferation of microorganisms. Wound drains may be ports of microorganism entry. Microorganisms in the wound bed continue the inflammatory phase of wound healing and delay wound resolution; aseptic technique must be strictly observed to reduce the risk of infection.[4]
- Pouching is an effective means of collecting wound and fistula drainage.[9] Suction may be used with pouching systems to pull fluid away from the wound bed.
- Excessive wound drainage is removed to allow for wound healing to occur without tissue congestion, microorganism proliferation, and skin maceration.[11]
- Excessive wound drainage may need to be calculated into the assessment of a patient's daily intake and output. At a minimum, it is necessary to note how often dressings or pads are being changed to track excessive exudate.

- Negative-pressure wound therapy (see Procedure 118, Negative-Pressure Wound Therapy) stimulates tissue growth and promotes wound healing. The closed system also provides active withdrawal of excessive wound fluid to assist in the management of exudating wounds.[4,7]
- Assess the patient's nutritional needs, specifically for protein along with consideration of micronutrients such as vitamins A, C, and D and trace elements such as copper, zinc, and selenium, with exudating wounds.[8]
- Excessive wound exudate production may result in the loss of up to 100 g of protein daily in wound exudate.[2,8] Nutritional supplementation of protein is necessary for wound healing.

DRESSING DETERMINATION

A wide variety of dressings are available for the clinician to use to manage exudate produced by wounds. Inappropriate dressing selection may exacerbate wound management.[4-6,15-17,22,23] Superabsorbent dressings are wound dressings are used for moderately to highly exuding wounds[24] and are designed to create an optimum moist wound bed.[4,10,11,13,21] These include the following:

- Alginates: absorbent wound care dressings containing sodium and calcium fibers derived from seaweed. The dressing forms into a gel when in contact with fluid.
- Foams: absorbent dressing containing a hydrophilic polyurethane or silicone foam. The dressing is designed for granulating wounds of various sizes and etiologies.
- Hydrocolloids: absorbent dressing containing gel-forming agents to absorb and control exudate in an adhesive compound.
- Silicone: absorbent dressing coated with soft silicone as an adhesive or wound contact layer. A variety of silicone dressings are available and selected based on wound characteristics.
- Superabsorbent: dressings made from polymers that absorb and lock away excessive exudate.
- Antibacterial: dressings containing antibacterial substances such as honey or silver.
- Antiseptics: dressings containing antiseptics such as polyhexanide biguanide and chlorohexidine.

EQUIPMENT

- Nonsterile gloves and face mask with eye shield
- Sterile gloves and gowns
- Sterile gauze (4 × 4 pads); abdominal pad (e.g., ABD) or other selective absorptive dressings as indicated
- Sterile water or normal saline (NS) solution for cleansing
- Liquid skin barrier, skin barrier wafers, paste, powder and sealant, or hydrocolloid to protect periwound surface
- Drainage bag or pouch: ostomy-type appliance
- Hypoallergenic tape

Additional equipment, to have available as needed, includes the following:

- Clean scissors or forceps
- Desiccant powder
- Antiseptic wipes for cleaning the reservoir port and tubing extending from the wound site
- Graduated container of appropriate size

PATIENT AND FAMILY EDUCATION

- Explain the procedure and the reason for changing the wound dressing; educate the patient regarding potential pain and odor during the procedure. ***Rationale:*** Patient anxiety and discomfort are decreased.
- Discuss the patient's role in the dressing-change procedure and maintenance of wound drains or pouches. ***Rationale:*** Patient cooperation is elicited; patient is prepared for wound management at discharge.

PATIENT ASSESSMENT AND PREPARATION

Patient Assessment

- Monitor for signs and symptoms of wound infection, including the following. ***Rationale:*** Early detection of infection facilitates prompt and appropriate interventions.

- ❖ Erythema
- ❖ Edema
- ❖ Increased pain
- ❖ Elevated temperature and white blood cell count
- ❖ Changes in wound drainage: amount, color, odor
- ❖ Increased pressure or tenderness at the wound site
- Assess the patency of the wound drainage system. ***Rationale:*** Drains are frequently soft and pliable and thus can easily become kinked or blocked if wound drainage is fibrous in composition. Pouches with drainage systems may also become blocked with fibrous wound drainage; patency of the system is needed to ensure that the wound drainage system moves exudate away from the wound.

Patient Preparation

- Verify the correct patient with two identifiers. ***Rationale:*** Before performing a procedure, the nurse should ensure the correct identification of the patient for the intended intervention.
- Ensure that the patient understands the preprocedural teaching. Answer questions as they arise, and reinforce information as needed. ***Rationale:*** Understanding of previously taught information is evaluated and reinforced.
- Follow institutional standards for assessing pain. Administer analgesia as prescribed. ***Rationale:*** Identifies the need for pain interventions.
- Place the patient in the position of optimal comfort and visualization for dressing the wound. ***Rationale:*** Facilitates visualization and enhances patient tolerance of the procedure.
- Optimize lighting in the room and provide privacy for the patient. ***Rationale:*** These measures allow for optimal wound assessment and patient comfort.

Procedure	for Management of Wound Exudate With Drains and Pouches		
Steps	Rationale		Special Considerations
Dressing Wounds with Drains 1. 🔲 2. 🔲 3. Remove the old dressing.	Maintains clean technique; standard precautions.		Use caution with dressing removal to ensure that drains are not dislodged.
4. Remove nonsterile gloves, and wash hands.			
5. Establish a sterile field.	Maintains a sterile area for dressing supplies. The procedure for acute wounds should be completed with aseptic technique.		No evidence exists to support the use of sterile technique when changing dressings on chronic wounds.
6. Cleanse and irrigate the wound (see Procedure 116, Cleansing, Irrigating, Culturing, and Dressing an Open Wound) as indicated.	Removes contaminated drainage and debris from the wound.		Irrigation of wound drains should be performed only if indicated and only by the provider.[2,9]

Procedure	for Management of Wound Exudate With Drains and Pouches—*Continued*	
Steps	Rationale	Special Considerations
7. Change gloves; open 4 × 4 gauze pads, and apply on top of the wound and around drains (Fig. 119.1). If a dry wound bed is desired, consider a desiccant powder. Avoid wrapping gauze around the drain site.	Gauze absorbs drainage to keep underlying skin dry; wrapping gauze around the drain may result in inadvertent drain removal with future dressing changes.	Drains are placed to remove excessive wound fluid. Apply a wound dressing capable of absorbing wound drainage and preventing moisture accumulation on surrounding healthy skin.[1,2,9] Jackson-Pratt and Hemovac drainage systems require emptying when they are half full of drainage or air (Fig. 119.3). After emptying, the drain is "recharged" by squeezing the bulb/reservoir to achieve negative suction.[19]

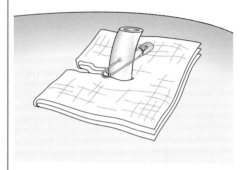

Figure 119.1   Dressing a wound with a drain.

8. If necessary, apply a secondary absorbent dressing (e.g., ABD, 4 × 4 gauze pads, foam dressing).	A secondary dressing absorbs drainage and protects clothing from drainage.	Wound exudate that leaks from the edges or the outer layer of the dressing (strike-through) creates a portal for bacteria to enter the wound. Dressings should be changed when they are 75% saturated or when strike-through is present.
9. Apply a liquid skin barrier to the periwound area, and allow to dry. Apply hypoallergenic tape across the wound dressing, extending approximately 2 inches beyond the dressing onto the skin. **(Level E*)**	When tape is used to secure dressings, frequent dressing changes may result in skin irritation or disruption from the adhesive tape. A liquid skin barrier protects periwound tissue from the mechanical irritation of tape.[2] Hypoallergenic tape is less traumatic to noninjured skin; extend tape beyond the dressing edges to anchor and secure the dressing well.	Assess the periwound edge for chemical and moisture irritation or skin breakdown from wound exudate.

Pouching a Wound With Exudate
1. HH
2. PE

3. If the current drainage pouch has an external opening, drain and measure the content volume and discard according to institutional protocols.	Maintains clean technique; standard precautions. Reduces transmission of microorganisms during dressing change; provides documentation of wound or fistula drainage.	Ensure that all needed supplies are obtained before removing the old pouching system and that adequate time is available to complete the entire procedure.
4. Gently remove the old drainage pouch; support the underlying skin with the fingertips while the drainage pouch is being removed; dispose of the pouch in an appropriate manner.	Prevents tissue trauma to the underlying skin.	A moist cloth may be applied to loosen the edges of the drainage pouch and assist with the removal process.

*Level E: Multiple case reports, theory-based evidence from expert opinions, or peer-reviewed professional organizational standards without clinical studies to support recommendations.

Steps	Rationale	Special Considerations
5. With wet (e.g., NS) gauze 4 × 4 pads, gently cleanse the wound site from the area of least contamination to greatest (see Procedure 116, Cleansing, Irrigating, Culturing, and Dressing an Open Wound); cleanse and dry the surrounding intact skin.	Maintains a clean wound environment; surrounding skin should be free from moisture.	Inspect periwound skin for signs of maceration.
6. If ordered, irrigate the wound or fistula (see Procedure 116, Cleansing, Irrigating, Culturing, and Dressing an Open Wound) as ordered.	Cleanses the wound bed; decreases the microorganism count.	Eye protection should be worn to prevent exposure to potential contaminants.
7. With the wrapper from the wound drainage pouch or wafer, create a template by drawing or measuring the wound or fistula edge onto the wrapper; cut out the center of the pattern on the wound skin barrier and the drainage pouch (cut the pattern slightly larger than the tracing).	Irregular shapes and sizes of draining wounds are difficult to estimate; tracing the wound onto the wrapper allows for a better fit, with less potential for leaking on intact surrounding skin, and increases patient comfort by eliminating unsuccessful application attempts.	
8. Apply a skin barrier (e.g., wafer, liquid, paste, and sealant). **(Level E*)**	Assists in providing a good seal for the drainage pouch.	A good seal is important to prevent moisture or wound exudate undermining the dressing, creating skin maceration, and creating a pathway for microorganisms.
9. Remove the adhesive paper from the drainage pouch; apply the drainage pouch over the wound, and with gentle, even pressure, secure the pouch edges to the skin barrier (Fig. 119.2).	Gentle, even pressure helps ensure a better seal from the drainage pouch to the skin barrier; care must be taken to avoid development of wrinkles during pouch application; wrinkles in the pouch barrier create a leak, and fluid is not contained within the drainage pouch.[2]	If wrinkles are present, sealant paste may be added to the drainage pouch edges to fill spaces created by the wrinkles. Position the pouch to maximize movement of the exudate away from the wound, keeping in mind that patient positioning may change after the procedure. Carefully monitor the wound management system for leaks. If a leak develops, initiate a wound management change. Trapped effluent can cause denudation within a short period.[6]

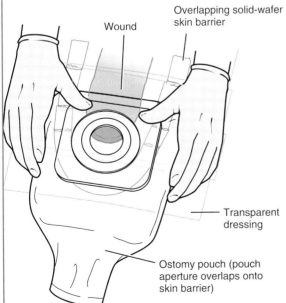

Wound

Overlapping solid-wafer skin barrier

Transparent dressing

Ostomy pouch (pouch aperture overlaps onto skin barrier)

Figure 119.2   Pouching a wound

*Level E: Multiple case reports, theory-based evidence from expert opinions, or peer-reviewed professional organizational standards without clinical studies to support recommendations.

UNIT VII

Procedure continues on following page

Procedure | for Management of Wound Exudate With Drains and Pouches—*Continued*

Steps	Rationale	Special Considerations

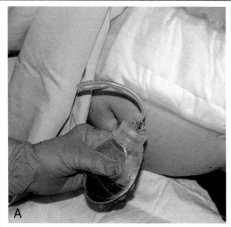 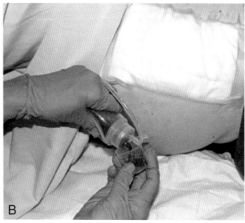

Figure 119.3 Jackson-Pratt drain. **A,** Drainage tubes and reservoir. **B,** Emptying the drainage reservoir. *(From Cooper K, Gosnell K: Foundations and adult health nursing, ed 9, 2023, Elsevier.)*

Steps	Rationale	Special Considerations
10. Close the drainage pouch; wound exudate may be allowed to collect in the pouch, or suction may be attached to the end of the pouch to pull fluid away from the wound into a more distant collection container. **(Level D*)**	The type and amount of drainage coming from a wound determine whether or not suction is added to the drainage pouch.[2]	If suction is not used, empty the appliance regularly. Excessive exudate may create tension within the pouch, causing it to loosen the appliance.

*Level D: Peer-reviewed professional and organizational standards with the support of clinical study recommendations.

Expected Outcomes

- Selected dressing will absorb and retain excess exudate and will prevent skin excoriation
- Drains remain intact and patent
- Pouching system effectively collects and directs exudate away from wound bed
- Surrounding skin is dry and free from excessive wound drainage moisture (maceration)
- Wound drainage exit sites are clean and dry without signs of infection or irritation
- Wound healing is enhanced because of effective wound drainage removal
- Wound drainage decreases in volume (over time) and is absent of foul odor or undesirable color
- Selected treatment plan will facilitate patient comfort and improve quality of life

Unexpected Outcomes

- Wound drain becomes dislodged, blocked, or kinked
- Skin erosion or maceration occurs around the wound edges
- Wound drain (if present) is dislodged during dressing or pouching procedure
- Wound is not healing efficiently because management of wound drainage is not effective
- Wound infection is suspected because of inadequate removal of wound drainage that allowed for bacterial growth

Procedure continues on following page

Patient Monitoring and Care

Steps	Rationale	Reportable Conditions
		These conditions should be reported to the provider if they persist despite nursing interventions. • Erythema • Edema • Increase or change in pain • Elevated temperature and white blood cell count • Changes in wound drainage: amount, color, odor • Increased pressure or tenderness at the wound site
1. Observe for signs of wound infection.	Drains assist with the removal of excessive fluid but also provide a portal of entry for microorganisms.[7]	
2. Assess for patency of the wound drainage system and effective seal of the pouching system.	Drains are frequently soft and pliable and thus can easily become kinked or blocked if wound drainage is fibrous in composition. Leakage from the pouch or secondary dressing may lead to maceration of the periwound skin.	• Wound drainage suddenly decreasing in amount or stopping • Periwound skin breakdown
3. Monitor the amount of wound drainage relative to patient intake and output.	Excessive wound drainage may cause a fluid imbalance, necessitating intravenous or oral fluid replacements.	• Tachycardia • Hypotension • Oliguria • Increasing amounts of drainage • Laboratory analysis suggestive of hypoalbuminemia
4. Monitor caloric and protein intake in the presence of heavily draining wounds. Draining wounds also lose micronutrients and can slow wound healing. Consider supplements, and initiate a nutritional consult as needed.	Excessive wound drainage may result in the loss of 100 g of protein per day. Adequate protein must be replaced for wound healing.[8]	
1. Follow institutional standards for assessing pain. Administer analgesia as prescribed.	Identifies the need for pain interventions.	• Continued pain despite pain interventions

Documentation

Documentation should include the following:
- Patient and family education
- Premedication given, patient tolerance of the procedure, and response to pain medication
- Wound cleansing, irrigation (if performed), and dressing change completed, with date and time
- Description of wound bed, drains, pouch (suction pressure if applied), surrounding skin, and characteristics of wound exudate (color, amount, odor)
- Dressing applied
- Unexpected outcomes
- Nursing interventions

UNIT VII

References and Additional Readings

For a complete list of references and additional readings for this procedure, scan this QR code with your smartphone, or visit https://www.elsevier.com/__data/assets/pdf_file/0008/1319894/Chapter0119.pdf.

120 Fecal Containment Devices and Bowel Management Systems

Matthew Golbitz

PURPOSE A fecal containment device (FCD) consists of an external collection pouch that is fitted over the patient's anus to drain liquid or semiliquid stool. A bowel management system (BMS), also referred to as a *stool management system* or *fecal management system,* is a fully enclosed system designed to collect liquid or semiliquid stool in acutely or critically ill patients with fecal incontinence. Containment of feces by utilizing these devices may assist with the prevention or treatment of incontinence-associated dermatitis (IAD), pressure injuries, contamination of perineal wounds, and infection.

PREREQUISITE NURSING KNOWLEDGE

- Fecal incontinence is described as the involuntary discharge or seepage of liquid, semiliquid, or solid stool from the rectum.[5]
- Acutely and critically ill patients are at high risk of fecal incontinence related to administration of a variety of medications (e.g., antimicrobial, cardiovascular, central nervous system, and gastrointestinal agents), enteral feedings, disease processes (e.g., gastrointestinal disease, hepatic disease, spinal cord trauma), and enterotoxins (e.g., *Clostridium difficile*).[23]
- Patients with fecal incontinence and immobility are considered to be at increased risk of developing IAD.[10,15]
- Incontinence-associated dermatitis (IAD) is erythema and inflammation of the skin that results from contact of urine or stool with perineal or perigenital skin and often occurs in conjunction with pressure, shear force, and friction force and leads to pressure injuries.[6,10,17]
- Excessive moisture changes the skin's protective pH increases the permeability of the skin, thereby decreasing its protective function.[16] Perineal skin damage may progress rapidly and ranges in severity, presenting with erythema, edema, weeping, denuded skin, injury, and pain.[6,10,16,23]
- The goal of the healthcare team is to provide appropriate treatment and services to achieve or maintain as much normal function and quality of life as possible to each incontinent patient.[13] A valid and reliable pressure injury risk assessment tool should be used to assess a patient's risk on admission and consistently throughout the hospitalization.[16]
- Although it is well established that excessive moisture and incontinence, especially fecal incontinence, significantly increases the patient's risk of IAD and pressure injuries, research evidence to guide fecal containment practice is limited.[6,23]

- There is increasing evidence that use of an FCD and BMS may reduce the frequency of IAD and pressure injury development in critically or acutely ill patients.[5,7] Furthermore, use of a BMS may reduce the spread or cross-contamination of *C. difficile*.[7,9,17] BMS use may result in decreased patient mortality and morbidity (reduced development of skin breakdown and infection, decreased hospital length of stay) and decreased use of hospital resources (e.g., reduced linen use, decreased nursing time requirements).[7,9]
- A BMS may have a special port for obtaining fecal samples, which also helps prevent cross-contamination.[1,3,4,8]
- Management of fecal incontinence should include the following elements:
  - Identification and treatment of the diarrhea. If the source of fecal incontinence cannot be eliminated, drug therapy may be used; however, the effectiveness of these drugs is not known because randomized studies have focused on the management of chronic diarrhea in outpatients rather than acute diarrhea in hospitalized patients.[23,24]
  - Meticulous perineal skin care. Skin cleansing should be performed promptly after each incontinent episode with a cleanser specifically indicated for perineal skin. Avoid soap and water. Most soap is a mixture of alkali and fatty acids, and its pH tends to be higher than that of normal skin, which can disrupt the skin's protective properties. However, the pH of a majority of perineal cleansers is closer to that of healthy skin.[6,15]
  - Apply a moisturizer with skin protectant. Moisturizers help hydrate intact skin, replace oils in the skin, and soothe skin irritation. Moisturizers that contain petrolatum, lanolin, dimethicone, or zinc can provide a protective barrier to protect and soothe denuded areas.[13,15,23]
  - Use absorbent underpads that wick effluent away from the skin and allow for air circulation between the patient's skin and support surface. Avoid the use of

- adult incontinence briefs that trap moisture against the skin. Change underpads frequently.[13]
  - ❖ Consider application of an FCD or BMS.
- FCDs adhere directly to the perianal skin, moving feces away from the skin and into a drainage container. The device can remain in place for 1 to 2 days without leaking.[14] If the device is well adhered and not leaking, it may remain in place longer if clinically indicated. Care must be taken during removal of the device to prevent skin trauma or tears.
- The general consensus in the literature is that the FCD offers many advantages over adult incontinence briefs and balloon rectal catheters and is the least invasive method of fecal containment. However, the manual dexterity required in the application of an FCD may require training and has been found to be more cumbersome compared with other methods of fecal containment.[14]
- At times, devices not intended for management of fecal incontinence have been used. Adaptation of a device for an unapproved use may be associated with patient injury and concerns of increased liability if a problem arises.[13,24] The clinician should use fecal containment systems that are approved by the U.S. Food and Drug Administration (FDA) rather than adapting devices for the management of liquid feces.[13]
- BMSs are FDA-approved devices that consist of a rectal catheter that is inserted into the rectum, held in place by means of an inflatable balloon or a flexible indwelling diverter, and left in the rectal vault for up to 29 days for the diversion of liquid and semiliquid stool into a collection system[1,3,4,8] (Figs. 120.1 and 120.2). The overall function and guidelines for use of the various BMSs are similar. However, the healthcare provider should review the manufacturer's instructions for the particular device before use. Early research suggests that these devices successfully divert feces, allowing for perineal skin protection and healing.[5,7]

- Manufacturer-specific contraindications for BMS[1,3,4,8,12] include the following:
  - ❖ Allergies to product components (e.g., silicone)
  - ❖ Patients younger than 18 years of age
  - ❖ Anal/rectal canal strictures, stenosis, or injury
  - ❖ Impaction that cannot be dislodged or formed stool in the rectal vault
  - ❖ Lack of adequate anal/sphincter control or tone
  - ❖ Rectal or prostate surgery within the previous 6 weeks or colon surgery within the past year
  - ❖ Confirmed anal/rectal tumor
  - ❖ Iμμυνοχompromised status
  - ❖ Recent myocardial infarction
  - ❖ Rectal mucosal disease or compromised rectal wall integrity (e.g., proctitis, severe hemorrhoids, inflammation of the rectum)
  - ❖ Complaints of unresolved pain or discomfort after BMS insertion
- Adverse events reported in the literature include the following[1,3,4,8,12,18,19,20,21]:
  - ❖ Autonomic dysreflexia in patients with a spinal cord injury
  - ❖ Decreased rectal sphincter tone
  - ❖ Rectal perforation
  - ❖ Gastrointestinal hemorrhage
  - ❖ Ischemic pressure necrosis and injury of the rectal mucosa
  - ❖ Abdominal distension and/or bowel obstruction
  - ❖ Persistent rectal pain
  - ❖ Sepsis
- A BMS should be used with caution with the following[1,3,4,6,12,20,21]:
  - ❖ Patients who have a tendency to bleed easily due to anticoagulation/antiplatelet therapy or underlying coagulation disorders. Check PT, INR, PTT, and platelets.
  - ❖ Patients with inflammatory bowel disease.
- If blood is present in the rectum, ensure that there is no evidence of pressure necrosis from the device. Discontinuation of use of the device is recommended if evident. Notify the physician of any signs of bleeding.[1,3,4,8]
- Follow the manufacturer's guidelines when using ointments or lubricants with a petroleum base as they may compromise the integrity of the BMS device.[1,3,4,8]

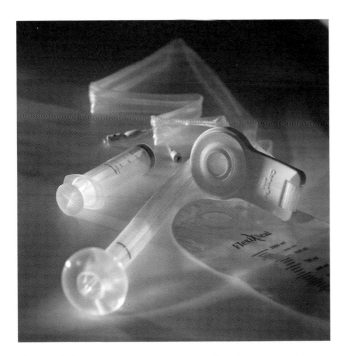

Figure 120.1 Flexi-Seal FMS *(ConvaTec, Skillman, NJ. Copyright 1996, 2010 Covidien. Courtesy Covidien.)*

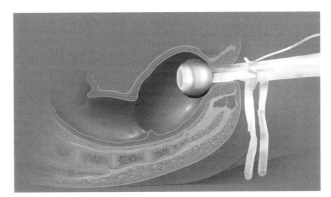

Figure 120.2 ActiFlow Indwelling Bowel Catheter. *(Courtesy Hollister, Inc., Libertyville, IL.)*

UNIT VII

EQUIPMENT

- Nonsterile gloves
- Personal protective equipment (i.e., gowns and face protection)
- Water
- Water-soluble lubricant
- FCD or BMS
- Absorbent underpads
- Skin-cleansing solution
  Additional equipment to have available as needed includes the following:
- Scissors

PATIENT AND FAMILY EDUCATION

- Explain the procedure and rationale for application of an FCD or insertion of a BMS. ***Rationale:*** Patient and family anxiety and discomfort may be decreased.
- Discuss goals of bowel management program and expected benefits of the intervention. ***Rationale:*** The patient is prepared for placement of the BMS, possible odors, and perineal skin and wound care interventions.

PATIENT ASSESSMENT AND PREPARATION

Patient Assessment

- Review the patient's medical record, and discuss medical history with the patient for possible contraindications before BMS placement. ***Rationale:*** This avoids possible complications associated with placement of the device.
- Evaluate the consistency of fecal contents; contents must be liquid to semiliquid to flow through the BMS. ***Rationale:*** Liquid fecal consistency is important to prevent occlusion of the device.
- Assess the perineal skin for the presence of open areas and pressure injuries, and apply moisture barrier creams. ***Rationale:*** A BMS may be used to prevent and treat IAD, and additional skin care products may be indicated to assist in perineal skin healing.[22]
- Evaluate the patient's need for analgesia or sedation. ***Rationale:*** The patient may tolerate the procedure more comfortably.

Patient Preparation

- Verify the correct patient with two identifiers. ***Rationale:*** Before performing a procedure, the nurse should ensure the correct identification of the patient for the intended intervention.
- Ensure that the patient and family understand the preprocedural teaching. Answer questions as they arise, and reinforce information as needed. ***Rationale:*** Understanding of previously taught information is evaluated and reinforced.
- Optimize lighting in the room, and provide privacy for the patient. ***Rationale:*** These interventions facilitate visualization and enhance patient tolerance of the procedure.

Procedure	for Fecal Containment Device and Bowel Management System	
Steps	Rationale	Special Considerations

Several fecal containment devices are commercially available. General principles for placement of the device are consistent among systems; however, the healthcare provider should read and follow manufacturer-specific recommendations for placement of the device. The procedure is most effectively performed with two healthcare professionals.

Fecal Containment Devices

Steps	Rationale	Special Considerations
1. 🅷🅷		
2. 🅿🅴		
3. Position the patient in the left lateral position with the upper knee slightly flexed.[11] **(Level D*)**	Assists with visualization and comfort of the patient for placement.	
4. Cleanse the perineal area with a no-rinse, pH-balanced cleansing solution. Allow the skin to dry thoroughly.[11] **(Level D*)**	Evaluates skin for presence of breakdown. The FCD adheres better to clean, dry skin.	Do not apply the device if the perineal skin is not intact. Consider clipping hair to facilitate better adherence.[11]
5. Separate the patient's buttocks. If recommended by the manufacturer, a no-sting skin protectant barrier solution can be applied and allowed to dry.[11,14] **(Level D*)**	Application of the FCD usually requires two experienced healthcare professionals to correctly position the patient and apply the device correctly.[11,14]	Avoid the use of adhesive products that can cause discomfort or irritation to delicate perineal tissue. Follow the manufacturer's instructions for specifics on application and tips for better adherence.
6. Remove protective wrap, and firmly apply the FCD around the anus. **(Level M*)**	Firm pressure and body heat allows the adhesive backing of the FCD to adhere more effectively to the skin.	The healthcare professional may need to adjust the opening of the FCD to fit comfortably yet snugly around the anal opening.

*Level M: Manufacturer's recommendations only.
*Level D: Peer-reviewed professional and organizational standards with the support of clinical study recommendations.

Procedure continues on following page

Procedure	for Fecal Containment Device and Bowel Management System—*Continued*

Steps	Rationale	Special Considerations
7. Attach the collection bag to the distal opening of the FCD, and place it in a dependent position. **(Level M*)**	The collection device moves the fecal material away from the skin.	Unless contraindicated, position the patient in the side-lying position, and avoid placing the patient's weight on the device.
8. Monitor the volume, consistency, and color of fecal material. Fecal output must be evaluated as part of the patient's overall output assessment.	If diarrhea is excessive, fluids and electrolytes may be lost in the feces, resulting in dehydration and electrolyte imbalances.	
9. Change the FCD if leaking is noted or if the stool is too thick to pass through the device; if diarrhea has resolved, consider discontinuing use.	An adequate seal is necessary for effective performance of the FCD and protection of perineal skin.	Gently remove the FCD to avoid tearing skin. Use a nonirritating, no-sting adhesive remover to assist with removal of the device.
10. Discard used supplies.	Maintains infection-control practices and decreases contamination.	
11. 🖐		
Bowel Management System		
1. 🖐		
2. 🄿🄴		
3. Administer prescribed analgesia or sedation agents if ordered.	May assist patient tolerance of the procedure.	
4. Position the patient in the left lateral position with the upper knee slightly flexed.[1,3,4,8] **(Level D*)**	Assists with visualization and comfort of the patient for placement.	
5. Apply water-soluble lubricant to a gloved finger, and perform a manual digital rectal examination.[22] **(Level D*)**	Evaluates the rectal vault for impacted stool and rectal tone.	Perform digital disimpaction before continuing with placement of the BMS. The device may not be retained if rectal tone is poor.
6. Remove anything else from the rectum, such as temperature probes. **(Level M*)**	Prevents trauma and improper placement of the device.	
7. Cleanse the perineal area with a no-rinse, pH-balanced cleansing solution.	Allows for better visualization of the skin and thus evaluation for the presence of breakdown.	
8. Open the BMS kit, and connect the pieces according to the manufacturer's instructions. **(Level M*)**	The functionality of the device should be assessed before placement.[1,3,4,8]	
9. Apply water-soluble lubricant to the distal end of the BMS. With slow, gentle pressure, advance the balloon through the anal sphincter. **(Level M*)**	Lubricant assists with insertion of the device gently through the anus and into the rectal vault.	Do not advance the BMS if resistance is felt.
10. Inflate the BMS balloon with water or normal saline solution per the instruction guidelines. **(Level M*)**	Water or normal saline solution may be used to inflate the balloon and hold the device in place.	The manufacturer may include prepackaged syringes. Do not exceed the manufacturer's recommended volume for balloon inflation. Additional fluid volume in the balloon can increase the amount of pressure on the intestinal mucosa, which may contribute to decreased rectal sphincter tone, rectal perforation, gastrointestinal hemorrhage, ischemic pressure necrosis, rectal mucosa injury, abdominal distension, and/or sepsis[1,3,4,8,12,20,21]

*Level M: Manufacturer's recommendations only.
*Level D: Peer-reviewed professional and organizational standards with the support of clinical study recommendations.

UNIT VII

Procedure | for Fecal Containment Device and Bowel Management System—*Continued*

Steps	Rationale	Special Considerations
11. Gently pull the BMS back to ensure that the balloon is in the rectum and positioned against the rectal floor (Fig. 120.3). **(Level M*)**	The device should rest on the rectal floor to collect fecal material and provide a seal.	Some BMS manufacturers have a position indicator noted on the drainage tubing that should be visible after insertion.[1,3,4,8]

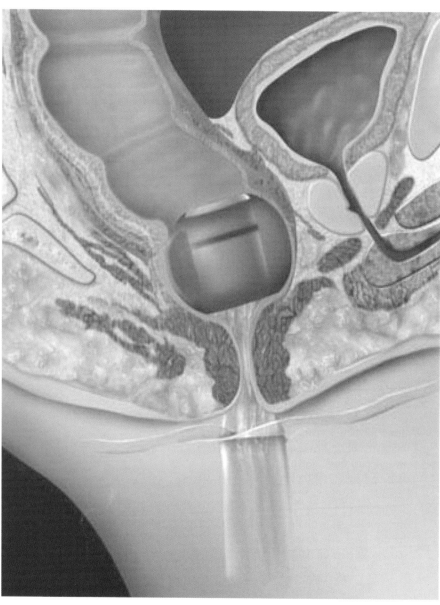

Figure 120.3 Correct placement of a bowel management system in the rectum. *(Courtesy Hollister, Inc., Libertyville, IL.)*

Steps	Rationale	Special Considerations
12. Position the drainage bag in a dependent position. Ensure that there is no traction on the drainage bag or tubing. Secure the tubing and drainage bag.	Allows for effective flow of fecal material. Prevents traumatic removal and possible damage to the rectal mucosa.	Unless contraindicated, position the patient in the side-lying position, and avoid placing the patient's body weight on the device tubing.
13. Evaluate the consistency of the fecal material. Stool should be liquid to semiliquid. The BMS may be irrigated with water as necessary to ensure patency.[1,3,4,7] **(Level M*)**	Allows for effective flow of fecal material.	Slight leakage or smear of feces is often unavoidable. Do not exceed the manufacturer's recommendations for fluid volume in the balloon[1,3,4,8,12,20,21]

*Level M: Manufacturer's recommendations only.

Procedure continues on following page

Procedure for Fecal Containment Device and Bowel Management System—*Continued*

Steps	Rationale	Special Considerations
14. Discard used supplies. Remove protective equipment and gloves, and discard in an appropriate receptacle.	Maintains infection-control practices.	
15. 🔲		

Expected Outcomes

- Containment of liquid feces
- Perineal skin remains intact or, if compromised before placement of BMS, healing of skin is evident
- Intake and output balance are maintained

Unexpected Outcomes

- Injury to anal sphincter or rectal vault
- Fluid and electrolyte imbalances
- Infection
- Pressure necrosis
- Loss of sphincter tone
- Perineal skin breakdown

Patient Monitoring and Care

Steps	Rationale	Reportable Conditions
		These conditions should be reported to the provider if they persist despite nursing interventions.
1. Assess the patient's perineal skin for fecal drainage. Check the location of the tubing of the BMS with each reposition, especially in the perineum. **(Level C*)**	Continued assessment of the patient for IAD and development of pressure injury is essential because these conditions may prolong hospitalization.[2,6,10,15,22]	- Foul drainage or odor - Worsening erythema and edema - Pain - Elevated temperature - Elevated white blood cell count
2. Monitor fluid and electrolyte balance.	If diarrhea is excessive, fluids and electrolytes may be lost in the feces, resulting in dehydration and electrolyte imbalances.	- Output greater than intake - Abnormal electrolyte laboratory analysis - Signs and symptoms of electrolyte imbalances (e.g., cardiac ectopy, neuromuscular symptoms), tachycardia, decreased urine output, thirst, signs and symptoms of dehydration
3. Evaluate the amount and consistency of fecal drainage.	Migration of the catheter or change in the fecal consistency may indicate obstruction or occlusion of the BMS.	Sudden change in amount of fecal drainage or consistency
4. Follow institutional standards for assessing pain. Administer analgesia as prescribed.	Identifies the need for pain interventions.	Continued pain despite pain interventions
5. Assess indications for maintaining BMS.	As the frequency and amount of liquid bowel movements begin to slow, the BMS may be removed to prevent anal sphincter atony, expulsion, traumatic removal, or pressure injury.[22]	- Development of pressure injury - Accidental expulsion of BMS due to poor anal sphincter tone - Traumatic removal - Any signs of rectal bleeding

*Level C: Qualitative studies, descriptive or correlational studies, integrative reviews, systematic reviews, or randomized controlled trials with inconsistent results.

UNIT VII

Documentation

Documentation should include the following:
- Patient and family education
- Description of perineal skin condition
- Patency of BMS
- Description and volume of feces
- Patient tolerance of procedure
- Progression of perineal wound healing
- Unexpected outcomes
- Pain assessment, interventions, effectiveness, and insertion date

References and Additional Readings

For a complete list of references and additional readings for this procedure, scan this QR code with your smartphone, or visit https://www.elsevier.com/__data/assets/pdf_file/0009/1319895/Chapter0120.pdf.

PROCEDURE

121

Percutaneous Endoscopic Gastrostomy, Gastrostomy, and Jejunostomy Tube Care

Carly D. Byrne

PURPOSE Gastrostomy, percutaneous endoscopic gastrostomy (PEG), and jejunostomy tubes provide long-term access to the gastrointestinal (GI) tract for nutrition and require ongoing maintenance and care.

PREREQUISITE NURSING KNOWLEDGE

- Knowledge of the anatomy and physiology of the upper and lower GI system.
- Patients who require supplemental enteral nutritional support for longer than 4 weeks or patients who cannot have enteral tubes passed orally or nasally because of anatomy or surgery are candidates for long-term enteral access.[3,6]
- Use of a PEG tube is the most common technique for providing long-term enteral access. There are multiple techniques for PEG tube insertion.[1,6] The procedure generally takes place in an endoscopy or radiology department and is performed by a gastroenterologist, surgeon, radiologist, or medical intensivist. Patients generally require a local anesthetic but may also require other sedative agents.[1,6]
- PEG tubes are large-bore catheters that range from 18F to 22F and have a mushroom-shaped, curved end in the stomach and a two-port distal end to instill enteral nutrition, medications, and fluid. Commercial PEG tubes have disks, perpendicular to the tube, to hold the device close to the skin and lessen the shift of the tube in and out of the skin (Fig. 121.1).
- Relative contraindications for PEG placement include the following:[4]
  - Previous gastric resection
  - Tumors that block the passage of the endoscope
  - Massive ascites
  - Morbid obesity
  - Esophageal or gastric varices
  - Esophageal stricture or narrowing
- Some gastrostomy tubes have a balloon in the intestinal lumen that is inflated with sterile water instead of a mushroom-shaped end. This balloon prevents inadvertent dislocation. The distal end of the tube has an infusion port and a port for balloon instillation (Fig. 121.2). Balloons should be checked weekly to evaluate for leakage and to change the water.[1] Tubes should be changed per the

manufacturer's recommendations; some may not require replacement for up to 3 to 9 months.[1]
- A jejunostomy tube, which does not have a balloon or a mushroom-shaped end, is indicated in patients who are at risk for aspiration or unable to tolerate enteral feedings into the stomach. These tubes are routinely sutured in place for stability (Fig. 121.3). Jejunostomy tubes are generally smaller bore compared with gastrostomy tubes and therefore are more susceptible to occlusion.[8] These tubes are generally in place for 6 to 9 months.[1]
- If a PEG or gastrostomy tube is inadvertently removed, reinsertion of the tube is a routine procedure at the bedside after the tunnel and stoma are healed (approximately 2 to 6 weeks after insertion). If the tube requires replacement before establishment of a well-formed tract or stoma, replacement should be performed using endoscopic or image-guided radiography, as there is a risk for the stomach and anterior abdominal wall to separate from each other, which would place the patient at risk for infection or peritonitis.[6]
- Because these tubes all enter through the abdominal wall, skin care at the insertion site is important for skin integrity and prevention of infection.
- Individualized patient nutrition goals should be determined in consultation with the interdisciplinary team. The nutrition plan is developed on the basis of the collaborative assessment of the nurse, dietitian, and physician or advanced practice nurse and in partnership with the patient and family, if possible.[2]

EQUIPMENT

- Cotton-tipped swabs
- Gauze pads (4 × 4 regular and 4 × 4 drain cut)
- Gloves, nonsterile
- Mild soap
- Protective skin barrier (e.g., vitamins A and D ointment or other commercial topical moisture barrier products)

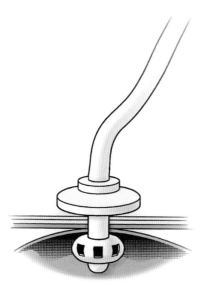

Figure 121.1   Percutaneous endoscopic gastrostomy.

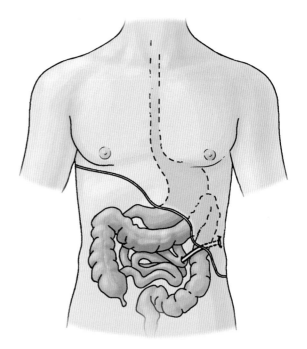

Figure 121.3   Jejunostomy tube placement.

explanation provides the patient and family with important information and may decrease patient and family anxiety.
* Explain that long-term enteral access catheters can be removed when oral intake meets the needs of the patient. ***Rationale***: This information may serve as a goal for the patient to consume more via the oral route.
* Aspiration is a continued risk when the patient is positioned flat. ***Rationale:*** Gastric residual volume can reflux and create a risk for pulmonary aspiration.

PATIENT ASSESSMENT AND PREPARATION

Patient Assessment

* Perform hand hygiene, and don gloves.
* Introduce yourself to the patient.
* Verify the correct patient with two identifiers.
* Perform a GI assessment. Note the presence of abdominal distension, bowel sounds, flatus, and bowel movements. Determine whether the patient has had diarrhea, constipation, or signs of GI dysfunction. ***Rationale:*** A patient needs a functional gut to receive enteral nutrition.
* Assess for feeding tube migration.
   * Ensure that the numeric markings on the tube at the exit site are consistent with what is documented in the patient's record initially and over time.
   * Assess to determine if the tube has migrated inward or outward. Marking measurements may decrease or increase over time depending on the patient's condition (e.g., weight gain, weight loss, swelling, ascites).
   * If a marking is at or below zero, tube feedings should be discontinued or withheld, and a provider should be notified immediately, as this may indicate that the tube is internally dislodged and in the peritoneum.
   * Notify the provider for any concerns about tube migration.

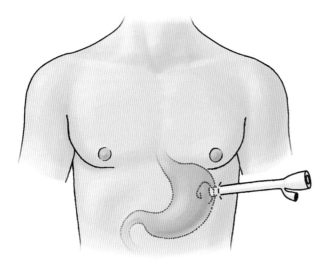

Figure 121.2   Gastrostomy tube.

* Silk tape (or paper tape if patient has a sensitivity to silk tape)
* Commercial horizontal or vertical stabilization device

PATIENT AND FAMILY EDUCATION

* Explain the purpose for the tube to the patient and family. ***Rationale:*** Engaging with the patient and family provides an opportunity for them to be engaged in their care, and information may decrease patient and family anxiety.
* Explain the reason for skin care assessment and tube maintenance. ***Rationale:*** This informs the patient and family of what to expect and may be an opportunity to encourage them to participate in care.
* Stress the importance of not pulling on the tube. ***Rationale:*** Unnecessary pain and skin irritation may be avoided. Accidental discontinuation of the tube may also be avoided.
* Explain that oral nutrition may be possible even if the patient has a long-term enteral access catheter. ***Rationale:*** This

- Assess skin condition at the exit site of the feeding tube at the stoma; signs and symptoms of infection are on the bullet list below. ***Rationale:*** Intact skin integrity is a defense against infection. Early assessment of signs of infection promotes early, appropriate intervention.
  - ❖ Site redness or edema
  - ❖ Warmth
  - ❖ Purulent drainage
  - ❖ Pain or tenderness
  - ❖ Fever
- Remove gloves, and perform hand hygiene.

Patient Preparation

- Verify the correct patient with two identifiers. ***Rationale:*** Patients should be correctly identified before any intended intervention.
- Assess the patient and family's understanding of the procedure, answer questions as they arise, and reinforce information as needed. ***Rationale:*** Engaging with the patient and family ensures that they are included in the plan of care and provides an opportunity to ensure understanding.
- Assist the patient to a position of comfort while ensuring that the stoma tube is easily accessible.

Procedure for Percutaneous Endoscopic Gastrostomy, Gastrostomy, or Jejunostomy Tube Care		
Steps	**Rationale**	**Special Considerations**
1. 🅷🅷		
2. 🅿🅴		
3. Moisten gauze pads and two cotton-tipped applicators with mild soap and warm water.[4] **(Level E*)**	Soap and water cleanse the skin surface at the stoma.[4]	Avoid the use of hydrogen peroxide as it can cause skin irritation and is cytotoxic to cells.
4. Cleanse the tube and stoma	The tube and stoma should be cleansed at least daily.[4]	
A. Wipe the area closest to the tube (stoma) with the cotton-tipped applicators and proximal skin with the moistened gauze.	Moisture under the bumper can erode skin at the tract.[2]	
B. Rinse with water.	After PEG placement, bumpers should be left in place for the first 4 days.[2,6] Four days after PEG placement, allow approximately 0.5–1.5 cm between the bumper and skin to maintain proper tension to reduce the risk of skin erosion, buried bumper syndrome, or infection.[2,6]	
C. Displace the bumper to ensure cleaning and drying next to the skin at the stoma.		
D. Verify that the bumper is not too tight against the skin. One fingerbreadth should fit between the bumper and the skin. **(Level E*)**		
5. Dry the skin and stoma thoroughly with a dry gauze pad.	Prevents chafing and skin maceration.	
6. If significant moisture is found on the skin around the stoma, use cotton-tipped applicators to apply a protective skin barrier (e.g., vitamin A and D ointment or other commercial topical moisture barrier product) in a circular motion around the stoma.[7] **(Level E*)**	Protective barrier ointment provides a moisture barrier for skin and assists wound healing.	Increased moisture can cause a fungal infection that may require a topical medication application for treatment. If purulent drainage is persistent, collaborate with the physician or advanced practice nurse to obtain an order for an antimicrobial ointment, and apply it after skin cleansing.
7. Apply a foam or glycerin hydrogel dressing (or, if for a PEG, a single 4 × 4 split gauze if there is no available foam and hydrogel dressing available) around the tube, and secure it with tape along the edges. Change the dressing every 12 hours or per your organization's practice. The dressing should also be changed when soiled or moist.[2,4] **(Level E*)**	The dressing absorbs moisture from the stoma. If no drainage is present, the gauze may be left off.[4] If available, use a foam or glycerin hydrogel dressing instead of gauze. Hydrogel dressings have been shown to decrease the number of peristomal infections, and dressing changes can be extended to 7 days.[2]	Do not apply an occlusive dressing as this can lead to skin breakdown and stoma maceration.[4]

*Level E: Multiple case reports, theory-based evidence from expert opinions, or peer-reviewed professional organizational standards without clinical studies to support recommendations.

UNIT VIII

Procedure continues on following page

Procedure	**for Percutaneous Endoscopic Gastrostomy, Gastrostomy, or Jejunostomy Tube Care—*Continued***	
Steps	Rationale	Special Considerations
8. Anchor the tube to the skin at an adjacent area on the abdomen if the insertion site of the tube is well healed.	Reduces tension on the tube and avoids stoma erosion.[2]	If PEG tube anchoring is to an adjacent area on the abdomen (including an abdominal binder), ensure it is done in a manner that external bumpers are not causing pressure points to skin around the stoma.
9. The bumper (flange) should be rotated to avoid skin damage from repeated taping.[2] **(Level E*)**	Ensure that there are no pressure points on the skin to reduce the risk of device-related pressure ulcers.[2]	
10. Remove **PE**, and discard used supplies.		
11. **HH**		
12. **PE**		
13. Initiate enteral feedings as prescribed. A. Ensure that the correct tubing is used. B. Identify and confirm the enteral nutrition label.[3] C. Trace the tubing or catheter from the patient to the point of origin before connecting or reconnecting an infusion at any transition point (e.g., changing a setting or adding additional feeds to a bag) and as part of the handoff process.[5] D. Label the enteral tubing and feeding per your organization's practice.[5] **(Level E*)**	Tubing and pumps that are specifically designed for enteral feedings should be used only. Use of IV tubing or IV pumps has caused serious errors resulting in patient harm.[5]	Do not force connections.[5]
14. Elevate the head of bed 30–45 degrees.[3]	Risk of aspiration is reduced when the head of the bed is elevated.	
15. Flush the feeding tube with:[3] A. 15 mL of purified or sterile water before and after the administration of medications. B. 30 mL of purified or sterile water after gastric residual measurements and before and after feedings C. 30 mL of purified or sterile water every 4 hours during continuous feedings.[3] **(Level E*)**	The most common causes of a clogged tube are related to insufficient flushing.[1,2] **(Level C*)**	Tube clogging is more likely to occur with thick enteral feeds, use of bulking agents, and medications.[2] Repeated gastric residual volumes should be avoided to decrease the risk of tube clogging.[2]
16. Initiate feedings as ordered and in accordance with the organization's practice.		Gastric residual volume (GRV) is no longer frequently used as part of routine care for patients on enteral nutrition. For organizations that still obtain GRVs, withholding enteral nutrition for a GRV <500 mL in the absence of other signs and symptoms of intolerance should be avoided.[3]
17. Remove **PE**, and discard used supplies.		

* Level C: Qualitative studies, descriptive or correlational studies, integrative reviews, systematic reviews, or randomized controlled trials with inconsistent results.

*Level E: Multiple case reports, theory-based evidence from expert opinions, or peer-reviewed professional organizational standards without clinical studies to support recommendations.

Expected Outcomes

- Intact skin at the stoma of the long-term enteral access device (EAD)
- Long-term enteral access for enteral feeding and fluid administration remains patent

Unexpected Outcomes

- Infection or ulceration at the stoma[2,7]
- Tube removal by patient or accidental dislodgment with patient movement[7]
- Buried bumper syndrome[1,2]
- Peritonitis[7]
- Peristomal leakage[2,7]
- Colonic perforation[7]
- Bleeding[2,7]
- Fistulas (colonic and gastrocutaneous)[2,7]
- Tube malfunction, clogged tube, and degradation of the tube[1,2,7]
- Nonhealing stoma[7]

Patient Monitoring and Care

Steps	Rationale	Reportable Conditions
		These conditions should be reported to the provider if they persist despite nursing interventions. • Erosion of the stoma • Signs and symptoms of infection
1. Regularly assess the integrity of the skin and quality of drainage from the stoma per your organization's practice with any changes or as needed.	Intact skin is the first line of prevention against infection.	
2. Ensure that the PEG tube has an external disk or bumper positioned approximately 0.5–1.5 cm above the skin.[4,7] **(Level E*)**	The disk/bumper helps prevent excess movement of the tube in and out of the skin. If the disk exerts excess pressure, tissue injury may occur.[4,7]	• Pressure injury adjacent to the stoma • Removal of the tube by the patient • Clogging of the device • Buried bumper
3. For PEG and gastrostomy tubes, rotate the external tube daily and then weekly once the stoma has fully healed.[2,4] **(Level E*)**	Jejunostomy tubes should not be rotated; rotating these tubes can cause twisting and knotting of the tube in the jejunem.[1]	
4. If the tube is prematurely removed before the tract healing, apply a sterile dressing, and notify the provider immediately.[6] **(Level E*)**	A tube removed before the tract is established is a potential surgical emergency and may necessitate immediate return to the operating room or endoscopy suite for repair and replacement.[6] Inform the physician or advanced practice nurseso he or she can determine the urgency of replacement. The immediate response may be to place a replacement commercial tube or Foley catheter in the tract. This should be performed with caution following organizational standards.[3] Tubes with established tracts can be replaced by the nurse at the bedside with a tube of comparable size and length.	• Removal of the EAD

*Level E: Multiple case reports, theory-based evidence from expert opinions, or peer-reviewed professional organizational standards without clinical studies to support recommendations.

Procedure continues on following page

UNIT VIII

Patient Monitoring and Care —*Continued*

Steps	Rationale	Reportable Conditions
5. Evaluate and monitor the condition of the tube with ongoing use. Follow organizational policy regarding tube replacement.[3] **(Level E*)** 6. If necessary, carry out interventions to unclog the enteral feeding tube:[3] **(Level E*)** A. Instill warm purified or sterile water from a 30- to 60-mL syringe into the EAD, and apply a gentle back-and-forth motion to the syringe plunger. B. If water does not resolve the clog, consider consulting with the provider regarding use of an uncoated pancreatic enzyme solution. C. As a last resort, consider using an enzyme-containing declogging kit if available within the organization.	Routine tube changes are not necessary. Tube changes should be considered when there is device failure, tube degradation, or nonhealing ulcer formation.	• Tube degradation • Nonhealing ulcer at the stoma site • Fistula formation • Tube failure, including occlusion. • Obstruction that is not relieved.

*Level E: Multiple case reports, theory-based evidence from expert opinions, or peer-reviewed professional organizational standards without clinical studies to support recommendations.

Documentation

Documentation should include the following:
- Patient and family education
- Condition of the stoma
- Any treatment rendered related to site complications
- Tube patency
- Pain assessment, interventions, and effectiveness
- Type of tube and distance of the tube from the adapter to the entrance into the skin
- Unexpected outcomes
- Nursing interventions

References and Additional Readings

For a complete list of references and additional readings for this procedure, scan this QR code with your smartphone, or visit https://www.elsevier.com/__data/assets/pdf_file/0010/1319896/Chapter0121.pdf.

UNIT VIII

122 Small-Bore Feeding Tube Insertion and Nursing Care

Carly D. Byrne

PURPOSE A small-bore feeding tube is inserted to provide access to the gastrointestinal tract for the patient who is unable to orally consume adequate calories.[6,9] The tube can be used for administration of nutrition, fluid, and medications.

PREREQUISITE NURSING KNOWLEDGE

- The gastrointestinal (GI) tract should be functioning for gastric feedings to be digested and absorbed. Bowel sounds may not be audible, yet the GI tract is functional, and enteral nutrition can be instituted safely and effectively and be well tolerated. GI findings that may affect the normal functioning of the tract and preclude gastric feeding include bowel obstruction, paralytic ileus, and some fistulas.
- Small-bore feeding tubes may be placed in either the stomach or in the small intestine. While postpyloric placement is more difficult, it may be the most appropriate for specific patient populations who are at a higher risk for aspiration.[9]
- Often, small-bore feeding tubes can be placed at the bedside blindly.[1,3,6,9] Procedural risks associated with blindly inserting a small-bore feeding tube include aspiration, GI tract perforation, pneumothorax, and circulatory or respiratory compromise.
- The gold standard for confirming tube placement is via radiograph. Proper tube placement should be confirmed before initiating feedings or administering medications.[1,2,5]
- Small-bore feeding tubes are preferable over large-bore nasogastric tubes during the course of critical illness, as they present a lower risk for sinusitis and tissue necrosis in the nares.
- Patients may still be able to have simultaneous oral intake if they are able to safely swallow and protect their airway.
- Both weighted (tubes with an enlarged tip, filled with tungsten) and unweighted (bolus tip) small-bore nasogastric tubes are available. A prepackaged guidewire is typically already in the lumen to assist advancement of the tube within the length of the esophagus, stomach, and past the pyloric sphincter. After successful placement, the guidewire should be removed and discarded. The size of tubes ranges from 6F to 12F. They are radiopaque along the entire length of the tube. External markings provide accurate insertion depth. Organizations should select products and/or adopt practices to ensure that feeding ports are in compatible with intravenous syringes.
- Contraindications for insertion of a nasogastric feeding tube are basilar skull fracture, maxillofacial disorders, transsphenoidal surgical approaches, uncorrected coagulation disorders, and some esophageal and gastric abnormalities.[9]

- Small-bore feeding tubes are not designed for drainage of gastric contents. If gastric decompression is desired, a large-bore nasogastric tube should be placed. See Procedure 100, Nasogastric and Orogastric Tube Placement and Removal for nasogastric tube placement.
- It is important to review and follow organizational standards regarding insertion of a small-bore feeding tube.

EQUIPMENT

- Commercial securement device (internal or external) or tape
- Emesis basin
- Enteral access device, as appropriate
- Nonsterile gloves
- Permanent marker
- Protective pad or towel
- Skin-preparation agent
- Small-bore feeding tube
- Water, purified or sterile
- Water-soluble lubricant (if tube is not prelubricated)
- Large cup of drinking water and straw, if clinically appropriate
- Capnography, if available
- pH paper, if available

PATIENT AND FAMILY EDUCATION

- Provide the patient and family with an explanation of the essential role adequate nutrition plays in promoting recovery from illness and wound healing and also how the tube can help provide adequate nutritional intake. *Rationale:* Explanation engages the patient and family in the plan of care and may allay patient and family anxiety.
- Explain the steps of the procedure and how the patient can assist with the passage of the tube, including positioning and swallowing when cued. *Rationale:* Engaging the patient provides the patient with a sense of control and may help facilitate insertion.
- Describe the typical sensations experienced during feeding tube insertion (including stimulation of patients gag reflex). *Rationale:* Explanation may alleviate anxiety.
- Reinforce the importance of using care when changing position or getting out of bed once the tube is placed. *Rationale:* Emphasis may aid in preventing inadvertently dislodging of the tube.

- Explain the reason for one or more radiographs after tube insertion. *Rationale:* Knowledge may decrease anxiety and fear of the unknown.
- Discuss the reasons for not pulling at the tube once it has been placed and secured. *Rationale:* Leaving the tube in place avoids the need for reinsertion and another radiograph for verification. Dislodging the tube can increase the risk of aspiration.

PATIENT ASSESSMENT AND PREPARATION

Patient Assessment

- Assess the patient for the presence of contraindications for nasal placement of small-bore feeding tubes, including head or neck cancer or surgery; recent basilar skull fracture; history of transsphenoidal surgery, including pituitary resection; facial, nasal, or sinus trauma; esophageal cancer; and severe clotting abnormalities.[6,9] *Rationale:* These conditions carry a high risk for complications from passage of the tube through the nasopharyngeal area. Intracranial placement of small-bore feeding tubes has occurred with the nasal approach in patients with basilar skull fracture. The orogastric route is a safer alternative in this situation.
- Assess GI function. *Rationale:* A functional GI tract is essential for safe and effective tube feeding. The integrity and function of the GI tract guide decisions regarding the optimal location for delivery of nutrients (gastric vs. post-pyloric tip position).

Patient Preparation

- Verify the correct patient with two identifiers. *Rationale:* Patients should be correctly identified before any intended intervention.
- Assess the patient and family's understanding of the procedure, answer questions as they arise, and reinforce information as needed. *Rationale:* Engaging with the patient and family ensures that they are included in the plan of care and provides an opportunity to ensure understanding.
- If the patient has an existing large-bore feeding tube, assess for continued need. If no longer clinically warranted, discontinue the tube before placing a small-bore tube. *Rationale:* In some cases, the large-bore tube may remain in place to allow gastric decompression while postpyloric feeding is administered through the nasoenteric tube. If there is a need to discontinue the large-bore tube, the large-bore tube should be discontinued before insertion of the small-bore tube to avoid any risk for dislodgment of the small-bore tube.
- Perform oral care to moisten the mucosa. Suction the oropharyngeal area of excess secretions. *Rationale:* A moist, cleared oropharyngeal area facilitates patient comfort and passage of the tube.

Procedure	**for Small-Bore Feeding Tube Insertion and Care**	
Steps	Rationale	Special Considerations
1. **HH**		
2. **PE**		
3. Verfiy the correct patient with two identifiers.		
4. Encourage the patient to sit in an upright position and tip the head forward, if not contraindicated. If the patient can tolerate upright positioning, position the patient laterally to the right side for insertion of the tube. Ensure that the patient is in a comfortable position.[6] **(Level E*)**	Proper positioning helps facilitate passage of the tube into the esophagus.	
5. Estimate the depth of tube insertion.	Measuring allows the provider to determine the length of the portion of the feeding tube that will need to be advanced into the naris during the insertion procedure for the tip of the tube to reach the patient's stomach.	
A. For nasogastric tube placement: i. Measure the tube from the tip of nose to the earlobe and then from the earlobe to the xiphoid process. Add an additional 10 cm, and mark the tube with the permanent marker.[8] **(Level D*)**	Adding an additional 10cm helps ensure gastric tube placement.[8]	

*Level D: Peer-reviewed professional and organizational standards with the support of clinical study recommendations.

*Level E: Multiple case reports, theory-based evidence from expert opinions, or peer-reviewed professional organizational standards without clinical studies to support recommendations.

Procedure for Small-Bore Feeding Tube Insertion and Care—*Continued*

Steps	Rationale	Special Considerations

B. For postpyloric tube placement:
  i. Measure the tube from the tip of the nose to the earlobe, and then from the earlobe to the xiphoid process.
  ii. Add 20–30 cm of length to the tube, and mark the tube with permanent marker.[7] **(Level E*)**		

6. Place the protective pad or towel on the patient as appropriate.	Laying a protective pad across the patient's chest protects their clothing from any possible soiling that may occur.	
7. Lubricate the tip of the tube with purified or sterile water if the tube is prelubricated. Consider flushing the tube before insertion to lubricate the stylet. **(Level M*)**	Water activates a lubricant on the surface of the tube to facilitate passage through the nares. Flushing the tube eases the removal of the stylet once in place.	If the tube does not have self-lubrication, a water-soluble lubricant can be applied to the tube for patient comfort.
8. Insert the tip of the tube into either naris; advance to the posterior pharynx until resistance is met.[9] **(Level D*)**	Once the tube is advanced through the naris, the oropharynx is reached and the tube meets resistance. Coughing may indicate that the tube has entered the airway, the tube should be withdrawn into the nasopharynx before advancement of the tube.[9]	If coughing occurs or if the patient's oxygen saturation falls as the tube is advanced, withdraw it until breathing and oxygenation return to baseline before trying to advance the tube further.[5]
9. Ask the patient to swallow. If the patient can cooperate and safely swallow, give small sips of water to attempt to trigger the swallow reflex and ease tube passage.[9] **(Level E*)**	Swallowing immediately assists passage of the tube into the esophagus.[9]	
10. As the patient swallows, advance the tube to the predetermined marking for either gastric or postpyloric placement. Do not remove the guidewire. **(Level M*)**	The initial swallow gets the tube into the esophagus, and the nurse can advance it to the desired position without repeated swallowing.	If the patient is unconscious or unable to assist, do not attempt to use water orally to pass the tube.
11. Using tape, temporarily secure the tube to the patient's face. If using a guidewire, do not remove the guidewire until tube placement is confirmed.		• The guidewire may be left in and removed after radiographic verification. • The stylet should never be reinserted while the tube is in the patient.
12. If the desired placement is in the stomach, use two or more of the following methods to predict tube location or placement.[1,5] **(Level B*)** A. Observe for signs of respiratory distress. B. Use capnography if available. C. Measure the pH of aspirate from the tube if pH strips are available. D. Obtain aspirate, and observe if the aspirate is consistent with gastric contents.	Using two or more methods may help predict proper tube placement.[1,5]	

*Level B: Well-designed, controlled studies with results that consistently support a specific action, intervention, or treatment.
*Level D: Peer-reviewed professional and organizational standards with the support of clinical study recommendations.
*Level E: Multiple case reports, theory-based evidence from expert opinions, or peer-reviewed professional organizational standards without clinical studies to support recommendations.
*Level M: Manufacturer's recommendations only.

Procedure continues on following page

UNIT VIII

Procedure for Small-Bore Feeding Tube Insertion and Care—*Continued*

Steps	Rationale	Special Considerations
13. Remove **PE**, and discard used supplies.		
14. **HH**		
15. Obtain a chest or abdominal radiograph to confirm that tube placement is in the intended location. **(Level A*)**	Radiograph is considered the gold standard and safest way to ensure correct placement.[2,5]	Never use air bolus or water bubbling method to verify tube location as these methods have been proven to be unreliable.[1,2,5] **(Level B*)**
16. **HH**		
17. **PE**		
18. If postpyloric placement was intended but unsuccessful, position the patient on the right side (if not already) for several hours, and recheck the location via radiography until the tube migrates past the pylorus.[2] If the tube does not migrate, consult with the provider to determine whether a prokinetic agent can be administered. Repeat the radiograph until postpyloric placement is achieved and confirmed via radiograph.	Right-sided positioning and peristalsis may help pass the tube through the pylorus.[1] Prokinetic agents may help assist in moving the tube through the pyloric sphincter.[2]	The ideal tube tip location is at the fourth portion of the duodenum or in the jejunum. High doses of metoclopramide should be used with caution, as it can lead to tardive dyskinesia.
19. Once tube placement is confirmed, remove the guidewire if one was used by holding the tube securely at the naris with one hand and pulling gently on the guidewire with the other hand.		
20. Ensure that the exit site of the tube is marked at the naris with a permanent marker.[2,4]	Marking the tube at the exit site allows for frequent assessment of tube displacement.[2,4]	
21. Apply a skin preparation to the nose and securing surface of the nose/face; allow it to dry.[5] **(Level E*)**	Prepares the surface of skin to help with the tape adhering.	Using a skin preparation agent can reduce the risk for skin breakdown.
22. Secure the tube in place using a commercial fixation device or tape, while avoiding any excess pressure on the skin. If tape is used, tape the tube securely to the nose with one-half of a 3-cm strip. The lower portion of the tape is then split up to the tip of the nose and wrapped around the tube.	Avoiding excess pressure on the skin mitigates the risk of skin breakdown.	Consider using a commercial tube fixation device if it is available.[6]
23. Remove **PE**, and discard used supplies.		
24. **HH**		

*Level A: Meta-analysis of quantitative studies or metasynthesis of qualitative studies with results that consistently support a specific action, intervention, or treatment (including systematic review of randomized controlled trials).

*Level B: Well-designed, controlled studies with results that consistently support a specific action, intervention, or treatment.

*Level E: Multiple case reports, theory-based evidence from expert opinions, or peer-reviewed professional organizational standards without clinical studies to support recommendations.

Expected Outcomes

- The distal tip of tube is placed in either the stomach or the small bowel.
- Patient tolerates enteral feedings, medications, and fluid.
- The tube remains patent.
- No skin injury is associated with tube placement.
- The patient is able to swallow oral foods and fluids while the small-bore feeding tube is in place, if allowed.

Unexpected Outcomes

- Coughing or dyspnea, indicating potential bronchial placement[3,6]
- Pneumothorax from inadvertent pleural placement[3]
- Tube coiled in the esophagus or posterior pharynx[9]
- Esophageal tear resulting from trauma of the passing tube[9]
- Epistaxis or sinusitis[6,9]
- Tube dislodging during therapy, necessitating removal and new tube placement
- Clogging of the enteral tube with medication fragments or enteral formula[9]
- Skin injury associated with placement[9]

Patient Monitoring and Care

Steps	Rationale	Reportable Conditions
		These conditions should be reported to the provider if they persist despite nursing interventions.
1. Monitor the patient's tolerance to tube placement.	Agitation may inhibit successful placement. A change in tube length can indicate that the tip of the tube may be in an unintended location.[2] Coughing, vomiting, or respiratory symptoms may indicate tube dislodgment or aspiration.[2]	• Inability to tolerate tube placement, self-extubation, or agitation • Persistent coughing, vomiting, dyspnea, or decrease in oxygen saturation • Patient removal of the tube, requiring reassessment and replacement of the tube
2. Assess the oral cavity, and perform oral care per organizational standards.	Mouth breathing dries secretions, encouraging bacterial growth and mucosal breakdown.	• Ulceration • Foul odor
3. Monitor the insertion site of the tube for redness, swelling, drainage, bleeding, or skin breakdown.[8]	Many critically ill patients have fragile skin and have associated conditions that predispose them to skin breakdown. Frequent monitoring and subsequent repositioning of the tube can prevent serious damage.	• Redness • Swelling • Drainage • Bleeding • Ulceration or signs of skin breakdown at the insertion site
4. Regularly assess the tube every 4 hours to ensure that it has remained in its intended position.[1,2,5] **(Level B*)** Retape the tube, or replace the commercial securement device as needed if it becomes loose or soiled.	A decrease in tube length at the point of insertion may indicate that the tube is no longer in correct placement and may be higher up in the GI tract. Radiographic confirmation may be needed.[2,5]	• Concerns related to tube displacement
5. Monitor and assess the patient during periods of persistent coughing, vomiting, and agitation and if the patient requires vigorous suctioning.[5]	Coughing and vomiting may force the tube up the GI tract and place the patient at risk for aspiration.	• Agitation, persistent coughing or vomiting, dyspnea, or agitation

*Level B: Well-designed, controlled studies with results that consistently support a specific action, intervention, or treatment.

UNIT VIII

Procedure continues on following page

Patient Monitoring and Care —*Continued*

Steps	Rationale	Reportable Conditions
6. Frequently flush the feeding tube with: A. 15 mL of purified or sterile water following medication administration.[2] B. 30 mL of water before or after feedings and every 4 hours during continuous feeds.[2]	Frequent flushing helps maintain the patency of the tube.[2]	
7. If necessary, carry out interventions to unclog the enteral feeding tube:[2] A. Instill the 30–60 mL syringe into the enteral access device, and apply a gentle back-and-forth motion to the syringe plunger. B. If water does not resolve the clog, consider consulting with the provider to use an uncoated pancreatic enzyme solution. C. Consider using an enzyme-containing declogging kit if available within the organization.		• Obstruction that is not relieved
8. Assess and treat pain as clinically appropriate.		

Documentation

Documentation should include the following:
- The type, size, and location of the tube inserted
- Patient tolerance to the procedure
- The length (in centimeters) of the tube at the naris or lip
- Radiographic confirmation of the tube position
- Unexpected outcomes and any associated nursing interventions to provide support
- Nursing interventions
- Medications administered per organizational requirements
- Patient and family education

References and Additional Readings

For a complete list of references and additional readings for this procedure, scan this QR code with your smartphone, or visit https://www.elsevier.com/__data/assets/pdf_file/0011/1319897/Chapter0122.pdf

123 Small-Bore Feeding Tube Insertion Using Guidance Systems

Jacqueline Crawford and Heather M. Etzl

PURPOSE The use of electromagnetic technology can assist with safe bedside placement of small-bore nasoenteric feeding tubes. The guidance system helps avoid intubation of the pulmonary system and facilitates postpyloric placement of these tubes.[10,12,21]

PREREQUISITE NURSING KNOWLEDGE

- Upper respiratory and gastrointestinal anatomy and physiology.
- Correct placement of the receiver unit is required to provide an accurate tracing of the tube path.
- Proficiency in assessing the lungs and abdomen.
- Clinical and technical competence in placement of small-bore feeding tubes and in use of electromagnetic guidance devices.[6,18]
- Recognition of risk factors associated with placement errors during insertion of small-bore feeding tubes including endotracheal intubation, advanced age, altered level of consciousness, and diminished reflexes for airway protection.[22]
- An understanding of the benefits of enteral nutrition, including indications for postpyloric placement.[9,17]
- When small-bore feeding tube placement is clinically contraindicated.

EQUIPMENT

- Feeding tube placement device (Fig. 123.1)
- Small-bore feeding tube with electromagnetic transmitting stylet
- Irrigation tray
- 50-mL or larger enteral compatible syringe
- Water (tap water or sterile water based on institutional policy)
- Nonsterile gloves
- Water-soluble lubricant
- Water-absorbent barrier to protect the patient's clothing
- Tape or other securing device

Additional equipment, to have available as needed, includes the following:

- Gowns, goggles
- Viscous lidocaine (optional)
- Stethoscope

PATIENT AND FAMILY EDUCATION

- Explain the essential role adequate nutritional status plays in promoting wound healing and recovery from illness. *Rationale:* Explanation may elicit cooperation and allay patient and family anxiety.
- Explain why a feeding tube is needed to ensure adequate nutritional intake. *Rationale:* Explanation may elicit cooperation and facilitate tube insertion.
- Outline the steps of the procedure and the patient's role during feeding tube insertion (e.g., positioning, swallowing as instructed). *Rationale:* Patient cooperation may facilitate insertion.
- Describe the typical sensations experienced during feeding tube insertion. *Rationale:* Explanation may alleviate anxiety and promote patient cooperation.
- Reinforce the importance of using care when changing position or getting out of bed once the tube is placed. *Rationale:* Emphasis may aid in preventing inadvertent dislodgment of the tube.

PATIENT ASSESSMENT AND PREPARATION

Patient Assessment

- Verify that the patient has no implanted medical devices that may be affected by electromagnetic fields. *Rationale:* The electromagnetic guidance system is generally contraindicated for patients with implanted medical devices because of the potential for electromagnetic interference to affect the function of the implanted device or the electromagnetic guidance system. However, no contraindication exists specifically for defibrillators and pacemakers.[3]
- Assess the patient for the presence of absolute contraindications for nasal placement of small-bore feeding tubes without direct visualization, including recent basilar skull fracture; history of transsphenoidal surgery; facial, nasal, or sinus trauma; bariatric surgery; or severe clotting abnormalities. *Rationale:* These conditions carry a high

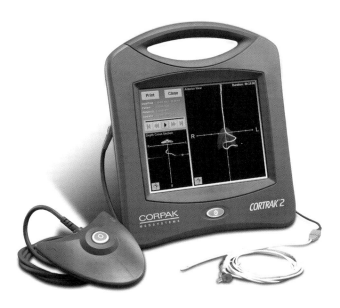

Figure 123.1   The Cortrak 2 Enteral Access System. *(Used with permission from Avanos Medical, Alpharetta, GA.)*

risk for complications from passage of the tube through the nasopharyngeal area. Intracranial placement of small-bore feeding tubes has occurred with the nasal approach in patients with basilar skull fracture. The orogastric route is a safer alternative in this situation.[7,14,20]

- Insertion of small-bore feeding tubes in a patient with a history of bariatric surgery requires direct visualization via fluoroscopy or endoscopy because of the risk of perforation at anastomosis sites at staple lines.[5,23,19]
- Evaluate the patient for relative contraindications to nasal or oral placement of a small-bore feeding tube, including esophageal varices with recent bleeding or ligation within 72 hours; esophageal obstruction; recent esophageal surgery or esophageal stent; history of gastrointestinal surgery with altered anatomical pathways; gastroesophageal reflux; hiatal hernia; gastroparesis (unless feeding postpyloric); nasal polyps or other septal abnormalities; sinusitis; and minor to moderate clotting abnormalities. ***Rationale:***

These conditions carry a relative risk for complications from passage of the tube through the nasopharyngeal route. Placement of the tube may still be undertaken if the assessment of benefit outweighs the risk.[7,13,16,20]

- Assess gastrointestinal function. ***Rationale:*** A functional gastrointestinal tract is essential for safe and effective tube feeding. The integrity and function of the gastrointestinal tract guide decisions regarding the optimal location for delivery of nutrients (gastric vs. postpyloric tip position).[12]

Patient Preparation

- Verify the correct patient with two identifiers. ***Rationale:*** Before performing a procedure, the nurse should ensure the correct identification of the patient for the intended intervention.
- Ensure that the patient and family understand the preprocedural teaching. Answer questions as they arise, and reinforce information as needed. ***Rationale:*** Understanding of previously taught information is evaluated and reinforced.
- Ensure that informed consent has been obtained if required by hospital policy. ***Rationale:*** Informed consent protects the rights of the patient and allows the patient to make a competent decision.
- Perform a preprocedural verification and time-out, if nonemergent. ***Rationale:*** This ensures patient safety.
- Assess the need to remove any existing large-bore feeding tube. ***Rationale:*** In some cases, the large-bore tube may remain in place to allow gastric decompression while delivery of enteral formula takes place in the small intestine. When the large-bore tube is to be replaced by a small-bore tube, the larger tube should be removed before the new tube is passed to avoid dislodging the small-bore tube during removal of the large-bore tube.
- If ordered, administer a prokinetic agent such as metoclopramide or erythromycin 10 minutes before the procedure to aid in postpyloric tube placement. Metoclopramide is used with caution because prolonged administration at higher doses is associated with the development of tardive dyskinesia. ***Rationale:*** Enhanced gastric motility facilitates passage of the tube distal to the pylorus.[5,16]

Procedure **for Small-Bore Feeding Tube Insertion Using an Electromagnetic Guidance System**

Steps	Rationale	Special Considerations
1. 🔲		
2. 🔲		
3. Place a water-absorbent barrier to protect the patient's clothing.	Prepares for the procedure.	
4. Assist the patient to the supine position with the head of the bed elevated to at least 30 degrees unless contraindicated.[7]	The patient should be positioned as straight as possible for accurate tracking of the feeding tube. This position helps facilitate the initial advancement of the tube into the esophagus.	
5. Activate the electromagnetic device.	Provides power.	Hold the button until the power is on.
6. Allow the unit to perform a self-test for about 5 seconds.	Prepares the equipment.	If a fault is detected, the receiver unit will flash red. The fault is cleared and receiver functionality verified by unplugging and replugging the receiver from the monitor.
7. Log in by typing your username and password.	Prepares the equipment.	Log in and username procedures are determined by organizational policy.
8. Press "New Placement."	Prepares the equipment.	
9. Enter patient information; follow institutional standards.	The device can store a record of the insertion for future reference.	
10. Place the leading foot of the receiver unit over the patient's xiphoid process. The receiver unit cord will be directed toward the patient's feet (Fig. 123.2).	The receiver unit must be parallel to the spine and centered along the midline to ensure reliable tracking of the tube during placement. Incorrect placement of the receiver alters the appearance of the tracing, making it difficult to interpret the path viewed on the screen.	A weighted band is available to place over the receiver unit for added stability. The receiver can be propped into position with a wedge or cloth to keep the receiver unit parallel to the spine. Do not reposition the receiver unit once it has been correctly placed on the xiphoid process. Movement of the receiver unit alters the alignment and the relationship of the track displayed on the monitor unit.

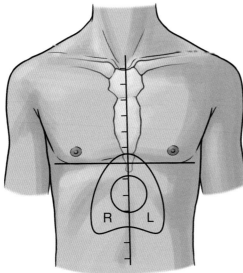

Figure 123.2 Receiver unit placement. *(Used with permission from Avanos Medical, Alpharetta, GA.)*

UNIT VIII

Procedure continues on following page

Procedure	for Small-Bore Feeding Tube Insertion Using an Electromagnetic Guidance System—*Continued*	
Steps	Rationale	Special Considerations
11. Flush the feeding tube with water, and dip the tip of the tube in water. Cap the medication port. Move the stylet a few centimeters in and out of the tube. Ensure that the stylet is firmly seated in the feeding tube.	If the stylet is moving within the tube during insertion, the tracing on the monitor is inaccurate. Water activates a lubricant that has been applied to the internal and external surface of the tube. This ensures that the stylet moves freely out of the tube once the desired position is achieved.	Observe for patency or leaks in the tube during flushing.
12. Connect the proximal end of the feeding tube transmitter stylet to the stylet interconnect cable on the monitor unit, connecting arrow to arrow.	The feeding tube uses a special electromagnetic stylet that transmits a signal during tube insertion.	Arrows that appear on both the stylet and the cable connectors will only fit together one way, acting as a guide to prevent damage to the equipment during connection.
13. Lubricate the distal end of the tube with water-soluble jelly. Note that viscous lidocaine may be used if prescribed by the physician or advanced practice nurse.[15] **(Level A*)**	Minimizes mucosal injury, facilitates insertion, and promotes patient comfort.	Oil-soluble lubricants should not be used because they are not absorbed by the pulmonary mucosa and may cause complications.
14. Insert the feeding tube into the nares, and advance the tube gently along the base of the nostril.		
15. After inserting the feeding tube to the back of the patient's throat (approximately 10 cm), press "Start" either on the monitor unit or the central button on the receiver unit to begin to view the tube tip position.	An "Out of Range" message appears on the screen if the unit is started prematurely. Resistance at approximately 25 cm may indicate contact with the piriform sinus and would require retraction of the tube and gentle readvancement.[2]	If the "Out of Range" message still appears at 30–35 cm, the tube is likely coiled in the mouth or throat. A receiver unit self-test is done, and the monitor indicates that the receiver is working before the tube tip is displayed. Withdraw the tube, and reinsert according to the aforementioned instructions.
16. Ask the patient to swallow if able. Advance the tube to coincide with the swallowing maneuver. If allowed, give the patient sips of water or ice chips.	Swallowing assists passage of the tube into the esophagus.	If the patient is unable to swallow, position the patient's chin to his or her chest if feasible to assist with passage of the tube into the esophagus.

*Level A: Meta-analysis of quantitative studies or meta-synthesis of qualitative studies with results that consistently support a specific action, intervention, or treatment (including systematic review of randomized controlled trials).

Procedure for Small-Bore Feeding Tube Insertion Using an Electromagnetic Guidance System—*Continued*

Steps	Rationale	Special Considerations
17. Follow the path of the tube tip by the tracing of the illuminated dot on the view screen and the depth tracing on the depth cross-section view (Fig. 123.3). The lateral screen can also be used to monitor depth (Fig. 123.4).[3] **(Level M*)**	The depth cross-section and lateral screens show the distance of the tube tip from the sternum. The relatively posterior anatomical location of the esophagus and the duodenum is reflected by greater depth of these structures in relation to the stomach. A deviation from the expected path may indicate a placement error.[2,3]	During the placement procedure or placement review, the operator is presented with touch screen buttons (toggle buttons) that allow toggling between the major view and the minor view. Before or during the placement process, the operator can press one of the toggle buttons in the major view portion of the screen to toggle the major view between the anterior view (default) and the lateral view. When the lateral view is displayed in the major view pane, the anterior view is displayed in the minor view pane, and the minor toggle button is disabled. When the major view is toggled, the minor view pane returns to the view displayed before the initial toggle of the major view. During placement, while the anterior view is displayed in the major view portion of the screen, the operator can press the toggle button in the minor view portion to toggle the minor view between the depth cross-section and the lateral views.[2,3]

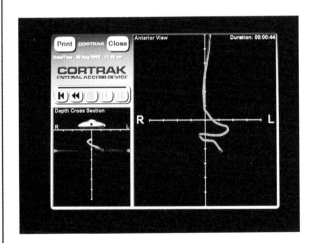

Figure 123.3 CORTRAK screen display, anterior and depth cross-section views. *(Used with permission from Avanos Medical, Alpharetta, GA.)*

*Level M: Manufacturer's recommendations only.

Procedure continues on following page

UNIT VIII

Procedure | **for Small-Bore Feeding Tube Insertion Using an Electromagnetic Guidance System—*Continued***

Steps	Rationale	Special Considerations

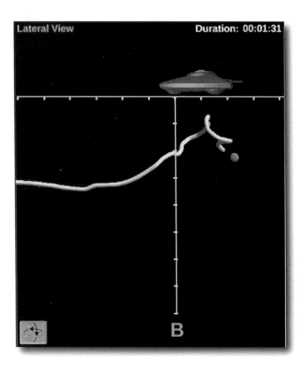

Figure 123.4   Lateral view, major screen. *(Used with permission from Avanos Medical, Alpharetta, GA.)*

Steps	Rationale	Special Considerations
18. If the patient develops coughing or has signs or symptoms of respiratory distress or if the tracing veers sharply into the upper right or left quadrant at approximately 35–40 cm, slowly retract the feeding tube to 15 cm to erase the track, and restart the placement procedure.[2,3] **(Level M*)**	This finding may indicate a tube in the bronchus. Slowly pulling back the feeding tube clears the tracing of the placement attempt. A new track is visible as the placement resumes. If resistance is met, do not continue to push the tube. Withdraw the feeding tube at this point, and then continue to advance the feeding tube down the esophagus and into the stomach.	Restarting the device is not necessary. The feeding tube should slide down the esophagus easily. Median distance from the naris to the tracheoesophageal junction is about 20 cm.[7,11] The length of tube needed to reach the stomach is approximately 60 cm; additional length is needed for postpyloric placement.[11]
19. If the feeding tube tip is not moving forward as the tube is inserted, slowly retract the feeding tube until the colored dot begins to move, and then proceed with placement.[2,3]	This may indicate that the tube is coiling rather than advancing. Coiled loops behind the transmitter are not visible on the monitor. The pathway through the stomach should resemble a backward C shape. If gastric placement is desired, the procedure is complete.	
20. If postpyloric placement is the goal, continue advancing the tube across midline. Assess configuration of the display pattern (pathway and depth) to determine whether the tube is appropriately positioned in the postpyloric region (see Fig. 123.3).[2,3] **(Level M*)**	The pathway through the duodenum often resembles a smaller, forward C shape. When the depth indicator is several notches below the horizontal axis, duodenal tube tip location is likely.	Instilling a bolus of air into the tube when the tip is nearing the pylorus may facilitate relaxation of the pylorus and aid in passage into the small bowel. A duodenum that is more posterior may show an upward curve in the anterior view before the tube passes farther into the duodenum.
21. Press "End" on the monitor display or the orange button on the receiver. **(Level M*)**	Stops the recording or timing of the insertion procedure.	

*Level M: Manufacturer's recommendations only.

Procedure **for Small-Bore Feeding Tube Insertion Using an Electromagnetic Guidance System—*Continued***

Steps	Rationale	Special Considerations
22. At this point, the stylet may or may not be removed. Save the stylet in a clean bag (see **Step 29**).	The feeding tube is well visualized using radiography with or without the stylet in place; the stylet that comes with the tube may be reinserted to check tube position.	The U.S. Food and Drug Administration approved reinsertion of the transmitting stylet for periodic confirmation of tip location.[2,3]
23. Secure the feeding tube with tape or a commercial fixation device.	Decreases the risk of inadvertent removal or change in position of the tube.	Avoid undue pressure on the naris from the tube to prevent skin breakdown. The tube should be secured floating approximately 1 cm below the naris. Consider the use of a nasal bridle system to secure the tube against accidental removal with use of a loop of plastic tubing through one naris, around the vomer bone, and back out of the other naris. The feeding tube is secured to this bridle.[4]
24. Press "Print" to obtain a tracing of the placement (Fig. 123.5).	The tracing can be used as part of confirming placement and documentation per institutional policy.	If the alternate depth view printout is desired, toggle during playback to allow printing of the depth cross-section or lateral view.
25. Disconnect the transmitting stylet from the interconnect cable.	The procedure is complete.	
26. Press "Close" on the monitor unit; press "Shutdown."	The procedure is complete.	Do not use the orange button to power off.

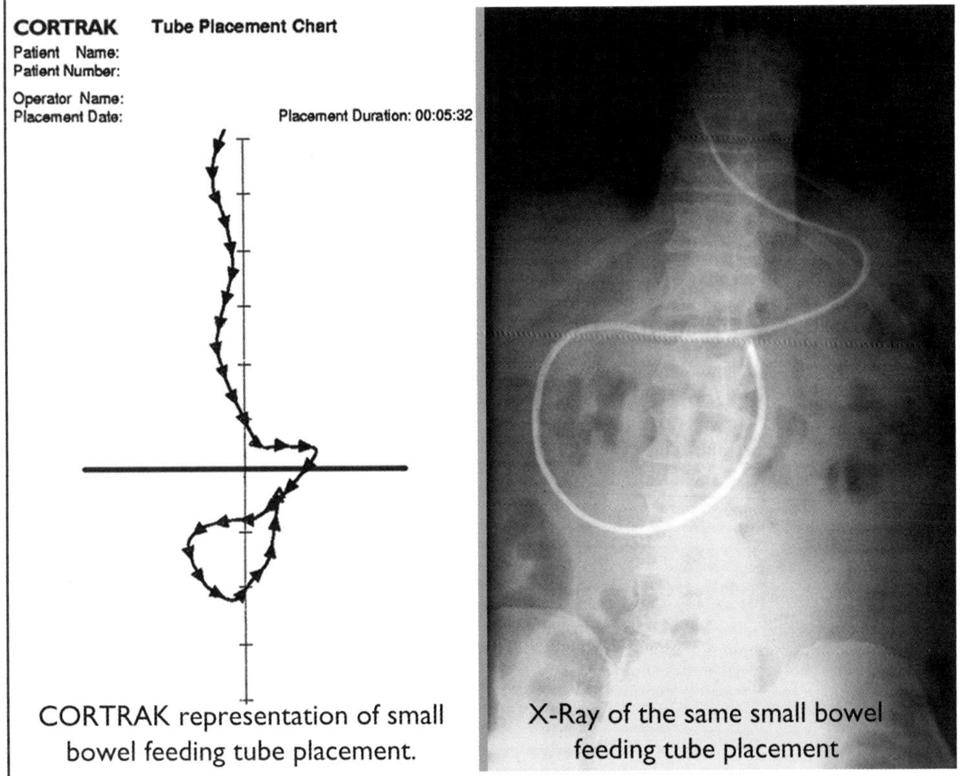

CORTRAK Tube Placement Chart

Patient Name:
Patient Number:

Operator Name:
Placement Date: Placement Duration: 00:05:32

CORTRAK representation of small bowel feeding tube placement.

X-Ray of the same small bowel feeding tube placement

Figure 123.5 Comparison of x-ray with CORTRAK 2 EAS printout. *(Used with permission from Avanos Medical, Alpharetta, GA.)*

UNIT VIII

Procedure continues on following page

Steps	Rationale	Special Considerations
27. Obtain radiographic confirmation of correct placement of the tube before its initial use for feedings or medication administration.[1] **(Level A*)**	Radiographic confirmation with abdominal radiography is the gold standard for determining the exact tube position after insertion.[1,6,18] The tip of the tube usually is not visible on chest radiography. Some evidence indicates that well-trained and experienced clinicians can achieve a high level of success in placing feeding tubes when a Cortrak device is used. Successful use of this device is dependent on the user's familiarity and dexterity with the device.[6,18]	Gastric auscultation of an air bolus through the tube, aspiration of fluid from the tube, and placement of the proximal end of the feeding tube under water while observing for bubbles are all unreliable methods to confirm placement in the gastrointestinal tract.[1] Numerous cases have been reported in which clinicians failed to recognize placement of feeding tubes in the respiratory tract while using Cortrak guidance; some of these have been associated with fatal outcomes.[1,18]
28. When proper location of the feeding tube is confirmed, flush with 5–10 mL of water if not flushed before insertion.[2,3] **(Level M*)**	Activates internal lubrication to allow easier removal of the stylet.	Failure to flush the feeding tube for stylet removal may damage the feeding tube.
29. Remove the stylet before administering feedings.[2,3] **(Level M*)**	The stylet can be reinserted into its original tube while attached to the system to reverify the tube's position.	Clean the stylet with an alcohol swab, and store it in the bag provided by the manufacturer for this use. Label it with the patient's identification.
30. Note the centimeter marking on the tube at the tip of the patient's nose to identify the depth of tube placement.[16,18]	A simple bedside assessment for displacement is to monitor the tube for a change in the external length.[16,18]	This information lets other healthcare providers know whether the tube has been inadvertently pulled out of position. Rethreading of the stylet requires attachment of the electromagnetic transmitter stylet to the Cortrak system.
31. Remove **PE**, and discard used supplies.		
32. **HH**		
33. Ensure that the system components are cleaned.[3] **(Level M*)**	Prepares for future use.	Prevents microbial cross-contamination between patients.

*Level A: Meta-analysis of quantitative studies or meta-synthesis of qualitative studies with results that consistently support a specific action, intervention, or treatment (including systematic review of randomized controlled trials).
*Level M: Manufacturer's recommendations only.

Expected Outcomes

- The distal tip of the feeding tube rests in the stomach or small intestine
- The patient tolerates enteral feeding at rates that meet established goals
- The patient is able to swallow oral foods and fluids while the small-bore tube is in place, if appropriate
- The small-bore tube accepts enteral feedings, medications, and fluid

Unexpected Outcomes

- Coughing, dyspnea, oxygen desaturation, and restlessness/anxiety indicate potential pulmonary placement
- Pneumothorax from inadvertent pleural placement
- Pulmonary aspiration of gastric contents
- Epistaxis or esophageal injury during passage of the tube
- Inadvertent tube dislodgment
- Skin irritation or breakdown at the nose
- Occluded feeding tube
- Sinusitis or otitis media

Patient Monitoring and Care

Steps	Rationale	Reportable Conditions
		These conditions should be reported to the provider if they persist despite nursing interventions.
1. Monitor the length of the tube in the patient and tolerance to tube placement.[16,8]	Placement may be difficult in agitated patients. A change in tube length can indicate that the tip of the tube may be in an unintended location. Coughing, vomiting, or respiratory symptoms may indicate tube dislodgment or aspiration.[1]	• Inability to tolerate tube placement • Inadvertent removal of the tube (partial or complete) • Coughing, vomiting, dyspnea, or decrease in oxygen saturation
2. Assess the oral cavity, and perform oral care per institutional standards.	Mouth breathing dries secretions, encouraging bacterial growth and mucosal breakdown.	
3. Ensure that the tube is secured in a way that avoids pressure on the naris. Assess the insertion site for drainage, bleeding, redness, swelling, or ulceration.	Pressure from the tube can compromise blood flow to the tissue and cause skin damage and infection.	• Drainage • Bleeding • Redness • Swelling • Ulceration
4. Follow institutional standards for assessing pain. Administer analgesia as prescribed.	Identifies the need for pain interventions.	• Continued pain despite pain interventions.

Documentation

Documentation should include the following:
- Type and size of the tube inserted
- Length of tube inserted per the tube's measurement marking at the naris
- Patient response to the insertion
- Unexpected outcomes
- Radiographic confirmation of the tube position and printed tracings per institutional requirements
- Nursing interventions
- Medications administered
- Patient and family education

References and Additional Readings

For a complete list of references and additional readings for this procedure, scan this QR code with your smartphone, or visit https://www.elsevier.com/__data/assets/pdf_file/0012/1319898/Chapter0123.pdf.

UNIT VIII

PROCEDURE

124 Thermoregulation: Heating, Cooling, and Targeted Temperature Management

Nancy Freeland

PURPOSE An external surface blanket, a hydrogel pad temperature-management device, an internal intravascular warming and cooling device, or a semi-invasive esophageal thermal regulation device may be used to increase or decrease the body temperature.[12,14] All of these devices may be used to regulate patient temperature or as therapeutic treatment modalities to reduce body temperature after acute injury (e.g., global cerebral ischemia, cardiac arrest, or hypoxia), thereby decreasing cellular oxygen consumption and intracranial pressure. Decreasing cerebral blood flow improves the discrepancy between oxygen supply and oxygen demand.[3,4]

PREREQUISITE NURSING KNOWLEDGE

- The hypothalamus is the primary thermoregulatory center for the body and where the central sensors for the body core temperature are located; it maintains normothermia through internal regulation of heat production or heat loss. Information is sent from the brain, spinal cord, deep abdominal and thoracic tissue, and thermosensors underneath the skin to the hypothalamus.[13]
- In the preoptic area of the hypothalamus, thermosensitive neurons incorporate information from the peripheral and blood receptors and compare it with the body's set point. The body reacts when there is a difference between the set point and the actual temperature.
- Through a negative feedback loop, warm and cold sensory neurons respond to feedback from the peripheral sensors and balance their signals to maintain a set point of 37.0°C (98.6°F).[6,24]
- When the thermal area of the hypothalamus senses heat gain or a warmer temperature than the set point, the body vasodilates and sweats to assist in lowering the body temperature. Conversely, when the neurons sense a temperature below the set point (heat loss), vasoconstriction and shivering occur to increase catabolism, conserve heat, and raise body temperature.[6,24]
- The body has the following mechanisms to dissipate heat:
  - Conduction occurs when heat is lost by direct transfer from one surface to a second adjacent cooler object.[5,7]
  - Convection occurs when heat is transferred from a surface to surrounding air.[5,7]
  - Radiation occurs when heat (thermal energy) is transferred through air or space between separated surfaces without direct contact between the objects.[5,7]
  - Evaporation occurs when heat loss accompanies water evaporated from the skin and respiratory tract to the surrounding air.[5,7]
- Knowledge of terms associated with temperature (Table 124.1).
- Alterations in thermoregulation can result from a primary central nervous system injury or disease (e.g., subarachnoid hemorrhage, traumatic brain injury, spinal cord injury, or neoplasm) and metabolic conditions (e.g., diabetes mellitus, toxic levels of ethanol alcohol or other drugs such as barbiturates and phenothiazine agents).
- Body temperature is the measurement of the presence or absence of heat. Body heat is generated, conserved, redistributed, or dissipated during all physiological processes. Factors such as age, circadian rhythm, and hormones influence body temperature.
- Body temperature may be measured with a variety of thermometers and at several body sites. Electronic or digital thermometers are used to obtain rectal, oral, and axillary temperatures. Thermistors within catheters or probes measure rectal, nasopharyngeal, esophageal, bladder, brain, and pulmonary artery temperatures. Infrared thermometers measure tympanic membrane and temporal artery temperatures. Choose the method of temperature monitoring that best meets the patient's clinical condition and obtains results that are reliable, accurate, and safe to support clinical decisions.[26,32]
- When assessing body temperature, some basic aspects must be considered that influence normal thermoregulation, such as age, gender, and site of measurement.
- The best evaluation of body temperature uses the core temperature; it is the least influenced by environmental and other factors and maintains a stable temperature.[24]
- The most accurate core temperature monitoring methods are intravascular (e.g., pulmonary artery catheter), esophageal, and bladder.[32,34,37]

TABLE 124.1	Terms Associated With Temperature
Term	**Definition**
Normothermia/ euthermia	Optimal range of body temperature associated with health.
Hypothermia	Subnormal core body temperature equal to or below 35°C.[22]
Induced hypothermia	Intentional reduction of body temperature to decrease the cerebral metabolic rate of oxygen, intracranial pressure, and cerebral blood volume, thereby improving the oxygen supply-and-demand mismatch.[29] This may be accomplished by surface means (transfer of heat from the skin to the cooling device) or central means (circulatory heat exchange in a cardiopulmonary bypass machine or cooling catheter)
Targeted temperature management	Targeted temperature management is a clinical treatment strategy to control core body temperature (target temperature) for a certain duration to reduce secondary brain injury.[17]
Fever	Fever is a response to either endogenous or exogenous pyrogens or to direct effects on the hypothalamic temperature-control centers.[26]
Hyperthermia	The body temperature is out of control due to failed thermoregulation. The body temperature is high, usually resulting from infection, medication, or head injury.[25,19]

TABLE 124.2	Bedside Shivering Assessment Scale (BSAS)[13]

Score	Term	Description
0	None	No shivering noted on palpation of masseter, neck, or chest wall, and no electrophysiological evidence of shivering (using electrocardiographs)
1	Mild	Shivering localized to neck or thorax only
2	Moderate	Shivering involves gross movement of the upper extremities (in addition to neck and thorax)
3	Severe	Shivering involves gross movements of trunk, upper extremities, and lower extremities

TABLE 124.3	Techniques to Increase Heat Gain

Mechanism of Heat Transfer	Techniques to Increase Heat Gain
Radiation	Warming lights, warm environment, room temperature, blankets
Conduction	Warm blankets, circulating water blanket, continuous arteriovenous rewarming, cardiopulmonary bypass
Convection	Thermal fans, circulating air blanket
Evaporation	Head and body covers; warm, humidified oxygen

- The pulmonary artery catheter is the best representation of core temperature and the gold standard for clinical thermometry.[14,24,26,30,37]
- Regardless of method and site chosen, the same site and same method should be used repeatedly to trend the serial measurements during the application of warming or cooling therapy.[6,22]
- Shivering is an involuntary shaking of the body generated to maintain thermal homeostasis. Shivering causes rhythmic tremors that result in skeletal muscle contraction and is a normal physiological mechanism to generate heat production.[1,8,13]
  - ❖ Early detection of shivering can be accomplished by palpating the mandible and feeling a humming vibration. Electrocardiographic artifacts from skeletal muscle movement are seen on the bedside monitor. If not detected early, shivering can progress from visible twitching of the head or neck to visible twitching of the pectorals or trunk, and then to generalized shaking of the entire body and teeth chattering.[1]
  - ❖ The Bedside Shivering Assessment Scale (BSAS) is a simple and reliable tool for evaluating the metabolic stress of shivering (Table 124.2).[1,13,27]
  - ❖ Shivering may be visible on the Bispectral Index Monitor in the form of an increase in electromyogram activity (see Procedure 83, Signal Processed Electroencephalography).
  - ❖ Shivering increases the metabolic rate, carbon dioxide (CO_2) production, resting energy expenditure, oxygen consumption, and myocardial work, and it lowers brain tissue oxygen levels.[1,13,27]
  - ❖ The overall metabolic consequences of shivering may eliminate many of the clinical benefits of temperature control.[1,27]

- At a body temperature <35°C, the basal metabolic rate can no longer supply sufficient body heat, and an exogenous source of heat is needed.
- Table 124.3 outlines techniques to increase heat gain.
- Hypothermia may be categorized as mild (34°C to 35.9°C), moderate (30°C to 33.9°C), or severe/deep (<30°C).[4] The American Heart Association (AHA) recommends that if ventricular fibrillation or ventricular tachycardia is present with severe hypothermia, defibrillation should be attempted. The value of subsequent defibrillations is uncertain; therefore active rewarming should occur, and the AHA suggests that it may be reasonable to further defibrillate, following the basic life support (BLS) algorithm.[23]
- Hypothermia may be caused by an increase in heat loss, a decrease in heat production, an alteration in thermoregulation, and a variety of clinical conditions.
- An increase in heat loss may occur from the following:[7]
  - ❖ Accidental (e.g., cold water drowning)
  - ❖ Environmental exposure
  - ❖ Induced vasodilation caused by high levels of ethanol alcohol, barbiturates, phenothiazines, or general anesthesia
  - ❖ Central nervous system dysfunction (e.g., spinal cord injury)
  - ❖ Dermal dysfunction (e.g., burns)
  - ❖ Iatrogenic conditions (e.g., administration of cold intravenous fluids, hemodialysis, cardiopulmonary bypass)
  - ❖ Trauma
- A decrease in heat production is associated with the following:
  - ❖ Endocrine conditions (e.g., hypothyroidism)
  - ❖ Malnutrition
  - ❖ Diabetic ketoacidosis

- ❖ Neuromuscular insufficiency (e.g., resulting from a pharmacological paralysis caused by a neuromuscular blocking agent or anesthetic agent)
- Clinical conditions associated with hypothermia are sepsis, hepatic coma, prolonged cardiac arrest, and systemic inflammatory response syndrome.
- Severe hypothermia may mimic death; resuscitative efforts should be initiated despite the absence of vital signs.
- Rewarming for cardiac arrest survivors who have undergone therapeutic hypothermia should not occur faster than 0.25°C to 0.50°C per hour.[4,25,31,32] Rapid rewarming can cause rewarming acidosis, electrolyte shifts, shivering, and hypovolemic shock.
- Rapid rewarming could cause an increase in insulin sensitivity and electrolyte disorders caused by shifts from the intracellular to the extracellular compartment.[10,37]
- Rapid rewarming could lead to loss of some or even all the protective effects of hypothermia.[10,15,32]
- Studies have suggested that there could be a detrimental effect of post–targeted temperature management fever on outcome, so careful control of body temperature for at least 48 hours following the end of rewarming is mandatory. Rewarming acidosis results from the increase in CO_2 production associated with the temperature increase and from the return of accumulated acids in the peripheral circulation to the heart.[10,15,32]
- Rewarming shock occurs when hypothermic vasoconstriction masks hypovolemia. If the patient's circulating volume is insufficient during rewarming vasodilation, sudden decreases in blood pressure, systemic vascular resistance, and preload occur. In cases of severe to profound hypothermia, peripheral rewarming with external devices should be used with extreme caution. Core methods of rewarming should be considered.
- Hyperthermia occurs when the thermoregulatory system of the body absorbs or produces more heat than it can dissipate.[15]
- Malignant hyperthermia is a rare, life-threatening hereditary condition of the skeletal muscle that occurs on exposure to a triggering agent or agents.[18,19,38]
  - ❖ The triggering agents commonly associated with malignant hyperthermia are volatile anesthetic agents, particularly halogenated inhalation anesthetics and/or the depolarizing muscle relaxant succinylcholine.[19,38]
  - ❖ Malignant hyperthermia involves instability of the muscle cell membrane, which causes a sudden increase in myoplasmic calcium and skeletal muscle contractures.
  - ❖ The earliest indication of malignant hyperthermia is an increase in end-tidal carbon dioxide level or hyperventilation while breathing spontaneously. Additional symptoms could include tachycardia, supraventricular or ventricular arrhythmia, masseter spasm, or generalized muscular rigidity.[18,28,38]
  - ❖ A rapid temperature increase of 1°C every several minutes may occur, and this rapid rise is more significant in diagnosing malignant hyperthermia than a peak temperature. The treatment of hyperthermia should be either use of an internal cooling device or a specific surface cooling device.[19,28]
  - ❖ Treatment includes discontinuation of the triggering agent and administration of a muscle relaxant (e.g.,

dantrolene sodium). The muscle relaxant inhibits the release of calcium from the sarcoplasmic reticulum without affecting calcium uptake.[28] Refer to hospital protocol for storage and administration of muscle relaxant.

- Heat stroke is characterized as a rectal temperature greater than 40°C (104°F) and central nervous system dysfunction. It occurs when the outdoor temperature and humidity are excessive, and heat is transferred to the body. Increased humidity prevents the body from cooling by evaporation. Other signs of heat stroke include hypotension, tachycardia, tachypnea, mental status changes from confusion to coma, and possibly seizures. The skin is hot and dry, and sweating may occur. Initial interventions include support of airway, breathing, and circulation. Rapid cooling of the patient is the main treatment priority, with a goal of reducing the temperature to 38.9°C (102°F) as soon as possible.
- Fever occurs in response to a pyrogen and is defined as a temperature greater than 38.3°C.[11] During fever, the hypothalamus retains its function, and shivering and diaphoresis occur to gain or lose body heat. Fever may be an adaptive response and may be considered beneficial in the absence of neurological disease processes. However, a febrile state increases the heart rate and metabolic rate and may be detrimental to a critically ill patient. The question of whether to reduce or treat a fever remains unanswered and must be based on the patient's physical and hemodynamic stability and provider preference.[11]
  - ❖ Fever worsens neurological outcome and increases mortality in neurological patients.[24]
  - ❖ It is thought that fever occurs in approximately 50% of patients in the intensive care unit and is associated with adverse outcomes, including death with high fever.[11]
- Some external warming or cooling devices transfer warmth or coolness to the patient via conduction. Warmed or cooled fluids circulate through coils or channels in a thermal blanket or pad that is commonly placed under the patient.
- Additional warming and cooling systems are available. Hydrogel pads or external wraps can be placed on the patient's skin in the trunk and upper leg regions. These external systems are controlled through a feedback loop system with a core temperature (e.g., a bladder probe, an esophageal probe) that is attached to a central console and automatically regulates the temperature according to programmed temperature target points. The feedback of patient temperature is compared with the set target temperature, and the circulating water temperature is adjusted to ensure that the target temperature is maintained.
- Other external devices transfer warmth to the patient via convection. A device used for warming blows warm air through microperforations on the underside of a blanket that is placed over the patient. The air is directed through the blanket onto the patient's skin.
- The esophageal cooling device induces body temperature change through heat transfer between the esophagus and heart/major vessels. The vena cava, aorta, and left atrium lie near the esophagus, leading to efficient heat exchange with the central circulation.[12] Similar to the external warming and cooling systems, these devices are attached to a console that automatically regulates the temperature according to programmed temperature target points. The

feedback of patient temperature is compared with the set target temperature, and the circulating water temperature is adjusted to ensure that the target temperature is maintained.

- Specific information about controls, alarms, troubleshooting, and safety features is available from each manufacturer and must be understood by the nurse before using the equipment.

EQUIPMENT

- Warming or cooling device
- Sheet or bath blanket
- Nonsterile gloves
- Temperature probe, cable, and module to monitor the patient's temperature (varies based on the type of site and thermometer selected and available)
- Hydrogel pads, external wraps or blankets needed by the equipment that will be used
- Cardiac monitoring (see Procedure 49)
- Appropriate skin-care products (refer to hospital policy)
Additional equipment to have available as needed includes the following:
- Hemodynamic monitoring (see Procedure 59)
- Sterile or distilled water (see manufacturer's recommendations)
- Intravascular cooling/warming central venous catheter
- Start-up tubing kit
- Console, including cable for monitoring temperature
- Central venous catheter insertion tray
- Antiseptic solution
- Sterile drape
- Masks with eye shields, hair cover, sterile gloves, and sterile gowns
- Occlusive dressing
- Antimicrobial (e.g., chlorhexidine gluconate–impregnated disc/dressing)
- Normal saline solution
- Esophageal cooling device
- Waterproof tape or securement device
- Water-soluble lubricant

PATIENT AND FAMILY EDUCATION

- Explain the reason for the use of a warming or cooling device and standard of care, including monitoring of temperature, expected length of therapy, comfort measures, and parameters for discontinuation of the device. *Rationale:* Explanation encourages the patient and family to ask questions and verbalize concerns about the procedure.
- Assess the patient and family understanding of the warming or cooling therapy. *Rationale:* Clarification and reinforcement of information are needed during times of stress and anxiety.
- Encourage the patient to notify the nurse of any discomfort. If the patient is unable to verbalize discomfort, look for signs and symptoms of discomfort such as grimacing, restlessness, and diaphoresis. *Rationale:* Identification of discomfort facilitates early intervention and promotes comfort.

PATIENT ASSESSMENT AND PREPARATION

Patient Assessment

- Assess risk factors, medical history, the cause of the patient's underlying condition, and the type and the length of temperature exposure. *Rationale:* Assessment assists in anticipating, recognizing, and responding to the patient's responses and potential side effects of therapy.
- Assess the patient's medication therapy. *Rationale:* Medications such as vasopressors and vasodilators may affect heat transfer, increase the potential for skin injury, and contribute to an adverse hemodynamic response.
- Obtain a core temperature (e.g., pulmonary artery, esophageal, bladder). *Rationale:* Assessment determines baseline temperature and determines when a warming or cooling device is needed.
- Obtain vital signs and hemodynamic values. *Rationale:* Assessment determines baseline cardiovascular data. Initially, tachycardia and hypertension can occur because of cutaneous vasoconstriction and shivering with attempts at heat conservation.[4,9] Rewarming may cause hypotension from vasodilatation.[4,9]
- Monitor the patient's cardiac rhythm. *Rationale:* Monitoring determines the baseline cardiac rhythm. Most common and well-known electrocardiographic changes include presence of J (Osborn) waves, interval prolongation, and atrial and ventricular arrhythmias.[5] Tachycardia and hypertension may occur as a result of cutaneous vasoconstriction, and shivering may occur as the patient attempts to conserve heat.[4] Once patients begin to cool, bradycardia is the most common arrhythmia, together with PR prolongation, sinus bradycardia, and even junctional or ventricular escape rhythms. Bradycardia should be treated only if it is associated with hypotension. Hypothermia also prolongs the QT interval.[3,4] Tachycardia and ventricular dysrhythmias may occur if the patient is hyperthermic.[4]
- Assess the patient's electrolyte, glucose, arterial blood gas, and coagulation study results. *Rationale:* Alterations in temperature balance may result in acid-base imbalance, coagulopathy, electrolyte imbalance, glycemic imbalance, and hypoxemia.[9,17] Close monitoring of metabolic parameters with careful consideration of replacement during cooling and warming therapy is necessary.[9,17]
- Assess the patient's level of consciousness and neurological function. *Rationale:* Assessment determines baseline neurological status. A change in mental status, level of consciousness, or impaired neurological function may occur because of an undesirable high or low temperature or from the condition causing the alteration in mental status. Fatigue, muscle incoordination, poor

judgment, weakness, hallucinations, lethargy, and stupor may occur with hypothermia. Seizures may occur with hyperthermia.

- Assess the patient's ventilatory function. ***Rationale:*** Hypoventilation, suppression of cough, and mucociliary reflexes associated with hypothermia may lead to hypoxemia, atelectasis, and pneumonia. Hypothermia shifts the oxygenation-dissociation curve to the left, and less oxygen is released from oxyhemoglobin to the tissues. Because of peripheral vasoconstriction, digit-based pulse oximetry is often unreliable. Hyperthermia shifts the oxygenation dissociation curve to the right, and oxygen is readily released from oxyhemoglobin.[30,31]
- Assess the patient's bowel sounds, abdomen, and gastrointestinal function. ***Rationale:*** Assessment determines baseline status. Patients with hypothermia may develop ileus because of decreased intestinal motility. Vomiting and diarrhea may occur with hyperthermia.
- Assess the patient's skin integrity. ***Rationale:*** Assessment provides baseline data. Patients treated with therapeutic hypothermia should be considered at high risk for pressure ulcer development and should be managed accordingly. The hypothermia may not as such increase the risk for pressure ulcers, but combined with the severity of the underlying illness, it may be more likely.[2]

Patient Preparation

- Ensure that the patient and family understand the preprocedural education. Answer questions as they arise, and reinforce information as needed. ***Rationale:*** Understanding of previously taught information is evaluated and reinforced.
- Verify the correct patient with two identifiers. ***Rationale:*** Before performing a procedure, the nurse should ensure the correct identification of the patient for the intended intervention.
- If a warm air device will be used, remove the patient's gown and top sheet. ***Rationale:*** The warm air device works via convection and should be in direct contact with the patient's skin for optimal results.
- If the patient is unintentionally hypothermic, cover the patient's head with a blanket, towel, or aluminum cap. ***Rationale:*** This action minimizes additional heat loss.
- Ensure that informed consent has been obtained for insertion of an intravascular catheter. ***Rationale:*** Informed consent protects the rights of the patient and makes a competent decision possible for the patient; however, in emergency circumstances, time may not allow for the consent form to be signed.
- Perform a preprocedure verification and time out with placement of an intravascular catheter, if nonemergent. ***Rationale:*** Ensures patient safety.

Procedure for External Warming/Cooling Devices

Steps	Rationale	Special Considerations
Procedure for Obtaining Core Temperatures		
1. HH		
2. PE		
3. Pulmonary artery:		
A. Connect the cardiac output temperature cable from the bedside monitor to the pulmonary artery catheter.	Measures the temperature of the blood in the pulmonary artery.	Invasive placement risk for infection or puncture-related complications.
B. Observe the temperature display on the bedside monitor.	Provides a temperature value.	
4. Bladder:		
A. Connect the bladder temperature cable from the bedside monitor to the bladder probe.	Measures the temperature of the urine in the patient's bladder.	The accuracy of bladder temperatures may be influenced by urine flow rate.[16,26]
B. Observe the temperature display on the bedside monitor.	Provides a temperature value.	Refer to manufacturer's guidelines, and follow institutional policy regarding whether the temperature-sensing indwelling urinary catheter is magnetic resonance imaging safe.

Procedure for External Warming/Cooling Devices—*Continued*		
Steps	Rationale	Special Considerations
1. Esophageal: A. Assess the patient for contraindications to placement of an esophageal temperature probe for temperature monitoring.	Ensures that the esophageal temperature probe is inserted safely.	Follow institutional policy regarding whether nurses can insert esophageal temperature probes. Contraindications for placement of the esophageal temperature probe include patients with known esophageal strictures or who have a history of esophageal cancer, esophageal perforation, and end-stage liver disease and varicies.[24] If resistance is met, withdraw the probe, and gently advance it again; this may indicate tracheal intubation of the probe. Never force the probe. If the patient exhibits signs of respiratory distress, such as coughing or gasping, immediately withdraw the temperature probe.
B. Measure from the opening of the patient's mouth to the earlobe and from the earlobe to the upper part of the sternum (manubrium), about two finger widths below the sternal notch for accurate probe placement. Mark the measurement on the tube. Lubricate the tip of the catheter with water-soluble lubricant.	Correct measurement for probe placement is necessary for accurate core temperature monitoring. Eases insertion of the probe.	
C. Insert the esophageal temperature probe into the oral cavity, and advance it.	Initiates the procedure.	
D. Continue to advance the catheter until the placement marked on the probe reaches the patient's lips.	Positions the probe.	
E. Secure the esophageal temperature sensor to the patient.	Reduces the risk of inadvertent displacement.	
F. Connect the cable from the esophageal probe to the bedside monitor.	Measures the esophageal temperature.	
G. Observe the temperature display on the bedside monitor.	Provides a temperature value.	
H. Placement may be verified with radiography.[21]	Most catheters have a radiopaque tip that is visible on a radiograph.	
I. Discard used supplies in appropriate receptacles.	Safely discards supplies.	

Procedure for Intravascular Warming/Cooling Devices

Initiation of a Warming or Cooling Device

1. Plug the device into a grounded outlet.	Establishes a power source.	
2. **HH**		
3. **PE**		
4. Select a method for continuously monitoring the patient's core temperature.[31] (**Level D***)	"Core" body temperature should be measured using a probe placed in the bladder, the esophagus, or a vessel (artery or vein). These approaches give the closest approximation to brain temperature.[30,34]	Some warming or cooling devices have an adapter for connecting a temperature probe from the patient directly to the device.

Use of Traditional Warming or Cooling Fluid Device

1. Place a dry, absorbent sheet between the patient and the blanket when using all-vinyl blankets. (**Level M***)	A dry, absorbent sheet placed between the patient and the hypothermia/hyperthermia blanket provides a sanitary barrier and absorbs perspiration. It also promotes more uniform distribution of heat.	Avoid applying additional sheets or blankets because efficient heating or cooling occurs with maximal contact between the thermal pad and the patient's skin.

*Level D: Peer-reviewed professional and organizational standards with the support of clinical study recommendations.
*Level M: Manufacturer's recommendations only.

Procedure continues on following page

UNIT IX

Procedure | for External Warming/Cooling Devices—*Continued*

Steps	Rationale	Special Considerations
2. Vinyl blankets with nonwoven fabric surfaces do not require an absorbent sheet when using the nonwoven side. (**Level M***)		
3. Fill the reservoir in the unit to the indicated full level. Follow manufacturer's recommendations on water type.	The reservoir must contain enough water for the machine to function properly.	
4. Attach the hoses to the circulating fluid blanket.	Allows the flow of warmed or cooled water to the blanket.	
A. Check that the clamps are closed before connecting the hoses from the device to the blanket.	Prevents water leakage.	
B. After connecting the hoses, ensure that all connections are tight before unclamping the hoses.		
C. Check for kinks in the hoses.		
5. Press the start switch on.	Activates the device.	
6. Set the controls.		Follow institutional standards regarding the use of manual or automatic modes.
A. Manual control of blanket temperature.		
i. Press the manual control switch on.		
ii. Choose the set point for the temperature of the circulating fluid based on the prescribed patient body temperature and the manufacturer's directions.	The device maintains the circulating fluid in the blanket at the temperature set point.	The patient's temperature must be continuously monitored (**Level M***)
iii. Turn the warming or cooling device off when the desired temperature is reached.	The temperature goal is achieved.	Closely monitor the patient's temperature for fluctuation.
B. Automatic control of patient temperature.		
i. Connect the patient temperature probe to the unit before pressing a control mode switch.	Prevents triggering of the temperature probe alarm.	Most warming or cooling devices sound an alarm if the probe relays a low temperature; this may be indicative of probe dislodgment.
ii. Select the automatic mode and the set point based on the prescribed patient body temperature and the manufacturer's directions.	In the automatic mode, the unit warms or cools the circulating fluid in the blanket based on the set point (desired temperature) for the patient. A temperature probe connected to the unit monitors the patient's temperature.	The unit operates only if the patient's temperature probe is connected to the unit. Lights on the display panel indicate whether the unit is heating or cooling at any given time.
iii. Obtain the patient's temperature from the readout on the display unit.	Indicates the patient's temperature.	

*Level M: Manufacturer's recommendations only.

Procedure for External Warming/Cooling Devices—*Continued*

Steps	Rationale	Special Considerations
iv. Verify the patient's temperature with another source, and compare it with the readout on the device's display unit.	Ensures that the warming or cooling device's temperature probe is functioning and correlates with the patient's temperature obtained with another method.	
v. When the desired patient temperature is reached, the warming or cooling device will maintain that set point temperature until the machine is turned off.	The temperature goal is achieved.	May continue to monitor the patient's temperature by pressing on the "monitor only" switch.

Warming or Cooling Fluid Devices That Use Hydrogel Pads or External Wraps

Steps	Rationale	Special Considerations
1. Apply the adhesive hydrogel pads or the external wraps to the body per manufacturer's recommendations.	The pads or the wraps should cover approximately 40% of the patient.	Pads and wraps should be placed over clean, dry, intact skin. Inspect and prepare skin according to institutional standards.
2. Connect the hoses from the pads or wraps to the warming or cooling fluid device.	Prepares the system.	
3. Set the patient's target temperature as prescribed.	Sets the desired temperature.	
4. Activate the automatic mode.	The system will automatically adjust to achieve the target temperature.	
5. Set the time to target per institutional standards.	Prepares the system.	
6. Follow the provider's orders and the manufacturer's recommendations for warming/cooling device maintenance.	Ensures safe patient monitoring.	

Use of a Warm Air Device

Steps	Rationale	Special Considerations
1. Remove the patient's gown, sheet, and blankets. Then place the circulating air blanket on top of the patient.	Prepares the equipment.	
2. Place a cotton blanket or sheet over the circulating air blanket.	Aids in keeping the air blanket in place.	Maintains privacy.
3. Connect the air blanket to the hose attached to the device.	The blanket inflates as air flows from the hose into it.	
4. Turn on the device, and select the temperature of the air that will flow through the blanket.	The device warms the patient by directing warm airstreams directly onto the patient's skin.	The patient's temperature should be monitored based on the manufacturer's recommendations or institution policy. (**Level M***)

After the Warming or Cooling System Is Initiated

Steps	Rationale	Special Considerations
1. Discard used supplies in an appropriate receptacle.	Removes and safely discards used supplies.	
2. 🅷🅷		

*Level M: Manufacturer's recommendations only.

Procedure continues on following page

UNIT IX

Procedure for Intravascular Warming/Cooling Devices

Steps	Rationale	Special Considerations
1. Assist the provider with insertion of the intravascular catheter (see Procedure 74, Central Venous Catheter Insertion [Perform]).	Facilitates the insertion process.	
2. Connect the tubing from the warming or cooling fluid device to the intravascular catheter.	Prepares the system.	
3. Set the patient's target temperature as ordered by the provider.	Sets the desired temperature.	
4. Select the treatment mode.	Sets the desired mode of therapy.	
5. Activate the warming or cooling system.	Initiates the system.	
6. If the intravascular catheter device includes lumens for intravenous fluid administration, maintain patency with intravenous fluids or saline solution flush as ordered.	Provides venous access for intravenous fluids and medication administration.	Follow manufacturer's recommendations for warming/cooling device maintenance.
7. Follow the provider's orders for desired patient temperature therapy, duration of therapy, and monitoring parameters.	Ensure safe patient monitoring.	
8. Ensure that a postinsertion chest x-ray is obtained if the catheter was placed in the subclavian or internal jugular vein.	Confirms placement.	
9. Discard used supplies in appropriate receptacles.	Removes and safely discards used supplies; safely removes sharp objects.	
10. 🅷🅷		

Procedure for Semi-invasive Esophageal Warming/Cooling Devices

Steps	Rationale	Special Considerations
1. 🅷🅷		
2. 🅿🅴		
3. Obtain a measurement for placement by extending the esophageal tube from the patient's lips to the earlobe and then from the earlobe to the tip of the xiphoid process. Mark the location on the tube. (**Level M***)	Approximates the length of the tube to insert.	
4. Fill the reservoir in the unit to the indicated full level. Follow the manufacturer's recommendations on water type.	The reservoir must contain enough water for the machine to function properly.	
5. Place a Foley thermistor and/or rectal temperature probe, and connect one to the heating or cooling device.	Ensure continuous temperature monitoring.	A second temperature source is recommended for verification and may be connected to the patient monitor. An esophageal temperature source will not be accurate utilizing this device. (**Level M***)

*Level M: Manufacturer's recommendations only.

Procedure for Semi-invasive Esophageal Warming/Cooling Devices—*Continued*

Steps	Rationale	Special Considerations
6. Connect the esophageal tube to the appropriate heating or cooling device hoses, power on the unit, set the patient target temperature according to hospital protocol, and place the heating or cooling device in automatic mode.	Sets the desired temperature and allows the flow of warmed or cooled water to the tube.	A second temperature source is recommended for verification and may be connected to the patient monitor. The tube must have fluid circulating to allow ease of insertion into the esophagus.
7. Inspect the tube before placement.	Ensures that there are no leaks or deformities with the tube.	
8. Lubricate the esophageal tube generously with water-soluble lubricant before insertion. **(Level M*)**	The lubricant facilitates passage of the tube through the oropharynx and esophagus.	
9. Place the patient as flat as tolerated, and insert the esophageal temperature management device using gentle pressure posteriorly and downward through the mouth, past the oropharynx, and into the esophagus.		A gentle jaw thrust may be required to assist passage of the device.
10. Advance the device with light pressure until the required length of tube has been inserted. Secure the bite block in place.		
11. Confirm placement of the esophageal temperature management device in accordance with hospital protocol. **(Level D*)**	Radiographic verification is the recommended method to ensure correct placement.	
12. Secure with a securement device or tape in accordance with hospital protocol.		Ensure that the tube and tube set connections are not in contact with the patient's skin as direct contact between the tube and exposed skin may cause shivering.
13. Discard used supplies in appropriate receptacles.	Removes and safely discards used supplies.	

*Level M: Manufacturer's recommendations only.
*Level D: Peer-reviewed professional and organizational standards with the support of clinical study recommendations.

Expected Outcomes

- External warming or cooling device applied
- Desirable core body temperature achieved

Unexpected Outcomes

- Inability to achieve desired core body temperature
- Hemodynamic instability
- Cardiac dysrhythmias
- Acid-base, electrolyte, glucose, and coagulation imbalance
- Intolerable discomfort
- Shivering
- Skin injury

UNIT IX

Patient Monitoring and Care

Steps	Rationale	Reportable Conditions
		These conditions should be reported to the provider if they persist despite nursing interventions.
1. Perform a physical assessment of all systems frequently and as needed.	Alterations in temperature affect every system. The condition that caused the change in temperature may worsen or be refractory to treatment.	• Significant changes in assessment
2. Continuously monitor the patient's temperature.[34,36]	Assesses the patient's response to warming or cooling. Some institutions require two methods of monitoring the patient's temperature when cooling or warming. At least one should have audible alarms for temperatures above and below the desired limit. Follow institutional policy.	• Continued hypothermia or hyperthermia (temperature outside of prescribed target temperature)
3. Measure the patient's blood pressure as frequently as indicated by the patient's condition and according to institutional standards.	Vasodilation occurs with rewarming, and vasoconstriction may occur with cooling. Maintains perfusion and prevents recurrent hypotension.	• Hypotension or hypertension
4. Palpate the patient's mandible for a humming vibration, and observe for shivering.	Aids in early detection and prompt treatment of shivering. Shivering may contribute to the inability to maintain core temperature goals.	• Shivering • Decreased mixed venous oxygenation saturation • Continued shivering despite prescribed medications
5. Examine the patient's skin condition hourly. Follow the manufacturer's recommendations for assessing the patient's skin under hydrogel pads and external wraps (e.g., at least every 4 hours). **(Level M*)**	Detects signs or symptoms of skin irritation so the temperature of the device can be adjusted, or padding can be placed between the skin and the device.	• Signs or symptoms of skin irritation or injury
6. Continuously monitor the patient's cardiac rate and rhythm.	Detects cardiac dysrhythmias associated with warming or cooling therapy.	• Cardiac dysrhythmias
7. Obtain arterial blood gas results as prescribed and as indicated. Continuously monitor the patient's oxygen saturation and end-tidal carbon dioxide as prescribed.	Detects hypoxemia and acid-base imbalances. Maintains adequate oxygenation and minimizes fraction of inspired oxygen.	• Decreased oxygen saturation • Elevated partial pressure of oxygen in arterial blood • Elevated or decrease partial pressure of carbon dioxide in arterial blood • Abnormal arterial blood gas results
8. Obtain blood samples as prescribed.	Detects electrolyte shifts associated with warming and cooling therapy.	• Hyperkalemia/hypokalemia • Alterations in magnesium and phosphate levels • Hyperglycemia[17] • Coagulation study results[17]
9. Assess for venous thromboembolism (VTE) in vessels that contain intravascular cooling/warming devices.[17,21] **(Level C*)**	Intravascular cooling devices have been associated with increased risk of VTE.[17,21]	• VTE or pulmonary emboli
10. Follow institutional standards for assessing pain. Administer analgesia as prescribed.	Identifies the need for pain interventions.	• Continued pain despite pain interventions

*Level C: Qualitative studies, descriptive or correlational studies, integrative reviews, systematic reviews, or randomized controlled trials with inconsistent results.
*Level M: Manufacturer's recommendations only.

Documentation

Documentation should include the following:
- Patient and family education
- Patient's temperature and site(s) of temperature assessment
- Vital signs, cardiac rhythm, and hemodynamic status
- Physical assessment findings
- Neurological examination findings
- Skin assessment and/or preventive measures
- Mechanical ventilator settings
- Post-insertion chest radiograph (intravascular devices placed in the subclavian or internal jugular veins; confirm secure airway)
- Acid-base, electrolyte, glucose, lactate, and coagulation assessment and interventions
- Type of warming or cooling device used
- Mode of cooling or warming device (automatic or manual), patient's set point or water temperature (as required by institutional standards)
- Time external warming or cooling is initiated and terminated
- Pain assessment, interventions, and effectiveness of interventions
- Sedation assessment, interventions, and effectiveness of interventions
- Shiver assessment, interventions, and effectiveness of interventions
- Unexpected outcomes
- Additional interventions

References and Additional Readings

For a complete list of references and additional readings for this procedure, scan this QR code with your smartphone, or visit https://www.elsevier.com/__data/assets/pdf_file/0004/1319899/Chapter0124.pdf

UNIT IX

125 Prevention of Immobility-Related Complications: Kinetic Therapy (Continuous Lateral Rotation Therapy and Lateral Rotation Therapy) and Ambulation of Acute and Critically Ill Patients

Jan Powers and Kellie Girardot

PURPOSE Immobility in acutely and critically ill patients is a significant problem. Complications related to immobility can lead to increased morbidity and mortality as a result of pneumonia, pressure injuries, venous stasis, urinary stasis, and decreased muscle mass. Mobility can be viewed across a continuum. For patients who are immobile and unable to get out of bed, in-bed activities are essential. This can also include continuous rotational therapies, such as kinetic therapy. The term *kinetic therapy* (KT) refers to a 40-degree or greater rotation.[20,41] KT includes lateral turning 40 to 62 degrees on each side. KT provides dynamic rotation and benefits pulmonary status by enhancing mobilization and removal of pulmonary secretions and assisting in preventing and treating complications of immobility. Continuous lateral rotation therapy (CLRT) involves the use of dynamic rotation of a support surface delivered via a specialized overlay or bed to continuously rotate the patient side to side. CLRT is similar to KT, but the degree of turn is less than 40 degrees. Lateral rotation therapy is used for patients with traumatic injury, such as an unstable spine injury, those requiring traction, and those who need aggressive rotation therapy. As soon as patients are hemodynamically stable, it is imperative to progress their activity with the goal of out-of-bed activity and ambulation as soon as possible. Progressive upright mobility allows the patient to progress along a continuum of increased activity levels as tolerated. The purpose of this procedure is to clearly delineate nursing interventions that will help prevent immobility-related complications.

PREREQUISITE NURSING KNOWLEDGE

- The concepts of safe patient handling.
- The physiological effects of immobility on body systems and the negative impact of immobility in critically ill patients, including the following:
  - ❖ Respiratory: decreased movement of secretions,[31] decreased respiratory motion,[31] increased risk of atelectasis,[31] increased risk of pneumonia,[10,31] increased risk of pulmonary embolism,[31] and increased ventilator days[9,43,54]
  - ❖ Integumentary: increase risk of pressure injuries[30] and increased dependent edema[31]
  - ❖ Cardiovascular: decreased blood volume,[31] increased resting heart rate,[31,53] cardiac deconditioning,[31] orthostatic intolerance,[31,53] and increased risk of deep venous thrombosis[10]
  - ❖ Neurological: increased incidence of delirium,[9,19,21,31,43,45] depression,[31] and anxiety[30,31]
  - ❖ Skeletal muscle: intensive care unit (ICU)-acquired weakness[9,21,37,39] and decreased function[8,9,21,32,43,45,47,54]
  - ❖ Psychological: poor quality of life[9,18,54]
  - ❖ Other: increased ICU and hospital length of stay[9,18,19,30,37,39,47] and increased hospital cost[37,54]
  - ❖ Gastrointestinal: constipation and fecal impaction
  - ❖ Metabolic: glucose intolerance
  - ❖ Genitourinary stasis[52]

CONTINUOUS LATERAL ROTATION THERAPY

CLRT involves continuous turning of the patient on the bed with lateral rotations. CLRT involves the use of dynamic rotation of a support surface delivered via a specialized overlay or bed to continuously rotate the patient laterally from side to side. CLRT is a therapy that focuses on strategically and continuously repositioning the patient. CLRT may reduce the impact of extended bed rest by providing frequent repositioning to prevent pulmonary complications and the breakdown of tissue under pressure.[28]

Patients who are mechanically ventilated have an increased risk of hospital-acquired conditions (HACs) such as ventilator-associated pneumonia (VAP) and hospital-acquired pressure injury (HAPI). CLRT has been shown to reduce HAC incidence.[28] A cost-effectiveness analysis found CLRT to be highly cost-effective compared with standard care by preventing HACs that seriously harm patients in the ICU.[28] Patients should be placed on a lateral rotation support surface as soon as possible to prevent the negative effects of immobility and possible pulmonary complications.[4,20,52] Rotation therapy may be useful for preventing and treating respiratory complications in selected critically ill patients and decreases the incidence of pneumonia but has no effect on duration of mechanical ventilation, number of days in the ICU, or hospital mortality.[22]

PREREQUISITE NURSING KNOWLEDGE

- Principles for prevention of pressure-induced injury, including high-risk areas for tissue injury associated with friction, shearing, pressure, and moisture in the critically ill patient.[12,13] Pressure points and locations where moisture or incontinence may occur require special attention to prevent skin breakdown. Prolonged external pressure over bony prominences, shear and friction forces, and excessive moisture increase the risk of pressure injury.[12,13,40]
- Pressure injury may occur while a patient is on a specialty surface. Assess all at-risk areas of the patient's skin, especially the face, ears, occiput, shoulders, heals, and coccyx areas.
- Interventions to prevent ventilator-acquired pneumonia.[2,11,38] CLRT is an adjunct treatment and should not be the sole therapy instituted to prevent VAP.[2,22]
- Indications for CLRT include critically ill patients who are at a higher risk of pulmonary complications, such as the following:
  - ❖ Patients at risk for VAP
  - ❖ Patients with increasing ventilator support requirements refractory to standard treatment
  - ❖ Fraction of inspired oxygen (Fio$_2$) greater than 50% for 1 hour or longer[20,48]
  - ❖ Positive end-expiratory pressure (PEEP) greater than 8 cm H$_2$O[48]
  - ❖ Patients who have the following clinical indications for acute lung injury or adult respiratory distress syndrome:
    - ○ Partial pressure of arterial oxygen (Pao$_2$) to fraction of inspired oxygen (Fio$_2$) ratio less than 300)[20,44,48]
    - ○ Presence of bilateral opacities or infiltrates via chest radiograph[22,48]
    - ○ Presence of atelectasis via chest radiograph[22,48]
- Contraindications for CLRT, such as the following:
  - ❖ Unstable spine or pelvic injury until the injury is stabilized[48]
  - ❖ Long bone fractures and/or traction[48]
  - ❖ Unstable intracranial pressure (greater than 20 mm Hg)[48]
- CLRT should be used cautiously with the following:
  - ❖ Extreme agitation and/or motion sickness[48]
  - ❖ Immediate postoperative period following open heart surgery[48]
  - ❖ Multiple rib fractures[46,48]
  - ❖ Bronchospasm[48]
  - ❖ Uncontrollable diarrhea[48]
- Because of the lack of evidence for specific therapy parameters, the degree of rotation and time interval should be set per institution protocols.[22] The degree of rotation is set individually on each side; it may be intermittent or constant, or it may provide unilateral or bilateral rotation, depending on patient condition. For example, if a patient does not tolerate turning to the left side, the surface may be programmed for a shorter time interval or lesser degree of rotation on that side.
- Components necessary for maximal patient benefit include initiation of therapy within 48 hours of intubation and continuous rotation for more than 18 hours per day.[48,52]
- Potential physiological changes that occur during CLRT. Changes in patient's hemodynamics or oxygen saturation during rotation are often the result of the patient's underlying disease process.[48] If hemodynamic and/or oxygenation changes occur, the patient's oxygenation, respiratory rate, ventilator settings, arterial blood gas levels, adequacy of volume resuscitation, cardiac performance, vascular tone, and other appropriate parameters should be assessed, and the need for additional intervention should be evaluated.[49]
- Potential complications associated with CLRT may include disconnection or dislodgement of intravascular catheters, intolerance to rotation, adverse effects on intracranial pressure, and dysrhythmias.[22,48]
- Several support surfaces are available for CLRT. Identify the type of continuous lateral rotation therapy used at the individual institution, whether a framed surface or added overlay, and follow the manufacturer's guidelines. Refer to institutional protocols for types of support surfaces that may be used.
- Manufacturer-specific guidelines for implementing CLRT should be reviewed before the patient is placed on the support surface/bed frame.
- Daily evaluation of the patient's response to CLRT and assessment of continued need for CLRT are required. Criteria for discontinuation may include resolution of indications for therapy.

UNIT IX

EQUIPMENT

- Nonsterile gloves
- Sheet, slide board, mechanical lifts or other transitioning device to assist with moving a patient onto a surface
- Appropriate CLRT surface
- Phone number and name of company representative; keep this in an easily accessible area of the chart in the event the bed malfunctions

PATIENT AND FAMILY EDUCATION

- Explain to the patient and family the adverse effects of pulmonary complications and consequences of immobility. *Rationale:* Explanation encourages understanding when a different bed surface is needed based on the risk assessment of the patient. The patient and family are able to ask questions.
- Explain the purpose of CLRT, properties of the support surface, and possible risks involved with treatment. *Rationale:* Understanding and cooperation are increased when patients and families understand the purpose of therapy.

PATIENT ASSESSMENT AND PREPARATION

Patient Assessment

- Assessment of the patient's respiratory status, including breath sounds, respiratory rate, cough, oxygen saturation, arterial blood gas, chest radiograph, and mental status.

Rationale: This provides an initial and ongoing evaluation of effectiveness of CLRT on body systems.

- Assessment of the patient's skin, including evidence of pressure injury or other alterations. *Rationale:* This provides baseline and ongoing skin status data.
- Assessment of the patient's vascular system, including hemodynamic stability, presence of lower extremity edema, and deep venous thrombosis. *Rationale:* This provides baseline and ongoing vascular status data.
- Discuss goals for pressure redistribution and CLRT with the prescribing provider. *Rationale:* The properties of the CLRT support surface are evaluated to match patient factors.

Patient Preparation

- Ensure that the patient and family understand the pre-procedural teaching. Answer questions as they arise, and reinforce information as needed. *Rationale:* Understanding previously taught clinical information and rationale is evaluated and reinforced.
- Evaluate the properties of the support surface to meet pulmonary needs. *Rationale:* Support surface selection should match the clinical indication for patient therapy.
- Verify the correct patient with two identifiers. *Rationale:* Before performing a procedure, the nurse should ensure the correct identification of the patient for the intended intervention.
- Ensure that adequate personnel are available to assist when moving the patient to the new surface. Place the patient in the supine position with the head of the bed elevated 30 degrees (if not medically contraindicated) in preparation for a move to a specialty surface. *Rationale:* This potentiates transfer of the patient from one bed to another.

Procedure	Continuous Lateral Rotation Therapy		
Steps	**Rationale**		**Special Considerations**
1. 🄷🄷			
2. 🄿🄴			
3. Ensure that the bed is locked in the horizontal position, the drive is disengaged, and the brake is on.	Ensures patient and staff safety.		Align both surfaces side by side at a comfortable height for staff to move the patient to the new surface, ensuring that both surfaces are locked and will not move on patient transfer.
4. With use of a draw sheet, lift, or other transfer device, move the patient to the center of the surface while maintaining body alignment.	Shearing of the patient's skin and/or patient or staff injury may be avoided.		Do not leave the patient unattended at any time during patient transfer.
5. Transfer the patient to the center of the bed, aligning the patient using guides on the surface or per the manufacturer's instructions.	Ensures proper positioning of the patient for rotation.		If using a specialty mattress overlay, it is recommended to place the mattress on the bed frame and then transfer the patient to the new surface.

Procedure	Continuous Lateral Rotation Therapy—*Continued*	
Steps	**Rationale**	**Special Considerations**
6. Utilize all securement straps and supports to ensure that the patient is held safely in place and to prevent shearing over potential areas of friction.	Prevents unexpected outcomes and promotes patient safety.	
7. Ensure that all invasive tubing and lines are free from obstruction or risk of dislodgement.		
8. Initiate therapy per provider order or institutional protocols.		
9. Monitor the patient through an entire rotational cycle to assess for ventilation or hemodynamic changes. Ensure that invasive tubing and lines remain free from obstruction or risk of dislodgement.	Ensures that the patient remains safe and tolerates rotation.	Consider longer time intervals or a decreased angle initially to allow the patient to increase tolerance to rotation.[48]
10. Discard any used supplies, and remove **PE**.		
11. **HH**		

Expected Outcomes

- Improved pulmonary function
- Absence of VAP
- Intact skin integrity, wound healing, absence of friction and shearing, absence of excessive skin moisture or dryness
- Improved peripheral circulation
- Improved urinary elimination

Unexpected Outcomes

- Desaturation with rotation
- Hemodynamic instability with rotation
- Dislodgement of invasive lines
- Development of worsening pulmonary status
- Development of urinary tract infection
- Friction, shearing, motion sickness, agitation, disorientation, and falls from lateral movement of the support surface if the patient is not strapped in properly
- Pressure ulcer formation or further deterioration of existing pressure ulcers

Patient Monitoring and Care

Steps	Rationale	Reportable Conditions
		These conditions should be reported to the provider if they persist despite nursing interventions.
1. Cardiopulmonary resuscitation (CPR): Identify the CPR valve or deflate surface to the bed frame. If it has a foam base, place a back board under the patient. Begin CPR.	A flat, firm surface is needed for effective CPR.	- Need for CPR

Procedure continues on following page

Patient Monitoring and Care —*Continued*

Steps	Rationale	Reportable Conditions
2. Assess the patient's pulmonary function.	Lateral rotational movement provides continuous postural drainage and mobilization of secretions.[51]	• Adventitious breath sounds • Decreased respiratory rate and depth • Cough • Cyanosis • Dyspnea • Nasal flaring • Decreased oxygen saturation • Abnormal blood gases • Decreased mental acuity • Restlessness • Abnormal chest radiograph results
3. Assess the skin for evidence of breakdown by manually repositioning the patient at least every 2 hours. Closely monitor pressure point areas (occiput, sacrum, and heels) or areas that may rub against support surfaces with rotation (axilla, groin/inner thighs, face/ears, and/or feet) per hospital policy. Consider applying a protective dressing to areas prone to shearing.[27,35,51]	The patient continues to be at risk for skin breakdown and pressure ulcer development. Ensure that routine skin assessments continue throughout rotation therapy.	• Development of pressure injuries, skin breakdown, or worsening of wounds
4. Assess the patient's vascular circulation.	Lateral rotational movement discourages venous stasis.	• Edema, decreased or absent pulses, discoloration, and/or pain
5. Assess the patient for urinary retention.	Lateral rotational movement decreases urinary stasis.	• Decreased urine output • Bladder distention
6. Monitor the patient's tolerance and hemodynamic goals.	Lateral rotational movement may alter hemodynamics because of the degree of rotation and changes in transducer positioning.[49]	• Intolerance to the device • Vital signs consistently below or above desired goals/parameters
7. Follow institutional standards for assessing pain. Administer analgesia as prescribed.	Identifies the need for pain interventions.	• Continued pain despite pain interventions
8. Maintain in motion for 18 of 24 hours.[49]	Provides proper rotation and adequate mobility.	• Inability to tolerate rotation therapy angle and time frame
9. Determine when therapy should be discontinued. Reassess need every 24 hours.[49]	Lateral rotation therapy is no longer required.	

Documentation

Documentation should include the following:
- Patient and family education
- Date and time therapy instituted
- Rationale for use of lateral rotation therapy surface
- Number of hours the patient is in rotation mode per 24 hours and the degree of rotation achieved
- Complete a full skin assessment per institutional policy and as needed
- Status of wound healing if applicable
- The patient's response to therapy
- Any unexpected outcomes and interventions performed

LATERAL ROTATION SURFACE

Purpose

The lateral rotation surface is a unique kinetic therapy surface that can be perceived to be technically challenging and requires a coordinated effort for use. This rotation therapy is ideal for patients with traumatic injuries such as unstable spine injuries or fractures requiring traction and for patients who need aggressive rotation therapy. The lateral rotation surface is a kinetic therapy surface that does not incorporate low air loss into its technology, but if the patient is in continuous motion (rotation), pressure over bony prominences may be relieved during the continuous turning therapy. However, because of the aggressive degree of the turn, possible shear and friction injuries of the skin can occur during rotation, especially if the patient is not secured adequately with side packs.

PREREQUISITE NURSING KNOWLEDGE

- The lateral rotation therapy bed is based on a platform that provides rotation and pressure relief by continuous rotation. The use of this therapy includes frequent assessments of patient skin and the safety of lines, drains, and tubes.[6,24]
- The lateral rotation therapy surface can be used for patients who require spinal immobilization and the prevention of complications due to immobility.[4,22,36,41]
  - ❖ Preventive interventions, such as providing skin protectants, monitoring nutrition, containing excessive moisture, and preventing shearing and friction, are indicated with the use of the lateral rotation therapy surface.
  - ❖ Layers of linen placed on the surface should be limited to allow maximal benefit of the surface for the patient's skin.

- For maximal benefit, the support surface should be in rotation more than 18 hours per day and at optimal rotation.[20,24,41]
  - ❖ The support surface should provide continuous rotation at varying degrees.
  - ❖ Serial skin assessments are required when patients are on rotation therapy surfaces, per institutional protocols.
  - ❖ The clinician should evaluate the patient's tolerance of kinetic therapy and consider sedation and analgesics as appropriate.
- Indications include critically ill patients who are at a higher risk of pulmonary complications such as the following:
  - ❖ Patients with increasing ventilatory support requirements
  - ❖ Patients who have clinical indications for acute lung injury or adult respiratory distress syndrome.[4,20,52]
  - ❖ Worsening Pao_2-to-Fio_2 ratio
  - ❖ Presence of bilateral opacities or infiltrates via chest radiograph concomitant with pulmonary edema
  - ❖ Refractory hypoxemia
- When ordering kinetic therapy, the clinician should assess the properties of the pressure redistribution surface and evaluate patient skin/tissue redistribution needs (i.e., moisture control, pressure redistribution).
- Trauma diagnosis and spinal cord injury should be understood. Pressure injury–related risks associated with traumatic and spinal cord injury should be understood related to prolonged immobility.[4,20,52] Low air-loss surfaces are contraindicated for patients with unstable spine or pelvic injuries until the injury is stabilized. The lateral rotation therapy surface may be used with spinal injuries; additional care is necessary when placing patients with unstable spinal cord injuries or those with pelvic instability on a lateral rotation therapy surface that has a firm, flat surface. Cervical traction and skeletal traction may be used with a lateral rotation therapy surface (see Procedure 91, Cervical Traction and Stabilization: Assist and Nursing Care).
- A lateral rotation therapy bed is shown in Figure 125.1.

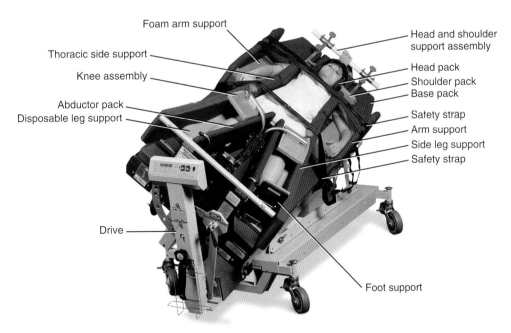

Foam arm support
Thoracic side support
Knee assembly
Abductor pack
Disposable leg support
Drive
Head and shoulder support assembly
Head pack
Shoulder pack
Base pack
Satety strap
Arm support
Side leg support
Safety strap
Foot support

Figure 125.1 RotoRest Delta Advanced Kinetic Therapy bed. *(Photo used with permission by Arjo Inc.)*

UNIT IX

- Noted principles in caring for a patient receiving kinetic therapy on a lateral rotation therapy bed include technical and clinical competence in the following:
  - The surface below the patient and the positioning packs consist of pressure-redistributing foam and a pad of nonliquid polymer gel with a low-friction, low-shear nylon fabric with moisture-permeable backing cover that does not absorb body fluids.
  - The gel pads prevent the patient from bottoming out and transfer body heat evenly; they are radiographically transparent.
  - The bed provides continuous, slow, side-to-side turning of the patient by rotating the bed frame. Keeping the patient in maximal rotation assists with prevention of skin breakdown and provides the most effective therapy for pulmonary indications. The bed can turn up to 62 degrees on each side, either intermittently or constantly, providing unilateral or bilateral rotation.
  - The amount of time the patient is held at the rotation limit before rotating in the opposite direction can be adjusted from 7 seconds to 30 minutes.
  - Head and shoulder packs provide cervical stability but should not be used as the primary means of stabilizing cervical spine fractures. Cervical traction, halo, and vest or internal fixation may be required. Lateral arm and leg hatches facilitate range of motion.
  - Hatches underneath the bed (located in the cervical, thoracic, and rectal areas) provide access for skin care, catheter maintenance, and bladder and bowel management. Do not open thoracic and sacral hatches at the same time.
  - The bed has a built-in scale with a maximal patient weight of 300 pounds.[12] The overall width of the bed is 34 inches with a height of 94 inches.
  - An optional vibrator pack is available to provide chest physiotherapy to further mobilize pulmonary secretions.

EQUIPMENT

- Nonsterile gloves
- Sheet or slide board to assist with moving the patient onto the surface
- Transparent or foam protective dressings for areas prone to friction or shearing
- Appropriate support surface and positioning packs for the lateral rotation therapy surface

PATIENT AND FAMILY EDUCATION

- Explain to the patient and family the adverse effects of critical illness and immobility, including pulmonary complications, tissue pressure, and excessive moisture of the skin. *Rationale:* Providing an explanation promotes understanding of the need for prevention, interventional strategies, and the specialty devices that are utilized based on patient risk assessment. The patient and family are able to share understanding of the plan of care and ask questions.

- Describe the goals of lateral rotation therapy and how the therapy can aid in maintaining patient alignment in patients with spinal injuries. *Rationale:* The patient and family are able to share understanding of the plan of care and ask questions.
- Explain how the therapy can serve as both a prevention and an interventional care strategy. *Rationale:* Understanding and cooperation are increased.
- Explain to the patient and family the pulmonary benefit of rotation in promoting dynamic movement of pulmonary secretions. *Rationale:* Facilitates understanding of the role of pulmonary secretion mobilization in critically ill patients.

PATIENT ASSESSMENT AND PREPARATION

Patient Assessment

- Assess the patient's risk for a pressure injury with an evidence-based practice assessment tool (i.e., Braden score). *Rationale:* Valid assessment tools assist in the identification of patient risk for alterations in skin.
- Assess the patient's skin for evidence of pressure injury formation or alterations in skin on admission and throughout care based on institutional standards. *Rationale:* This provides baseline and ongoing skin status data.
- Assess and ensure hemodynamic stability; assess for the presence of edema in the lower extremities and the potential for thromboembolism. *Rationale:* This provides baseline data for serial assessment and if necessary to treat the adverse effects of immobility.
- Assess the patient's pulmonary status to include the quality and presence of adventitious breath sounds, the rate and depth of respirations, cough, cyanosis, dyspnea, arterial blood gas results, chest radiograph, mental status, and restlessness. *Rationale:* This provides baseline data for additional comparisons. Lateral movement provides postural drainage, mobilizes secretions, and enhances air exchange.
- Assess the patient's bladder for complications associated with urinary stasis from immobility to include the presence of bladder distention, incomplete bladder emptying, or urinary infrequency. *Rationale:* Baseline data are provided before implementation of lateral movement that decreases urinary stasis and associated complications.
- Discuss goals for rotation therapy with the interprofessional team as part of the daily plan of care. *Rationale:* The principles of therapy are evaluated to match patient factors related to type of injury, moisture, and need for redistribution of pressure on skin and wounds.
- Reassess every 12 to 24 hours for the need to continue, change, or discontinue rotation therapy. *Rationale:* Reevaluation of the benefit of the therapy is important in creating an individualized plan of care.

Patient Preparation

- Ensure that the patient and family understand the preprocedural teaching. Answer questions as they arise, and reinforce information as needed. *Rationale:* Understanding of previously taught clinical information and rationale is evaluated and reinforced.

- Evaluate the properties of the support surface to meet pulmonary needs, skin factors related to the type of injury, moisture, and need for redistribution of pressure on skin and wounds. Order and inspect the bed functions before the patient is placed on the surface. *Rationale:* The support surface selection should match the clinical indication for patient therapy. Relief of external pressure may decrease the risk of pressure injury formation and facilitate wound healing.

- Verify the correct patient with two identifiers. *Rationale:* Before performing a procedure, the nurse should ensure the correct identification of the patient for the intended intervention.

- Organize moving the patient to the special surface, ensuring that adequate personnel are available. *Rationale:* This potentiates transfer of the patient from one bed to another.

Procedure for Kinetic Therapy With a Lateral Rotation Surface

Steps	Rationale	Special Considerations
1. Obtain the bed that will be used for kinetic lateral rotation.	Rental beds may require a provider's order.	These beds are U.S. Food and Drug Administration (FDA) regulated. Ensures that the properties of the specialty surface meet the patient's specific needs.
2. Follow the manufacturer's guidelines for setting up the bed to include patient height, weight, and rotation settings.	Prepares the equipment.	The lateral rotation therapy surface is considered more challenging to use and thus is described in this section.
3. **HH**		
4. **PE**		
Prepare for Patient Placement		
5. Ensure that the bed is locked in the horizontal position and that the drive is disengaged.	Ensures patient safety.	
6. Check all hatches to ensure that they are properly latched; be sure castors are locked.	Prevents unplanned movement of the bed.	
7. Zero the bed scale system.	Prepares the bed for patient daily weight.	
8. Prepare the surface: A. Remove all vertical packs. B. Cover support brackets with a washcloth. C. Slide thoracic and foot packs to the side and ends of the unit. D. Consider routing for any patient-specific drains/tubes.	Allows for smooth transfer of the patient onto the bed and protects the patient from discomfort. Prepares for safe management of lines, drains, and tubes.	
Prepare for Patient Transfer and Positioning With the Lateral Rotation Surface		
1. Using a draw sheet, lift, or slide board, gently move the patient to the center of the surface while maintaining body alignment.	Bouncing of the patient can result in skin abrasions and progression of injury.	Pillar bars can be covered with a towel or folded paper sheet to avoid the possibility of abrasion. Assess the security of all lines, drains, and tubes to accommodate a full 62-degree turn.
2. Center the patient on the bed by aligning the nose, umbilicus, and pubis with the center posts. Align both head and shoulder pack posts vertically and horizontally.	Facilitates proper balance. Rotating to one side indicates that the patient is not centered.	Traction equipment may be installed once the patient is centered.

Procedure continues on following page

UNIT IX

Procedure **for Kinetic Therapy With a Lateral Rotation Surface**—*Continued*		
Steps	Rationale	Special Considerations
3. Pack installation for one side of the patient is repeated and mirrored on the opposite side.	Packs are the main supporting apparatus. Packs provide support to prevent lateral movement within the bed, which can lead to skin breakdown.	Packs and supports are labeled for the patient's right and left sides.
4. Install shoulder and head pack assemblies by sliding onto the head and shoulder posts. Slide the head and shoulder packs inward to lightly touch the patient's head.	Provides support and protects the ears from pressure. Proper shoulder and head support help prevent lateral movement within the bed, which can lead to ear skin breakdown and cervical injury.	Maintain a 1-inch (2.54-cm) clearance from the shoulder; pass the hand between the shoulder and pack to verify the clearance. Verify that the pack is not pressing against the ears. If cervical traction causes the patient to slide up on the bed during rotation, place the patient in the reverse Trendelenburg position.
5. Place thoracic side supports in appropriate holes provided in the frame, and ensure that they are tightened securely. Lock cam handles to hold the pack in position.	Provides support to prevent lateral movement within the bed, which may lead to shearing skin injury.	The holes in the frame in which the side supports fit are near the surface of the base packs. Packs are labeled "Right" and "Left." The thicker side of the pack is always against the patient. Ensure that packs are placed snuggly to the patient's torso to prevent sliding and potential shearing of the skin. Maintain a 1-inch (2.54-cm) clearance between the end of the pack and the axilla.
6. Adjust the knee assembly to a position slightly above the patient's knee. Lock cam handles to hold the pack in position.	Provides support.	
7. Place the disposable leg support under the thigh and calf so it fits under the ankle and knee but not beneath the heel.	Decreases external pressure on the heels.	Leg supports should be changed with excessive moisture or when soiled.
8. Place the foot supports in the foot bracket assembly. The assembly should be positioned so the footrest is in anatomical position. Tighten the foot assembly. Lock the cam handles to hold the position.	Maintains each foot in proper anatomical position and prevents migration.	The foot supports should not be left in place for longer than 2 hours at a time. A schedule of 2 hours on and 2 hours off should be maintained continuously. Side-to-side motion does not relieve pressure on the soles of the feet.
9. Install the abductor packs into the preset metal brackets.	Provides support.	Adjust and lower if extra space is required at the groin.
10. Place the side leg supports snugly against the patient's hips. Lock the cam handles to hold the position.	Provides support.	
11. Install the knee pack by pressing the pin on the support tube while inserting the support tube into the knee pack assembly. Tighten the knob to hold the assembly in position.	Prevents pressure on the knee.	Maintain a 1-inch (2.54-cm) clearance between the foam and the skin. Knee packs can be adjusted to allow for variation in abduction and flexion of the patient's legs. They maintain proper posture of the lower limbs in the patient with spasticity, discouraging contracture formation.

Procedure | **for Kinetic Therapy With a Lateral Rotation Surface—*Continued***

Steps	Rationale	Special Considerations
12. Install the disposable foam arm supports.	Ensures that the patient's hands are in a position of function and that the ulnar nerve and elbows are protected.	Disposable arm supports should be changed with excessive moisture or when soiled.
13. Secure the arm supports in the holes provided on the frame.	Provides support and promotes safety.	
14. Place a hand on the patient's shoulder, and adjust the shoulder pack to lightly touch your hand.	Prevents pressure injury.	A 1-inch (2.54-cm) clearance should always exist between the patient's shoulders and the shoulder packs.
15. Verify that all packs are in position, all hatches are closed, all cam handles are locked, and brakes are locked.	Provides support.	Remove any obstructions from the area that may impede the unit rotation cycle.
16. Fasten the restraining straps. Safety straps must be in place at all times. One safety strap is used to hold down the shoulder assembly. Place the other strap across the hip region.	Prevents falls and patient injury.	
17. Initiate therapy.	Determine whether the equipment and positioning works.	Observe the patient through a full rotation cycle; ensure that all packs are appropriately set, pressure points are protected, drains and lines are not pulled or pinched during rotation, and there are no obstructions during the cycle.
18. Monitor patient hemodynamics with rotation therapy.	Determines the patient's response to therapy.	Changes in hemodynamics are expected; monitor the patient's tolerance and hemodynamic goals (e.g., urine output, mentation, mean arterial pressure, intracranial pressure). The patient may need time to acclimate to kinetic therapy. Interpret vital signs with knowledge of fixed transducer variation caused by degree of rotation (i.e., level may change, providing false data).
19. Remove **PE**, and discard used supplies.	Reduces transmission of microorganisms; standard precautions.	
20. **HH**		

Expected Outcomes

- Maximal pulmonary function achieved
- Intact skin integrity, absence of friction and shear injuries, absence of excessive skin moisture or dryness
- Improved peripheral circulation
- Improved urinary elimination

Unexpected Outcomes

- Development of worsening pulmonary status
- Friction, shearing, motion sickness, agitation, disorientation, and falls from lateral movement of the table if the patient is not strapped in properly
- Pressure injury formation or further deterioration of existing pressure injuries
- Desaturation or hemodynamic instability with rotation
- Dislodged invasive lines or tubes
- Development of urinary tract infection

Patient Monitoring and Care

Steps	Rationale	Reportable Conditions
		These conditions should be reported to the provider if they persist despite nursing interventions. • Need for emergency care
1. To initiate cardiopulmonary resuscitation (CPR): A. Return the bed to the horizontal position by disengaging rotation and manually rotating. B. Pull the crank arm handle (the clutch), and lock it in place with the lock. C. Follow the manufacturer's guidelines regarding if a back board is needed for CPR.	A flat, firm surface is necessary for CPR.	
2. Evaluate the patient's existing pressure areas and injuries, wounds, flaps, and grafts for evidence of healing according to institutional protocols. Monitor skin regularly, and provide extra attention to any pressure points and locations where moisture or incontinence may occur.	Relief of external pressure facilitates healing.	• New breakdown • Impaired healing
3. Assess the skin for evidence of pressure (especially on the occiput, sacrum, and heels), friction, shearing, or moisture per hospital policy. Consider applying a protective dressing to areas prone to friction or shearing (i.e., transparent semiocclusive, hydrocolloid, or foam dressing).	The kinetic therapy surface alone does not protect from pressure injury formation. Ensure that adequate skin assessment continues throughout therapy.	• Development of pressure injury or skin breakdown
4. Evaluate the patient's peripheral vascular circulation. Follow hospital policy for prevention of thromboembolism.	Lateral movement discourages venous stasis.	• Edema • Decreased or absent pulses • Discoloration • Pain
5. Evaluate the patient's pulmonary function.	Lateral movement provides continuous postural drainage and mobilization of secretions.	• Adventitious breath sounds • Decreased respiratory rate and depth • Cough • Cyanosis • Dyspnea • Decreased oxygen saturation • Abnormal blood gases • Decreased mental acuity • Restlessness • Abnormal chest radiograph results
6. Evaluate the patient for urinary retention.	Lateral movement decreases urinary stasis.	• Decreased urine output • Bladder distention

Patient Monitoring and Care —*Continued*

Steps	Rationale	Reportable Conditions
7. Evaluate the patient's acceptance of and adaptation to the device (motion sickness, agitation, disorientation).	Increases cooperation and decreases anxiety.	• Intolerance to device
8. Monitor patient's tolerance and hemodynamic goals (e.g., urine output, mentation, mean arterial pressure, intracranial pressure). The patient may need time to acclimate to kinetic therapy.	Lateral movement may alter hemodynamics because of the degree of rotation (turn) and changes in transducer positioning.	• Increased or decreased blood pressure • Increased or decreased heart rate • Elevation in intracranial pressure
9. Follow institutional standards for assessing pain. Administer analgesia as prescribed.	Identifies the need for pain interventions.	• Continued pain despite pain interventions
10. Maintain the bed in motion for 18 hours of every 24-hour period.[6] The target rotation on a kinetic therapy surface is 62 degrees.	Provides proper rotation and adequate mobility. The surface is not pressure relieving if unable to turn; the patient is at great risk for pressure injury.	• Inability to rotate as per schedule
11. Maintain safety straps and positioning packs at all times.	Prevents falls and patient injury.	• Falls or injury
12. Maintain a schedule for foot supports: 2 hours on and 2 hours off continuously.	Side-to-side movement does not relieve pressure on the soles of the feet.	• Breakdown on the soles of the feet
13. Determine when therapy should be discontinued. Reassess need every 12- to 24-hour period.	Lateral rotation therapy is no longer required.	• Need for discontinuation of therapy

Documentation

Documentation should include the following:
- Patient and family education
- Date and time therapy is instituted
- Rationale for use of lateral rotation therapy surface
- Number of hours patient is in rotation mode per 24-hour period and degree of rotation achieved
- Patient tolerance of therapy
- Safety straps in place and bed alarms engaged
- Complete skin assessments of pressure areas and wound assessments per institutional standards and as necessary
- Status of wound healing, if applicable
- Patient's response to therapy
- Any unexpected outcomes and interventions performed

AMBULATION OF CRITICALLY ILL PATIENTS

Purpose

Early progressive mobility beginning within 48 hours of ICU admission is safe and feasible, and it results in improved outcomes for critically ill patients, including those on mechanical ventilation.[8-10,15,16,18,19,21,23,25,26,30,32,34,37,39,43,45,47,54] Mobility that progresses to ambulation, when appropriate, should be a priority of nursing care.[17]

PREREQUISITE NURSING KNOWLEDGE

- Principles of progressive mobility. Progressive mobility adapts with improving levels of patient function, decreases the time until the patient is out of bed, and improves outcomes.[9,37] Use of a nurse-driven mobility protocol can increase the rate of patient ambulation in the ICU.[17]
- Indications for ambulation include the following[3]:
  ❖ The patient tolerates being in the chair position.
  ❖ The patient can move the legs against gravity.
  ❖ The patient tolerates full or partial weight bearing.
  ❖ The patient can stand and pivot to a chair.

UNIT IX

- Contraindications for ambulation include the following:
  - Heart rate less than 40 beats/min[9,14,43] or greater than 130 beats/min[9,14,50]
  - Systolic blood pressure less than 90 mm Hg[3,9,14,26,50] or greater than 200 mm Hg[9,14,45,50]
  - Mean arterial pressure less than 65 mm Hg[1,9,17,37,43,45] or greater than 110 mm Hg[1,9,14,34,43]
  - Administration of a new vasopressor agent[21,37]; requirement of two or more vasopressors[14,50]
  - Acute myocardial infarction,[10,34,37] active cardiac ischemia,[9,14,17,21,42,43] or acute or unstable angina[10]
  - Cardiac index less than 2.0 L/min/m²[.25]
  - Dysrhythmia requiring new medications[17,21,25,37] or unstable rhythm[7,17,50]
  - Intra-aortic balloon[42,50]
  - Active bleeding[7,14,18,42,50]
  - Oxygen saturation less than 88%[3,9,14,17,26,37,43]
  - Respiratory rate less than 5 beats/min[9,14,26,43] or greater than 40 beats/min[9,14,21,26,43]
  - Fio_2 greater than 60%[14,17,21,25,26,34,50]
  - Positive end-expiratory pressure greater than 10 cm H_2O[10,14,26,34]
  - Unsecure airway,[21,26,43] nasotracheal intubation[10,21]
  - Unstable fracture or spine instability[10,14,42]
  - Increased intracranial pressure greater than 15 mm Hg[14,21,42]
- Use caution during ambulation for the following:
  - Increased agitation, RASS greater than +2[21,42]
  - Acute deep venous thrombosis[29,33]
  - Continuous dialysis
  - Femoral lines
- Signs of intolerance to ambulation include the following:
  - Sustained heart rate less than 40 beats/min, greater than 130 beats/min, or 20% from baseline[9]
  - Systolic blood pressure less than 90 mm Hg or greater than 200 mm Hg[9,34]
  - MAP less than 65 mm Hg or greater than 110 mm Hg[9]
  - Sustained respiratory rate greater than 40 beats/min,[9,21] less than 5 beats/min, or 20% from baseline[9]
  - Oxygen saturation less than 88% for 1 minute[9]
  - Ventilator asynchrony[9,21]
  - Concern for airway device integrity[9]
  - Development of any contraindications[9,21]
- Potential adverse events associated with ambulation include the following:
  - Fall[9,21,32]
  - Tube dislodgement[9,14,21,32]
  - Cardiac or respiratory event[9,15,21]
  - Hemodynamic instability[14,16]

EQUIPMENT

- Gait belt
- Portable ventilator and/or Ambu bag
- IV pump on wheels
- Portable monitor
- ICU platform walker
- Mechanical lift, ambulation shorts

PATIENT AND FAMILY EDUCATION

- Explain to the patient and family the adverse effects of immobility. **Rationale:** Explanation encourages cooperation and willingness to participate.
- Explain the purpose and possible risks of ambulation. **Rationale:** Explanation helps the patient and family understand the benefits of ambulation while also informing them of the possible risks.
- Explain to the patient and family what will happen, and let the patient know how he or she can help. **Rationale:** This allows the patient and family the opportunity to ask questions and provides the patient the opportunity to help with positioning.

PATIENT ASSESSMENT AND PREPARATION

Patient Assessment

- Determine the patient's baseline level of activity. **Rationale:** Patients who are unable to walk (i.e., wheelchair-bound) should not be expected to walk during the acute hospital stay, and appropriate assistive devices (i.e., walker or cane) should be provided for patients requiring such devices before admission.
- Review the medical record for activity orders and restrictions. **Rationale:** A patient with a bed rest order cannot be ambulated.[21] Activity restrictions, such as non–weight-bearing status, must be maintained.[17]
- Patient's level of cooperation. **Rationale:** A patient who does not respond to verbal commands may be unable to ambulate.[14,21]
- Assess for contraindications. **Rationale:** If contraindications are present or it is unsafe to ambulate, other forms of mobility may be considered.
- Assess the patient's physical readiness for ambulation (i.e., mobility level, ability to bear weight). **Rationale:** The patient must be physically able to ambulate to ensure the patient's safety.[3,23,32]
  - A mobility assessment tool, such as the Banner Mobility Assessment Tool, may be used.[5]
- Assess pain level using an organization-approved pain scale. **Rationale:** Pain should be addressed before ambulating to help prevent or minimize pain.[23]
- Assess the environment for potential threats to patient safety. **Rationale:** The floor should be free from slip or trip hazards to maintain patient safety.
- Assess all lines and tubes, including the endotracheal tube (ETT) or tracheostomy tube, to ensure that they are secure. **Rationale:** Securing all lines and tubes prevents accidental dislodgement.[23]
- For patients with an ETT, assess the centimeter mark at the lip before and after ambulation. **Rationale:** This ensures that no movement of the tube has occurred.

Patient Preparation

- Verify the correct patient with two identifiers. **Rationale:** Before performing a procedure, the nurse should ensure the correct identification of the patient for the intended intervention.

- Administer pain medication as indicated. ***Rationale:*** Ambulation timed to coincide with medication peak effectiveness will help prevent or minimize pain.[23]
- Assemble an adequate number of staff to help. ***Rationale:*** A multidisciplinary approach is necessary to ensure success and safety.[45,47]
- Ensure that each staff member has a clear understanding of his or her role during the ambulation episode. ***Rationale:*** Having clear roles ensures patient safety throughout the procedure.[23]

- Gather the necessary equipment, including mobility aids and emergency equipment. ***Rationale:*** Emergency equipment should be immediately available for use if an emergency should occur.[23]
- Ensure that the surface the patient will walk on is clean and dry. Remove any objects obstructing the pathway. ***Rationale:*** An area free from obstruction prevents falls and ensures adequate space to perform ambulation.[23]
- Obtain baseline vital signs. ***Rationale:*** Baseline vital signs are necessary to monitor for signs of intolerance.[18,19]

Procedure for Ambulation of Critically Ill Patients

Steps	Rationale	Special Considerations
1. **HH**		
2. **PE**		
3. Ensure that the bed is in a low position and the brakes are applied.	This prepares the work environment.	
4. Move the IV pole and lines to the side you are getting up on (the side toward the vent).	Prevents inadvertent dislodgement.	

5. Assist the patient to a dangling position on the side of the bed (toward the vent).
  a. Turn the patient onto the side facing the direction he or she will exit the bed.
  b. With one arm behind the patient's shoulders and one arm behind the patient's knees, assist the patient to a sitting position while bringing the feet to the floor.
	Prepares the patient to be moved. Helps the patient sit up and move legs off the bed at the same time. If the patient remains alert, the patient demonstrates trunk control, and vital signs remain within acceptable parameters, it is safe to continue.[18,19]	If the patient appears weak or unsteady, return the patient to the laying position in the bed.

6. Ensure that all lines are accounted for and have enough slack.	Caution should be taken to prevent lines from disconnecting.[26]	
7. Place nonslip or slip-resistant footwear on the patient's feet.	Proper footwear prevents accidental falls.	
8. Apply a gait belt, if required.		
9. Place the patient on a portable ventilator, if indicated.		For mechanically ventilated patients, the respiratory therapist's role is to maintain airway and ventilation during ambulation.
10. Assist the patient to a standing position A. If using a gait belt, grasp it on both sides, and use it to help "pull" the patient up.	If the patient remains alert, the patient demonstrates trunk control, and vital signs remain in acceptable parameters, it is safe to continue.[18,19]	If the patient appears weak or unsteady, return the patient to the bed or chair.

Procedure continues on following page

Procedure for Ambulation of Critically Ill Patients—*Continued*

Steps	Rationale	Special Considerations
11. Allow the patient to stand until balance is achieved.	If the patient remains alert, the patient demonstrates trunk control, and vital signs remain in acceptable parameters, it is safe to continue.[18,19]	If the patient appears weak or unsteady, return him/her to the bed or chair. If the patient is unable to stand with the assistance of two staff individuals, a gait harness (ambulation shorts) may be used to assist with ambulation.[23]
12. Stand on the patient's unaffected side.	Provides assistance without blocking the patient.	
13. Take a few steps forward with the patient. A. If using a gait belt, grasp the belt in the middle of the patient's back. B. If the patient does not require a gait belt, place the hand closest to the patient around the upper arm.	Grasping the belt in the middle of the back provides support at the waist so the patient's center of gravity remains midline.	
14. If able, continue ambulating per the goal distance.	The goal distance should align with the specific goals of treatment for the individual patient and should be increased with each ambulation session.[23]	
15. Instruct the patient to look ahead and lift each foot off of the ground.		
16. Match your steps to the patient's.	Allowing the patient to set the pace prevents falls.	
17. Return the patient to the bed or chair. A. Have patient stand with the back of the knees touching the bed or chair. B. If using a gait belt, grasp it on both sides to assist the patient into a sitting position. C. If not using a gait belt, assist the patient to a sitting position.		
18. Remove the gait belt.		
19. Obtain vital signs.		
20. Assess, treat, and reassess pain.		
21. Document the procedure in the patient's medical record.	Promotes clear communication among healthcare providers.	

Expected Outcomes

- Patient ambulates without episode of injury.
- Patient is able to ambulate without excessive fatigue or dizziness.
- Patient demonstrates the correct gait.

Unexpected Outcomes

- Patient is unable to ambulate.
- Patient falls.
- Patient demonstrates incorrect gait.
- Patient or healthcare team member sustains an injury.

Patient Monitoring and Care

Steps	Rationale	Reportable Conditions
		These conditions should be reported to the provider if they persist despite nursing interventions.
1. Assess for lightheadedness, dizziness, or faintness. A. If the patient becomes lightheaded or dizzy, lay the patient on their back on the bed. If the patient experiences these symptoms and also is pale or diaphoretic, recheck the heart rate and blood pressure. Do not continue.	Orthostatic hypotension and vertigo can occur when a patient has been immobile for any given amount of time. A patient with orthostatic hypotension or vertigo could fall.	• Change in level of consciousness • Hemodynamic instability
2. Observe for signs of intolerance	If the patient remains alert, the patient demonstrates trunk control, and vital signs remain in acceptable parameters, it is safe to continue.[18,19] Mobilization may need to temporarily cease because of the patient's physiological response.[23]	• Hemodynamic instability • Cardiac or respiratory event • Tube dislodgement • Fall

Documentation

Documentation should include the following:
- Patient and family education
- Patient's progress toward goals
- Type of assistive device used
- Amount of assistance required
- Distance walked, or steps taken
- Activity tolerance
- Unexpected outcomes and related interventions

References and Additional Readings

For a complete list of references and additional readings for this procedure, scan this QR code with your smartphone, or visit https://www.elsevier.com/__data/assets/pdf_file/0005/1319900/Chapter0125.pdf.

UNIT IX

126 Intrahospital Transport of Critically Ill Patients

Paula Halcomb

PURPOSE Intrahospital transport involves the transfer of a critically ill patient from one diagnostic treatment or inpatient area within the hospital to another, for example radiology. Intrahospital transport of critically ill patients is associated with risk of adverse events. Transport for diagnostic examinations and procedures is a necessary part of patient care. Standardized procedures can reduce the risk and incidence of and improve response to adverse events. Patients can be safely transported with the use of appropriate equipment, properly trained staff, and adherence to defined protocols.[10]

PREREQUISITE NURSING KNOWLEDGE

- Transport of critically ill patients for procedures and diagnostic examinations is necessary for treatments, surgeries, and diagnostic procedures that cannot be performed in the unit or emergency department but are required to dictate or alter the course of care. As a result, patients are frequently transported to and from the emergency department, operating room, procedural and diagnostic areas, and intensive care units. Multiple factors contribute to the risk of transporting critically ill patients, including technical or equipment issues, team skill and preparation, severity of patient condition, and the distance and time traveled. Critically ill patients have an inherently higher risk of iatrogenic injury because of the severity of their illness or injury, the acuity of their condition and resulting interventions and medications needed for care, and the volume of equipment needed to stabilize their condition. Physiological stress from transport alone may precipitate respiratory, neurological, and hemodynamic instability. Additional sedation and pain medication may be required.[1,2,3,5,6,8,18,23]
- Serious or critical adverse events are those that create a change in patient condition that requires intervention. Adverse events include but are not limited to: hypoxia or other changes in respiratory status that may require intubation or changes in ventilator settings, increased intracranial pressure, hypotension or need for increased vasoactive support, cardioversion, need for volume or cardiopulmonary resuscitation, and inadvertent removal of airway or central lines. Critically ill cardiovascular and neurological patients are at risk for accidental dislodgement or thrombosis of support lines for vascular access, drive lines for extracorporeal membrane oxygenation and ventricular assist devices, chest tubes, and intracranial pressure monitoring.[6,12,23,31]
- Adverse events are often precipitated by lack of planning, inadequate equipment or equipment maintenance, improperly trained staff, and lack of sufficient staff resources. These issues can lead to equipment failure and staff failure to follow protocols. Higher rates of adverse events occur during off shifts and are incrementally associated with the severity of the patient's illness. Some physiological changes are to be expected related to patient response to stress from transport; however, these can be anticipated and proactively managed to prevent further compromise. Often the equipment available for transport is not designed to meet the needs for transport, which results in mishaps related to workarounds. Environmental factors such as space restrictions, long transport distance, and lack of resources for dealing with emergencies may also play a role in adverse events.[10,13,23,33]
- Iatrogenic complications, adverse events, and injuries sustained as a result of transport (not patient disease or an injury process) are often underreported. Categories of events include equipment malfunction or failure, inadequate monitoring, incorrect use of equipment, clinical deterioration, communication failure, and accidental dislodgement of a line or tube, among others. Examples of equipment-related events include inadequate battery life or equipment malfunction/failure on infusion pumps, monitoring equipment, and transport ventilators as well as lack of MRI-compatible equipment and other issues. Lack of or inadequate communication among team members and the receiving department or delays in transport or diagnostic area availability are examples of organizational events. During transport, accidental dislodgement of lines and tubes, inadequate supply of continuous infusions, and clinical deterioration are common examples of adverse events. Events can occur during preparation for transport, during transport, during transfer to another bed or table for a procedure or examination, or during return to the original location and transfer to nontransport equipment. These events are estimated to occur in up to 70% to 86% of all intrahospital transports. The need for therapeutic intervention has been noted in up to 80% of adverse events.[1-4,6-9,23,28]
- Some facilities utilize rapid response or specialized transport teams to increase the safety and efficiency of transport.

Structured team briefing along with use of checklists can increase safety and reduce error during transport (Fig. 126.1).[3,7,8,11,23,25,27,35,38]

- Risk factors for adverse events during intrahospital transport include high severity of illness or injury severity score, ventilation with positive end-expiratory pressure (PEEP) of greater than 6 cm H_2O, sedation before transport, multiple lines and tubes, and vasoactive or antiarrhythmic infusions. Failure of technology and team dynamics also plays a role.[3,7,8,38]

- Tracking of events through some type of formal reporting system and debriefing with involved personnel is an essential quality improvement strategy. This type of tracking enables healthcare institutions to trend issues, follow up on problems, and determine education and interventions needed to decrease harm.[2,7-9]

- Healthcare organizations should imbed structures to support education and performance for healthcare professionals regarding transport of critically ill patients. Education and standardized workflow may mitigate the risk and improve the response to adverse events during transport. Standardized procedures, organization and education of staff, standard equipment, and use of checklists for intrahospital transport can reduce the incidence of adverse events from iatrogenic causes and improve patient outcomes. Incident debriefing can be especially useful as a tool to prevent recurrence of adverse events due to equipment or staff failure.[2,4,7,8,14,23,25,38]

- Preplanning should be an integral part of the transport process. Checklists for transport of critically ill patients include many items covering preparation for transport, the transport process and equipment, monitoring during transport and any diagnostic study or procedure, return to the unit of origin, and transfer back to standard in-room equipment. Extremely critical unstable patients benefit from a credentialed provider being part of the transport team. Handoff and clear two-way communication among transport team members as well as the receiving area is included. Battery capability and life of any equipment should be considered.[7,8,13,23,33,38]

- For mechanically ventilated patients, transport ventilators are recommended over bag-valve-mask devices if possible because of the risk of inconsistent ventilation with bag-valve-mask devices. Capnography in mechanically ventilated patients is essential to detect inadequate ventilation and adequacy of airway position. In spontaneously breathing patients, capnography is useful in detecting apnea and hypoventilation. Monitoring of certain physiological variables should be maintained during transport including but not limited to monitoring of respiratory rate, pulse oximetry, capnography, electrocardiography (ECG), blood pressure, and external ventricular drains. Patients at risk for hypothermia or hyperthermia should have their temperatures monitored.[5,10,13,68]

- Although many facilities may not have the resources for specialized transport teams, there is evidence to support that specialized transport teams are associated with quicker transport times and more favorable patient outcomes.[6]

EQUIPMENT

- Personal protective equipment including protective goggles
- Bag-valve-mask device
- Full oxygen tank with Christmas tree if applicable
- PEEP valve
- Transport ventilator with fully charged battery if applicable
- Transport monitor with charged battery
  - ❖ Noninvasive blood pressure cuff and cables
  - ❖ Invasive pressure-monitoring modules and cable
  - ❖ Continuous ECG leads and cables
  - ❖ Defibrillator with hands-free pads and pacing capability, if desired
  - ❖ Capnography monitoring with cable
- Thermometer if applicable
- Infusion pumps with charged batteries if applicable
- Additional bags of continuous drips if need is anticipated
- Pain/sedation and or resuscitation medications if need is anticipated
- Additional lengths of intravenous (IV) tubing if need is anticipated
- Normal saline flushes

PATIENT AND FAMILY EDUCATION

- Assess the patient's and family's level of understanding about the condition and reason for the transport and procedure if the clinical situation permits. *Rationale:* This assessment identifies the patient's and family's knowledge deficits concerning the patient's condition, the procedure, the expected benefits, and the potential risks. It also allows time for questions to clarify information and voice concerns. Explanations decrease patient anxiety and enhance cooperation.

- Explain the purpose of the transport to the patient and/or family. Outline the steps taken to ensure patient safety, and give a realistic time estimate for the trip. Assure the patient and family that they will be updated as soon as the transport is completed. *Rationale:* Knowledge and the opportunity to have questions addressed may ease anxiety.

PATIENT ASSESSMENT AND PREPARATION

Patient Assessment

- Review the patient's medical record for medical history and history of present illness. *Rationale:* Knowledge of the patient condition and history allows the nurse to anticipate potential safety issues with transport.

- Perform a physical assessment including neurological status (including mobility and sensation of extremities in the case of spine precautions), breath sounds, and vital signs immediately before transport. *Rationale:* Baseline assessment is essential to recognize changes in patient condition during and after transport.

Intrahospital Transport Checklist

Patient Name:	DOB:	Age:
MRN:	Location:	Code Status:
Isolation:	Allergies:	
Admission Diagnosis:		

Transport Team: RN   RT   Provider if applicable   NCT/ Transporter   Hard Chart

Trauma
- C-spine
- Log roll
- Spinal/cervical precautions
- Traction/ External Fixator:
- Ortho or Neuro Provider for transport
- Long Bone/ Pelvic fracture stabilized
- RASS
- EMV/GCS _____
- Pupils: (L)_____ (R)_____
- Pupils: Reactive/ Non-reactive
- Wounds controlled appropriately

Airway/ Breathing
- ETT @ _____
- ETT secured @_____ teeth/nare
- Trach # _____
- Trach secured with trach tie
- Obturator/Extra trach for Transport
- 2 full oxygen tanks
- Bilateral Breath sounds present
- ET suction immediately prior to transport if needed
- Noninvasive ventilation CPAP/BiPAP

Monitoring:
- Vital Signs
  - T: _____
  - P: _____
  - R: _____
  - BP: _____ / _____
- BP: Invasive/ Non-invasive
- SaO2
- ETCO2
- ECG
- Vent settings
  - FIO2: _____
  - PEEP: _____
  - Rate: _____
  - Mode: _____

Lines/ Drains
- A-line zero/ functioning properly
- IV/ IO Access _____
- Central Line Access_____
- ICP drain secure
- Chest Tube secure
- NGT/ OGT
- Feeding Tube
- Restraints
- F/C emptied & secured

Infusions/ Drips / Medications
- Blood Products
- Sedatives _____
- Vasopressors _____
- Inotropes _____
- Fluids _____
- NMBA _____
- Analgesics _____
- Antiarrhythmics _____
- Emergency Meds or additional sedatives, analgesics or NMBAs if anticipated

Figure 126.1   Intrahospital checklist examples.

Equipment

    Defibrillator
    Portable ventilator
    FULL Oxygen tank
    Ambu-bag with Peep valve and facemask
    Cardiac monitor
    Stethoscope
    CVC/ PA zero
    Temporary pacemaker connected capturing/ sensing appropriately

    All equipment fully charged functioning battery
    All equipment functioning properly

Safety Considerations

    Blankets/heat loss measures in place
    Emergency airway equipment
    Consider discontinuing insulin drip or taking glucose and glucometer for transport
    Moving/handling plan for safe transfer with mobility precautions communicated (slider, 6 people lift, etc.)
    MRI compatible equipment and IV tubing if applicable
    MRI safety screening for patient and staff if applicable
    Dressing considerations for hyperbaric chamber
    If chest tube present, can patient tolerate CT to H_2O SEAL DURING TRANSPORT AND/OR DIAGNOSTIC PROCEDURE?
    If unable to tolerate H_2O seal utilize portable suction
    Intubation bag
    Consider provider accompaniment for:
        Unstable C-spine fracture
        Peep >10cm/ FiO_2 100%
        Rapid infuser in use
        Difficult airway
        Mechanical circulatory support (IABP, FCMO, CPS)
        Unstable arrythmia

Figure 126.1 cont'd

- Ensure that the airway is secured and stable. Verify the location of the endotracheal tube at the nare or teeth. Verify that the tracheostomy tube is secured with protective dressing under the trach plate. Rationale: Adequate tube securement is essential in preventing inadvertent airway and line removal during transport.
- Ensure that IV lines are covered with occlusive dressings and that the tubing is securely fastened and of adequate length for transport. **Rationale:** Inadvertent line dislodgements are a significant safety risk during transport.
- Ensure that continuous IV infusions have adequate volume for the trip and any delays that may occur. Verify the rate and dose of all IV infusions. Note the depth of the central venous catheter/and/or pulmonary artery catheter.
- Ensure that all tubes and drains are secured. Note the depth and drainage when applicable. Rationale: Inadvertent tube and line dislodgement or removal causes potential patient harm.

Patient Preparation

- Verify the correct patient with two identifiers before transport and before any diagnostic examination or procedure. Include the patient in the identification process if

UNIT IX

communicative. Have patient labels available. Rationale: Before performing a procedure, the nurse should ensure the correct identification of the patient for the intended intervention. Labels may be needed for supply or the blood bank.

- Verify that all team members are ready for transport and aware of all safety issues and precautions and that all lines, drains, and airways are secured for transport. Rationale: Closed-loop communication is an essential method to ensure safe patient handling and that all team members are ready to begin transport.

Procedure	**for Intrahospital Transport of Critically Ill Patients**	
Steps	**Rationale**	**Special Considerations**

1. **HH**
2. **PE**
3. Gather and inspect the functionality and battery life of all equipment planned for use during transport. Employ a transport checklist if your facility has one (see Fig. 126.1). All equipment batteries should be tested before leaving the patient's room:
   A. Transport monitor with defibrillator and pacing capability, invasive pressure monitoring, oximetry, and continuous waveform capnography. Defibrillator pads and monitoring cables present.
   B. Transport ventilator battery fully charged.
   C. Infusion pumps with batteries fully charged.
4. Ensure that the oxygen tank is full, the bag-valve-mask device is functional, the PEEP valve is set appropriately, and the airway (endotracheal tube/tracheostomy) is secured (endotracheal tube position documented before transport).
   A. Ensure that the transport ventilator is working and the patient's ventilation is stable before leaving the patient's room.
5. Ensure that all IV access is secured (depth in centimeters noted before transport for central lines), flushed, and patent.
   A. Tubing is long enough for transport.
   B. Drips have adequate volume for trip and potential delays.
6. Ensure that the Foley catheter, drains, and chest tubes are secured.
   A. Document the depth of drains before transport if applicable (e.g., PEG depth, CT depth)
7. Assess mobility restrictions and document.
   A. If spines are not cleared, ensure that cervical collar placement is adequate.
   B. Inform the team of the logroll and transfer board process.
8. Consider pain/sedation medication or emergency medications if the patient is not on continuous infusion.

Helps prevent adverse events related to equipment failure, which is a primary cause of events during transport.[7,10,13,33] (**Levels A, B, D***) Ensuring that equipment is on and functioning appropriately helps reduce the risk of adverse events.[7,10,13,33] (**Levels A, B, D***) Securing lines and documenting their location informs the nurse if accidental dislodgement has occurred, which is essential in predicting issues with medication administration.[7,10,13,33]

(**Level A, B, D***) Securing drains and documenting their location informs the nurse if accidental dislodgement has occurred, which is essential in preventing potential adverse events.[7,10,13,33]

(**Level A, B, D***) Critically ill patients, especially trauma or surgical patients, may have mobility restrictions. It is essential that the team is aware of restrictions as a whole and employs closed-loop communication to ensure optimal patient safety.

Pain may make the patient more agitated and precipitate adverse events such as accidental removal of lines or tubes. Agitation may precipitate adverse vital sign changes during transport.

Extremely critical patients may benefit from a provider that has demonstrated competency with airway management and line placement accompanying the transport team.

Expected Outcomes

- Transport to desired location and back with no adverse events.

Unexpected Outcomes

- Deterioration in patient condition (e.g., hypotension, increased intracranial pressure, hypoxemia, cardiac arrhythmia)
- Inadvertent airway or drain dislodgement
- Inadvertent line dislodgement
- Respiratory or cardiac arrest

Patient Monitoring and Care

Steps	Rationale	Reportable Conditions
		These conditions should be reported to the provider if they persist despite nursing interventions.
1. Monitor vital signs with continuous ECG, invasive pressures if applicable, pulse oximetry, and capnography.	Movement from transport may stress the patient and precipitate hemodynamic compromise.	Report deterioration in vital signs to the provider immediately.
2. Assess the position of the airway, drains, and IV access during transport.	Inadvertent dislodgement of lines, drains, or an airway can cause critical patient compromise.	Report movement or dislodgement of the airway or lines/drains to the provider immediately.
3. Upon return to unit, perform full a physical assessment and vital signs. A. Assess the position of the airway. B. Assess the position of lines and drains. C. Ensure that all equipment is plugged into a functional outlet with generator backup. D. Ensure that all invasive monitoring lines are zeroed and have adequate waveforms. E. Ensure that all continuous medications are still infusing and that the rate is correct. F. Perform a neurological examination including movement of extremities if applicable.	Transport can be stressful on the patient. Full assessment ensures that the patient is stable and that the airway and lines are in the appropriate position.	Report changes in airway or line position, changes in physical assessment, or adverse vital signs to the provider immediately.

Documentation

Documentation should include the following:
- Vital signs
- Physical assessment
- Neurological assessment
- Patient response to transport/diagnostic examination
- Family education and communication
- Patient education if applicable based on patient condition
- Unexpected outcomes and interventions required
- Communication with provider
- Medications or nursing interventions required during or as a result of transport

References and Additional Readings

For a complete list of references and additional readings for this procedure, scan this QR code with your smartphone, or visit https://www.elsevier.com/__data/assets/pdf_file/0006/1319901/Chapter0126.pdf

UNIT IX

Index

Page numbers followed by "*f*" indicate figures, "*t*" indicate tables, and "*b*" indicate boxes.

INDEX

INDEX